	Hydroxyzine	Meperidine	Metoclopramide	Midazolam	Morphine	Nalbuphine	Pentazocine	Pentobarbital	Perphenazine	Prochlorperazine	Promazine	Promethazine	Ranitidine	Scopolamine Hbr	Secobarbital	Thiethylperazine
	C	C	C	C	C	C	C	C	C	C	C	C	C	C	I	
	C	C	C	C	C		C	I	C	C		C		C	I	C
	C	C	C	C	C		C	I	C	C	C	C	C	C	I	
								I							I	
	I	I	I		I	I	I	I	I	I	I	I		I	I	I
	I	C	C	I	C		C	I	C	I	I	I	C	C	I	
	C	C	C	C	C		C	I	C	C	C	C	C	C	I	
	C	C	C		C	C	C	I	C	C	C	C		C	I	
	C	C	C		C		C	I	C	C	C	C	C	C	I	
	C	C			C		I	I		C	C	C	C	C	I	
		I			I		I					I				
		C	C		C	C	C	I		C	C	C	I	C	I	
	C		C		I		C	I	C	C	C	C	C	C	I	
	C	C			C		C		C	C	C	C	C	C	I	
	C		C		C	C		I	I	I	C	C	I	C		C
	C	I	C				C	I	C	C	C	C	C	C	I	
	C							I		C		C	C	C	I	C
	C	C	C		C			I	C	C	C	C	C	C	I	
	I	I			I	I	I		I	I	I	I		C	I	
		C	C		C		C	I		C		C	C	C	I	I
	C	C	C		C	C	C	I	C		C	C	C	C	I	
	C	C	C		C		C	I		C		C		C	I	
	C	C	C		C	C	C	I	C	C	C		C	C	I	
		C	C	I	C	C	C		C	C		C		C		C
	C	C	C		C	C	C	C	C	C	C	C	C		I	
	I	I	I		I	I	I	I	I	I	I	I		I		I
						C			I				C		I	

Parenteral compatibility occurs when two or more drugs are successfully mixed without liquefaction, deliquescence, or precipitation.

Mosby's

1997 Nursing Drug Reference

Linda Skidmore-Roth, R.N., M.S.N., N.P.

Formerly, Nursing Faculty,
New Mexico State University,
Las Cruces, New Mexico;
El Paso Community College,
El Paso, Texas

Mosby

St. Louis Baltimore Boston Carlsbad Chicago Naples New York
Philadelphia Portland London Madrid Mexico City Singapore
Sydney Tokyo Toronto Wiesbaden

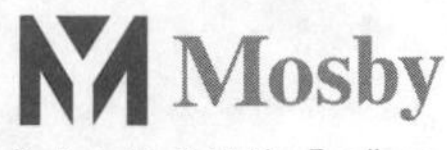

A Times Mirror Company

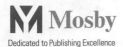

Vice President and Publisher: Nancy Coon
Editor: Robin Carter
Developmental editor: Liz Fathman
Project manager: Carol Sullivan Weis
Senior production editor: Christine Schwepker
Designer: Sheilah Barrett
Manufacturing manager: Betty Richmond
Cover design: Rokusek Design

A NOTE TO THE READER

The authors and publisher have made every attempt to check dosages and nursing content for accuracy. Because the science of pharmacology is continually advancing, our knowledge base continues to expand. Therefore we recommend that the reader always check product information for changes in dosage or administration before administering any medication. This is particularly important with new or rarely used drugs.

Printed in the United States of America
Editing, production, and composition by Graphic World, Inc.
Printing/binding by Rand McNally

Mosby–Year Book, Inc.
11830 Westline Industrial Drive
St. Louis, Missouri 63146

ISSN 1044-8470
ISBN 0-8151-7909-X

96 97 98 99 00 / 9 8 7 6 5 4 3 2 1

Consultants

Barbara A. Brunow, R.N., M.S.N.
Instructor, Providence Hospital, School of Nursing,
Sandusky, Ohio

Connie L. Bush, R.N., M.S.
Associate Professor, Nursing,
Niagara County Community College,
Sanborn, New York

Judy E. Davidson, R.N., M.S., C.C.R.N.
Clinical Nurse Specialist,
University of California San Diego Medical Center,
San Diego, California

Jane Doyle, R.N., B.S.N., M.S., M.B.A.
Nursing Faculty,
Mount Wachusett Community College,
Gardner, Massachusetts

Laurel A. Eisenhauer, R.N., Ph.D.
Professor of Nursing,
Boston College School of Nursing,
Chestnut Hill, Massachusetts

Tim Engelhardt, B.Sc., Pharm.D.
Manager, Pharmacy Services,
Calgary District Hospital Group,
Calgary, Alberta

Theresa M. Hulub, R.N., M.S.Ed., M.S.N.
Professor of Nursing Education,
Niagara County Community College,
Sanborn, New York

Kimberly A. Hunter, Pharm.D.
Assistant Professor of Pharmacy Practice,
Washington State University College of Pharmacy;
Geriatric Clinical Pharmacist,
Sacred Heart Medical Center,
Spokane, Washington

Jon E. Lewis, B.A., Ph.D.
Senior Research Scientist and Director,
Respiratory Diseases,
Marion Merrell Dow Research Institute,
Cincinnati, Ohio

Edwina A. McConnell, R.N., Ph.D.
Independent Nurse Consultant,
Madison, Wisconsin

Rosemary A. Pine, R.N., M.S.N.
Assistant Professor of Nursing,
Department Chair, ADN Program,
Houston Baptist University,
Houston, Texas

Mary Quintas, R.N.
Miles Community College,
Department of Nursing,
Miles City, Montana

Roberta Roynayne, R.N., B.Sc.N., M.Sc.
Assistant Professor,
University of Ottawa,
School of Nursing,
Ottawa, Ontario

Carol Ruscin, R.N., B.S.
Level I Faculty,
Baptist Medical System,
School of Nursing,
Little Rock, Arkansas

Lori Schoonover, Pharm.D.
Assistant Professor, Pharmacy,
Washington State University,
Spokane, Washington

Roberta J. Secrest, Ph.D., Pharm.D., R.Ph.
Associate Scientist,
Marion Merrell Dow Research Institute,
Cincinnati, Ohio

John R. White, Jr., Pharm.D.
Assistant Professor,
Washington State University,
College of Pharmacy,
Spokane, Washington

Preface

Since the first publication of *Mosby's Nursing Drug Reference* in 1988, more than 100 U.S. and Canadian pharmacists and consultants have closely reviewed the book's content. Today, *Mosby's 1997 Nursing Drug Reference* has been completely revised and updated with the addition of more than 1800 new drug facts—including 11 new drugs recently approved by the FDA. Nursing considerations have been revised and hundreds of newly researched side effects, adverse reactions, precautions, interactions, contraindications, and IV therapy facts have been added. To keep our readers up-to-date, monographs for the most recently FDA-approved drugs have been included. Also, for the first time, drugs have been identified as prescription (℞) and over-the-counter (OTC) in the monograph headings. New drug monographs in the book include ***acarbose,*** used to treat diabetes mellitus; ***bicalutamide,*** an antineoplastic used to treat prostatic cancer; ***mycophenolate mofetil,*** an immunosuppressive used for organ transplantation; ***lamivudine,*** an antiviral for HIV infections; and ***nalmefene,*** an opioid antagonist.

Although drug references abound, few are truly portable and geared specifically for clinical use by the practicing nurse or student. The guiding principle behind this reference is to provide a book that allows easy access to drug information and nursing considerations that specifically tell the nurse what to do in terms consistent with the nursing process. Every detail—down to the paper, typeface, cover, binding, color, and appendixes—is carefully chosen with the user in mind.

More than 1300 generic and 4500 trade medications, alphabetized by generic name, are included. Trade names are given for all medications commonly used in the United States and Canada. Drugs available only in Canada are identified by an asterisk. The following information is provided, whenever possible, for safe and effective administration of each drug:

Pronunciations: Pronunciations are provided to help the nursing student master the more complex generic names.

Functional and chemical classifications: All known broad functional and chemical classifications are given. These classifications allow the nurse to see similarities and dissimilarities among drugs in the same functional but different chemical classes.

Controlled-substance schedule: Schedules are included for the United States (I, II, III, IV, V) and Canada (F, G).

Combination products: These products have been integrated into the monographs and organized according to main ingredient.

Action: Pharmacologic properties are described in concise terms. Action is discussed to the cellular level when known.

Uses: Provides drug application.

Investigational uses: Provides drug applications for those uses that may be encountered in practice, but are not yet FDA-approved.

Dosages and routes: All available and approved dosages and routes are given for adult, pediatric, and geriatric patients.

Available forms: All available forms—including tablets, capsules, extended-release, injectables (IV, IM, SC), solutions, creams, ointments, lotions, gels, shampoos, elixirs, suspensions, suppositories, sprays, aerosols, and lozenges—are provided.

Side effects/adverse reactions: Grouped by body system, common side effects are *italicized,* and life-threatening reactions are in ***bold italic type,*** allowing the nurse to quickly identify common and life-threatening reactions.

Contraindications: Contraindications are instances in which a medication should absolutely not be given. When the FDA has assigned pregnancy safety category D or X, it appears here.

Precautions: Special precautionary steps are given here, including FDA pregnancy safety categories A, B, and C.

Pharmacokinetics: Metabolism, distribution, and elimination are provided for all dosage forms, if known.

Interactions: This section includes confirmed drug, food, and smoking interactions. The reaction is listed first, followed by the drug or nutrient causing that interaction, when applicable.

Compatibilities: Syringe, Y-site, and additive compatibilities have been added to the text for the new edition.

Lab test interferences: When known, lab test interferences are provided.

Nursing considerations: Highlighted nursing considerations are organized to foster use of the nursing process: Assess, Administer, Perform/provide, Evaluate, and Teach patient/family. Nursing considerations are consistently grouped under these headings to help the nurse group interventions that can be used for planning nursing care.

Treatment of overdose: Drugs and treatment for overdoses are provided for appropriate drugs.

The following appendixes are included to further enhance the usability of this reference: selected new drugs, controlled substances, FDA pregnancy categories, commonly used antibiotics in adults and children, formulas for drug calculations, nomogram for calculation of body surface area, weights and equivalents, home care medication record, bibliography, and abbreviations. Drug-to-drug and drug-to-solution IV compatibility charts have been printed immediately inside the front and back covers for quick access.

I am indebted to the nursing and pharmacology consultants who reviewed the manuscript and galley pages and thank them for their criticism and encouragement. I would also like to thank Robin Carter and Liz Fathman, my editors, whose active encouragement and enthusiasm have made this book better than it might otherwise have been. I am likewise grateful to Christine Carroll Schwepker, Carol Sullivan Weis, and Graphic World, Inc. for the coordination of the production process, and Sheilah Barrett for her creativity and cooperative spirit. In addition, I want to extend a special note of gratitude to Don Ladig, who has supported and encouraged my efforts since the inception of this project.

Linda Skidmore-Roth

Contents

Drug categories, 1

Alpha-adrenergic blockers, 1
Anesthetics—general/local, 2
Antacids, 3
Antianginals, 5
Anticholinergics, 6
Anticoagulants, 8
Anticonvulsants, 10
Antidepressants, 11
Antidiabetics, 13
Antidiarrheals, 15
Antidysrhythmics, 16
Antifungals (systemic), 18
Antihistamines, 20
Antihypertensives, 21
Antiinfectives, 23
Antineoplastics, 25
Antiparkinson agents, 28
Antipsychotics, 29
Antituberculars, 31
Antitussives/expectorants, 32
Antivirals, 34
Barbiturates, 35
Benzodiazepines, 37
Beta-adrenergic blockers, 38
Bronchodilators, 40
Calcium channel blockers, 41
Cardiac glycosides, 43
Cholinergics, 44
Cholinergic blockers, 46
Corticosteroids, 47
Diuretics, 49
Histamine (H_2) antagonists, 51
Immunosuppressants, 52
Laxatives, 53
Narcotics, 55
Neuromuscular blocking agents, 57
Nonsteroidal antiinflammatories, 58
Salicylates, 59
Thrombolytics, 61
Thyroid hormones, 63
Vasodilators, 64
Vitamins, 66

Individual drugs, 67

Appendixes

A. Selected new drugs, 1101
B. Controlled substance chart, 1112
C. FDA pregnancy categories, 1112
D. Commonly used antibiotics in adults and children, 1113
E. Formulas for drug calculations, 1115
F. Nomogram for calculation of body surface area, 1116
G. Weights and equivalents, 1117
H. Home care medication record, 1118
I. Bibliography, 1119
J. Abbreviations, 1120

Index, 1123

ALPHA-ADRENERGIC BLOCKERS

Action: Acts by binding to α-adrenergic receptors, causing dilation of peripheral blood vessels. Lowers peripheral resistance, resulting in decreased blood pressure.

Uses: Used for pheochromocytoma, prevention of tissue necrosis and sloughing associated with extravasation of IV vasopressors.

Side effects/adverse reactions: The most common side effects are hypotension, tachycardia, nasal stuffiness, nausea, vomiting, and diarrhea.

Contraindications: Hypersensitive reactions may occur, and allergies should be identified before these products are given. Patients with myocardial infarction, coronary insufficiency, angina, or other evidence of coronary artery disease should not use these products.

Pharmacokinetics: Onset, peak, and duration vary among products.

Interactions: Vasoconstrictive and hypertensive effects of epinephrine are antagonized by α-adrenergic blockers.

Possible nursing diagnoses:

- Altered tissue perfusion *[uses]*
- Risk of injury *[adverse reactions]*
- Sleep pattern disturbance *[adverse reactions]*

NURSING CONSIDERATIONS

Assess:

- Electrolytes: K, Na, Cl, CO_2
- Weight daily, I&O
- B/P lying, standing before starting treatment, q4h thereafter
- Nausea, vomiting, diarrhea
- Skin turgor, dryness of mucous membranes for hydration status

Administer:

- Starting with low dose, gradually increasing to prevent side effects
- With food or milk for GI symptoms

Evaluate:

- Therapeutic response: decreased B/P, increased peripheral pulses

Teach patient/family:

- To avoid alcoholic beverages
- To report dizziness, palpitations, fainting
- To change position slowly or fainting may occur
- To take drug exactly as prescribed
- To avoid all OTC products (cough, cold, allergy) unless directed by prescriber

Generic names

phenoxybenzamine (p. 841)

phentolamine (p. 844)

ANESTHETICS—GENERAL/LOCAL

Action: Anesthetics (general) act on the CNS to produce tranquilization and sleep before invasive procedures. Anesthetics (local) inhibit conduction of nerve impulses from sensory nerves.

Uses: General anesthetics are used to premedicate for surgery, induction and maintenance in general anesthesia. For local anesthetics, refer to individual product listing for indications.

Side effects/adverse reactions: The most common side effects are dystonia, akathisia, flexion of arms, fine tremors, drowsiness, restlessness, and hypotension. Also common are chills, respiratory depression, and laryngospasm.

Contraindications: Persons with CVA, increased intracranial pressure, severe hypertension, cardiac decompensation should not use these products, since severe adverse reactions can occur.

Precautions: Anesthetics (general) should be used with caution in the elderly, cardiovascular disease (hypotension, bradydysrhythmias), renal disease, liver disease, Parkinson's disease, children <2 yr. The precaution for anesthetics (local) is pregnancy.

Pharmacokinetics: Onset, peak, and duration vary widely among products. Most products are metabolized in the liver and excreted in urine.

Interactions: MAOIs, tricyclics, phenothiazines may cause severe hypotension or hypertension when used with local anesthetics. CNS depressants will potentiate general and local anesthetics.

Possible nursing diagnoses:

General:

- Risk of injury *[adverse reactions]*
- Knowledge deficit *[teaching]*

Local:

- Pain *[uses]*
- Knowledge deficit *[teaching]*

NURSING CONSIDERATIONS

Assess:

- VS q10min during IV administration, q30min after IM dose

Administer:

- Anticholinergic preoperatively to decrease secretions
- Only with crash cart, resuscitative equipment nearby

Perform/provide:

- Quiet environment for recovery to decrease psychotic symptoms

Evaluate:

- Therapeutic response: maintenance of anesthesia, decreased pain

Generic names (Injectables only)

General anesthetics
droperidol (p. 399)
etomidate (p. 445)
fentanyl (p. 457)
fentanyl/droperidol (p. 458)
fentanyl transdermal (p. 459)
ketamine (p. 593)
methohexital (p. 682)
procaine (p. 889)
tetracaine (p. 1004)

Local anesthetics
chloroprocaine (p. 257)
etidocaine (p. 442)
lidocaine (p. 611)
mepivacaine (p. 663)
midazolam (p. 714)
propofol (p. 901)
thiopental (p. 1015)

ANTACIDS

Action: Antacids are basic compounds that neutralize gastric acidity and decrease the rate of gastric emptying. Products are divided into those containing aluminum, magnesium, calcium, or a combination of these.
Uses: Hyperacidity is decreased by antacids in conditions such as peptic ulcer disease, reflux esophagitis, gastritis, and hiatal hernia.
Side effects/adverse reactions: The most common side effect caused by aluminum-containing antacids is constipation, which may lead to fecal impaction and bowel obstruction. Diarrhea occurs often when magnesium products are given. Alkalosis may occur when systemic products are used. Constipation occurs more frequently than laxation with calcium carbonate. The release of CO_2 from carbonate-containing antacids causes belching, abdominal distention, and flatulence. Sodium bicarbonate may act as a systemic antacid and produce systemic electrolyte disturbances and alkalosis. Calcium carbonate and sodium bicarbonate may cause rebound hyperacidity and milk-alkali syndrome. Alkaluria may occur when products are used on a long-term basis, particularly in persons with abnormal renal function.
Contraindications: Sensitivity to aluminum or magnesium products may cause hypersensitive reactions. Aluminum products should not be used by persons sensitive to aluminum; magnesium products should not be used by persons sensitive to magnesium. Check for sensitivity before administering.
Precautions: Magnesium products should be given cautiously to patients with renal insufficiency and during pregnancy and lactation. Sodium content of antacids may be significant; use with caution for patients with hypertension, CHF, or those on a low-sodium diet.
Pharmacokinetics: Duration is 20-40 min. If ingested 1 hr after meals, acidity is reduced for at least 3 hr.

Interactions: Drugs whose effects may be increased by some antacids: quinidine, amphetamines, pseudoephedrine, levodopa, valproic acid, dicumarol. Drugs whose effects may be decreased by some antacids: cimetadine, corticosteroids, ranitidine, iron salts, phenothiazines, phenytoin, digoxin, tetracyclines, ketoconazole, salicylates, isoniazid.

Possible nursing diagnoses:

- Pain *[uses]*
- Constipation *[adverse reactions]*
- Diarrhea *[adverse reactions]*

NURSING CONSIDERATIONS

Assess:

- Aggravating and alleviating factors of epigastric pain or hyperacidity; identify the location, duration, and characteristics of epigastric pain
- GI symptoms, including constipation, diarrhea, abdominal pain; if severe abdominal pain with fever occurs, these drugs should not be given
- Renal symptoms, including increasing urinary pH, electrolytes

Administer:

- All products with an 8-oz glass of water to ensure absorption in the stomach
- Another antacid if constipation occurs with aluminum products

Evaluate:

- The therapeutic effectiveness of the drug; absence of epigastric pain and decreased acidity should occur

Teach patient/family:

- Not to take other drugs within 1-2 hr of antacid administration, since antacids may impair absorption of other drugs

---

Generic names

aluminum hydroxide (p. 95)
bismuth subsalicylate (p. 178)
calcium carbonate (p. 200)
dihydroxyaluminum (p. 373)
magaldrate (p. 634)
magnesium oxide (p. 635)
sodium bicarbonate (p. 957)

ANTIANGINALS

Action: The antianginals are divided into the nitrates, calcium channel blockers, and β-adrenergic blockers. The nitrates dilate coronary arteries, causing decreased preload, and dilate systemic arteries, causing decreased afterload. Calcium channel blockers dilate coronary arteries, decrease SA/AV node conduction. β-Adrenergic blockers decrease heart rate so that myocardial O_2 use is decreased. Dipyridamole selectively dilates coronary arteries to increase coronary blood flow.

Uses: Antianginals are used in chronic stable angina pectoris, unstable angina, vasospastic angina. Some (i.e., calcium channel blockers and β-blockers) may be used for dysrhythmias and in hypertension.

Side effects/adverse reactions: The most common side effects are postural hypotension, headache, flushing, dizziness, nausea, edema, and drowsiness. Also common are rash, dysrhythmias, and fatigue.

Contraindications: Persons with known hypersensitivity, increased intracranial pressure, or cerebral hemorrhage should not use some of these products.

Precautions: Antianginals should be used with caution in postural hypotension, pregnancy, lactation, children, renal disease, and hepatic injury.

Pharmacokinetics: Onset, peak, and duration vary widely among coronary products. Most products are metabolized in the liver and excreted in urine.

Interactions: Please check individual monographs, since interactions vary widely among products.

Possible nursing diagnoses:

- Altered tissue perfusion: cardiopulmonary *[uses]*
- Pain *[uses]*
- Risk of injury *[uses]*
- Knowledge deficit *[teaching]*
- Decreased cardiac output *[adverse reactions]*

NURSING CONSIDERATIONS

Assess:

- Orthostatic B/P, pulse
- Pain: duration, time started, activity being performed, character
- Tolerance if taken over long period
- Headache, light-headedness, decreased B/P; may indicate a need for decreased dosage

Perform/provide:

- Storage protected from light, moisture; place in cool environment

Evaluate:
- Therapeutic response: decrease, prevention of anginal pain

Teach patient/family:
- To keep tabs in original container
- Not to use OTC products unless directed by prescriber
- To report bradycardia, dizziness, confusion, depression, fever
- To take pulse at home, advise when to notify prescriber
- To avoid alcohol, smoking, sodium intake
- To comply with weight control, dietary adjustments, modified exercise program
- To carry Medic Alert ID to identify drug that you are taking, allergies
- To make position changes slowly to prevent fainting

Generic names

Nitrates
amyl nitrite (p. 128)
erythrityl (p. 419)
isosorbide (p. 584)
nitroglycerin (p. 762)
pentaerythritol (p. 821)

β-Adrenergic blockers
atenolol (p. 139)
dipyridamole (p. 382)
metoprolol (p. 704)
nadolol (p. 734)
propranolol (p. 904)

Calcium channel blockers
amlodipine (p. 110)
bepridil (p. 169)
diltiazem (p. 373)
nicardipine (p. 756)
nifedipine (p. 760)
verapamil (p. 1082)

ANTICHOLINERGICS

Action: Anticholinergics inhibit the muscarinic actions of acetylcholine at receptor sites in the autonomic nervous system; anticholinergics are also known as antimuscarinic drugs.

Uses: Anticholinergics are used for a variety of conditions: gastrointestinal anticholinergics are used to decrease motility (smooth muscle tone) in the GI, biliary, and urinary tracts and for their ability to decrease gastric secretions (propantheline, glycopyrrolate); decreasing involuntary movements in parkinsonism (benztropine, trihexyphenidyl); bradydysrhythmias (atropine); nausea and vomiting (scopolamine); and as cycloplegic mydriatics (atropine, hematropine, scopalamine, cyclopentolate, tropicamide).

Side effects/adverse reactions: The most common side effects are dry mouth, constipation, urinary retention, urinary hesitancy, headache, and dizziness. Also common is paralytic ileus.

Contraindications: Persons with narrow-angle glaucoma, myasthenia gravis, or GI/GU obstruction should not use some of these products.

Precautions: Anticholinergics should be used with caution in patients who are elderly, pregnant, or lactating or in those with prostatic hypertrophy, CHF, or hypertension; use with caution in presence of high environmental temperature.

Pharmacokinetics: Onset, peak, and duration vary widely among products. Most products are metabolized in the liver and excreted in urine.

Interactions: Increased anticholinergic effects may occur when used with MAOIs and tricyclic antidepressants and amantadine. Anticholinergics may cause a decreased effect of phenothiazines and levodopa.

Possible nursing diagnoses:

- Decreased cardiac output *[uses]*
- Constipation *[adverse reactions]*
- Knowledge deficit *[teaching]*

NURSING CONSIDERATIONS

Assess:

- I&O ratio; retention commonly causes decreased urinary output
- Urinary hesitancy, retention; palpate bladder if retention occurs
- Constipation; increase fluids, bulk, exercise if this occurs
- For tolerance over long-term therapy, dose may need to be increased or changed
- Mental status: affect, mood, CNS depression, worsening of mental symptoms during early therapy

Administer:

- Parenteral dose with patient recumbent to prevent postural hypotension
- With or after meals to prevent GI upset; may give with fluids other than water
- Parenteral dose slowly; keep in bed for at least 1 hr after dose; monitor vital signs
- After checking dose carefully; even slight overdose can lead to toxicity

Perform/provide:

- Storage at room temp
- Hard candy, frequent drinks, sugarless gum to relieve dry mouth

Evaluate:

- Therapeutic response: decreased secretions, absence of nausea and vomiting

Teach patient/family:

- To avoid driving or other hazardous activities; drowsiness may occur
- To avoid OTC medication: cough, cold preparations with alcohol, antihistamines unless directed by prescriber

Generic names

atropine (p. 143)
belladonna alkaloids (p. 161)
benztropine (p. 167)
biperiden (p. 176)
clidinium (p. 283)
cyclopentolate (p. 314)
dicyclomine (p. 359)
glycopyrrolate (p. 507)
homatropine (p. 529)
hyoscyamine (p. 548)
mepenzolate (p. 657)
methantheline (p. 674)
methscopolamine (p. 687)
procyclidine (p. 893)
propantheline (p. 900)
scopolamine (p. 945)
scopolamine (transdermal) (p. 947)
trihexyphenidyl (p. 1057)
tropicamide (p. 1068)

ANTICOAGULANTS

Action: Anticoagulants interfere with blood clotting by preventing clot formation.

Uses: Anticoagulants are used for deep-vein thrombosis, pulmonary emboli, myocardial infarction, open-heart surgery, disseminated intravascular clotting syndrome, atrial fibrillation with embolization, transfusion, and dialysis.

Side effects/adverse reactions: The most serious adverse reactions are hemorrhage, agranulocytosis, leukopenia, eosinophilia, and thrombocytopenia, depending on the specific product. The most common side effects are diarrhea, rash, and fever.

Contraindications: Persons with hemophilia, leukemia with bleeding, peptic ulcer disease, thrombocytopenic purpura, blood dyscrasias, acute nephritis, and subacute bacterial endocarditis should not use these products.

Precautions: Anticoagulants should be used with caution in alcoholism, elderly, and pregnancy.

Pharmacokinetics: Onset, peak, and duration vary widely among products. Most products are metabolized in the liver and excreted in urine.

Interactions: Salicylates, steroids, and nonsteroidal antiinflammatories will potentiate the action of anticoagulants. Anticoagulants may cause serious effects; please check individual monographs.

Possible nursing diagnoses:

- Altered tissue perfusion *[uses]*
- Risk of injury *[side effects]*
- Knowledge deficit *[teaching]*

NURSING CONSIDERATIONS

Assess:

- Blood studies (Hct, platelets, occult blood in stools) q3mo
- Partial prothrombin time, which should be 1½-2 × control PPT qd, also APTT, ACT
- B/P, watch for increasing signs of hypertension
- Bleeding gums, petechiae, ecchymosis, black tarry stools, hematuria
- Fever, skin rash, urticaria
- Needed dosage change q1-2wk

Administer:

- At same time each day to maintain steady blood levels
- Do not massage area or aspirate when giving SC injection; give in abdomen between pelvic bone, rotate sites; do not pull back on plunger; leave in for 10 sec; apply gentle pressure for 1 min
- Without changing needles
- Avoiding all IM injections that may cause bleeding

Perform/provide:

- Storage in tight container

Evaluate:

- Therapeutic response: decrease of deep vein thrombosis

Teach patient/family:

- To avoid OTC preparations that may cause serious drug interactions unless directed by prescriber
- That drug may be held during active bleeding (menstruation), depending on condition
- To use soft-bristle toothbrush to avoid bleeding gums, avoid contact sports, use electric razor
- To carry a Medic Alert ID identifying drug taken
- To report any signs of bleeding: gums, under skin, urine, stools

---

Generic names

dalteparin (p. 325)
enoxaprin (p. 409)
heparin (p. 524)
warfarin (p. 1092)

ANTICONVULSANTS

Action: Anticonvulsants are divided into the barbiturates (p. 35), benzodiazepines (p. 37), hydantoins, succinimides, and miscellaneous products. Barbiturates and benzodiazepines are discussed in separate sections. Hydantoins act by inhibiting the spread of seizure activity in the motor cortex. Succinimides act by inhibiting spike and wave formation; they also decrease amplitude, frequency, duration, and spread of discharge in seizures.

Uses: Hydantoins are used in generalized tonic-clonic seizures, status epilepticus, and psychomotor seizures. Succinimides are used for absence (petit mal) seizures. Barbiturates are used in generalized tonic-clonic and cortical focal seizures.

Side effects/adverse reactions: Bone marrow depression is the most life-threatening adverse reaction associated with hydantoins or succinimides. The most common side effects are GI symptoms. Other common side effects for hydantoins are gingival hyperplasia and CNS effects such as nystagmus, ataxia, slurred speech, and mental confusion.

Contraindications: Hypersensitive reactions may occur, and allergies should be identified before these products are given.

Precautions: Persons with renal or hepatic disease should be watched closely.

Pharmacokinetics: Onset, peak, and duration vary widely among products. Most products are metabolized in the liver and excreted in urine, bile, and feces.

Interactions: Decreased effects of estrogens, oral contraceptives (hydantoins).

Possible nursing diagnoses:

- Risk of injury *[uses]*
- Noncompliance *[teaching]*
- Sleep pattern disturbance *[adverse reactions]*

NURSING CONSIDERATIONS

Assess:

- Renal function studies, including BUN, creatinine, serum uric acid, urine creatinine clearance before and during therapy
- Blood studies: RBC, Hct, Hgb, reticulocyte counts qwk for 4 wk then qmo
- Hepatic studies: AST (SGOT), ALT (SGPT), bilirubin, creatinine
- Mental status, including mood, sensorium, affect, behavorial changes; if mental status changes, notify prescriber
- Eye problems, including need for ophthalmic exam before, during, and after treatment (slit lamp, funduscopy, tonometry)

- Allergic reaction, including red raised rash; if this occurs, drug should be discontinued
- Blood dyscrasia, including fever, sore throat, bruising, rash, jaundice
- Toxicity, including bone marrow depression, nausea, vomiting, ataxia, diplopia, cardiovascular collapse, Stevens-Johnson syndrome

Administer:

- With food, milk to decrease GI symptoms

Perform/provide:

- Good oral hygiene is important for hydantoins

Evaluate:

- Therapeutic response, including decreased seizure activity; document on patient's chart

Teach patient/family:

- To carry ID card or Medic Alert bracelet stating drugs taken, condition, prescriber's name, phone number
- To avoid driving, other activities that require alertness

Generic names

Hydantoins
ethotoin (p. 440)
mephenytoin (p. 661)
phensuximide (p. 841)
phenytoin (p. 849)

Succinimides
ethosuximide (p. 439)
methsuximide (p. 688)
phensuximide (p. 841)

Miscellaneous
acetazolamide (p. 72)
carbamazepine (p. 207)
clonazepam (p. 291)
diazepam (p. 352)
felbamate (p. 353)
gabapentin (p. 494)
lamotrigine (p. 600)
magnesium sulfate (p. 638)
paraldehyde (p. 804)
paramethadione (p. 806)
phenacemide (p. 834)
phenobarbital (p. 838)
primidone (p. 885)
trimethadione (p. 1059)
valproate (p. 1076)

ANTIDEPRESSANTS

Action: Antidepressants are divided into the tricyclics, MAOIs, and miscellaneous antidepressants. The tricyclics work by blocking reuptake of norepinephrine and serotonin into nerve endings and increasing action of norepinephrine and serotonin in nerve cells. MAOIs act by increasing concentrations of endogenous epinephrine, norepinephrine, serotonin, dopamine in storage sites in CNS by inhibition of MAO; increased concentration reduces depression.

Uses: Antidepressants are used for depression and in some cases enuresis in children.

Side effects/adverse reactions: The most serious adverse reactions are paralytic ileus, acute renal failure, hypertension, and hypertensive crisis, depending on the specific product. Common side effects are dizziness, drowsiness, diarrhea, dry mouth, retention, and orthostatic hypotension.

Contraindications: The contraindications to antidepressants are convulsive disorders, prostatic hypertrophy, severe renal, hepatic, cardiac disease depending on the type of medication.

Precautions: Antidepressants should be used cautiously in suicidal patients, severe depression, schizophrenia, hyperactivity, diabetes mellitus, pregnancy, and the elderly.

Pharmacokinetics: Onset, peak, and duration vary widely among products. Most products are metabolized in the liver and excreted in urine.

Interactions: Please check individual monographs, since interactions vary widely among products.

Possible nursing diagnoses:

- Ineffective individual coping *[uses]*
- Risk of injury *[uses/adverse reactions]*
- Knowledge deficit *[teaching]*

NURSING CONSIDERATIONS

Assess:

- B/P (lying, standing), pulse q4h; if systolic B/P drops 20 mm Hg, hold drug, notify prescriber; take vital signs q4h in patients with cardiovascular disease
- Blood studies: CBC, leukocytes, differential, cardiac enzymes if patient is receiving long-term therapy
- Hepatic studies: AST (SGOT), ALT (SGPT), bilirubin, creatinine
- Weight qwk; appetite may increase with drug
- EPS, primarily in elderly: rigidity, dystonia, akathisia
- Mental status: mood, sensorium, affect, suicidal tendencies, increase in psychiatric symptoms: depression, panic
- Urinary retention, constipation; constipation is more likely to occur in children, elderly
- Withdrawal symptoms: headache, nausea, vomiting, muscle pain, weakness; do not usually occur unless drug was discontinued abruptly
- Alcohol consumption; if alcohol is consumed, hold dose until morning

Administer:

- Increased fluids, bulk in diet if constipation, urinary retention occur
- With food or milk for GI symptoms
- Gum, hard candy, or frequent sips of water for dry mouth

Perform/provide:

• Storage in tight container at room temp; do not refreeze

• Assistance with ambulation during beginning therapy, since drowsiness, dizziness occur

• Safety measures including siderails primarily in elderly

• Checking to see PO medication swallowed

Evaluate:

• Therapeutic response: decreased depression

Teach patient/family:

• That therapeutic effects may take 2-3 wk

• To use caution in driving, other activities requiring alertness because of drowsiness, dizziness, blurred vision

• To avoid alcohol ingestion, other CNS depressants

• Not to discontinue medication quickly after long-term use; may cause nausea, headache, malaise

• To wear sunscreen or large hat, since photosensitivity may occur

---

Generic names

Tricyclics
amitriptyline (p. 109)
amoxapine (p. 115)
clomipramine (p. 290)
desipramine (p. 335)
doxepin (p. 393)
imipramine (p. 555)
nortriptyline (p. 770)
protriptyline (p. 908)
trimipramine (p. 1064)

Miscellaneous
bupropion (p. 191)
fluoxetine (p. 478)
fluvoxamine (p. 486)
maprotiline (p. 640)
nefazodone (p. 748)
paroxetine (p. 809)
sertraline (p. 952)
trazodone (p. 1044)
venlafaxine (p. 1080)

MAOIs
isocarboxazid (p. 579)
phenelzine (p. 837)
tranylcypromine (p. 1043)

ANTIDIABETICS

Action: Antidiabetics are divided into the insulins that decrease blood sugar, phosphate, and potassium and increase blood pyruvate and lactate; and oral antidiabetics that cause functioning β-cells in the pancreas to release insulin, improve the effect of endogenous and exogenous insulin.

Uses: Insulins are used for ketoacidosis and diabetes mellitus types I (IDDM) and II (NIDDM); oral antidiabetics are used for stable adult-onset diabetes mellitus type II (NIDDM).

Side effects/adverse reactions: The most common side effect of insulin and oral antidiabetics is hypoglycemia. Other adverse reactions to oral antidiabetics include blood dyscrasias, hepatotoxicity, and rarely, cholestatic jaundice. Adverse reactions to insulin products include allergic responses and more rarely, anaphylaxis.

Contraindications: Hypersensitive reactions may occur, and allergies should be identified before these products are given. Oral antidiabetics should not be used in juvenile or brittle diabetes, diabetic ketoacidosis, severe renal disease, or severe hepatic disease.

Precautions: Oral antidiabetics should be used with caution in the elderly, in cardiac disease, pregnancy, lactation, and in the presence of alcohol.

Pharmacokinetics: Onset, peak, and duration vary widely among products. Oral antidiabetics are metabolized in the liver, with metabolites excreted in urine, bile, and feces.

Interactions: Interactions vary widely among products. Check individual monograph for specific information.

Possible nursing diagnoses:

- Altered nutrition: more than body requirements *[uses]*

NURSING CONSIDERATIONS

Assess:

- Blood, urine glucose levels during treatment to determine diabetes control (oral products)
- Fasting blood glucose, 2 hr PP (60-100 mg/dl normal fasting level) (70-130 mg/dl normal 2-hr level)
- Hypoglycemic reaction that can occur during peak time

Administer:

- Insulin after warming to room temp by rotating in palms to prevent lipodystrophy from injecting cold insulin
- Human insulin to those allergic to beef or pork
- Oral antidiabetic 30 min before meals

Perform/provide:

- Rotation of injection sites when giving insulin; use abdomen, upper back, thighs, upper arm, buttocks; rotate sites within one of these regions; keep a record of sites

Evaluate:

- Therapeutic response, including decrease in polyuria, polydipsia, polyphagia, clear sensorium, absence of dizziness, stable gait

Teach patient/family:

- To avoid alcohol and salicylates except on advice of prescriber
- Symptoms of ketoacidosis: nausea, thirst, polyuria, dry mouth, decreased B/P, dry, flushed skin, acetone breath, drowsiness, Kussmaul respiration

• Symptoms of hypoglycemia: headache, tremors, fatigue, weakness; and that candy or sugar should be carried to treat hypoglycemia
• To test urine for glucose/ketones tid if this drug is replacing insulin
• To continue weight control, dietary restrictions, exercise, hygiene

Generic names

acetohexamide (p. 74)
chlorpropamide (p. 265)
glipizide (p. 502)
glyburide (p. 504)
insulin, regular (p. 565)
insulin, regular concentrated (p. 566)
insulin, zinc suspension (Lente) (p. 568)
insulin, zinc suspension extended (ultralente) (p. 569)
insulin, zinc suspension, prompt (semilente) (p. 570)
metformin (p. 671)
tolbutamide (p. 1038)

ANTIDIARRHEALS

Action: Antidiarrheals work by various actions, including direct action on intestinal muscles to decrease GI peristalsis; or by inhibiting prostaglandin synthesis responsible for GI hypermotility; by acting on mucosal receptors responsible for peristalsis; or by decreasing water content of stools.

Uses: Antidiarrheals are used for diarrhea of undetermined causes.

Side effects/adverse reactions: The most serious adverse reactions of some products are paralytic ileus, toxic megacolon, and angioneurotic edema. The most common side effects are constipation, nausea, dry mouth, and abdominal pain.

Contraindications: Persons with severe ulcerative colitis, pseudomembranous colitis with some products.

Precautions: Antidiarrheals should be used with caution in the elderly, pregnancy, lactation, children, dehydration.

Pharmacokinetics: Onset, peak, and duration vary widely among products. Most products are metabolized in the liver and excreted in urine.

Interactions: Please check individual monographs, since interactions vary widely among products.

Possible nursing diagnoses:

• Diarrhea *[uses]*
• Constipation *[adverse reactions]*
• Fluid volume deficit *[adverse reactions]*
• Knowledge deficit *[teaching]*

NURSING CONSIDERATIONS

Assess:

- Electrolytes (K, Na, Cl) if on long-term therapy
- Bowel pattern before; for rebound constipation after termination of medication
- Response after 48 hr; if no response, drug should be discontinued
- Dehydration in children

Administer:

- For 48 hr only

Evaluate:

- Therapeutic response: decreased diarrhea

Teach patient/family:

- To avoid OTC products
- Not to exceed recommended dose

Generic names

bismuth subsalicylate (p. 178)
difenoxin (p. 364)
kaolin/pectin (p. 593)
loperamide (p. 625)
opium tincture (p. 778)

ANTIDYSRHYTHMICS

Action: Antidysrhythmics are divided into four classes and miscellaneous antidysrhythmics:

- Class I increases the duration of action potential and effective refractory period and reduces disparity in the refractory period between a normal and infarcted myocardium; further subclasses include Ia, Ib, Ic
- Class II decreases the rate of SA node discharge, increases recovery time, slows conduction through the AV node, and decreases heart rate, which decreases O_2 consumption in the myocardium
- Class III increases the duration of action potential and the effective refractory period
- Class IV inhibits calcium ion influx across the cell membrane during cardiac depolarization; decreases SA node discharge, decreases conduction velocity through the AV node
- Miscellaneous antidysrhythmics include those such as adenosine, which slows conduction through the AV node, and digoxin, which decreases conduction velocity and prolongs the effective refractory period in the AV node

Uses: These products are used for PVCs, tachycardia, hypertension, atrial fibrillation, angina pectoris.

Side effects/adverse reactions: Side effects and adverse reactions vary widely among products.

Contraindications: Contraindications vary widely among products.

Precautions: Precautions vary widely among products.

Pharmacokinetics: Onset, peak, and duration vary widely among products.

Interactions: Interactions vary widely among products; check individual monograph for specific information.

Possible nursing diagnoses:

- Decreased cardiac output *[uses]*
- Altered tissue perfusion: cardiopulmonary *[uses]*
- Diarrhea *[adverse reactions]*
- Impaired gas exchange *[adverse reactions]*

NURSING CONSIDERATIONS

Assess:

- ECG continuously to determine drug effectiveness, PVCs or other dysrhythmias
- IV infusion rate to avoid causing nausea, vomiting
- For dehydration or hypovolemia
- B/P continuously for hypotension, hypertension
- I&O ratio
- Serum potassium
- Edema in feet and legs daily

Evaluate:

- Therapeutic response, including decrease in B/P in hypertension; decreased B/P, edema, moist rales in CHF

Teach patient/family:

- To comply with dosage schedule, even if patient is feeling better
- To report bradycardia, dizziness, confusion, depression, fever

Generic names

Class I
moricizine (p. 727)

Class Ia
disopyramide (p. 383)
procainamide (p. 888)
quinidine (p. 923)

Class Ib
lidocaine (p. 611)
mexiletine (p. 709)
phenytoin (p. 849)
tocainide (p. 1030)

Class Ic
flecainide (p. 465)
indecainide (p. 559)
propafenone (p. 899)

Class II
acebutolol (p. 67)
esmolol (p. 424)
propranolol (p. 904)
sotalol (p. 962)

Class III
amiodarone (p. 107)
bretylium (p. 180)

Class IV
verapamil (p. 1082)

Miscellaneous
adenosine (p. 81)
atropine (p. 143)
digoxin (p. 368)

ANTIFUNGALS (SYSTEMIC)

Action: Antifungals act by increasing cell membrane permeability in susceptible organisms by binding sterols and decreasing potassium, sodium, and nutrients in the cell.

Uses: Antifungals are used for infections of histoplasmosis, blastomycosis, coccidiomycosis, cryptococcosis, aspergillosis, phycomycosis, candidiasis, sporotrichosis causing severe meningitis, septicemia, and skin infections.

Side effects/adverse reactions: The most serious adverse reactions include renal tubular acidosis, permanent renal impairment, anuria, oliguria, hemorrhagic gastroenteritis, acute liver failure, and blood dyscrasias. Some common side effects include hypokalemia, nausea, vomiting, anorexia, headache, fever, and chills.

Contraindications: Persons with severe bone depression or hypersensitivity should not use these products.

Precautions: Antifungals should be used with caution in renal disease, pregnancy, and hepatic disease.

Pharmacokinetics: Onset, peak, and duration vary widely among products. Most products are metabolized in the liver and excreted in urine.

Interactions: Please check individual monographs, since interactions vary widely among products.

Possible nursing diagnoses:

- Risk of infection *[uses]*
- Risk of injury *[adverse reactions]*
- Knowledge deficit *[teaching]*

NURSING CONSIDERATIONS

Assess:

- VS q15-30min during first infusion; note changes in pulse, B/P
- I&O ratio; watch for decreasing urinary output, change in specific gravity; discontinue drug to prevent permanent damage to renal tubules
- Blood studies: CBC, K, Na, Ca, Mg q2wk
- Weight weekly; if weight increases over 2 lb/wk, edema is present; renal damage should be considered
- For renal toxicity: increasing BUN, if >40 mg/dl or if serum creatinine >3 mg/dl; drug may be discontinued or dosage reduced
- For hepatotoxicity: increasing AST, ALT, alk phosphatase, bilirubin
- For allergic reaction: dermatitis, rash; drug should be discontinued, antihistamines (mild reaction) or epinephrine (severe reaction) administered
- For hypokalemia: anorexia, drowsiness, weakness, decreased reflexes, dizziness, increased urinary output, increased thirst, paresthesias
- For ototoxicity: tinnitus (ringing, roaring in ears), vertigo, loss of hearing (rare)

Administer:

- IV using in-line filter (mean pore diameter >1 μm) using distal veins; check for extravasation, necrosis q8h
- Drug only after C&S confirms organism, drug needed to treat condition; make sure drug is used in life-threatening infections

Perform/provide:

- Protection from light during infusion, cover with foil
- Symptomatic treatment as ordered for adverse reactions: aspirin, antihistamines, antiemetics, antispasmodics
- Storage protected from moisture and light; diluted sol is stable for 24 hr

Evaluate:

- Therapeutic response: decreased fever, malaise, rash, negative C&S for infecting organism

Teach patient/family:

- That long-term therapy may be needed to clear infection (2 wk-3 mo depending on type of infection)

Generic names

amphotericin B (p. 123)
fluconazole (p. 467)
flucytosine (p. 468)
griseofulvin (p. 511)
itraconazole (p. 590)
ketoconazole (p. 594)
miconazole (p. 711)
nystatin (p. 772)

ANTIHISTAMINES

Action: Antihistamines compete with histamines for H_1-receptor sites. They antagonize in varying degrees most of the pharmacologic effects of histamines.

Uses: Products are used to control the symptoms of allergies, rhinitis, and pruritus.

Side effects/adverse reactions: Most products cause drowsiness; however, two of the newer products, astemizole and terfenadine, produce little, if any, drowsiness. Other common side effects are headache and thickening of bronchial secretions. Serious blood dyscrasias may occur, but are rare. Urinary retention, GI effects occur with many of these products.

Contraindications: Hypersensitivity to H_1-receptor antagonists occurs rarely. Patients with acute asthma and lower respiratory tract disease should not use these products, since thick secretions may result. Other contraindications include narrow-angle glaucoma, bladder neck obstruction, stenosing peptic ulcer, symptomatic prostatic hypertrophy, newborn, lactation.

Precautions: These products must be used cautiously in conjunction with intraocular pressure, since they increase intraocular pressure. Caution should also be used in patients with renal and cardiac disease, hypertension, and seizure disorders, pregnancy, lactation and in the elderly.

Pharmacokinetics: Onset varies from 20-60 min, with duration lasting 4-12 hr. In general, pharmacokinetics vary widely among products.

Interactions: Barbiturates, narcotics, hypnotics, tricyclic antidepressants, or alcohol can increase CNS depression when taken with antihistamines.

Possible nursing diagnoses:

- Ineffective airway clearance *[uses]*

NURSING CONSIDERATIONS

Assess:

- I&O ratio; be alert for urinary retention, frequency, dysuria; drug should be discontinued if these occur
- CBC during long-term therapy, since hemolytic anemia, although rare, may occur

• Blood dyscrasias: thrombocytopenia, agranulocytosis (rare)
• Respiratory status, including rate, rhythm, increase in bronchial secretions, wheezing, chest tightness
• Cardiac status, including palpitations, increased pulse, hypotension

Administer:
• With food or milk to decrease GI symptoms; absorption may be decreased slightly
• Whole (sustained release tabs)

Perform/provide:
• Hard candy, gum, frequent rinsing of mouth for dryness

Evaluate:
• Therapeutic response, including absence of allergy symptoms, itching

Teach patient/family:
• To notify prescriber if confusion, sedation, hypotension occur
• To avoid driving, other hazardous activity if drowsiness occurs
• To avoid concurrent use of alcohol, other CNS depressants
• To discontinue a few days before skin testing

Generic names

acrivastine/pseudoephedrine (p. 76)
astemizole (p. 138)
azatadine (p. 148)
brompheniramine (p. 185)
budesonide (p. 187)
chlorpheniramine (p. 261)
clemastine (p. 282)
cyproheptadine (p. 319)
dexchlorpheniramine (p. 344)
diphenydramine (p. 378)
loratadine (p. 627)
promethazine (p. 898)
terfenadine (p. 1000)
trimeprazine (p. 1058)
tripelennamine (p. 1065)
triprolidine (p. 1067)

ANTIHYPERTENSIVES

Action: Antihypertensives are divided into angiotensin-converting enzyme (ACE) inhibitors, β-adrenergic blockers, calcium channel blockers, centrally acting adrenergics, diuretics, peripherally acting antiadrenergics, and vasodilators. β-Blockers, calcium channel blockers, and diuretics are discussed in separate sections. Angiotensin-converting enzyme inhibitors act by selectively suppressing renin-angiotensin I to angiotensin II; dilation of arterial and venous vessels occurs. Centrally acting adrenergics act by inhibiting the sympathetic vasomotor center in the CNS that reduces impulses in the sympathetic nervous system; blood pressure, pulse rate, and cardiac output decrease. Peripherally acting antiadrenergics inhibit sympathetic vasoconstriction by inhibiting release of norepinephrine and/or depleting norepinephrine stores in adrenergic nerve endings. Vasodilators act on arteriolar smooth muscle by producing direct relaxation or vasodilation; a reduction in blood pressure, with concomitant increases in heart rate and cardiac output, occurs.

Uses: Used for hypertension and for heart failure not responsive to conventional therapy. Some products are used in hypertensive crisis, angina, and for some cardiac dysrhythmias.

Side effects/adverse reactions: The most common side effects are marked hypotension, bradycardia, tachycardia, headache, nausea, and vomiting. Side effects and adverse reactions may vary widely between classes and specific products.

Contraindications: Hypersensitive reactions may occur, and allergies should be identified before these products are given. Antihypertensives should not be used in patients with heart block or in children.

Precautions: Antihypertensives should be used with caution in the elderly, in dialysis patients, and in the presence of hypovolemia, leukemia, and electrolyte imbalances.

Pharmacokinetics: Onset, peak, and duration vary widely among products. Most products are metabolized in the liver, with metabolites excreted in urine, bile, and feces.

Interactions: Interactions vary widely among products; check individual monograph for specific information.

Possible nursing diagnoses:

- Altered tissue perfusion *[uses]*
- Decreased cardiac output *[uses]*
- Diarrhea *[adverse reactions]*
- Impaired gas exchange *[adverse reactions]*

NURSING CONSIDERATIONS

Assess:

- Blood studies: neutrophil; decreased platelets occur with many of the products
- Renal studies: protein, BUN, creatinine; watch for increased levels that may indicate nephrotic syndrome; obtain baselines in renal and liver function studies before beginning treatment
- Edema in feet and legs daily
- Allergic reaction, including rash, fever, pruritus, urticaria: drug should be discontinued if antihistamines fail to help
- Symptoms of CHF: edema, dyspnea, wet rales, B/P
- Renal symptoms: polyuria, oliguria, frequency

Perform/provide:

- Supine or Trendelenburg position for severe hypotension

Evaluate:

• Therapeutic response, including decrease in B/P in hypotension; decreased B/P, edema, moist rales in CHF

Teach patient/family:

• To comply with dosage schedule, even if feeling better

• To rise slowly to sitting or standing position to minimize orthostatic hypotension

Generic names

Angiotensin-converting enzyme inhibitors
benazepril (p. 162)
enalapril (p. 407)
fosinopril (p. 490)
perindopril (p. 826)
quinapril (p. 920)
ramipril (p. 927)
spirapril (p. 964)

Centrally acting adrenergics
clonidine (p. 293)
guanabenz (p. 513)
guanfacine (p. 516)
methyldopa (p. 690)

Peripherally acting antiadrenergics
guanadrel (p. 514)
guanethidine (p. 515)
prazosin (p. 879)
reserpine (p. 930)
terazosin (p. 996)

Vasodilators
diazoxide (p. 354)
hydralazine (p. 530)
minoxidil (p. 718)
nitroprusside (p. 764)

Antiadrenergic
combined alpha/beta blocker—labetalol (p. 598)

ANTIINFECTIVES

Action: Antiinfectives are divided into several groups, which include but are not limited to penicillins, cephalosporins, aminoglycosides, sulfonamides, tetracyclines, monobactam, erythromycins, and quinolones. These drugs act by inhibiting the growth and replication of susceptible bacterial organisms.

Uses: Used for infections of susceptible organisms. These products are effective against bacterial, rickettsial, and spirochete infections.

Side effects/adverse reactions: The most common side effects are nausea, vomiting, and diarrhea. Adverse reactions include bone marrow depression and anaphylaxis.

Contraindications: Hypersensitivity reactions may occur, and allergies should be identified before these products are given. Cross-sensitivity can

occur between products of different classes (penicillins or cephalosporins). Many persons allergic to penicillins are also allergic to cephalosporins.
Precautions: Antiinfectives should be used with caution in persons with renal and liver disease.
Pharmacokinetics: Onset, peak, and duration vary widely among products. Most products are metabolized in the liver, and metabolites are excreted in urine, bile, and feces.
Interactions: Interactions vary widely among products; check individual monograph for specific information.
Possible nursing diagnoses:
- Risk of infection *[uses]*
- Diarrhea *[adverse reactions]*

NURSING CONSIDERATIONS

Assess:
- Nephrotoxicity, including increased BUN, creatinine
- Blood studies: AST (SGOT), ALT (SGPT), CBC, Hct, bilirubin; test monthly if patient is on long-term therapy
- Bowel pattern qd; if severe diarrhea occurs, drug should be discontinued
- Urine output; if decreasing, notify prescriber; may indicate nephrotoxicity
- Allergic reaction, including rash, fever, pruritus, urticaria; drug should be discontinued
- Bleeding: ecchymosis, bleeding gums, hematuria, stool guaiac daily
- Overgrowth of infection: perineal itching, fever, malaise, redness, pain, swelling, drainage, rash, diarrhea, change in cough, sputum

Administer:
- For 10-14 days to ensure organism death, prevention of superinfection
- After C&S completed; drug may be taken as soon as culture is taken

Evaluate:
- Therapeutic response, including absence of fever, fatigue, malaise, draining wounds

Teach patient/family:
- To comply with dosage schedule, even if feeling better
- To report sore throat, bruising, bleeding, joint pain; may indicate blood dyscrasias (rare)

Generic names

Aminoglycosides
amikacin (p. 98)
azithromycin (p. 150)
clarithromycin (p. 281)
gentamicin (p. 499)
kanamycin (p. 591)
neomycin (p. 749)
netilmicin (p. 753)
streptomycin (p. 971)
tobramycin (p. 1032)

Cephalosporins
cefaclor (p. 217)
cefadroxil (p. 218)
cefamandole (p. 219)
cefazolin (p. 221)
cefixime (p. 222)
cefmetazole (p. 223)
cefonicid (p. 225)
cefoperazone (p. 226)
ceforanide (p. 227)
cefotaxime (p. 229)
cefprozil (p. 235)
cefuroxime (p. 240)
cephalexin (p. 242)
cephalothin (p. 243)
cephapirin (p. 245)
cephradine (p. 247)
moxalactam (p. 729)

Penicillins
amoxicillin/clavulanate (p. 117)
ampicillin/sulbactam (p. 125)
azlocillin (p. 152)
bacampicillin (p. 154)
cloxacillin (p. 297)
dicloxacillin (p. 358)
imipenem/cilastatin (p. 554)
methicillin (p. 678)
mezlocillin (p. 710)
nafcillin (p. 736)
oxacillin (p. 781)
penicillin G benzathine (p. 813)
penicillin G potassium (p. 815)
penicillin G procaine (p. 817)
penicillin G sodium (p. 818)
penicillin V (p. 820)
piperacillin (p. 858)
ticarcillin (p. 1025)
ticarcillin/clavulanate (p. 1027)

Sulfonamides
sulfasalazine (p. 983)
sulfisoxazole (p. 986)

Tetracyclines
demeclocycline (p. 334)
doxycycline (p. 397)
minocycline (p. 717)
oxytetracycline (p. 795)
tetracycline (p. 1006)

ANTINEOPLASTICS

Action: Antineoplastics are divided into alkylating agents, antimetabolites, antibiotic agents, hormonal agents, and miscellaneous agents. Alkylating agents act by cross-linking strands of DNA. Antimetabolites act by inhibiting DNA synthesis. Antibiotic agents act by inhibiting RNA synthesis and by delaying or inhibiting mitosis. Hormones alter the effects of androgens, luteinizing hormone, follicle-stimulating hormone, and estrogen by changing the hormonal environment.
Uses: Uses vary widely among products and classes of drugs. They are

used to treat leukemia, Hodgkin's disease, lymphomas, and other tumors throughout the body.

Side effects/adverse reactions: Most products cause thrombocytopenia, leukopenia, and anemia, and if these reactions occur, the drug may have to be stopped until the problem is corrected. Other side effects include nausea, vomiting, glossitis, and hair loss. Some products also cause hepatotoxicity, nephrotoxicity, and cardiotoxicity.

Contraindications: Hypersensitive reactions may occur, and allergies should be identified before these products are given. Also, persons with severe liver and kidney disease should not use these products unless the benefits outweigh the risks.

Precautions: Persons with bleeding, severe bone marrow depression, or renal or hepatic disease should be watched closely.

Pharmacokinetics: Onset, peak, and duration vary widely among products. Most products cross the placenta and are excreted in breast milk and in urine.

Interactions: Toxicity may occur when used with other antineoplastics or radiation.

Possible nursing diagnoses:

- Risk of infection *[adverse reactions]*
- Altered nutrition: less than body requirements *[adverse reactions]*
- Altered oral mucous membrane *[adverse reactions]*

NURSING CONSIDERATIONS

Assess:

- CBC, differential, platelet count weekly; withhold drug if WBC is <4000 or platelet count is <75,000; notify prescriber of results
- Renal function studies, including BUN, creatinine, serum uric acid, and urine creatinine clearance before and during therapy
- I&O ratio; report fall in urine output of 30 ml/hr
- Monitor temp q4h (may indicate beginning infection)
- Liver function tests before and during therapy (bilirubin, AST [SGOT], ALT [SGPT], LDH) as needed or monthly
- Bleeding, including hematuria, guaiac, bruising or petechiae, mucosa, or orifices q8h; obtain prescription for viscous Xylocaine (lidocaine)
- Yellowing of skin, sclera, dark urine, clay-colored stools, itchy skin, abdominal pain, fever, diarrhea
- Edema in feet, joint pain, stomach pain, shaking
- Inflammation of mucosa, breaks in skin

Administer:

- Checking IV site for irritation; phlebitis
- Epinephrine for hypersensitivity reaction
- Antibiotics for prophylaxis of infection

Perform/provide:

- Strict asepsis, protective isolation if WBC levels are low
- Comprehensive oral hygiene, using careful technique and soft-bristle brush

Evaluate:

- Therapeutic response, including decreased tumor size

Teach patient/family:

- To report signs of infection, including increased temp, sore throat, malaise
- To report signs of anemia, including fatigue, headache, faintness, shortness of breath, irritability
- To report bleeding and avoid use of razors or commercial mouthwash

---

Generic names

Alkylating agents
busulfan (p. 193)
carboplatin (p. 209)
carmustine (p. 213)
chlorambucil (p. 250)
cisplatin (p. 277)
cyclophosphamide (p. 315)
dacarbazine (p. 322)
lomustine (p. 623)
mechlorethamine (p. 646)
melphalan (p. 654)
streptozocin (p. 972)
thiotepa (p. 1018)
uracil mustard (p. 1071)

Antimetabolites
cytarabine (p. 320)
doxorubicin (p. 395)
etoposide (p. 446)
fludarabine (p. 469)
fluorouracil (p. 476)
mercaptopurine (p. 665)
thioguanine (6-TG) (p. 1014)

Antibiotic agents
bleomycin (p. 181)
dactinomycin (p. 324)
daunorubicin (p. 331)
methotrexate (p. 683)
mitomycin (p. 720)
mitoxantrone (p. 723)
plicamycin (p. 865)

Hormonal agents
aminoglutethimide (p. 104)
estramustine (p. 429)
flutamide (p. 486)
goserelin acetate (p. 510)
leuprolide (p. 602)
megestrol (p. 653)
mitotane (p. 722)
tamoxifen (p. 992)
testolactone (p. 1001)

Miscellaneous
altretamine (p. 93)
asparaginase (p. 134)
cladribine (p. 279)
interferon alfa-2A (p. 571)
interferon alfa-2B (p. 571)
pentostatin (p. 827)
procarbazine (p. 890)
vinblastine (p. 1084)
vincristine (p. 1086)
vinorelbine (p. 1088)

ANTIPARKINSON AGENTS

Action: Antiparkinson agents are divided into cholinergics and dopamine agonists. Cholinergics work by blocking or competing at central acetylcholine receptors; dopamine agonists work by decarboxylation to dopamine or by activation of dopamine receptors; monoamine oxidase type B inhibitors work by increasing dopamine activity by inhibiting MAO type B activity.

Uses: Antiparkinson agents are used alone or in combination for patients with Parkinson's disease.

Side effects/adverse reactions: Side effects and adverse reactions vary widely among products. The most common side effects include involuntary movements, headache, numbness, insomnia, nightmares, nausea, vomiting, dry mouth, and orthostatic hypotension.

Contraindications: Persons with hypersensitivity, narrow-angle glaucoma, and undiagnosed skin lesions should not use these products.

Precautions: Antiparkinson agents should be used with caution in pregnancy, lactation, children, renal, cardiac, hepatic disease, and affective disorder.

Pharmacokinetics: Onset, peak, and duration vary widely among products. Most products are metabolized in the liver and excreted in urine.

Interactions: Please check individual monographs, since interactions vary widely among products.

Possible nursing diagnoses:

- Risk of injury *[uses]*
- Risk of impaired mobility *[uses]*
- Knowledge deficit *[teaching]*

NURSING CONSIDERATIONS

Assess:

- B/P, respiration
- Mental status: affect, mood, behavioral changes, depression, complete suicide assessment

Administer:

- Drug up until NPO before surgery
- Adjust dosage depending on patient response
- With meals; limit protein taken with drug
- Only after MAOIs have been discontinued for 2 wk

Perform/provide:

- Assistance with ambulation, during beginning therapy
- Testing for diabetes mellitus, acromegaly if on long-term therapy

Evaluate:

• Therapeutic response: decrease in akathisia, increased mood

Teach patient/family:

• To change positions slowly to prevent orthostatic hypotension

• To report side effects: twitching, eye spasm; indicate overdose

• To use drug exactly as prescribed; if drug is discontinued abruptly, parkinsonian crisis may occur

Generic names

amantadine (p. 96)
benztropine (p. 167)
biperiden (p. 176)
bromocriptine (p. 184)
carbidopa/levodopa (p. 208)
levodopa (p. 605)
procyclidine (p. 893)
selegiline (p. 950)
trihexyphenidyl (p. 1057)

ANTIPSYCHOTICS

Action: Antipsychotics/neuroleptics are divided into several subgroups: phenothiazines, thioxanthenes, butyrophenones, dibenzoxazepines, dibenzodiazepines, and indolones and other heterocyclic compounds. Although chemically different, these subgroups share many pharmacologic and clinical properties. All antipsychotics work to block postsynaptic dopamine receptors in the brain that are responsible for psychotic behavior, including hallucinations, delusions, and paranoia.

Uses: Antipsychotic behavior is decreased in conditions such as schizophrenia, paranoia, and mania. These agents are also effective for severe anxiety, intractable hiccups, nausea, vomiting, behavioral problems in children, and before surgery for relaxation.

Side effects/adverse reactions: The most common side effects include EPS such as pseudoparkinsonism, akathisia, dystonia, and tardive dyskinesia, which may be controlled by use of antiparkinsonian agents. Serious adverse reactions such as hypotension, agranulocytosis, cardiac arrest, and laryngospasm have occurred. Other common side effects include dry mouth and photosensitivity.

Contraindications: Persons with liver damage, severe hypertension or coronary disease, cerebral arteriosclerosis, blood dyscrasias, bone marrow depression, parkinsonism, severely depressed persons, narrow-angle glaucoma, children <12 yr, or persons withdrawing from alcohol or barbiturates should not use antipsychotics until these conditions are corrected.

Precautions: Caution must be used when antipsychotics are given to the elderly, since metabolism is slowed and adverse reactions can occur rapidly. Hepatic and renal disease may cause poor metabolism and excretion of the drug. Seizure threshold is decreased with these products; increases in the dose of anticonvulsants may be required. Persons with diabetes mellitus, prostatic hypertrophy, chronic respiratory disease, and peptic ulcer disease should be monitored closely.

Pharmacokinetics: Onset, peak, and duration vary widely with different products and routes. Products are metabolized by the liver, are excreted in urine as metabolites, are highly bound to plasma proteins, cross the placenta, and enter breast milk. Half-life can be extended over 3 days.

Interactions: Because other CNS depressants can cause oversedation, these combinations should be used carefully. Anticholinergics may decrease the therapeutic actions of phenothiazines and also cause increased anticholinergic effects.

Possible nursing diagnoses:

- Altered thought processes *[uses]*
- Sensory-perceptual alterations *[uses]*

NURSING CONSIDERATIONS

Assess:

- Bilirubin, CBC, liver function studies qmo, since these drugs are metabolized in the liver and excreted in urine
- I&O ratio: palpate bladder if low urinary output occurs, since urinary retention occurs with many of these products
- Affect, orientation, LOC, reflexes, gait, coordination, sleep pattern disturbances
- Dizziness, faintness, palpitations, tachycardia on rising
- B/P lying and standing; wide fluctuations between lying and standing B/P may require dosage or product change, since orthostatic hypotension is occurring
- EPS, including akathisia, tardive dyskinesia, pseudoparkinsonism

Administer:

- Antiparkinsonian agent if EPS occur
- Liquid concentrates mixed in glass of juice or cola, since taste is unpleasant; avoid contact with skin when preparing liquid concentrate or parenteral medications

Perform/provide:

- Supervised ambulation until stabilized on medication; do not involve in strenuous exercise program because fainting is possible; patient should not stand still for long periods
- Increased fluids to prevent constipation
- Sips of water, candy, gum for dry mouth

Evaluate:
• Therapeutic response: decrease in excitement, hallucinations, delusions, paranoia, reorganization of thought patterns, speech

Teach patient/family:
• To rise from sitting or lying position gradually, since fainting may occur
• To remain lying down for at least 30 min after IM injections
• To avoid hot tubs, hot showers, or tub baths, since hypotension may occur
• To wear a sunscreen or protective clothing to prevent burns
• To take extra precautions during hot weather to stay cool; heat stroke can occur
• To avoid driving, other activities requiring alertness until response to medication is known
• That drowsiness or impaired mental/motor activity is evident the first 2 wk, but tends to decrease over time

---

Generic names

Phenothiazines
chlorpromazine (p. 262)
fluphenazine (p. 481)
mesoridazine (p. 668)
perphenazine (p. 831)
prochlorperazine (p. 892)
promazine (p. 895)
thioridazine (p. 1016)
thiothixene (p. 1020)
trifluoperazine (p. 1053)

Butyrophenone
haloperidol (p. 521)

Miscellaneous
loxapine (p. 631)
molindone (p. 725)
risperidone (p. 937)

ANTITUBERCULARS

Action: Antituberculars act by inhibiting RNA or DNA, or interfering with lipid and protein synthesis, thereby decreasing tubercle bacilli replication.
Uses: Antituberculars are used for pulmonary tuberculosis.
Side effects/adverse reactions: They vary widely among products. Most products can cause nausea, vomiting, anorexia, and rash. Serious adverse reactions include renal failure, nephrotoxicity, ototoxicity, and hepatic necrosis.
Contraindications: Persons with severe renal disease or hypersensitivity should not use these products.
Precautions: Antituberculars should be used with caution with pregnancy, lactation, and hepatic disease.
Pharmacokinetics: Onset, peak, and duration vary widely among products. Most products are metabolized in the liver and excreted in urine.

Interactions: Please check individual monographs, since interactions vary widely among products.

Possible nursing diagnoses:

- Risk of infection *[uses]*
- Risk of injury *[adverse reactions]*
- Knowledge deficit *[teaching]*
- Noncompliance *[teaching]*

NURSING CONSIDERATIONS

Assess:

- Signs of anemia: Hct, Hgb, fatigue
- Liver studies qwk: ALT (SGPT), AST (SGOT), bilirubin
- Renal status before, qmo: BUN, creatinine, output, specific gravity, urinalysis
- Hepatic status: decreased appetite, jaundice, dark urine, fatigue

Administer:

- For some of these agents on empty stomach, 1 hr ac (only for isoniazid and rifampin) or 2 hr pc
- Antiemetic if vomiting occurs
- After C&S is completed; qmo to detect resistance

Evaluate:

- Therapeutic response: decreased symptoms of TB, culture negative

Teach patient/family:

- That compliance with dosage schedule, duration is necessary
- That scheduled appointments must be kept; relapse may occur
- To avoid alcohol while taking drug
- To report flulike symptoms: excessive fatigue, anorexia, vomiting, sore throat; unusual bleeding, yellowish discoloration of skin/eyes

Generic names

capreomycin (p. 203)
cycloserine (p. 317)
ethambutol (p. 435)
ethionamide (p. 438)
isoniazid (p. 582)
kanamycin (p. 591)
pyrazinamide (p. 913)
rifabutin (p. 933)
rifampin (p. 934)
streptomycin (p. 971)

ANTITUSSIVES/EXPECTORANTS

Action: Antitussives act by suppressing the cough reflex by direct action on the cough center in the medulla. Expectorants act by liquefying and reducing the viscosity of thick, tenacious secretions.

Uses: Antitussives/expectorants are used to treat cough occurring in pneumonia, bronchitis, TB, cystic fibrosis, and emphysema; as an adjunct in atelectasis (expectorants); and nonproductive cough (antitussives).
Side effects/adverse reactions: The most common side effects are drowsiness, dizziness, and nausea.
Contraindications: Some products are contraindicated in hypothyroidism, iodine sensitivity, pregnancy, and lactation.
Precautions: Some products should be used cautiously in asthmatic, elderly, and debilitated patients.
Pharmacokinetics: Onset, peak, and duration vary widely among products. Some products are metabolized in the liver and excreted in urine.
Interactions: Please check individual monographs since interactions vary widely among products.
Possible nursing diagnoses:
- Ineffective breathing pattern *[uses]*
- Ineffective airway clearance *[uses]*
- Knowledge deficit *[teaching]*

NURSING CONSIDERATIONS
Assess:
- Cough: type, frequency, character (including sputum)

Administer:
- Decreased dose to elderly patients; their metabolism may be slowed

Perform/provide:
- Increased fluids to liquefy secretions
- Humidification of patient's room

Evaluate:
- Therapeutic response: absence of cough

Teach patient/family:
- To avoid driving, other hazardous activities until patient is stabilized on this medication
- To avoid smoking, smoke-filled rooms, perfumes, dust, environmental pollutants, cleaners that increase cough

---

Generic names

acetylcysteine (p. 75)
ammonium (p. 111)
benzonatate (p. 165)
codeine (p. 300)
dextromethorphan (p. 348)
diphenhydramine (p. 378)
guaifenesin (p. 512)
hydrocodone (p. 533)
potassium iodide (p. 872)
terpin hydrate (p. 1000)

ANTIVIRALS

Action: Antivirals act by interfering with DNA synthesis that is needed for viral replication.

Uses: Antivirals are used for mucocutaneous herpes simplex virus, herpes genitalis (HSV_1, HSV_2), advanced HIV infections, herpes simplex virus encephalitis, varicella-zoster encephalomyelitis.

Side effects/adverse reactions: Serious adverse reactions are fatal metabolic encephalopathy, blood dyscrasias, and acute renal failure. Common side effects are nausea, vomiting, anorexia, diarrhea, headache, vaginitis, and moniliasis.

Contraindications: Persons with hypersensitivity, herpes zoster in immunosuppressed individuals should not use these products.

Precautions: Antivirals should be used with caution in renal disease, liver disease, lactation, pregnancy, and dehydration.

Pharmacokinetics: Onset, peak, and duration vary widely among products. Most products are metabolized in the liver and excreted in urine.

Interactions: Please check individual monographs, since interactions vary widely among products.

Possible nursing diagnoses:

- Risk of infection *[uses]*
- Risk of injury *[adverse reactions]*
- Knowledge deficit *[teaching]*

NURSING CONSIDERATIONS

Assess:

- Signs of infection, anemia
- I&O ratio; report hematuria, oliguria, fatigue, weakness; may indicate nephrotoxicity; check for protein in urine during treatment
- Any patient with compromised renal system, since drug is excreted slowly in poor renal system function; toxicity may occur rapidly
- Liver studies: AST (SGOT), ALT (SGPT)
- Blood studies: WBC, RBC, Hct, Hgb, bleeding time; blood dyscrasias may occur; drug should be discontinued
- Renal studies: urinalysis, protein, BUN, creatinine, CrCl
- C&S before drug therapy; drug may be taken as soon as culture is taken; repeat C&S after treatment
- Bowel pattern before, during treatment; if severe abdominal pain with bleeding occurs, drug should be discontinued
- Skin eruptions: rash, urticaria, itching
- Allergies before treatment, reaction of each medication; record allergies on chart in bright red letters

Administer:

- Increased fluids to 3 L/day to decrease crystalluria when given IV

Perform/provide:

- Storage at room temp for up to 12 hr after reconstitution
- Adequate intake of fluids (2 L) to prevent deposit in kidneys

Evaluate:

- Therapeutic response: absence of control of infection

Teach patient/family:

- That drug does not cure infection, just controls symptoms
- To report sore throat, fever, fatigue; could indicate superinfection
- That drug must be taken in equal intervals around the clock to maintain blood levels for duration of therapy
- To notify prescriber of side effects of bruising, bleeding, fatigue, malaise; may indicate blood dyscrasias

---

Generic names

acyclovir (p. 78)
amantadine (p. 96)
didanosine (p. 360)
famciclovir (p. 450)
foscarnet (p. 488)
ganciclovir (p. 496)
rimantadine (p. 935)
stavudine (p. 968)
vidarabine (p. 1084)
zalcitabine (p. 1095)
zidovudine (p. 1096)

BARBITURATES

Action: Barbiturates act by decreasing impulse transmission to the cerebral cortex.

Uses: All forms of epilepsy can be controlled, since the seizure threshold is increased. Uses also include febrile seizures in children, sedation, insomnia, hyperbilirubinemia, chronic cholestasis with some of these products. Ultra-short-acting barbiturates are used as anesthetics.

Side effects/adverse reactions: The most common side effects are drowsiness and nausea. Serious adverse reactions such as Stevens-Johnson syndrome and blood dyscrasias may occur with high doses and long-term treatment.

Contraindications: Hypersensitivity may occur, and allergies should be identified before administering. Barbiturates are identified as pregnancy category D and should not be used in pregnancy. Other contraindications include porphyria and marked impairment of liver function.

Precautions: Caution must be used when these products are given to the elderly or debilitated; usually smaller doses are needed, since metabolism is slowed. Persons with renal and hepatic disease may show delayed excretion. Barbiturates may produce excitability in children.

Pharmacokinetics: Onset of action can be slow, up to 1 hr, with a peak of 8 hr and a duration of 3-10 hr. These drugs are metabolized by the liver, excreted by the kidneys, cross the placenta, and enter breast milk.

Interactions: Increased CNS depressant effect may occur with alcohol, MAOIs, sedatives, or narcotics. These products should be used together cautiously. Oral anticoagulants, corticosteroids, griseofulvin, quinidine, oral contraceptives, and theophylline may show a decreased effect when used with barbiturates.

Possible nursing diagnoses:

- Sleep pattern disturbance *[uses]*
- Risk of injury *[adverse reactions]*

NURSING CONSIDERATIONS

Assess:

- Hepatic and renal studies: AST (SGOT), ALT (SGPT), bilirubin, creatinine, LDH, alkaline phosphatase, BUN if patient is on long-term therapy, since these products are metabolized and excreted by the liver and kidney
- Blood studies: CBC, hematocrit, hemoglobin, and prothrombin time if patient is on long-term therapy, since these products increase the possibility of bleeding and blood dyscrasias
- Barbiturate toxicity: hypotension, pulmonary constriction; cold, clammy skin; cyanosis of lips; insomnia; nausea; vomiting, hallucinations, delirium, weakness

Evaluate:

- Therapeutic response, including appropriate sedation or seizure control

Teach patient/family:

- That physical dependency may result when used for extended periods (45-90 days, depending on dose)
- To avoid driving, activities that require alertness, since drowsiness and dizziness may occur
- To abstain from alcohol or other psychotropic medications unless directed by prescriber
- Not to discontinue medication abruptly after long-term use; withdrawal symptoms will occur

---

Generic names

amobarbital (p. 113)
mephobarbital (p. 662)
pentobarbital (p. 825)
phenobarbital (p. 838)
secobarbital (p. 947)
talbutal (p. 991)
thiopental (p. 1015)

BENZODIAZEPINES

Action: Benzodiazepines potentiate the effects of γ-aminobutyrate (GABA), including any other inhibitory transmitters in the CNS, resulting in decreased anxiety.

Uses: Anxiety is relieved in conditions such as phobic disorders. Benzodiazepines are also used for acute alcohol withdrawal to relieve the possibility of delirium tremens, and some products are used before surgery for relaxation.

Side effects/adverse reactions: The most common side effects are dizziness, drowsiness, blurred vision, and orthostatic hypotension. Most adverse effects are mediated through the CNS. There is a risk of physicial dependence and abuse.

Contraindications: Hypersensitivity, acute narrow-angle glaucoma, children <6 months, liver disease (clonazepam), lactation (diazepam).

Precautions: Caution must be used when these products are given to the elderly or debilitated; usually smaller doses are needed, since metabolism is slowed. Persons with renal and hepatic disease may show delayed excretion. Clonazepam may increase incidence of seizures.

Pharmacokinetics: Onset of action is ½-1 hr, with a peak of 1-2 hr and a duration of 4-6 hr. These drugs are metabolized by the liver, excreted by the kidneys, cross the placenta, and enter breast milk.

Interactions: Increased CNS depressant effect may occur with other CNS depressants. These products should be used together cautiously. Alcohol should not be used; fatal reactions can occur. The serum concentration and toxicity of digoxin may be increased.

Possible nursing diagnoses:

- Anxiety *[uses]*
- Risk of injury *[adverse reactions]*

NURSING CONSIDERATIONS

Assess:

- B/P (lying, standing), pulse; if systolic B/P drops 20 mm Hg, hold drug, notify prescriber; orthostatic hypotension is severe
- Hepatic and renal studies: AST (SGOT), ALT (SGPT), bilirubin, creatinine, LDH, alkaline phosphatase
- Physical dependency, withdrawal symptoms, including headache, nausea, vomiting, muscle pain, weakness after long-term use

Administer:

- With food or milk for GI symptoms; may give crushed if patient is unable to swallow medication whole

Evaluate:
- Therapeutic response, including relaxation or decreased anxiety

Teach patient/family:
- That drug should not be used for everyday stress or long-term; not to take more than prescribed amount, since drug is habit forming
- To avoid driving and activities that require alertness, since drowsiness and dizziness occur
- To abstain from alcohol, other psychotropic medications unless directed by prescriber
- Not to discontinue medication abruptly after long-term use; withdrawal symptoms will occur

---

Generic names

alprazolam (p. 89)
chlordiazepoxide (p. 255)
clonazepam (p. 291)
diazepam (p. 352)
flurazepam (p. 484)
halazepam (p. 518)
lorazepam (p. 627)
midazolam (p. 714)
oxazepam (p. 786)
prazepam (p. 877)
quazepam (p. 918)
temazepam (p. 994)
triazolam (p. 1051)

BETA-ADRENERGIC BLOCKERS

Action: β-Blockers are divided into selective and nonselective blockers. Nonselective blockers produce a fall in blood pressure without reflex tachycardia or reduction in heart rate through a mixture of β-blocking effects; elevated plasma renins are reduced. Selective β-blockers competitively block stimulation of β_1-receptors in cardiac smooth muscle; these drugs produce chronotropic and inotropic effects.

Uses: β-Blockers are used for hypertension, ventricular dysrhythmias, and prophylaxis of angina pectoris.

Side effects/adverse reactions: The most common side effects are orthostatic hypotension, bradycardia, diarrhea, nausea, vomiting. Serious adverse reactions include blood dyscrasias, bronchospasm, and CHF.

Contraindications: Hypersensitive reactions may occur, and allergies should be identified before these products are given. β-Adrenergic blockers should not be used in heart block, CHF, or cardiogenic shock.

Precautions: β-Blockers should be used with caution in the elderly or in renal and thyroid disease, COPD, CAD, diabetes mellitus, pregnancy, or asthma.

Pharmacokinetics: Onset, peak, and duration vary widely among products. Most products are metabolized in the liver, with metabolites excreted in urine, bile, and feces.

Interactions: Interactions vary widely among products; check individual monograph for specific information.

Possible nursing diagnoses:

- Altered tissue perfusion *[uses]*
- Decreased cardiac output *[uses]*
- Diarrhea *[adverse reactions]*
- Impaired gas exchange *[adverse reactions]*

NURSING CONSIDERATIONS

Assess:

- Renal studies, including protein, BUN, creatinine; watch for increased levels that may indicate nephrotic syndrome; obtain baselines in renal and liver function studies before beginning treatment
- I&O, weight daily
- B/P during beginning treatment and periodically thereafter, pulse q4h, note rate, rhythm, quality
- Apical/radial pulse before administration; notify prescriber of significant changes
- Edema in feet and legs daily

Administer:

- PO ac, hs, tablets may be crushed or swallowed whole
- Reduced dosage in renal dysfunction

Evaluate:

- Therapeutic response, including decrease in B/P in hypertension, decreased B/P, edema, moist rales in CHF

Teach patient/family:

- To comply with dosage schedule, even if feeling better
- To rise slowly to sitting or standing position to minimize orthostatic hypotension
- To report bradycardia, dizziness, confusion, depression, fever
- To take pulse at home; advise when to notify prescriber
- To comply with weight control, dietary adjustment, modified exercise program
- To wear support hose to minimize effects of orthostatic hypotension
- Not to discontinue drug abruptly; taper over 2 wk; may precipitate angina

Generic names

Selective β_1 receptor blockers
acebutolol (p. 67)
atenolol (p. 139)
esmolol (p. 424)
metoprolol (p. 704)

Nonselective β_1 and β_2 blockers
carteolol (p. 214)
nadolol (p. 734)
pindolol (p. 856)
propranolol (p. 904)
timolol (p. 1029)

Combined α_1, β_1, and β_2 receptor blocker
labetalol (p. 598)

BRONCHODILATORS

Action: Bronchodilators are divided into anticholinergics, α/β-adrenergic agonists, β-adrenergic agonists, and phosphodiesterase inhibitors. Anticholinergics act by inhibiting interaction of acetylcholine at receptor sites on bronchial smooth muscle; α/β-adrenergic agonists by relaxing bronchial smooth muscle and increasing diameter of nasal passages; β-adrenergic agonists by action on β_2-receptors, which relaxes bronchial smooth muscle; phosphodiesterase inhibitors by blocking phosphodiesterase increase cAMP, which mediates smooth muscle relaxation in the respiratory system.

Uses: Bronchodilators are used for bronchial asthma, bronchospasm associated with bronchitis, emphysema, or other obstructive pulmonary diseases, Cheyne-Stokes respirations, prevention of exercise-induced asthma.

Side effects/adverse reactions: The most common side effects are tremors, anxiety, nausea, vomiting, and irritation in throat. The most serious adverse reactions include bronchospasm and dyspnea.

Contraindications: Persons with hypersensitivity, narrow-angle glaucoma, tachydysrhythmias, and severe cardiac disease should not use some of these products.

Precautions: Bronchodilators should be used with caution in lactation, pregnancy, hyperthyroidism, hypertension, prostatic hypertrophy, and seizure disorders.

Pharmacokinetics: Onset, peak, and duration vary widely among products. Most products are metabolized in the liver and excreted in urine.

Interactions: Please check individual monographs, since interactions vary widely among products.

Possible nursing diagnoses:

- Ineffective airway clearance *[uses]*
- Activity intolerance *[uses]*

• Risk of injury *[adverse reactions]*
• Knowledge deficit *[teaching]*

NURSING CONSIDERATIONS

Assess:

• Respiratory function: vital capacity, forced expiratory volume, ABGs, lung sounds, heart rate and rhythm

Administer:

• After shaking, exhale, place mouthpiece in mouth, inhale slowly, hold breath, remove, exhale slowly
• Gum, sips of water for dry mouth
• PO with meals to decrease gastric irritation

Perform/provide:

• Storage in light-resistant container, do not expose to temps over 86° F (30° C)

Evaluate:

• Therapeutic response: absence of dyspnea, wheezing

Teach patient/family:

• Not to use OTC medications; extra stimulation may occur
• Use of inhaler; review package insert with patient
• To avoid getting aerosol in eyes
• To wash inhaler in warm water qd and dry
• To avoid smoking, smoke-filled rooms, persons with respiratory infections

---

Generic names

albuterol (p. 83)
aminophylline (p. 105)
atropine (p. 143)
bitolterol (p. 180)
dyphylline (p. 401)
ephedrine (p. 411)
epinephrine (p. 412)
ethylnorepinephrine (p. 441)
ipratropium (p. 577)
isoetharine (p. 580)
isoproterenol (p. 583)
metaproterenol (p. 670)
oxtriphylline (p. 788)
pirbuterol (p. 862)
terbutaline (p. 998)
theophylline (p. 1010)

CALCIUM CHANNEL BLOCKERS

Action: These products act by inhibiting calcium ion influx across the cell membrane in cardiac and vascular smooth muscle. This action produces relaxation of coronary vascular smooth muscle, dilates coronary arteries, slows SA/AV node conduction, and dilates peripheral arteries.

Uses: These products are used for chronic stable angina pectoris, vasospastic angina, dysrhythmias, hypertension, and unstable angina.
Side effects/adverse reactions: The most common side effects are dysrhythmias and edema. Also common are headache, fatigue, drowsiness, and flushing.
Contraindications: Persons with 2nd or 3rd degree heart block, sick sinus syndrome, hypotension of <90 mm Hg systolic, Wolff-Parkinson-White syndrome or cardiogenic shock should not use these products, since worsening of those conditions may occur.
Precautions: CHF may worsen, since edema may be increased. Hypotension may worsen, since B/P is decreased. Patients with renal and liver disease should use these products cautiously, since they are metabolized in the liver and excreted by the kidneys.
Pharmacokinetics: Onset, peak, and duration vary widely with route of administration. Drugs are metabolized by the liver and excreted in the urine primarily as metabolites.
Interactions: Increased levels of digoxin and theophylline may occur when used with these products. Increased effects of β-blockers and antihypertensives may occur with calcium channel blockers.
Possible nursing diagnoses:
- Altered tissue perfusion: cardiopulmonary *[uses]*
- Decreased cardiac output *[adverse reactions]*

NURSING CONSIDERATIONS

Assess:
- Cardiac system, including B/P, pulse, respirations, ECG intervals (PR, QRS, QT)

Administer:
- PO before meals and hs

Evaluate:
- Therapeutic response, including decreased anginal pain, decreased B/P, dysrhythmias

Teach patient/family:
- How to take pulse before taking drug; patient should record or graph pulses to identify changes
- To avoid hazardous activities until stabilized on this drug, since dizziness occurs frequently
- Need for compliance to all areas of medical regimen, including diet, exercise, stress reduction, drug therapy

Generic names

diltiazem (p. 373)
felodipine (p. 454)
nicardipine (p. 756)
nifedipine (p. 760)
verapamil (p. 1082)

CARDIAC GLYCOSIDES

Action: Products act by inhibiting sodium and potassium ATPase and then making more calcium available to activate contracted proteins. Cardiac contractility and cardiac output are increased.
Uses: These products are used for CHF, atrial fibrillation, atrial flutter, atrial tachycardia, and rapid digitalization in these disorders.
Side effects/adverse reactions: The most common side effects are cardiac disturbances, headache, hypotension, GI symptoms. Also common are blurred vision and yellow-green halos.
Contraindications: Hypersensitive reactions may occur, and allergies should be identified before these products are given. Also, persons with ventricular tachycardia, ventricular fibrillation, and carotid sinus syndrome should not use these products.
Precautions: Persons with acute MI and those who have or may develop serum potassium, calcium, or magnesium imbalances should use these products cautiously. Also, persons with AV block, severe respiratory disease, hypothyroidism, renal and liver disease, and the elderly should exercise caution when these drugs are prescribed.
Pharmacokinetics: Onset, peak, and duration vary widely with the route of administration. Digitoxin is inactivated by the liver, and inactive metabolites are excreted in urine. Digoxin is excreted in urine mainly as the parent drug and metabolites.
Interactions: Toxicity may occur when used with diuretics, succinylcholine, quinidine, and thioamines. Increased blood levels may occur with propantheline bromide, spironolactone, quinidine, verapamil, aminoglycosides (PO), amiodarone, anticholinergics, and quinine. Diuretics may increase toxicity.
Possible nursing diagnoses:
- Altered tissue perfusion: cardiopulmonary *[uses]*
- Decreased cardiac output *[adverse reactions]*

NURSING CONSIDERATIONS

Assess:
- Cardiac system, including B/P, pulse, respirations, and increased urine output

• Apical pulse for 1 min before giving drug; if pulse <60, take again in 1 hr; if <60, notify prescriber
• Electrolytes, including K, Na, Cl, Mg; renal function studies, including BUN and creatinine; and blood studies, including AST (SGOT), ALT (SGPT), bilirubin
• I&O ratio, daily weights
• Monitor therapeutic drug levels

Administer:
• K supplements if ordered for K levels <3 mg/dl

Evaluate:
• Therapeutic response, including decreased weight, edema, pulse, respiration, and increased urine output

Teach patient/family:
• How to take pulse before taking drug; patient should record or graph pulse to identify changes
• To avoid hazardous activities until stabilized on this drug, since dizziness occurs frequently
• Need for compliance to all areas of medical regimen, including diet, exercise, stress reduction, drug therapy

Generic names

digitoxin (p. 367)
digoxin (p. 368)

CHOLINERGICS

Action: Cholinergics act by preventing destruction of acetylcholine, which increases concentration at sites where acetylcholine is released; this exaggerates the effects of acetylcholine and facilitates transmission of impulses across myoneural junction. Cholinergics may also act by stimulating receptors for acetylcholine.

Uses: Cholinergics are used for myasthenia gravis, as antagonists of nondepolarizing neuromuscular blockade, postoperative bladder distention and urinary distention, postoperative ileus.

Side effects/adverse reactions: The most serious adverse reactions are respiratory depression, bronchospasm, constriction, laryngospasm, respiratory arrest, convulsions, and paralysis. The most common side effects are nausea, diarrhea, and vomiting.

Contraindications: Persons with obstruction of the intestine or renal system should not use these products.

Precautions: Caution should be used in patients with bradycardia, hy-

potension, seizure disorders, bronchial asthma, coronary occlusion, hyperthyroidism, lactation, and children.
Pharmacokinetics: Onset, peak, and duration vary widely among products. Most products are metabolized in the liver and excreted in urine.
Interactions: Please check individual monographs, since interactions vary widely among products.
Possible nursing diagnoses:
- Altered urinary elimination *[uses]*
- Ineffective breathing pattern *[uses]*
- Knowledge deficit *[teaching]*
- Noncompliance *[teaching]*

NURSING CONSIDERATIONS

Assess:
- VS, respiration q8h
- I&O ratio; check for urinary retention or incontinence
- Bradycardia, hypotension, bronchospasm, headache, dizziness, convulsions, respiratory depression; drug should be discontinued if toxicity occurs

Administer:
- Only with atropine sulfate available for cholinergic crisis
- Only after all other cholinergics have been discontinued
- Increased doses if tolerance occurs
- Larger doses after exercise or fatigue
- On empty stomach for better absorption

Perform/provide:
- Storage at room temp

Evaluate:
- Therapeutic response: increased muscle strength, hand grasp, improved muscle gait, absence of labored breathing (if severe)

Teach patient/family:
- That drug is not a cure; it only relieves symptoms (myasthenia gravis)
- To wear Medic Alert ID specifying myasthenia gravis, drugs taken

---

Generic names

bethanechol (p. 174)
edrophonium (p. 405)
neostigmine (p. 752)
physostigmine (p. 852)
pyridostigmine (p. 914)

CHOLINERGIC BLOCKERS

Action: Cholinergic blockers inhibit or block acetylcholine at receptor sites in the autonomic nervous system.

Uses: Many products are used to decrease secretions before surgery, to reverse neuromuscular blockade, and to decrease motility of GI, biliary, urinary tracts. Other products are used for parkinsonian symptoms, including dystonia associated with neuroleptic drugs.

Side effects/adverse reactions: The most common side effects are dryness of the mouth and constipation, which can be prevented by frequent rinsing of the mouth and increasing water and bulk in the diet.

Contraindications: Hypersensitivity can occur, and allergies should be identified before administering these products. Persons with GI and GU obstruction should not use these products, since constipation and urinary retention may occur. They are also contraindicated in angle-closure glaucoma and myasthenia gravis.

Precautions: Caution must be used when these products are given to the elderly, since metabolism is slowed. Also, persons with tachycardia or prostatic hypertrophy should use these products with caution.

Pharmacokinetics: Onset, peak, and duration vary with route.

Interactions: Increase in anticholinergic effect occurs when used with narcotics, barbiturates, antihistamines, MAOIs, phenothiazines, amantadine.

Possible nursing diagnoses:

- Impaired physical mobility *[uses]*
- Pain *[uses]*

NURSING CONSIDERATIONS

Assess:

- I&O ratio; be alert for urinary retention, frequency, dysuria; drug should be discontinued if these occur
- Urinary hesitancy, retention; palpate bladder if retention occurs
- Constipation; increase fluids, bulk, exercise
- For tolerance over long-term therapy, dose may have to be increased or changed
- Mental status: affect, mood, CNS depression, worsening of mental symptoms during early therapy

Administer:

- With food or milk to decrease GI symptoms
- Parenteral dose with patient recumbent to prevent postural hypotension; give parenteral dose slowly, monitoring vital signs

Perform/provide:

• Hard candy, gum, frequent rinsing of mouth for dryness

Evaluate:

• Therapeutic response, including absence of cramps and EPS

Teach patient/family:

• To avoid driving, other hazardous activity if drowsiness occurs

• To avoid concurrent use of cough, cold preparations with alcohol, antihistamines unless directed by prescriber

• To use with caution in hot weather, since medication may increase susceptibility to heat stroke

---

Generic names

atropine (p. 143)
benztropine (p. 167)
biperiden (p. 176)
glycopyrrolate (p. 507)
procyclidine (p. 893)
scopolamine (p. 945)
trihexyphenidyl (p. 1057)

CORTICOSTEROIDS

Action: Corticosteroids are divided into glucocorticoids and mineralocorticoids. Glucocorticoids decrease inflammation by the suppression of migration of polymorphonuclear leukocytes, fibroblasts, increased capillary permeability, and lysosomal stabilization. They also have varied metabolic effects and modify the body's immune responses to many stimuli. Mineralocorticoids act by increasing resorption of sodium by increasing hydrogen and potassium excretion in the distal tubule.

Uses: Glucocorticoids are used to decrease inflammation and for immunosuppression. In addition, some products may be given for allergy, adrenal insufficiency, or cerebral edema. Mineralocorticoids are given for adrenal insufficiency or adrenogenital syndrome.

Side effects/adverse reactions: The most common side effects include change in behavior, including insomnia and euphoria; GI irritation, including peptic ulcer; metabolic reactions, including hypokalemia, hyperglycemia, and carbohydrate intolerance; and sodium and fluid retention. Most adverse reactions are dose dependent.

Contraindications: Hypersensitivity may occur and should be identified before administering. Since these products mask infection, they should not be used in systemic fungal infections or amebiasis. Mothers taking pharmacologic doses of corticosteroids should not nurse.

Precautions: Caution must be used when these products are prescribed for diabetic patients, since hyperglycemia may occur. Also, patients with glaucoma, seizure disorders, peptic ulcer, impaired renal function, CHF, hypertension, ulcerative colitis, or myasthenia gravis should be monitored closely if corticosteroids are given. Use with caution in children and the elderly and during pregnancy.

Pharmacokinetics: For oral preparations the onset of action occurs between 1 and 2 hr, and duration can be up to 2 days, with a half-life of 2-4 days. Pharmacokinetics vary widely among products. These products cross the placenta and appear in breast milk.

Interactions: Decreased corticosteroid effect may occur with barbiturates, rifampin, phenytoin; corticosteroid dose may have to be increased. There is a possibility of GI bleeding when used with salicylates, indomethacin. Steroids may reduce salicylate levels. When using with digitalis glycosides, potassium-depleting diuretics, and amphotericin, serum potassium levels should be monitored.

Possible nursing diagnoses:

- Risk of infection *[adverse reactions]*
- Body-image disturbance *[adverse reactions]*
- Risk for violence: self-directed (suicide) *[adverse reactions]*

NURSING CONSIDERATIONS

Assess:

- Potassium, blood sugar, urine glucose while on long-term therapy; hypokalemia and hyperglycemia are common
- Weight daily; notify prescriber of weekly gain >5 lb, since these products alter fluid and electrolyte balance
- I&O ratio; be alert for decreasing urinary output and increasing edema
- Plasma cortisol levels during long-term therapy (normal level is 138-635 nmol/L SI U when drawn at 8 AM)
- Infection, including increased temperature, WBC, even after withdrawal of medication; drug masks symptoms of infection
- Adrenal insufficiency: nausea, anorexia, fatigue, dizziness, dyspnea, weakness, joint pain
- Potassium depletion, including paresthesias, fatigue, nausea, vomiting, depression, polyuria, dysrhythmias, weakness
- Mental status, including affect, mood, behavioral changes, aggression; if severe personality changes occur, including depression, drug may have to be tapered and then discontinued

Administer:

- With food or milk to decrease GI symptoms

Evaluate:

- Therapeutic response, including decreased inflammation

Teach patient/family:

- That ID as steroid user should be carried
- Not to discontinue this medication abruptly, or adrenal crisis can result
- Teach patient all aspects of drug use, including cushingoid symptoms
- That single daily or alternate-day doses should be taken in the morning before 9 AM (for replacement therapy)
- To take with meals or a snack

Generic names

Glucocorticoids
beclomethasone (p. 159)
betamethasone (p. 171)
cortisone (p. 306)
dexamethasone (p. 340)
flunisolide (p. 473)
hydrocortisone (p. 534)
hydrocortisone sodium phosphate (p. 535)
methylprednisolone (p. 695)
paramethasone (p. 807)
prednisolone (p. 880)
prednisone (p. 883)
rimexolone (p. 936)
triamcinolone (p. 1047)

Mineralocorticoid
fludrocortisone (p. 471)

DIURETICS

Action: Diuretics are divided into subgroups: thiazides and thiazide-like diuretics, loop diuretics, carbonic anhydrase inhibitors, osmotic diuretics, and potassium-sparing diuretics. Each one of these subgroups has its own mechanism of action. Thiazides and thiazide-like diuretics increase excretion of water and sodium by inhibiting resorption in the early distal tubule. Loop diuretics inhibit resorption of sodium and chloride in the thick ascending limb of the loop of Henle. Carbonic anhydrase inhibitors increase sodium excretion by decreasing sodium-hydrogen ion exchange throughout the renal tubule. Carbonic anhydrase inhibitors also decrease secretion of aqueous humor in the eye and thus decrease intraocular pressure. Osmotic diuretics increase the osmotic pressure of glomerular filtrate, thus decreasing net absorption of sodium. The potassium-sparing diuretics interfere with sodium resorption at the distal tubule, thus decreasing potassium excretion.

Uses: Blood pressure is reduced in hypertension; edema is reduced in CHF; intraocular pressure is decreased in glaucoma.

Side effects/adverse reactions: Hypokalemia, hyperuricemia, and hyperglycemia occur most frequently with thiazide diuretics. Aplastic anemia, blood dyscrasias, volume depletion, and dehydration may occur when thiazide-like diuretics, loop diuretics, or carbonic anhydrase inhibitors are given. Side effects and adverse reactions vary widely for the miscellaneous products.

Contraindications: Persons with electrolyte imbalances (Na, Cl, K), dehydration, or anuria should not be given these products until the problem is corrected.

Precautions: Caution must be used when diuretics are given to the elderly, since electrolyte disturbances and dehydration can occur rapidly. Hepatic and renal disease may cause poor metabolism and excretion of the drug.

Pharmacokinetics: Onset, peak, and duration vary widely among the different subgroups of these drugs.

Interactions: Cholestyramine and colestipol will decrease the absorption of thiazide diuretics. Concurrent use of thiazides with diazoxide may increase hyperuricemia, hyperglycemia, and antihypertensive effects of thiazides. Ototoxicity may occur when loop diuretics are used with aminoglycosides. Thiazide and loop diuretics may increase therapeutic and toxic effects of lithium.

Possible nursing diagnoses:

- Fluid volume excess *[uses]*
- Decreased cardiac output *[adverse reactions]*

NURSING CONSIDERATIONS

Assess:

- Weight, I&O daily to determine fluid loss; check skin turgor for dehydration
- Electrolytes: K, Na, Cl; include BUN, blood sugar, CBC, serum creatinine, blood pH, ABGs, uric acid, Ca; electrolyte imbalances may occur quickly
- B/P lying, standing; postural hypotension may occur, since fluid loss occurs from intravascular spaces first
- Signs of metabolic alkalosis, including drowsiness and restlessness
- Signs of hypokalemia with some products, including postural hypotension, malaise, fatigue, tachycardia, leg cramps, weakness

Administer:

- In AM to avoid interference with sleep if using drug as a diuretic
- K replacement if K is less than 3.0 mg/dl

Evaluate:

- Therapeutic response: improvement in edema of feet, legs, sacral area daily if medication is being used in CHF; improvement in B/P if medication is being used as a diuretic; improvement in intraocular pressure if medication is being used to decrease aqueous humor in the eye

Teach patient/family:

- To take drug early in the day (diuretic) to prevent nocturia

Generic names

Thiazides
chlorothiazide (p. 259)
hydrochlorothiazide (p. 532)

Thiazide-like
chlorthalidone (p. 266)
indapamide (p. 558)
metolazone (p. 703)

Loop
bumetanide (p. 188)
ethacrynate (p. 433)
furosemide (p. 492)
torsemide (p. 1041)

Carbonic anhydrase inhibitors
acetazolamide (p. 72)
methazolamide (p. 675)

Potassium-sparing
amiloride (p. 98)
spironolactone (p. 966)
triamterene (p. 1050)

Osmotic
mannitol (p. 639)
urea (p. 1072)

HISTAMINE H_2 ANTAGONISTS

Action: Histamine H_2 antagonists act by inhibiting histamine at H_2 receptor site in parietal cells, which inhibits gastric acid secretion.

Uses: Histamine H_2 antagonists are used for short-term treatment of duodenal and gastric ulcers and maintenance therapy for duodenal ulcer; gastroesophageal reflux disease.

Side effects/adverse reactions: The most serious adverse reactions are agranulocytosis, thrombocytopenia, neutropenia, aplastic anemia, exfoliative dermatitis. The most common side effects are confusion (not with ranitidine), headache, and diarrhea.

Contraindications: Persons with hypersensitivity should not use these products.

Precautions: Caution should be used in pregnancy, lactation, child <16 yr, organic brain syndrome, hepatic disease, renal disease.

Pharmacokinetics: Onset, peak, and duration vary widely among products. Most products are metabolized in the liver and excreted in urine.

Interactions: Antacids interfere with absorption of histamine H_2 antagonists. Check individual monographs for other interactions.

Possible nursing diagnoses:

- Pain *[uses]*
- Risk of injury *[bleeding]*
- Knowledge deficit *[teaching]*

NURSING CONSIDERATIONS

Assess:

- Gastric pH (>5 should be maintained)
- I&O ratio, BUN, creatinine

Administer:

- With meals for prolonged drug effect
- Antacids 1 hr before or 1 hr after cimetidine
- IV slowly; bradycardia may occur; give over 30 min

Perform/provide:

- Storage of diluted sol at room temp for up to 48 hr

Evaluate:

- Therapeutic response: decreased pain in abdomen

Teach patient/family:

- That gynecomastia, impotence may occur, but are reversible
- To avoid driving, other hazardous activities until patient is stabilized on this medication
- To avoid black pepper, caffeine, alcohol, harsh spices, extremes in temp of food
- To avoid OTC preparations: aspirin, cough, cold preparations
- That drug must be continued for prescribed time to be effective
- To report bruising, fatigue, malaise; blood dyscrasias may occur

---

Generic names

cimetidine (p. 273)
famotidine (p. 450)
ranitidine (p. 929)

IMMUNOSUPPRESSANTS

Action: Immunosuppressants act by inhibiting lymphocytes (T).

Uses: Most products are used for organ transplants to prevent rejection.

Side effects/adverse reactions: The most serious adverse reactions are albuminuria, hematuria, proteinuria, renal failure, and hepatotoxicity. The most common side effects are overgrowth of oral *Candida,* gum hyperplasia, tremors, and headache. The most serious adverse reactions for azathioprine are hematologic (leukopenia and thrombocytopenia) and GI (nausea and vomiting). There is a risk of secondary infection.

Contraindications: Products are contraindicated in hypersensitivity.

Precautions: Caution should be used in severe renal disease, severe hepatic disease, and pregnancy.

Pharmacokinetics: Onset, peak, and duration vary widely among products. Most products are metabolized in the liver and excreted in urine.

Interactions: Please check individual monographs, since interactions vary widely among products.

Possible nursing diagnoses:

- Risk of infection *[adverse reactions]*
- Risk of injury *[uses]*
- Knowledge deficit *[teaching]*

NURSING CONSIDERATIONS

Assess:

- Renal studies: BUN, creatinine at least qmo during treatment, 3 mo after treatment
- Liver function studies: alk phosphatase, AST (SGOT), ALT (SGPT), bilirubin
- Drug blood levels during treatment
- Hepatotoxicity: dark urine, jaundice, itching, light-colored stools; drug should be discontinued

Administer:

- For several days before transplant surgery
- With meals for GI upset or drug mixed with chocolate milk
- With oral antifungal for *Candida* infections

Evaluate:

- Therapeutic response: absence of rejection

Teach patient/family:

- To report fever, chills, sore throat, fatigue, since serious infections may occur
- To use contraceptive measures during treatment, for 12 wk after ending therapy

Generic names

azathioprine (p. 149)
cyclosporine (p. 318)
muromonab CD3 (p. 732)
tacrolimus (p. 990)

LAXATIVES

Action: Laxatives are divided into bulk products, lubricants, osmotics, saline laxative stimulants, and stool softeners. Bulk laxatives work by absorbing water and expanding to increase moisture content and bulk in the stool. Lubricants increase water retention in the stool, causing reabsorption of water in the bowel. Stimulants act by increasing peristalsis by direct effect on the intestine. Saline draws water into the intestinal lumen.

Osmotics increase distention and promote peristalsis. Stool softeners reduce surface tension of liquids of the bowel.

Uses: Laxatives are used as a preparation for bowel and rectal exam, constipation, and stool softener.

Side effects/adverse reactions: The most common side effects are nausea, abdominal cramps, and diarrhea.

Contraindications: Persons with GI obstruction, perforation, gastric retention, toxic colitis, megacolon, abdominal pain, nausea, vomiting, or fecal impaction should not use these products.

Precautions: Caution should be used in rectal bleeding, large hemorrhoids, and anal excoriation.

Pharmacokinetics: Onset, peak, and duration vary among products.

Interactions: Please check individual monographs, since interactions vary widely among products.

Possible nursing diagnoses:

- Constipation *[uses]*
- Diarrhea *[adverse reactions]*
- Knowledge deficit *[teaching]*

NURSING CONSIDERATIONS

Assess:

- Blood, urine electrolytes if drug is used often by patient
- I&O ratio: to identify fluid loss
- Cause of constipation; identify whether fluids, bulk, or exercise is missing from lifestyle
- Cramping, rectal bleeding, nausea, vomiting; if these symptoms occur, drug should be discontinued

Administer:

- Alone only with water for better absorption; do not take within 1 hr of antacids, milk, or cimetidine

Evaluate:

- Therapeutic response: decrease in constipation

Teach patient/family:

- To swallow tabs whole; not to chew
- Not to use laxatives for long-term therapy; bowel tone will be lost
- That normal bowel movements do not always occur daily
- Not to use in presence of abdominal pain, nausea, vomiting
- To notify prescriber of abdominal pain, nausea, vomiting
- To notify prescriber if constipation is unrelieved or of symptoms of electrolyte imbalance: muscle cramps, pain, weakness, dizziness

Generic names

Bulk laxatives
calcium polycarbophil (p. 203)
methylcellulose (p. 689)
psyllium (p. 911)

Lubricants
mineral oil (p. 716)

Osmotic agents
glycerin (p. 506)
lactulose (p. 600)

Saline laxatives
magnesium salts (p. 638)
sodium biphosphate/phosphate (p. 958)

Stimulants
bisacodyl (p. 177)
cascara (p. 216)
phenolphthalein (p. 840)
senna (p. 951)

Stool softeners
docusate (p. 387)

NARCOTICS

Action: Narcotics act by depressing pain impulse transmission at the spinal cord level by interacting with opioid receptors. Products are divided into opiates and nonopiates.

Uses: Most products are used to control moderate to severe pain and are used before and after surgery.

Side effects/adverse reactions: GI symptoms, including nausea, vomiting, anorexia, constipation, and cramps are the most common side effects. Other common side effects include light-headedness, dizziness, sedation. Serious adverse reactions such as respiratory depression, respiratory arrest, circulatory depression, and increased intracranial pressure may result but are less common and usually dose dependent.

Contraindications: Hypersensitive reactions occur frequently. Check for sensitivity before administering. These drugs should not be used if narcotic addiction is suspected, and they are also contraindicated in acute bronchial asthma and upper airway obstruction.

Precautions: Caution must be used when these products are given to persons with an addictive personality, since the possibility of addiction is so great. Also, they may worsen intracranial pressure. Persons with severe heart disease, hepatic or renal disease, respiratory conditions, or seizure disorders should be monitored closely for worsening condition.

Pharmacokinetics: Onset of action is immediate by IV route and rapid by IM and PO routes. Peak occurs from 1-2 hr, depending on route, with a duration of 2-8 hr. These agents cross the placenta and appear in breast milk.

Interactions: Barbiturates, other narcotics, hypnotics, antipsychotics, or alcohol can increase CNS depression when taken with narcotics.

Possible nursing diagnoses:

- Pain *[uses]*
- Impaired gas exchange *[adverse reactions]*

NURSING CONSIDERATIONS

Assess:

- I&O ratio; be alert for urinary retention, frequency, dysuria; drug should be discontinued if these occur
- Respiratory dysfunction, including respiratory depression, rate, rhythm, character; notify prescriber if respirations are <12/min
- CNS changes: dizziness, drowsiness, hallucinations, euphoria, LOC, pupil reaction
- Allergic reactions: rash, urticaria
- Need for pain medication; use pain scoring

Administer:

- With antiemetic if nausea or vomiting occurs
- When pain is beginning to return; determine dosage interval by response

Perform/provide:

- Assistance with ambulation; patient should not be ambulating during drug peak

Evaluate:

- Therapeutic response, including decrease in pain

Teach patient/family:

- To report any symptoms of CNS changes, allergic reactions, or shortness of breath
- That physical dependency may result when used for extended periods
- That withdrawal symptoms may occur, including nausea, vomiting, cramps, fever, faintness, anorexia
- To avoid alcohol and other CNS depressants

Generic names

alfentanil (p. 86)
buprenorphine (p. 189)
butorphanol (p. 195)
codeine (p. 300)
dezocine (p. 351)
fentanyl (p. 457)
fentanyl transdermal (p. 459)
hydromorphone (p. 538)
levorphanol (p. 608)
meperidine (p. 658)
methadone (p. 672)
morphine (p. 728)
nalbuphine (p. 738)
oxycodone (p. 790)
oxymorphone (p. 793)
pentazocine (p. 823)
propoxyphene (p. 903)

NEUROMUSCULAR BLOCKING AGENTS

Action: Neuromuscular blocking agents are divided into depolarizing and nondepolarizing blockers. They act by inhibiting transmission of nerve impulses by binding with cholinergic receptor sites.

Uses: Neuromuscular blocking agents are used to facilitate endotracheal intubation and skeletal muscle relaxation during mechanical ventilation, surgery, or general anesthesia.

Side effects/adverse reactions: The most serious adverse reactions are prolonged apnea, bronchospasm, cyanosis, respiratory depression, and malignant hyperthermia. The most common side effects are bradycardia and decreased motility.

Contraindications: Persons who are hypersensitive should not be given this product.

Precautions: Caution should be used in pregnancy, thyroid disease, collagen disease, cardiac disease, lactation, children <2 yr, electrolyte imbalances, dehydration, neuromuscular disease (myasthenia gravis), and respiratory disease.

Pharmacokinetics: Onset, peak, and duration vary widely among products. Most products are metabolized in the liver and excreted in urine.

Interactions: Aminoglycosides potentiate neuromuscular blockade. See individual monographs.

Possible nursing diagnoses:

- Ineffective breathing pattern *[uses]*
- Risk of injury *[adverse reactions]*
- Knowledge deficit *[teaching]*

NURSING CONSIDERATIONS

Assess:

- For electrolyte imbalances (K, Mg); may lead to increased action of this drug
- Vital signs (B/P, pulse, respirations, airway) q15min until fully recovered; rate, depth, pattern of respirations, strength of hand grip
- I&O ratio; check for urinary retention, frequency, hesitancy
- Recovery: decreased paralysis of face, diaphragm, leg, arm, rest of body
- Allergic reactions: rash, fever, respiratory distress, pruritus; drug should be discontinued

Administer:

- Using nerve stimulator by anesthesiologist to determine neuromuscular blockade
- Anticholinesterase to reverse neuromuscular blockade

• IV undiluted over 1-2 min (only by qualified person, usually an anesthesiologist)

Perform/provide:

• Storage in light-resistant, cool area

• Reassurance if communication is difficult during recovery from neuromuscular blockade

Evaluate:

• Therapeutic response: paralysis of jaw, eyelid, head, neck, rest of body

Generic names

atracurium (p. 142)
doxacurium (p. 390)
gallamine (p. 495)
metocurine (p. 702)
mivacurium (p. 724)
pancuronium (p. 802)
pipecuronium (p. 857)
succinylcholine (p. 974)
tubocurarine (p. 1069)
vecuronium (p. 1079)

NONSTEROIDAL ANTIINFLAMMATORIES

Action: Nonsteroidals decrease prostaglandin synthesis by inhibiting an enzyme needed for biosynthesis.

Uses: Nonsteroidal antiinflammatories are used to treat mild to moderate pain, osteoarthritis, rheumatoid arthritis, and dysmenorrhea.

Side effects/adverse reactions: The most serious adverse reactions are nephrotoxicity (dysuria, hematuria, oliguria, azotemia), blood dyscrasias, and cholestatic hepatitis. The most common side effects are nausea, abdominal pain, anorexia, dizziness, and drowsiness.

Contraindications: Persons with hypersensitivity, asthma, severe renal disease, and severe hepatic disease should not use these products.

Precautions: Caution should be used in pregnancy, lactation, children, bleeding disorders, GI disorders, cardiac disorders, hypersensitivity to other antiinflammatory agents, and the elderly.

Pharmacokinetics: Onset, peak, and duration vary widely among products. Most products are metabolized in the liver and excreted in urine.

Interactions: Please check individual monographs, since interactions vary widely among products.

Possible nursing diagnoses:

• Chronic pain *[uses]*

• Impaired physical mobility *[uses]*

• Knowledge deficit *[teaching]*

• Noncompliance *[teaching]*

NURSING CONSIDERATIONS

Assess:

- Renal, liver, blood studies: BUN, creatinine, AST (SGOT), ALT (SGPT), Hgb, before treatment, periodically thereafter
- Audiometric, ophthalmic examination before, during, and after treatment
- For eye, ear problems: blurred vision, tinnitus; may indicate toxicity

Administer:

- With food to decrease GI symptoms; however, best to take on empty stomach to facilitate absorption

Perform/provide:

- Storage at room temp

Evaluate:

- Therapeutic response: decreased pain, stiffness in joints, decreased swelling in joints, ability to move more easily

Teach patient/family:

- To report blurred vision, ringing, roaring in ears; may indicate toxicity
- To avoid driving, other hazardous activities if dizziness, drowsiness occur, especially elderly
- To report change in urine pattern, increased weight, edema, increased pain in joints, fever, blood in urine; indicate nephrotoxicity
- That therapeutic effects may take up to 1 mo

Generic names

diclofenac (p. 357)
etodolac (p. 444)
fenoprofen (p. 456)
flurbiprofen (p. 485)
ibuprofen (p. 549)
indomethacin (p. 560)
ketoprofen (p. 595)
ketorolac (p. 596)
meclofenamate (p. 649)
mefenamic (p. 652)
nabumetone (p. 733)
naproxen (p. 745)
oxyphenbutazone (p. 794)
phenylbutazone (p. 845)
piroxicam (p. 863)
sulindac (p. 987)
tolmetin (p. 1039)

SALICYLATES

Action: Salicylates have analgesic, antipyretic, and antiinflammatory effects. The antiinflammatory and analgesic activities may be mediated through the inhibition of prostaglandin synthesis. Antipyretic action results from inhibition of the hypothalamic heat-regulating center.

Uses: The primary uses of salicylates are relief of mild to moderate pain and fever and in inflammatory conditions such as arthritis, thromboembolic disorders, and rheumatic fever.

Side effects/adverse reactions: The most common side effects are GI symptoms and rash. Serious blood dyscrasias and hepatotoxicity may result when used for long periods at high doses. Tinnitus or impaired hearing may indicate that blood salicylate levels are reaching or exceeding the upper limit of the therapeutic range.

Contraindications: Hypersensitivity to salicylates is common. Check for sensitivity before administering. Persons with bleeding disorders, GI bleeding, and vit K deficiency should not use these products, since salicylates increase prothrombin time. Children should not use these products, since salicylates have been associated with Reye's syndrome.

Precautions: Caution is needed when salicylates are given to patients with anemia, hepatic or renal disease, or Hodgkin's disease. Caution should also be exercised in pregnancy and lactation.

Pharmacokinetics: Onset of action occurs in 15-30 min, with a peak of 1-2 hr and a duration up to 6 hr. These drugs are metabolized by the liver and excreted by the kidneys.

Interactions: Increased effects of anticoagulants, insulin, methotrexate, heparin, valproic acid, and oral sulfonylureas may occur when used with salicylates. Aspirin may decrease serum concentrations of nonsteroidal antiinflammatory agents.

Possible nursing diagnoses:

- Pain *[uses]*
- Impaired physical mobility *[uses]*
- Activity intolerance *[uses]*
- Sensory/perceptual alteration: auditory *[adverse reactions]*
- Thermoregulation *[uses]*

NURSING CONSIDERATIONS

Assess:

- Hepatic and renal studies: AST (SGOT), ALT (SGPT), bilirubin, creatinine, LDH, alk phosphatase, BUN if patient is on long-term therapy, since these products are metabolized and excreted by the liver and kidney
- Blood studies: CBC, hematocrit, hemoglobin, and prothrombin time if patient is on long-term therapy, since these products increase the possibility of bleeding and blood dyscrasias
- Hepatotoxicity: dark urine, clay-colored stools, yellowing of skin, sclera, itching, abdominal pain, fever, diarrhea, which may occur with long-term use
- Ototoxicity: tinnitus, ringing, roaring in ears; audiometric testing is needed before and after long-term therapy

Administer:

- With food or milk to decrease gastric irritation; give 30 min before or 1 hr after meals with a full glass of water

Evaluate:

- Therapeutic response/including decreased pain, fever

Teach patient/family:

- That blood sugar levels should be monitored closely if patient is diabetic
- Not to exceed recommended dosage; acute poisoning may result
- That therapeutic response takes 2 wk in arthritis
- To avoid use of alcohol, since GI bleeding may result
- To notify prescriber of ringing in the ears or persistent GI pain
- To take with full glass of H_2O to reduce risk of lodging in esophagus

Generic names

aspirin (p. 136)
choline salicylate (p. 270)
magnesium salicylate (p. 637)
salsalate (p. 942)
sodium thiosalicylate (p. 960)

THROMBOLYTICS

Action: Thrombolytics act by activating conversion of plasminogen to plasmin (fibrinolysin): plasmin is able to break down clots (fibrin).
Uses: Thrombolytics are used to treat deep vein thrombosis, pulmonary embolism, arterial thrombosis, arterial embolism, arteriovenous cannula occlusion, lysis of coronary artery thrombi after MI, acute evolving transmural MI.
Side effects/adverse reactions: Serious adverse reactions include GI, GU, intracranial retroperitoneal bleeding, and anaphylaxis. The most common side effects are decreased Hct, urticaria, headache, and nausea.
Contraindications: Persons with hypersensitivity, active bleeding, intraspinal surgery, neoplasms of the CNS, ulcerative colitis/enteritis, severe hypertension, renal disease, hepatic disease, hypocoagulation, COPD, subacute bacterial endocarditis, rheumatic valvular disease, cerebral embolism/thrombosis/hemorrhage, intraarterial diagnostic procedure or surgery (10 days), and recent major surgery should not use these products.
Precautions: Caution should be used in arterial emboli from left side of heart and pregnancy.
Pharmacokinetics: Onset, peak, and duration vary widely among products. Most products are metabolized in the liver and excreted in urine.
Interactions: Please check individual monographs, since interactions vary widely among products.
Possible nursing diagnoses:

- Risk of injury *[uses]*

NURSING CONSIDERATIONS

Assess:

- VS, B/P, pulse, resp, neuro signs, temp at least q4h, temp >104° F (40° C) are indicators of internal bleeding; cardiac rhythm following intracoronary administration; systolic pressure increase of >25 mm Hg should be reported to prescriber
- For neurologic changes that may indicate intracranial bleeding
- Retroperitoneal bleeding: back pain, leg weakness, diminished pulses
- Allergy: fever, rash, itching, chill; mild reaction may be treated with antihistamines
- For bleeding during 1st hr of treatment: hematuria, hematemesis, bleeding from mucous membranes, epistaxis, ecchymosis
- Blood studies (Hct, platelets, PTT, PT, TT, APTT) before starting therapy; PT or APTT must be less than ×2 control before starting therapy; TT or PT q3-4h during treatment

Administer:

- As soon as thrombi identified; not useful for thrombi over 1 wk old
- Cryoprecipitate or fresh, frozen plasma if bleeding occurs
- Loading dose at beginning of therapy; may require increased loading doses
- Heparin after fibrinogen level is over 100 mg/dl. Heparin infusion to increase PTT to 1.5-2 × baseline for 3-7 days
- About 10% patients have high streptococcal antibody titers requiring increased loading doses
- IV therapy using 0.8 μm filter

Perform/provide:

- Storage of reconstituted drug in refrigerator; discard after 24 hr
- Bed rest during entire course of treatment
- Avoidance of venous or arterial puncture, inj, rectal temp
- Treatment of fever with acetaminophen or aspirin
- Pressure for 30 sec to minor bleeding sites; inform prescriber if this does not attain hemostasis; apply pressure dressing

Evaluate:

- Therapeutic response: resolution of thrombosis, embolism

Generic names

alteplase (p. 92)
anistreplase (p. 129)
streptokinase (p. 969)
urokinase (p. 1074)

THYROID HORMONES

Action: Acts by increasing metabolic rates, resulting in increased cardiac output, O_2 consumption, body temp, blood volume, growth, development at cellular level, respiratory rate, enzyme system activity.
Uses: Products are used for thyroid replacement.
Side effects/adverse reactions: The most common side effects include insomnia, tremors, tachycardia, palpitations, angina, dysrhythmias, weight loss, and changes in appetite. Serious adverse reactions include thyroid storm.
Contraindications: Persons with adrenal insufficiency, myocardial infarction, or thyrotoxicosis should not use these products.
Precautions: The elderly and patients with angina pectoris, hypertension, ischemia, cardiac disease, or diabetes mellitus or insipidus should be watched closely when using these products. Caution should be used in pregnancy (A) and lactation.
Pharmacokinetics: Pharmacokinetics vary widely among products; check specific monographs.
Interactions:
- Impaired absorption of thyroid products may occur when administered with cholestyramine (separate by 4-5 hr)
- Increased effects of anticoagulants, sympathomimetics, tricyclic antidepressants, catecholamines may occur
- Decreased effects of digitalis, glycosides, insulin, hypoglycemics may occur
- Decreased effects of thyroid products may occur with estrogens

Possible nursing diagnoses:
- Knowledge deficit *[teaching]*
- Noncompliance *[teaching]*
- Body image disturbance *[adverse reactions]*

NURSING CONSIDERATIONS

Assess:
- B/P, pulse before each dose
- I&O ratio
- Weight qd in same clothing, using same scale, at same time of day
- Height, growth rate if given to a child
- T_3, T_4, which are decreased; radioimmunoassay of TSH, which is increased; ratio uptake, which is decreased if patient is on too low a dosage of medication
- Increased nervousness, excitability, irritability; may indicate overdosage, usually after 1-3 wk of treatment

• Cardiac status: angina, palpitation, chest pain, change in VS

Administer:

• At same time each day to maintain drug level

• Only for hormone imbalances, not to be used for obesity, male infertility, menstrual conditions, lethargy

Perform/provide:

• Removal of medication 4 wk before RAIU test

Evaluate:

• Therapeutic response: absence of depression; increased weight loss; diuresis; pulse; appetite; absence of constipation; peripheral edema; cold intolerance; pale, cool, dry skin; brittle nails; alopecia; coarse hair; menorrhagia; night blindness; paresthesias; syncope; stupor; coma; rosy cheeks

Teach patient/family:

• That hair loss will occur in child and is temporary

• To report excitability, irritability, anxiety; indicates overdose

• Not to switch brands unless directed by prescriber

• That hypothyroid child will show almost immediate behavior/personality change

• That treatment drug is not to be taken to reduce weight

• To avoid OTC preparations with iodine; read labels

• To avoid iodine food, iodinized salt, soybeans, tofu, turnips, some seafood, some bread

Generic names

levothyroxine (T_4) (p. 609)
liothyronine (T_3) (p. 617)
liotrix (p. 618)
thyroglobulin (p. 1022)
thyroid USP (p. 1023)
thyrotropin (TSH) (p. 1025)

VASODILATORS

Action: Vasodilators have various modes of action. Please check individual monograph for specific action.

Uses: Vasodilators are used to treat intermittent claudication, arteriosclerosis obliterans, vasospasm and muscular ischemia, ischemic cerebral vascular disease, hypertension, and angina.

Side effects/adverse reactions: The most common side effects are headache, nausea, hypotension or hypertension, and ECG changes.

Contraindications: Some drugs are contraindicated in acute MI, paroxysmal tachycardia, and thyrotoxicosis.

Precautions: Caution should be used in uncompensated heart disease or peptic ulcer disease.

Pharmacokinetics: Onset, peak, and duration vary widely among products. Most products are metabolized in the liver and excreted in urine.
Interactions: Please check individual monographs, since interactions vary widely among products.
Possible nursing diagnoses:
- Decreased cardiac output *[uses]*
- Altered tissue perfusion: cardiovascular/pulmonary *[uses]*
- Knowledge deficit *[teaching]*

NURSING CONSIDERATIONS

Assess:
- Bleeding time in individuals with bleeding disorders
- Cardiac status: B/P, pulse, rate, rhythm, character; watch for increasing pulse

Administer:
- With meals to reduce GI symptoms

Perform/provide:
- Storage in tight container at room temp

Evaluate:
- Therapeutic response: ability to walk without pain, increased temp in extremities, increased pulse volume

Teach patient/family:
- That medication is not cure; may need to be taken continuously
- That it is necessary to quit smoking to prevent excessive vasoconstriction
- That improvement may be sudden, but usually occurs gradually over several weeks
- To report headache, weakness, increased pulse, as drug may have to be decreased or discontinued
- To avoid hazardous activities until stabilized on medication; dizziness may occur

---

Generic names

amyl nitrite (p. 128)
cyclandelate (p. 311)
dipyridamole (p. 382)
hydralazine (p. 530)
isoxsuprine (p. 588)
minoxidil (p. 718)
papaverine (p. 803)
tolazoline (p. 1036)

VITAMINS

Action: Action varies widely among products and classes; check specific monographs.
Uses: Vitamins are used to correct and prevent vitamin deficiencies.
Side effects/adverse reactions: There are no side effects or adverse reactions with the water-soluble vitamins (C, B). However, fat-soluble vitamins (A, D, E, K) may accumulate in the body and cause adverse reactions (see specific monographs).
Contraindications: Hypersensitive reactions may occur, and allergies should be identified before these products are given.
Pharmacokinetics: Onset, peak, and duration vary widely among products; check individual monograph for specific information.
Possible nursing diagnoses:
- Nutrition, less than body requirements *[uses]*

NURSING CONSIDERATIONS
Administer:
- PO with food for better absorption

Perform/provide:
- Storage in tight, light-resistant container

Evaluate:
- Therapeutic response: no vitamin deficiency

Teach patient/family:
- Not to take more than prescribed amount

Generic names

Fat-soluble
menadione/menadiol sodium diphosphate (vitamin K_3) (p. 656)
phytonadione (p. 853)
vitamin A (p. 1089)
vitamin D (p. 1090)
vitamin E (p. 1092)

Water-soluble
ascorbic acid (C) (p. 133)
cyanocobalamin hydroxocobalimin (B_{12}) (p. 310)
pyridoxine (B_6) (p. 916)
riboflavin (B_2) (p. 930)
thiamine (B_1) (p. 1012)

Miscellaneous
multivitamins (p. 731)

A

acebutolol (℞)

(a-ce-byoot'oh-lole)

Monitan*, Rhotral*, Sectral

Func. class.: Antihypertensive, beta blocker, antidysrhythmic

Action: Competitively blocks stimulation of β-adrenergic receptor within vascular smooth muscle; produces chronotropic, inotropic activity (decreases rate of SA node discharge, increases recovery time), slows conduction of AV node, decreases heart rate, which decreases O_2 consumption in myocardium; also decreases renin-aldosterone-angiotensin system at high doses, inhibits β-2 receptors in bronchial system (high doses)

Uses: Mild to moderate hypertension, sinus tachycardia, persistent atrial extrasystoles, tachydysrhythmias, prophylaxis of angina pectoris

Investigational uses: Prophylaxis of MI, treatment of angina pectoris, tremor, mitral valve prolapse, thyrotoxicosis, idiopathic hypertrophic subaortic stenosis

Dosage and routes:

Hypertension

• *Adult:* PO 400 mg qd or in 2 divided doses; may be increased to desired response

Ventricular dysrhythmia

• *Adult:* PO 200 mg bid, may increase gradually, usual range 600-1200 mg daily

Available forms: Caps 200, 400 mg; tabs 200, 400 mg*

Side effects/adverse reactions:

CV: ***Profound hypotension, bradycardia, CHF,*** *cold extremities, postural hypotension,* ***2nd or 3rd degree heart block***

CNS: Insomnia, fatigue, dizziness, mental changes, memory loss, hallucinations, depression, lethargy, drowsiness, strange dreams, catatonia

GI: Nausea, diarrhea, vomiting, ***mesenteric arterial thrombosis, ischemic colitis***

INTEG: Rash, fever, alopecia

HEMA: ***Agranulocytosis, thrombocytopenia, purpura***

EENT: Sore throat, dry burning eyes

GU: Impotence

ENDO: Increased hypoglycemic response to insulin

RESP: ***Bronchospasm,*** dyspnea, wheezing

Contraindications: Hypersensitivity to β-blockers, cardiogenic shock, heart block (2nd, 3rd degree), sinus bradycardia, CHF, cardiac failure

Precautions: Major surgery, pregnancy (B), lactation, diabetes mellitus, renal disease, thyroid disease, COPD, asthma, well-compensated heart failure, aortic, mitral valve disease

Pharmacokinetics:

PO: Onset 1-1½ hr, peak 2-4 hr, duration 10-12 hr; half-life 6-7 hr, excreted unchanged in urine, protein binding 5%-15%

Interactions:

• Increased hypotension, bradycardia: reserpine, hydralazine, methyldopa, prazosin, anticholinergics

• Decreased antihypertensive effects: indomethacin

• Increased hypoglycemic effect: insulin

• Decreased bronchodilation: theophyllines, β_2 agonists

Lab test interferences:

Interference: Glucose/insulin tolerance tests

Increase: Uric acid, K, triglyceride, lipoproteins

NURSING CONSIDERATIONS

Assess:

• B/P during beginning treatment,

periodically thereafter; pulse q4h; note rate, rhythm, quality

• Apical/radial pulse before administration; notify prescriber of any significant changes (pulse <50 bpm); signs of CHF (dyspnea, crackles, weight gain, jugular vein distension)

• Baselines in renal, liver function tests before therapy begins

• Edema in feet, legs daily: monitor I&O

• Skin turgor, dryness of mucous membranes for hydration status, especially elderly

Administer:

• PO ac, hs, tablet may be crushed or swallowed whole; give with food to prevent GI upset

• Reduced dosage in renal dysfunction

Perform/provide:

• Storage protected from light, moisture; place in cool environment

Evaluate:

• Therapeutic response: decreased B/P after 1-2 wk; decreased dysrhythmias

Teach patient/family:

• Not to discontinue drug abruptly, taper over 2 wk; may cause precipitate angina if stopped abruptly; do not double dose; if a dose is missed, take as soon as remembered up to 4 hr before next dose

• Not to use OTC products containing α-adrenergic stimulants (such as nasal decongestants, OTC cold preparations) unless directed by prescriber

• To report bradycardia, dizziness, confusion, depression, fever

• To take pulse at home, advise when to notify prescriber

• To avoid alcohol, smoking, sodium intake

• To comply with weight control, dietary adjustments, modified exercise program

• To carry Medic Alert ID to identify drug, allergies

• To avoid hazardous activities if dizziness is present

• To report symptoms of CHF: difficult breathing, especially on exertion or when lying down, night cough, swelling of extremities

• That if diabetic, monitor blood glucose; hyperglycemia, hypoglycemia occur

Treatment of overdose: Lavage, IV atropine for bradycardia, IV theophylline for bronchospasm, digitalis, O_2, diuretic for cardiac failure, hemodialysis, IV glucose for hyperglycemia, IV diazepam (or phenytoin) for seizures

* Available in Canada only

acetaminophen (OTC)

(a-seat-a-mee'noe-fen)

Abenol*, Aceta, Actamin, Aminofen, Acetaminophen Uniserts, Anacin-3 Infant's Drops, Anacin-3 Maximum Strength, Apacet, Apo-Acetaminophen*, Aspirin Free Pain Relief, Atasol*, Banesin, Campain*, Children's Feverall, Dapa Extra Strength, Datril Extra Strength, Dolane, Dorcol Children's Fever and Pain Reducer, Exdol*, Genapap Extra Strength, Genapap Infant's Drops, Geners Extra Strength, Halenol Children's, Junior Strength Feverall, Liquiprin Elixir, Liquiprin Infant Drops, Meda Cap, Myapap Drops, Oraphen-PD, Panadol, Panadol Infant's Drops, Panex 500, Parten, Pedric, Phenaphen Caplets, Redutemp, Robigesic*, Rounax*, St. Joseph Aspirin-free Infant Drops, Tapanol Extra Strength, Tempra, Tempra Drops, Tylenol, Tylenol Caplets, Tylenol Extra Strength, Tylenol Infant's Drops, Ty-Pap, Ty-Tab, Valadol, Valorin

Func. class.: Nonnarcotic analgesic, antipyretic

Chem. class.: Nonsalicylate, paraaminophenol derivative

Combination products: Bancap: acetaminophen 325 mg with butalbital 50 mg; Bromo-seltzer: acetaminophen 325 mg/capful measure with citric acid 2.224 g/capful measure, sodium bicarbonate 2.871 g/capful measure; Capital with Codeine: acetaminophen 120 mg/5 ml with codeine 12 mg/5 ml; Codalan No. 1: acetaminophen 500 mg with caffeine 30 mg, codeine phosphate 8 mg; Codalan No. 2: acetaminophen 500 mg with caffeine 30 mg, codeine phosphate 15 mg; Codalan No. 3: acetaminophen 500 mg with caffeine 30 mg, codeine phosphate 30 mg; Congespirin, Aspirin-Free: acetaminophen 81 mg with phenylephrine HCl 81 mg; Empracet with Codeine Phosphate 60 mg No. 4, Tylenol with Codeine No. 4: acetaminophen 300 mg with codeine phosphate 60 mg; Endccon, Phenapap No. 2: phenylpropanolamine HCl 25 mg with acetaminophen 325 mg; Esgic, Fioricet: acetaminophen 325 mg with butalbital 50 mg, caffeine 40 mg; Excedrin: acetaminophen 194 mg with aspirin 227 mg, caffeine 33 mg, buffers; Excedrin Extra Strength: aspirin 250 mg with acetaminophen 250 mg, caffeine 65 mg; Excedrin P.M.: acetaminophen 500 mg with diphenhydramine citrate 38 mg; Gemnisyn: acetaminophen 325 mg with aspirin 325 mg; Midol PMS Caplets: acetaminophen 500 mg with pamabrom 25 mg, pyrilamine maleate 15 mg; Naldegisic: acetaminophen 325 mg with pseudoephedrine HCl 15 mg; Pamprin: acetaminophen 325 mg with pamabrom 25 mg, pyrilamine maleate 12.5 mg; Pamprin Maximum Cramp Relief: acetaminophen 500 mg with pamabrom 25 mg, pyrilamine maleate 15 mg; Paracet Forte: chlorzoxazone 250 mg, acetaminophen 300 mg; Percogesic: acetaminophen 325 mg with phenyltoloxamine citrate 30 mg; Phenaphen with Codeine No. 2: acetaminophen 325 mg with codeine phosphate 15 mg; Phenaphen with Codeine No. 2, Proval No. 3: codeine 30 mg with acetaminophen 325 mg; Phenaphen with Codeine No. 3, Proval No. 2: acetaminophen 325 mg with codeine phosphate 30 mg; Phenaphen with Codeine No. 4: acetaminophen 325 mg with codeine phosphate 60 mg; Phenaphen-650 with Codeine: acetaminophen 650 mg with codeine phosphate 30 mg; Phrenilin: acetaminophen 325 mg with butalbital 50 mg; Phrenilin Forte: acetaminophen 650 mg, butalbital 50 mg; Phrenilin with Codeine No. 3: acetaminophen 325 mg, butalbital 50 mg, codeine phosphate 30 mg; Sine-Aid: acetaminophen 325 mg, pseudoephedrine HCl 30 mg; Sine-Aid Extra Strength Caplets, Tylenol Sinus Maximum Strength Caplets: acetaminophen 500 mg, pseudoephedrine HCl 30 mg; Sine-Off Extra Strength, Sinutab: acetaminophen 500 mg, pseudoephedrine HCl 30 mg; Sinubid: acetaminophen 600 mg, phenylpropanolamine HCl 100 mg, phenyltoloxamine citrate 66 mg; Sinutab Maximum Nighttime: acetaminophen 167 mg/5 ml, diphenhydramine HCl 8.3 mg/5 ml, pseudoephedrine HCl 10 mg/5 ml; Sinutab II Maximum, Tylenol maximum strength sinus: acetaminophen 500 mg, pseudoephedrine HCl 30 mg; SK-APAP with Codeine, Tylenol with Codeine No. 2: codeine 5 mg with acetaminophen 300 mg; Trendar: acetaminophen 325 mg with pamabrom 25 mg; Tylenol with Codeine No. 1: acetaminophen 300 mg with codeine phosphate 7.5 mg; Tylenol with Codeine No. 2: acetaminophen 300 mg with codeine phosphate 15 mg; Tylenol with Codeine No. 3: acetaminophen 300 mg with codeine phosphate 30 mg; Tylenol with Codeine No. 4: acetaminophen 300 mg with codeine phosphate 60 mg; Tylox: acetaminophen 500 mg with oxycodone HCl 5 mg

Action: May block pain impulses peripherally that occur in response to inhibition of prostaglandin synthesis; does not possess antiinflammatory properties; antipyretic action results from inhibition of prostaglandins in the CNS (hypothalamic heat-regulating center)

Uses: Mild to moderate pain or fever

Dosage and routes:

- *Adult and child >10 yr:* PO 325-650 mg q4h prn, not to exceed 4 g/day; REC: 325-650 mg q4h prn, not exceed 4 g/day
- *Child 0-3 mo:* 40 mg/dose
- *Child 4-11 mo:* 80 mg/dose
- *Child <1 yr:* PO/REC 15-60 mg/dose q4-6h, not to exceed 65 mg/kg/day
- *Child 1-2 yr:* PO/REC 60 mg/dose
- *Child 2-3 yr:* PO/REC 120 mg/dose
- *Child 3-4 yr:* PO/REC 180 mg/dose
- *Child 4-5 yr:* PO/REC 240 mg/dose
- *Child 5-10 yr:* PO/REC 325 mg/dose

Available forms: Rectal supp 120, 125, 325, 600, 650 mg; chewable tabs 80, 160 mg; caps 500 mg; elix 120, 160, 325 mg/5 ml; liq 160 mg/5 ml, 500 mg/15ml; sol 100 mg/1 ml, 120 mg/2.5 ml; granules 80 mg/packet, 80 mg/cap; Tabs 160, 325, 500, 650 mg

Side effects/adverse reactions:

SYST: ***Anaphylaxis***

HEMA: ***Leukopenia, neutropenia, hemolytic anemia (long-term use), thrombocytopenia, pancytopenia***

CNS: Stimulation, drowsiness

GI: Nausea, vomiting, abdominal pain, ***hepatotoxicity***

INTEG: Rash, urticaria, ***angioedema***

TOXICITY: ***Cyanosis, anemia, neutropenia, jaundice, pancytopenia, CNS stimulation, delirium followed***

* Available in Canada only

by vascular collapse, convulsions, coma, death

Contraindications: Hypersensitivity, intolerance to tartrazine (yellow dye #4), alcohol, table sugar, saccharin

Precautions: Anemia, hepatic disease, renal disease, chronic alcoholism, pregnancy (B), elderly, lactation

Pharmacokinetics: Well absorbed PO, rectal absorption varies

PO: Onset 10-30 min, peak ½-2 hr, duration 3-4 hr

REC: Onset slow, peak 1-2 hr, duration 3-4 hr; 85%-90% metabolized by liver, excreted by kidneys; metabolites may be toxic if overdose occurs; widely distributed, crosses placenta, excreted in breast milk, half-life 1-4 hr)

Interactions:

- Increased effects of chloramphenicol
- Decreased effects of acetaminophen: cholestyramine, oral contraceptives, anticholinergics, colestipol
- Increased effect of acetaminophen: diflunisal, caffeine
- Severe hypothermia: phenothiazines
- Increased chance of hepatotoxicity: alcohol

Lab test interferences:

Interference: Chemstrip G, Dextrostix, Visidex II

NURSING CONSIDERATIONS

Assess:

- Liver function studies: AST, ALT, bilirubin, creatinine prior to therapy if long-term therapy is anticipated
- Renal function studies: BUN, urine creatinine, occult blood, albumin, if patient is on long-term therapy; presence of blood or albumin indicates nephritis
- Blood studies: CBC, pro-time if patient is on long-term therapy
- I&O ratio; decreasing output may indicate renal failure (long-term therapy)
- For fever and pain: type of pain, location, intensity, duration
- Mucosa, fingernail beds for cyanosis; inquire about dyspnea, vertigo, headache, weakness; symptoms indicate methemoglobinemia; notify prescriber immediately
- For chronic poisoning: rapid, weak pulse; dyspnea; cold, clammy extremities; report immediately to prescriber
- Hepatotoxicity: dark urine; clay-colored stools; yellowing of skin, sclera; itching, abdominal pain; fever; diarrhea if patient is on long-term therapy
- Allergic reactions: rash, urticaria; if these occur, drug may have to be discontinued

Administer:

- To patient crushed or whole; chewable tablets may be chewed; give with full glass of water
- With food or milk to decrease gastric symptoms if needed

Perform/provide:

- Storage of suppositories <80° F (27° C)

Evaluate:

- Therapeutic response: absence of pain, fever

Teach patient/family:

- Not to exceed recommended dosage; acute poisoning with liver damage may result. Acute toxicity includes symptoms of nausea, vomiting, abdominal pain; prescriber should be notified immediately.
- To read label on other OTC drugs; many contain acetaminophen and may cause toxicity if taken concurrently
- To recognize signs of chronic overdose: bleeding, bruising, malaise, fever, sore throat

• That urine may become dark brown as a result of phenactin (metabolite of acetaminophen)
• To notify prescriber for pain or fever lasting over 3 days

Treatment of overdose: Drug level, gastric lavage, activated charcoal; administer oral acetylcysteine to prevent hepatic damage (see acetylcysteine monograph), monitor for bleeding

acetazolamide (℞)

(a-set-a-zole′a-mide)

Acetazolam*, acetazolamide, AK-Zol, Dazamide, Diamox, Diamox Sequels, Hydrazol/ Diamox Parenteral

Func. class.: Diuretic; carbonic anhydrase inhibitor

Chem. class.: Sulfonamide derivative

Action: Inhibits carbonic anhydrase activity in proximal renal tubules to decrease reabsorption of water, sodium, potassium, bicarbonate; decreases carbonic anhydrase in CNS, increasing seizure threshold; able to decrease aqueous humor in eye, which lowers intraocular pressure

Uses: Open-angle glaucoma, narrow-angle glaucoma (preoperatively, if surgery delayed), epilepsy (petit mal, grand mal, mixed), edema in CHF, drug-induced edema, acute mountain sickness

Investigational uses: Prevention of uric acid/cystine renal stones

Dosage and routes:

Closed-angle glaucoma

• *Adult:* PO/IM/IV 250 mg q4h or 250 mg bid, to be used for short-term therapy

Open-angle glaucoma

• *Adult:* PO/IM/IV 250 mg-1 g/day in divided doses for amounts over 250 mg

Edema

• *Adult:* IM/IV 250-375 mg/day in AM
• *Child:* IM/IV 5 mg/kg/day in AM

Seizures

• *Adult:* PO/IM/IV 8-30 mg/kg/day, usual range 375-1000 mg/day
• *Child:* PO/IM/IV 8-30 mg/kg/day in divided doses tid or qid, or 300-900 mg/m^2/day, not to exceed 1.5 g/day

Mountain sickness

• *Adult:* PO 250 mg q8-12h

Renal stones

• *Adult:* PO 250 mg hs

Available forms: Tabs 125, 250 mg; caps sust rel 500 mg; inj IM/IV 500 mg

Side effects/adverse reactions:

GU: Frequency, polyuria, ***uremia,*** glucosuria, hematuria, dysuria, crystalluria, renal calculi

CNS: Drowsiness, paresthesia, anxiety, depression, headache, dizziness, confusion, stimulation, fatigue, ***convulsions,*** sedation, nervousness

GI: Nausea, vomiting, anorexia, constipation, diarrhea, melena, weight loss, ***hepatic insufficiency,*** taste alterations

EENT: Myopia, tinnitus

INTEG: Rash, pruritus, urticaria, fever, ***Stevens-Johnson syndrome,*** photosensitivity

ENDO: Hyperglycemia

HEMA: ***Aplastic anemia, hemolytic anemia, leukopenia, agranulocytosis, thrombocytopenia, purpura, pancytopenia***

META: Hypokalemia, hyperchloremic acidosis

Contraindications: Hypersensitivity to sulfonamides, severe renal disease, severe hepatic disease, electrolyte imbalances (hyponatremia,

* Available in Canada only

hypokalemia), hyperchloremic acidosis, Addison's disease, long-term use in narrow-angle glaucoma, COPD

Precautions: Hypercalciuria, pregnancy (C), lactation

Pharmacokinetics:

PO: Onset 1-1½ hr, peak 2-4 hr, duration 6-12 hr

PO–SUS REL: Onset 2 hr, peak 8-12 hr, duration 18-24 hr

IV: Onset 2 min, peak 15 min, duration 4-5 hr, 65% absorbed if fasting (oral), 75% absorbed if given with food; half-life 2½-5½ hr; excreted unchanged by kidneys (80% within 24 hr), crosses placenta

Interactions:

- Increased action of amphetamines, procainamide, quinidine, tricyclics, flecainide, ephedrine, pseudoephedrine
- Increased excretion of barbiturates, ASA, lithium
- Toxicity: salicylates
- Hypokalemia: with other diuretics, corticosteroids, amphotericin B

Additive compatibility: Cimetidine

Lab test interferences:

False positive: Urinary protein, 17 hydroxysteroid

Increase: Blood glucose levels, bilirubin, blood ammonia, calcium, chloride

Decrease: Urine citrate, K

NURSING CONSIDERATIONS

Assess:

- Weight daily, I&O daily to determine fluid loss; effect of drug may be decreased if used qd
- Rate, depth, rhythm of respiration, effect of exertion
- B/P lying, standing; postural hypotension may occur
- Electrolytes: K, Na, chloride; also BUN, blood sugar, CBC, serum creatinine, blood pH, ABGs, liver function tests

Administer:

- After diluting 500 mg in >5 ml sterile H_2O for injection; direct IV—give at 100-500 mg/min; may be diluted further in LR, D_5W, $D_{10}W$ 0.45% NaCl, 0.9% NaCl, or Ringer's Sol and infused over 4-8 hr; use within 24 hr of dilution.
- PO or IV if possible; IM administration is painful
- In AM to avoid interference with sleep if using drug as diuretic
- K replacement if K level is less than 3.0
- With food if nausea occurs; absorption may be decreased slightly

Perform/provide:

- Storage in dark, cool area; use reconstituted solution within 24 hr

Evaluate:

- Therapeutic response: improvement in edema of feet, legs, sacral area daily if medication is being used in CHF; or decrease in aqueous humor if medication is being used in glaucoma

Teach patient/family:

- To take exactly as prescribed; if dose is missed, take as soon as remembered; do not double dose
- To increase fluid intake by 2-3 L/day unless contraindicated; to rise slowly from lying or sitting position
- To notify prescriber if sore throat, unusual bleeding, bruising, paresthesias, tremors, flank pain, or skin rash occurs
- To use sunscreen to prevent photosensitivity
- To avoid hazardous activities if drowsiness occurs

Treatment of overdose: Lavage if taken orally; monitor electrolytes; administer dextrose in saline; monitor hydration, CV, renal status

acetohexamide (℞)

(a-set-oh-hex'a-mide)

acetohexamide, Dimelor*, Dymelor

Func. class.: Antidiabetic

Chem. class.: Sulfonylurea (1st generation)

Action: Causes functioning β-cells in pancreas to release insulin, leading to drop in blood glucose levels; may improve binding between insulin and insulin receptors or increase number of insulin receptors with prolonged administration. May also reduce basal hepatic glucose secretion. Not effective if patient lacks functioning β-cells

Uses: Stable adult-onset diabetes mellitus (type II), NIDDM

Dosage and routes:

• *Adult:* PO 250 mg-1.5 g/day; usually given before breakfast unless large dose is required; then dose is divided in two

Available forms: Tabs 250, 500 mg scored

Side effects/adverse reactions:

CNS: Headache, weakness, tinnitus, fatigue, dizziness, vertigo

GI: Nausea, vomiting, diarrhea, ***hepatotoxicity, jaundice,*** heartburn

HEMA: ***Leukopenia, thrombocytopenia, agranulocytosis, aplastic anemia, hemolytic anemia,*** increased AST, ALT, alk phosphatase

INTEG: Rash, allergic reactions, pruritus, urticaria, eczema, photosensitivity, erythema

ENDO: ***Hypoglycemia,*** hyponatremia

Contraindications: Hypersensitivity to sulfonylureas, juvenile or brittle diabetes, renal failure

Precautions: Pregnancy (C), elderly, cardiac disease, renal disease, hepatic disease, thyroid disease, severe hypoglycemic reactions

Pharmacokinetics:

PO: Completely absorbed by GI route, onset 1 hr, peak 2-4 hr, duration 12-24 hr, half-life 6-8 hr, metabolized in liver, excreted in urine (active metabolites, unchanged drug)

Interactions:

• Increased hypoglycemic effects: oral anticoagulants, salicylates, sulfonamides, nonsteroidal antiinflammatories, guanethidine, methyldopa, MAOIs, chloramphenicol, insulin, cimetidine

• Decreased action of acetohexamide: calcium channel blockers, corticosteroids, oral contraceptives, thiazide diuretics, thyroid preparations, estrogens, phenobarbital, phenothiazines, phenytoin, rifampin, sympathomimetics

• Decreased effect of both drugs: diazoxide

NURSING CONSIDERATIONS

Assess:

• Hypoglycemic/hyperglycemic reaction that can occur soon after meals

Administer:

• Drug 30 min before meals

Perform/provide:

• Storage in tight container in cool environment

Evaluate:

• Therapeutic response: decrease in polyuria, polydipsia, polyphagia, clear sensorium, absence of dizziness, stable gait

Teach patient/family:

• To check for symptoms of cholestatic jaundice: dark urine, pruritus, yellow sclera; if these occur, prescriber should be notified

• To use capillary blood glucose test or Chemstrip 3 ×/day

• Symptoms of hypo/hyperglycemia, what to do about each

• That drug must be continued on

* Available in Canada only

daily basis; explain consequence of discontinuing drug abruptly

• To take drug in morning to prevent hypoglycemic reactions at night, to take as prescribed; if dose is missed, take when remembered

• To avoid OTC medications unless directed by prescriber

• That diabetes is lifelong illness; that this drug is not a cure

• That all food included in diet plan must be eaten to prevent hypoglycemia

• To carry Medic Alert ID for emergency purposes, carry a glucagon emergency kit

Treatment of overdose: Glucose 25 g IV, via dextrose 50% sol, 50 ml or 1 mg glucagon

---

acetylcysteine (℞)

(a-se-til-sis'tay-een)

Airbron*, Mucomyst, Mucosal

Func. class.: Mucolytic, antidote-acetaminophen

Chem. class.: Amino acid L-cysteine

Action: Decreases viscosity of secretions by breaking disulfide links of mucoproteins; increases hepatic glutathione, which is necessary to inactivate toxic metabolites in acetaminophen overdose

Uses: Acetaminophen toxicity; bronchitis; pneumonia; cystic fibrosis; emphysema; atelectasis; tuberculosis; complications of thoracic, cardiovascular surgery; diagnosis in bronchial lab tests

Dosage and routes:

Mucolytic

• *Adult and child:* INSTILL 1-2 ml (10%-20% sol) q1-4h prn or 3-5 ml (20% sol) or 6-10 ml (10% sol) tid or qid

Acetaminophen toxicity

• *Adult and child:* PO 140 mg/kg, then 70 mg/kg q4h × 17 doses to total of 1330 mg/kg

Available forms: Sol 10%, 20%

Side effects/adverse reactions:

CNS: Dizziness, drowsiness, headache, fever, chills

GI: Nausea, stomatitis, constipation, vomiting, anorexia, ***hepatotoxicity***

EENT: Rhinorrhea, tooth damage

CV: Hypotension

INTEG: Urticaria, rash, fever, clamminess

RESP: ***Bronchospasm,*** burning, ***hemoptysis,*** chest tightness

Contraindications: Hypersensitivity, increased intracranial pressure, status asthmaticus

Precautions: Hypothyroidism, Addison's disease, CNS depression, brain tumor, asthma, hepatic disease, renal disease, COPD, psychosis, alcoholism, convulsive disorders, lactation, pregnancy (B)

Pharmacokinetics:

INH/INSTILL: Onset 1 min, duration 5-10 min, metabolized by liver, excreted in urine

Interactions:

• Do not use with iron, copper, rubber

• Do not mix with antibiotics: tetracycline, chlortetracycline, oxytetracycline, erythromycin, lactobionate, amphotericin-B, sodium ampicillin; iodized oil, chymotrypsin, trypsin, hydrogen peroxide

NURSING CONSIDERATIONS

Assess:

• Cough: type, frequency, character, including sputum

• Rate, rhythm of respirations, increased dyspnea; discontinue if bronchospasm occurs

• Antidotal use: decrease in hepatic encephalopathy

• VS, cardiac status including checking for dysrhythmias, increased rate, palpitations
• ABGs for increased CO_2 retention in asthma patients
• Antidotal use: liver function tests, acetaminophen levels; inform prescriber if dose is vomited or vomiting is persistent

Administer:
• Store in refrigerator: use within 96 hr of opening
• Before meals ½-1 hr for better absorption, to decrease nausea
• 20% solutions diluted with NS or water for injection; may give 10% solution undiluted
• Only after patient clears airway by deep breathing, coughing
• Antidotal use: give within 24 hr; give with cola or soft drink to disguise taste; can be given with H_2O through tubes; use within 1 hr
• By syringe 2-3 doses of 1-2 ml of 20% or 2-4 ml of 10% solution
• Decreased dose to elderly patients; their metabolism may be slowed
• Gum, hard candy, frequent rinsing of mouth for dryness of oral cavity
• Only if suction machine is available

Perform/provide:
• Storage in refrigerator after opening
• Assistance with inhaled dose: bronchodilator if bronchospasm occurs
• Mechanical suction if cough insufficient to remove excess bronchial secretions

Evaluate:
• Therapeutic response: absence of purulent secretions when coughing; absence of hepatic damage in acetaminophen toxicity

Teach patient/family:
• To avoid driving, other hazardous activities until patient is stabilized on this medication
• To avoid alcohol, other CNS depressants; will enhance sedating properties of this drug
• That unpleasant odor will decrease after repeated use
• That discoloration of solution after bottle is opened does not impair its effectiveness
• To avoid smoking, smoke-filled rooms, perfume, dust, environmental pollutants, cleaners

acrivastine/pseudoephedrine (℞)

(ac-ri-vas'teen)
Semprex-D
Func. class.: Antihistamine
Chem. class.: H_1-histamine antagonist

Action: Acts on blood vessels, GI, respiratory system by competing with histamine for H_1-receptor site; decreases allergic response by blocking pharmacologic effects of histamine; less sedation rate than with other antihistamines; causes increased heart rate, vasodilation, increased secretions

Uses: Rhinitis, allergy symptoms, chronic idiopathic urticaria

Dosage and routes:
• *Adult, child >12 yr:* PO 8 mg q4-6h

Available forms: Caps 8, 60 mg

Side effects/adverse reactions:
GU: Dysmenorrhea
RESP: Cough, pharyngitis
GI: Nausea, dry mouth
CNS: Headache, dizziness, nervousness, insomnia

Contraindications: Hypersensitivity to this drug or triprolidine, severe hypertension, cardiac disease

Precautions: Pregnancy (B), lactation, elderly, children, respiratory

* Available in Canada only

disease, hypertension, diabetes mellitus, ischemic heart disease, increased intraocular pressure, prostate hypertrophy

Pharmacokinetics: Metabolized by the liver excreted in kidneys, feces; half-life 1½ hr, peak 1-1½ hr, duration 12 hr

Interactions:

- Increased CNS depression: alcohol, narcotics, sedatives, hypnotics
- Hypertensive crisis: MAO inhibitors

Lab test interferences:

False negative: Skin allergy tests (discontinue antihistamine 3 days prior to testing)

NURSING CONSIDERATIONS

Assess:

- Respiratory status: rate, rhythm, increase in bronchial secretions, wheezing, chest tightness; provide fluids to 2 L/day to decrease thickness of secretions

Administer:

- With food, fluid for GI symptoms

Perform/provide:

- Storage in tight, light-resistant container

Evaluate:

- Therapeutic response: absence of running or congested nose, rashes

Teach patient/family:

- All aspects of drug use; to avoid driving, other hazardous activity if drowsy; to avoid alcohol, other CNS depressants that may potentiate effect
- Not to exceed recommended dose
- To use hard candy, gum, or frequent rinsing of mouth for dryness

Treatment of overdose: Administer ipecac syrup or lavage, diazepam, vasopressors, barbiturates (short-acting)

activated charcoal (OTC)

Acta-Char, Acta-Char Liquid-A, Actidose-Aqua, Aqueous-Charcodote*, Charac-50*, Insta-Char, Insta-Char Aqueous Suspension, Liqui-Char, Liqu-Char, Superchar, Charcoaide, Charcocaps, Charcodote, Charcotabs, Digestalin

Func. class.: Antiflatulent/antidote

Action: Binds poisons, toxins, irritants; increases adsorption in GI tract; inactivates toxins and binds until excreted

Uses: Flatulence, poisoning, dyspepsia, distention, deodorant in wounds, diarrhea

Dosage and routes:

Poisoning

- *Adult and child:* PO 30-100 g or 1 g/kg, minimum dose 30 g/250 ml of water, may give 20-40 g q6h for 1-2 days in severe poisoning

Flatulence/dyspepsia

- *Adult:* PO 520-975 mg pc up to 4.16 g/day

Available forms: Powder 15, 30, 40, 120, 125, 240 g/container; oral susp 12.5 g/60 ml, 15 g/72 ml, 15 g/120 ml, 25 g/120 ml, 30 g/120 ml, 50 g/240 ml; Canada 15 g/120 ml, 25 g/125 ml, 50 g/225 ml, 50 g/250 ml

Side effects/adverse reactions:

GI: Nausea, black stools, vomiting, constipation, diarrhea

Contraindications: Hypersensitivity to this drug, unconsciousness, semiconsciousness, poisoning of cyanide, mineral acids, alkalies

Pharmacokinetics:

PO: Excreted in feces

Interactions:

- Decreased effectiveness of both drugs: ipecac, laxatives

• Do not mix with dairy products

NURSING CONSIDERATIONS

Assess:

• Respiration, pulse, B/P to determine charcoal effectiveness if taken for barbiturate/narcotic poisoning

Administer:

• After inducing vomiting unless vomiting contraindicated (i.e., cyanide or alkalies)

• After mixing with water, fruit juice, or sorbitol to form thick syrup; do not use dairy products to mix charcoal

• Repeat dose if vomiting occurs soon after dose

• After spacing at least 1 hr before or after other drugs, or absorption will be decreased

• With a laxative to promote elimination

• Alone; do not administer with ipecac

• Through a nasogastric tube if patient unable to swallow

• Keeping container tightly closed to prevent absorption of gases

Evaluate:

• Therapeutic response: LOC-alert (poisoning)

Teach patient/family:

• That stools will be black

• How to prevent further poisonings

acyclovir (topical) (℞)

(ay-sye′kloe-ver)

Zovirax

Func. class.: Local antiinfective

Chem. class.: Antiviral

Action: Interferes with viral DNA replication

Uses: Simple mucocutaneous herpes simplex, in immunocompromised clients with initial herpes genitalis

Dosage and routes:

• *Adult and child:* TOP apply to all lesions q3h while awake, 6 times/day × 1 wk

Available forms: TOP oint 5% (50 mg/g)

Side effects/adverse reactions:

INTEG: Rash, urticaria, stinging, burning, pruritus, vulvitis

Contraindications: Hypersensitivity

Precautions: Pregnancy (C), lactation

NURSING CONSIDERATIONS

Assess:

• Allergic reaction: burning, stinging, swelling, redness, rash, vulvitis, pruritus

Administer:

• Using finger cot or rubber glove to prevent further infection

• Enough medication to cover lesions completely

• After cleansing with soap, water before each application; dry well

Perform/provide:

• Storage at room temperature in dry place

Evaluate:

• Therapeutic response: decrease in size, number of lesions

Teach patient/family:

• Not to use in eyes or when there is no evidence of infection

• To apply with glove to prevent further infection

• To avoid use of OTC creams, ointments, lotions unless directed by prescriber

• To use medical asepsis (hand washing) before, after each application and avoid contact with eyes

• To adhere strictly to prescribed regimen to maximize successful treatment outcome

• To begin taking drug when symptoms arise

acyclovir (℞)

(ay-sye'kloe-ver)

Zovirax

Func. class.: Antiviral

Chem. class.: Acyclic purine nucleoside analog

Action: Interferes with DNA synthesis by conversion to acyclovir triphosphate, causing decreased viral replication, time of lesional healing

Uses: Mucocutaneous herpes simplex virus, herpes genitalis (HSV-1, HSV-2), herpes zoster

Dosage and routes:

Herpes simplex

• *Adult and child >12 yr:* IV INF 5 mg/kg over 1 hr q8h × 5 days

• *Child <12 yr:* IV INF 250 mg/ m^2 over 1 hr q8h × 5 days

Genital herpes

• *Adult:* PO 200 mg q4h 5×/day while awake for 5 days to 6 mo depending on whether initial, recurrent, or chronic

Herpes simplex encephalitis

• *Adult IV:* 10 mg/kg over 1 hr q8h × 7 days

• *Child >6 mo:* IV 500 mg/m^2 q8h × 10 days

Herpes zoster

• *Adult:* PO 800 mg × 5 days IV 5 mg/kg q8h

Children with immunosuppression:

• *Child >2 yr:* 20 mg/kg qid × 5 days

Available forms: Tabs, caps 200 mg; inj IV 500 mg

Side effects/adverse reactions:

CNS: Tremors, confusion, lethargy, hallucinations, ***convulsions,*** *dizziness, headache,* encephalopathic changes

GI: Nausea, vomiting, diarrhea, increased ALT, AST, abdominal pain, glossitis, colitis

GU: ***Oliguria, proteinuria, hematuria,*** vaginitis, moniliasis, ***glomerulonephritis, acute renal failure,*** changes in menses, polydypsia

EENT: Gingival hyperplasia

INTEG: Rash, urticaria, pruritus, pain or phlebitis at IV site, unusual sweating, alopecia

MS: Joint pain, leg pain, muscle cramps

Contraindications: Hypersensitivity

Precautions: Lactation, hepatic disease, renal disease, electrolyte imbalance, dehydration, pregnancy (C)

Pharmacokinetics:

IV: Peak 1 hr, half-life 20 min-3 hr (terminal); metabolized by liver, excreted by kidneys as unchanged drug (95%); crosses placenta; absorbed minimally (PO), distributed widely; crosses placenta, CSF concentrations are 50% plasma

PO: onset unknown, peak 1½-2 hours, terminal half-life 3½ hours

Interactions:

• Increased neurotoxicity, nephrotoxicity: aminoglycosides, amphotericin, interferon, probenecid, methotrexate, zidovudine

Solution compatibilities: D_5W, LR, or NaCl (D_5 0.9% NaCl, 0.9% NaCl) solutions

Y-site compatibilities: Amikacin, ampicillin, cefamandole, cefazolin, cefonicid, cefoperazone, ceforanide, cefotaxime, cefoxitin, ceftazidime, ceftizoxime, ceftriaxone, cefuroxime, cephapirin, chloramphenicol, cimetidine, clindamycin, co-trimoxazole, dexamethasone sodium phosphate, dimenhydrinate, diphenhydramine, erythromycin lactobionate, gentamicin, heparin, hydrocortisone sodium succinate, hydromorphone, imipenem/ cilastatin, lorazepam, magnesium sulfate, meperidine, methylprednisolone sodium succinate, metoclopramide, metronidazole, morphine, multivitamin infusion, nafcillin, oxacillin, penicillin G potassium, pentobarbital, perphenazine, piperacillin, potassium chloride, ranitidine, sodium bicarbonate, tetracycline, theophylline, ticarcillin, tobramycin, vancomycin, zidovudine

NURSING CONSIDERATIONS

Assess:

• Signs of infection, anemia

• I&O ratio; report hematuria, oliguria, fatigue, weakness; may indicate nephrotoxicity; check for protein in urine during treatment

• Any patient with compromised renal system, since drug is excreted slowly in poor renal system function; toxicity may occur rapidly

• Liver studies: AST, ALT

• Blood studies: WBC, RBC, Hct, Hgb, bleeding time; blood dyscrasias may occur; drug should be discontinued

• Renal studies: urinalysis, protein, BUN, creatinine, CrCl

• C&S before drug therapy; drug may be taken as soon as culture is taken; repeat C&S after treatment; determine the presence of other sexually transmitted diseases

• Bowel pattern before, during treatment; if severe abdominal pain with bleeding occurs, drug should be discontinued

• Skin eruptions: rash, urticaria, itching

• Allergies before treatment, reaction of each medication; place allergies on chart in bright red letters

Administer:

• Increased fluids to 3 L/day to decrease crystalluria when given IV

• After reconstituting with 10 ml compatible solution/500 mg of drug, concentration of 50 mg/ml, shake, use within 12 hr (<7 mg/ml); give over at least 1 hr (constant rate) by infusion pump to prevent nephrotoxicity; do not reconstitute with sol containing benzyl alcohol in neonates

• Lower dose in acute or chronic renal failure

Perform/provide:

• Storage at room temperature for up to 12 hr after reconstitution; if refrigerated, sol may show a precipitate that clears at room temperature

• Adequate intake of fluids (2 L) to prevent deposit in kidneys

Evaluate:

• Therapeutic response: absence of itching, painful lesions; crusting and healed lesions

Teach patient/family:

• To take as prescribed; if dose is missed, take as soon as remembered up to 1 hr before next dose; do not double dose

• That drug may be taken orally before infection occurs; drug should be taken when itching or pain occurs, usually before eruptions

• That partners need to be told that patient has herpes; they can become infected; condoms must be worn to prevent reinfections

• That drug does not cure infection, just controls symptoms and does not prevent infection to others

• To report sore throat, fever, fatigue; may indicate superinfection

• That drug must be taken in equal intervals around the clock to maintain blood levels for duration of therapy

• To notify prescriber of side effects of bruising, bleeding, fatigue, malaise; may indicate blood dyscrasias

• To seek dental care during treatment to prevent gingival hyperplasia

---

* Available in Canada only

Treatment of overdose: Discontinue drug, hemodialysis, resuscitate if needed

adenosine (℞)

(a-den'oh-seen)

Adenocard

Func. class.: Antidysrhythmic

Chem. class.: Endogenous nucleoside

Action: Slows conduction through AV node, can interrupt reentry pathways through AV node, and can restore normal sinus rhythm in patients with paroxysmal supraventricular tachycardia (PSVT)

Uses: PSVT

Dosage and routes:

• *Adult:* IV BOL 6 mg; if conversion to normal sinus rhythm does not occur within 1-2 min, give 12 mg by rapid IV BOL; may repeat 12 mg dose again in 1-2 min

Available forms: Inj 3 mg/ml

Side effects/adverse reactions:

GI: Nausea, metallic taste, throat tightness, groin pressure

RESP: Dyspnea, chest pressure, hyperventilation

CNS: Lightheadedness, dizziness, arm tingling, numbness, apprehension, blurred vision, headache

CV: Chest pain, ***atrial tachydysrhythmias,*** sweating, palpitations, hypotension, *facial flushing*

Contraindications: Hypersensitivity, 2nd or 3rd degree heart block, AV block, sick sinus syndrome, atrial flutter, atrial fibrillation, ventricular tachycardia

Precautions: Pregnancy (C), lactation, children, asthma, elderly

Pharmacokinetics: Cleared from plasma in <30 sec, half-life 10 sec

Interactions:

• Increased effects of adenosine: dipyridamole

• Decreased activity of adenosine; theophylline or other methylxanthines (caffeine)

• Higher degree of heart block: carbamazepine

Lab test interferences:

Increase: Liver function tests

NURSING CONSIDERATIONS

Assess:

• Cardiac status continually

• B/P continuously for fluctuations

• I&O ratio, electrolytes (K, Na, Cl)

• Cardiac status: B/P, pulse, respiration, ECG intervals (PR, QRS, QT)

• Respiratory status: rate, rhythm, lung fields for rales, watch for respiratory depression

• CNS effects: dizziness, confusion, psychosis, paresthesias, convulsions; drug should be discontinued

• Lung fields, bilateral rales may occur in CHF patient

• Increased respiration, increased pulse; drug should be discontinued

Administer:

• IV bolus undiluted; give 6 mg or less over 1 min; if using an IV line, use port near insertion site, flush with normal saline (50 ml)

Perform/provide

• Storage at room temperature; sol should be clear; discard unused drug

Evaluate:

• Therapeutic response: decreased anginal pain, decreased B/P, dysrhythmias, decreased heart rate

Treatment of overdose: Defibrillation, vasopressor for hypotension

albumin, normal serum 5%/25% (℞)

(al-byoo'min)

Albuminar 5%, Albutein 5%, Buminate 5%, Plasbumin 5%, Albuminar 25%, Albutein 25%, Buminate 25%, Plasbumin-25%

Func. class.: Blood derivative

Chem. class.: Placental human plasma

Action: Exerts oncotic pressure, which expands volume of circulating blood and maintains cardiac output

Uses: Restores plasma volume in burns, hyperbilirubinemia, shock, hypoproteinemia, prevention of cerebral edema, cardiopulmonary bypass procedures, ARDS

Dosage and routes:

Burns

• *Adult:* IV dose to maintain plasma albumin at 30-50 g/L, use 5% sol initially, then 25% sol after 24 hr

Shock

• *Adult:* IV 500 ml of 5% sol q30 min, as needed

• *Child:* ¼-½ adult dose in nonemergencies

Hypoproteinemia

• *Adult:* IV 1000-2000 ml of 5% sol qd, not to exceed 5-10 ml/min or 25-100 g of 25% sol qd, not to exceed 3 ml/min, titrated to patient response

Hyperbilirubinemia/erythroblastosis fetalis

• *Infant:* IV 1 g of 25% sol/kg before transfusion

Available forms: Inj IV 50, 250 mg/ml (5%, 25%)

Side effects/adverse reactions:

GI: Nausea, vomiting, increased salivation

INTEG: Rash, urticaria

CNS: Fever, chills, flushing, headache

RESP: Altered respirations, ***pulmonary edema***

CV: Fluid overload, hypotension, erratic pulse, tachycardia

Contraindications: Hypersensitivity, CHF, severe anemia, renal insufficiency

Precautions: Decreased salt intake, decreased cardiac reserve, lack of albumin deficiency, hepatic disease, renal disease, pregnancy (C)

Pharmacokinetics: In hyponutrition states, metabolized as protein/energy source.

Solution compatibilities: 0.9% NaCl, D_5W, D_5/0.9% NaCl, D_5/0.45%, D_5/LR, LR

Lab test interferences:

False increase: Alk phosphatase

NURSING CONSIDERATIONS

Assess:

• Blood studies Hct, Hgb; if serum protein declines, dyspnea, hypoxemia can result

• Decreased B/P, erratic pulse, respiration

• I&O ratio: urinary output may decrease

• CVP, pulmonary wedge pressure will increase if overload occurs

• Allergy: fever, rash, itching, chills, flushing, urticaria, nausea, vomiting, hypotension, requires discontinuation of infusion, use of new lot if therapy reinstituted

• CVP reading: distended neck veins indicate circulatory overload; shortness of breath, anxiety, insomnia, expiratory rales, frothy blood-tinged cough, cyanosis indicate pulmonary overload

Administer:

• IV slowly, to prevent fluid overload; dilute with NS for injection or D_5W; 5% may be given undiluted; 25% may be given diluted or undi-

* Available in Canada only

luted, give over 4 hr, use infusion pump

Perform/provide:

• Adequate hydration before, during administration

• Check type of albumin; some stored at room temperature, some need to be refrigerated

Evaluate:

• Therapeutic response: increased B/P, decreased edema, increased serum albumin levels; increased plasma protein

albuterol (℞)

(al-byoo′ter-ole)

albuterol, Gen-Salbutamol*, Novosalmol*, Proventil, Proventil Repetabs, Salbutamol*, Ventolin, Ventolin Rotacaps, Ventodisk*, Volmax*

Func. class.: Adrenergic β_2 agonist

Action: Causes bronchodilation by action on β_2 (pulmonary) receptors by increasing levels of cAMP, which relaxes smooth muscle; produces bronchodilation, CNS, cardiac stimulation, as well as increased diuresis and gastric acid secretion; longer acting than isoproterenol

Uses: Prevention of exercise-induced asthma, bronchospasm, prevention of premature labor

Investigational uses: Hyperkalemia in dialysis patients

Dosage and routes:

To prevent exercise-induced asthma

• *Adult:* INH 2 puffs 15 min before exercising, NEB/LPPB 5 mg tid-qid

Bronchospasm

• *Adult:* INH 1-2 puffs q4-6h PO 2-4 mg tid-qid, not to exceed 8 mg

Available forms: Aerosol 90 µg/actuation; tabs 2, 4 mg; syr 2 mg/5 ml; cont rel 4, 8 mg

Side effects/adverse reactions:

CNS: Tremors, anxiety, insomnia, headache, dizziness, stimulation, *restlessness,* hallucinations, flushing, irritability

EENT: Dry nose, irritation of nose and throat

CV: Palpitations, tachycardia, hypertension, angina, hypotension, dysrhythmias

GI: Heartburn, nausea, vomiting

MS: Muscle cramps

Contraindications: Hypersensitivity to sympathomimetics, tachydysrhythmias, severe cardiac disease

Precautions: Lactation, pregnancy (C), cardiac disorders, hyperthyroidism, diabetes mellitus, hypertension, prostatic hypertrophy, narrow-angle glaucoma, seizures, exercise-induced bronchospasm (aerosol) in children <12 years

Pharmacokinetics: Well absorbed PO, extensively metabolized in the liver, excreted in urine, crosses placenta, breast milk, blood-brain barrier

PO: Onset ½ hr, peak 2½ hr, duration 4-6 hr, half-life 2½ hr

PO-ER: Onset ½ hour; peak 2-3 hr; duration 12 hr

INH: Onset 5-15 min, peak 1-1½ hr, duration 4-6 hr, half-life 4 hr

Interactions:

• Increased action of aerosol bronchodilators

• Increased action of albuterol: tricyclic antidepressants, MAOIs, other adrenergics

• May inhibit action of albuterol: other β-blockers

NURSING CONSIDERATIONS

Assess:

• Respiratory function: vital capacity, forced expiratory volume, ABGs, lung sounds, heart rate and rhythm (baseline)

• That patient has not received theophylline therapy before giving dose

• Client's ability to self-medicate
• For evidence of allergic reactions

Administer:

• After shaking, exhale, place mouthpiece in mouth, inhale slowly, hold breath, remove, exhale slowly
• Gum, sips of water for dry mouth
• PO with meals to decrease gastric irritation
• Syrup to children (no alcohol, sugar)

Perform/provide:

• Storage in light-resistant container, do not expose to temperatures over 86° F (30° C)

Evaluate:

• Therapeutic response: absence of dyspnea, wheezing after 1 hr, improved airway exchange, improved ABGs

Teach patient/family:

• To use exactly as prescribed; take missed dose when remembered, alter schedule
• Not to use OTC medications; extra stimulation may occur
• Use of inhaler; review package insert with patient; use demonstration, return demonstration
• To avoid getting aerosol in eyes; blurring may result
• To wash inhaler in warm water qd and dry
• To avoid smoking, smoke-filled rooms, persons with respiratory infections
• That paradoxic bronchospasm may occur and to stop drug immediately
• To limit caffeine products such as chocolate, coffee, tea, and colas

Treatment of overdose: Administer a β_2-adrenergic blocker

aldesleukin (interleukin-2, IL-2) (℞)

(al-dess'loo-kin)

Proleukin

Func. class.: Miscellaneous antineoplastic

Chem. class.: Interleukin-2, human recombinant

Action: Enhancement of lymphocyte mitogenesis and stimulation of IL-2-dependent cell lines; enhancement of lymphocyte cytotoxicity; induction of killer cell activity; induction of interferon γ-production; results in activation of cellular immunity, cytokines and inhibition of tumor growth

Uses: Metastatic renal cell carcinoma in adults

Dosage and routes:

• *Adult:* IV INF 600,000 IU/kg (0.037 mg/kg) q8h over 15 min × 14 doses; off 9 days, repeat schedule for another 14 doses, for a max of 28 doses/course

Available forms: Powder for inj, lyophilized

Side effects/adverse reactions:

CV: Hypotension, sinus tachycardia, dysrhythmias, bradycardia, PVCs, PACs, myocardial ischemia, ***myocardial infarction, cardiac arrest***

RESP: Pulmonary congestion, dyspnea, ***pulmonary edema, respiratory failure,*** tachypnea, pleural effusion, wheezing

GI: Nausea, vomiting, diarrhea, stomatitis, anorexia, GI bleeding, dyspepsia, constipation, ***intestinal perforation***/ileus, jaundice, ascites

HEMA: Anemia, ***thrombocytopenia, leukopenia, coagulation disorders, leukocytosis, eosinophilia***

CNS: Mental status changes, dizziness, sensory dysfunction, syncope,

* Available in Canada only

motor dysfunction, fever, chills, headache

GU: ***Oliguria/anuria, proteinuria, hematuria,*** dysuria, ***renal failure***

INTEG: Pruritus, erythema, rash, dry skin, ***exfoliative dermatitis,*** purpura, petechiae, urticaria

MS: Arthralgia, myalgia

SYST: Infection

Contraindications: Hypersensitivity, abnormal thallium stress test or pulmonary function tests, organ allografts

Precautions: CNS metastases, bacterial infections, renal/hepatic disease, pregnancy (C), lactation, children, anemia, thrombocytopenia

Pharmacokinetics: Renal elimination half-life 85 min

Interactions:

• Potentiate hypotension: antihypertensives

• Reduced antitumor effectiveness: corticosteroids

• Increased toxicity: aminoglycosides, indomethacin, cytotoxic chemotherapy, methotrexate, asparaginase, doxorubicin

• Do not mix with any other drug

Lab test interferences:

Increase: Bilirubin, BUN, serum creatinine, transaminase, alk phosphatase; hypomagnesemia, acidosis hypocalcemia, hypophosphatemia, hypokalemia, hyperuricemia, hypoalbuminemia, hypoproteinemia, hyponatremia, hyperkalemia, alkalosis

NURSING CONSIDERATIONS

Assess:

• CBC, differential, platelet count weekly; withhold drug if WBC is $<4000/mm^3$ or platelet count is $<75{,}000/mm^3$; notify prescriber of these results

• Capillary leak syndrome including a drop in mean arterial pressure (2-12 hr after initiating therapy); hypotension and hypoperfusion will occur

• Renal function studies: BUN, serum uric acid, urine CrCl, electrolytes before, during therapy

• I&O ratio; report fall in urine output to <30 ml/hr

• Monitor temperature q4h; fever may indicate beginning infection

• Liver function tests before, during therapy: bilirubin, AST, ALT, alk phosphatase as needed or monthly

• ECG; watch for ST-T wave changes, low QRS and T, possible dysrhythmias (sinus tachycardia, PVCs)

• Baselines in pulmonary function; document FEV >2 L or ≥75% prior to therapy

• Stress thallium study prior to therapy; document normal ejection fraction, unimpaired wall motion

• Bleeding: hematuria, guaiac, bruising or petechiae, mucosa or orifices q8h

• Food preferences; list likes, dislikes

• Inflammation of mucosa, breaks in skin

• Buccal cavity q8h for dryness, sores, ulceration, white patches, oral pain, bleeding, dysphagia

• Alkalosis if severe vomiting is present

• Local irritation, pain, burning at injection site

• GI symptoms: frequency of stools, cramping

• Acidosis, signs of dehydration: rapid respirations, poor skin turgor, decreased urine output, dry skin, restlessness, weakness

• Cardiac status: B/P, pulse, character, rhythm, rate, ABGs, ECG

Administer:

• Hydrocortisone, dexamethasone or sodium bicarbonate (1 mEq/1 ml)

for extravasation, apply ice compresses
• Antiemetic 30-60 min before giving drug to prevent vomiting
• IV after diluting 22 million IU (1.3 mg)/1.2 ml sterile H_2O for inj at site of vial and swirl, do not shake; dilute dose with 50 ml D_5W and give over 15 min; use plastic bag; do not use an in-line filter, give through Y-tube or 3-way stopcock
• Topical or systemic analgesics for pain
• Transfusion for anemia
• Antispasmodic for GI symptoms

Perform/provide:
• Strict hand-washing technique, gloves, protective clothing
• Liquid diet: carbonated beverage, gelatin (Jell-O) may be added if patient is not nauseated or vomiting
• Rinsing of mouth tid-qid with water, club soda; brushing of teeth bid-tid with soft brush or cotton-tipped applicators for stomatitis; use unwaxed dental floss
• Storage in refrigerator of diluted drug; do not freeze; administer within 48 hr; bring to room temperature before infusing; discard unused portion

Evaluate:
• Therapeutic response: decreased tumor size, spread of malignancy

Teach patient/family:
• To use a nonhormonal contraceptive method during therapy
• To report any complaints, side effects to nurse or prescriber
• To avoid foods with citric acid, hot or rough texture
• To report any bleeding, white spots, ulcerations in mouth to prescriber; tell patient to examine mouth qd
• To avoid crowds and persons with infections when granulocyte count is low

alfentanil (℞)

(al-fen′ta-nil)
Alfenta, Rapifen*
Func. class.: Narcotic analgesic
Chem. class.: Opiate, synthetic

Controlled Substance Schedule II
Action: Inhibits ascending pain pathways in limbic system, thalamus, midbrain, hypothalamus
Uses: In combination with other drugs in general anesthesia, as a primary anesthetic in general surgery
Dosage and routes:
Anesthesia <30 min
Combination
• *Adult:* IV 8-50 μg/kg, may increase by 3-15 μg/kg
Anesthetic induction
• *Adult:* IV 3-5 μg/kg, then 0.5-1.5 μg/kg/min; total dose is 8-40 μg/kg
Anesthesia 30-60 min
Induction
• *Adult:* IV 20-50 μg/kg
Maintenance
• *Adult:* IV 5-15 μg/kg; may give up to 75 μg/kg total dose
Continuous anesthesia >45 min
Induction
• *Adult:* IV 50-75 μg/kg
Maintenance
• *Adult:* IV 0.5-3.0 μg/kg/min; rate should be decreased by 30%-50% after 1 hr maintenance inf; may be increased to 4 μg/kg/min or bol doses of 7 μg/kg
Induction of anesthesia >45 min
• *Adult:* IV 130-245 μg/kg, then 0.5-1.5 μg/kg/min or general anesthesia
Available forms: Inj 500 μg/ml
Side effects/adverse reactions:
CNS: Drowsiness, dizziness, confusion, headache, sedation, euphoria, delirium, agitation, anxiety
GI: Nausea, vomiting, anorexia, constipation, cramps, dry mouth
GU: Urinary retention, dysuria

* Available in Canada only

INTEG: *Rash,* urticaria, bruising, flushing, diaphoresis, pruritus
EENT: Tinnitus, blurred vision, miosis, diplopia
CV: Palpitation, bradycardia, change in B/P, facial flushing, syncope, asystole
RESP: ***Respiratory depression, apnea***
MS: Rigidity
Contraindications: Child <12 yr, hypersensitivity
Precautions: Pregnancy (C), lactation, increased intracranial pressure, acute MI, severe heart disease, renal disease, hepatic disease, asthma, respiratory conditions, convulsive disorders, elderly
Pharmacokinetics: Half-life 1-2 hr, 90% bound to plasma proteins, duration 30 min
Interactions:
• Respiratory depression, hypotension, profound sedation: alcohol, sedative, hypnotics, or other CNS depressants, antihistamines, phenothiazines
Solution compatibilities: LR, 0.9% NaCl, D_5W, D_5/0.9% NaCl
Lab test interferences:
Increase: Amylase

NURSING CONSIDERATIONS

Assess:
• I&O ratio, check for decreasing output; may indicate urinary retention, especially in elderly
• CNS changes: dizziness, drowsiness, hallucinations, euphoria, LOC, pupil reaction
• Allergic reactions: rash, urticaria
• Respiratory dysfunction: respiratory depression, character, rate, rhythm: notify prescriber if respirations are <12/min; CV status: bradycardia, syncope
• Use pain scoring to determine pain perception
Administer:
• Direct IV over 1½-3 min; use tuberculin syringe
• Cont IV by diluting 20 ml of drug in 230 ml of diluent (40 μg/ml); discontinue inf 15 min before surgery is completed
Perform/provide:
• Storage in light-resistant area at room temperature
Evaluate:
• Therapeutic response: maintenance of anesthesia
Teach patient/family:
• Tell patient to call for assistance when ambulating or smoking; drowsiness, dizziness may occur
• Advise patient to make position changes slowly to prevent orthostatic hypotension
Treatment of overdose: Nalaxone HCl 0.2-0.8 mg IV, O_2, IV fluids, vasopressors

---

alglucerase (℞)

(all-gloo-ser′ase)
Ceredase
Func. class.: Enzyme

Action: Catalyzes the breakdown of glucocerebroside, which accumulates in macrophages primarily in the liver, spleen, and bone marrow in Gaucher's disease
Uses: Long-term enzyme replacement for a confirmed diagnosis of type I Gaucher's disease
Dosage and routes:
• *Adult and child:* IV 60 U/kg diluted in up to 100 ml of 0.9% NaCl given over 1-2 hr; dose is repeated q2wk, but may be given QOD or as infrequently as q4wk; dose should be adjusted downward at intervals of 3-6 mo
Available forms: Inj 80 IU/ml
Side effects/adverse reactions:
CNS: Fever, malaise, chills

GI: Nausea, vomiting, diarrhea, abdominal discomfort
INTEG: Pain on injection, burning and swelling at site of injection
Contraindications: Hypersensitivity
Precautions: Pregnancy (C), lactation
Pharmacokinetics: Steady-state enzymatic activity occurs within 60 min after a single injection; elimination half-life 4-20 min

NURSING CONSIDERATIONS

Assess:

- GI status: transient nausea, vomiting, abdominal discomfort
- Hypersensitive reactions; rashes and local injection site reactions may occur
- For increased fluid retention in cardiac disease

Administer:

- By IV infusion over 1-2 hr
- Dilute 60 U/kg in up to 10 ml of 0.9% NaCl

Perform/provide:

- Storage in refrigerator; do not freeze; do not shake, as this may inactivate the drug

Evaluate:

- Therapeutic response: Reduction of splenomegaly and hepatomegaly; improvement of hematologic deficiencies, reduced cachexia and wasting in children

Teach patient/family:

- To use only as directed by prescriber
- To report unusual side effects and avoid all other medications unless prescribed

allopurinol (℞)

(al-oh-pure'i-nole)
allopurinol, Apo Allopurinol*, Lopurin, Purimol*, Zyloprim
Func. class.: Antigout drug
Chem. class.: Xanthene oxidase inhibitor

Action: Inhibits the enzyme xanthine oxidase, reducing uric acid synthesis
Uses: Chronic gout, hyperuricemia associated with malignancies, recurrent calcium oxalate calculi
Dosage and routes:
Gout/hyperuricemia

- *Adult:* PO 200-600 mg qd depending on severity, not to exceed 800 mg/day
- *Child 6-10 yr:* 300 mg qd
- *Child <6 yr:* 150 mg qd

Impaired renal function

- *Adult:* PO 200 mg qd when CrCl is 20 to 10 ml/min

Recurrent calculi

- *Adult:* PO 200-300 mg qd

Uric acid nephropathy prevention

- *Adult:* PO 600-800 mg qd × 2-3 days

Available forms: Tabs 100, 300 mg
Side effects/adverse reactions:
HEMA: ***Agranulocytosis, thrombocytopenia, aplastic anemia, pancytopenia, leukopenia, bone marrow depression, eosinophilia***
CNS: Headache, drowsiness, neuritis, paresthesia
GI: Nausea, vomiting, anorexia, malaise, metallic taste, cramps, peptic ulcer, diarrhea, stomatitis
MISC: Myopathy, arthralgia, hepatomegaly, ***cholestatic jaundice, renal failure***
EENT: Retinopathy, cataracts, epistaxis
INTEG: Fever, chills, dermatitis, pru-

* Available in Canada only

ritus, purpura, erythema, ecchymosis, alopecia

Contraindications: Hypersensitivity

Precautions: Pregnancy (B), lactation, renal disease, hepatic disease, children

Pharmacokinetics:

PO: Peak 2-4 hr; excreted in feces, urine, half-life 2-3 hr, terminal half-life 18-30 hr

Interactions:

- Increased action of oral anticoagulants, chlorpropamide, cyclophosphamide, hydantoin, theophylline, vidarabine, ACE inhibitors
- Decreased effects of probenecid
- Rash: ampicillin, amoxicillin
- Increased hypersensitivity: thiazide diuretics
- Decreased effects of allopurinol: aluminum salts

Lab test interferences:

Increase: AST/ALT, alk phosphatase

Decrease: Hct/Hgb, leukocytes, serum glucose

NURSING CONSIDERATIONS

Assess:

- Uric acid levels q2wk; uric acid levels should be 6 mg/dl
- CBC, AST, BUN, creatinine before starting treatment, monthly
- I&O ratio; increase fluids to prevent stone formation
- Nutritional status: discourage organ meat, sardines, salmon, legumes, gravies (high-purine foods)

Administer:

- With meals, to prevent GI symptoms
- A few days before antineoplastic therapy

Evaluate:

- Therapeutic response: decreased pain in joints, decreased stone formation in kidney

Teach patient/family:

- To take as prescribed; if dose is missed, take as soon as remembered; do not double dose
- To increase fluid intake to 3-4 L/day
- To report skin rash, stomatitis, malaise, fever, aching; drug should be discontinued
- To avoid hazardous activities if drowsiness or dizziness occurs
- To avoid alcohol, caffeine; will increase uric acid levels
- To avoid large doses of vitamin C; kidney stone formation may occur
- To maintain a diet enhancing urine alkalinity, e.g., milk

alprazolam (℞)

(al-pray′zoe-lam)

Apo-Alpraz*, Novo-Alprazol*, Nu-Alpraz*, Xanax

Func. class.: Sedative/hypnotic

Chem. class.: Benzodiazepine

Controlled Substance Schedule IV

Action: Depresses subcortical levels of CNS, including limbic system, reticular formation

Uses: Anxiety, panic disorders, anxiety with depressive symptoms

Dosage and routes:

- *Adult:* PO 0.25-0.5 mg tid, not to exceed 4 mg/day in divided doses
- *Geriatric:* PO 0.25 mg bid-tid

Available forms: Tabs 0.25, 0.5, 1, 2 mg

Side effects/adverse reactions:

CNS: Dizziness, drowsiness, confusion, headache, anxiety, tremors, stimulation, fatigue, depression, insomnia, hallucinations

GI: Constipation, dry mouth, nausea, vomiting, anorexia, diarrhea

INTEG: Rash, dermatitis, itching

CV: Orthostatic hypotension, ***ECG changes, tachycardia,*** hypotension

EENT: Blurred vision, tinnitus, mydriasis

Contraindications: Hypersensitivity to benzodiazepines, narrow-angle glaucoma, psychosis, pregnancy (D), lactation, child <18 yr

Precautions: Elderly, debilitated, hepatic disease, renal disease

Pharmacokinetics:

PO: Onset 30 min, peak 1-2 hr, duration 4-6 hr, therapeutic response 2-3 days; metabolized by liver, excreted by kidneys; crosses placenta, breast milk; half-life 12-15 hr

Interactions:

- Increased toxicity: benzodiazepines
- Increased CNS depression: anticonvulsants, alcohol, antihistamines, sedative/hypnotics
- Decreased action of alprazolam: disulfiram, cimetidine
- Decreased action of levodopa

Lab test interferences:

Increase: AST/ALT, serum bilirubin

False increase: 17-OHCS

Decrease: RAIU

NURSING CONSIDERATIONS

Assess:

- B/P lying, standing; pulse; if systolic B/P drops 20 mm Hg, hold drug, notify prescriber
- Blood studies: CBC during long-term therapy; blood dyscrasias have occurred rarely
- Hepatic studies: AST, ALT, bilirubin, creatinine, LDH, alk phosphatase
- I&O; may indicate renal dysfunction
- For indications of increasing tolerance and abuse
- Mental status: mood, sensorium, affect, sleeping pattern, drowsiness, dizziness, especially in elderly
- Physical dependency, withdrawal symptoms: anxiety, panic attacks, agitation, convulsions, headache, nausea, vomiting, muscle pain, weakness
- Suicidal tendencies

Administer:

- With food or milk for GI symptoms
- Crushed if patient is unable to swallow medication whole
- Sugarless gum, hard candy, frequent sips of water for dry mouth

Perform/provide:

- Assistance with ambulation during beginning therapy; drowsiness/dizziness occurs
- Safety measures, including side rails
- Check that PO medication has been swallowed

Evaluate:

- Therapeutic response: decreased anxiety, restlessness, sleeplessness

Teach patient/family:

- Not to double doses; take exactly as prescribed; if dose is missed, take within 1 hr as scheduled
- That drug may be taken with food
- Not to use for everyday stress or longer than 3 mo unless directed by prescriber; not to take more than prescribed amount; may be habit forming
- To avoid OTC preparations unless approved by prescriber
- To avoid driving, activities that require alertness, since drowsiness may occur
- To avoid alcohol ingestion or other psychotropic medications unless directed by prescriber
- Not to discontinue medication abruptly after long-term use
- To rise slowly or fainting may occur, especially elderly
- That drowsiness may worsen at beginning of treatment

Treatment of overdose: Lavage, VS, supportive care

alprostadil (℞)

(al-pros'ta-dil)

Caverject, PGEI, prostaglandin E_1, Prostin VR Pediatric, Prostin VR*

Func. class.: Hormone

Chem. class.: Prostaglandin E_1

Action: Relaxes smooth muscles of ductus arteriosus; results in increased O_2 content throughout body; causes erection by dilation of cavernosal arteries and relaxation of trabecular muscle, this leads to the trapping of blood

Uses: To maintain patent ductus arteriosus (temporary treatment), erectile dysfunction

Dosage and routes:

Patent ductus arteriosus:

• *Infants:* IV INF 0.1 µg/kg/min, until desired response, then reduce to lowest effective amount, 0.4 µg/kg/min not likely to produce greater beneficial effects

Erectile dysfunction of vasculogenic or mixed etiology, psychogenic

• *Men:* Intracavernosal 2.5 µg may increase by 2.5 µg; may then increase by 5-10 µg until adequate response occurs

Available forms: Inj IV 500 µg/ml; lyopholized powder for inj 11.9 µg at 10 µg/ml

Side effects/adverse reactions:

MISC: ***Sepsis,*** hypokalemia, ***peritonitis,*** hypoglycemia, hyperkalemia

RESP: ***Apnea, bradypnea, wheezing, respiratory depression***

HEMA: ***DIC*** (disseminated intravascular coagulation), ***thrombocytopenia,*** anemia, ***bleeding***

CNS: Fever, ***convulsions,*** lethargy, hypothermia, stiffness, hyperirritability, ***cerebral bleeding***

GI: Diarrhea, regurgitation, hyperbilirubinemia

GU: Oliguria, hematuria, ***anuria***

CV: ***Bradycardia, tachycardia,*** *hypotension,* ***CHF, ventricular fibrillation, shock,*** flushing, ***cardiac arrest,*** edema

Local (Caverject): Penile pain, prolonged erection, penile fibrosis, penile rash, edema, hematoma, ecchymosis

Systems (Caverject): Headache, dizziness, flu symptoms, sinusitis, nasal congestion, hypertension, back pain, prostatic disorder

Contraindications: ***Hypersensitivity,*** respiratory distress syndrome (RDS)

Precautions: Bleeding disorders

Pharmacokinetics: Up to 80% metabolized in lungs, excreted in urine (metabolites)

Interactions:

• Do not mix in sol or syringe with other drugs; compatibility not known

NURSING CONSIDERATIONS

Assess:

• ABGs, arterial pH, arterial pressure, continuous ECG; if arterial pressure decreases, reduce or stop drug

• Apnea and bradycardia; if these occur, discontinue drug

• Increased pH, B/P, output, decreased ratio of PA to AP (restricted systemic blood flow)

Administer:

• Only with emergency equipment available and by trained clinicians

• After diluting with NS or D_5W injection to a concentration of 500 µg/ml, dilute further with 0.9% NaCl, D_5W; 500 µg of drug/250 ml of dilute = 2 µg/ml; 0.1 µg/kg/min run at 0.05 ml/kg/min, use infusion pump

Perform/provide:

• Arterial pressure measurement during infusion

• Refrigeration for drug; discard all mixed unused portion

Evaluate:

• Therapeutic response: increased PO_2 (cyanotic heart disease); erection

Teach patient/family:

• About diagnosis, prognosis, treatment

• Method for self-injection (erectile disorder), amount to be used, disposal of needle

Treatment of overdose: Discontinue drug, provide supportive measures

alteplase (℞)

(al′te-plase)

Activase, Activase rt-PA*, tissue plasminogen activator, t-Pa

Func. class.: Antithrombotic

Chem. class.: Tissue plasminogen activator (TPA)

Action: Produces fibrin conversion of plasminogen to plasmin; able to bind to fibrin, convert plasminogen in thrombus to plasmin, which leads to local fibrinolysis, limited systemic proteolysis

Uses: Lysis of obstructing thrombi associated with acute MI; although not currently approved, alteplase will be used for other conditions requiring thrombolysis, i.e., PE, DUT, unclotting arteriovenous shunts

Dosage and routes:

• *Adult:* IV a total of 100 mg; 6-10 mg given IV BOL over 1-2 min, 60 mg given over first hour, 20 mg given over second hour, 20 mg given over third hour; or 1.25 mg/kg given over 3 hr for smaller patients

Available forms: Powder for inj 20 mg (11.6 million IU)/vial, 50 mg (29 million IU)/vial

Side effects/adverse reactions:

SYST: ***GI, GU, intracranial, retroperitoneal bleeding,*** *surface bleeding*

CV: ***Sinus bradycardia, ventricular tachycardia, accelerated idioventricular rhythm***

INTEG: Urticaria, rash

Contraindications: Hypersensitivity, active internal bleeding, recent CVA, severe uncontrolled hypertension, intracranial/intraspinal surgery/trauma, aneurysm

Precautions: Pregnancy (C), lactation, children

Pharmacokinetics: Cleared by liver, 80% cleared within 10 min of drug termination

Interactions:

• Increased bleeding: heparin, acetylsalicylic acid, dipyridamole

Y-site compatibility: Lidocaine

Lab test interferences:

Increase: PT, APTT, TT

NURSING CONSIDERATIONS

Assess:

• VS, B/P, pulse, respirations, neurologic signs, temperature at least q4h; temperature >104° F (40° C) indicates internal bleeding; monitor rhythm closely; ventricular dysrhythmias may occur with hyperfusion; monitor heart, breath sounds, neuro status, peripheral pulses

• For bleeding during first hour of treatment: hematuria, hematemesis, bleeding from mucous membranes, epistaxis, ecchymosis; guaiac all body fluids, stools

• Allergy: fever, rash, itching, chills; mild reaction may be treated with antihistamines

• Blood studies (Hct, platelets, PTT, PT, TT, APTT) before starting therapy; PT or APTT must be less than 2 × control before starting therapy TT or PT q3-4h during treatment

* Available in Canada only

Administer:
- After reconstituting with provided diluent, add appropriate amount of sterile water for injection (no preservatives) 20 mg vial/20 ml or 50 mg vial/50 ml to make 1 mg/ml, mix by slow inversion or dilute with NaCl, D_5W to a concentration of 0.5 mg/ml; 1.5 to <0.5 mg/ml may result in precipitation of drug; use 18G needle; flush line with NaCl after administration
- Heparin therapy after thrombolytic therapy is discontinued, TT, ACT, or APTT less than 2 × control (about 3-4 hr)
- Reconstituted IV solution within 8 hr
- Within 6 hr of coronary occlusion for best results

Perform/provide:
- Avoidance of invasive procedures, injection, rectal temperature
- Pressure for 30 sec to minor bleeding sites; 30 min to sites of atrial puncture, followed by pressure dressing; inform prescriber if this does not attain hemostasis; apply pressure dressing
- Storage of powder at room temperature or refrigerate; protect from excessive light

Evaluate:
- Therapeutic response: lysis of thrombi

Teach patient/family:
- Purpose and expected results of treatment

altretamine (℞)
(al-tret'a-meen)
Hexalen, hexamethylmelamine
Func. class.: Misc. antineoplastic
Chem. class.: S-triazine derivative (formerly known as hexamethylmelamine)

Action: Products of metabolism form covalent adducts with tissue macromolecules including DNA, which may be responsible for cytotoxicity; activity is not cell cycle phase specific

Uses: Palliative treatment of recurrent, persistent ovarian cancer following first-line treatment with cisplatin or alkylating agent-based combination

Dosage and routes:
- *Adult:* PO 260 mg/m^2/day for 14 or 21 days in a 28-day cycle; give in 4 divided doses after meals and at hs

Available forms: Caps 50 mg

Side effects/adverse reactions:
GI: Nausea, anorexia, vomiting, increased alk phosphatase, ***hepatic toxicity***
CNS: Peripheral sensory neuropathy, fatigue, ***seizures,*** mood disorders, disorders of consciousness, ataxia, dizziness, vertigo
HEMA: ***Leukopenia, thrombocytopenia, anemia***
GU: Increased BUN, serum creatinine
INTEG: Rash, pruritus, alopecia

Contraindications: Hypersensitivity, severe bone marrow depression, severe neurologic toxicity

Precautions: Pregnancy (D), lactation, children

Pharmacokinetics:
PO: Well absorbed orally, rapidly

metabolized in liver, metabolites excreted in urine; peak ½-3 hr

Interactions:

• Possible increased toxicity of altretamine: cimetidine

• Severe orthostatic hypotension: MAOI

NURSING CONSIDERATIONS

Assess:

• CBC, differential, platelet count weekly, withhold drug if WBC is <2000 or platelet count is <75,000 or granulocyte count is <1000/ mm^3; notify prescriber of results

• Renal function studies: BUN, serum uric acid, urine CrCl before, during therapy

• I&O ratio; report fall in urine output of 30 ml/hr

• Temperature q4h; may indicate beginning infection

• Liver function tests before, during therapy (bilirubin, AST, ALT, LDH) as needed or monthly

Administer:

• Antacid before oral agent, give drug after meals, at hs

• Antiemetic 30-60 min before giving drug to prevent vomiting

• Antibiotics for prophylaxis of infection

Perform/provide:

• Strict medical asepsis, protective isolation if WBC levels are low

Evaluate:

• Therapeutic response: decreased tumor size, spread of malignancy

Teach patient/family:

• To report signs of infection: increased temperature, sore throat, flu symptoms

• To report signs of anemia: fatigue, headache, faintness, shortness of breath, irritability

• To report bleeding; avoid use of razors, commercial mouthwash

• To avoid use of aspirin products, ibuprofen

• That hair may be lost during therapy; a wig or hairpiece may make patient feel better; new hair may be different in color, texture (rare)

aluminum acetate (OTC)

Bluboro Powder, Boropak Powder, Burow's Solution, Domeboro, Modified Burow's Solution, Pedi-boro Soak Paks

Func. class.: Astringent

Chem. class.: Aluminum product

Action: Maintains skin acidity, which is protective to skin surface

Uses: Skin irritation, inflammation, athlete's foot, insect bites, poison ivy, eczema, acne, rash, bruises, pruritus (anal)

Dosage and routes:

• *Adult and child:* TOP apply for 15-30 min q4-8h (1:10-40); gargle use 1:10 sol prn

Available forms: Solution, cream*

Side effects/adverse reactions:

INTEG: Irritation, increasing inflammation

Contraindications: Tight, occlusive dressing

Interactions:

• Inhibits action of topical collagenase ointment

• Decreased action of aluminum acetate: soap

NURSING CONSIDERATIONS

Assess:

• Area of body to receive topical application, irritation, rash, breaks, dryness

Administer:

• 1 pk/1 pt H_2O (1:10-40 H_2O)

Perform/provide:

• Wet dressings using only loose-fitting dressing

* Available in Canada only

Evaluate:
- Therapeutic response: decreased skin irritation

Teach patient/family:
- To discontinue use if irritation occurs
- To avoid using near eye area
- To retain otic preparation for 2-3 min

aluminum hydroxide (OTC)

AlternaGEL, Alternagel, Alu-Cap, Alugel*, Aluminum Hydroxide, Aluminum Hydroxide Gel, Alu-Tab, Amphojel, Basaljel*, Concentrated Aluminum Hydroxide

Func. class.: Antacid

Chem. class.: Aluminum product

Action: Neutralizes gastric acidity, binds phosphates in GI tract; these phosphates are excreted

Uses: Antacid, hyperphosphatemia in chronic renal failure

Dosage and routes:
- *Adult:* SUSP 5-10 ml 1 hr pc, hs; PO 600 mg 1 hr pc, hs, chewed with milk or water

Hyperphosphatemia in renal failure
- *Adult:* SUSP 500 mg-2 g bid-qid

Available forms: Caps 475, 500 mg; tabs 300, 500 mg; chewable tabs 600 mg; susp (4%) 600 mg/5 ml; liq 320 mg/5 ml, 600 mg/5 ml

Side effects/adverse reactions:

GI: Constipation, anorexia, ***obstruction,*** fecal impaction

META: Hypophosphatemia, hypercalciuria

Contraindications: Hypersensitivity to this drug or aluminum products

Precautions: Elderly, fluid restriction, decreased GI motility, GI obstruction, dehydration, renal disease, sodium-restricted diets, pregnancy (C), lactation

Pharmacokinetics:

PO: Onset 20-40 min, excreted in feces

Interactions:
- Decreased effectiveness of tetracyclines, anticholinergics, phenothiazines, isoniazid, quinidine, phenytoin, digitalis, iron salts, warfarin, ketoconazole; separate by at least 2 hr

NURSING CONSIDERATIONS

Assess:
- Phosphate levels, since drug is bound in GI system
- Hypophosphatemia: anorexia, weakness, fatigue, bone pain, hyporeflexia
- Constipation; increase bulk in diet if needed
- Phosphate levels, urinary pH, Ca^{++}, electrolytes

Administer:
- Laxatives or stool softeners if constipation occurs, especially elderly
- After shaking liquid
- By nasogastric tube if patient unable to swallow
- With small amount of water or milk

Evaluate:
- Therapeutic response: absence of pain, decreased acidity

Teach patient/family:
- To increase fluids to 2 L/day unless contraindicated, measures to prevent constipation
- To avoid phosphate foods (most dairy products, eggs, fruits, carbonated beverages) during drug therapy
- Not to use for prolonged periods in patients with low serum phosphate or if on a low-sodium diet
- To add cheese, corn, pasta, plums, prunes, lentils after drug is discontinued

• Stools may appear white or speckled
• To check with prescriber after 2 wk of self-prescribed antacid use

amantadine (℞)

(a-man'ta-deen)
amantadine HCl, Symadine, Symmetrel
Func. class.: Antiviral, antiparkinsonian agent
Chem. class.: Tricyclic amine

Action: Prevents uncoating of nucleic acid in viral cell, preventing penetration of virus to host; causes release of dopamine from neurons
Uses: Prophylaxis or treatment of influenza type A, extrapyramidal reactions, parkinsonism, respiratory tract infections
Investigational uses: Neuroleptic malignant syndrome, cocaine dependency, enuresis
Dosage and routes:
Influenza type A
• *Adult and child >12 yr:* PO 200 mg/day in single dose or divided bid
• *Child 9-12 yr:* PO 100 mg bid
• *Child 1-9 yr:* PO 4.4-8.8 mg/kg/day divided bid-tid, not to exceed 200 mg/day
Extrapyramidal reaction/parkinsonism
• *Adult:* PO 100 mg bid, up to 400 mg/day in EPS; give for 1 wk, then 100 mg as needed up to 400 mg in parkinsonism
Available forms: Caps 100 mg; syr 50 mg/5 ml
Side effects/adverse reactions:
CNS: Headache, dizziness, drowsiness, fatigue, anxiety, psychosis, depression, hallucinations, tremors, ***convulsions***
CV: Orthostatic hypotension, ***CHF***
INTEG: Photosensitivity, dermatitis
EENT: Blurred vision
HEMA: ***Leukopenia***
GI: Nausea, vomiting, constipation, dry mouth
GU: Frequency, retention
Contraindications: Hypersensitivity, lactation, child <1 yr, pregnancy (C), eczematic rash
Precautions: Epilepsy, CHF, orthostatic hypotension, psychiatric disorders, hepatic disease, renal disease, peripheral edema
Pharmacokinetics:
PO: Onset 48 hr, half-life 24 hr, not metabolized, excreted in urine (90%) unchanged, crosses placenta, excreted in breast milk
Interactions:
• Increased anticholinergic response: atropine, other anticholinergics
• Increased CNS stimulation: CNS stimulants
• Decreased renal excretion of amantadine: triamterene, hydrochlorothiazide

NURSING CONSIDERATIONS
Assess:
• I&O ratio; report frequency, hesitancy
• CHF, confusion, mottling of skin
• Bowel pattern before, during treatment
• Skin eruptions, photosensitivity after administration of drug
• Respiratory status: rate, character, wheezing, tightness in chest
• Allergies before initiation of treatment, reaction of each medication; place allergies on chart in bright red letters
• Signs of infection
Administer:
• Before exposure to influenza; continue for 10 days after contact
• At least 4 hr before hs to prevent insomnia
• After meals for better absorption, to decrease GI symptoms

* Available in Canada only

• In divided doses to prevent CNS disturbances: headache, dizziness, fatigue, drowsiness

Perform/provide:

• Storage in tight, dry container

Evaluate:

• Therapeutic response: absence of fever, malaise, cough, dyspnea in infection; tremors, shuffling gait in Parkinson's disease

Teach patient/family:

• To change body position slowly to prevent orthostatic hypotension

• About aspects of drug therapy: need to report dyspnea, weight gain, dizziness, poor concentration, dysuria, behavioral changes

• To avoid hazardous activities if dizziness, blurred vision occurs

• To take drug exactly as prescribed; parkinsonian crisis may occur if drug is discontinued abruptly; do not double dose; if a dose is missed, do not take within 4 hr of next

• To avoid alcohol

Treatment of overdose: Withdraw drug, maintain airway, administer epinephrine, aminophylline, O_2, IV corticosteroids, physostigmine

amcinonide (℞)

(am-sin'oh-nide)

Cyclocort

Func. class.: Topical corticosteroid

Chem. class.: Synthetic fluorinated agent, group II potency

Action: Antipruritic, antiinflammatory

Uses: Psoriasis, eczema, contact dermatitis, pruritus

Dosage and routes:

• *Adult and child:* Apply to affected area bid-tid; rub completely into skin

Available forms: Cream 0.1%; oint 0.1%

Side effects/adverse reactions:

INTEG: Burning, dryness, itching, irritation, acne, folliculitis, hypertrichosis, perioral dermatitis, hypopigmentation, atrophy, striae, miliaria, allergic contact dermatitis, secondary infection

Contraindications: Hypersensitivity to corticosteroids, fungal infections

Precautions: Pregnancy (C), lactation, viral infections, bacterial infections

NURSING CONSIDERATIONS

Assess:

• Temperature, worsening of rash; if fever develops, drug should be discontinued

• For systemic absorption: increased temperature, inflammation, irritation

Administer:

• Only to affected areas; do not get in eyes

• Medication, then cover with occlusive dressing (only if prescribed), seal to normal skin, change q12h; systemic absorption may occur

• Only to dermatoses; do not use on weeping, denuded, or infected area

Perform/provide:

• Cleansing before application of drug

• Treatment for a few days after area has cleared

• Storage at room temperature

Evaluate:

• Therapeutic response: absence of severe itching, patches on skin, flaking

Teach patient/family:

• To avoid sunlight on affected area; burns may occur

• To discontinue drug, notify prescriber if local irritation or fever develops

amikacin (℞)

(am-i-kay′sin)

amikacin sulfate, Amikin

Func. class.: Antibiotic

Chem. class.: Aminoglycoside

Action: Interferes with protein synthesis in bacterial cell by binding to ribosomal subunit, which causes misreading of genetic code; inaccurate peptide sequence forms in protein chain, causing bacterial death

Uses: Severe systemic infections of CNS, respiratory, GI, urinary tract, bone, skin, soft tissues caused by *P. aeruginosa, E. coli, Enterobacter, Acinetobacter, Providencia, Citrobacter, Staphylococcus, Serratia, Proteus, Klebsiella* pneumonia

Dosage and routes:

Severe systemic infections

• *Adult and child:* IV INF 15 mg/kg/day in 2-3 divided doses q8-12h in 100-200 ml D_5W over 30-60 min, not to exceed 1.5 g; decreased doses are needed in poor renal function as determined by blood levels, renal function studies; IM 15 mg/kg/day in divided doses q8-12h

• *Neonates:* IV INF 10 mg/kg initially, then 7.5 mg/kg q12h in D_5W over 1-2 hr

Severe urinary tract infections

• *Adults:* IM 250 mg bid

• *Adults with poor renal function:* 7.5 mg/kg initially, then increased as determined by blood levels, renal function studies

Available forms: Inj IM, IV 50, 250 mg/ml

Side effects/adverse reactions:

GU: ***Oliguria, hematuria, renal damage, azotemia, failure, nephrotoxicity***

CNS: Confusion, depression, numbness, tremors, ***convulsions,*** muscle twitching, ***neurotoxicity,*** dizziness, vertigo, tinnitus

EENT: ***Ototoxicity,*** deafness, visual disturbances

HEMA: ***Agranulocytosis, thrombocytopenia, leukopenia, eosinophilia, anemia***

GI: Nausea, vomiting, anorexia, increased ALT, AST, bilirubin, hepatomegaly, ***hepatic necrosis,*** splenomegaly

CV: Hypotension or hypertension, palpitations

INTEG: Rash, burning, urticaria, dermatitis, alopecia

Contraindications: Mild to moderate infections, hypersensitivity to aminoglycosides

Precautions: Neonates, mild renal disease, pregnancy (D), myasthenia gravis, lactation, hearing deficits, Parkinson's disease, elderly

Pharmacokinetics:

IM: Onset rapid, peak 1-2 hr

IV: Onset immediate, peak 1-2 hr; plasma half-life 2-3 hr; not metabolized, excreted unchanged in urine, crosses placental barrier

Interactions:

• Increased ototoxicity, neurotoxicity, nephrotoxicity: other aminoglycosides, amphotericin B, polymyxin, vancomycin, ethacrynic acid, furosemide, mannitol, methoxyflurane, cisplatin, cephalosporins

• Increased neuromuscular blockade, respiratory depression: anesthetics, nondepolarizing neuromuscular blockers, succinylcholine

• Do not mix in sol or syr: carbenicillin, ticarcillin, amphotericin B, cephalothin, erythromycin, heparin, ampicillin, cefazolin, chlorothiazide, phenytoin, thiopental, vit B complex with C, warfarin, methicillin

NURSING CONSIDERATIONS

Assess:

• Weight before treatment; calculation of dosage is usually based on ideal body weight but may be calculated on actual body weight

- I&O ratio; urinalysis daily for proteinuria, cells, casts; report sudden change in urine output
- VS during infusion; watch for hypotension, change in pulse
- IV site for thrombophlebitis including pain, redness, swelling q30 min; change site if needed; apply warm compresses to discontinued site
- Serum peak, drawn at 30-60 min after IV infusion or 60 min after IM injection, trough level drawn just before next dose; peak 20-30 min; peak serum level, trough <8 h; adjust dosage per levels
- Urine pH if drug is used for UTI; urine should be kept alkaline
- Renal impairment by securing urine for CrCl testing, BUN, serum creatinine; lower dosage should be given in renal impairment (CrCl <80 ml/min)
- Deafness by audiometric testing, ringing, roaring in ears, vertigo; assess hearing before, during, after treatment
- Dehydration: high specific gravity, decrease in skin turgor, dry mucous membranes, dark urine
- Overgrowth of infection, including increased temperature, malaise, redness, pain, swelling, perineal itching, diarrhea, stomatitis, change in cough, sputum
- C&S before starting treatment to identify organism
- Vestibular dysfunction: nausea, vomiting, dizziness, headache; drug should be discontinued if severe
- Injection sites for redness, swelling, abscesses; use warm compresses at site

Administer:

- IV, dilute 500 mg of drug/100-200 ml of IV D_5W, D_5NaCl or 0.9% NaCl and give over ½-1hr; flush after administration with D_5W or 0.9% NaCl
- IM injection in large muscle mass; rotate injection sites
- In evenly spaced doses to maintain blood level
- Bicarbonate to alkalinize urine if ordered for UTI, as drug is most active in alkaline environment

Perform/provide:

- Adequate fluids of 2-3 L/day, unless contraindicated, to prevent irritation of tubules
- Flush of IV line with NS or D_5W after infusion
- Supervised ambulation, other safety measures with vestibular dysfunction

Evaluate:

- Therapeutic response: absence of fever, draining wounds, negative C&S after treatment

Teach patient/family:

- To report headache, dizziness, symptoms for overgrowth of infection, renal impairment
- To report loss of hearing, ringing, roaring in ears or feeling of fullness in head

Treatment of hypersensitivity: Hemodialysis, exchange transfusion in the newborn, monitor serum levels of drug, may give ticarcillin or carbenicillin

amiloride (℞)

(a-mill'oh-ride)

amiloride HCl, Midamor

Func. class.: Potassium-sparing diuretic

Chem. class.: Pyrazine

Action: Acts primarily on distal tubule, secondarily by inhibiting reabsorption of sodium, H_2O, and increasing potassium retention

Uses: Edema in CHF in combination with other diuretics, for hypertension, adjunct with other diuretics to maintain potassium

Dosage and routes:

• *Adult:* PO 5 mg qd, may be increased to 10-20 mg qd if needed

Available forms: Tab 5 mg

Side effects/adverse reactions:

GU: Polyuria, dysuria, frequency, impotence

ELECT: Acidosis, hyponatremia, ***hyperkalemia,*** hypochloremia

CNS: Headache, dizziness, fatigue, weakness, paresthesias, tremor, depression, anxiety

GI: Nausea, diarrhea, dry mouth, *vomiting, anorexia,* cramps, constipation, abdominal pain, jaundice, bleeding

EENT: Loss of hearing, tinnitus, blurred vision, nasal congestion, increased intraocular pressure

INTEG: Rash, pruritus, alopecia, urticaria

MS: Cramps, joint pain

CV: Orthostatic hypotension, dysrhythmias, angina

HEMA: ***Agranulocytopenia, leukopenia, thrombocytopenia*** (rare)

Contraindications: Anuria, hypersensitivity, hyperkalemia, impaired renal function

Precautions: Dehydration, pregnancy (B), diabetes, acidosis, lactation

Pharmacokinetics:

PO: Onset 2 hr, peak 6-10 hr, duration 24 hr; excreted in urine, feces, half-life 6-9 hr

Interactions:

• Enhanced action of antihypertensives; lithium toxicity may be provoked

• Hyperkalemia: other potassium-sparing diuretics, potassium products, ACE inhibitors, salt substitutes

Lab test interferences:

Interfere: GTT

NURSING CONSIDERATIONS

Assess:

• Weight, I&O daily to determine fluid loss; effect of drug may be decreased if used qd

• Rate, depth, rhythm of respiration, effect of exertion

• B/P lying, standing; postural hypotension may occur

• Electrolytes: K, Na, Cl; glucose (serum), BUN, CBC, serum creatinine, blood pH, ABGs

• Improvement in CVP q8h

• Signs of drowsiness, restlessness

• Rashes, temperature elevation qd

• Confusion, especially in elderly; take safety precautions if needed

Administer:

• In AM to avoid interference with sleep if using drug as a diuretic

• With food; if nausea occurs, absorption may be decreased slightly

Evaluate:

• Therapeutic response: improvement in edema of feet, legs, sacral area daily if medication is being used in CHF

Teach patient/family:

• To take as prescribed; if dose is missed, take when remembered within 1 hr of next dose

• About adverse reactions: muscle cramps, weakness, nausea, dizziness, blurred vision

• To take with food or milk for GI symptoms

• To take early in day to prevent nocturia

• To avoid potassium-rich foods: oranges, bananas; salt substitutes, dried fruits

Treatment of overdose: Lavage if taken orally, monitor electrolytes, administer sodium bicarbonate for

* Available in Canada only

K^+ >6.5 mEq/L, monitor hydration, CV, renal status

amino acid injection (℞)

(a-mee′noe)

FreAmine HBC, HepatAmine

Func. class.: Nitrogen product

Action: Needed for anabolism to maintain structure, decrease catabolism, promote healing

Uses: Hepatic encephalopathy, cirrhosis, hepatitis, nutritional support in cancer

Dosage and routes:

• *Adult:* IV 80-120 g/day; 500 ml of amino acids/500 ml D_{50} given over 24 hr

Available forms: Inj IV many strengths, types

Side effects/adverse reactions:

CNS: Dizziness, headache, confusion, ***loss of consciousness***

CV: Hypertension, ***CHF, pulmonary edema***

GI: Nausea, vomiting, liver fat deposits, abdominal pain

GU: Glycosuria, osmotic diuresis

ENDO: Hyperglycemia, rebound hypoglycemia, electrolyte imbalances, hyperosmolar syndrome, hyperosmolar hyperglycemic nonketotic syndrome, alkalosis, acidosis, hypophosphatemia, hyperammonemia, dehydration, hypocalcemia

INTEG: Chills, flushing, warm feeling, rash, urticaria, extravasation necrosis, phlebitis at injection site

Contraindications: Hypersensitivity, severe electrolyte imbalances, anuria, severe liver damage, maple syrup urine disease, PKU

Precautions: Renal disease, pregnancy (C), lactation, children, diabetes mellitus, CHF

Y-site compatibilities: Cefamandole, cefazolin, cefoperazone, cefotaxime, cefoxitin, cephalothin, cephapirin, chloramphenicol, clindamycin, digoxin, dobutamine, dopamine, doxycycline, erythromycin lactobionate, fat emulsion, foscarnet, furosemide, gentamicin, isoproterenol, kanamycin, lidocaine, meperidine, methicillin, mezlocillin, miconazole, morphine, nafcillin, netilmicin, norepinephrine, oxacillin, penicillin G potassium, piperacillin, sargramostim, ticarcillin, tobramycin, urokinase, vancomycin

NURSING CONSIDERATIONS

Assess:

• Electrolytes (K, Na, Ca, Cl, Mg), blood glucose, ammonia, phosphate, ketones

• Renal, liver function studies: BUN, creatinine, ALT (SGOT), AST (SGPT), bilirubin

• Injection site for extravasation: redness along vein, edema at site, necrosis, pain, hard tender area; site should be changed immediately

• Monitor respiratory function q4h: auscultate lung fields bilaterally for crackles, respirations, quality, rate, rhythm

• Monitor temperature q4h for increased fever, indicating infection; if infection suspected, infusion is discontinued, tubing bottle cultured

• Monitor for impending hepatic coma: asterixis, confusion, uremic fetor, lethargy

• Urine glucose q6h using Chemstrips, which are not affected by infusion substances

• Hyperammonemia: nausea, vomiting, malaise, tremors, anorexia, convulsions

Administer:

• Up to 40% protein and dextrose (up to 12.5%) via peripheral vein; stronger solutions require central IV administration

• TPN only mixed with dextrose to promote protein synthesis
• Immediately after mixing in pharmacy under strict aseptic technique using laminar flowhood, use infusion pump, in-line filter (0.22 μm) unless mixed with fat emulsion and dextrose (3 in 1)
• Using careful monitoring technique; do not speed up infusion; pulmonary edema, glucose overload will result

Perform/provide:
• Storage depends on type of solution; consult manufacturer
• Changing dressing and IV tubing to prevent infection q24-48h

Evaluate:
• Therapeutic response: weight gain, decrease in jaundice in liver disorders, increased LOC

Teach patient/family:
• Reason for use of TPN
• If chills, sweating are experienced, report at once
• About infusion pump and blood glucose monitoring

amino acid solution (℞)

Aminosyn, Aminosyn II, Aminosyn-PF, FreAmine III, Novamine, Travasol, Trophmine

Func. class.: Nitrogen product

Action: Needed for anabolism to maintain structure, decrease catabolism, promote healing

Uses: Nutritional support in cancer, trauma, intestinal obstruction, short bowel syndrome, severe malabsorption

Dosage and routes:
• *Adult:* IV 1-1.5 g/kg/day titrated to patient's needs
• *Child:* IV 2-3 g/kg/day titrated to patient's needs

Available forms: Inj IV many types, strengths

Side effects/adverse reactions:
CNS: Dizziness, headache, confusion, ***loss of consciousness***
CV: Hypertension, ***CHF, pulmonary edema***
GI: Nausea, vomiting, liver fat deposits, abdominal pain, jaundice
GU: Glycosuria, osmotic diuresis
ENDO: Hyperglycemia, rebound hypoglycemia, electrolyte imbalances, hyperosmolar syndrome, hyperosmolar hyperglycemic nonketotic syndrome, alkalosis, acidosis, hypophosphatemia, hyperammonemia, dehydration, hypocalcemia
INTEG: Chills, flushing, warm feeling, rash, urticaria, extravasation necrosis, phlebitis at injection site

Contraindications: Hypersensitivity, severe electrolyte imbalances, anuria, severe liver damage, maple syrup urine disease, PKU

Precautions: Renal disease, pregnancy (C), lactation, children, diabetes mellitus, CHF

Y-site compatibilities: Cefamandole, cefazolin, cefoperazone, cefotaxime, cefoxitin, cephalothin, cephapirin, chloramphenicol, clindamycin, digoxin, dobutamine, dopamine, doxycycline, erythromycin lactobionate, fat emulsion, foscarnet, furosemide, gentamicin, isoproterenol, kanamycin, lidocaine, meperidine, methicillin, mezlocillin, miconazole, morphine, nafcillin, netilmicin, norepinephrine, oxacillin, penicillin G potassium, piperacillin, sargramostim, ticarcillin, tobramycin, urokinase, vancomycin

NURSING CONSIDERATIONS

Assess:
• Electrolytes (K, Na, Ca, Cl, Mg), blood glucose, ammonia, phosphate

• Renal, liver function studies: BUN, creatinine, ALT (SGOT), AST (SGPT), bilirubin
• Injection site for extravasation: redness along vein, edema at site, necrosis, pain, hard tender area; site should be changed immediately
• Monitor respiratory function q4h: auscultate lung fields bilaterally for crackles, respirations, quality, rate, rhythm
• Monitor temperature q4h for increased fever, indicating infection; if infection suspected, discontinue infusion, culture tubing, bottle
• Urine glucose q6h using Tes-Tape, Clinistix, which are not affected by infusion substances; blood glucose is preferred testing method
• Hyperammonemia: nausea, vomiting, malaise, tremors, anorexia, convulsions

Administer:
• Up to 40% protein and dextrose (up to 12.5%) via peripheral vein; stronger solutions require central IV administration, use infusion pump
• TPN only mixed with dextrose to promote protein synthesis
• Immediately after mixing in pharmacy under strict aseptic technique using laminar flow hood, use infusion pump, in-line filter (0.22 μm) unless mixed with fat emulsion and dextrose (3 in 1)
• Using careful monitoring technique; do not speed up infusion; pulmonary edema, glucose overload will result

Perform/provide:
• Storage depends on type of solution; consult label
• Changing dressing and IV tubing to prevent infection q24-48h

Evaluate:
• Therapeutic response: weight gain, decrease in jaundice in liver disorders, increased serum albumin

Teach patient/family:
• Reason for use of TPN
• Any chills, sweating should be reported at once
• About infusion pump and blood glucose monitoring

aminocaproic acid (℞)

(a-mee-noe-ka-proe′ik)

Amicar, aminocaproic acid, EACA

Func. class.: Hemostatic

Chem. class.: Synthetic monoaminocarboxylic acid

Action: Inhibits fibrinolysis by inhibiting plasminogen activator substances

Uses: Hemorrhage from hyperfibrinolysis, adjunctive therapy in hemophilia

Investigational uses: Prevention of recurrent subarachnoid hemorrhage

Dosage and routes:
• *Adult:* PO/IV 5 g loading dose, then 1-1.25 g q1h if needed, not to exceed 30 g/day

Available forms: Inj IV 250 mg/ml; tab 500 mg; syr 250 mg/ml

Side effects/adverse reactions:

GU: Dysuria, frequency, oliguria, ***renal failure,*** ejaculatory failure, menstrual irregularities

GI: Nausea, vomiting, abdominal cramps, diarrhea

INTEG: Rash

CNS: Headache, dizziness, malaise, fatigue, hallucinations, delirium, psychosis, ***convulsions,*** weakness

HEMA: ***Thrombosis***

CV: ***Dysrhythmias,*** orthostatic hypotension, bradycardia

EENT: Tinnitus, nasal congestion, conjunctival suffusion

Contraindications: Hypersensitivity, abnormal bleeding, postpartum bleeding, DIC, upper urinary tract bleeding, new burns

Precautions: Neonates/infants, mild or moderate renal disease, hepatic disease, thrombosis, cardiac disease, pregnancy (C), lactation

Pharmacokinetics:

PO/IV: Peak 2 hr, excreted by kidneys as unmetabolized drug, rapidly absorbed

Interactions:

- Increased coagulation: estrogens, oral contraceptives
- Do not mix with sodium lactate in solution

Lab test interferences:

Increased: K^+, CPK

NURSING CONSIDERATIONS

Assess:

- I&O; if urinary output decreases, notify prescriber and stop drug
- Blood studies: coagulation factors, platelets, protamine coagulation test for extravascular clotting, thrombophlebitis
- B/P, pulse for increase
- Drug level: 0.13 mg/ml is required to decrease fibrinolysis
- Creatine phosphokinase, urinalysis
- Allergy: fever, rash, itching, jaundice
- Myopathy: if weakness, fever, myoglobinemia, or oliguria, discontinue drug
- Bleeding: mucous membrane, epistaxis, ecchymosis, petechiae, hematuria, hematemesis

Administer:

- Give IV loading dose over 30 min to avoid hypotension
- IV after dilution with 4-5 g/250 ml NS, D_5W, LR, give over 1 hr; may give by continuous infusion after loading dose(s) of 1 g/hr diluted in 50-100 ml of compatible solutions; use infusion pump; do not give by direct IV

Perform/provide:

- Storage in tight container in cool environment; do not freeze

Evaluate:

- Therapeutic response: decreased bleeding

Teach patient/family:

- To report any signs of bleeding (gums, under skin, urine, stools, emesis) or myopathy
- To change position slowly to decrease orthostatic hypotension
- Proper administration for 8-10 days following dental procedure in hemophilia
- To inform physicians and dentists that drug is being taken
- To change position slowly

---

aminoglutethimide (℞)

(a-meen-noe-gloo-teth′i-mide)

Cytadren

Func. class.: Antineoplastic, adrenal steroid inhibitor

Chem. class.: Hormone

Action: Acts by inhibiting DNA, RNA, protein synthesis; is derived from *Streptomyces verticillus;* replication is decreased by binding to DNA, which causes strand splitting; phase specific in G_2 and M phases; blocks biosynthesis of all steroid hormones (cortisol, androgens, progestins)

Uses: Suppression of adrenal function in Cushing's syndrome, metastatic breast cancer, adrenal cancer

Investigational uses: Advanced prostate cancer, metastatic postmenopausal breast cancer

Dosage and routes:

- *Adult:* PO 250 mg qid at 6 hr intervals, may increase by 250 mg/day q1-2wk, not to exceed 2 g/day

Available forms: Tabs 250 mg

---

* Available in Canada only

Side effects/adverse reactions:
GI: Nausea, vomiting, anorexia, ***hepatotoxicity***
INTEG: Rash, pruritus, hirsutism
CV: ***Hypotension,*** *tachycardia*
CNS: Drowsiness, morbilliform skin rash, dizziness, headache, lethargy
Contraindications: Hypersensitivity, hypothyroidism, pregnancy (D)
Precautions: Renal disease, hepatic disease, respiratory disease
Pharmacokinetics: Half-life 13 hr, metabolized in liver, excreted in urine, crosses placenta
Interactions:
• Accelerated metabolism: dexamethasone

NURSING CONSIDERATIONS
Assess:
• Renal function studies: BUN, serum uric acid, urine CrCl, electrolytes before, during therapy
• I&O ratio; report fall in urine output of 30 ml/hr
• Monitor temperature q4h; may indicate beginning infection
• Liver function tests before, during therapy (bilirubin, AST, ALT, LDH) as needed or monthly
• RBC, Hct, Hgb, since these may be decreased
• Food preferences; list likes, dislikes
• Inflammation of mucosa, breaks in skin
• Yellowing of skin, sclera, dark urine, clay-colored stools, itchy skin, abdominal pain, fever, diarrhea
• Symptoms indicating severe allergic reaction: rash, pruritus, urticaria, purpuric skin lesions, itching, flushing
Administer:
• Antacid before oral agent; give last dose of the day after evening meal before bedtime
• Local or systemic drugs for infection if indicated
Perform/provide:
• Special skin care
• Liquid diet, including cola, Jell-O; dry toast or crackers as ordered may be added if patient is not nauseated or vomiting
• Nutritious diet with iron and vitamin supplements as ordered
Evaluate:
• Therapeutic response: decrease in size of tumor or decrease in Cushing's syndrome
Teach patient/family:
• To report any complaints, side effects to nurse or prescriber
• That masculinization can occur, is reversible after discontinuing treatment
• To avoid self-administration of adjuvant corticosteroids
• That drowsiness may occur and to avoid driving or operating heavy machinery

aminophylline (℞)

(am-in-off'i-lin)
Amoline, Corophyllin*, Palaron*, Phyllocontin, Truphylline
Func. class.: Spasmolytic
Chem. class.: Xanthine, ethylenediamide

Action: Relaxes smooth muscle of respiratory system by blocking phosphodiesterase, which increases cyclic AMP. Increased cyclic AMP alters intracellular calcium ion movements; produces bronchodilation, increased pulmonary blood flow, relaxation of respiratory tract
Uses: Bronchial asthma, bronchospasm, Cheyne-Stokes respirations
Investigational uses: Apnea in infancy for respiratory/myocardial stimulation
Dosage and routes:
• *Adult:* PO 500 mg, then 250-500

mg q6-8h; CONT IV 0.3-0.9 mg/kg/hr (maintenance); RECT 500 mg q6-8h

• *Child:* PO 7.5 mg/kg, then 3-6 mg/kg q6-8h; IV 7.5 mg/kg, then 3-6 mg/kg q6-8h injected over 5 min; do not exceed 25 mg/min; may give loading dose of 5.6 mg/kg over ½ hr; CONT IV 1 mg/kg/hr (maintenance); for children/infants use drug without preservative or alcohol

• *Neonates:* IV/PO 1 mg/kg initially for plasma increases of each 2 μg/ml, then 1 mg/kg q6h

Available forms: Inj IV, IM, rectal supp 250, 500 mg; rectal sol 300 mg/5 ml; elix 250 mg/5 ml; oral liq 105 mg/5 ml; tabs 100, 200 mg, tabs con-rel 225 mg; tabs sust-rel 300 mg

Side effects/adverse reactions:

CNS: Anxiety, restlessness, insomnia, *dizziness,* ***convulsions,*** headache, light-headedness, muscle twitching

CV: Palpitations, sinus tachycardia, hypotension, flushing, dysrhythmias, increased respiratory rate

GI: Nausea, vomiting, anorexia, diarrhea, bitter taste, dyspepsia, anal irritation (suppositories), epigastric pain

RESP: Increased rate

INTEG: Flushing, urticaria, *rectal supp (irritation)*

GU: Urinary frequency

Contraindications: Hypersensitivity to xanthines, tachydysrhythmias

Precautions: Elderly, CHF, cor pulmonale, hepatic disease, active peptic ulcer disease, diabetes mellitus, hyperthyroidism, hypertension, children, pregnancy (C), lactation, glaucoma, prostatic hypertrophy

Pharmacokinetics: Well absorbed PO, extended rel well absorbed slowly, rectal supp is erratic, rectal sol is absorbed quickly; metabolized by liver (caffeine); excreted in urine; crosses placenta; appears in breast milk

Half-life: 3-12 hr; half-life increased in geriatric patients, hepatic disease, CHF

PO: Onset ¼ hr, peak 1-2 hr, duration 6-8 hr

PO-ER: Unknown, peak 4-7 hr, duration 8-12 hr

IV: Onset rapid, duration 6-8 hr

REC: Onset erratic, peak 1-2 hr, duration 6-8 hr

Interactions:

• Increased action of aminophylline: cimetidine, propranolol, erythromycin, troleandomycin

• Dysrhythmias: halothane

• May increase effects of anticoagulants

• Cardiotoxicity: β-blockers

• Increased elimination: smoking

• Increased toxicity: erythromycin, influenza vaccine, oral contraceptives, glucocorticoids, disulfiram

• Decreased effects of lithium

• Decreased effects of: rifampin, barbiturates, adrenergics, ketoconazole

Syringe compatibilities: Heparin, metoclopramide, pentobarbital, thiopental

Y-site compatibilities: Amrinone, atracurium, cimetidine, enalaprilat, foscarnet, heparin sodium with hydrocortisone sodium succinate, morphine, netilmicin, pancuronium, potassium chloride, ranitidine, tolazoline, vecuronium

Additive compatibilities: Amobarbital, bretylium, calcium, gluconate, chloramphenicol, dexamethasone, diphenhydramine, dopamine, erythromycin lactobionate, esmolol, heparin, hydrocortisone, lidocaine, methyldopate, metronidazole, pentobarbital, potassium chloride, ranitidine, secobarbital, sodium bicarbonate, sodium iodide, terbutaline, verapamil

Lab test interferences:

Increased: Plasma free fatty acids

NURSING CONSIDERATIONS

Assess:

- Theophylline blood levels (therapeutic level is 10-20 μg/ml); toxicity may occur with small increase above 20 μg/ml, especially elderly
- Monitor I&O; diuresis occurs; dehydration may result in elderly or children
- Whether theophylline was given recently (24 hr)
- Respiratory rate, rhythm, depth; auscultate lung fields bilaterally; notify prescriber of abnormalities
- Allergic reactions: rash, urticaria; if these occur, drug should be discontinued

Administer:

- PO after meals to decrease GI symptoms; absorption may be affected with a full glass of water; do not crush or chew enteric-coated or ER tabs
- IV after diluting in 5% dextrose to decrease burning sensation at injection site; only clear solutions
- May be diluted for IV INF in 100-200 ml in D_5W, $D_{10}W$, $D_{20}W$, 0.9% NaCl, 0.45% NaCl, LR
- Avoid IM injection; pain, LR and tissue damage may occur
- Only clear sol; flush IV line before dose
- Rectal dose if patient is unable to take PO; retain rectal dose for ½ hour

Perform/provide:

- Storage of diluted solution for 24 hr if refrigerated

Evaluate:

- Therapeutic response: decreased dyspnea, respiratory stimulation in infancy, clear lung fields bilaterally

Teach patient/family:

- To take doses as prescribed, not to skip dose, not to double dose
- To check OTC medications, current prescription medications for ephedrine; will increase CNS stimulation; not to drink alcohol or caffeine products (tea, coffee, chocolate, colas)
- To avoid hazardous activities; dizziness may occur
- If GI upset occurs, to take drug with 8 oz water; avoid food, since absorption may be decreased
- To remain in bed 15-20 min after rectal suppository is inserted to avoid removal
- To notify prescriber of toxicity: insomnia, anxiety, nausea, vomiting, rapid pulse, convulsions
- To notify prescriber of change in smoking habit; a change in dose may be required
- To increase fluids to 2 L/day to decrease secretion viscosity

---

amiodarone (℞)

(am-ee-oh'da-rone)

Cordarone

Func. class.: Antidysrhythmic (class III)

Chem. class.: Iodinated benzofuran derivative

Action: Prolongs duration of action potential and effective refractory period, noncompetitive α- and β-adrenergic inhibition

Uses: Severe ventricular tachycardia, supraventricular tachycardia, ventricular fibrillation not controlled by first-line agents

Dosage and routes:

- *Adult:* PO loading dose 800-1600 mg/day 1-3 wk; then 600-800 mg/day 1 mo; maintenance 200-600 mg/day

Available forms: Tabs 200 mg

Side effects/adverse reactions:
CNS: Headache, dizziness, involuntary movement, tremors, peripheral neuropathy, malaise, fatigue, ataxia, paresthesias, insomnia
GI: Nausea, vomiting, diarrhea, abdominal pain, anorexia, constipation, ***hepatotoxicity***
CV: Hypotension, bradycardia, ***sinus arrest, CHF,*** *dysrhythmias,* ***SA node dysfunction***
INTEG: Rash, photosensitivity, blue-gray skin discoloration, alopecia, spontaneous ecchymosis
EENT: Blurred vision, halos, photophobia, ***corneal microdeposits,*** dry eyes
ENDO: Hyperthyroidism or hypothyroidism
MS: Weakness, pain in extremities
RESP: ***Pulmonary fibrosis,*** pulmonary inflammation
MISC: Flushing, abnormal taste or smell, edema, abnormal salivation, coagulation abnormalities
Precautions: Goiter, Hashimoto's thyroiditis, SN dysfunction, 2nd or 3rd degree AV block, electrolyte imbalances, pregnancy (C), bradycardia, lactation
Pharmacokinetics:
PO: Onset 1-3 wk, peak 2-10 hr; half-life 15-100 days; metabolized by liver, excreted by kidneys
Interactions:
- Bradycardia: β-blockers, calcium channel blockers
- Increased levels of digitalis, quinidine, procainamide, flecainide, disopyramide, phenytoin
- Increased anticoagulant effects: warfarin
- Bradycardia, arrest: lidocaine

NURSING CONSIDERATIONS
Assess:
- I&O ratio; electrolytes: (K, Na, Cl)
- Liver function studies: AST (SGOT), ALT (SGPT), bilirubin, alk phosphatase
- ECG continuously to determine drug effectiveness, measure PR, QRS, QT intervals, check for PVCs, other dysrhythmias
- For dehydration or hypovolemia
- B/P continuously for hypotension, hypertension
- For rebound hypertension after 1-2 hr
- CNS symptoms: confusion, psychosis, numbness, depression, involuntary movements; if these occur, drug should be discontinued
- Hypothyroidism: lethargy, dizziness, constipation, enlarged thyroid gland, edema of extremities, cool, pale skin
- Hyperthyroidism: restlessness, tachycardia, eyelid puffiness, weight loss, frequent urination, menstrual irregularities, dyspnea, warm, moist skin
- Pulmonary toxicity: dyspnea, fatigue, cough, fever, chest pain; drug should be discontinued
- Cardiac rate, respiration: rate, rhythm, character, chest pain

Administer:
- Reduced dosage slowly with ECG monitoring

Evaluate:
- Therapeutic response: decrease in ventricular tachycardia, supraventricular tachycardia or fibrillation

Teach patient/family:
- To take this drug as directed; avoid missed doses
- To use sunscreen or stay out of sun to prevent burns
- To report side effects immediately
- That skin discoloration is usually reversible
- That dark glasses may be needed for photophobia

Treatment of overdose: O_2, artificial ventilation, ECG, administer do-

* Available in Canada only

pamine for circulatory depression, administer diazepam or thiopental for convulsions, isoproterenol

amitriptyline (℞)

(a-mee-trip'ti-leen)

amitriptylline HCl, Amitril, Apo-Amitriptyline*, Elavil, Emitrip, Endep, Enovil, Levate*, Meravil*, Novotriptyn*, Rolavil*

Func. class.: Antidepressant—tricyclic

Chem. class.: Tertiary amine

Action: Blocks reuptake of norepinephrine, serotonin into nerve endings, increasing action of norepinephrine, serotonin in nerve cells

Uses: Major depression

Investigational uses: Chronic pain management

Dosage and routes:

- *Adult:* PO 50-100 mg hs, may increase to 200 mg qd, not to exceed 300 mg/day; IM 20-30 mg qid, or 80-120 mg hs
- *Adolescent/geriatric:* PO 30 mg/day in divided doses, may be increased to 150 mg/day

Available forms: Tabs 10, 25, 50, 75, 100, 150 mg; inj IM 10 mg/ml

Side effects/adverse reactions:

HEMA: ***Agranulocytosis, thrombocytopenia, eosinophilia, leukopenia***

CNS: Dizziness, drowsiness, confusion, headache, anxiety, tremors, stimulation, weakness, insomnia, nightmares, EPS (elderly), increased psychiatric symptoms, seizures

GI: Diarrhea, dry mouth, nausea, vomiting, ***paralytic ileus,*** increased appetite, cramps, epigastric distress, jaundice, ***hepatitis,*** stomatitis

GU: Retention

INTEG: Rash, urticaria, sweating, pruritus, photosensitivity

CV: Orthostatic hypotension, ***ECG changes, tachycardia, hypertension,*** palpitations

EENT: Blurred vision, tinnitus, mydriasis, ophthalmoplegia

Contraindications: Hypersensitivity to tricyclic antidepressants, recovery phase of myocardial infarction

Precautions: Suicidal patients, convulsive disorders, prostatic hypertrophy, schizophrenia, psychosis, severe depression, increased intraocular pressure, narrow-angle glaucoma, urinary retention, cardiac disease, hepatic disease, renal disease, hyperthyroidism, electroshock therapy, elective surgery, child <12 yr, pregnancy (C), lactation, elderly

Pharmacokinetics:

PO/IM: Onset 45 min, peak 2-12 hr, therapeutic response 2-3 wk; metabolized by liver, excreted in urine, feces, crosses placenta, excreted in breast milk, half-life 10-50 hr

Interactions:

- Decreased effects of guanethidine, clonidine, indirect acting sympathomimetics (ephedrine)
- Increased effects of direct acting sympathomimetics (epinephrine), alcohol, barbiturates, benzodiazepines, CNS depressants
- Hyperpyretic crisis, convulsions, hypertensive episode: MAOI (pargyline [Eutonyl])

Lab test interferences:

Increase: Serum bilirubin, blood glucose, alk phosphatase

Decrease: VMA, 5-HIAA

False increase: Urinary catecholamines

NURSING CONSIDERATIONS

Assess:

- B/P lying, standing; pulse q4h; if systolic B/P drops 20 mm Hg, hold drug, notify prescriber; take vital signs q4h in patients with cardiovascular disease

• Blood studies: CBC, leukocytes, differential, cardiac enzymes if patient is receiving long-term therapy
• Hepatic studies: AST (SGOT), ALT (SGPT), bilirubin
• Weight qwk; appetite may increase with drug
• ECG for flattening of T wave, bundle branch block, AV block, dysrhythmias in cardiac patients
• EPS primarily in elderly: rigidity, dystonia, akathisia
• Mental status: mood, sensorium, affect, suicidal tendencies; increase in psychiatric symptoms: depression, panic
• Urinary retention, constipation; constipation is most likely to occur in children and elderly
• Withdrawal symptoms: headache, nausea, vomiting, muscle pain, weakness; do not usually occur unless drug was discontinued abruptly
• Alcohol consumption; if alcohol is consumed, hold dose until morning

Administer:
• Increased fluids, bulk in diet if constipation, urinary retention occur, especially elderly
• With food or milk for GI symptoms
• Crushed if patient is unable to swallow medication whole
• Dosage hs if oversedation occurs during day; may take entire dose hs; elderly may not tolerate once/day dosing
• Gum, hard sugarless candy, or frequent sips of water for dry mouth

Perform/provide:
• Storage at room temperature; do not freeze
• Assistance with ambulation during beginning therapy, since drowsiness/dizziness occurs
• Safety measures, including side rails, primarily in elderly
• Checking to see PO medication swallowed

Evaluate:
• Therapeutic response: decrease in depression, absence of suicidal thoughts

Teach patient/family:
• To take medication as directed; do not double dose
• That therapeutic effects may take 2-3 wk
• To use caution in driving, other activities requiring alertness because of drowsiness, dizziness, blurred vision; to avoid rising quickly from sitting to standing, especially elderly
• To avoid alcohol ingestion, other CNS depressants
• Not to discontinue medication quickly after long-term use: may cause nausea, headache, malaise
• To wear sunscreen or large hat, since photosensitivity occurs

Treatment of overdose: ECG monitoring, induce emesis, lavage, activated charcoal, administer anticonvulsant

amlodipine (℞)

(am-loe'di-peen)
Norvasc
Func. class.: Calcium channel blocker
Chem. class.: Dihydropyridine

Action: Inhibits calcium ion influx across cell membrane during cardiac depolarization; produces relaxation of coronary vascular smooth muscle, peripheral vascular smooth muscle; dilates coronary vascular arteries; increases myocardial oxygen delivery in patients with vasospastic angina

Uses: Chronic stable angina pectoris, hypertension, vasospastic angina

Dosage and routes:

Angina

• *Adult:* PO 5-10 mg qd

Hypertension

• *Adult:* PO 5 mg qd initially, may increase up to 10 mg/day

Available forms: Tabs 2.5, 5, 10 mg

Side effects/adverse reactions:

CV: Dysrhythmia, edema, bradycardia, hypotension, palpitations, syncope, AV block

GI: Nausea, vomiting, diarrhea, gastric upset, constipation, abdominal cramps, flatulence, anorexia

GU: Nocturia, polyuria, ***acute renal failure***

INTEG: Rash, pruritus, urticaria, hair loss

CNS: Headache, fatigue, dizziness, anxiety, depression, insomnia, paresthesia, somnolence, asthenia

OTHER: Flushing, nasal congestion, sweating, shortness of breath, sexual difficulties, muscle cramps, cough, weight gain, tinnitus, epistaxis

Contraindications: Sick sinus syndrome, 2nd or 3rd degree heart block, hypotension less than 90 mm Hg systolic, hypersensitivity

Precautions: CHF, hypotension, hepatic injury, pregnancy (C), lactation, children, renal disease, elderly

Pharmacokinetics:

PO: Onset not determined, peak 6-12 hr, half-life 30-50 hr; metabolized by liver, excreted in urine (90% as metabolites)

Interactions:

• Increased effects of digitalis, neuromuscular blocking agents, theophylline, prazosin, β-blockers, fentanyl

NURSING CONSIDERATIONS

Assess:

• Cardiac status: B/P, pulse, respiration, ECG

Administer:

• Once a day

Evaluate:

• Therapeutic response: decreased anginal pain, decreased B/P

Teach patient/family:

• To take drug as prescribed, do not double or skip dose

• To avoid hazardous activities until stabilized on drug, dizziness is no longer a problem

• To limit caffeine consumption

• To avoid OTC drugs unless directed by prescriber

• To comply in all areas of medical regimen: diet, exercise, stress reduction, drug therapy

• To notify prescriber of irregular heart beat, shortness of breath, swelling of feet and hands, pronounced dizziness, constipation, nausea, hypotension

Treatment of overdose: Defibrillation, β-agonists, IV calcium inotropic agents, diuretics, atropine for AV block, vasopressor for hypotension

ammonium chloride

(PO-OTC, IV-℞)

Func. class.: Acidifier

Chem. class.: Ammonium ion

Action: Lowers urinary pH, liberates hydrogen and chloride ions in blood and extracellular fluid with decreased pH and correction of alkalosis

Uses: Alkalosis (metabolic), systemic and urinary acidifier, expectorant, diuretic

Dosage and routes:

Alkalosis

• *Adult and child:* IV INF 0.9-1.3 ml/min of a 2.14% sol, not to exceed 5 ml/min

Acidifier

- *Adult:* PO 4-12 g/day in divided doses
- *Child:* PO 75 mg/kg/day in divided doses

Expectorant

- *Adult:* PO 250-500 mg q2-4h as needed

Available forms: Tabs 500 mg, 1 g; inj IV 0.4, 5 mEq/ml

Side effects/adverse reactions:

CNS: Drowsiness, headache, confusion, stimulation, tremors, *twitching, hyperreflexia,* ***tetany,*** *EEG changes*

CV: Bradycardia, dysrhythmias, bounding pulse

GU: Glycosuria, thirst

GI: Gastric irritation, nausea, vomiting, anorexia, diarrhea

INTEG: Rash, pain at infusion site

META: Acidosis, hypokalemia, hyperchloremia, hyperglycemia

RESP: ***Apnea,*** irregular respirations, hyperventilation

Contraindications: Hypersensitivity, severe hepatic disease, severe renal disease

Precautions: Severe respiratory disease, cardiac edema, respiratory acidosis, infants, pregnancy (C), lactation, children, elderly

Pharmacokinetics:

PO: Absorbed in 3-6 hr; metabolized in liver, excreted in urine and feces

Interactions:

- Increased toxicity: PAS
- Decreased effects of: amphetamines, tricyclic antidepressants, salicylates, sulfonylureas
- Increased risk of systemic acidosis: spironolactone

Additive compatibilities: Amikacin, aminophylline, sodium bicarbonate

Lab test interferences:

Increase: Blood ammonia, AST/ALT

Decrease: Serum Mg, urine urobilinogen

NURSING CONSIDERATIONS

Assess:

- Respiratory rate, rhythm, depth; notify prescriber of abnormalities that may indicate acidosis
- Electrolytes and CO_2, chloride before and during treatment
- Urine pH, urinary output, urine glucose, specific gravity during beginning treatment
- I&O ratio, report large increases or decreases
- For CNS symptoms: confusion, twitching, hyperreflexia, stimulation, headache that may indicate ammonia toxicity
- For cardiac dysrhythmias
- For respiratory symptoms: hyperventilation

Administer:

- PO with meals if GI symptoms occur
- IV slowly to avoid pain at infusion site and toxicity
- After diluting sol to 2.14% (IV), each 20-ml vial must be further diluted by adding 1-2 vials/500-1000 ml of compatible sol given at 5 ml/min or less; KCl 20-40 mEq/L may be added to the infusion; for infants dilute 1 ml of drug/5-10 ml of diluent
- With water for expectorant, not compatible with milk or other alkaline solutions

Evaluate:

- Therapeutic response: decreasing metabolic alkalosis or increasing urinary acidity or diuresis, productive cough

Teach patient/family:

- To increase potassium in diet: bananas, oranges, cantaloupe, honeydew, spinach, potatoes, dry fruit

---

* Available in Canada only

amobarbital (℞)

(am-oh-bar′bi-tal)

amobarbital sodium, Amytal, Amytal Sodium, Amytal Sodium Pulvules, Novamobarb*

Func. class.: Sedative hypnotic-barbiturate (intermediate acting)

Chem. class.: Amylobarbitone

Controlled Substance Schedule II (USA), Schedule G (Canada)

Action: Depresses activity in brain cells primarily in reticular activating system in brain stem; also selectively depresses neurons in posterior hypothalamus, limbic structures; able to decrease seizure activity by inhibition of impulses in CNS; depresses REM sleep

Uses: Sedation, preanesthetic sedation, insomnia, anticonvulsant, adjunct in psychiatry, hypnotic

Dosage and routes:

Preanesthetic sedation

- *Adult:* PO/IM 200 mg 1-2 hr preoperatively
- *Child:* up to 100 mg

Sedation

- *Adult:* PO 30-50 mg bid or tid, may be 15-120 mg bid-qid
- *Child:* PO 2 mg/kg/day in 4 divided doses

Anticonvulsant/psychiatry

- *Adult:* IV 65-500 mg given over several min, not to exceed 100 mg/min; not to exceed 1 g
- *Child* <6 yr: IV/IM 3-5 mg/kg over several min

Insomnia

- *Adult:* PO/IM 65-200 mg hs, not to exceed 5 ml in one site
- *Child:* IM 3-5 mg/kg at hs, not to exceed 5 ml in one site

Available forms: Tabs 30, 50, 100 mg; caps 65, 200 mg; powder for inj IM, IV 250, 500 mg/vial

Side effects/adverse reactions:

CNS: Lethargy, drowsiness, hangover, dizziness, stimulation in the elderly and children, lightheadedness, physical dependence, CNS depression, mental depression, slurred speech

GI: Nausea, vomiting, diarrhea, constipation

INTEG: Rash, urticaria, pain, abscesses at injection site, ***angioedema,*** thrombophlebitis, ***Stevens-Johnson syndrome***

CV: Hypotension, bradycardia

RESP: ***Depression, apnea, laryngospasm, bronchospasm***

HEMA: ***Agranulocytosis, thrombocytopenia, megaloblastic anemia*** (long-term treatment)

Contraindications: Hypersensitivity to barbiturates, respiratory depression, addiction to barbiturates, severe liver impairment, porphyria, pregnancy (D), lactation

Precautions: Anemia, lactation, hepatic disease, renal disease, hypertension, elderly, acute/chronic pain

Pharmacokinetics:

PO: Onset 45-60 min, duration 6-8 hr

IV: Onset 5 min, duration 3-6 hr

Metabolized by liver, excreted by kidneys (inactive metabolites), crosses placenta, highly protein bound, excreted in breast milk, half-life 16-40 hr

Interactions:

- Increased CNS depression: alcohol, MAOIs, sedative, narcotics, general anesthetics, antipsychotics
- Decreased effect of oral anticoagulants, corticosteroids, griseofulvin, quinidine, oral contraceptives, estrogens
- May increase or decrease phenytoin levels
- Increased half-life of doxycycline

• Incompatible in sol with cefazolin, cephalothin, chlorpromazine, cimetidine, clindamycin, codeine, dimenhydrinate, droperidol, hydrocortisone, hydroxyzine, insulin, levarterenol, levorphanol, meperidine, methadone, morphine, pentazocine, penicillin G, phytonadione, procaine, prochlorperazine, streptomycin, tetracycline, thiamine, trifluoperazine, vancomycin in sol or syringe

Lab test interferences:

False increase: Sulfobromophthalein

NURSING CONSIDERATIONS

Assess:

• VS q30 min after parenteral route for 2 hr

• Blood studies: Hct, Hgb, RBCs, serum folate, vit D (if on long-term therapy); pro-time in patients receiving anticoagulants

• Hepatic studies: AST (SGOT), ALT (SGPT), bilirubin; if increased, drug is usually discontinued

• Mental status: mood, sensorium, affect, memory (long, short), especially elderly

• Physical dependency: more frequent requests for medication, shakes, anxiety; elderly may be more sensitive due to decreased metabolism

• Barbiturate toxicity: hypotension; pulmonary constriction; cold, clammy skin; cyanosis of lips; CNS depression; nausea; vomiting; hallucinations; delirium; weakness; coma, pupillary constriction; mild symptoms may occur in 8-12 hr without drug

• Respiratory dysfunction: respiratory depression, character, rate, rhythm; hold drug if respirations are <10/min or if pupils are dilated

• Blood dyscrasias: fever, sore throat, bruising, rash, jaundice, epistaxis

Administer:

• After removal of cigarettes, to prevent fires

• Deep IM injection in large muscle mass to prevent tissue sloughing, abscesses, no more than 5 ml/site

• After trying conservative measures for insomnia

• After diluting each 125 mg/1.25 ml, give by direct IV at a rate of 100 mg or less/1 min (adult), or 60 mg/min child; titrate slowly to desired response with sterile water for injection to a concentration of 100 mg/ml; inject within 30 min of preparation; do not shake solution or use cloudy solution; use large vein; may cause thrombosis, extravasation

• IV only with resuscitative equipment available, administer at <100 mg/min (only by qualified personnel)

• ½-1 hr before hs for expected sleeplessness

• On empty stomach for best absorption

Perform/provide:

• Assistance with ambulation after receiving dose

• Safety measures: side rails, nightlight, call bell within easy reach

• Checking to see PO medication swallowed

Evaluate:

• Therapeutic response: ability to sleep at night, decreased amount of early morning awakening if taking drug for insomnia, or decrease in number, severity of seizures if taking drug for seizure disorder

Teach patient/family:

• To take as directed; do not double dose

• That hangover is common

• That drug is indicated only for short-term treatment of insomnia and is probably ineffective after 2 wk

* Available in Canada only

• That physical dependency may result when used for extended time (45-90 days, depending on dose)
• To avoid driving, other activities requiring alertness
• To avoid alcohol ingestion, CNS depressants; serious CNS depression may result
• Not to discontinue medication quickly after long-term use; drug should be tapered over 1 wk
• To tell all prescribers that a barbiturate is being taken
• That withdrawal insomnia may occur after short-term use; do not start using drug again; insomnia will improve in 1-3 nights; may experience increased dreaming
• That effects may take 2 nights for benefits to be noticed
• Alternative measures to improve sleep: reading, exercise several hours before hs, warm bath, warm milk, TV, self-hypnosis, deep breathing

Treatment of overdose: Lavage, activated charcoal, warming blanket, vital signs, hemodialysis, alkalinize urine; give IV volume expanders, IV fluids

amoxapine (℞)

(a-mox'a-peen)
amoxapine, Asendin
Func. class.: Antidepressant—tricyclic
Chem. class.: Dibenzoxazepine derivative—secondary amine

Action: Blocks reuptake of norepinephrine, serotonin into nerve endings, increasing action of norepinephrine, serotonin in nerve cells

Uses: Depression

Dosage and routes:
• *Adult:* PO 50 mg tid, may increase to 100 mg tid on 3rd day of therapy; not to exceed 300 mg/day unless lower doses have been given for at least 2 wk, may be given daily dose hs, not to exceed 600 mg/day in hospitalized patients

Available forms: Tabs 10, 25, 50, 75, 100, 150 mg

Side effects/adverse reactions:
HEMA: ***Agranulocytosis, thrombocytopenia, eosinophilia, leukopenia***
CNS: Dizziness, drowsiness, confusion, headache, anxiety, tremors, stimulation, weakness, insomnia, nightmares, EPS (elderly), increased psychiatric symptoms, paresthesia, impairment of sexual functioning
GI: Diarrhea, dry mouth, constipation, nausea, vomiting, ***paralytic ileus,*** increased appetite, cramps, epigastric distress, jaundice, ***hepatitis,*** stomatitis
GU: Retention, ***acute renal failure***
INTEG: Rash, urticaria, sweating, pruritus, photosensitivity
CV: Orthostatic hypotension, ECG changes, tachycardia, ***hypertension,*** palpitations
EENT: Blurred vision, tinnitus, mydriasis, ophthalmoplegia

Contraindications: Hypersensitivity to tricyclic antidepressants, recovery phase of myocardial infarction, convulsive disorders, prostatic hypertrophy

Precautions: Suicidal patients, severe depression, increased intraocular pressure, narrow-angle glaucoma, urinary retention, cardiac disease, hepatic disease, hyperthyroidism, electroshock therapy, elective surgery, elderly, pregnancy (C)

Pharmacokinetics:
PO: Steady state 7 days; metabolized by liver, excreted by kidneys, crosses placenta, half-life 8 hr

Interactions:
• Decreased effects of guanethidine,

clonidine, indirect-acting sympathomimetics (ephedrine)
• Increased effects of direct-acting sympathomimetics (epinephrine), alcohol, barbiturates, benzodiazepines, CNS depressants
• Hyperpyretic crisis, convulsions, hypertensive episode: MAOI (pargyline [Eutonyl])

Lab test interferences:
Increase: Serum bilirubin, blood glucose, alk phosphatase
False increase: Urinary catecholamines
Decrease: VMA, 5-HIAA

NURSING CONSIDERATIONS

Assess:
• B/P lying, standing; pulse q4h; if systolic B/P drops 20 mm Hg, hold drug, notify prescriber; take vital signs q4h in patients with cardiovascular disease
• Blood studies: CBC, leukocytes, differential, cardiac enzymes if patient is receiving long-term therapy
• Hepatic studies: AST (SGOT), ALT (SGPT), bilirubin
• Weight qwk, appetite may increase with drug
• ECG for flattening of T wave, bundle branch block, AV block, dysrhythmias in cardiac patients
• EPS primarily in elderly: rigidity, dystonia, akathisia
• Mental status: mood, sensorium, affect, suicidal tendencies, increase in psychiatric symptoms: depression, panic
• Urinary retention, constipation; constipation is more likely to occur in children, elderly
• Withdrawal symptoms: headache, nausea, vomiting, muscle pain, weakness; do not usually occur unless drug was discontinued abruptly
• Alcohol consumption; if alcohol is consumed, hold dose until morning

Administer:
• Increased fluids, bulk in diet if constipation, urinary retention occur, especially in elderly
• With food or milk for GI symptoms
• Crushed if patient is unable to swallow medication whole
• Dosage hs if oversedation occurs during day; may take entire dose hs; elderly may not tolerate once/day dosing
• Gum, hard candy, or frequent sips of water for dry mouth

Perform/provide:
• Storage at room temperature; do not freeze
• Assistance with ambulation during beginning therapy, since drowsiness/dizziness occurs
• Safety measures including side rails primarily for elderly
• Check to see PO medication swallowed

Evaluate:
• Therapeutic response: decreased depression, absence of suicidal thoughts

Teach patient/family:
• To take as directed, not to double dose
• That therapeutic effects may take 2-3 wk
• To use caution in driving or other activities requiring alertness because of drowsiness, dizziness, blurred vision
• To avoid alcohol ingestion, other CNS depressants
• Not to discontinue medication quickly after long-term use; may cause nausea, headache, malaise
• To wear sunscreen or large hat, since photosensitivity occurs

Treatment of overdose: ECG monitoring, induce emesis, lavage, activated charcoal, administer anticonvulsant

amoxicillin/clavulanate potassium (℞)

(a-mox-i-sill'in)

Augmentin, Clavulin*

Func. class.: Broad-spectrum antibiotic

Chem. class.: Aminopenicillin-β lactamase inhibitor

Action: Interferes with cell wall replication of susceptible organisms; the cell wall, rendered osmotically unstable, swells and bursts from osmotic pressure; combination increases spectrum of activity against β-lactamase resistance organisms

Uses: Sinus infections, pneumonia, otitis media, skin, UTI; effective for strains of *E. coli, P. mirabilis, H. influenzae, E. faecalis, S. pneumoniae,* and some β-lactamase-producing organisms

Dosage and routes:

- *Adult:* PO 250-500 mg q8h depending on severity of infection
- *Child:* PO 20-40 mg/kg/day in divided doses q8h

Available forms: Tabs 250, 500 mg; chew tabs 125, 250 mg; powder for oral susp 125, 250 mg/5 ml

Side effects/adverse reactions:

HEMA: Anemia, ***bone marrow depression, granulocytopenia, leukopenia, eosinophilia,*** thrombocytopenic purpura

GI: Nausea, diarrhea, vomiting, increased AST, ALT, abdominal pain, glossitis, colitis, black tongue, pseudomembranous colitis

GU: Oliguria, proteinuria, hematuria, *vaginitis, moniliasis,* ***glomerulonephritis***

CNS: Headache, fever

META: Hyperkalemia, hypokalemia, alkalosis, hypernatremia

Contraindications: Hypersensitivity to penicillins

Precautions: Pregnancy (B), lactation, hypersensitivity to cephalosporins; neonates

Interactions:

- Increased amoxicillin concentrations: aspirin, probenecid

Pharmacokinetics:

PO: Peak 2 hr, duration 6-8 hr; half-life 1-1⅓ hr, metabolized in liver, excreted in urine, crosses placenta, enters breast milk

Lab test interferences:

False positive: Urine glucose, urine protein

NURSING CONSIDERATIONS

Assess:

- I&O ratio; report hematuria, oliguria, since penicillin in high doses is nephrotoxic
- Any patient with a compromised renal system, since drug is excreted slowly in poor renal system function; toxicity may occur
- Liver studies: AST (SGOT), ALT (SGPT)
- Blood studies: WBC, RBC, Hgb & Hct, bleeding time
- Renal studies: urinalysis, protein, blood
- Culture, sensitivity before drug therapy; drug may be given as soon as culture is taken
- Bowel pattern before, during treatment
- Skin eruptions after administration of penicillin to 1 wk after discontinuing drug
- Respiratory status: rate, character, wheezing, tightness in chest
- Allergies before initiation of treatment, reaction of each medication; place allergies on chart in bright red

Administer:

- After C&S completed
- Only as directed 2 (250 mg tab) are ≠ to 1 (500 mg tab) due to strength of clavulanate

Perform/provide:

- Adrenaline, suction, tracheostomy

set, endotracheal intubation equipment on unit
• Adequate intake of fluids (2 L) during diarrhea episodes
• Scratch test to assess allergy after securing order from prescriber; usually done when penicillin is only drug of choice
• Storage refrigerated for 2 wk or room temperature for 1 wk
Evaluate:
• Therapeutic response: absence of fever, draining wounds
Teach patient/family:
• To take as prescribed, not to double dose
• Aspects of drug therapy: need to complete entire course of medication to ensure organism death (10-14 days); culture may be taken after completed course of medication
• To report sore throat, fever, fatigue (may indicate a superinfection or agranulocytosis); vaginal candidiasis
• That drug must be taken in equal intervals around the clock to maintain blood levels
• To wear or carry a Medic Alert ID if allergic to penicillins
• To notify nurse of diarrhea
Treatment of hypersensitivity: Withdraw drug, maintain airway, administer epinephrine, aminophylline, O_2, IV corticosteroids for anaphylaxis

amoxicillin (℞)

(a-mox-i-sill'in)
amoxicillin, Amoxil, Amoxil Pediatric Drops, Apo-Amoxi*, Novamoxin*, Nu-Amoxi*, Polymox, Polymox Drops, Trimox 125, Trimox 250, Trimox 500, Wymox
Func. class.: Broad-spectrum antibiotic
Chem. class.: Aminopenicillin

Action: Interferes with cell wall replication of susceptible organisms; the cell wall, rendered osmotically unstable, swells and bursts from osmotic pressure
Uses: Effective for gram-positive cocci *(S. aureus, S. pyogenes, E. faecalis, S. pneumoniae),* gram-negative cocci *(N. gonorrhoeae, N. meningitidis),* gram-positive bacilli *(C. diphtheriae, L. monocytogenes),* gram-negative bacilli *(H. influenzae, E. Coli, P. mirabilis, Salmonella, Shigella)*
Investigational uses: Lyme disease
Dosage and routes:
Systemic infections
• *Adult:* PO 750 mg-1.5 g qd in divided doses q8h
• *Child:* PO 20-40 mg/kg/day in divided doses q8h
Gonorrhea/urinary tract infections
• *Adult:* PO 3 g given with 1 g probenecid as a single dose
Available forms: Caps 250, 500 mg; chew tabs 125, 250 mg; powder for oral susp 50, 125, 250 mg/5 ml
Side effects/adverse reactions:
HEMA: Anemia, increased bleeding time, ***bone marrow depression, granulocytopenia***
GI: Nausea, vomiting, diarrhea, increased AST (SGOT), ALT (SGPT), abdominal pain, glossitis, colitis, ***pseudomembranous colitis***

* Available in Canada only

CNS: Headache, fever
SYST: ***Anaphylaxis, respiratory distress***
Contraindications: Hypersensitivity to penicillins
Precautions: Pregnancy (B), lactation, hypersensitivity to cephalosporins; neonates
Interactions:
• Increased amoxicillin concentrations: aspirin, probenecid
• Decreased effectiveness of oral contraceptives
• Amoxicillin-induced skin rash: allopurinol
Pharmacokinetics:
PO: Peak 2 hr, duration 6-8 hr; half-life 1-1⅓ hr, metabolized in liver, excreted in urine, crosses placenta, enters breast milk
Lab test interferences:
False positive: Urine glucose, urine protein

NURSING CONSIDERATIONS

Assess:
• I&O ratio; report hematuria, oliguria, since penicillin in high doses is nephrotoxic
• Any patient with a compromised renal system, since drug is excreted slowly in poor renal system function; toxicity may occur rapidly
• Liver studies: AST (SGOT), ALT (SGPT)
• Blood studies: WBC, RBC, Hgb & Hct, bleeding time
• Renal studies: urinalysis, protein, blood
• Culture, sensitivity before drug therapy; drug may be given as soon as culture is taken
• Bowel pattern before, during treatment
• Skin eruptions after administration of penicillin to 1 wk after discontinuing drug
• Respiratory status: rate, character, wheezing, tightness in the chest
• Allergies before initiation of treatment, reaction of each medication; place allergies on chart in bright red
Administer:
• After C&S completed
Perform/provide:
• Adrenaline, suction, tracheostomy set, endotracheal intubation equipment on unit
• Adequate intake of fluids (2 L) during diarrhea episodes
• Scratch test to assess allergy after securing order from prescriber; usually done when penicillin is only drug of choice
• Storage in tight container; after reconstituting, oral suspension refrigerated for 2 wk or stored at room temperature for 1 wk
Evaluate:
• Therapeutic response: absence of fever, draining wounds
Teach patient/family:
• To take as prescribed, not to double dose
• Aspects of drug therapy: need to complete entire course of medication to ensure organism death (10-14 days); culture may be taken after completed course of medication
• To report sore throat, fever, fatigue, diarrhea (may indicate a superimposed infection or agranulocytopenia)
• That drug must be taken in equal intervals around the clock to maintain blood levels; take on empty stomach with a full glass of water
• To wear or carry a Medic Alert ID if allergic to penicillins
Treatment of anaphylaxis: Withdraw drug, maintain airway, administer epinephrine, aminophylline, O_2, IV corticosteroids

amphetamine (℞)

(am-fet'a-meen)
amphetamine sulfate
Func. class.: Cerebral stimulant
Chem. class.: Amphetamine

Controlled Substance Schedule II
Action: Increases release of norepinephrine, dopamine in cerebral cortex to reticular activating system
Uses: Narcolepsy, exogenous obesity, attention deficit disorder
Dosage and routes:
Narcolepsy
• *Adult:* PO 5-60 mg qd in divided doses
• *Child >12 yr:* PO 10 mg qd increasing by 10 mg/day at weekly intervals
• *Child 6-12 yr:* PO 5 mg qd increasing by 5 mg/wk, max 60 mg/day
Attention deficit disorder
• *Child >6 yr:* PO 5 mg qd-bid increasing by 5 mg/day at weekly intervals
• *Child 3-6 yr:* PO 2.5 mg qd increasing by 2.5 mg/day at weekly intervals
Obesity
• *Adult:* PO 5-30 mg in divided doses 30-60 min before meals
Available forms: Tabs 5, 10 mg; long-acting capsules 5, 10 mg
Side effects/adverse reactions:
CNS: Hyperactivity, insomnia, restlessness, talkativeness, dizziness, headache, chills, stimulation, dysphoria, irritability, aggressiveness, tremor, dependence, addiction
GI: Nausea, vomiting, anorexia, dry mouth, diarrhea, constipation, weight loss, metallic taste, cramps
GU: Impotence, change in libido
CV: Palpitations, tachycardia, hypertension, dysrhythmias, decreased heart rate
INTEG: Urticaria
Contraindications: Pregnancy (X), hypersensitivity to sympathomimetic amines, hyperthyroidism, hypertension, glaucoma, severe arteriosclerosis, drug abuse, cardiovascular disease, anxiety, lactation
Precautions: Gilles de la Tourette's disorder, lactation, child <3 yr
Pharmacokinetics:
PO: Onset 30 min, peak 1-3 hr, duration 4-20 hr, metabolized by liver, excreted by kidneys, crosses placenta, breast milk, half-life 10-30 hr
Interactions:
• Hypertensive crisis: MAOIs or within 14 days of MAOIs or furazolidone
• Increased effect of amphetamine: acetazolamide, antacids, sodium bicarbonate urinary alkalinizers
• Decreased effect of amphetamine: barbiturates, tricyclics, urinary acidifiers (ascorbic acid, ammonium chloride)
• Decreased effect of guanethidine

NURSING CONSIDERATIONS
Assess:
• VS, B/P, since this drug may reverse antihypertensives; check patients with cardiac disease more often
• CBC, urinalysis, in diabetes: blood sugar, urine sugar; insulin changes may be required, since eating will decrease
• Height; growth rate in children may be decreased
• Mental status: mood, sensorium, affect, stimulation, insomnia; aggressiveness may occur
• Physical dependency; should not be used for extended time; dose should be discontinued gradually
• Withdrawal symptoms: headache, nausea, vomiting, muscle pain, weakness
• Drug tolerance will develop after long-term use

• Dosage should not be increased if tolerance develops
Administer:
• At least 6 hr before hs to avoid sleeplessness
• For obesity only if patient is on weight-reduction program that includes dietary changes, exercise; patient will develop tolerance, and weight loss won't occur without additional methods; give 30-60 min before meals
• Gum, hard candy, frequent sips of water for dry mouth
Evaluate:
• Therapeutic response: decreased activity in attention deficit disorder; absence of sleeping during day in narcolepsy; decrease in weight
Teach patient/family:
• Do not double dose; if dose is missed, take up to 6 hr before hs
• To decrease caffeine consumption (coffee, tea, cola, chocolate), which may increase irritability, stimulation
• To avoid OTC preparations unless approved by prescriber
• To taper off drug over several weeks, or depression, increased sleeping, lethargy may occur
• To avoid alcohol ingestion
• To avoid hazardous activities until patient is stabilized on medication
• To get needed rest; patients will feel more tired at end of day
Treatment of overdose: Administer fluids, hemodialysis, peritoneal dialysis, antihypertensives for increased B/P; ammonium Cl for increased excretion

A

amphotericin B (℞)

(am-foe-ter'i-sin)
amphotericin B, Fungizone IV
Func. class.: Antifungal
Chem. class.: Amphoteric polyene

Combination products: Mysteclin F: amphotericin B 25 mg/5 ml with tetracycline equivalent to tetracycline HCl 25 mg/5 ml; Mysteclin-F: amphotericin B 50 mg with tetracycline equivalent to tetracycline HCl 250 mg

Action: Increases cell membrane permeability in susceptible organisms by binding sterols; decreases potassium, sodium, and nutrients in cell
Uses: Histoplasmosis, blastomycosis, coccidioidomycosis, cryptococcosis, aspergillosis, phycomycosis, candidiasis, sporotrichosis causing severe meningitis, septicemia, skin infections
Dosage and routes:
• *Adult and child:* IV INF 1 mg/250 ml D_5W (0.1 mg/ml) over 2-4 hr or 0.25 mg/kg/day over 6 hr; may be increased gradually up to 1 mg/kg/day, not to exceed 1.5 mg/kg; INTRATHECAL 25 μg/0.1 ml diluted in 10-20 ml CSF given by barbotage 2-3 times a wk, gradually increased to 0.5 mg q48-72 hr
Candida infection of GI tract
Adults: 100 mg PO qid × 2 wk
Candida oral infection
1 loz qid × 7-14 days; allow 1 loz to dissolve slowly in mouth
Available forms: Powder for inj 50 mg
Side effects/adverse reactions:
EENT: Tinnitus, deafness, diplopia, blurred vision

INTEG: Burning, irritation, pain, necrosis at injection site with extravasation, flushing, dermatitis, skin rash (topical route)
CNS: Headache, fever, chills, peripheral nerve pain, paresthesias, peripheral neuropathy, ***convulsions,*** dizziness
GU: Hypokalemia, azotemia, hyposthenuria, ***renal tubular acidosis,*** nephrocalcinosis, ***permanent renal impairment, anuria, oliguria***
GI: Nausea, vomiting, anorexia, diarrhea, cramps, ***hemorrhagic gastroenteritis, acute liver failure***
MS: ***Arthralgia, myalgia,*** generalized pain, weakness, weight loss
HEMA: Normochromic, normocytic anemia, ***thrombocytopenia, agranulocytosis, leukopenia, eosinophilia,*** hypokalemia, hyponatremia, hypomagnesemia
Contraindications: Hypersensitivity, severe bone marrow depression
Precautions: Renal disease, pregnancy (B), lactation
Pharmacokinetics:
IV: Peak 1-2 hr, initial half-life 24 hr, metabolized in liver, excreted in urine (metabolites), breast milk, highly bound to plasma proteins; penetrates poorly CSF, bronchial secretions, aqueous humor, muscle, bone
Interactions:
- Increased nephrotoxicity: other nephrotoxic antibiotics (aminoglycosides, cisplatin, vancomycin, cyclosporine, polymixin B)
- Increased hypokalemia: corticosteroids, digitalis, skeletal muscle relaxants
- Antagonism: miconazole

Syringe compatibility: Heparin
Y-site compatibility: Zidovudine
Additive compatibilities: Heparin, hydrocortisone, methylprednisolone, sodium bicarbonate

NURSING CONSIDERATIONS
Assess:
- VS q15-30min during first infusion; note changes in pulse, B/P
- I&O ratio; watch for decreasing urinary output, change in specific gravity; discontinue drug to prevent permanent damage to renal tubules
- Blood studies: CBC, K, Na, Ca, Mg q2wk, BUN, creatinine weekly
- Weight weekly; if weight increases over 2 lb/wk, edema is present; renal damage should be considered
- For renal toxicity: increasing BUN, serum creatinine; if BUN is >40 mg/dl or if serum creatinine >3 mg/dl, drug may be discontinued or dosage reduced
- For hepatotoxicity: increasing AST (SGOT), ALT (SGPT), alk phosphatase, bilirubin
- For allergic reaction: dermatitis, rash; drug should be discontinued, antihistamines (mild reaction) or epinephrine (severe reaction) administered
- For hypokalemia: anorexia, drowsiness, weakness, decreased reflexes, dizziness, increased urinary output, increased thirst, paresthesias
- For ototoxicity: tinnitus (ringing, roaring in ears) vertigo, loss of hearing (rare)

Administer:
- After diluting 50 mg/10 ml sterile water (no preservatives) or NS, (5 mg-1 ml) shake, dilute with 500 ml of solution to concentration of 0.1 mg/ml
- Test dose of 1 mg/20 ml D_5W; give over 10-30 min
- IV using in-line filter (mean pore diameter >1 µm) using distal veins; check for extravasation, necrosis q8h; use an infusion pump; administer over 6 hr; rapid infusion may result in circulation collapse
- Drug only after C&S confirms organism, drug needed to treat con-

dition; make sure drug is used in life-threatening infections

Perform/provide:

- Protection from light during infusion, cover with foil
- Symptomatic treatment as ordered for adverse reactions: aspirin, antihistamines, antiemetics, antispasmodics
- Storage, protected from moisture and light; diluted solution is stable for 24 hr at room temperature

Evaluate:

- Therapeutic response: decreased fever, malaise, rash, negative C&S for infecting organism

Teach patient/family:

- That long-term therapy may be needed to clear infection (2 wk-3 mo depending on type of infection)

---

amphotericin B (topical) (℞)

(am-foe-ter'i-sin)

Fungizone

Func. class.: Local antiinfective

Chem. class.: Antifungal (polyene)

Action: Increases cell membrane permeability in susceptible organisms by binding sterols

Uses: Cutaneous, mucocutaneous infections caused by *Candida*

Dosage and routes:

- *Adult and child:* TOP bid-qid for 7-21 days or longer if needed

Available forms: Cream, lotion, oint 3%

Side effects/adverse reactions:

INTEG: Urticaria, stinging, burning, dry skin, pruritus, contact dermatitis, erythema, staining of nail lesions

Contraindications: Hypersensitivity

Precautions: Pregnancy (B), lactation

NURSING CONSIDERATIONS

Assess:

- Allergic reaction: burning, stinging, swelling, redness

Administer:

- Enough medication to cover lesions completely; apply liberally and rub thoroughly into affected area
- After cleansing with soap, water before each application, dry well (as ordered)

Perform/provide:

- Storage at room temperature in dry place

Evaluate:

- Therapeutic response: decrease in size, number of lesions

Teach patient/family:

- That skin and clothing may become discolored
- To apply with glove to prevent further infection; not to cover with occlusive dressing
- To avoid use of OTC creams, ointments, lotions unless directed by prescriber
- To use medical asepsis (hand washing) before, after each application to prevent further infection
- To continue even if condition improves
- To report increased itching, burning, rash, redness; ointment may irritate most hairy areas

ampicillin (℞)

(am-pi-sill'in)

Ampicin*, Amcill, D-Amp*, Apo-Ampi*, Nu-Ampi*, Novo Ampicillin*, Omnipen, Polycillin, Omnipen-N, Polycillin-N, Supen, Totacillin, Totacillin-N

Func. class.: Broad-spectrum antibiotic

Chem. class.: Aminopenicillin

Action: Interferes with cell wall replication of susceptible organisms; the cell wall, rendered osmotically unstable, swells, bursts from osmotic pressure

Uses: Effective for gram-positive cocci *(S. aureus, S. pyogenes, E. faecalis, S. pneumoniae),* gram-negative cocci *(N. gonorrhoeae, N. meningitidis),* gram-negative bacilli *(H. influenzae, P. mirabilis, Salmonella, Shigella, L. monocytogenes),* gram-positive bacilli

Dosage and routes:

Systemic infections

• *Adult:* PO 1-2 g qd in divided doses q6h; IV/IM 2-8 g qd in divided doses q4-6h

• *Child:* PO 50-100 mg/kg/day in divided doses q6h; IV/IM 100-200 mg/kg/day in divided doses q6h

Meningitis

• *Adult:* IV 8-14 g/day in divided doses q3-4h

• *Child:* IV 200-300 mg/kg/day in divided doses q3-4h

Gonorrhea

• *Adult:* PO 3.5 g given with 1 g probenecid as a single dose

Available forms: Powder for inj IV, IM 125, 250, 500 mg, 1, 2, 10 g; IV inf 500 mg, 1, 2 g; caps 250, 500 mg; powder for oral susp 100/1 ml, 125, 250, 500 mg/5 ml

Side effects/adverse reactions:

INTEG: Rash, urticaria

HEMA: Anemia, increased bleeding time, ***bone marrow depression, granulocytopenia***

GI: Nausea, vomiting, diarrhea

GU: Oliguria, proteinuria, hematuria, *vaginitis, moniliasis,* ***glomerulonephritis***

CNS: Lethargy, hallucinations, anxiety, depression, twitching, ***coma, convulsions***

Contraindications: Hypersensitivity to penicillins

Precautions: Pregnancy (B), lactation; hypersensitivity to cephalosporins; neonates

Pharmacokinetics:

PO: Peak 2 hr

IV: Peak 5 min

IM: Peak 1 hr

Half-life 50-110 min; metabolized in liver, excreted in urine, bile, breast milk, crosses placenta

Interactions:

• Possible increased bleeding: oral anticoagulants

• Increased ampicillin concentrations: aspirin, probenecid

• Decreased effectiveness of oral contraceptives

• Increased ampicillin-induced skin rash: allopurinol

Syringe compatibilities: Chloramphenicol, colistimethate, heparin, procaine, lidocaine

Y-site compatibilities: Acyclovir, cyclophosphamide, enalaprilat, esmolol, famotidine, fludarabine, foscarnet, heparin, hydromorphone, regular insulin, labetalol, magnesium sulfate, melphalan, meperidine, morphine, perphenazine, phytonadione, potassium chloride, tolazoline, vitamin B with C

Additive compatibilities: Clindamycin, erythromycin, floxacillin, furosemide, verapamil

Lab test interferences:

False positive: Urine glucose, urine protein

* Available in Canada only

NURSING CONSIDERATIONS

Assess:

- I&O ratio; report hematuria, oliguria, since penicillin in high doses is nephrotoxic
- Any patient with compromised renal system, since drug is excreted slowly in poor renal system function; toxicity may occur
- Liver studies: AST (SGOT), ALT (SGPT)
- Blood studies: WBC, RBC, Hgb & Hct, bleeding time
- Renal studies: urinalysis, protein, blood
- Culture, sensitivity before drug therapy; drug may be taken as soon as culture is taken
- Bowel pattern before, during treatment
- Skin eruptions after administration of penicillin to 1 wk after discontinuing drug
- Respiratory status: rate, character, wheezing, tightness in chest
- Allergies before initiation of treatment; reaction of each medication; place allergies on chart in bright red

Administer:

- After diluting with sterile H_2O 0.9-1.2 ml/125 mg drug, administer over 3-5 min (up to 500 mg), 10-15 min (>500 mg) by direct IV; may be diluted in 50 ml or more of D_5W, D_5 ½ NaCl to a concentration of 30 mg/ml or less; IV sol is stable for 1 hr; give at prescribed rate
- After C&S completed
- On empty stomach for best absorption (1-2 hr ac or 2-3 hr pc)

Perform/provide:

- Adrenaline, suction, tracheostomy set, endotracheal intubation equipment on unit
- Adequate intake of fluids (2 L) during diarrhea episodes
- Scratch test to assess allergy after securing order from prescriber; usually done when penicillin is only drug of choice
- Storage in tight container; after reconstituting, oral suspension refrigerated for 2 wk or stored at room temperature for 1 wk

Evaluate:

- Therapeutic response: absence of temperature, draining wounds

Teach patient/family:

- To take oral penicillin on empty stomach with full glass of water
- Aspects of drug therapy: need to complete entire course of medication to ensure organism death (10-14 days); culture may be taken after completed course of medication
- To report sore throat, fever, fatigue, diarrhea (may indicate superinfection); report rash or other signs of allergy
- That drug must be taken in equal intervals around the clock to maintain blood levels
- To wear or carry a Medic Alert ID if allergic to penicillins

Treatment of anaphylaxis: Withdraw drug, maintain airway, administer epinephrine, aminophylline, O_2, IV corticosteroids

ampicillin, sulbactam (℞)

Unasyn

Func. class.: Broad-spectrum antibiotic

Chem. class.: Aminopenicillin with β-lactamase inhibitor

Action: Interferes with cell wall replication of susceptible organisms; the cell wall, rendered osmotically unstable, swells, bursts from osmotic pressure; combination extends spectrum of activity by β-lactamase inhibition

Uses: Skin infections, pneumonia *(S. aureus, E. coli, Klebsiella, P. mirabilis, B. fragilis, H. influenza, Enterobacter, A. calcoaceticus)*, intraabdominal infections *(Enterobacter, Klebsiella, Bacteroides, E. coli)* gynecologic infections *(E. coli, Bacteroides)*

Dosage and routes:

• *Adult:* IV 1 g ampicillin, 0.5 g sulbactam to 2 g ampicillin and 1 g sulbactam q6h, not to exceed 4 g/day sulbactam

Available forms: Powder for inj 1.5 g (1 g ampicillin, 0.5 g sulbactam), 3.0 g (2 g ampicillin, 1 g sulbactam)

Side effects/adverse reactions:

HEMA: Anemia, increased bleeding time, ***bone marrow depression, granulocytopenia***

GI: Nausea, vomiting, diarrhea, increased AST (SGOT), ALT (SGPT), abdominal pain, glossitis, colitis

GU: Oliguria, proteinuria, hematuria, *vaginitis, moniliasis,* ***glomerulonephritis***

CNS: Lethargy, hallucinations, anxiety, depression, twitching, ***coma, convulsions***

Contraindications: Hypersensitivity to penicillins

Precautions: Pregnancy (C), lactation, hypersensitivity to cephalosporins, neonates

Pharmacokinetics:

IV: Peak 5 min; half-life 50-110 min; little metabolized in liver, 75% to 85% of both drugs excreted in urine, diffuses to breast milk, crosses placenta

Interactions:

• Increased ampicillin concentration: aspirin, probenecid

Y-site compatibilities: Enalaprilat, famotidine, fluconazole, regular insulin, meperidine, morphine, paclitaxel

Lab test interferences:

False positive: Urine glucose, urine protein

NURSING CONSIDERATIONS

Assess:

• Bowel pattern before, during treatment

• Respiratory status: rate, character, wheezing, tightness in chest

• I&O ratio; report hematuria, oliguria, since penicillin in high doses is nephrotoxic

• Any patient with compromised renal system, since drug is excreted slowly in poor renal system function; toxicity may occur rapidly

• Liver studies: AST (SGOT), ALT (SGPT)

• Blood studies: WBC, RBC, Hct, Hgb, bleeding time

• Renal studies: urinalysis, protein, blood

• C&S before drug therapy; drug may be given as soon as culture is taken

• Skin eruptions after administration of ampicillin 1 wk after discontinuing drug

• Allergies before initiation of treatment; reaction of each medication; report allergies on chart in red

Administer:

• IV after diluting 1.5 g/4 ml or more sterile H_2O for inj (375 mg/ml); allow to stand until foaming stops; dilute further in 50 ml or more of D_5W, NaCl, administer within 1 hr after reconstitution; give as an intermittent inf over 15-30 min

• After C&S completed; on empty stomach

Perform/provide:

• Adrenaline, suction, tracheostomy set, endotracheal intubation equipment on unit for possible anaphylaxis

• Adequate intake of fluids (2 L) during diarrhea episodes

• Scratch test to assess allergy after securing order from prescriber; usually done when penicillin is only drug choice
• Storage in tight container, out of light

Evaluate:

• Therapeutic response: absence of fever, draining wounds, negative C&S

Teach patient/family:

• To report sore throat, fever, fatigue (may indicate superinfection)
• To wear or carry Medic Alert ID if allergic to penicillin products

Treatment of anaphylaxis: Withdraw drug, maintain airway, administer epinephrine, aminophylline, O_2, IV corticosteroids

---

amrinone (℞)

(am′ri-none)
Inocor

Func. class.: Cardiac inotropic agent

Chem. class.: Bipyrimidine derivative

Action: Positive inotropic agent with vasodilator properties; reduces preload and afterload by direct relaxation of vascular smooth muscle, increases cardiac output

Uses: Short-term management of CHF that has not responded to other medication; can be used with digitalis

Dosage and routes:

• *Adult:* IV BOL 0.75 mg/kg given over 2-3 min; start inf of 5-10 μg/kg/min; may give another bol 30 min after start of therapy, not to exceed 10 mg/kg total daily dose
• *Infant:* IV 3-4.5 mg/kg in divided doses, then start inf of 10 μg/kg/min
• *Neonates:* IV 3-4.5 mg/kg in divided doses, then start inf of 3-5 μg/kg/min

Available forms: Inj 5 mg/ml

Side effects/adverse reactions:

HEMA: ***Thrombocytopenia***

CV: Dysrhythmias, hypotension, headache, chest pain

GI: Nausea, vomiting, anorexia, abdominal pain, ***hepatotoxicity, ascites,*** jaundice, hiccups

INTEG: Allergic reactions, burning at injection site

RESP: Pleuritis, ***pulmonary densities, hypoxemia***

Contraindications: Hypersensitivity to this drug or bisulfites, severe aortic disease, severe pulmonic valvular disease, acute MI

Precautions: Lactation, pregnancy (C), children, renal disease, hepatic disease, atrial flutter/fibrillation, elderly

Pharmacokinetics:

IV: Onset 2-5 min, peak 10 min, duration variable; half-life 4-6 hr, metabolized in liver, excreted in urine as drug and metabolites 60%-90%

Interactions:

• Excessive hypotension: antihypertensives
• Additive effect: cardiac glycosides

Y-site compatibilities: Aminophylline, atropine, bretylium, calcium chloride, cimetidine, dobutamine, dopamine, epinephrine, hydrocortisone sodium succinate, isoproterenol, lidocaine, metaraminol bitartrate, methylprednisolone sodium succinate, nitroglycerin, nitroprusside, norepinephrine, phenylephrine, potassium chloride, procainamide, verapamil

NURSING CONSIDERATIONS

Assess:

• B/P and pulse q5min during infusion; if B/P drops 30 mm Hg, stop infusion and call prescriber

• Electrolytes: K, S, Cl, Ca; renal function studies: BUN, creatinine; blood studies: platelet count
• ALT (SGOT), AST (SGPT), bilirubin daily
• I&O ratio and weight qd; diuresis should increase with continuing therapy
• If platelets are <150,000/mm³, drug is usually discontinued and another drug started
• Extravasation; change site q48h

Administer:
• Do not mix directly with glucose solutions; chemical reaction occurs over 24 hr; precipitate forms if amrinone and furosemide come in contact
• Into running dextrose infusion through Y-connector or directly into tubing; may give undiluted over 2-3 min or dilute with NS to 1-3 mg/ml, run at prescribed rate
• By infusion pump for doses other than bolus
• Potassium supplements if ordered for potassium levels <3.0

Evaluate:
• Therapeutic response: increased cardiac output, decreased PCWP, adequate CVP, decreased dyspnea, fatigue, edema, ECG

Treatment of overdose: Discontinue drug, support circulation

---

amyl nitrite (℞)

(am'il)

amyl nitrite, Amyl Nitrite Aspirols, Amyl Nitrite Vaporole

Func. class.: Coronary vasodilator

Chem. class.: Nitrite

Action: Relaxes vascular smooth muscle; may dilate coronary blood vessels, resulting in reduced venous return, decreased cardiac output; reduces preload, afterload, which decreases left ventricular end diastolic pressure, systemic vascular resistance; converts hemoglobin to methemoglobin, which is able to bind cyanide

Uses: Acute angina pectoris, cyanide poisoning

Investigational uses: Cardiac murmur diagnosis

Dosage and routes:

Angina
• Adult: INH 0.18-0.3 ml as needed, 1-6 inhalations from 1 cap, may repeat in 3-5 min

Cyanide poisoning
• Adult: INH 0.3 ml ampule inhaled 15 sec until preparation of sodium nitrite infusion is ready

Available forms: Inh pearls 0.18, 0.3 ml

Side effects/adverse reactions:

CV: Postural hypotension, ***tachycardia, cardiovascular collapse,*** palpitations

CNS: Headache, dizziness, weakness, syncope

GI: Nausea, vomiting, abdominal pain

INTEG: Flushing, pallor, sweating

MISC: Muscle twitching, ***hemolytic anemia, methemoglobinemia***

Contraindications: Hypersensitivity to nitrites, severe anemia, increased intracranial pressure, hypertension, pregnancy (X)

Precautions: Lactation, children, drug abuse, head injury, cerebral hemorrhage, hypotension

Pharmacokinetics:

INH: Onset 30 sec, duration 3-5 min; metabolized by liver, ⅓ excreted in urine, half-life 1-4 min

Interactions:
• Increased hypotension: alcohol, β-blockers, antihypertensive

---

NURSING CONSIDERATIONS

Assess:

- B/P supine and sitting, pulse during treatment until stable
- For drug tolerance: the need for more medication for each attack
- For postural hypotension, headache during treatment, which are common side effects because of vasodilation

Administer:

- After wrapping, crushing ampule to avoid cuts
- Ordered analgesic if headache develops
- To patient who is sitting or lying down during treatment; keep head low, take deep breaths, which will decrease dizziness
- Drug, and have patient rest for 15 min

Perform/provide:

- Storage in light-resistant area in cool environment or refrigerate

Evaluate:

- Therapeutic response: relief of chest pain (angina)

Teach patient/family:

- To keep a record of angina attacks and what aggravates condition; prolonged chest pain may indicate MI: seek emergency treatment
- That medication may explode in presence of flame
- To take several deep breaths despite foul odor
- To make position changes slowly to prevent orthostatic hypotension
- To keep drug out of reach of children and in secure place, as there is high abuse potential

anistreplase (APSAC) (℞)

(an-ih-strep'layz)

aniosoylated plasminogen, Eminase

Func. class.: Thrombolytic enzyme

Chem. class.: Anisolated plasminogen streptokinase activator complex

Action: Promotes thrombolysis by promoting conversion of plasminogen to plasmin

Uses: Management of acute MI; although not yet approved, anistreplase will also be used for other conditions requiring thrombolysis, i.e., PE, DUT, unclotting arteriovenous shunts.

Dosage and routes:

- *Adult:* IV 30 U over 2-5 min as soon as possible after onset of symptoms

Available forms: Powder, lyophilized 30 U/vial

Side effects/adverse reactions:

HEMA: Decreased Hct, ***GI, GU, intracranial, retroperitoneal,*** surface bleeding, ***thrombocytopenia***

INTEG: Rash, urticaria, phlebitis at site, itching, flushing

CNS: Headache, fever, sweating, agitation, dizziness, paresthesia, tremor, vertigo

GI: Nausea, vomiting

RESP: Altered respirations, dyspnea, ***bronchospasm, lung edema***

MS: Low back pain, arthralgia

CV: Hypotension, dysrhythmias, conduction disorders

SYST: ***Anaphylaxis***

Contraindications: Hypersensitivity, active internal bleeding, intraspinal or intracranial surgery, neoplasms of CNS, severe hypertension, cerebral embolism/thrombosis/hemorrhage

Precautions: Arterial emboli from left side of heart, pregnancy (B), ulcerative colitis/enteritis, renal disease, hepatic disease, hypocoagulation, COPD, subacute bacterial endocarditis, rheumatic valvular disease, intraarterial diagnostic procedure or surgery (10 days), recent major surgery, lactation

Pharmacokinetics: Half-life 105 min

Interactions:

• Increased bleeding potential: aspirin, indomethacin, phenylbutazone, anticoagulants

• Do not mix with any other sol or drug

Lab test interferences:

Increase: PT, APTT, TT

Decrease: Fibrinogen, plasminogen

NURSING CONSIDERATIONS

Assess:

• VS, B/P, pulse, respirations, neurologic signs, temperature at least q4h, temp >104° F (40° C) or indicators of internal bleeding, cardiac rhythm after intracoronary administration

• Allergy: fever, rash, itching, chills; mild reaction may be treated with antihistamines

• Bleeding during 1st hr of treatment (hematuria, hematemesis, bleeding from mucous membranes, epistaxis, ecchymosis)

• Blood studies (Hct, platelets, PTT, PT, TT, APTT) before starting therapy; PT or APTT must be less than 2 × control before starting therapy; TT or PT q3-4h during treatment

Administer:

• Reconstitute single-dose vial/5 ml sterile water for injection (not bacteriostatic water), and roll (not shake) to enhance reconstitution; give over 2-5 mins by direct IV; give within 6 hr of thrombi identification for best results

• Cryoprecipitate or fresh frozen plasma if bleeding occurs

• Heparin therapy after thrombolytic therapy is discontinued, TT or APTT less than 2 × control (about 3-4 hr)

• About 10% of patients have high streptococcal antibody titers, requiring increased loading doses

Perform/provide:

• Bed rest during entire course of treatment; handle patient as little as possible during therapy

• Storage of powder in refrigerator; use within 30 min after reconstitution

• Avoid invasive procedures: inj, rectal temperature

• Treat fever with acetaminophen

• Pressure of 30 sec to minor bleeding sites, 30 min to sites of arterial puncture followed by dressing; inform prescriber if hemostasis not attained; apply pressure dressing

Evaluate:

• Therapeutic response: absence of thrombi formation in MI, improved ventricular function

antihemophilic factor (AHF) (℞)

(an-tee-hee-moe-fill′ik)

antihemophilic factor, Humate-P, Kogenate, profilate OSD, Recombinate, Monoclate-P, Profilate HP, Hemofil M, Koate H.T., Koate H.S., Kryobulin VH*, Monoclate

Func. class.: Hemostatic

Chem. class.: Factor VIII

Action: Necessary for clotting; activates factor X in conjunction with activated factor IX; transforms prothrombin to thrombin

* Available in Canada only

Uses: Hemophilia A, patients with acquired circulating factor VIII inhibitors, factor VIII deficiency

Dosage and routes:

Massive hemorrhage

- *Adult/child:* IV 40-50 U/kg, then 20-25 U/kg q8-12h

Bleeding (frank, overt)

- *Adult/child:* IV 15-25 U/kg, then 8-15 U/kg q8-12h × 4 days

Hemorrhage near vital organs

- *Adult/child:* IV 15 U/kg, then 8 U/kg q8h × 2 days, then 4 U/kg q8h × 2 days

Minor hemorrhage

- *Adult/child:* IV 8-10 u/kg/q24 hr × 2-3 days or 8 U/kg q12h × 2 days, then q24h × 2 days

Joint bleeding

- *Adult/child:* IV 5-10 U/kg q8-12h × 1-2 days

Available forms: Inj IV 250, 500, 1000, 1500 U/vial (number of units noted on label)

Side effects/adverse reactions:

GI: Nausea, vomiting, abdominal cramps, jaundice, ***viral hepatitis***

INTEG: Rash, flushing, *urticaria,* stinging at injection site

CNS: Headache, *lethargy, chills, fever, flushing*

HEMA: ***Thrombosis, hemolysis, AIDS***

CV: Hypotension, tachycardia

RESP: ***Bronchospasm***

Contraindications: Hypersensitivity, monoclonal antibody-derived factor VIII

Precautions: Neonates/infants, hepatic disease, blood types A, B, AB, pregnancy (C), factor VIII inhibitor

Pharmacokinetics:

IV: Half-life 4 hr, terminal 15 hr

Interactions:

- Do not admix with other drugs

NURSING CONSIDERATIONS

Assess:

- Blood studies (coagulation factors assay by % normal: 5% prevents spontaneous hemorrhage, 30%-50% for surgery, 80%-100% for severe hemorrhage)
- I&O, urine color; notify physician if urine becomes orange, red
- Pulse: discontinue infusion if significant increase
- Hct, Coombs' test with blood types A, B, AB
- Test for factor VIII inhibitors before starting treatment, may require concomitant antiinhibitor coagulant complex therapy
- Allergy: fever, rash, itching, jaundice; give diphenhydramine HCl (Benadryl), continue therapy if reaction is mild
- Blood group of patient, donors (if applicable; most factor VIII not from specific blood group donors)
- Bleeding: ankles, knees, elbows, other joints

Administer:

- After rotating gently to mix
- IV slowly, plastic syringe to reconstitute, and administer; adheres to glass; use another needle as a vent when reconstituting
- After dilution with warm NS, D_5W, LR, give within 3 hr
- IV INF: give at ≤2 ml/min if concentration exceeds 34 U/ml or over 3 min if concentration is less than 34 U/ml

Perform/provide:

- Storage in refrigerator; do not freeze; after reconstitution, do not refrigerate; give within 3 hr

Evaluate:

- Therapeutic response: absence of bleeding

Teach patient/family:

- To report any signs of bleeding: gums, under skin, urine, stools, emesis; review methods to prevent bleeding
- To avoid salicylates (increase bleeding tendencies)

• To prepare, administer factor VIII concentrates at first sign of danger
• To advise health professionals of treatment for hemophilia
• Signs of viral hepatitis, AIDS
• That immunization for hepatitis B may be given first
• To report hives, urticaria, chest tightness, hypotension; may be monoclonal antibody-derived factor VIII
• To be checked q2-3mo for HIV screen
• To carry ID describing disease process

antithrombin III, human (℞)

ATnativ, Kybernin, Thrombate III

Func. class.: Antithrombin

Chem. class.: Pooled human plasma

Action: Inactivates thrombin and the activated forms of factors IX, X, XI, XII, resulting in inhibition of coagulation

Uses: Hereditary antithrombin III deficiency in connection with surgical or obstetric procedures or for thromboembolism

Dosage and routes: Dosage is individualized. After first dose, antithrombin III level should increase to about 120% of normal; thereafter maintain at levels >80%; this is usually achieved by administering maintenance doses q24h

Available forms: Lyophilized powder, 50 ml infusion bottles containing 500 IU antithrombin III with 10 ml sterile water for injection; 1000 IU/0.2 ml sterile H_2O for inj

Side effects/adverse reactions:

SYST: Bleeding, surface bleeding, ***anaphylaxis,*** vasodilatory effects

Precautions: Pregnancy (C), lactation, children

Pharmacokinetics: Unknown

Interactions:

• Increased anticoagulant effect: heparin
• Do not administer with other drugs in syringe or solutions

NURSING CONSIDERATIONS

Assess:

• VS, B/P, pulse, respirations, neurologic signs, temperature at least q4h, temperature 104° F (40° C) or indicators of internal bleeding, cardiac rhythm
• For neurologic changes that may indicate intracranial bleeding
• Retroperitoneal bleeding: back pain, leg weakness, diminished pulses

Administer:

• Heparin after fibrinogen level is over 100 mg/dl; heparin infusion to increase PTT to 1.5-2 × baseline for 3-7 days
• After reconstituting 500 IU/10 ml of NS or D_5W; do not shake; rotate to dissolve; allow to warm to room temperature; use within 3 hr of reconstitution; give 50 IU or less/min; do not exceed 100 IU/min
• IV therapy using 0.22 or 0.45 microfilter

Perform/provide:

• Bed rest during entire course of treatment
• Avoidance of venous or arterial puncture, inj, rectal temperature
• Treatment of fever with acetaminophen or aspirin

Evaluate:

• Therapeutic response: absence of thrombi formation

ascorbic acid (vit C) (OTC)

(a-skor'bic)

Apo-C*, ascorbic acid, Ascorbicap, Ascorbic Acid Caplets, Cecon, Cemill, Cenolate, Cetane, Cevalin, Cevi-Bid, Ce-Vi-Sol, C-Crystals, Cebid Timecelles, Cotane, Dull-C, Flavorcee, N'ice Vitamin C Drops, Redoxon*, Sunkist Vitamin C, Vita-C

Func. class.: Vit C, water-soluble vitamin

Action: Needed for wound healing, collagen synthesis, antioxidant, carbohydrate metabolism

Uses: Vit C deficiency, scurvy, delayed wound and bone healing, chronic disease, urine acidification, before gastrectomy

Investigational uses: Acidification of urine, common cold prevention

Dosage and routes:

Scurvy

- *Adult:* PO/SC/IM/IV 100 mg-500 mg qd, then 50 mg or more qd
- *Child:* PO/SC/IM/IV 100-300 mg qd, then 35 mg or more qd

Wound healing/chronic disease/fracture

- *Adult:* SC/IM/IV/PO 200-500 mg qd
- *Child:* SC/IM/IV/PO 100-200 mg added doses

Urine acidification

- *Adult:* 4-12 g qd in divided doses

Available forms: Tabs 25, 50, 100, 250, 500, 1000, 1500 mg; tabs effervescent 1000 mg; tabs chewable 100, 250, 500 mg; tabs timed release 500, 750, 1000, 1500 mg; caps timed release 500 mg; crys 4 g/tsp; powd 4 g/tsp; liq 35 mg/0.6 ml; sol 100 mg/ml; syr 20 mg/ml, 500 mg/5 ml; inj SC, IM, IV 100, 250, 500 mg/ml

Side effects/adverse reactions:

CNS: Headache, insomnia, dizziness, fatigue, flushing

GI: Nausea, vomiting, diarrhea, anorexia, heartburn, cramps

GU: Polyuria, urine acidification, oxalate or urate renal stones

HEMA: ***Hemolytic anemia in patients with G6PD***

Contraindications: None significant

Precautions: Gout, pregnancy (A)

Pharmacokinetics:

PO, INJ: Metabolized in liver, unused amounts excreted in urine (unchanged) and metabolites, crosses placenta, breast milk

Interactions:

- Increased effects of salicylates, oral contraceptives
- Increased side effects of PAS, digitalis, sulfonamides
- Decreased effects of phenothiazines, disulfiram, amphetamines, heparin, coumarin (massive doses)

Syringe compatibility: Metoclopramide

Additive compatibilities: Amikacin, calcium chloride, calcium gluceptate, calcium gluconate, cephalothin, chloramphenicol, chlorpromazine, colistimethate, cyanocobalamin, diphenhydramine, heparin, kanamycin, methicillin, methyldopate, penicillin G potassium, polymyxin B, prednisolone, procaine, prochlorperazine, promethazine, tetracycline, verapamil

Lab test interferences:

- *False positive:* negatives in glucose tests
- *False negative:* occult blood

NURSING CONSIDERATIONS

Assess:

- I&O ratio
- Ascorbic acid levels throughout

treatment if continued deficiency is suspected
• Nutritional status: citrus fruits, vegetables
• Injection sites for inflammation

Administer:
• Undiluted by direct IV 100 mg over at least 1 min
• By IV INF diluted with D_5W, D_5NaCl, NS, LR, Ringer's, sodium lactate and given over 15 min

Evaluate:
• Therapeutic response: absence of anorexia, irritability, pallor, joint pain, hyperkeratosis, petechiae, poor wound healing

Teach patient/family:
• Necessary foods in diet
• That if oral contraceptives are taken, increased levels of vit C are needed
• That smoking decreases vit C levels, not to exceed prescribed dose; increases will be excreted in urine, except time release

asparaginase (℞)

(a-spar'a-gin-ase)
Elspar, Kidrolase*
Func. class.: Antineoplastic
Chem. class.: *E. coli* enzyme

Action: Indirectly inhibits protein synthesis in tumor cells; without amino acid, DNA, RNA synthesis is halted; asparagine, protein synthesis is halted; G_1 phase of cell cycle specific; a nonvesicant

Uses: Acute lymphocytic leukemia in combination with other antineoplastics

Dosage and routes:
In combination
• *Adult:* IV 1000 IU/kg/day × 10 days given over 30 min; IM 6000 IU/m^2/day

Sole induction
• *Adult:* IV 200 IU/kg/day × 28 days

Available forms: Inj 10,000 IU

Side effects/adverse reactions:
SYST: ***Anaphylaxis, hypersensitivity***
HEMA: ***Thrombocytopenia, leukopenia, myelosuppression, anemia, decreased clotting factors***
GI: *Nausea, vomiting, anorexia, cramps, stomatitis,* ***hepatotoxicity, pancreatitis***
GU: Urinary retention, ***renal failure,*** glycosuria, polyuria, azotemia, uric acid neuropathy
INTEG: *Rash,* urticaria, chills, fever
ENDO: Hyperglycemia
RESP: ***Fibrosis, pulmonary infiltrate***
CV: Chest pain
CNS: Neuritis, dizziness, headache, ***coma,*** depression, fatigue, confusion, hallucinations

Contraindications: Hypersensitivity, infants, pregnancy (D), lactation, pancreatitis

Precautions: Renal disease, hepatic disease

Pharmacokinetics: Half-life 4-9 hr, terminal 1.4-1.8 hr

Interactions:
• Decreased action of methotrexate
• Do not use with radiation
• Increased toxicity: vincristine, prednisone
• Synergism in combination with cytarabine, 6-azauridine
• Considered incompatible with other drugs or sol

Lab test interferences:
Decrease: Thyroid function tests

NURSING CONSIDERATIONS

Assess:
• For signs and symptoms of pancreatitis (nausea, vomiting, severe abdominal pain), anaphylaxis (bronchospasm, dyspnea), cyanosis
• CBC, differential, platelet count weekly; withhold drug if WBC is

* Available in Canada only

<4000 or platelet count is <75,000; notify prescriber of these results

• Pulmonary function tests, chest x-ray studies before, during therapy; chest x-ray film should be obtained q2wk during treatment

• Renal function studies: BUN, serum uric acid, ammonia urine CrCl, electrolytes before, during therapy

• I&O ratio; report fall in urine output of 30/ml/hr

• Monitor temperature q4h; may indicate beginning infection

• Liver function tests before, during therapy (bilirubin, AST [SGOT], ALT [SGPT], LDH) as needed or monthly

• RBC, Hct, Hgb, since these may be decreased

• Serum, urine glucose levels

• Bleeding: hematuria, guaiac, bruising or petechiae, mucosa or orifices q8h

• Dyspnea, rales, nonproductive cough, chest pain, tachypnea fatigue, increased pulse, pallor, lethargy, swelling around eyes or lips; anaphylaxis may occur

• Food preferences; list likes, dislikes

• Yellowing of skin and sclera, dark urine, clay-colored stools, itchy skin, abdominal pain, fever, diarrhea

• Local irritation, pain, burning, discoloration at injection site

• Symptoms indicating severe allergic reaction: rash, pruritus, urticaria, purpuric skin lesions, itching, flushing, dyspnea

• Frequency of stools, characteristics: cramping, acidosis; signs of dehydration: rapid respirations, poor skin turgor, decreased urine output, dry skin, restlessness, weakness

Administer:

• After intradermal skin testing and desensitization, give 0.1 ml (2 IU) intradermally after reconstituting with 5 ml sterile H_2O or 0.9% NaCl for injection; then add 0.1 ml of reconstituted drug to 9.9 ml diluent (20 IU/ml); observe for 1 hr, check for wheal

• Allopurinol or sodium bicarbonate to reduce uric acid levels, alkalinization of urine

• IV infusion using 21G, 23G, 25G needle; administer by slow IV infusion via Y-tube or 3-way stopcock of flowing D_5W or NS infusion over 30 min after diluting 10,000 IU/5 ml of sterile H_2O or 0.9% NaCl (no preservatives) (2000 IU/ml); use of filter may be necessary if fibers are present

• Transfusion for anemia

• Antispasmodic

Perform/provide:

• Deep-breathing exercises with patient 3-4 × day; place in semi-Fowler's position

• Increase fluid intake to 2-3 L/day to prevent urate deposits, calculi formation

• Diet low in purines: absence of organ meats (kidney, liver), dried beans, peas to maintain alkaline urine

• Rinsing of mouth 3-4 × day with water, club soda

• Brushing of teeth 2-3 × day with soft brush or cotton-tipped applicators for stomatitis; use unwaxed dental floss

• Warm compresses at injection site for inflammation

• Nutritious diet with iron, vitamin supplements

• HOB raised to facilitate breathing

Evaluate:

• Therapeutic response: decreased exacerbations in ALL

Teach patient/family:

• To report any complaints or side effects to nurse or prescriber

• To report any changes in breathing or coughing

Treatment of anaphylaxis: Administer epinephrine, diphenhydramine, IV corticosteroids

aspirin (OTC)

(as'pir-in)

acetylsalicylic acid Ancasal*, Apo-ASA*, Apo-Asen*, Arthrinol*, Arthrisin*, A.S.A., Aspergum, Aspirin*, Atria S.R.*, Bayer, Bayer Children's Aspirin, Easprin, Ecotrin, Ecotrin Maximum Strength, 8-Hour Bayer Timed Release, Empirin, Entrophen*, Genprin, Maximum Bayer, Norwich Extra-Strength, Novasen*, Sal-Adult*, Sal-Infant*, St. Joseph Children's, Supasa*, Therapy Bayer, ZORprin

Func. class.: Nonnarcotic analgesic, nonsteroidal antiinflammatory, antipyretic, antiplatelet

Chem. class.: Salicylate

Combination products: A.S.A. and Codeine Compound No. 3 Pulvules: codeine 30 mg with aspirin 380 mg, caffeine 30 mg; Ascriptin with Codeine No. 2: aspirin 325 mg with codeine phosphate 15 mg, buffers; Ascriptin with Codeine No. 3: aspirin 325 mg with codeine phosphate 30 mg, buffers; Axotal: aspirin 650 mg with butalbital 50 mg; B-A-C: aspirin 650 mg with butalbital 50 mg, caffeine 40 mg, buffers; B-A-C No. 3: aspirin 325 mg with butalbital 50 mg, caffeine 40 mg, codeine phosphate 30 mg, buffers; BC Powder: aspirin 650 mg with caffeine 32 mg, salicylamide 195 mg; Darvon Compound Pulvules: aspirin 389 mg with caffeine 32.4 mg, propoxyphene HCl 32 mg; Darvon Compound-65 Pulvules, Dolene Compound-65, SK-65-Compound: aspirin 389 mg with caffeine 32.4 mg with propoxyphene HCl 65 mg; Darvon with A.S.A. Pulvules: aspirin 325 mg with propoxyphene HCl 65 mg; Darvon-N and A.S.A.: aspirin 325 mg with propoxyphene napsylate 100 mg; Empirin with Codeine 15 mg No. 2: codeine 15 mg with aspirin 325 mg; Empirin with Codeine 60 mg No. 4: aspirin 325 mg with codeine phosphate 60 mg; Equagesic, Equazine-M, Mepro-Analgesic, Mepor Compound, Micrainin: aspirin 325 mg with meprobamate 200 mg; Fiorinal: aspirin 325 mg with butalbital 50 mg, caffeine 40 mg; Fiorinal with Codeine No. 1: aspirin 325 mg with butalbital 50 mg, caffeine 40 mg, codeine phosphate 7.5 mg; Fiorinal with Codeine No. 2: aspirin 325 mg with butalbital 50 mg, caffeine 40 mg, and codeine phosphate 15 mg; Fiorinal with Codeine No. 3: aspirin 325 mg with butalbital 50 mg, caffeine 40 mg, codeine phosphate 30 mg; Midol Caplets: aspirin 454 mg with caffeine 32.4 mg, cinnamedrine HCl 14.9 mg; Percodan-Demi: aspirin 325 mg with oxycodone HCl 2.25 mg, oxycodone terephthalate 0.19 mg; Trigesic: aspirin 230 mg with acetaminophen 125 mg, caffeine 30 mg; Vanquish Caplets: aspirin 227 mg with acetaminophen 194 mg, caffeine 30 mg, buffers

Action: Blocks pain impulses in CNS that occur in response to inhibition of prostaglandin synthesis; antipyretic action results from vasodilation of peripheral vessels; decreases platelet aggregation

Uses: Mild to moderate pain or fever including rheumatoid arthritis, osteoarthritis, thromboembolic disorders, transient ischemic attacks in men, rheumatic fever, postmyocardial infarction, prophylaxis of myocardial infarction

* Available in Canada only

Dosage and routes:

Arthritis

• *Adult:* PO 2.6-5.2 g/day in divided doses q4-6h

• *Child:* PO 90-130 mg/kg/day in divided doses q4-6h

Pain/fever

• *Adult:* PO/REC 325-650 mg q4h prn, not to exceed 4 g/day

• *Child:* PO/REC 40-100 mg/kg/day in divided doses q4-6h prn

Thromboembolic disorders

• *Adult:* PO 325-650 mg/day or bid

Transient ischemic attacks

• *Adult:* PO 650 mg qid or 325 mg qid

Available forms: Tabs 65, 81, 325, 500, 650, 975 mg; chewable tabs 81 mg; caps 325, 500 mg; tabs controlled-release 800 mg; tabs time-release 650 mg; supp 60, 120, 125, 130, 195, 200, 300, 325, 600, 650 mg, 1.2 g; cream; gum 227.5 mg

Side effects/adverse reactions:

HEMA: ***Thrombocytopenia, agranulocytosis, leukopenia, neutropenia, hemolytic anemia,*** increased pro-time, aPTT, bleeding time

CNS: Stimulation, drowsiness, dizziness, confusion, ***convulsion,*** headache, flushing, hallucinations, ***coma***

GI: Nausea, vomiting, ***GI bleeding,*** diarrhea, heartburn, anorexia, ***hepatitis***

INTEG: Rash, urticaria, bruising

EENT: Tinnitus, hearing loss

CV: Rapid pulse, pulmonary edema

RESP: Wheezing, hyperpnea

ENDO: Hypoglycemia, hyponatremia, hypokalemia

Contraindications: Hypersensitivity to salicylates, tartrazine (FDC yellow dye #5), GI bleeding, bleeding disorders, children <12 yr, children with flulike symptoms, pregnancy (D), lactation, Vit K deficiency, peptic ulcer

Precautions: Anemia, hepatic disease, renal disease, Hodgkin's disease, pre/postoperatively

Pharmacokinetics: Well absorbed PO; enteric and rectal products may be erratic

PO: Onset 15-30 min, peak 1-2 hr, duration 4-6 hr

REC: Onset slow, duration 4-6 hr; Metabolized by liver, inactive metabolites excreted by kidneys, crosses placenta, excreted in breast milk, half-life 1-3½ hr; up to 30 hrs in large doses

Interactions:

• Decreased effects of aspirin: antacids, steroids, urinary alkalizers

• Increased bleeding: alcohol, heparin, valproic acid, plicamycin, cefamandole

• Increased effects of anticoagulants, insulin, methotrexate, thrombolytic agents, penicillins, phenytoin, valproic acid, oral hypoglycemics, sulfonamides

• Increased salicylate levels: urinary acidifiers

• Decreased effects of probenecid, spironolactone, sulfinpyrazone, sulfonylamides

• Toxic effects: PABA, furosemide, carbonic anhydrase inhibitors

• Decreased blood sugar levels: salicylates

• Gastric ulcer: steroids, antiinflammatories, nonsteroidal antiinflammatories

• Ototoxicity: vancomycin

Lab test interferences:

Increase: Coagulation studies, liver function studies, serum uric acid, amylase, CO_2, urinary protein

Decrease: Serum K, PBI, cholesterol

Interfere: Urine catecholamines, pregnancy test, urine glucose tests (Clinistix, Tes-Tape)

NURSING CONSIDERATIONS

Assess:

• Liver function studies: AST

(SGOT), ALT (SGPT), bilirubin, creatinine if patient is on long-term therapy
• Renal function studies: BUN, urine creatinine if patient is on long-term therapy
• Blood studies: CBC, Hct, Hgb, pro-time if patient is on long-term therapy
• I&O ratio; decreasing output may indicate renal failure (long-term therapy)
• Hepatotoxicity: dark urine, clay-colored stools, yellowing of skin, sclera, itching, abdominal pain, fever, diarrhea if patient is on long-term therapy
• Allergic reactions: rash, urticaria; if these occur, drug may have to be discontinued
• Renal dysfunction: decreased urine output
• Ototoxicity: tinnitus, ringing, roaring in ears; audiometric testing needed before, after long-term therapy
• Visual changes: blurring, halos; corneal, retinal damage
• Edema in feet, ankles, legs
• Drug history; many drug interactions
• Pain: Location, duration, type, intensity, prior to dose and 1 hour after
• Musculoskeletal status: ROM prior to dose
• Fever; length of time and related symptoms

Administer:
• To patient crushed or whole; chewable tablets may be chewed (do not crush enteric product)
• With food or milk to decrease gastric symptoms; give 30 min before or 2 hr after meals

Evaluate:
• Therapeutic response: decreased pain, inflammation, fever

Teach patient/family:
• To report any symptoms of hepatotoxicity, renal toxicity, visual changes, ototoxicity, allergic reactions, bleeding (long-term therapy)
• To take with 8 oz H_2O and sit upright for ½ hour after dose
• Not to exceed recommended dosage; acute poisoning may result
• To read label on other OTC drugs; many contain aspirin
• That the therapeutic response takes 2 wk (arthritis)
• To report tinnitus, confusion, diarrhea, sweating, hyperventilation
• To avoid alcohol ingestion; GI bleeding may occur
• That patients who have allergies may develop allergic reactions
• To avoid buffered or effervescent products
• Not to be given to children; Reye's syndrome may develop

Treatment of overdose: Lavage, activated charcoal, monitor electrolytes, VS

astemizole (℞)

(a-stem'i-zole)
Hismanal
Func. class.: Antihistamine
Chem. class.: H_1-histamine antagonist

Action: Acts on blood vessels, GI, respiratory system by competing with histamine for H_1-receptor site; decreases allergic response by blocking pharmacologic effects of histamine

Uses: Rhinitis, allergy symptoms

Dosage and routes:
• *Adult and child >12 yr:* PO 10 mg qd; to reduce time to steady state may take 30 mg day 1, 20 mg day 2, followed by 10 mg daily

Available forms: Tabs 10 mg

A

Side effects/adverse reactions:
GU: Frequency, dysuria, urinary retention, impotence
HEMA: ***Hemolytic anemia, thrombocytopenia, leukopenia, agranulocytosis, pancytopenia***
RESP: Thickening of bronchial secretions, dry nose, throat
GI: Nausea, diarrhea, abdominal pain, vomiting, constipation
CNS: Headache, stimulation, drowsiness, sedation, fatigue, confusion, blurred vision, tinnitus, restlessness, tremors, paradoxical excitation in children or elderly
INTEG: Rash, eczema, photosensitivity, urticaria
CV: Hypotension, palpitations, bradycardia, tachycardia, ***dysrhythmias*** (rare)

Contraindications: Hypersensitivity, newborn or premature infants, lactation, severe hepatic disease

Precautions: Pregnancy (C), elderly, children, respiratory disease, narrow-angle glaucoma, prostatic hypertrophy, bladder neck obstruction, asthma, elderly

Pharmacokinetics:
PO: Peak 1-2 hr, 97% bound to plasma proteins; half-life is biphasic 3½ hr, 16-23 hr

Interactions:
- Increased CNS depression: alcohol, other CNS depressants, procarbazine
- Increased anticholinergic effects: MAOIs
- Decreased action of oral anticoagulants
- Serious CV reactions: ketoconazole, itraconazole, erythromycin
- Avoid use with antifungals, macrolide antibiotics

Lab test interferences:
False negative: Skin allergy tests

NURSING CONSIDERATIONS

Assess:
- I&O ratio: be alert for urinary retention, frequency, dysuria, especially elderly; drug should be discontinued if these occur
- CBC during long-term therapy
- Respiratory status: rate, rhythm, increase in bronchial secretions, wheezing, chest tightness

Administer:
- On empty stomach 1 hr before or 2 hr after meals

Perform/provide:
- Hard candy, gum, frequent rinsing of mouth for dryness
- Storage in tight, light-resistant container

Evaluate:
- Therapeutic response: absence of running or congested nose or rashes

Teach patient/family:
- All aspects of drug use; to notify prescriber if confusion, sedation, hypotension occur
- To avoid driving, other hazardous activity if drowsiness occurs
- To avoid alcohol, other CNS depressants
- Not to exceed recommended dose; dysrhythmias may occur

Treatment of overdose: Administer ipecac syrup or lavage, diazepam, vasopressors, barbiturates (short-acting)

---

atenolol (℞)

(a-ten'oh-lole)

Apo-Atenol*, atenolol, Novo-Atenol*, Tenormin

Func. class.: Antihypertensive, antianginal

Chem. class.: β-Blocker, β-1, 2 blocker (high doses)

Combination products: Tenoretic 50: atenolol 50 mg with chlorthalidone 25 mg; Tenorectic 100: atenolol 100 mg with chlorthalidone 25 mg

Action: Competitively blocks stimulation of β-adrenergic receptor within vascular smooth muscle; produces negative chronotropic activity, positive inotropic activity (decreases rate of SA node discharge, increases recovery time), slows conduction of AV node, decreases heart rate, decreases O_2 consumption in myocardium; also decreases renin-aldosterone-angiotensin system at high doses, inhibits β-2 receptors in bronchial system at higher doses

Uses: Mild to moderate hypertension, prophylaxis of angina pectoris, suspected or known myocardial infarction

Investigational uses: Dysrhythmia, mitral valve prolapse, pheochromocytoma, hypertrophic cardiomyopathy, vascular headaches, thyrotoxicosis, tremors

Dosage and routes:

• *Adult:* IV 5 mg, repeat in 10 min if initial dose is well tolerated, then start PO dose 10 min after last IV dose

• *Adult:* PO 50 mg qd, increasing q1-2wk to 100 mg qd; may increase to 200 mg qd for angina

Available forms: Tabs 50, 100 mg

Side effects/adverse reactions:

CV: ***Profound hypotension, bradycardia, CHF,*** *cold extremities, postural hypotension, 2nd or 3rd degree heart block*

CNS: Insomnia, fatigue, dizziness, mental changes, memory loss, hallucinations, depression, lethargy, drowsiness, strange dreams, catatonia

GI: Nausea, diarrhea, vomiting, ***mesenteric arterial thrombosis, ischemic colitis***

INTEG: Rash, fever, alopecia

HEMA: ***Agranulocytosis, thrombocytopenia, purpura***

EENT: Sore throat, dry burning eyes

GU: Impotence

ENDO: Increased hypoglycemic response to insulin

RESP: ***Bronchospasm,*** dyspnea, wheezing

Contraindications: Hypersensitivity to β-blockers, cardiogenic shock, 2nd or 3rd degree heart block, sinus bradycardia, CHF, cardiac failure

Precautions: Major surgery, pregnancy (C), lactation, diabetes mellitus, renal disease, thyroid disease, COPD, asthma, well-compensated heart failure

Pharmacokinetics:

PO: Peak 2-4 hr; half-life 6-7 hr, excreted unchanged in urine, protein binding 5%-15%

Interactions:

• Increased hypotension, bradycardia: reserpine, hydralazine, methyldopa, prazosin, anticholinergics, digoxin

• Decreased antihypertensive effects: indomethacin

• Increased hypoglycemic effect: insulin

• Mutual inhibition: sympathomimetics (cough, cold preparations)

• Decreased bronchodilation: theophyllines, β_2-agonists

• Paradoxical hypertension: clonidine

• Incompatible with any other drug in sol or syringe

Lab test interferences:

Interference: Glucose/insulin tolerance tests

NURSING CONSIDERATIONS

Assess:

• I&O, weight daily

• B/P, pulse q4h; note rate, rhythm, quality

• Apical/radial pulse before administration; notify prescriber of any significant changes

• Baselines in renal, liver function tests before therapy begins

• Edema in feet, legs daily

• Skin turgor, dryness of mucous membranes for hydration status

Administer:

• PO ac, hs, tablet may be crushed or swallowed whole

• Reduced dosage in renal dysfunction

• IV undiluted by direct IV over 5 min or diluted in 10-50 ml of D_5W, D_5/NaCl, or NS and give as an infusion at prescribed rate

Perform/provide:

• Storage protected from light, moisture; placed in cool environment

Evaluate:

• Therapeutic response: decreased B/P after 1-2 wk

Teach patient/family:

• Not to discontinue drug abruptly; taper over 2 wk

• Not to use OTC products unless directed by prescriber

• To report bradycardia, dizziness, confusion, depression, fever

• To take pulse at home; advise when to notify prescriber

• To avoid alcohol, smoking, sodium intake

• To comply with weight control, dietary adjustments, modified exercise program

• To carry Medic Alert ID to identify drug that you are taking, allergies

• To avoid hazardous activities if dizziness is present

Treatment of overdose: Lavage, IV atropine for bradycardia, IV theophylline for bronchospasm, digitalis, O_2, diuretic for cardiac failure, hemodialysis

(a-t

Mepro

Func. cla

Chem. class..

derivative, analo

Action: Interferes wit

synthesis in protozoa

Uses: *Pneumocystis carini*

tions not sensitive to trimethop

sulfamethoxazole

Dosage and routes:

• *Adult:* 750 mg with food tid for 21 days

Available forms: Tabs 250 mg

Side effects/adverse reactions:

CV: Hypotension

HEMA: Anemia, leukopenia

INTEG: Pruritus, urticaria, rash, oral monilia

GI: Nausea, vomiting, diarrhea, anorexia, increased AST and ALT, acute pancreatitis, constipation, abdominal pain

CNS: Dizziness, headache, anxiety

META: Hyperkalemia, hyperglycemia, hyponatremia

Contraindications: Hypersensitivity or history of developing life-threatening allergic reactions to any component of the formulation

Precautions: Blood dyscrasias, hepatic disease, diabetes mellitus, pregnancy (C), lactation, children, elderly

Pharmacokinetics: Excreted unchanged in feces (94%), highly protein bound

Interactions:

Use caution when administering concurrently with other highly plasma protein–bound drugs with narrow therapeutic indices

NURSING CONSIDERATIONS

Assess:

• Blood studies, blood glucose, ACBC, platelets

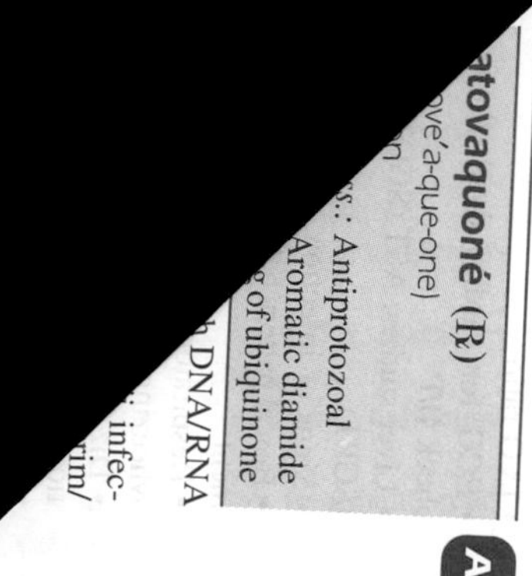

notify all people giving drugs

Administer:

- With food because of increased absorption of the drug and higher plasma concentrations

Evaluate:

- Therapeutic response: decreased temperature, ability to breathe

Teach patient/family:

- To report sore throat, fever, fatigue; may indicate superinfection
- To take with food to increase plasma concentrations

---

atracurium (℞)

(a-tra-cyoor′ee-um)

Tracrium

Func. class.: Neuromuscular blocker (nondepolarizing)

Chem. class.: Biquaternary ammonium ester

Action: Inhibits transmission of nerve impulses by binding with cholinergic receptor sites, antagonizing action of acetylcholine

Uses: Facilitation of endotracheal intubation, skeletal muscle relaxation during mechanical ventilation, surgery, or general anesthesia

Dosage and routes:

- *Adult:* IV BOL 0.4-0.5 mg/kg, then

ng/kg 20-45 min after needed for prolonged

orms: Inj IV 10 mg/ml

/adverse reactions:

cardia, tachycardia, increase B/P

onged apnea, broncho-anosis, respiratory de-

eased secretions

sh, flushing, pruritus, ur-

lications: Hypersensi-

ons: Pregnancy (C), cardiac disease, lactation, children <2 yr, electrolyte imbalances, dehydration, neuromuscular disease, respiratory disease

Pharmacokinetics:

IV: Onset 2 min, duration 20-60 min; half-life 2 min, 29 min (terminal), excreted in urine, feces (metabolites), crosses placenta

Interactions:

- Increased neuromuscular blockade: aminoglycosides, clindamycin, lincomycin, quinidine, local anesthetics, polymyxin antibiotics, lithium, narcotic analgesics, thiazides, enflurane, isoflurane
- Dysrhythmias: theophylline

Y-site compatibilities: Aminophylline, cefazolin, cefuroxime, cimetidine, cotrimoxazole, dobutamine, dopamine, epinephrine, esmolol, fentanyl, gentamicin, heparin, hydrocortisone sodium succinate, isoproterenol, lorazepam midazolam, morphine, nitroglycerine, ranitidine, sodium nitroprusside, vancomycin

NURSING CONSIDERATIONS

Assess:

- For electrolyte imbalances (K, Mg); may lead to increased action of this drug
- Vital signs (B/P, pulse, respirations, airway) until fully recovered;

---

* Available in Canada only

rate, depth, pattern of respirations, strength of hand grip
• I&O ratio; check for urinary retention, frequency, hesitancy
• Recovery: decreased paralysis of face, diaphragm, leg, arm, rest of body
• Allergic reactions: rash, fever, respiratory distress, pruritus; drug should be discontinued

Administer:
• Using nerve stimulator by anesthesiologist to determine neuromuscular blockade
• Anticholinesterase to reverse neuromuscular blockade
• IV undiluted by direct IV over 5 min, or diluted in 10-50 ml of D_5W, ½ NaCl or NS and give as an infusion at prescribed rate, administered
• By slow IV over 1-2 min (only by qualified person); do not administer IM
• Only slightly discolored solution

Perform/provide:
• Storage in light-resistant area
• Reassurance if communication is difficult during recovery from neuromuscular blockade

Evaluate:
• Therapeutic response: paralysis of jaw, eyelid, head, neck, rest of body

Treatment of overdose: Edrophonium or neostigmine, atropine, monitor VS; mechanical ventilation

atropine (℞)

(a'troe-peen)
Atropair, Atro-Pen, Atropisol, Isopto-Atropine, I-Tropina, Minims Atopine*, Ocu-Tropine

Func. class.: Anticholinergic parasympatholytic

Chem. class.: Belladonna alkaloid

Combination products: Atropine, Demerol Injection: meperidine HCl 50 mg/ml with atropine sulfate 0.4 mg/ml; Atropine, Demerol Injection: meperidine HCl 75 mg/ml with atropine sulfate 0.4 mg/ml

Action: Blocks acetylcholine at parasympathetic neuroeffector sites; increases cardiac output, heart rate by blocking vagal stimulation in heart; dries secretions by blocking vagus

Uses: Bradycardia, bradydysrhythmia, anticholinesterase insecticide poisoning, blocking cardiac vagal reflexes, decreasing secretions before surgery, antispasmodic with GU, biliary surgery, bronchodilator

Dosage and routes:

Bradycardia/bradydysrhythmias
• *Adult:* IV BOL 0.5-1 mg given q3-5min, not to exceed 2 mg
• *Child:* IV BOL 0.01-0.03 mg/kg up to 0.4 mg or 0.3 mg/m^2; may repeat q4-6h

Insecticide poisoning
• *Adult and child:* IM/IV 2 mg qh until muscarinic symptoms disappear, may need 6 mg qh

Presurgery
• *Adult:* SC/IM/IV 0.4-0.6 mg before anesthesia
• *Child:* SC 0.1-0.4 mg 30 min before surgery

Available forms: Inj 0.05, 0.1, 0.3, 0.4, 0.5, 0.8, 1 mg/ml, 2 mg/0.7 ml autoinjector tabs 0.4 mg; tabs sol 0.4, 0.6 mg

Side effects/adverse reactions:
GU: Retention, hesitancy, impotence, dysuria
CNS: Headache, dizziness, involuntary movement, confusion, psychosis, anxiety, coma, flushing, drowsiness, insomnia, weakness
GI: Dry mouth, nausea, vomiting, abdominal pain, anorexia, constipation, paralytic ileus, abdominal distention, altered taste
CV: Hypotension, paradoxical bradycardia, angina, PVCs, hypertension, tachycardia, ectopic ventricular beats
INTEG: Rash, urticaria, contact dermatitis, dry skin, flushing
EENT: Blurred vision, photophobia, glaucoma, eye pain, pupil dilation, nasal congestion
MISC: Suppression of lactation, decreased sweating

Contraindications: Hypersensitivity to belladonna alkaloids, angle-closure glaucoma, GI obstructions, myasthenia gravis, thyrotoxicosis, ulcerative colitis, prostatic hypertrophy, tachycardia/tachydysrhythmias, asthma, acute hemorrhage, hepatic disease, myocardial ischemia

Precautions: Pregnancy (C), renal disease, lactation, CHF, tachydysrhythmias, hyperthyroidism, COPD, hepatic disease, child <6 yr, hypertension, elderly, intraabdominal infections, Down syndrome, spastic paralysis, gastric ulcer

Pharmacokinetics: Well absorbed PO, IM, SC; half-life 13-40 hours, excreted by kidneys unchanged (70%-90% in 24 hr); metabolized in liver, 40%-50% crosses placenta, excreted in breast milk
IV: Peak 2-4 min, duration 4-6 hr
IM/SC: Onset 15-50 min; peak 30 min, duration 4-6 hr
PO: Onset ½ hour; peak ½-1 hr; duration 4-6 hr

Interactions:
- Decreases effect of atropine; antacids
- Decreased effects of phenothiazines
- Increased anticholinergic effects of anticholinergics, tricylic antidepressants, amantadine, MAOIs, quinidine

Syringe compatibilities: Benzquinamide, butorphanol, chlorpromazine, cimetidine, dimenhydrinate, diphenhydramine, droperidol, fentanyl, glycopyrrolate, heparin, hydromorphone, hydroxyzine, meperidine, metoclopramide, midazolam, morphine, nalbuphine, pentazocine, prochlorperazine, promazine, promethazine, propiomazine, ranitidine, scopolamine

Y-site compatibilities: Amrinone, famotidine, heparin, hydrocortisone sodium succinate, nafcillin, potassium chloride

Additive compatibilities: Dobutamine, netilmicin, sodium bicarbonate, verapamil

NURSING CONSIDERATIONS

Assess:
- I&O ratio; check for urinary retention, daily output
- ECG for ectopic ventricular beats, PVC, tachycardia
- For bowel sounds; check for constipation
- Respiratory status: rate, rhythm, cyanosis, wheezing, dyspnea, engorged neck veins
- Increased intraocular pressure: eye pain, nausea, vomiting, blurred vision, increased tearing
- Cardiac rate: rhythm, character, B/P continuously
- Allergic reaction: rash, urticaria

Administer:
- IV undiluted or diluted with 10 ml sterile H_2O, give at 0.6 mg/min,

* Available in Canada only

give through Y-tube or 3-way stopcock; do not add to IV sol; may cause paradoxical bradycardia lasting 2 min
• Increased bulk, water in diet if constipation occurs
• PO ½ hour ac
• IM; atropine flush may occur in children and is not harmful

Perform/provide:
• Sugarless hard candy, gum, frequent rinsing of mouth for dryness

Evaluate:
• Therapeutic response: decreased dysrhythmias, increased heart rate, secretions, GI, GU spasms, bronchodilation

Teach patient/family:
• To report blurred vision, chest pain, allergic reactions
• Not to perform strenuous activity in high temperatures; heat stroke may result
• To take as prescribed; not to skip doses
• Not to operate machinery if drowsiness occurs
• Not to take OTC products without approval of prescriber

Treatment of overdose: O_2, artificial ventilation, ECG; administer dopamine for circulatory depression; administer diazepam or thiopental for convulsions; assess need for antidysrhythmics

atropine (optic) (℞)

(a'troe-peen)

Atropine-1, Atropine Care Ophthalmic, Atropine Sulfate Ophthalmic, Atropine Sulfate S.O.P., Atropisol, Isopto Atropine

Func. class.: Mydriatic

Chem. class.: Belladonna alkaloid

Action: Blocks response of iris sphincter muscle, ciliary muscle of the lens to cholinergic stimulation, resulting in dilation, paralysis of accommodation

Uses: Iritis, cycloplegic refraction

Dosage and routes:
• *Adult:* INSTILL SOL 1-2 gtt of a 1% sol qd-tid for iritis or 1 hr before refracting (cycloplegic refraction); INSTILL OINT bid-tid
• *Child:* INSTILL SOL 1-2 gtt of a 0.5% sol qd-tid for iritis or bid × 1-3 days before exam (cycloplegic refraction); INSTILL OINT qd-bid 2-3 days before exam

Available forms: Oint 1%; sol 0.5%, 1%, 2%

Side effects/adverse reactions:

SYST: Tachycardia, confusion, fever, flushing, dry skin, dry mouth, abdominal discomfort, headache, irritability (infants: bladder distention, irregular pulse, respiratory depression)

EENT: Photophobia, blurred vision, increased intraocular pressure, conjunctivitis

Contraindications: Hypersensitivity, infants <3 mo, open or narrow-angle glaucoma, conjunctivitis

Precautions: Elderly, pregnancy, lactation, Down syndrome, children

Pharmacokinetics:

INSTILL: Peak 30-40 min (mydriasis), 60-180 min (cycloplegia), duration 6-12 days

NURSING CONSIDERATIONS

Assess:
• Eye pain; discontinue use if pain occurs

Evaluate:
• Therapeutic response: decrease in inflammation (iritis) or cycloplegic refraction

Teach patient/family:
• To report change in vision; blurring or loss of sight; trouble breathing; sweating; flushing
• Method of instillation: pressure on

lacrimal sac for 1 min; do not touch dropper to eye
- That blurred vision will decrease with repeated use of drug
- Not to do hazardous things until able to see
- To omit next instillation if side effects are present
- To wait 5 min to use other drops
- Not to blink more than usual

auranofin (℞)

(au-rane′oh-fin)
Ridaura
Func. class.: Antiinflammatory
Chem. class.: Active gold compound (29%)

Action: Antiinflammatory action unknown; may decrease phagocytosis, lysosomal activity, or prostaglandin synthesis; decreases concentration of rheumatoid factor, immunoglobulins
Uses: Rheumatoid arthritis
Dosage and routes:
- *Adult:* PO 6 mg qd or 3 mg bid; may increase to 9 mg/day after 3 mo

Available forms: Caps 3 mg
Side effects/adverse reactions:
HEMA: ***Thrombocytopenia, agranulocytosis, aplastic anemia, leukopenia, eosinophilia, neutropenia***
INTEG: Rash, pruritus, dermatitis, ***exfoliative dermatitis***, urticaria, alopecia, photosensitivity
CNS: Dizziness, confusion, hallucinations, ***seizures,*** EEG abnormalities
GI: Diarrhea, abdominal cramping, stomatitis, nausea, vomiting, enterocolitis, anorexia, flatulence, metallic taste, dyspepsia, jaundice, increased AST, ALT, glossitis, gingivitis, melena, constipation
GU: ***Proteinuria, hematuria,*** increased BUN, creatinine, vaginitis
MISC: Iritis, corneal ulcers, gold deposits in ocular tissues
RESP: ***Interstitial pneumonitis, fibrosis,*** cough, dyspnea
Contraindications: Hypersensitivity to gold, necrotizing enterocolitis, bone marrow aplasia, child <6 yr, lactation, pulmonary fibrosis, exfoliative dermatitis, blood dyscrasias, recent radiation therapy, renal/hepatic disease, marked hypertension, uncontrolled CHF
Precautions: Elderly, CHF, diabetes mellitus, allergic conditions, ulcerative colitis, renal disease, liver disease, pregnancy (C)
Pharmacokinetics:
PO: Absorbed by GI tract, peak 2 hr, steady state 8-16 wk, excreted in urine, feces
Interactions:
- Do not use with penicillamine or antimalarials
- May increase levels of phenytoin

Lab test interferences:
False positive: TB test
NURSING CONSIDERATIONS
Assess:
- Respiratory status: dyspnea, wheezing; if respiratory problems occur, drug should be discontinued
- I&O ratio
- Urine: hematuria, proteinuria; increased BUN, creatinine may require decrease in dosage
- Platelet counts qmo; drug should be discontinued if <100,000/mm^3
- Hepatic test: ALT (SGOT), AST (SGPT), alk phosphatase
- Diarrhea stools; if severe, drug should be discontinued
- Allergy: rash, dermatitis, pruritus; drug should be discontinued if any of these occur
- Gold toxicity: decreased Hgb, WBC <4000/mm^3, granulocytes <1500/mm^3, platelets <150,000/mm^3, severe diarrhea, stomatitis, hematuria, rash, itching, proteinuria

Administer:
- Bid or may give as single dose qAM with food or drink

Evaluate:
- Therapeutic response: ability to move joints with less pain

Teach patient/family
- That drug must be taken as prescribed to be useful, to obtain lab work monthly
- That diarrhea is common, but if blood appears in stools or urine, notify prescriber at once; that patient should check for bruising, petechiae, bleeding gums
- To report abnormal skin conditions, stomatitis, fatigue, jaundice; may indicate blood dyscrasias
- To avoid exposure to sunlight or ultraviolet light; to use sunscreen to prevent burns
- That therapeutic effect may take 3-4 mo
- To use dilute hydrogen peroxide for mild stomatitis, avoid hot spicy foods, food with high acidic content; use soft toothbrush, rinse more frequently, floss daily
- That contraception should be used during treatment

aurothioglucose/ gold sodium thiomalate (℞)

(aur-oh-thye-oh-gloo′kose)
Solganal/Myochrysine

Func. class.: Antiinflammatory
Chem. class.: Active gold compound (50%)

Action: Antiinflammatory action unknown; may decrease phagocytosis, lysosomal activity, prostaglandin synthesis

Uses: Rheumatoid arthritis, psoriatic arthritis

Dosage and routes:
- *Adult:* IM 10 mg, then 25 mg qwk × 2-3 wk, then 50 mg/wk until total of 1 g is administered, then 25-50 mg q3-4wk if there is improvement without toxicity (aurothioglucose) total of 800 mg-1 g
- *Adult:* IM 10 mg, then 25 mg after 1 wk, then 50 mg qwk for total of 14-20 doses, then 50 mg q2wk × 4, then 50 mg q3wk × 4, then 50 mg qmo for maintenance (gold sodium thiomalate)
- *Child 6-12 yr:* IM 1 mg/kg/wk × 20 wk, or ¼ of adult dose (aurothioglucose)
- *Child:* IM 1 mg/kg/wk × 20 wk, then q3-4wk if improvement without toxicity (gold sodium thiomalate) not to exceed 2.5 mg

Available forms: IM inj 50 mg/ml, 25 mg/ml

Side effects/adverse reactions:

EENT: Iritis, corneal ulcers

HEMA: ***Thrombocytopenia, agranulocytosis, aplastic anemia, leukopenia, eosinophilia, neutropenia***

INTEG: Rash, pruritus, dermatitis, urticaria, alopecia, photosensitivity, ***exfoliative dermatitis, angioedema***

GI: Stomatitis, nausea, vomiting, metallic taste, jaundice, ***hepatitis,*** diarrhea, cramping, flatulence

GU: Proteinuria, hematuria, ***nephrosis, tubular necrosis***

RESP: Interstitial pneumonitis, pharyngitis, ***pulmonary fibrosis***

CNS: Dizziness, EEG abnormalities, ***encephalitis,*** confusion, hallucinations

CV: Bradycardia, rapid pulse

SYST: ***Anaphylaxis***

Contraindications: Hypersensitivity to gold, systemic lupus erythematosus, uncontrolled diabetes mellitus, marked hypertension, recent radiation therapy, CHF, lactation, renal disease, liver disease

Precautions: Decreased tolerance in elderly, children, blood dyscrasias, pregnancy (C)
Pharmacokinetics:
IM: Peak 4-6 hr; half-life 3-27 days; excreted in urine, feces; half-life increases up to 168 days with 11th dose
Interactions:
- Increased blood dyscrasias: antimalarials, cytotoxic agents, immunosuppressants, oxyphenbutazone, phenylbutazone, penicillamine

Lab test interferences:
False positive: TB test

NURSING CONSIDERATIONS

Assess:
- Respiratory status: dyspnea, wheezing; if respiratory problems occur, drug should be discontinued
- I&O ratio
- For pregnancy before administration; do not give in pregnancy
- Urine: hematuria, proteinuria, increased BUN, creatinine may require decrease in dosage
- Platelet counts qmo; drug should be discontinued if <100,000/mm^3
- Hepatic test: ALT, AST, alk phosphatase
- Diarrhea stools; if severe, drug should be discontinued
- Allergy: rash, dermatitis, pruritus; drug should be discontinued if any of these occur
- Gold toxicity: decreased Hgb, WBC <4000/mm^3, granulocytes <1500/mm^3, platelets <150,000/mm^3, severe diarrhea, stomatitis, hematuria, rash, itching, proteinuria

Administer:
- Bid or may give as single dose qAM
- Deep IM, never IV
- Slowly, keep patient recumbent for 10 min after injection, monitor for transient reaction

Evaluate:
- Therapeutic response: ability to move joints with less pain

Teach patient/family
- That drug must be taken as prescribed to be useful
- To obtain lab work monthly
- That diarrhea is common, but if blood appears in stools or urine, notify prescriber at once; that patient should check for bruising, petechiae, bleeding gums
- To report skin conditions, stomatitis, fatigue, jaundice, which may indicate blood dyscrasias; report fever, chills, which may indicate infection
- That therapeutic effect may take 3-4 months
- To use dilute hydrogen peroxide for mild stomatitis, avoid hot spicy foods, food with high acidic content; use soft toothbrush, rinse more frequently
- That contraception should be used during treatment
- To use sunscreen to prevent burns

---

azatadine (℞)

(a-za'ta-deen)
Optimine
Func. class.: Antihistamine
Chem. class.: Piperidine H_1-receptor antagonist

Action: Acts on blood vessels, GI, respiratory system by competing with histamine for H_1-receptor site; decreases allergic response by blocking histamine
Uses: Allergy symptoms, rhinitis, chronic urticaria
Dosage and routes:
- *Adult:* PO 1-2 mg bid, not to exceed 4 mg/day

Available forms: Tabs 1 mg
Side effects/adverse reactions:
CNS: Dizziness, drowsiness, poor coordination, fatigue, anxiety, eu-

phoria, confusion, paresthesia, neuritis, sweating, chills

CV: Hypotension, palpitations, tachycardia

RESP: Increased thick secretions, wheezing, chest tightness

HEMA: ***Thrombocytopenia, agranulocytosis, hemolytic anemia***

GI: Constipation, dry mouth, nausea, vomiting, anorexia, diarrhea

INTEG: Rash, urticaria, photosensitivity

GU: Retention, dysuria, frequency, impotence

EENT: Blurred vision, dilated pupils, tinnitus, nasal stuffiness, dry nose, throat, mouth

Contraindications: Hypersensitivity to H_1-receptor antagonist, acute asthma attack, lower respiratory tract disease, child <12 yr

Precautions: Increased intraocular pressure, renal disease, cardiac disease, bronchial asthma, seizure disorder, stenosed peptic ulcers, hyperthyroidism, prostatic hypertrophy, bladder neck obstruction, pregnancy (B), lactation, elderly

Pharmacokinetics:

PO: Peak 4 hr; metabolized in liver, excreted by kidneys, crosses placenta, crosses blood-brain barrier, minimally bound to plasma proteins, half-life 9-12 hr

Interactions:

- Increased CNS depression: barbiturates, narcotics, hypnotics, tricyclic antidepressants, alcohol
- Decreased effect of oral anticoagulants, heparin
- Increased effect of azatadine: MAOIs

Lab test interferences:

False negative: Skin allergy tests

NURSING CONSIDERATIONS

Assess:

- I&O ratio; be alert for urinary retention, frequency, dysuria, especially elderly; drug should be discontinued if these occur
- CBC during long-term therapy
- Blood dyscrasias: thrombocytopenia, agranulocytosis; these occur rarely
- Respiratory status: rate, rhythm, increase or thickening in bronchial secretions, wheezing, chest tightness

Administer:

- With meals if GI symptoms occur; absorption may slightly decrease

Perform/provide:

- Hard candy, gum, frequent rinsing of mouth for dryness
- Storage in tight container at room temperature

Evaluate:

- Therapeutic response: absence of running or congested nose; rash

Teach patient/family:

- All aspects of drug use; to notify prescriber if confusion, sedation, or hypotension occurs
- To avoid driving or other hazardous activities if drowsiness occurs
- To avoid concurrent use of alcohol, other CNS depressants

Treatment of overdose: Administer ipecac syrup or lavage, diazepam, vasopressors, barbiturates (short-acting)

azathioprine (℞)

(ay-za-thye′oh-preen)

Imuran

Func. class.: Immunosuppressant

Chem. class.: Purine analog

Action: Produces immunosuppression by inhibiting purine synthesis in cells

Uses: Renal transplants to prevent graft rejection, refractory rheumatoid arthritis, refractory ITP, glomerulonephritis, nephrotic syndrome, bone marrow transplant

Dosage and routes:

Prevention of rejection

• *Adult and child:* PO, IV 3-5 mg/kg/day, then maintenance (PO) of at least 1-2 mg/kg/day

Refractory rheumatoid arthritis

• *Adult:* PO 1/mg/kg/day, may increase dose after 2 mo by 0.5 mg/kg/day, not to exceed 2.5 mg/kg/day

Available forms: Tabs 50 mg; inj IV 100 mg

Side effects/adverse reactions:

GI: Nausea, vomiting, stomatitis, esophagitis, ***pancreatitis, hepatotoxicity, jaundice***

HEMA: ***Leukopenia, thrombocytopenia, anemia, pancytopenia***

INTEG: Rash

MS: Arthralgia, muscle wasting

Contraindications: Hypersensitivity, pregnancy (D), lactation

Precautions: Severe renal disease, severe hepatic disease

Pharmacokinetics: Metabolized in liver, excreted in urine (active metabolite), crosses placenta

Interactions:

• Increased action of azathioprine: allopurinol

• Do not admix with other drugs

NURSING CONSIDERATIONS

Assess:

• Blood studies: Hgb, WBC, platelets during treatment monthly; if leukocytes are <3000/mm^3, drug should be discontinued

• Liver function studies: alk phosphatase, AST (SGOT), ALT (SGPT), bilirubin

• Hepatotoxicity: dark urine, jaundice, itching, light-colored stools; drug should be discontinued

Administer:

• IV after diluting 100 mg/10 ml of sterile H_2O for inj; rotate to dissolve; may further dilute with 50 ml or more saline or glucose in saline

• For several days before transplant surgery

• All medications PO if possible, avoiding IM injections, since bleeding may occur

• With meals to reduce GI upset

Evaluate:

• Therapeutic response: absence of graft rejection, immunosuppression in autoimmune disorders

Teach patient/family:

• That therapeutic response may take 3-4 mo in rheumatoid arthritis

• To report fever, rash, severe diarrhea, chills, sore throat, fatigue, since serious infections may occur

• To use contraceptive measures during treatment, for 12 wk after ending therapy

• To avoid crowds to reduce risk of infection

---

azithromycin (℞)

(ay-zith′row-my-sin)

Zithromax

Func. class.: Antibacterial

Chem. class.: Macrolide (azalide) antibiotic

Action: Binds to 50S ribosomal subunits of susceptible bacteria and suppresses protein synthesis; much greater spectrum of activity than erythromycin

Uses: Mild to moderate infections of the upper respiratory tract, lower respiratory tract; uncomplicated skin and skin structure infections caused by *M. catarrhalis, S. pneumoniae, S. pyogenes, S. aureus, S. agalactiae, M. pneumoniae, H. influenzae, Clostridium, L. pneumophila;* nongonococcal urethritis or cervicitis due to *C. trachomatis*

* Available in Canada only

Dosage and routes:
• *Adult:* PO 500 mg on day 1, then 250 mg qd on days 2-5 for a total dose of 1.5 g; may give a one-time dose of 1 g for chlamydial infections

Available forms: Caps 250

Side effects/adverse reactions:
INTEG: Rash, urticaria, pruritus, photosensitivity
CV: Palpitations, chest pain
CNS: Dizziness, headache, vertigo, somnolence
GI: Nausea, vomiting, diarrhea, ***hepatotoxicity,*** abdominal pain, stomatitis, heartburn, dyspepsia, flatulence, melena, ***cholestatic jaundice***
GU: Vaginitis, moniliasis, nephritis

Contraindications: Hypersensitivity to azithromycin or erythromycin

Precautions: Pregnancy (C), lactation, hepatic, renal, cardiac disease, elderly, children <16 yrs

Pharmacokinetics: Peak 12 hr, duration 24 hr, half-life 11-57 hr, excreted in bile, feces, urine primarily as unchanged drug

Interactions:
• Increased effects of oral anticoagulants, digoxin, theophylline, methylprednisolone, cyclosporine, bromocriptine, disopyramide, triazolam, carbamazepine
• Decreased action of clindamycin
• Toxicity: carbamazepine, terfenadine
• Dysrhythmias: astemizole, terfenadine
• Decreased absorption of azithromycin: food, aluminium, magnesium antacids

Lab test interferences:
False increase: 17-OHCS/17-KS, AST (SGOT), ALT (SGPT)
Decrease: Folate assay

NURSING CONSIDERATIONS

Assess:
• I&O ratio; report hematuria, oliguria in renal disease
• Liver studies: AST (SGOT), ALT (SGPT)
• Renal studies: urinalysis, protein, blood
• C&S before drug therapy; drug may be taken as soon as culture is taken; C&S may be repeated after treatment
• Bowel pattern before, during treatment
• Skin eruptions, itching
• Respiratory status: rate, character, wheezing, tightness in chest; discontinue drug if these occur
• Allergies before treatment, reaction of each medication; place allergies on chart in bright red, notify all people giving drugs

Administer:
• Adequate intake of fluids (2 L) during diarrhea episodes

Perform/provide:
• Storage at room temperature

Evaluate:
• Therapeutic response: C&S negative for infection; decreased signs of infection

Teach patient/family:
• To take with 8 oz H_2O; not to take with food; take 1 hr before or 2 hr after meals; do not take with fruit juices
• To report sore throat, fever, fatigue; may indicate superinfection
• Not to take aluminum/magnesium-containing antacids simultaneously with this drug
• To notify nurse of diarrhea stools, dark urine, pale stools, yellow discoloration of eyes or skin, severe abdominal pain
• To take at evenly spaced intervals; complete dosage regimen

Treatment of hypersensitivity: Withdraw drug, maintain airway, administer epinephrine, aminophylline, O_2, IV corticosteroids

azlocillin (℞)

(az-loe-sill'in)

Azlin

Func. class.: Broad-spectrum antibiotic

Chem. class.: Extended-spectrum penicillin

Action: Interferes with cell wall replication of susceptible organisms; the cell wall, rendered osmotically unstable, swells, bursts from osmotic pressure; a β-lactam antibiotic

Uses: Lower respiratory infections, skin, bone, bacterial septicemia, urinary tract infections, yaws; effective for gram-positive bacilli *(C. perfringens, C. tetani),* gram-negative bacilli *(Bacteroides, P. aeruginosa, E. coli, H. influenzae, P. mirabilis)*

Dosage and routes:

• *Adult:* IV 100-350 mg/kg/day in 4-6 divided doses, max 24 g

Cystic fibrosis

• *Child:* IV 75 mg/kg q4h, max total dose 24 g

Available forms: Powder for inj 2, 3, 4 g

Side effects/adverse reactions:

HEMA: Anemia, increased bleeding time, ***bone marrow depression, granulocytopenia***

GI: Nausea, vomiting, diarrhea, increased AST, ALT, abdominal pain, glossitis, colitis

GU: Oliguria, proteinuria, hematuria, *vaginitis, moniliasis,* ***glomerulonephritis***

CNS: Lethargy, hallucinations, anxiety, depression, twitching, ***coma, convulsions***

META: Hypokalemia, alkalosis, hypernatremia

Contraindications: Hypersensitivity to penicillins

Precautions: Pregnancy (B), lactation, hypersensitivity to cephalosporins, neonates

Pharmacokinetics: Half-life 55-70 min, metabolized in liver, excreted in urine, bile, breast milk (small amount), crosses placenta

Interactions:

• Decreased antimicrobial effectiveness of azlocillin: tetracyclines, erythromycins

• Increased azlocillin concentrations: aspirin, probenecid

• Incompatible in sol with aminoglycosides, amphotericin B, chloramphenicol, lincomycin, oxytetracycline, polymyxin B, promethazine, tetracycline, vit B with C

Lab test interferences:

False positive: Urine glucose, urine protein

Decrease: Uric acid

NURSING CONSIDERATIONS

Assess:

• I&O ratio; report hematuria, oliguria, since penicillin in high doses is nephrotoxic

• Any patient with compromised renal system, since drug is excreted slowly in poor renal system function; toxicity may occur rapidly

• Liver studies: AST (SGOT), ALT (SGPT)

• Blood studies: WBC, RBC, Hgb, Hct, bleeding time

• Renal studies: urinalysis, protein, blood

• Culture, sensitivity before drug therapy; drug may be given as soon as culture is taken

• Bowel pattern before, during treatment

• Skin eruptions after administration of penicillin to 1 wk after discontinuing drug

• Respiratory status: rate, character, wheezing, tightness in chest

• Allergies before initiation of treatment; reaction of each medication; place allergies on chart in bright red

Administer:
• IV after reconstituting 1 g/10 ml of D_5W, NS, or sterile water, shake
• After further dilution in 50-100 ml of compatible solution, give over 30 min; change IV site q48h
• After C&S completed
• Slowly (direct IV) over 5 min to prevent chest discomfort
Perform/provide:
• Adrenaline, suction, tracheostomy set, endotracheal intubation equipment on unit
• Adequate intake of fluids (2 L) during diarrhea episodes
• Scratch test to assess allergy after securing order from physician; usually done when penicillin is only drug of choice
• Storage in cool environment; solution is stable for 24 hr at room temperature
Evaluate:
• Therapeutic response: absence of fever, draining wounds
Teach patient/family:
• That culture may be taken after completed course of medication
• To report sore throat, fever, fatigue (may indicate superinfection)
• To wear or carry a Medic Alert ID if allergic to penicillins
• To notify nurse of diarrhea
Treatment of anaphylaxis: Withdraw drug, maintain airway, administer epinephrine, aminophylline, O_2, IV corticosteroids

aztreonam (℞)
(az-tree'oh nam)
Azactam
Func. class.: Misc antibiotic
Chem. class.: Monobactam

Action: Inhibits organisms by inhibiting bacterial cell wall synthesis, which causes death of organism (bactericidal)
Uses: Urinary tract infection; septicemia; skin, muscle, bone infection; and other infections caused by gram-negative organisms
Dosage and routes:
Urinary tract infections
• *Adult:* IV/IM 500 mg-1 g q8-12h
Systemic infections
Adult: IV/IM 1-2 g q8-12h
Severe systemic infections
Adult: IV/IM 2 g q6-8h; do not exceed 8 g/day
Continue treatment for 48 hr after negative culture or until patient is asymptomatic
Available forms: Powder for inj 500 mg, 1, 2 g
Side effects/adverse reactions:
HEMA: Anemia, increased bleeding time, ***bone marrow depression, granulocytopenia***
GI: Nausea, vomiting, diarrhea, increased AST (SGOT), ALT (SGPT), abdominal pain, glossitis, colitis
CNS: Lethargy, hallucinations, anxiety, depression, twitching, ***coma, convulsions,*** malaise
EENT: Tinnitus, diplopia, nasal congestion
GU: Vaginal candidiasis, vaginitis, breast tenderness
Contraindications: Hypersensitivity to this drug, penicillins, cephalosporins
Precautions: Pregnancy (B), lactation, children, impaired renal, hepatic function, elderly
Pharmacokinetics:
IV: Peak immediate, trough 8 hr
IM: Peak 1 hr
Half-life: 1.7 hr; half-life prolonged in renal disease; protein binding 56%; metabolized by liver; excreted in urine; small amounts appear in breast milk, placenta

Interactions:
• Decreased effect of both drugs: β-lactamase antibiotics (cefoxitin, imipenem)
• Incompatible with nafcillin, metronidazole, cephradine
• Increased nephrotoxicity: aminoglycosides
Syringe compatibility: Clindamycin
Y-site compatibilities: Ciprofloxacin, enalaprilat, foscarnet, melphalan, ondansetron, vinorelbine, zidovudine
Additive compatibilities: Cefazolin, ciprofloxacin, clindamycin, gentamicin, tobramycin

NURSING CONSIDERATIONS
Assess:
• Signs of bruising, bleeding, anemia
• Bowel pattern before, during treatment
• Respiratory status: rate, character, wheezing, tightness in chest
• I&O ratio; report hematuria, oliguria, since this drug in high doses is nephrotoxic
• Any patient with compromised renal system, since drug is excreted slowly in poor renal system function; toxicity may occur rapidly
• Liver studies: AST (SGOT), ALT (SGPT)
• Blood studies: WBC, RBC, Hgb, Hct, bleeding time
• Renal studies: urinalysis, protein, blood
• Skin eruptions after administration of drug to 1 wk after discontinuing drug
• Allergies before initiation of treatment, reaction of medication; highlight allergies on chart
Administer:
• Direct IV after diluting with 6-10 ml sterile H_2O/15 ml drug; give over 3-5 min
• IV INF after diluting with 3 ml or more sterile H_2O/1 g drug; then dilute with 50-100 ml of D_5W, 0.9% NaCl solution; give over ½-1 hr, by Y-tube or 3-way stopcock; flush tubing before and after administration
• IM; dilute each g with at least 3 ml of 0.9% NaCl; give into large muscle
• Drug after C&S completed
Perform/provide:
• Adequate fluid intake (2 L) during diarrhea episodes
• Storage in refrigerator
Evaluate:
• Therapeutic response: absence of fever, purulent drainage, redness, inflammation
Teach patient/family:
• That culture may be taken after completed course of medication
• To report sore throat, fever, fatigue; may indicate superinfection

bacampicillin (℞)

(ba-kam-pi-sill'in)
Penglobe*, Spectrobid
Func. class.: Broad-spectrum antibiotic
Chem. class.: Aminopenicillin

Action: Interferes with cell wall replication of susceptible organisms; the cell wall, rendered osmotically unstable, swells, bursts from osmotic pressure; drug is hydrolyzed to ampicillin during absorption
Uses: Respiratory tract infections, skin, urinary tract infections; effective for gram-positive cocci *(E. faecalis, S. pneumoniae)*, gram-negative cocci *(N. gonorrhoeae)*, gram-negative bacilli *(E. coli, H. influenzae, P. mirabilis)*
Dosage and routes:
• *Adult:* PO 400-800 mg q12h
• *Child:* PO 25-50 mg/kg/day in divided doses q12h

* Available in Canada only

Available forms: Tabs 400 mg; powder for oral susp 125 mg/5 ml (equivalent to 87.5 mg ampicillin)

Side effects/adverse reactions:

HEMA: Anemia, increased bleeding time, ***bone marrow depression, granulocytopenia***

GI: Nausea, vomiting, diarrhea, increased AST (SGOT), ALT (SGPT), abdominal pain, glossitis, pseudomembranous colitis

GU: Oliguria, proteinuria, hematuria, *vaginitis, moniliasis,* ***glomerulonephritis***

CNS: Lethargy, hallucinations, anxiety, depression, twitching, ***coma, convulsions***

Contraindications: Hypersensitivity to penicillins

Precautions: Pregnancy (B), lactation, hypersensitivity to cephalosporins, neonates

Pharmacokinetics:

PO: Peak 30-60 min, duration 5-6 hr, half-life ½-1 hr, metabolized in liver, excreted in urine

Interactions:

- Increased bacampicillin concentrations: aspirin, probenecid
- Do not give with disulfiram

Lab test interferences:

False positive: Urine glucose, urine protein

Decrease: Uric acid

NURSING CONSIDERATIONS

Assess:

- I&O ratio; report hematuria, oliguria, since penicillin in high doses is nephrotoxic
- Any patient with compromised renal system, since drug is excreted slowly in poor renal system function; toxicity may occur
- Liver studies: AST (SGOT), ALT (SGPT)
- Blood studies: WBC, RBC, Hgb, Hct, bleeding time
- Renal studies: urinalysis, protein, blood
- Culture, sensitivity before drug therapy; drug may be given as soon as culture is taken
- Bowel pattern before, during treatment
- Skin eruptions after administration of penicillin to 1 wk after discontinuing drug
- Respiratory status: rate, character, wheezing, tightness in chest
- Allergies before initiation of treatment; reaction of each medication; report allergies on chart in bright red

Administer:

- After C&S completed
- Oral susp 1 hr before or 2 hr after meals

Perform/provide:

- Adrenaline, suction, tracheostomy set, endotracheal intubation equipment on unit
- Adequate intake of fluids (2 L) during diarrhea episodes
- Scratch test to assess allergy after securing order from physician; usually done when penicillin is only drug of choice
- Storage in dry tight container, oral suspension refrigerated for 2 wk or at room temperature for 1 wk

Evaluate:

- Therapeutic response: absence of fever, draining wounds

Teach patient/family:

- Aspects of drug therapy: culture may be taken after completed course of medication; patient must complete course of therapy
- To report sore throat, fever, fatigue (may indicate superinfection)
- To wear or carry a Medic Alert ID if allergic to penicillins
- To notify nurse of diarrhea
- That drug should be taken on an empty stomach, with a full glass of water

Treatment of hypersensitivity: Withdraw drug, maintain airway, administer epinephrine, aminophylline, O_2, IV corticosteroids

bacitracin (℞)

(bass-i-tray'sin)

Baci-IM, Bacitracin Sterile, Bacitracin U.S.P.

Func. class.: Antibacterial

Chem. class.: Bacillus subtilis derivative (polypeptide)

Action: Inhibits bacterial cell wall synthesis, interfering with osmotic pressure within cell

Uses: Staphylococcal pneumonia, empyema, pseudomembranous colitis

Dosage and routes:

- *Infants >2.5 kg:* IM 1,000 U/kg/day in divided doses q8-12h
- *Infants <2.5 kg:* IM 900 U/kg/day in divided doses q8-12h
- *Adults:* PO 20,000-25,000 U q6h × 7-10 days, IM 10,000-25,000 U q6h × 7-10 days

Available forms: Inj IM 10,000, 50,000 U

Side effects/adverse reactions:

INTEG: Rash, pain at injection site

GI: Nausea, vomiting, diarrhea

GU: ***Proteinuria, casts, azotemia***

Contraindications: Hypersensitivity, severe renal disease

Precautions: Pregnancy (C), lactation, renal disease

Pharmacokinetics: Peak 1-2 hr, duration >12 hr, metabolized in liver, excreted in urine

Interactions:

- Increased nephrotoxicity, neurotoxicity: aminoglycosides, polymyxin
- Increased neuromuscular blockade: nondepolarizing skeletal muscle relaxants, anesthetics

NURSING CONSIDERATIONS

Assess:

- I&O ratio; report oliguria, change in urinary output; high doses are nephrotoxic
- Any patient with compromised renal system; drug is excreted slowly in poor renal system function; toxicity may occur rapidly
- Renal studies: urinalysis, protein, blood, BUN, creatinine, urine pH (keep at 6.0)
- C&S before drug therapy; drug may be taken as soon as culture is taken; repeat C&S after treatment
- Bowel pattern before, during treatment; if severe diarrhea occurs, drug should be discontinued
- Skin eruptions, itching: rash, urticaria, erythema
- Respiratory status: rate, character, wheezing, tightness in chest, dyspnea on exertion
- Allergies before treatment, reaction of each medication; report allergies on chart in bright red; notify all people giving drugs

Administer:

- After reconstituting with NS
- IM in deep muscle mass; rotate injection site; do not give IV/SC

Perform/provide:

- Storage in refrigerator; protect from direct sunlight
- Adrenalin, suction, tracheostomy set, endotracheal intubation equipment on unit
- Adequate intake of fluids (2 L) during diarrhea episodes

Evaluate:

- Therapeutic response: absence of fever, cough, dyspnea, malaise

Teach patient/family:

- To report sore throat, fever, fatigue; may indicate superinfection

* Available in Canada only

bacitracin (ophthalmic) (℞)

(bass-i-tray'sin)

AK-Tracin, Bacitracin Ophthalmic

Func. class.: Antiinfective

Action: Inhibits cell wall synthesis in bacteria

Uses: Infection of eye

Dosage and routes:

- *Adult and child:* Apply to conjunctival sac bid-qid until desired response

Available forms: Oint 500 U/g

Side effects/adverse reactions:

EENT: Poor corneal wound healing, visual haze (temporary), overgrowth of nonsusceptible organisms

Contraindications: Hypersensitivity

Precautions: Antibiotic hypersensitivity, pregnancy (C), lactation

NURSING CONSIDERATIONS

Assess:

- Allergy: itching, lacrimation, redness, swelling

Administer:

- After washing hands; cleanse crusts or discharge from eye before application

Perform/provide:

- Storage at room temperature

Evaluate:

- Therapeutic response: absence of redness, inflammation, tearing

Teach patient/family:

- To use drug exactly as prescribed
- Not to use eye makeup, towels, washcloths, eye medication of others; reinfection may occur
- That drug container tip should not be touched to eye
- To report itching, increased redness, burning, stinging, swelling; drug should be discontinued
- That drug may cause blurred vision when ointment is applied

B

bacitracin (topical) (OTC)

(bass-i-tray'sin)

Baciguent, Bacitin*, Bacitracin

Func. class.: Local antiinfective

Chem. class.: Antibacterial

Action: Interferes with bacterial cell wall function by inhibiting protein synthesis

Uses: Topical staphylococci, streptococci

Dosage and routes:

- *Adult and child:* TOP bid-qid or more often if needed

Available forms: Oint 500 U/g

Side effects/adverse reactions:

INTEG: Rash, urticaria, stinging, burning, contact dermatitis

Contraindications: Hypersensitivity

Precautions: Pregnancy (C), lactation

NURSING CONSIDERATIONS

Assess:

- Allergic reaction: burning, stinging, swelling, redness
- For systemic effects and superimposed infections

Administer:

- After C&S is obtained, if lesion is weeping
- Enough medication to cover lesions completely
- After cleansing with soap, water before each application, dry well (as ordered)

Perform/provide:

- Storage at room temperature in dry place

Evaluate:

- Therapeutic response: decrease in size, number of lesions

Teach patient/family:

- To use medical asepsis (hand washing) before, after each application to prevent further infection
- To apply with glove or sterile swab to prevent further infection
- To avoid use of OTC creams, ointments, lotions unless directed by physician
- To watch for superinfections with long-term use or allergic reaction

baclofen (℞)

(bak'loe-fen)

Alpha-Baclofen*, baclofen, Lioresal, Lioresal DS, Lioresal Intrathecal

Func. class.: Skeletal muscle relaxant, central acting

Chem. class.: GABA chlorophenyl derivative

Action: Inhibits synaptic responses in CNS by decreasing GABA, which decreases neurotransmitter function; decreases frequency, severity of muscle spasms

Uses: Spinal cord injury, spasticity in multiple sclerosis

Dosage and routes:

- *Adult:* PO 5 mg tid × 3 days, then 10 mg tid × 3 days, then 15 mg tid × 3 days, then 20 mg tid × 3 days, then titrated to response, not to exceed 80 mg/day
- Intrathecal: use implantable intrathecal INF pump; use screening trial of 3 separate BOL doses if needed (50 μg/ml, 75 μg/1.5 ml, 100 μg/2 ml). Initial: double screening dose that produced result and give over 24 hr: increase by 10%-30% q24hr only. Maintenance: 1200-1500 μg/day

Available forms: Tabs 10, 20 mg; intrathecal injection 10 mg/20 ml (500 μg/ml), 10 mg/5 ml (2000 μg/ml)

Side effects/adverse reactions:

CNS: Dizziness, weakness, fatigue, drowsiness, headache, disorientation, insomnia, paresthesias, tremors

EENT: Nasal congestion, blurred vision, mydriasis, tinnitus

CV: Hypotension, chest pain, palpitations, edema

GI: Nausea, constipation, vomiting, increased AST (SGOT), alk phosphatase, abdominal pain, dry mouth, anorexia

GU: Urinary frequency

INTEG: Rash, pruritus

Contraindications: Hypersensitivity

Precautions: Peptic ulcer disease, renal disease, hepatic disease, stroke, seizure disorder, diabetes mellitus, pregnancy (C), lactation, elderly

Pharmacokinetics:

PO: Peak 2-3 hr, duration >8 hr, half-life 2½-4 hr, partially metabolized in liver, excreted in urine (unchanged)

INTRATHECAL: CSF levels with plasma levels 100 times oral route

Interactions:

- Increased CNS depression: alcohol, tricyclic antidepressants, narcotics, barbiturates, sedatives, hypnotics

Lab test interferences:

Increase: AST, alk phosphatase, blood glucose

NURSING CONSIDERATIONS

Assess:

- B/P, weight, blood sugar, and hepatic function periodically
- For increased seizure activity in epilepsy patient; this drug decreases seizure threshold
- I&O ratio; check for urinary retention, frequency, hesitancy
- ECG in epileptic patients; poor seizure control has occurred in patients taking this drug

* Available in Canada only

• Allergic reactions: rash, fever, respiratory distress
• Severe weakness, numbness in extremities
• Tolerance: increased need for medication, more frequent requests for medication, increased pain
• CNS depression: dizziness, drowsiness, psychiatric symptoms
• Dosage, as individual titration is required

Administer:
• With meals for GI symptoms
• Gum, frequent sips of water for dry mouth

Perform/provide:
• Storage in tight container at room temperature
• Assistance with ambulation if dizziness or drowsiness occurs

Evaluate:
• Therapeutic response: decreased pain, spasticity

Teach patient/family:
• Not to discontinue medication quickly; hallucinations, spasticity, tachycardia will occur; drug should be tapered off over 1-2 wk
• Not to take with alcohol, other CNS depressants
• To avoid hazardous activities if drowsiness or dizziness occurs
• To avoid using OTC medication: cough preparations, antihistamines, unless directed by prescriber
• To increase fluid intake >2 L/day

Treatment of overdose: Induce emesis of conscious patient, lavage, dialysis

beclomethasone (℞)

(be-kloe-meth′a-sone)
Beclo disk*, Becloforte Inhaler*, Beclovent Rotocaps*, Vancenase Nasal Inhaler, Vanceril
Func. class.: Corticosteroid, synthetic
Chem. class.: Glucocorticoid

Action: Prevents inflammation by depression of migration of polymorphonuclear leukocytes, fibroblasts, reversal of increased capillary permeability and lysosomal stabilization; does not suppress hypothalamus and pituitary function

Uses: Chronic asthma, rhinitis

Dosage and routes:
• *Adult:* INH 2-4 puffs tid-qid, not to exceed 20 inhalations/day
• *Child:* 6-12 yr: INH 1-2 puffs tid-qid, not to exceed 10 inhalations/day

Available forms: Aerosol 42 μg/actuation

Side effects/adverse reactions:
RESP: ***Bronchospasm***
GI: Dry mouth
EENT: Hoarseness, candidal infections of oral cavity, sore throat

Contraindications: Hypersensitivity, status asthmaticus (primary treatment), nonasthmatic bronchial disease; bacterial, fungal, viral infections of mouth, throat, lungs; children <3 yr

Precautions: Nasal disease/surgery, pregnancy (C), lactation

Pharmacokinetics:
INH: Onset 10 min, excreted in feces (metabolites), half-life 3-15 hr, crosses placenta, metabolized in lungs, liver, GI system

NURSING CONSIDERATIONS

Assess:
• Adrenal function periodically for HPA axis suppression

Administer:
- INH with water to decrease possibility of fungal infections
- Titrated dose, use lowest effective dose

Perform/provide:
- Gum, rinsing of mouth for dry mouth

Evaluate:
- Therapeutic response: decreased dyspnea, wheezing, dry rales on auscultation

Teach patient/family:
- That ID as steroid user should be carried
- To notify prescriber if therapeutic response decreases; dosage adjustment may be needed
- Proper administration technique
- To wash inhaler with warm water and dry after each use
- All aspects of drug usage, including cushingoid symptoms
- Symptoms of adrenal insufficiency: nausea, anorexia, fatigue, dizziness, dyspnea, weakness, joint pain, depression
- To keep drug out of children's reach

beclomethasone (nasal) (℞)

(be-kloe-meth'a-sone)

Beconase AQ Nasal, Beconase Inhalation, Vancenase AQ Nasal, Vancenase Nasal

Func. class.: Synthetic corticosteroid

Chem. class.: Beclomethasone diester

Action: Antiinflammatory, vasoconstrictive properties in nasal passages

Uses: Seasonal or perennial rhinitis

Dosage and routes:
- *Adult and child >12 yr:* INSTILL 1-2 sprays in each nostril bid-qid

Available forms: Aero 42 μg/spray

Side effects/adverse reactions:

EENT: Dryness, nasal irritation, burning, sneezing, secretions with blood, nasal ulcerations, ***perforation of nasal septum,*** *Candida* infection, earache, hoarseness

ENDO: ***Adrenal suppression***

INTEG: Rash, urticaria, pruritus

CNS: Headache, paresthesia

RESP: ***Acute status asthmaticus***

Contraindications: Hypersensitivity, systemic corticosteroid therapy

Precautions: Pregnancy (C), lactation, children <12, nasal ulcers, recurrent epistaxis respiration

Pharmacokinetics:

INSTILL: Readily absorbed; peak concentration, other data have not been determined

NURSING CONSIDERATIONS

Assess:
- Adrenal function periodically for HPA axis suppression
- Adrenal suppression: 17-KS, plasma cortisol for decreased levels
- Nasal passages during long-term treatment for changes in mucus

Administer:
- After cleaning aerosol top daily with warm water, dry thoroughly

Perform/provide:
- Storage in cool environment; do not puncture or incinerate container

Evaluate:
- Therapeutic response: decrease in runny nose

Teach patient/family:
- To clear nasal passages if sneezing attack occurs, repeat dose
- To continue using product even if mild nasal bleeding occurs; is usually transient
- Method of instillation after providing written instructions from manufacturer
- To clear nasal passages before administration; use decongestant if

needed; shake inhaler, invert, tilt head backward, insert nozzle into nostril, away from septum; hold other nostril closed and depress activator, inhale through nose, exhale through mouth

belladonna alkaloids (℞)

(bell-a-don'a)

Bellafoline

Func. class.: Gastrointestinal anticholinergic

Chem. class.: Belladonna alkaloid

Combination products: Barbidonna: belladonna alkaloids, atropine sulfate 0.025 mg, hyoscyamine sulfate 0.1286 mg, phenobarbital 16 mg, scopolamine hydrobromide 0.0074 mg; Barbidonna Elixir: belladonna alkaloids, atropine sulfate 0.034 mg/5 ml, hyoscyamine sulfate 0.0174 mg/5 ml, phenobarbital 21.6 mg/ml, scopolamine hydrobromide 0.01 mg/5 ml; Barbidonna No. 2: belladonna alkaloids, atropine sulfate 0.025 mg, hyoscyamine sulfate 0.1286 mg, phenobarbital 32 mg, scopolamine hydrobromide 0.0074 mg; Belap, Pheno-Bella: belladonna extract 10.8 mg (0.135 mg of alkaloids of belladonna leaf) with phenobarbital 16.2 mg; Bellalphen, Donnatal, Hyosophen: belladonna alkaloids, atropine sulfate 0.0194 mg, hyoscyamine sulfate 0.1037 mg, phenobarbital 16.2 mg, scopolamine hydrobromide 0.0065 mg; Belladenal-S: levorotatory belladonna alkaloids, malates 0.25 mg (of levorotatory belladonna alkaloids) with phenobarbital 50 mg; Butibel: belladonna extract 15 mg (0.187 mg of alkaloids of belladonna leaf) with butabarbital sodium 15 mg; Butibel Elixir: belladonna extract 15 mg (0.187 mg of alkaloids of belladonna leaf) with butabarbital sodium 15 mg; Chardonna-2: belladonna extract 15 mg (0.187 mg of alkaloids of belladonna leaf) with phenobarbital 15 mg; Donnatal: belladonna alkaloids, atropine sulfate 0.0194 mg, hyoscyamine sulfate 0.1037 mg, phenobarbital 32.4 mg, scopolamine hydrobromide 0.0065 mg; Donnatal Elixir, Hyosophen Elixir: belladonna alkaloids, atropine sulfate 0.0194 mg/5 ml, hyoscyamine sulfate 0.1037 mg/5 ml, phenobarbital 16.2 mg/5 ml, scopolamine hydrobromide 0.0065/5 ml; Donnatal Extentabs: belladonna alkaloids, atropine sulfate 0.0582 mg, hyoscyamine sulfate 0.3111 mg, phenobarbital 48.6 mg, scopolamine hydrobromide 0.0195; Donnatal, Hyosophen: belladonna alkaloids, atropine sulfate 0.0194 mg, hyoscyamine sulfate 0.1037 mg, phenobarbital 16.2 mg, scopolamine hydrobromide 0.0065 mg; Hybephen: belladonna alkaloids: atropine sulfate 0.0233 mg, hyoscyamine sulfate 0.1277 mg, phenobarbital 15 mg, scopolamine hydrobromide 0.0094 mg; Kinesed: belladonna alkaloids atropine sulfate 0.02 mg, hyoscyamine sulfate 0.12 mg, phenobarbital 16 mg, scopolamine hydrobromide 0.007 mg; Wyanoids: belladonna extract 15 mg (0.19 mg of alkaloids of belladonna leaf) with ephedrine 3 mg

Action: Inhibits muscarinic actions of acetylcholine at postganglionic parasympathetic neuron effector sites

Uses: Treatment of peptic ulcer disease, irritable bowel syndrome in combination with other drugs; for other GI disorders

Dosage and routes:
• *Adult:* PO 0.25-0.5 mg tid; SC 0.125-0.5 mg qd or bid
• *Child >6 yr:* PO 0.125-0.25 mg tid

Available forms: Tabs 0.25 mg; inj SC 0.5 mg/ml

Side effects/adverse reactions:
CNS: Confusion, stimulation in elderly, headache, insomnia, dizziness, drowsiness, anxiety, weakness, hallucination
GI: Dry mouth, constipation, ***paralytic ileus,*** heartburn, nausea, vomiting, dysphagia, absence of taste
GU: Hesitancy, retention, impotence
CV: Palpitations, tachycardia
EENT: Blurred vision, photophobia, mydriasis, cycloplegia, increased ocular tension
INTEG: Urticaria, rash, pruritus, anhidrosis, fever, allergic reactions, flushing

Contraindications: Hypersensitivity to anticholinergics, narrow-angle glaucoma, GI obstruction, myasthenia gravis, paralytic ileus, GI atony, toxic megacolon

Precautions: Hyperthyroidism, coronary artery disease, dysrhythmias, CHF, ulcerative colitis, hypertension, hiatal hernia, hepatic disease, renal disease, pregnancy (C), lactation, urinary obstruction

Pharmacokinetics:
PO: Duration 4-6 hr; metabolized by liver, excreted in urine, half-life 13-38 hr

Interactions:
• Increased anticholinergic effect: amantadine, tricyclic antidepressants, MAOIs
• Increased effect of nitrofurantoin
• Decreased effect of phenothiazines, levodopa

NURSING CONSIDERATIONS

Assess:
• VS, cardiac status: checking for dysrhythmias, increased rate, palpitations, flushing
• I&O ratio; check for urinary retention or hesitancy
• GI complaints: pain, bleeding (frank or occult), nausea, vomiting, anorexia, constipation

Administer:
• ½-1 hr ac for better absorption
• Decreased dose to elderly patients; their metabolism may be slowed
• Gum, hard candy, frequent rinsing of mouth for dryness of oral cavity

Perform/provide:
• Storage in tight container protected from light
• Increased fluids, bulk, exercise to decrease constipation

Evaluate:
• Therapeutic response: absence of epigastric pain, bleeding, nausea, vomiting

Teach patient/family:
• To avoid driving, other hazardous activities until stabilized on medication
• To avoid alcohol, other CNS depressants; will enhance sedating properties of this drug
• To avoid hot environments; heat stroke may occur; drug suppresses perspiration
• To use sunglasses when outside to prevent photophobia

---

benazepril (℞)

(ben-az′e-pril)
Lotensin
Func. class.: Antihypertensive
Chem. class.: Angiotensin-converting enzyme (ACE) inhibitor

Action: Selectively suppresses renin-angiotensin-aldosterone system; inhibits ACE, prevents conversion of angiotensin I to angiotensin II; results in dilation of arterial, venous vessels

Uses: Hypertension, alone or in combination with thiazide diuretics

Dosage and routes:

• *Adult:* PO 10 mg qd initially, then 20-40 mg/day divided bid or qd. Renal impairment: 5 mg qd with CrCl <30 ml/min/1.73 m^2, increase as needed to maximum of 40 mg/day

Available forms: Tabs 5, 10, 20, 40 mg

Side effects/adverse reactions:

CV: Hypotension, postural hypotension, syncope, palpitations, angina

GU: Increased BUN, creatinine, decreased libido, impotence, urinary tract infection

HEMA: ***Neutropenia, agranulocytosis***

INTEG: ***Angioedema,*** rash, flushing, sweating

RESP: Cough, asthma, bronchitis, dyspnea, sinusitis

META: Hyperkalemia, hyponatremia

GI: Nausea, constipation, vomiting, gastritis, melena

CNS: Anxiety, hypertonia, insomnia, paresthesia, headache, dizziness, fatigue

MS: Arthralgia, arthritis, myalgia

Contraindications: Hypersensitivity to ACE inhibitors, pregnancy (D), lactation, children

Precautions: Impaired renal, liver function, dialysis patients, hypovolemia, blood dyscrasias, CHF, COPD, asthma, elderly, bilateral renal artery stenosis

Pharmacokinetics:

PO: Peak ½-1 hr, serum protein binding 97%, half-life 10-11 hr, metabolized by liver (metabolites), excreted in urine

Interactions:

• Increased hypotension: diuretics, other antihypertensives, ganglionic blockers, adrenergic blockers
• Increased toxicity: vasodilators, hydralazine, prazosin, potassium-sparing diuretics, sympathomimetics, potassium supplements
• Decreased absorption: antacids
• Decreased antihypertensive effect: indomethacin
• Increased serum levels of digoxin, lithium
• Increased hypersensitivity: allopurinol

Lab test interferences:

False positive: Urine acetone

NURSING CONSIDERATIONS

Assess:

• Blood studies: neutrophils, decreased platelets
• B/P, orthostatic hypotension, syncope
• Renal studies: protein, BUN, creatinine; increased levels may indicate nephrotic syndrome
• Baselines in renal, liver function tests before therapy begins
• Potassium levels, although hyperkalemia rarely occurs
• Dipstick of urine for protein qd in first morning specimen; if protein is increased, a 24 hr urinary protein should be collected
• Edema in feet, legs daily
• Allergic reactions: rash, fever, pruritus, urticaria; drug should be discontinued if antihistamines fail to help
• Renal symptoms: polyuria, oliguria, frequency, dysuria

Administer:

• IV infusion of 0.9% NaCl (as ordered) to expand fluid volume if severe hypotension occurs

Perform/provide:

• Storage in tight container at 86° F (30° C) or less
• Supine or Trendelenburg position for severe hypotension

Evaluate:
- Therapeutic response: decrease in B/P

Teach patient/family:
- Not to discontinue drug abruptly
- Not to use OTC products (cough, cold, allergy) unless directed by physician; do not use salt substitutes containing potassium without consulting physician
- Importance of complying with dosage schedule, even if feeling better
- To rise slowly to sitting or standing position to minimize orthostatic hypotension
- To notify prescriber of mouth sores, sore throat, fever, swelling of hands or feet, irregular heartbeat, chest pain
- To report excessive perspiration, dehydration, vomiting, diarrhea; may lead to fall in B/P
- That drug may cause dizziness, fainting, light-headedness; may occur during 1st few days of therapy
- That drug may cause skin rash or impaired perspiration
- How to take B/P, and normal readings for age group

Treatment of overdose: 0.9% NaCl IV INF, hemodialysis

benzocaine (oral)

(OTC)

(ben'zoe-kane)

Anbesol Maximum Strength, Baby Anbesol, Children's Chloraseptic, Medamint, Orabase Baby, Oracin, Ora-Jel, Oratect, Spec-T Anesthetic, T-Caine, Tyrobenz

Func. class.: Topical local anesthetic

Chem. class.: Ester

Action: Inhibits conduction of nerve impulses from sensory nerves

Uses: Oral irritation, sore throat, toothache, cold sore, canker sore, sunburn, minor cuts, insect bites, pain, itching

Dosage and routes:
- *Adult and child >12 yr:* TOP apply to affected area; LOZ suck as needed

Available forms: Cream 1%, 5%; lotion 0.5%, 8%; oint 2%, 5%, 20%; sol 2.1%, 2.5%, 6.3%, 20%; lozenges 3, 5, 6.25, 10 mg; topical aerosol 20%; gel 6.3%, 7.5%, 10%, 20%

Side effects/adverse reactions:

EENT: Itching, irritation in ear

INTEG: Rash, urticaria

Contraindications: Hypersensitivity

Precautions: Pregnancy (C), lactation

Pharmacokinetics:

TOP: Peak 1 min, duration ½-1 hr

NURSING CONSIDERATIONS

Administer:
- To gums as needed for teething pain
- Lozenges for temporary sore throat pain

Perform/provide:
- Storage in tight, light-resistant container; do not freeze, puncture, or incinerate aerosol container

Evaluate:
- Affected area for redness, swelling, pain

Teach patient/family:
- To avoid contact with eyes
- Not to use for prolonged periods: use for <1 wk; if condition remains, physician should be contacted

* Available in Canada only

benzonatate (℞)

(ben-zoe'na-tate)

Tessalon Perles

Func. class.: Antitussive, non-narcotic

Chem. class.: Tetracaine derivative

Action: Inhibits cough reflex by anesthetizing stretch receptors in respiratory system, direct action on cough center in medulla

Uses: Nonproductive cough

Dosage and routes:

• *Adult and child:* PO 100 mg tid, not to exceed 600 mg/day

• *Child <10 yr:* PO 8 mg/kg in 3-6 divided doses

Available forms: Perles 100 mg

Side effects/adverse reactions:

CNS: Dizziness, drowsiness, headache

GI: Nausea, constipation, upset stomach

EENT: Nasal congestion, burning eyes

CV: Increased B/P, chest tightness, numbness

INTEG: Urticaria, rash, pruritus

Contraindications: Hypersensitivity

Precautions: Pregnancy (C), lactation

Pharmacokinetics:

PO: Onset 15-20 min, duration 3-8 hr, metabolized by liver, excreted in urine

NURSING CONSIDERATIONS

Assess:

• Cough: type, frequency, character including sputum

Perform/provide:

• Storage in tight, light-resistant containers

• Increased fluids, bulk, exercise to decrease constipation, liquefy sputum

• Chest percussion to bring up secretion if needed

Evaluate:

• Therapeutic response: absence of cough

Teach patient/family:

• To avoid driving, other hazardous activities until patient is stabilized on this medication

• Not to chew or break capsules; will anesthetize mouth

• To avoid smoking, smoke-filled rooms, perfumes, dust, environmental pollutants, cleaners

benzoyl peroxide (OTC)

(ben'zoe-ill per-ox'ide)

Acne-10, Acne-Aid, Ben-Aqua-5, Ben-Aqua-10, Benoxyl 5, Benoxyl 10, Benzoyl Peroxide, Benzac AC, Benzac W Wash 5, Benzac W Wash 10, Benzac W 2½, Benzac W 5, Benzac 5, Benzac 10, Benzac W 10, 5-Benzagel, 10-Benzagel, Brevoxyl, Clear By Design, Clearasil 10%, Clearasil Maximum Strength Acne Treatment, Cuticura Acne, Del Aqua-5, Del Aqua-10, Desquam-E, Desquam-X2.5, Desquam-X5, Desquam-X10, Desquam-X5 Wash, Desquam-X10 Wash, Dry and Clear, Dry and Clear Double Strength, Fostex 5% BPO, Fostex 10% BPO, Fostex 10% BPO Wash, Fostex 10% BPO Tinted, Luroxide, Oxy 5, Oxy 5 Tinted, Oxy 10, Oxy 10 Cover, Oxy 10 Wash, Pan Oxyl 5, Pan Oxyl 10, Pan Oxyl AQ 2½, Pan Oxyl AQ 5, Pan Oxyl AQ 10, Persa-Gel, Persa Gel W 5%, Persa Gel W 10%, pHisoAc BP, Propa P.H. Liquid Acne Soap, Theroxide, Theroxide Wash, Vanoxide, Xerac BP10, Xerac BP5, Zeroxin-5, Zeroxin-10

Func. class.: Antiacne medication

Action: Antibacterial activity, especially against predominant bacteria causing acne

Uses: Mild to moderate acne

Dosage and routes:

• *Adult and child:* TOP apply to affected area qd or bid

Available forms: Topical cleansers, lotions, creams, sticks, pads, gels, bars

Side effects/adverse reactions:

INTEG: Local skin irritation; stinging; warmth (dryness); scaling; erythema; edema; allergic, contact dermatitis

Contraindications: Hypersensitivity to benzoic acid derivatives

Precautions: Pregnancy (C), lactation, children <12 yr

Pharmacokinetics:

TOP: 50% absorbed through skin, metabolized to benzoic acid, excreted in urine as benzoate

Interaction:

• Skin irritation: tretinoin

NURSING CONSIDERATIONS

Assess:

• Area of body involved, including time involved, what helps or aggravates condition

• Allergic reaction: rash, irritation, scaling, dermatitis; discontinue use

Administer:

• With hand washing before and immediately after to avoid irritation

Perform/provide:

• Storage at room temperature

Evaluate:

• Therapeutic response: decreased amount of acne on body

Teach patient/family:

• To avoid application on normal skin, getting cream in eyes, nose, other mucous membranes

• To discontinue use if rash or irritation develops

• That transitory warmth or stinging may develop over treated area

• To expect dryness, peeling of treated area

• To avoid contact with hair, clothing; they may stain

• That cosmetics may be used over drug

• That dryness and peeling can be expected

* Available in Canada only

benzquinamide (℞)

(benz-kwin′a-mide)

Emete-Con

Func. class.: Antiemetic

Chem. class.: Benzoquinolize amide

Action: Acts centrally by blocking chemoreceptor trigger zone, which in turn acts on vomiting center

Uses: To inhibit nausea, vomiting associated with anesthetic, surgery

Dosage and routes:

• *Adult:* IM 50 mg or 0.5-1 mg/kg, may be repeated in 1 hr, then q3-4 hr prn; IV 25 mg or 0.2-0.4 mg/kg as a one-time dose

Available forms: Inj 50 mg/vial

Side effects/adverse reactions:

CNS: *Drowsiness,* fatigue, restlessness, tremor, headache, stimulation, dizziness, insomnia, twitching, excitement, nervousness, EPS

GI: Nausea, anorexia

CV: ***Premature atrial*** or ***ventricular contractions, atrial fibrillation,*** hypertension, hypotension

INTEG: Rash, urticaria, fever, chills, flushing, hives, shivering, sweating, temperature

EENT: Dry mouth, blurred vision, hiccups, salivation

Contraindications: Hypersensitivity, hypertension

Precautions: Children, pregnancy (C), lactation, elderly

Pharmacokinetics:

IM/IV: Onset 15 min, duration 3-4 hr, metabolized by liver, excreted in urine, feces, half-life 40 min

Syringe compatibilities: Atropine, droperidol/fentanyl, glycopyrrolate, hydroxyzine, ketamine, meperidine, midazolam, morphine, naloxone, pentazocine, propranolol, scopolamine

NURSING CONSIDERATIONS

Assess:

• Vital signs, B/P; check patients with cardiac disease more often; hypotension, hypertension, dysrhythmias may occur

• Observe for drowsiness; instruct patient not to drive, operate machinery

Administer:

• After reconstituting 50 mg of drug with 2.2 ml sterile water for injection to a concentration of 25 mg/ml; do not use NaCl. Direct IV 25 mg over ½-1 min by Y-tube or 3-way stopcock

• Reduced dosage if patient is receiving pressor drugs

Perform/provide:

• Storage of injection before, after reconstitution in light-resistant container, single-dose container

Evaluate:

• Therapeutic response: absence of nausea, vomiting

Treatment of overdose:

• Supportive care; atropine may be helpful

benztropine (℞)

(benz′troe-peen)

Apo-Benztropin*, Bensylate*, benztropine mesylate, Cogentin

Func. class.: Cholinergic blocker

Chem. class.: Tertiary amine

Action: Blockade of central acetylcholine receptors

Uses: Parkinson symptoms, EPS associated with neuroleptic drugs

Dosage and routes:

Drug-induced EPS

• *Adult:* IM/IV 1-4 mg qd-bid; give PO dose as soon as possible; PO 1-2 mg bid/tid, increase by 0.5 mg q5-6days

Parkinson symptoms

• *Adult:* PO 0.5-1 mg qd, increased 0.5 mg q5-6days titrated to patient response

Acute dystonic reactions

• *Adult:* IM/IV 1-2 mg, may increase to 1-2 mg bid (PO)

Available forms: Tabs 0.5, 1, 2 mg; inj IM, IV 1 mg/ml

Side effects/adverse reactions:

MS: Muscular weakness, cramping

INTEG: Rash, urticaria, dermatoses

MISC: Increased temperature, flushing, decreased sweating, hyperthermia, heat stroke, numbness of fingers

CNS: Confusion, anxiety, restlessness, irritability, delusions, hallucinations, headache, sedation, depression, incoherence, dizziness, memory loss

EENT: Blurred vision, photophobia, dilated pupils, difficulty swallowing, dry eyes, mydriasis, increased intraocular tension, angle-closure glaucoma

CV: Palpitations, tachycardia, hypotension, bradycardia

GI: Dryness of mouth, constipation, nausea, vomiting, abdominal distress, ***paralytic ileus,*** epigastric distress

GU: Hesitancy, retention, dysuria

Contraindications: Hypersensitivity, narrow-angle glaucoma, myasthenia gravis, GI/GU obstruction, child <3 yr, peptic ulcer, megacolon, prostate hypertrophy

Precautions: Pregnancy (C), elderly, lactation, tachycardia, liver, kidney disease, drug abuse history, dysrhythmias, hypotension, hypertension, psychiatric patients, children

Pharmacokinetics:

IM/IV: Onset 15 min, duration 6-10 hr

PO: Onset 1 hr, duration 6-10 hr

Interactions:

• Increased anticholinergic effect: antihistamines, phenothiazines, amantadine

• Decreased effect of levodopa

• Increased schizophrenic symptoms: haloperidol

• Incompatibilities: unknown

NURSING CONSIDERATIONS

Assess:

• I&O ratio; retention commonly causes decreased urinary output

• Parkinsonism, EPS: shuffling gait, muscle rigidity, involuntary movements

• Urinary hesitancy, retention; palpate bladder if retention occurs

• Constipation; increase fluids, bulk, exercise if this occurs

• For tolerance over long-term therapy; dose may have to be increased or changed

• Mental status: affect, mood, CNS depression, worsening of mental symptoms during early therapy

• Use caution in hot weather; drug may increase susceptibility to stroke by decreasing sweating

Administer:

• With or after meals to prevent GI upset; may give with fluids other than water

• At hs to avoid daytime drowsiness in patient with parkinsonism

• Undiluted IV (1 mg = 1 ml) dose at ≤1 mg/>1 min; keep in bed for at least 1 hr after dose

Perform/provide:

• Storage at room temperature

• Hard candy, frequent drinks, gum to relieve dry mouth

Evaluate:

• Therapeutic response: absence of involuntary movements

---

* Available in Canada only

Teach patient/family:

- Not to discontinue this drug abruptly; to taper off over 1 wk
- To avoid driving, other hazardous activities; drowsiness may occur
- To avoid OTC medication: cough, cold preparations with alcohol, antihistamines unless directed by prescriber

bepridil (℞)

(be'pri-dil)

Vascor

Func. class.: Calcium channel blocker

Action: Inhibits calcium ion influx across cell membrane during cardiac depolarization; produces relaxation of coronary vascular smooth muscle, dilates coronary arteries, decreases SA/AV node conduction, dilates peripheral arteries

Uses: Chronic stable angina, used alone or in combination with propranolol

Dosage and routes:

Angina

- *Adult:* 200-450 mg qd

Available forms: Tabs, film-coated, 200, 300, 400 mg

Side effects/adverse reactions:

CV: Dysrhythmia, edema, CHF, bradycardia, hypotension, palpitations, AV block

GI: Nausea, vomiting, diarrhea, gastric upset, constipation, increased liver function studies

GU: Nocturia, polyuria

CNS: Headache, fatigue, drowsiness, dizziness, anxiety, depression, weakness, insomnia, confusion, light-headedness, nervousness

Contraindications: Sick sinus syndrome, 2nd or 3rd degree heart block, Wolff-Parkinson-White syndrome, hypotension less than 90 mm Hg systolic, cardiogenic shock, history of serious ventricular dysrhythmias

Precautions: CHF, hypotension, hepatic injury, pregnancy (C), lactation, children, renal disease, idiopathic hypertropic subaortic stenosis (IHSS), concomitant β-blocker therapy

Pharmacokinetics: Peak 2-3 hr, 99% plasma protein bound, half-life 42 hr; completely metabolized in the liver and excreted in urine and feces

Interactions:

- Increased effects: β-blockers
- Decreased effects of lithium, rifampin
- Increased levels of digoxin

Lab test interferences:

Increase: Liver function tests, aminotransferase, CPK, LDH

NURSING CONSIDERATIONS

Assess:

- Cardiac status: B/P, pulse, respiration, ECG intervals (PR, QRS, QT), dysrhythmias

Administer:

- Before meals, hs

Evaluate:

- Therapeutic response: decreased anginal pain, decreased B/P

Teach patient/family:

- How to take pulse before taking drug; record or graph should be kept, use demonstration, return demonstration
- To avoid hazardous activities until stabilized on drug, dizziness no longer a problem
- To limit caffeine consumption
- To avoid OTC drugs unless directed by a prescriber
- Importance of compliance with all areas of medical regimen: diet, exercise, stress reduction, drug therapy

Treatment of overdose: Defibrillation, atropine for AV block, vasopressor for hypotension

beractant (℞)

(bear-ac'tant)

Survanta

Func. class.: Natural lung surfactant

Action: Replenishes surfactant and restores surface activity to the lungs in premature infants

Uses: Prevention and treatment (rescue) of respiratory distress syndrome in premature infants

Dosage and routes:

Intratracheal instill: 4 doses can be administered in the 1st 48 hrs of life; give doses no more frequently than q6h; each dose is 100 mg of phospholipids/kg birth weight (4 ml/kg)

Available forms: Susp 25 mg phospholipids/ml in 0.9% NaCl in single-use vials containing 8 ml susp

Side effects/adverse reactions:

Concurrent illnesses that have occurred during treatment are in bold

RESP: ***Pulmonary air leaks, pulmonary interstitial emphysema, apnea, pulmonary hemorrhage***

SYST: ***Patent ductus arteriosus, intracranial hemorrhage, severe intracranial hemorrhage, necrotizing enterocolitis, posttreatment sepsis, posttreatment infection,*** bradycardia, oxygen desaturation, pallor, vasoconstriction, hypotension, hypertension

Precautions: Bradycardia, rales, infections

Pharmacokinetics: Becomes lung associated within hours of administration

NURSING CONSIDERATIONS

Assess:

- Respiratory rate, rhythm, character, chest expansion, color, transcutaneous saturation, ABGs
- Endotracheal tube placement before dosing; for apnea after endotracheal administration
- Reflux of drug into the endotracheal tube during administration; stop drug if this occurs, and if needed, increase peak inspiratory pressure on the ventilator by 4-5 cm H_2O until tube is cleared
- Infant for repeat dosing using radiographic confirmation of RDS; repeat doses should be given as above; ventilator settings for repeat doses FIo_2 were decreased by 0.2 or amount to prevent cyanosis; ventilator rate of 30/min; inspiratory time <1 sec; if infant's pretreatment rate was >30, it was left unchanged during dosing; resume usual ventilator management after dosing

Administer:

- After suctioning
- By endotracheal administration only by persons trained in neonatal intubation and ventilation
- After using a No. 5 Fr end-hole catheter inserted into the endotracheal tube with the tip protruding just beyond the end of the endotracheal tube; shorten the catheter before insertion; do not insert the drug into the mainstem bronchus
- Divide each dose into quarters and administer with infant in different positions
- Determine dosing by weight of infant; slowly withdraw contents into plastic syringe through 20G needle; do not filter or shake; attach premeasured No. 5 Fr catheter to syringe; fill with drug and discard excess through catheter so only dose to be given remains in syringe
- For prevention dosing, stabilize, weigh, and intubate infant; give drug within 15 min of birth if possible; position infant and inject first quarter-dose through catheter over

2-3 sec; remove catheter and manually ventilate with O_2 to prevent cyanosis (60 bpm) and sufficient positive pressure to promote adequate air exchange and chest wall excursion
• For rescue dosing, give dosing as soon as infant is placed on ventilator after birth; immediately before administering dose, change ventilator settings to 60/min, inspiratory timc 0.5 sec, FIo_2 1; position infant and inject first quarter through catheter over 2-3 sec; remove catheter; return to mechanical ventilator
• Ventilate infant for >30 sec or until stable after prevention or rescue strategy; resposition for next dose; same procedure for subsequent dosing; do not suction for at least 1 hr after dosing unless airway obstruction is evident; resume ventilator therapy after dosing

Perform/provide:
• Reduction in peak ventilator inspiratory pressures immediatcly if chest expansion improves substantially after dose
• Reduction in FIo_2 in small, repeated steps when infant becomes pink and transcutaneous oxygen saturation is in excess of 95%; oxygen saturation should remain between 90% and 95%
• Suctioning of all infants before administration to prevent mucus plugging; if endotracheal tube obstruction is suspected, remove obstruction and replace tube immediately
• Storage in refrigeration; protect from light, warm to room temperature for >20 min or warm in hand >8 min before giving; do not use artificial warming methods; enter a vial only once; unopened, unused vials that have been warmed to room temperature may be rerefrigerated within 8 hr of warming; do not warm and return to refrigerator more than once

Evaluate:
• Therapeutic response: significant improvement in respiratory status

betamethasone/ betamethasone sodium phosphate/ betamethasone disodium phosphate/ betamethasone acetate/betamethasone sodium phosphate (℞)

(bay-ta-meth'a-sone)

Alphatrex*, Betacort, Betaderm*, Betatrex, Beta-Val Betnelan*, Celestone/Alphatrex, Betamethasone Dipropionate, Diprosone, Maxivate, Teladar/ Diprolene, Diprolene AF/Betamethasone Sodium Phosphate, Celestone Phosphate, Cel-U-Jec, Selestoject

Func. class.: Corticosteroid, synthetic

Chem. class.: Glucocorticoid, long-acting

Action: Decreases inflammation by suppressing migration of polymorphonuclear leukocytes, fibroblasts, reversal of increased capillary permeability and lysosomal stabilization

Uses: Immunosupression, severe inflammation, prevention of neonatal respiratory distress syndrome (by administration to mother)

Dosage and routes:
• *Adult:* PO 0.6-7.2 mg qd; IM/IV 0.6-7.2 mg qd in joint or soft tissue (sodium phosphate)
• *Pregnant adult:* IM 12 mg 36-48 hr, before premature delivery, then

same dose in 24 hr (betamethasone acetate)
Available forms: Tabs 0.6 mg; syr 0.6 mg/5 ml; inj 3, 4 mg/ml
Side effects/adverse reactions:
INTEG: Acne, poor wound healing, ecchymosis, bruising, petechiae
CNS: Depression, flushing, sweating, headache, ecchymosis, bruising, mood changes
CV: Hypertension, ***circulatory collapse, thrombophlebitis, embolism,*** tachycardia, ***necrotizing angiitis, CHF***
HEMA: ***Thrombocytopenia***
MS: Fractures, osteoporosis, weakness
GI: Diarrhea, nausea, abdominal distention, ***GI hemorrhage,*** *increased appetite,* ***pancreatitis***
EENT: Fungal infections, increased intraocular pressure, blurred vision
Contraindications: Psychosis, hypersensitivity, idiopathic thrombocytopenia, acute glomerulonephritis, amebiasis, fungal infections, nonasthmatic bronchial disease, child <2 yr, AIDS, TB
Precautions: Pregnancy (C), lactation, diabetes mellitus, glaucoma, osteoporosis, seizure disorders, ulcerative colitis, CHF, myasthenia gravis, renal disease, esophagitis, peptic ulcer
Pharmacokinetics:
PO: Onset 1-2 hr, peak 1 hr, duration 3 days
IM/IV: Onset 10 min, peak 4-8 hr, duration 1-1½ days
Metabolized in liver, excreted in urine as steroids, crosses placenta
Interactions:
• Decreased action of betamethasone: cholestyramine, colestipol, barbiturates, rifampin, ephedrine, phenytoin, theophylline
• Decreased effects of anticoagulants, anticonvulsants, antidiabetics, ambenonium, neostigmine, isoniazid, toxoids, vaccines, anticholinesterases, salicylates, somatrem
• Increased side effects: alcohol, salicylates, indomethacin, amphotericin B, digitalis, cyclosporine, diuretics
• Increased action of betamethasone: salicylates, estrogens, indomethacin, oral contraceptives, ketoconazole, macrolide antibiotics
Lab test interferences:
Increase: Cholesterol, sodium, blood glucose, uric acid, calcium, urine glucose
Decrease: Calcium, potassium, T_4, T_3, thyroid ^{131}I uptake test, urine 17-OHCS, 17-KS, PBI
False negative: Skin allergy tests

NURSING CONSIDERATIONS
Assess:
• Potassium, blood sugar, urine glucose while on long-term therapy; hypokalemia and hyperglycemia
• Weight daily; notify prescriber of weekly gain >5 lb
• B/P q4h, pulse; notify prescriber if chest pain occurs
• I&O ratio; be alert for decreasing urinary output and increasing edema
• Plasma cortisol levels during long-term therapy (normal level: 138-635 nmol/L SI units when drawn at 8 AM)
Administer:
• IV, only sodium phosphate product; give >1 min; may be given by IV INF in compatible sol
• After shaking suspension (parenteral)
• Titrated dose; use lowest effective dose
• IM injection deeply in large muscle mass, rotate sites, avoid deltoid, use 21G needle
• In one dose in AM to prevent adrenal suppression, avoid SC administration; may damage tissue

* Available in Canada only

• With food or milk to decrease GI symptoms

Perform/provide:

• Assistance with ambulation in patient with bone tissue disease to prevent fractures

Evaluate:

• Therapeutic response: ease of respirations, decreased inflammation

• Infection: increased temperature, WBC even after withdrawal of medication; drug masks infection symptoms

• Potassium depletion: paresthesias, fatigue, nausea, vomiting, depression, polyuria, dysrhythmias, weakness

• Edema, hypertension, cardiac symptoms

• Mental status: affect, mood, behavioral changes, aggression

Teach patient/family:

• That ID as steroid user should be carried

• To notify prescriber if therapeutic response decreases; dosage adjustment may be needed

• Not to discontinue abruptly; adrenal crisis can result

• To avoid OTC products: salicylates, alcohol in cough products, cold preparations unless directed by prescriber

• All aspects of drug usage including cushingoid symptoms

• Symptoms of adrenal insufficiency: nausea, anorexia, fatigue, dizziness, dyspnea, weakness, joint pain

betamethasone (℞)

(bay-ta-meth′a-sone)

Benisone, Uticort

Func. class.: Topical corticosteroid

Chem. class.: Synthetic fluorinated agent, group III potency

Action: Antipruritic, antiinflammatory

Uses: Psoriasis, eczema, contact dermatitis, pruritus

Dosage and routes:

• *Adult and child:* Apply to affected area qid

Available forms: Oint 0.025%; cream 0.025%; lotion 0.025%; gel 0.025%

Side effects/adverse reactions:

INTEG: Burning, dryness, itching, irritation, acne, folliculitis, hypertrichosis, perioral dermatitis, hypopigmentation, atrophy, striae, miliaria, allergic contact dermatitis, secondary infection

Contraindications: Hypersensitivity to corticosteroids, fungal infections

Precautions: Pregnancy (C), lactation, viral infections, bacterial infections

NURSING CONSIDERATIONS

Assess:

• Temperature; if fever develops, drug should be discontinued

• For systemic absorption: increased temperature, inflammation, irritation

Administer:

• Only to affected areas; do not get in eyes

• Medication, then cover with occlusive dressing (only if prescribed), seal to normal skin, change q12h; systemic absorption may occur

• Only to dermatoses; do not use on weeping, denuded, or infected area

Perform/provide:
- Cleansing before application of drug
- Treatment for a few days after area has cleared
- Storage at room temperature

Evaluate:
- Therapeutic response: absence of severe itching, patches on skin, flaking

Teach patient/family:
- To avoid sunlight on affected area; burns may occur

betamethasone valerate (℞)

(bay-ta-meth'a-sone)

Beta Cort*, Betaderm*, Betamethasone Valerate, Betatrex, Beta-Val, Valisone, Valisone Reduced Strength

Func. class.: Topical corticosteroid

Chem. class.: Synthetic fluorinated agent

Action: Possesses antipruritic, antiinflammatory actions

Uses: Psoriasis, eczema, contact dermatitis, pruritus

Dosage and routes:
- *Adult and child:* Apply to affected area qid

Available forms: Oint 0.1%; cream 0.01%, 0.1%; lotion 0.1%

Side effects/adverse reactions:

INTEG: Burning, dryness, itching, irritation, acne, folliculitis, hypertrichosis, perioral dermatitis, hypopigmentation, atrophy, striae, miliaria, allergic contact dermatitis, secondary infection

Contraindications: Hypersensitivity to corticosteroids, fungal infections

Precautions: Pregnancy (C), lactation, viral infections, bacterial infections

NURSING CONSIDERATIONS

Assess:
- Temperature; if fever develops, drug should be discontinued
- For systemic absorption: increased temperature, inflammation, irritation

Administer:
- Only to affected areas; do not get in eyes
- Medication, then cover with occlusive dressing (only if prescribed), seal to normal skin, change q12h; systemic absorption may occur
- Only to dermatoses; do not use on weeping, denuded, or infected area

Perform/provide:
- Cleansing before applying drug
- Treatment for a few days after area has cleared
- Storage at room temperature

Evaluate:
- Therapeutic response: absence of severe itching, patches on skin, flaking

Teach patient/family:
- To avoid sunlight on affected area; burns may occur

bethanechol (℞)

(be-than'e-kile)

bethanechol chloride, Duvoid, Myotonachol, Urebeth, Urecholine

Func. class.: Cholinergic stimulant

Chem. class.: Synthetic choline ester

Action: Stimulates muscarinic ACh receptors directly; mimics effects of parasympathetic nervous system stimulation; stimulates gastric motility, stimulates micturition

* Available in Canada only

Uses: Urinary retention (postoperative, postpartum), neurogenic atony of bladder with retention

Dosage and routes:

• *Adult:* PO 10-50 mg bid-qid; SC 2.5-10 mg tid qid prn

Test dose

• *Adult:* SC 2.5 mg repeated 15-30 min intervals × 4 doses to determine effective dose

Available forms: Tabs 5, 10, 25, 50 mg; inj SC 5 mg/ml

Side effects/adverse reactions:

INTEG: Rash, urticaria, flushing, increased sweating

CNS: Dizziness

GI: Nausea, bloody diarrhea, belching, vomiting, cramps, fecal incontinence

CV: Hypotension, bradycardia, orthostatic hypotension, reflex tachycardia, ***cardiac arrest, circulatory collapse***

GU: Urgency

RESP: ***Acute asthma, dyspnea***

EENT: Miosis, increased salivation, lacrimation, blurred vision

Contraindications: Hypersensitivity, severe bradycardia, asthma, severe hypotension, hyperthyroidism, peptic ulcer, parkinsonism, seizure disorders, CAD, coronary occlusion, mechanical obstruction, peritonitis, recent urinary or GI surgery

Precautions: Hypertension, pregnancy (C), lactation, child <8 yr, urinary retention

Pharmacokinetics:

PO: Onset 30-90 min, duration 1-6 hr

SC: Onset 5-15 min, duration 2 hr, excreted by kidneys

Interactions:

• Increased action of bethanechol: other cholinergics

• Hypotension: ganglionic blockers

• Decreased action of bethanechol: procainamide, quinidine

Lab test interferences:

Increase: AST, lipase/amylase, bilirubin, BSP

NURSING CONSIDERATIONS

Assess:

• B/P, pulse; observe after parenteral dose for 1 hr

• I&O ratio; check for urinary retention or incontinence

• Bradycardia, hypotension, bronchospasm, headache, dizziness, convulsions, respiratory depression; drug should be discontinued if toxicity occurs

Administer:

• Parenteral dose by SC route; use of IM, IV may result in cardiac arrest

• Only with atropine sulfate available for cholinergic crisis

• Only after all other cholinergics have been discontinued

• Increased doses if tolerance occurs

• To avoid nausea and vomiting, take on an empty stomach

Perform/provide:

• Storage at room temperature

• Bedpan/urinal if given for urinary retention

• Use of rectal tube if ordered, to increase passage of gas when used for abdominal distention

Evaluate:

• Therapeutic response: absence of urinary retention, abdominal distention

Teach patient/family:

• To take drug exactly as prescribed

• To make position changes slowly; orthostatic hypotension may occur

Treatment of overdose: Administer atropine 0.6-1.2 mg IV or IM (adult)

biperiden (℞)

(bye-per′i-den)

Akineton

Func. class.: Cholinergic blocker

Action: Centrally acting competitive anticholinergic

Uses: Parkinson symptoms, EPS secondary to neuroleptic drug therapy

Dosage and routes:

Extrapyramidal symptoms

• *Adult:* PO 2 mg qd-tid; IM/IV 2 mg q30min, if needed, not to exceed 8 mg/24 hr

Parkinson symptoms

• *Adult:* PO 2 mg tid-qid max 16 mg/24 hr

Available forms: Tabs 2 mg; inj IM/IV 5 mg/ml (lactate)

Side effects/adverse reactions:

CNS: Confusion, anxiety, restlessness, irritability, delusions, hallucinations, headache, sedation, depression, incoherence, dizziness, euphoria, tremors, memory loss

EENT: Blurred vision, photophobia, dilated pupils, difficulty swallowing, mydriasis, increased intraocular tension, angle-closure glaucoma

CV: Palpitations, tachycardia, postural hypotension, bradycardia

GI: Dryness of mouth, constipation, nausea, vomiting, abdominal distress, ***paralytic ileus***

GU: Hesitancy, retention, dysuria

MS: Weakness, cramping

INTEG: Rash, urticaria, dermatoses

MISC: Increased temperature, flushing, decreased sweating, hyperthermia, heat stroke, numbness of fingers

Contraindications: Hypersensitivity, narrow-angle glaucoma, myasthenia gravis, GI/GU obstruction, megacolon, stenosing peptic ulcers, prostatic hypertrophy

Precautions: Pregnancy (C), elderly, lactation, tachycardia, dysrhythmias, liver, kidney disease, drug abuse, hypotension, hypertension, psychiatric patients, children

Pharmacokinetics:

IM/IV: Onset 15 min, duration 6-10 hr

PO: Onset 1 hr, duration 6-10 hr

Interactions:

• Increased levels of digoxin, levodopa

• Increased schizophrenic symptoms: haloperidol

• Increased anticholinergic effect: antihistamines, phenothiazines, amantadine

• Incompatibilities are unknown

NURSING CONSIDERATIONS

Assess:

• I&O ratio; retention commonly causes decreased urinary output

• Parkinsonism, EPS: shuffling gait, muscle rigidity, involuntary movements

• Urinary hesitancy, retention; palpate bladder if retention occurs

• Constipation; increase fluids, bulk, exercise if this occurs

• For tolerance over long-term therapy; dose may have to be increased or changed

• Mental status: affect, mood, CNS depression, worsening of mental symptoms during early therapy

Administer:

• Parenteral dose with patient recumbent to prevent postural hypotension, give undiluted 2 mg or less/>1 min

• With or after meals to prevent GI upset; may give with fluids other than water

• At hs to avoid daytime drowsiness in patient with parkinsonism

Perform/provide:

• Storage at room temperature

• Hard candy, frequent drinks, gum to relieve dry mouth

* Available in Canada only

Evaluate:
• Therapeutic response: absence of involuntary movements
Teach patient/family:
• Use caution in hot weather; drug may increase susceptibility to stroke, decreases sweating
• Not to discontinue this drug abruptly; to taper off over 1 wk
• To avoid driving, other hazardous activities; drowsiness may occur
• To avoid OTC medication: cough, cold preparations with alcohol, antihistamines unless directed by prescriber

bisacodyl (OTC)

(bis-a-koe′dill)
Apo-Bisacodyl*, Bisacodyl, Bisacodyl Uniserts, Bisacolax*, Bisco-Lax, Dulcagen, Dulcolax, Fleet Bisacodyl Laxit*,
Func. class.: Laxative, stimulant
Chem. class.: Diphenylmethane

Action: Acts directly on intestine by increasing motor activity; thought to irritate colonic intramural plexus
Uses: Short-term treatment of constipation, bowel or rectal preparation for surgery, examination
Dosage and routes:
• *Adult:* PO 10-15 mg in PM or AM; may use up to 30 mg for bowel or rectal preparation; REC 10 mg; ENEMA 1.25 oz
• *Child >3 yr:* PO 5-10 mg
• *Child >2 yr:* REC 10 mg
• *Child <2 yr:* REC 5 mg
• *Child <6 yr:* ENEMA ½ contents of microenema
Available forms: Enteric coated tabs 5 mg; rec supp 10 mg
Side effects/adverse reactions:
CNS: Muscle weakness
GI: Nausea, vomiting, anorexia, cramps, diarrhea, rectal burning (suppositories)
META: Protein-losing enteropathy, alkalosis, hypokalemia, ***tetany,*** electrolyte, fluid imbalances
Contraindications: Hypersensitivity, rectal fissures, abdominal pain, nausea, vomiting, appendicitis, acute surgical abdomen, ulcerated hemorrhoids, acute hepatitis, fecal impaction, intestinal/biliary tract obstruction
Precautions: Pregnancy (C), lactation
Pharmacokinetics:
PO: Onset 6-10 min; acts within 6-12 hr
REC: Onset 15-16 min
Metabolized by liver; excreted in urine, bile, feces, breast milk
Interactions:
• Gastric irritation: antacids, milk, H_2 blockers

NURSING CONSIDERATIONS
Assess:
• Blood, urine electrolytes if drug is used often by patient
• I&O ratio to identify fluid loss
• Cause of constipation; identify whether fluids, bulk, or exercise missing from lifestyle
• Cramping, rectal bleeding, nausea, vomiting; if these symptoms occur, drug should be discontinued
Administer:
• Alone only with water for better absorption; do not take within 1 hr of other drugs or within 1 hr of antacids, milk, or cimetidine
• In AM or PM (oral dose)
Evaluate:
• Therapeutic response: decrease in constipation
Teach patient/family:
• To swallow tabs whole; not to chew
• Not to use laxatives for long-term therapy; bowel tone will be lost
• That normal bowel movements do not always occur daily

• Not to use in presence of abdominal pain, nausea, vomiting
• To notify prescriber if constipation is unrelieved or if symptoms of electrolyte imbalance occur: muscle cramps, pain, weakness, dizziness

bismuth subsalicylate (OTC)

(bis-meth)

Bismtral, Pepto-Bismol, Pepto-Bismol Maximum Strength

Func. class.: Antidiarrheal

Chem. class.: Salicylate

Action: Inhibits prostaglandin synthesis responsible for GI hypermotility; stimulates absorption of fluid and electrolytes

Uses: Diarrhea (cause undetermined), prevention of diarrhea when traveling

Dosage and routes:

• *Adult:* PO 30 ml or 2 tabs q30-60min, not to exceed 8 doses for >2 days
• *Child 10-14 yr:* PO 15 ml

Available forms: Chewable tabs 262 mg; susp 262 mg/15 ml

Side effects/adverse reactions:

HEMA: Increased bleeding time

GI: Increased fecal impaction (high doses), dark stools

CNS: Confusion, twitching

EENT: Hearing loss, tinnitus, metallic taste, blue gums, black tongue (chew tabs)

Contraindications: Child <3 yr

Precautions: Anticoagulant therapy

Pharmacokinetics:

PO: Onset 1 hr, peak 2 hr, duration 4 hr

Interactions:

• Increased side effects: alcohol, aminosalicyclic acid, carbonic anhydrase inhibitors
• Increased action of bismuth: ammonium chloride
• Decreased action of bismuth: antacids, corticosteroids
• Decreased action of uricosurics, indomethacin, antidiabetics, tetracyclines

Lab test interferences:

Interfere: Radiographic studies of GI system

NURSING CONSIDERATIONS

Assess:

• Skin turgor; shift if dehydration is suspected
• Electrolytes (K, Na, Cl) if diarrhea is severe or continues long term
• Bowel pattern before drug therapy, after treatment

Administer:

• But stop use if symptoms do not improve within 2 days or become worse, or if diarrhea is accompanied by high fever
• Increased fluids to rehydrate the patient

Evaluate:

• Therapeutic response: decreased diarrhea or absence of diarrhea when traveling

Teach patient/family:

• To chew or dissolve in mouth; do not swallow whole; shake liquid before using
• To avoid other salicylates unless directed by prescriber; not to give to children, possibility of Reye's syndrome
• That stools may turn black; tongue may darken; impaction may occur in debilitated patients

B

bisoprolol (℞)

(biss-op′proe-lol)
Zebeta
Func. class.: Antihypertensive
Chem. class.: β_1-blocker

Action: Preferentially and competitively blocks stimulation of β_1-adrenergic receptor within cardiac muscle; produces negative chronotropic and inotropic activity (decreases rate of SA node discharge, increases recovery time), slows conduction of AV node, decreases heart rate, which decreases O_2 consumption in myocardium; decreases renin-aldosterone-angiotensin system; inhibits β_2-receptors in bronchial and vascular smooth muscle at high doses

Uses: Mild to moderate hypertension

Investigational uses: Angina pectoris

Dosage and routes:

Hypertension

• *Adult:* PO 2.5-5 mg qd; may increase if necessary to 20 mg qd; may need to reduce dose in presence of renal or hepatic impairment

Available forms: Tabs 5, 10 mg

Side effects/adverse reactions:

MS: Joint pain, arthralgia

MISC: Facial swelling, weight gain, decreased exercise tolerance

CV: Ventricular dysrhythmias, profound hypotension, bradycardia, CHF, cold extremities, postural hypotension, 2nd or 3rd degree heart block

CNS: Vertigo, headache, insomnia, fatigue, dizziness, mental changes, memory loss, hallucinations, depression, lethargy, drowsiness, strange dreams, catatonia, peripheral neuropathy

GI: Nausea, diarrhea, vomiting, mesenteric arterial thrombosis, ischemic colitis, flatulence, gastritis, gastric pain

INTEG: Rash, fever, alopecia, pruritus, sweating

HEMA: Agranulocytosis, thrombocytopenia, purpura, eosinophilia

EENT: Sore throat, dry burning eyes

GU: Impotence, decreased libido

ENDO: Increased hypoglycemic response to insulin

RESP: Bronchospasm, dyspnea, wheezing, cough, nasal stuffiness

Contraindications: Hypersensitivity to β-blockers, cardiogenic shock, heart block (2nd, 3rd degree), sinus bradycardia, CHF, cardiac failure

Precautions: Major surgery, pregnancy (B), lactation, children, diabetes mellitus, renal or hepatic disease, thyroid disease, COPD, asthma, well-compensated heart failure, aortic or mitral valve disease, peripheral vascular disease, myasthenia gravis

Pharmacokinetics:

PO: Peak 2-4 hr; half-life 9-12 hr, 50% excreted unchanged in urine, protein binding 30%; metabolized in liver to inactive metabolites

Interactions:

• Increased hypotension, bradycardia: reserpine, hydralazine, methyldopa, quinidine, prazosin

• Decreased antihypertensive effects: indomethacin, nonsteroidal antiinflammatories, barbiturates, cholestyramine, colestipol, penicillins, salicylates

• Increased hypoglycemic effect: insulin

• Decreased bronchodilation: theophylline

• Decreased hypoglycemic effect of sulfonylureas

Lab test interferences:

Increase: AST and ALT

Interference: Glucose/insulin tolerance tests

NURSING CONSIDERATIONS

Assess:

• B/P during beginning treatment, periodically thereafter: pulse q4h: note rate, rhythm, quality

• Apical/radial pulse before administration; notify prescriber of any significant changes (pulse <60 bpm)

• Baselines in renal, liver function tests before therapy begins

• Edema in feet, legs daily

• Skin turgor, dryness of mucous membranes for hydration status, especially elderly

Administer:

• PO ac, hs tablet may be crushed or swallowed whole

• Reduced dosage in renal and hepatic dysfunction

Perform/provide:

• Storage protected from light, moisture; placed in cool environment

Evaluate:

• Therapeutic response: decreased B/P after 1-2 wk

Teach patient/family:

• Not to discontinue drug abruptly, taper over 2 wk, may cause precipitate angina

• Not to use OTC products containing α-adrenergic stimulants (such as nasal decongestants, OTC cold preparations) unless directed by prescriber

• To report bradycardia, dizziness, confusion, depression, fever

• To take pulse at home; advise when to notify prescriber

• To avoid alcohol, smoking, sodium intake

• To comply with weight control, dietary adjustments, modified exercise program

• To carry Medic Alert ID to identify drug taking, allergies

• To avoid hazardous activities if dizziness is present

• To report symptoms of CHF: difficult breathing, especially on exertion or when lying down, night cough, swelling of extremities

Treatment of overdose: Lavage, IV atropine for bradycardia, IV theophylline for bronchospasm, digitalis, O_2, diuretic for cardiac failure, hemodialysis, IV glucose for hyperglycemia, IV diazepam (or phenytoin) for seizures

---

bitolterol (℞)

(bye-tol′te-role)

Tornalate

Func. class.: Adrenergic β_2-agonist

Chem. class.: Acid ester of colterol

Action: Causes bronchodilation by action on β_2-receptors with increased synthesis of cAMP; relaxes bronchial smooth muscle; inhibits mast cell degranulation; stimulates cilia to remove secretions with very little effect on heart rate

Uses: Asthma, bronchospasm

Dosage and routes:

Inhaler

• *Adult and child >12 yr:* INH 2 puffs, wait 1-3 min before 3rd puff if needed, not to exceed 3 INH q6h or 2 INH q4h

Nebulization

• *Adult/Child >12 yr:* INH 0.5 ml (1 mg) tid by intermittent flow or 1.25 mg tid by continuous flow

Available forms: Aerosol 0.37 mg/actuation, 0.02% neb sol

Side effects/adverse reactions:

CNS: Tremors, anxiety, insomnia, headache, dizziness, stimulation, restlessness, hallucinations

EENT: Dry nose, irritation of nose and throat

CV: Palpitations, tachycardia, hy-

pertension, angina, hypotension
GI: Heartburn, nausea, vomiting, anorexia
MS: Muscle cramps
RESP: ***Bronchospasm,*** dyspnea
Contraindications: Hypersensitivity to sympathomimetics
Precautions: Lactation, pregnancy (C), cardiac disorders, hyperthyroidism, diabetes mellitus
Pharmacokinetics:
INH: Onset 3 min, peak ½-1 hr, duration 5-8 hr
Interactions:
• Increased action of aerosol bronchodilators
• Increased action of bitolterol: tricyclic antidepressants, MAOIs
• May inhibit action when used with other β-blockers

NURSING CONSIDERATIONS
Assess:
• Respiratory function: vital capacity, forced expiratory volume, ABGs
Administer:
• After shaking, exhale, place mouthpiece in mouth, inhale slowly, hold breath, remove, exhale slowly
• Gum, sips of water for dry mouth
Perform/provide:
• Storage in light-resistant container, do not expose to temperatures over 86° F (30° C)
Evaluate:
• Therapeutic response: absence of dyspnea, wheezing over 1 hr
Teach patient/family:
• Not to use OTC medications; extra stimulation may occur
• To use inhaler; review package insert with patient, provide demonstration, return demonstration
• To avoid getting aerosol in eyes
• To wash inhaler in warm water and dry qd
• On all aspects of drug; avoid smoking, smoke-filled rooms, persons with respiratory infections

Treatment of overdose: Administer a β_2-adrenergic blocker

B

bleomycin (℞)
(blee-oh-mye'sin)
BLM, Blenoxane
Func. class.: Antineoplastic, antibiotic
Chem. class.: Glycopeptide

Action: Inhibits synthesis of DNA, RNA, protein; derived from *Streptomyces verticillus;* replication is decreased by binding to DNA, which causes strand splitting; phase specific in the G_2 and M phases; a nonvesicant
Uses: Cancer of head, neck, penis, cervix, vulva of squamous cell origin, Hodgkin's disease, lymphosarcoma, reticulum cell sarcoma, testicular carcinoma
Dosage and routes:
• *Adult:* SC/IV/IM 0.25-0.5 U/kg 1-2 times/wk or 10-20 U/m^2, then 1 U/day or 5 U/wk; may also be given intraarterially; do not exceed total dose, 400 U in lifetime
Available forms: Inj IV, SC, IM, IA, intralesional, intracavity 15 units
Side effects/adverse reactions:
SYST: ***Anaphylaxis***
GI: Nausea, vomiting, anorexia, stomatitis, weight loss
INTEG: Rash, hyperkeratosis, nail changes, alopecia, fever and chills
RESP: ***Fibrosis,*** pneumonitis, wheezing, ***pulmonary toxicity***
CNS: Fever, chills
IDIOSYNCRATIC REACTION: Hypotension, confusion, fever, chills, wheezing
Contraindications: Hypersensitivity
Precautions: Renal, hepatic, respiratory disease, pregnancy (D)
Pharmacokinetics: Half-life 2 hr

when CrCl >35 ml/min half-life is increased in lower clearance, metabolized in liver, 50% excreted in urine (unchanged)

Interactions:

- Increased toxicity: other antineoplastics, radiation therapy
- Decreased serum digoxin levels: digoxin

Syringe compatibilities: Cisplatin, cyclophosphamide, doxorubicin, droperidol, fluorouracil, furosemide, heparin, leucovorin, methotrexate, metoclopramide, mitomycin, vinblastine, vincristine

Y-site compatibilities: Cisplatin, cyclophosphamide, doxorubicin, droperidol, fludarabine, fluorouracil, furosemide, heparin, leucovorin, melphalan, methotrexate, metoclopramide, mitomycin, ondansetron, paclitaxel, sargramostin, vinblastine, vincristine, vinorelbine

Additive compatibilities: Amikacin, cephapirin, dexamethasone sodium phosphate, diphenhydramine, fluorouracil, gentamicin, heparin, hydrocortisone sodium succinate, phenytoin, streptomycin, tobramycin, vincristine, vinblastine

Solution compatibilities: D_5W, 0.9% NaCl

NURSING CONSIDERATIONS

Assess:

- IM test dose
- Pulmonary function tests: chest x-ray film before and during therapy; should be obtained q2wk during treatment
- Temperature q4h; fever may indicate beginning infection
- Serum creatinine
- Dyspnea, rales, unproductive cough, chest pain, tachypnea, fatigue, increased pulse, pallor, lethargy
- Food preferences; list likes, dislikes
- Effects of alopecia and skin color on body image; discuss feelings about body changes
- Buccal cavity q8h for dryness, sores, ulceration, white patches, oral pain, bleeding, dysphagia
- Local irritation, pain, burning, discoloration at injection site
- Symptoms indicating severe allergic reaction: rash, pruritus, urticaria, purpuric skin lesions, itching, flushing
- Storage for 2 wk after reconstituting at room temperature; discard unused portions

Administer:

- IM/SC after reconstituting 5 U/1-5 ml sterile H_2O, D_5W, 0.9% NaCl, or bacteriostatic water for inj; do not use products containing benzyl alcohol when giving to neonates
- Direct IV after reconstituting 15 U or less/5 ml or more of D_5W or 0.9% NaCl; after further diluting with 50-100 ml D_5W or 0.9% NaCl, give 15 U or less/10 min through Y-tube or 3-way stopcock
- Two test doses 2-5 U before initial dose; monitor for anaphylaxis
- Antiemetic 30-60 min before giving drug to prevent vomiting, continue antiemetics 6-10 hr after treatment
- Topical or systemic analgesics for pain of stomatitis as ordered; antihistamines and antipyretics for fever and chills
- Intraarterial/IV injections over >10 min

Perform/provide:

- Deep breathing exercises with patient tid-qid; place in semi-Fowler's position
- Liquid diet: carbonated beverage; gelatin may be added if patient is not nauseated or vomiting
- Rinsing of mouth tid-qid with water, club soda; brushing of teeth with baking soda bid-tid with soft brush

or cotton-tipped applicators for stomatitis; use unwaxed dental floss
• HOB raised to facilitate breathing

Evaluate:
• Therapeutic response: decrease in size of tumor

Teach patient/family:
• To report any complaints, side effects to nurse or prescriber
• To report any changes in breathing, coughing, fever
• That hair may be lost during treatment and wig or hairpiece may make patient feel better; tell patient that new hair may be different in color, texture
• To avoid foods with citric acid, hot or rough texture
• To report any bleeding, white spots, ulcerations in mouth; to examine mouth qd and report symptoms

bretylium (℞)

(bre-til′ee-um)
Bretylate*, bretylium tosylate, Bretylol

Func. class.: Antidysrhythmic (Class III)
Chem. class.: Quaternary ammonium compound

Action: After a transient release of norepinephrine, inhibits further release by postganglionic nerve endings; prolongs duration of action potential and effective refractory period

Uses: Serious ventricular tachycardia, cardioversion, ventricular fibrillation; for short-term use only

Dosage and routes:

Severe ventricular fibrillation
• *Adult:* IV BOL 5 mg/kg, increase to 10 mg/kg repeated q15 min, up to 30 mg/kg; IV INF 1-2 mg/min or give 5-10 mg/kg over 10 min q6h (maintenance)

Ventricular dysrhythmias
• *Adult:* IV INF 500 mg diluted in 50 ml D_5W or NS, infuse over 10-30 min, may repeat in 1 hr, maintain with 1-2 mg/min or 5-10 mg/kg over 10-30 min q6h; IM 5-10 mg/kg undiluted; repeat in 1-2 hr if needed; maintain with same dose q6-8h

Available forms: Inj IV 50 mg/ml; 1, 2, 4 mg/ml prefilled syringes

Side effects/adverse reactions:
CNS: Syncope, dizziness, confusion, psychosis, anxiety
GI: Nausea, vomiting
CV: Hypotension, postural hypotension, bradycardia, angina, PVCs, substernal pressure, transient hypertension, precipitation of angina
RESP: ***Respiratory depression***

Contraindications: Hypersensitivity, digitalis toxicity, aortic stenosis, pulmonary hypertension, children

Precautions: Renal disease, pregnancy (C), lactation, children

Pharmacokinetics: Well absorbed by IM/IV routes
IV: Onset 5 min; duration 6-24 hr
IM: Onset ½-2 hr, duration 6-24 hr
Half-life 4-17 hr, excreted unchanged by kidneys (70%-80% in 24 hr), not metabolized

Interactions:
• Increased or decreased effects of bretylium: quinidine, procainamide, propranolol, other antidysrhythmics
• Hypotension: antihypertensives
• Toxicity: digitalis

Additive compatibilities: Aminophylline, calcium chloride, calcium gluconate, digoxine, dopamine, esmolol, regular insulin, lidocaine, potassium chloride, quinadine verapamil

Y-site compatibilities: Amrinone, dobutamine, famotidine, isoproterenol, ranitidine

Lab test interferences:
Decrease: Urinary epinephrine, uri-

nary norepinephrine, urinary VMA epinephrine

NURSING CONSIDERATIONS

Assess:

• ECG continuously to determine drug effectiveness, PVCs, other dysrhythmias

• IV inf rate to avoid causing nausea, vomiting

• For dehydration or hypovolemia

• B/P continuously for hypotension, hypertension; orthostatic hypotension; keep supine until hypotension subsides

• I&O ratio

• If systolic B/P <75 mm HG, notify prescriber

• For rebound hypertension after 1-2 hr

• Cardiac status: rate, rhythm, character, continuously

Administer:

• IV direct undiluted over 15-30 sec (ventricular fibrillation); may repeat in 15-30 min, not to exceed 30 mg/kg/24 hr

• IV INT INF by diluting 500 mg of drug/50 ml or more D_5W, 0.9% NaCl, D_5/0.45%, D_5/0.9% NaCl, D_5/Lr, LRONS, give over 15-30 min

• IV cont INF by diluting further; give at 1-2 mg diluted sol/min via infusion pump

• IM inj, rotate sites, inject <5 ml in any one site to prevent tissue necrosis, may repeat 1-2 hour

• Reduced dosage slowly with ECG monitoring, discontinue over 3-5 days, maintain on oral dysrhythmic

Perform/provide:

• Place patient in supine position unless otherwise ordered; assist with ambulation

• Have suction equipment available

Evaluate:

• Therapeutic response: absence of ventricular tachycardia, fibrillation

Teach patient/family:

• To make position changes slowly; orthostatic hypotension may occur

Treatment of overdose: O_2, artificial ventilation, ECG; administer dopamine for circulatory depression; administer diazepam or thiopental for convulsions

bromocriptine (℞)

(broe-moe-krip′teen)

Parlodel

Func. class.: Dopamine receptor agonist; ovulation stimulant

Chem. class.: Ergot alkaloid derivative

Action: Inhibits prolactin release by activating postsynaptic dopamine receptors; activation of striatal dopamine receptors may be reason for improvement in Parkinson's disease

Uses: Female infertility, Parkinson's disease, prevention of postpartum lactation, amenorrhea caused by hyperprolactinemia, acromegaly

Dosage and routes:

Hyperprolactinemic indications

• *Adult:* PO 1.25-2.5 mg with meals; may increase by 2.5 mg q3-7 days, usual 5-7.5 mg

Acromegaly

• *Adult:* PO 1.25-2.5 mg × 3 days hs; may increase by 1.25-2.5 mg q3-7 days; usual range 20-30 mg/day, max 100 mg/day

Postpartum lactation

• *Adult:* PO 2.5 mg qd-tid with meal × 14 or 21 days

Parkinson's disease

• *Adult:* PO 1.25 mg bid with meals, may increase q2-4 wk by 2.5 mg/day, not to exceed 100 mg qd

Available forms: Caps 5 mg; tabs 2.5 mg

Side effects/adverse reactions:

EENT: Blurred vision, diplopia, burning eyes, nasal congestion

CNS: Headache, depression, restlessness, anxiety, nervousness, confusion, ***convulsions,*** hallucinations, dizziness, fatigue, drowsiness, abnormal involuntary movements, psychosis
GU: Frequency, retention, incontinence, diuresis
GI: Nausea, vomiting, anorexia, cramps, constipation, diarrhea, dry mouth, GI hemorrhage
INTEG: Rash on face, arms, alopecia
CV: Orthostatic hypotension, decreased B/P, palpitation, extra systole, ***shock,*** dysrhythmias, bradycardia
Contraindications: Hypersensitivity to ergot, severe ischemic disease, pregnancy (D), severe peripheral vascular disease
Precautions: Lactation, hepatic disease, renal disease, children, pituitary tumors
Pharmacokinetics:
PO: Peak 1-3 hr, duration 4-8 hr, 90%-96% protein bound, half-life 3 hr, metabolized by liver (inactive metabolites), 85%-98% of dose excreted in feces
Interactions:
- Decreased action of bromocriptine: phenothiazines, imipramine, haloperidol, droperidol, amitriptyline
- Increased action of antihypertensives

Lab test interferences:
Increase: Growth hormone, AST (SGOT)/ALT (SGPT), CPK, BUN, uric acid, alk phosphatase, GGTP
NURSING CONSIDERATIONS
Assess:
- B/P; establish baseline, compare with other reading; this drug decreases B/P

Administer:
- With meal to prevent GI symptoms
- At hs so dizziness, orthostatic hypotension do not occur

Perform/provide:
- Storage at room temperature in tight container

Evaluate:
- Therapeutic response (Parkinson's disease): decreased dyskinesia, decreased slow movements, decreased drooling

Teach patient/family:
- To change position slowly to prevent orthostatic hypotension
- To use contraceptives during treatment with this drug; pregnancy may occur; to use methods other than oral contraceptives
- That therapeutic effect for Parkinson's disease may take 2 mo: galactorrhea, amenorrhea
- To avoid hazardous activity if dizziness occurs

brompheniramine (℞)

(brome-fen-ir'a-meen)
Bromphen, brompheniramine, Codimal-A, Cophene-B, Dehist, Diamine T.D., Dimetane, Dimetane Extentabs, Histaject, ND Stat, Nasahist-B
Func. class.: Antihistamine
Chem. class.: Alkylamine, H_1-receptor antagonist

Action: Acts on blood vessels, GI, respiratory system by competing with histamine for H_1-receptor site; decreases allergic response by blocking histamine
Uses: Allergy symptoms, rhinitis
Dosage and routes:
- *Adult:* PO 4-8 mg tid-qid, not to exceed 36 mg/day; TIME REL 8-12 mg bid-tid, not to exceed 36 mg/day; IM/IV/SC 5-20 mg q6-12h, not to exceed 40 mg/day

• *Child >6 yr:* PO 2 mg tid-qid, not to exceed 12 mg/day; IM/IV/SC 0.5 mg/kg/day divided tid or qid
• *Child <6 yr:* Only as directed by physician

Available forms: Tabs 4, 8, 12 mg; tabs, time rel 8, 12 mg; elix 2 mg/5 ml; inj IM/SC/IV 10, 100 mg/ml

Side effects/adverse reactions:

CNS: *Dizziness, drowsiness,* poor coordination, fatigue, anxiety, euphoria, confusion, paresthesia, neuritis

CV: Hypotension, palpitations, tachycardia

RESP: Increased thick secretions, wheezing, chest tightness

HEMA: ***Thrombocytopenia, agranulocytosis, hemolytic anemia***

GI: Dry mouth, nausea, vomiting, anorexia, constipation, diarrhea

INTEG: Photosensitivity

GU: Retention, dysuria, frequency, impotence

EENT: Blurred vision, dilated pupils, tinnitus, nasal stuffiness, dry nose, throat, mouth

Contraindications: Hypersensitivity to H_1-receptor antagonists, acute asthma attack, lower respiratory tract disease, child <6 yr

Precautions: Increased intraocular pressure, renal disease, cardiac disease, hypertension, bronchial asthma, seizure disorder, stenosed peptic ulcers, hyperthyroidism, prostatic hypertrophy, bladder neck obstruction, pregnancy (C), lactation

Pharmacokinetics:

PO: Peak 2-5 hr, duration to 48 hr; metabolized in liver, excreted by kidneys, excreted in breast milk, half-life 12-34 hr

Interactions:

• Increased CNS depression: barbiturates, narcotics, hypnotics, tricyclic antidepressants, alcohol
• Decreased effect of oral anticoagulants, heparin
• Increased drying effect: MAOIs
• Incompatible with aminophylline, insulins, pentobarbital

Lab test interferences:

False negative: Skin allergy tests

NURSING CONSIDERATIONS

Assess:

• I&O ratio; be alert for urinary retention, frequency, dysuria; drug should be discontinued if these occur
• CBC during long-term therapy
• Blood dyscrasias: thrombocytopenia, agranulocytosis (rare)
• Respiratory status: rate, rhythm, increase in bronchial secretions, wheezing, chest tightness

Administer:

• Direct IV undiluted or diluted with 10 ml 0.9% NaCl, given over 1 min or more
• IV INF by diluting in D_5W, 0.9% NaCl given at prescribed rate
• With meals if GI symptoms occur; absorption may slightly decrease

Perform/provide:

• Hard candy, gum, frequent rinsing of mouth for dryness
• Storage in tight container at room temperature

Evaluate:

• Therapeutic response: absence of running or congested nose or rashes

Teach patient/family:

• Not to crush or chew sustained release forms
• All aspects of drug use; to notify prescriber if confusion/sedation/hypotension occurs
• To avoid driving, other hazardous activities if drowsiness occurs
• To avoid use of alcohol, other CNS depressants while taking drug

Treatment of overdose: Administer ipecac syrup or lavage, diazepam, vasopressors, barbiturates (short-acting)

buclizine (℞)

(byoo'kli-zeen)
Bucladin-S, Softabs
Func. class.: Antiemetic, antihistamine, anticholinergic
Chem. class.: H_1-receptor antagonist (piperazine)

Action: Acts centrally by blocking chemoreceptor trigger zone, which in turn acts on vomiting center
Uses: Motion sickness, dizziness, nausea, vomiting
Dosage and routes:
• *Adult:* PO 25-50 mg prn ½ hr before travel; may be repeated q4-6h prn
Available forms: Tabs 50 mg
Side effects/adverse reactions:
CNS: *Drowsiness, dizziness,* fatigue, restlessness, headache, insomnia
GI: Nausea, anorexia, bitterness
EENT: Dry mouth, blurred vision
Contraindications: Hypersensitivity to cyclizines, shock
Precautions: Children, narrow-angle glaucoma, lactation, prostatic hypertrophy, elderly, pregnancy (C)
Pharmacokinetics:
PO: Duration 4-6 hr; other pharmacokinetics not known
NURSING CONSIDERATIONS
Assess:
• VS, B/P
• Signs of toxicity of other drugs or masking of symptoms of disease: brain tumor, intestinal obstruction
• Drowsiness, dizziness
Administer:
• Tablets may be swallowed whole, chewed, or allowed to dissolve
Evaluate:
• Therapeutic response: absence of dizziness, nausea, vomiting
Teach patient/family:
• To avoid hazardous activities, activities requiring alertness; dizziness may occur; instruct patient to request assistance with ambulation
• To avoid alcohol, depressants

budesonide (℞)

(byoo-des'o-nide)
Rhinocort
Func. class.: Glucocorticoid
Chem. class.: Nonhalogenated

Action: Prevents inflammation by depression of migration of polymorphonuclear leukocytes, fibroblasts, reversal of increased capillary permeability and lysosomal stabilization; does not suppress hypothalamus and pituitary function
Uses: Rhinitis, asthma
Dosage and routes:
• *Adult, child >12 yr:* Inh 400-600 μg/day; nasal: 200-400 μg/day
Available forms: Nasal aerosol 50 μg
Side effects/adverse reactions:
RESP: Nasal irritation, pharyngitis, cough, nasal bleeding
GI: Dry mouth, dyspepsia
INTEG: Itching, dermatitis
Contraindications: Hypersensitivity, status asthmaticus
Precautions: Pregnancy (C), lactation, elderly, child, TB, fungal, bacterial, systemic viral infections, ocular herpes simplex, nasal septal ulcers
Pharmacokinetics: Unknown
Interactions:
Increased effects: terbutaline
NURSING CONSIDERATIONS
Assess:
• Respiratory status: rate, rhythm, increase in bronchial secretions, wheezing, chest tightness; provide fluids to 2 L/day to decrease thickness of secretions; check for oral candidiasis

Administer:
- By inhalation; use scissors to open pouch

Perform/provide:
- Storage at 59°-86° F (15°-30° C); keep away from heat, open flame

Evaluate:
- Therapeutic response: absence of asthma, rhinitis

Teach patient/family:
- All aspects of drug use; to notify prescriber of pharyngitis, nasal bleeding
- Not to exceed recommended dose; adrenal suppression may occur

bumetanide (℞)

(byoo-met'a-nide)

Bumex

Func. class.: Loop diuretic

Chem. class.: Sulfonamide derivative

Action: Acts on ascending loop of Henle by increasing excretion of chloride, sodium

Uses: Edema in CHF, liver disease, renal disease (nephrotic syndrome), pulmonary edema, ascites (nephrotic syndrome), hypertension, anasarca

Investigational uses: May be used alone or as adjunct with antihypertensives such as spironolactone, triamterene

Dosage and routes:
- *Adult:* PO 0.5-2.0 mg qd; may give 2nd or 3rd dose at 4-5 hr intervals, not to exceed 10 mg/day; may be given on alternate days or intermittently; IV/IM 0.5-1.0 mg/day; may give 2nd or 3rd dose at 2-3 hr intervals, not to exceed 10 mg/day
- *Child:* PO, IM, IV 0.02-0.1 mg/kg q12h

Available forms: Tabs 0.5, 1, 2 mg; inj IV, IM 0.25 mg/ml

Side effects/adverse reactions:

GU: Polyuria, ***renal failure,*** glycosuria

ELECT: Hypokalemia, hypochloremic alkalosis, hypomagnesemia, hyperuricemia, hypocalcemia, hyponatremia, hyperglycemia

CNS: Headache, fatigue, weakness, vertigo

GI: Nausea, diarrhea, dry mouth, vomiting, anorexia, cramps, upset stomach, abdominal pain, ***acute pancreatitis, jaundice***

EENT: ***Loss of hearing,*** ear pain, tinnitus, blurred vision

INTEG: Rash, pruritus, purpura, ***Stevens-Johnson syndrome,*** sweating, photosensitivity

MS: Muscular cramps, arthritis, stiffness, tenderness

ENDO: Hyperglycemia

HEMA: ***Thrombocytopenia, agranulocytosis, neutropenia***

CV: ***Chest pain,*** hypotension, ***circulatory collapse,*** ECG changes, dehydration

Contraindications: Hypersensitivity to sulfonamides, anuria, hepatic coma, hypovolemia, lactation

Precautions: Dehydration, ascites, severe renal disease, pregnancy (C), hepatic cirrhosis

Pharmacokinetics:

PO: Onset ½-1 hr, duration 4 hr

IM: Onset 40 min, duration 4 hr

IV: Onset 5 min, duration 2-3 hr, excreted by kidneys, crosses placenta, excreted in breast milk

Interactions:
- Decreased diuretic effect: indomethacin, NSAIDs
- Ototoxicity: cisplatin, aminoglycosides, vancomycin
- Increased effect: antihypertensives
- Increased toxicity: lithium, nondepolarizing skeletal muscle relaxants, digitalis
- Decreased effects of antidiabetics

Y-site compatibilities: Amikacin, cisplatin, cyclophosphamide, dobutamine, fumotidine, dintrate, fludarabine, fluorouracil, foscarnet, heparin, hydrocortisone sodium succinate, kanamycin, leucovorin, methotrexate, mitomycin, potassium chloride, tobramycin, tolazoline, vitamin B complex with C

Syringe compatibilities: Cisplatin, cyclophosphamide, fluorouracil, heparin, leucovorin, methotrexate, mitomycin, vinblastine, vincristine

Additive compatibilities: Amikacin, aminophylline, amiodarone, ampicillin, atropine, flumetanide, calcium gluconate, cefumandole nafate, cefuroxime, cimetidine, cloxacillin, digoxin, epinephrine, heparin, isosorbide, kanamycin, lidocaine, morphine, nitroglycerin, ranitidine, sodium bicarbonate, tobramycin, verapamil

NURSING CONSIDERATIONS

Assess:

- Hearing with high IV doses
- Weight, I&O daily to determine fluid loss; effect of drug may be decreased if used qd
- Rate, depth, rhythm of respiration, effect of exertion
- B/P lying, standing; postural hypotension may occur
- Electrolytes: K, Na, Cl; include BUN, blood sugar, CBC, serum creatinine, blood pH, ABGs, uric acid, Ca, Mg
- Glucose in urine if patient is diabetic
- Improvement in edema of feet, legs, sacral area daily if medication is being used in CHF
- Improvement in CVP q8h
- Signs of metabolic alkalosis: drowsiness, restlessness
- Signs of hypokalemia: postural hypotension, malaise, fatigue, tachycardia, leg cramps, weakness
- Rashes, temperature elevation qd
- Confusion, especially in elderly; take safety precautions if needed
- For digitalis toxicity in patients taking digitalis products

Administer:

- Direct IV undiluted over at least 1 min through Y-tube or 3-way stopcock or heplock
- INT IV after dilution in LR, D_5W, 0.9% NaCl (rarely given by this method)
- In AM to avoid interference with sleep if using drug as a diuretic
- Potassium replacement if potassium is less than 3.0
- With food if nausea occurs; absorption may be decreased slightly

Evaluate:

- Therapeutic response: decreased edema, B/P

Teach patient/family:

- To increase fluid intake to 2-3 L/day unless contraindicated, to take K supplement, to rise slowly from lying or sitting position
- Adverse reactions: muscle cramps, weakness, nausea, dizziness
- To take with food or milk for GI symptoms
- To take early in day to prevent nocturia
- To use sunscreen to prevent photosensitivity

Treatment of overdose: Lavage if taken orally; monitor electrolytes; administer dextrose in saline; monitor hydration, CV, renal status

buprenorphine (℞)

(byoo-pre-nor′feen)

Buprenex

Func. class.: Narcotic analgesic

Chem. class.: Opiate, thebaine derivative

Controlled Substance Schedule V

Action: Depresses pain impulse

transmission at the spinal cord level by interacting with opioid receptors
Uses: Moderate to severe pain
Dosage and routes:
- *Adult:* IM/IV 0.3-0.6 mg q6h prn, reduce dosage in elderly

Available forms: Inj IM, IV 0.3 mg/ml (1 ml vials)
Side effects/adverse reactions:
CNS: Drowsiness, dizziness, confusion, headache, sedation, euphoria
GI: Nausea, vomiting, anorexia, constipation, cramps
GU: Increased urinary output, dysuria
INTEG: Rash, urticaria, bruising, flushing, diaphoresis, pruritus
EENT: Tinnitus, blurred vision, miosis, diplopia
CV: Palpitations, bradycardia, change in B/P
RESP: ***Respiratory depression***
Contraindications: Hypersensitivity, addiction (narcotic)
Precautions: Addictive personality, pregnancy (C), lactation, increased intracranial pressure, MI (acute), severe heart disease, respiratory depression, hepatic disease, renal disease
Pharmacokinetics:
IM: Onset 10-30 min, peak ½ hr, duration 3-4 hr
IV: Onset 1 min, peak 5 min, duration 2-5 hr
REC: Onset slow, duration 4-6 hr
Metabolized by liver; excreted by kidneys; crosses placenta; excreted in breast milk; half-life 2½-3½ hr; 96% bound to plasma proteins
Interactions:
- Effects may be increased with other CNS depressants: alcohol, narcotics, sedative/hypnotics, antipsychotics, skeletal muscle relaxants

Y-site compatibilities: Melphalan, vinorelbine
Syringe compatibility: Midazolam
Additive compatibilities: Atropine, diphenhydramine, droperidol, glycopyrrolate, haloperidol, hydroxyzine, promethazine, scopolamine

NURSING CONSIDERATIONS

Assess:
- I&O ratio; check for decreasing output; may indicate urinary retention
- CNS changes, dizziness, drowsiness, hallucinations, euphoria, LOC, pupil reaction
- Allergic reactions: rash, urticaria
- Respiratory dysfunction: respiratory depression, character, rate, rhythm; notify prescriber if respirations are <12/min
- Need for pain medication, tolerance

Administer:
- IV undiluted over 3-5 min, titrate to patient response
- With antiemetic if nausea, vomiting occur
- When pain is beginning to return; determine dosage interval by patient response

Perform/provide:
- Assistance with ambulation if needed

Evaluate:
- Therapeutic response: decrease in pain, absence of grimacing

Teach patient/family:
- To report any symptoms of CNS changes, allergic reactions
- That tolerance may result when used for extended periods

Treatment of overdose: Naloxone HCl (Narcan) 0.2-0.8 mg IV, O_2, IV fluids, vasopressors

* Available in Canada only

bupropion (℞)

(byoo-proe′pee-on)
Wellbutrin
Func. class.: Misc. antidepressant

Action: Inhibits reuptake of dopamine, serotonin, norepinephrine
Uses: Depression
Dosage and routes:
Adult: PO 100 mg bid initially, then increase after 3 days to 100 mg tid if needed; may increase after 1 month to 150 mg tid
Available forms: Tabs 75, 100 mg
Side effects/adverse reactions:
CNS: Headache, agitation, confusion, ***seizures,*** akathisia, delusions, insomnia, sedation, tremors
CV: Dysrhythmias, hypertension, palpitations, tachycardia, hypotension
GI: Nausea, vomiting, dry mouth, increased appetite, constipation
GU: Impotence, frequency, retention
INTEG: Rash, pruritus, sweating
EENT: Blurred vision, auditory disturbance
Contraindications: Hypersensitivity, seizure disorder, eating disorders
Precautions: Renal and hepatic disease, recent MI, cranial trauma, pregnancy (B), lactation, children
Pharmacokinetics: Onset 2-4 wk, half-life 12-14 hr; metabolized by liver
Interactions:
- Increased adverse reactions: levodopa, MAOIs, phenothiazines, tricyclic antidepressants, benzodiazepines, alcohol

NURSING CONSIDERATIONS
Assess
- Blood studies: CBC, leukocytes, differential, cardiac enzymes if patient is on long-term therapy
- Liver function tests before, during therapy: bilirubin, AST (SGOT), ALT (SGPT)
- ECG: watch for flattening of T wave, bundle branch block, AV block, dysrhythmias in cardiac patients
- Mental status: mood, sensorium, affect, suicidal tendencies, increase in psychiatric symptoms
- EPS primarily in elderly: akathisia
- Withdrawal symptoms: headache, nausea, vomiting, muscle pain, weakness if drug is discontinued abruptly
- Alcohol consumption: if alcohol is consumed, hold dose until morning

Administer:
- Increased fluids, bulk in diet if constipation occurs
- With food or milk for GI symptoms
- Gum, hard candy, or frequent sips of water for dry mouth

Perform/provide:
- Assistance with ambulation during beginning therapy, since sedation occurs
- Safety measures, including side rails, primarily in elderly
- Checking to see PO medication is swallowed

Evaluate:
- Therapeutic response: decreased depression, ability to function in daily activities, ability to sleep throughout the night

Teach patient/family:
- Therapeutic effects may take 2-4 wk
- To use caution in driving, other activities requiring alertness; sedation, blurred vision may occur

• To avoid alcohol ingestion, other CNS depressants
• Not to discontinue medication quickly after long-term use; may cause nausea, headache, malaise

Treatment of overdose: ECG monitoring; induce emesis, lavage, activated charcoal; administer anticonvulsant

buspirone (℞)

(byoo-spye'rone)
BuSpar
Func. class.: Antianxiety agent
Chem. class.: Azaspirodecanedione

Action: Acts by inhibiting the action of serotonin (5-HT)

Uses: Management and short-term relief of anxiety disorders

Dosage and routes:
• *Adult:* PO 5 mg tid; may increase by 5 mg/day q2-3d, not to exceed 60 mg/day

Available forms: Tabs 5, 10 mg

Side effects/adverse reactions:
CNS: Dizziness, headache, depression, stimulation, insomnia, nervousness, light-headedness, numbness, paresthesia, incoordination, tremors, excitement, involuntary movements, confusion, akathisia
GI: Nausea, dry mouth, diarrhea, constipation, flatulence, increased appetite, rectal bleeding
CV: Tachycardia, palpitations, hypotension, hypertension, ***CVA, CHF, MI***
EENT: Sore throat, tinnitus, blurred vision, nasal congestion, red, itching eyes, change in taste, smell
GU: Frequency, hesitancy, menstrual irregularity, change in libido
MS: Pain, weakness, muscle cramps, spasms
RESP: Hyperventilation, chest congestion, shortness of breath
INTEG: Rash, edema, pruritus, alopecia, dry skin
MISC: Sweating, fatigue, weight gain, fever

Contraindications: Hypersensitivity, child <18 yr

Precautions: Pregnancy (B), lactation, elderly, impaired hepatic/renal function

Interactions:
• Increased B/P: MAOIs; do not use together
• Increased effects: psychotropic drugs, alcohol (avoid use)
• Increased ALT: trazodone

NURSING CONSIDERATIONS

Assess:
• B/P (lying, standing), pulse; if systolic B/P drops 20 mm Hg, hold drug, notify prescriber
• Blood studies: CBC during long-term therapy; blood dyscrasias have occurred rarely
• Hepatic studies: AST (SGOT), ALT (SGPT), bilirubin, creatinine, LDH, alk phosphatase
• I&O; may indicate renal dysfunction
• Mental status: mood, sensorium, affect, sleeping pattern, drowsiness, dizziness
• Suicidal tendencies

Administer:
• With food or milk for GI symptoms
• Crushed if patient unable to swallow medication whole
• Sugarless gum, hard candy, frequent sips of water for dry mouth

Perform/provide:
• Assistance with ambulation during beginning therapy; drowsiness, dizziness occur
• Safety measures, including side rails, if drowsiness occurs

* Available in Canada only

- Check to see PO medication swallowed

Evaluate

- Therapeutic response: decreased anxiety, restlessness, sleeplessness

Teach patient/family:

- That drug may be taken with food
- To avoid OTC preparations unless approved by prescriber
- To avoid drinking, activities requiring alertness, since drowsiness may occur
- To avoid alcohol ingestion, other psychotropic medications, unless directed by prescriber
- Not to discontinue medication abruptly after long-term use
- To rise slowly or fainting may occur, especially elderly
- That drowsiness may worsen at beginning of treatment
- That 1-2 wk of therapy may be required before therapeutic effects occur

Treatment of overdose: Gastric lavage, VS, supportive care

busulfan (℞)

(byoo-sul'fan)

Myleran

Func. class.: Antineoplastic alkylating agent

Chem. class.: Nitrosurea

Action: Changes essential cellular ions to covalent bonding with resultant alkylation; this interferes with normal biologic function of DNA; activity is not phase specific; action is due to myelosuppression

Uses: Chronic myelocytic leukemia

Dosage and routes:

- *Adult:* PO 4-12 mg/day initially until WBC levels fall to 10,000/mm^3, then drug is stopped until WBC levels raise over 50,000/mm^3, then 1-3 mg/day
- *Child:* PO 0.06-0.12 mg/kg or 1.8-4.6 mg/m^2 day; dose is titrated to maintain WBC levels at 20,000/mm^3

Available forms: Tab 2 mg

Side effects/adverse reactions:

HEMA: ***Thrombocytopenia, leukopenia, pancytopenia, severe bone marrow depression***

GI: Nausea, vomiting, *diarrhea, weight loss*

GU: Impotence, sterility, amenorrhea, gynecomastia, ***renal toxicity,*** hyperuremia, adrenal insufficiency-like syndrome

INTEG: Dermatitis, hyperpigmentation, alopecia

RESP: ***Irreversible pulmonary fibrosis,*** pneumonitis

OTHER: ***Chromosomal aberrations***

Contraindications: Radiation, chemotherapy, lactation, pregnancy (3rd trimester) (D), blastic phase of chronic myelocytic leukemia, hypersensitivity

Precautions: Childbearing age men and women, leukopenia, thrombocytopenia, anemia, hepatotoxicity, renal toxicity

Pharmacokinetics: Well absorbed orally; excreted in urine; crosses placenta; excreted in breast milk

Interactions:

Increased toxicity: other antineoplastics or radiation

NURSING CONSIDERATIONS

Assess:

- CBC, differential, platelet count weekly; withhold drug if WBC is <4000 or platelet count is <75,000; notify prescriber of results
- Pulmonary function tests, chest x-ray films before, during therapy; chest film should be obtained q2wk during treatment
- Renal function studies: BUN, serum uric acid, urine CrCl before, during therapy

• I&O ratio; report fall in urine output <30 ml/hr
• Monitor for cold, fever, sore throat (may indicate beginning infection)
• For decreased hyperuricemia
• Bleeding: hematuria, guaiac, bruising or petechiae, mucosa or orifices q8h, no rectal temps
• Dyspnea, rales, unproductive cough, chest pain, tachypnea
• Food preferences; list likes, dislikes
• Edema in feet, joint, stomach pain, shaking
• Inflammation of mucosa, breaks in skin; use viscous xylocaine for oral pain

Administer:
• Antacid before oral agent, give drug after evening meal, before bedtime
• Antiemetic 30-60 min before giving drug to prevent vomiting
• Allopurinol or sodium bicarbonate to maintain uric acid levels, alkalinization of urine
• Antibiotics for prophylaxis of infection

Perform/provide:
• Comprehensive oral hygiene
• Strict medical asepsis, protective isolation if WBC levels are low
• Deep breathing exercises with patient tid-qid; place in semi-Fowler's position for pulmonary reactions
• Increase fluid intake to 2-3 L/day to prevent urate deposits, calculi formation
• Diet low in purines: organ meats (kidney, liver), dried beans, peas to maintain alkaline urine
• Storage in tight container

Evaluate:
• Therapeutic response: decreased exacerbations of chronic myelocytic leukemia

Teach patient/family:
• About protective isolation precautions
• To avoid use of products containing aspirin or ibuprofen, razors, commercial mouthwash
• To report signs of anemia, (fatigue, headache, irritability, faintness, shortness of breath)
• To report symptoms of bleeding (hematuria, tarry stools)
• That impotence or amenorrhea can occur, are reversible after discontinuing treatment
• To report any changes in breathing or coughing even several months after treatment

butoconazole (℞)

(byoo'toe-kone-a-zole)
Femstat
Func. class.: Local antiinfective
Chem. class.: Antifungal

Action: Binds sterols in fungal cell membrane, which increases permeability
Uses: Vulvovaginal infections caused by *Candida*
Dosage and routes:
• *Adult:* INTRA VAG 1 applicatorful hs × 3 days (nonpregnant), 6 days (2nd/3rd trimester pregnancy)
Available forms: Vaginal cream 2%
Side effects/adverse reactions:
GU: Rash, stinging, burning, vulvovaginal itching, soreness, swelling, discharge, finger itching
Contraindications: Hypersensitivity
Precautions: Pregnancy (C), lactation

NURSING CONSIDERATIONS
Assess:
• Allergic reaction: burning, stinging, itching, discharge, soreness
Administer:
• 1 applicatorful every night into vagina

* Available in Canada only

B

Perform/provide:
- Storage at room temperature in dry place

Evaluate:
- Therapeutic response: decrease in itching or white discharge

Teach patient/family:
- To use medical asepsis (handwashing) before, after each application
- That increased dreaming may occur
- To apply with applicator only
- To avoid use of any other vaginal product unless directed by physician; sanitary napkin may prevent soiling of undergarments
- To abstain from sexual intercourse until treatment is completed
- To notify prescriber if symptoms persist

---

butorphanol (℞)

(byoo-tor'fa-nole)

Stadol, Stadol NS

Func. class.: Narcotic analgesics

Chem. class.: Opiate

Action: Depresses pain impulse transmission at the spinal cord level by interacting with opioid receptors

Uses: Moderate to severe pain

Investigational uses: Migraine headache, pain

Dosage and routes:
- *Adult:* IM 1-4 mg q3-4h prn; IV 0.5-2 mg q3-4h prn; INTRANASAL, 1 spray in each nostril; may give another dose 1-1½ hr later; repeat if needed q3-4h

Available forms: Inj IM, IV 1, 2 mg/ml

Side effects/adverse reactions:

CNS: Drowsiness, dizziness, confusion, headache, sedation, euphoria, weakness, hallucinations

GI: Nausea, vomiting, anorexia, constipation, cramps

GU: Increased urinary output, dysuria, urinary retention

INTEG: Rash, urticaria, bruising, flushing, diaphoresis, pruritus

EENT: Tinnitus, blurred vision, miosis, diplopia

CV: Palpitations, bradycardia, change in B/P

RESP: ***Respiratory depression,*** pulmonary hypertension

Contraindications: Hypersensitivity, addiction (narcotic), CHF, myocardial infarction

Precautions: Addictive personality, pregnancy (B), lactation, increased intracranial pressure, respiratory depression, hepatic disease, renal disease, child <18 yr

Pharmacokinetics:

IM: Onset 10-30 min, peak ½ hr, duration 3-4 hr

IV: Onset 1 min, peak 5 min, duration 2-4 hr

Intranasal: Onset within 15 min, peak 1-2 hr, duration 4-5 hr

Metabolized by liver; excreted by kidneys; crosses placenta; excreted in breast milk; half-life 2½-3½ hr

Interactions:
- Effects may be increased with other CNS depressants: alcohol, narcotics, sedative/hypnotics, antipsychotics, skeletal muscle relaxants

Syringe compatibilities: Atropine, chlorpromazine, cimetidine, diphenhydramine, droperidol, fentanyl, hydroxyzine, meperidine, methotrimerprazine, metoclopramide, midazolam, morphine, pentazocine, perphenazine, prochlorperazine, promethazine, scopolamine, thiethylperazine

Y-site compatibilities: Enalaprilat, esmolol, fludarabine, melphalan, paclitaxel, sargramostim, vinorelbine

Lab test interferences:
Increase: Amylase

NURSING CONSIDERATIONS

Assess:
• I&O ratio; check for decreasing output; may indicate urinary retention
• For withdrawal symptoms in narcotic dependent patients: pulmonary embolus, vascular occlusion, abscesses, ulcerations
• CNS changes: dizziness, drowsiness, hallucinations, euphoria, LOC, pupil reaction
• Allergic reactions: rash, urticaria
• Respiratory dysfunction: respiratory depression, character, rate, rhythm; notify prescriber if respirations are <10/min
• Need for pain medication, physical dependence

Administer:
• IV undiluted at a rate of <2 mg/ >3-5 min, titrate to patient response
• IM deeply in large muscle mass
• With antiemetic if nausea, vomiting occur
• When pain is beginning to return; determine dosage interval by patient response

Perform/provide:
• Storage in light-resistant area at room temperature
• Assistance with ambulation
• Safety measures: side rails, nightlight, call bell within easy reach, especially elderly

Evaluate:
• Therapeutic response: decrease in pain

Teach patient/family:
• To report any symptoms of CNS changes, allergic reactions
• That physical dependency may result when used for extended periods
• That withdrawal symptoms may occur: nausea, vomiting, cramps, fever, faintness, anorexia

Treatment of overdose: Naloxone HCl (Narcan) 0.2-0.8 mg IV, O_2, IV fluids, vasopressors

calcifediol (℞)

(kal-si-fe-dye′ole)
Calderol
Func. class.: Vit D analog
Chem. class.: Sterol

Action: Increases intestinal absorption of calcium for bones; increases renal tubular absorption of phosphate; increases mobilization of calcium from bones, bone resorption

Uses: Metabolic bone disease with chronic renal failure, osteopenia, osteomalacia, hypocalcemia

Dosage and routes:
• *Adult:* PO 300-350 μg qwk divided into qd or qod doses; may increase q4wk

Available forms: Caps 20, 50 μg

Side effects/adverse reactions:
EENT: Tinnitus, conjunctivitis, photophobia, rhinorrhea
CNS: Drowsiness, headache, vertigo, fever, lethargy
GI: Nausea, diarrhea, vomiting, jaundice, anorexia, dry mouth, constipation, cramps, metallic taste
MS: Myalgia, arthralgia, decreased bone development
GU: Polyuria, hypercalciuria, hyperphosphatemia, hematuria
CV: Dysrhythmias

Contraindications: Hypersensitivity, hyperphosphatemia, hypercalcemia, vit D toxicity

Precautions: Pregnancy (C), renal calculi, lactation, CV disease

Pharmacokinetics:
PO: Peak 4 hr, duration 15-20 days; half-life 12-22 days

Interactions:
• Decreased absorption of calcife-

* Available in Canada only

diol: cholestyramine, colestipol HCl, mineral oil, fat-soluble vitamins
• Hypercalcemia: thiazide diuretics
• Cardiac dysrhythmias: cardiac glycosides
• Decreased effect of this drug: corticosteroids

Lab test interferences:
False increase: Cholesterol

NURSING CONSIDERATIONS

Assess:
• BUN, urinary calcium, AST, ALT, cholesterol, creatinine, uric acid, chloride, magnesium, electrolytes, urine pH, phosphate; may increase; calcium should be kept at 9-10 mg/dl, vit D 50-135 IU/dl, phosphate 70 mg/dl
• Alk phosphatase; may be decreased
• For increased blood level, since toxic reactions may occur rapidly
• For dry mouth, metallic taste, polyuria, bone pain, muscle weakness, headache, fatigue, tinnitus, change in LOC, irregular pulse, dysrhythmias, increased respirations, anorexia, nausea, vomiting, cramps, diarrhea, constipation; may indicate hypercalcemia
• Renal status: decreased urinary output (oliguria, anuria), edema in extremities, weight gain 5 lb, periorbital edema
• Nutritional status, diet for sources of vit D (milk, some seafood), calcium (dairy products, dark green vegetables), phosphates (dairy products)

Administer:
• PO may be increased q4wk depending on blood level

Perform/provide:
• Storage in tight, light-resistant containers at room temperature
• Restriction of sodium, potassium if required
• Restriction of fluids if required for chronic renal failure

Evaluate:
• Therapeutic response: calcium levels 9-10 mg/dl, decreasing symptoms of bone disease

Teach patient/family:
• The symptoms of hypercalcemia
• About foods rich in calcium

calcitonin (human) (℞)

(kal-si-toe'nin)
Cibacalcin
Func. class.: Parathyroid agents (calcium regulator)
Chem. class.: Polypeptide hormone

Action: Decreases bone resorption, blood calcium levels; increases deposits of calcium in bones
Uses: Paget's disease
Dosage and routes:
Paget's disease
• *Adult:* SC 0.5 mg/day initially; may require 0.5 mg bid × 6 mo, then decrease until symptoms reappear
Available forms: Inj (SC) 500 mg vial
Side effects/adverse reactions:
INTEG: Rash, flushing, pruritus of earlobes, edema of feet
CNS: Headache, tetany, chills, weakness, dizziness
GU: Diuresis
GI: Nausea, diarrhea, vomiting, anorexia, abdominal pain, salty taste, epigastric pain
MS: Swelling, tingling of hands
CV: Chest pressure
RESP: Dyspnea
Contraindications: Hypersensitivity
Precautions: Renal disease, children, lactation, osteogenic sarcoma, pregnancy (C)
Pharmacokinetics:
IM/SC: Onset 15 min, peak 4 hr,

duration 8-24 hr; metabolized by kidneys, excreted as inactive metabolites

NURSING CONSIDERATIONS

Assess:

• GI symptoms, polyuria, flushing, head swelling, tingling, headache; may indicate hypercalcemia

• Nutritional status; diet for sources of vit D (milk, some seafood), calcium (dairy products, dark green vegatables), phosphates

• BUN, creatinine, uric acid, chloride, electrolytes, urine pH, urinary calcium, magnesium, phosphate, urinalysis (calcium should be kept at 9-10 mg/dl, vit D 50-135 IU/dl), alk phosphatase baseline and q3-6mo

• Increased drug level, since toxic reactions occur rapidly; have calcium chloride on hand if calcium level drops too low; check for tetany

• Urine for sediment

Administer:

• By SC route only; rotate injection sites; use within 6 hr of reconstitution; give hs to minimize nausea, vomiting

Perform/provide:

• Store at <77° F (25° C); protect from light

Evaluate:

• Therapeutic response: calcium levels 9-10 mg/dl, decreasing symptoms of Paget's disease

Teach patient/family:

• Method of injection if patient will be responsible for self-medication

calcitonin (salmon) (℞)

(kal-si-toe'nin)

Calcimar, Miacalcin

Func. class.: Parathyroid agents (calcium regulator)

Chem. class.: Polypeptide hormone

Action: Decreases bone resorption, blood calcium levels; increases deposits of calcium in bones

Uses: Hypercalcemia, postmenopausal osteoporosis, Paget's disease

Dosage and routes:

Osteoporosis/Paget's disease

• *Adult:* SC/IM 100 IU qd, maintenance for Paget's disease 50-100 IU qd or qod

Hypercalcemia

• *Adult:* IM 4-8 IU/kg q6-12h

Available forms: Inj SC/IM 200 IU/ml

Side effects/adverse reactions:

INTEG: Rash, pruritus of earlobes, edema of feet

CNS: Headache, flushing, ***tetany,*** chills, weakness, dizziness

GU: Diuresis

GI: Nausea, diarrhea, vomiting, anorexia, abdominal pain, salty taste

MS: Swelling, tingling of hands

Contraindications: Hypersensitivity, children, lactation

Precautions: Renal disease, osteoporosis, pernicious anemia, Zollinger-Ellison syndrome, pregnancy (C)

Pharmacokinetics:

IM/SC: Onset 15 min, peak 4 hr, duration 8-24 hr; metabolized by kidneys, excreted as inactive metabolites

NURSING CONSIDERATIONS

Assess:

• BUN, creatinine, uric acid, chlo-

* Available in Canada only

ride, electrolytes, urine pH, urinary calcium, magnesium, phosphatase, urinalysis, calcitonin antibody formation (calcium should be kept at 9-10 mg/dl, vit D 50-135 IU/dl), alk phosphatase

- Increased level, since toxic reactions may occur rapidly
- Urine for sediment and casts
- History of allergies
- GI symptoms, polyuria, flushing, head swelling, tingling, headache; may indicate hypercalcemia
- Nutritional status; diet for sources of vit D (milk, some seafood), calcium (dairy products, dark green vegetables), phosphates
- Systemic allergic reaction to drug: skin test before 1st dose

Administer:

- After test dose of 10 IU/ml, 0.1 ml intradermally; watch 15 min; give only with epinephrine and emergency meds available
- IM injection in deep muscle mass slowly; rotate sites

Perform/provide:

- Storage in light-resistant area; refrigerate
- Restriction of sodium, potassium if required

Evaluate:

- Therapeutic response: calcium 9-10 mg/dl, decreasing symptoms of bone disease

Teach patient/family:

- To avoid OTC products
- To administer drug SC if patient will be responsible for self-medication
- Report difficulty swallowing or change in side effects immediately to physician

calcitriol (1,25-dihydroxycholecalciferol) (℞)

(kal-si-tyre'ole)

Calcijex, Rocaltrol Vitamin D_3

Func. class.: Parathyroid agents (calcium regulator)

Chem. class.: Vit D hormone

Action: Increases intestinal absorption of calcium, provides calcium for bones, increases renal tubular resorption of phosphate

Uses: Hypocalcemia in chronic renal disease, hypoparathyroidism, pseudohypoparathyroidism

Dosage and routes:

Hypocalcemia

- *Adult:* PO 0.25 μg qd, may increase by 0.25 μg/day q4-8wk, maintenance 0.25 μg qod-1 μg qd

Hypoparathyroidism/pseudohypoparathyroidism

- *Adult and child >1 yr:* PO 0.25 μg qd, may be increased q2-4wk; maintenance 0.25-2 μg qd

Available forms: Caps 0.25, 0.5 μg; inj 1 μg, 2 μg/ml

Side effects/adverse reactions:

CNS: Drowsiness, headache, vertigo, fever, lethargy

GI: Nausea, diarrhea, vomiting, jaundice, anorexia, dry mouth, constipation, cramps, metallic taste

MS: Myalgia, arthralgia, decreased bone development

GU: Polyuria, hypercalciuria, hyperphosphatemia, hematuria

Contraindications: Hypersensitivity, hyperphosphatemia, hypercalcemia, vit D toxicity

Precautions: Pregnancy (C), renal calculi, lactation, CV disease

Pharmacokinetics:

PO: Peak 4 hr, duration 15-20 days, half-life 3-6 hr

Interactions:
• Decreased absorption of calcitriol: cholestyramine, mineral oil
• Hypercalcemia: thiazide diuretics, calcium supplement
• Cardiac dysrhythmias: cardiac glycosides, verapamil
• Decreased effect of calcifediol: barbiturates, phenytoin, corticosteroids

Lab test interferences:
False increase: Cholesterol

NURSING CONSIDERATIONS

Assess:
• BUN, urinary calcium, AST (SGOT), ALT (SGPT), cholesterol, creatinine, albumin, uric acid, chloride, magnesium, electrolytes, urine pH, phosphate; may increase calcium, should be kept at 9-10 mg/dl, vit D 50-135 IU/dl, phosphate 70 mg/dl
• Alk phosphatase; may be decreased
• For increased drug level, since toxic reactions may occur rapidly
• For dry mouth, metallic taste, polyuria, bone pain, muscle weakness, headache, fatigue, change in LOC, dysrhythmias, increased respirations, anorexia, nausea, vomiting, cramps, diarrhea, constipation; may indicate hypercalcemia
• Renal status: decreased urinary output (oliguria, anuria), edema in extremities, weight gain 5-7 lb, periorbital edema
• Nutritional status, diet for sources of vit D (milk, some seafood); calcium (dairy products, dark green vegetables), phosphates (dairy products) must be avoided

Perform/provide:
• Storage protected from light, heat, moisture
• Restriction of sodium, potassium if required
• Restriction of fluids if required for chronic renal failure

Evaluate:
• Therapeutic response: calcium 9-10 mg/dl, decreasing symptoms of hypocalcemia, hypoparathyroidism

Teach patient/family:
• The symptoms of hypercalcemia
• About foods rich in calcium
• To avoid products with sodium: cured meats, dairy products, cold cuts, olives, beets, pickles, soups, meat tenderizers in chronic renal failure
• To avoid products with potassium: oranges, bananas, dried fruit, peas, dark green leafy vegetables, milk, melons, beans in chronic renal failure
• To avoid OTC products containing calcium, potassium, or sodium in chronic renal failure
• To avoid all preparations containing vit D
• To monitor weight weekly

calcium carbonate (OTC)

Alka-Mints, Amitone, Cal Carb-HD, Calci-Chew, Calci-Mix, Calciday 667, Calcium 600, Calcium Carbonate, Cal-Guard, Cal-Plus, Caltrate 600, Caltrate Jr., Chooz, Dicarbosil, Equilet, Gelcalc 600, Mallamint, Nephro-Calci, Os-Cal 500, Oystercal 500, Oysco 500, Oyst-Cal 500, Oyster Shell Calcium 500, Rolaids Calcium Rich, Tums, Tums E-X Extra Strength, Tums Extra Strength

Func. class.: Antacid, calcium supplement
Chem. class.: Calcium product

Action: Neutralizes gastric acidity
Uses: Antacid, calcium supplement; not suitable for chronic therapy

* Available in Canada only

Dosage and routes:
• *Adult:* PO 1 g 4-6 ×/day, chewed with water; SUSP 1 g 1 hr pc, hs
Available forms: Chewable tabs 350, 420, 500, 750 mg; tabs 650 mg; gum 500 mg; susp 1 g/5 ml
Side effects/adverse reactions:
GI: Constipation, anorexia, ***obstruction,*** nausea, vomiting, flatulence, diarrhea, rebound hyperacidity, eructation
CV: ***Hemorrhage, rebound hypertension***
META: Hypercalcemia, metabolic alkalosis
GU: Renal dysfunction, renal stones, ***renal failure***
Contraindications: Hypersensitivity, hypercalcemia, hyperparathyroidism, bone tumors
Precautions: Elderly, fluid restriction, decreased GI motility, GI obstruction, dehydration, renal disease, pregnancy (C), lactation
Pharmacokinetics:
PO: Onset 3 min, excreted in feces
Interactions:
• Increased plasma levels of quinidine, amphetamines
• Decreased levels of salicylates, calcium channel blockers, ketoconazole, tetracyclines, iron salts
• Hypercalcemia: thiazide diuretics
NURSING CONSIDERATIONS
Assess:
• Ca^+ (serum, urine), Ca^+ should be 8.5-10.5 mg/dl, urine Ca^+ should be 150 mg/day, monitor weekly
• Milk-alkali syndrome: nausea, vomiting, disorientation, headache
• Constipation; increase bulk in the diet if needed
• Hypercalcemia: headache, nausea, vomiting, confusion
Administer:
• As antacid 1 hr pc and hs
• As supplement 1½ hr pc and hs
• Only with regular tablets or capsules; do not give with enteric-coated tablets
• Laxatives or stool softeners if constipation occurs
Evaluate:
• Therapeutic response: absence of pain, decreased acidity
Teach patient/family:
• To increase fluids to 2 L unless contraindicated, to add bulk to diet for constipation
• Not to switch antacids unless directed by prescriber

calcium chloride/calcium gluceptate/calcium gluconate/calcium lactate (℞)

Func. class.: Electrolyte replacement—calcium product

Action: Cation needed for maintenance of nervous, muscular, skeletal, enzyme reactions, normal cardiac contractility, coagulation of blood; affects secretory activity of endocrine, exocrine glands
Uses: Prevention and treatment of hypocalcemia, hypermagnesemia, hypoparathyroidism, neonatal tetany, cardiac toxicity caused by hyperkalemia, lead colic, hyperphosphatemia, vit D deficiency
Dosage and routes:
Calcium chloride
• *Adult:* IV 500 mg-1 g q1-3 days as indicated by serum calcium levels, give at <1 ml/min; IAV 200-800 mg injected in ventricle of heart
• *Child:* IV 25 mg/kg over several min
Calcium gluceptate
• *Adult:* IV 5-20 ml; IM 2-5 ml
• *Newborn:* 0.5 ml/100 ml of blood transfused

Calcium gluconate

• *Adult:* PO 0.5-2 g bid-qid; IV 0.5-2 g at 0.5 ml/min (10% solution)

• *Child:* PO/IV 500 mg/kg/day in divided doses

Calcium lactate

• *Adult:* PO 325 mg-1.3 g tid with meals

• *Child:* PO 500 mg/kg/day in divided doses

Available forms: Many; check product listings

Side effects/adverse reactions:

INTEG: Pain, burning at IV site, severe venous thrombosis, necrosis, extravasation

HYPERCALCEMIA: Drowsiness, lethargy, muscle weakness, headache, constipation, ***coma,*** anorexia, nausea, vomiting, polyuria, thirst

CV: Shortened QT, heart block, hypotension, bradycardia, dysrthymias, ***cardiac arrest***

GI: Vomiting, nausea, constipation

Contraindications: Hypercalcemia, digitalis toxicity, ventricular fibrillation, renal calculi

Precautions: Pregnancy (C), lactation, children, renal disease, respiratory disease, cor pulmonale, digitalized patient, respiratory failure

Interactions:

• Increased dysrhythmias: digitalis glycosides

• Decreased action: calcium channel blockers

• Incompatible with amphotericin B, cephalothin, chlorpheniramine, chlortetracycline, digoxin, digitoxin, epinephrine, tetracycline, warfarin, $NaCO_3$, carbonate, phosphate, sulfate

Lab test interferences:

Increase: 11-OCHS

False decrease: Magnesium

Decrease: 17-OHCS

NURSING CONSIDERATIONS

Assess:

• ECG for decreased QT and T wave inversion: hypercalcemia, drug should be reduced or discontinued, consider cardiac monitoring

• Calcium levels during treatment (8.5-11.5 g/dl is normal level)

• Cardiac status: rate, rhythm, CVP, (PWP, PAWP if being monitored directly)

Administer:

• IV undiluted or diluted with equal amounts of NS for inj to a 5% sol, give 0.5-1 ml/min

• Through small-bore needle into large vein; if extravasation occurs, necrosis will result (IV); IM injection may cause severe burning, necrosis, tissue sloughing; warm sol to body temp before administering

• PO with or following meals to enhance absorption

Perform/provide:

• Seizure precautions: padded side rails, decreased stimuli, (noise, light); place airway suction equipment, padded mouth gag if Ca levels are low

• Store at room temperature

Evaluate:

• Therapeutic response: decreased twitching, paresthesias, muscle spasms, absence of tremors, convulsions, dysrhythmias, dyspnea, laryngospasm, negative Chvostek's sign, negative Trousseau's sign

Teach patient/family:

• To remain recumbent ½ hr after IV dose

• To add food high in vit D content

• To add calcium-rich foods to diet: dairy products, shellfish, dark green leafy vegetables; decrease oxalate-rich and zinc-rich foods: nuts, legumes, chocolate, spinach, soy

• To prevent injuries, avoid immobilization

calcium polycarbophil (OTC)

(pol-i-kar'boe-fil)

Fiber Norm, Mitrolan

Func. class.: Laxative

Chem. class.: Bulk-forming

Action: Attracts water, expands in intestine to increase peristalsis; also absorbs excess water in stool; decreases diarrhea

Uses: Constipation, irritable bowel syndrome (diarrhea), acute, nonspecific diarrhea

Dosage and routes:

• *Adult:* PO 1 g qd-qid prn, not to exceed 6 g/24 hr

• *Child 6-12 yr:* PO 500 mg bid prn, not to exceed 3 g/24 hr

• *Child 3-6 yr:* PO 500 mg bid prn, not to exceed 1.5 g/24 hr

Available forms: Chew tabs 500, 625, 1250 mg

Side effects/adverse reactions:

GI: ***Obstruction,*** abdominal distention, laxative dependency, flatus

Contraindications: Hypersensitivity, GI obstruction

Precautions: Pregnancy (C), lactation

Pharmacokinetics:

PO: Onset 12-24 min, peak 1-3 days

NURSING CONSIDERATIONS

Assess:

• Blood, urine electrolytes if used often

• I&O ratio to identify fluid loss

• Cause of constipation; identify whether fluids, bulk, or exercise is missing from lifestyle

• Cramping, rectal bleeding, nausea, vomiting; if these symptoms occur, drug should be discontinued

Administer:

• Alone for better absorption; do not take within 1 hr of other drugs

• In morning or evening (oral dose)

Evaluate:

• Therapeutic response: decreased constipation

Teach patient/family:

• Not to use laxatives for long-term therapy; bowel tone will be lost

• That normal bowel movements do not always occur daily

• Not to use in presence of abdominal pain, nausea, vomiting

• To notify physician if constipation unrelieved or if symptoms of electrolyte imbalance occur: muscle cramps, pain, weakness, dizziness

• To chew thoroughly and follow with water

capreomycin (℞)

(kap-ree-oh-mye'sin)

Capastat Sulfate

Func. class.: Antitubercular

Chem. class.: S. capreolus polypeptide antibiotic

Action: Inhibits RNA synthesis, decreases tubercle bacilli replication

Uses: Pulmonary TB as adjunct

Dosage and routes:

• *Adult:* IM 1 g qd × 2-4 mo, then 1 g 2-3 ×/wk × 18-24 mo, not to exceed 20 mg/kg/day; must be given with another antitubercular medication

Available forms: Powder for inj 1 g/10 ml vial

Side effects/adverse reactions:

INTEG: Pain, irritation, sterile abscess at injection site, rash, urticaria

CNS: Vertigo, fever, headache

EENT: Tinnitus, ***deafness, ototoxicity***

GU: ***Proteinuria,*** decreased CrCl, increased BUN, serum Cr, ***tubular necrosis,*** hypokalemia, alkalosis, ***hematuria, albuminuria, nephrotoxicity***

HEMA: ***Eosinophilia, leukocytosis, leukopenia***
Contraindications: Hypersensitivity
Precautions: Renal disease, hearing impairment, allergy history, hepatic disease, pregnancy (C), lactation
Pharmacokinetics:
IM: Peak 1-2 hr, half-life 4-6 hr; excreted in urine unchanged
Interactions:
• Increased renal toxicity: aminoglycosides, polymyxin, colistin, vancomycin
• Increased neuroblocking action: phenothiazine, tubocurarine, neostigmine
NURSING CONSIDERATIONS
Assess:
• Liver studies qwk: ALT, AST, bilirubin; potassium
• Renal status: before; qwk: BUN, creatinine, output, specific gravity, urinalysis
• Blood levels of drug
• Audiometric testing before, during, after treatment
• Ototoxicity: tinnitus, vertigo, change in hearing
• Hepatic status: decreased appetite, jaundice, dark urine, fatigue
Administer:
• After reconstituting with 2 ml NS or sterile water for injection, wait 2-3 min before giving
• With other antituberculars
• IM in large muscle mass; rotate sites
• Reduced dosage in renal impairment; if BUN >20 mg/dl, drug should be decreased or discontinued
Evaluate:
• Therapeutic response: decreased dyspnea, fatigue
Teach patient/family:
• That compliance with dosage schedule, duration is necessary
• Side effects, adverse reactions: hearing loss, change in urine or urinary habits

captopril (℞)
(kap′toe-pril)
Capoten
Func. class.: Antihypertensive
Chem. class.: Angiotensin-converting enzyme inhibitor

Combination products: Caposide 25/15: captopril 25 mg with hydrochlorothiazide 15 mg; Capozide 25/25: captopril 25 mg with hydrochlorothiazide 25 mg; Capozide 50/15: captopril 50 mg with hydrochlorothiazide 15 mg; Capozide 50/25: captopril 50 mg with hydrochlorothiazide 25 mg

Action: Selectively suppresses renin-angiotensin-aldosterone system; inhibits ACE; prevents conversion of angiotensin I to angiotensin II; results in dilation of arterial, venous vessels
Uses: Hypertension, heart failure not responsive to conventional therapy, left ventricular dysfunction after MI, diabetic nephropathy
Dosage and routes:
Malignant hypertension
• *Adult:* PO 25 mg increasing q2h until desired response, not to exceed 450 mg/day
Hypertension
• *Initial dose:* 25 mg bid-tid; may increase to 50 mg bid-tid at 1-2 wk intervals; usual range: 25-150 mg bid-tid; max 450 mg
CHF
• *Adult:* PO 12.5 mg bid-tid given with a diuretic; may increase to 50 mg bid-tid; after 14 days, may increase to 150 mg tid if needed

* Available in Canada only

LVD after MI
• *Adult:* PO 50 mg tid, may begin treatment 3 days after MI; give 6.25 mg as a single dose, then 12.5 mg tid, increase to 25 mg tid for several days, then to 50 mg tid
Diabetic nephropathy
• *Adult:* PO 25 mg tid
Available forms: Tabs 12.5, 25, 50, 100 mg
Side effects/adverse reactions:
CV: Hypotension, postural hypotension
GU: Impotence, dysuria, nocturia, proteinuria, ***nephrotic syndrome, acute reversible renal failure,*** polyuria, oliguria, frequency
HEMA: ***Neutropenia***
INT: Rash, *angioedema*
RESP: ***Bronchospasm,*** dyspnea, cough
META: Hyperkalemia
GI: Loss of taste
CNS: Fever, chills
Contraindications: Hypersensitivity, lactation, heart block, children, K-sparing diuretics, bilateral renal artery stenosis
Precautions: Dialysis patients, hypovolemia, leukemia, scleroderma, lupus erythematosus, blood dyscrasias, CHF, diabetes mellitus, renal disease, thyroid disease, COPD, asthma, pregnancy (C)
Pharmacokinetics:
PO: Peak 1 hr; duration 2-6 hr; half-life 6-7 hr; metabolized by liver (metabolites), excreted in urine; crosses placenta; excreted in breast milk
Interactions:
• Increased hypotension: diuretics, other antihypertensives, ganglionic blockers, adrenergic blockers
• Do not use with potassium-sparing diuretics, sympathomimetics, potassium supplements
Lab test interferences:
False positive: Urine acetone

NURSING CONSIDERATIONS
Assess:
• Blood studies: neutrophils, decreased platelets
• B/P
• Renal studies: protein, BUN, creatinine; watch for increased levels that may indicate nephrotic syndrome
• Baselines in renal, liver function tests before therapy begins
• K levels, although hyperkalemia rarely occurs
• Dipstick of urine for protein qd in first morning specimen; if protein is increased, a 24-hr urinary protein should be collected
• Edema in feet, legs daily
• Allergic reaction: rash, fever, pruritus, urticaria; drug should be discontinued if antihistamines fail to help
• Symptoms of CHF: edema, dyspnea, wet rales, B/P
• Renal symptoms: polyuria, oliguria, frequency
Administer:
• IV infusion of 0.9% NaCl (as ordered) to expand fluid volume if severe hypotension occurs
Perform/provide:
• Storage in tight container at 86° F (30° C) or less
• Supine or Trendelenburg position for severe hypotension
Evaluate:
• Therapeutic response: decrease in B/P in hypertension, decreased B/P, edema, moist rales (CHF)
Teach patient/family:
• To administer 1 hr before meals
• Not to discontinue drug abruptly
• Not to use OTC (cough, cold, or allergy) products unless directed by prescriber
• To avoid sunlight or wear sunscreen if in sunlight; photosensitivity may occur

• To comply with dosage schedule, even if feeling better
• To rise slowly to sitting or standing position to minimize orthostatic hypotension
• To notify prescriber of mouth sores, sore throat, fever, swelling of hands or feet, irregular heartbeat, chest pain, signs of angioedema
• That excessive perspiration, dehydration, vomiting; diarrhea may lead to fall in blood pressure—consult prescriber if these occur
• That dizziness, fainting, lightheadedness may occur during 1st few days of therapy
• That skin rash or impaired perspiration may occur
• How to take B/P

Treatment of overdose: 0.9% NaCl IV/INF; hemodialysis

carbachol (℞)

(kar'ba-kole)

Carboptic, Isopto Carbachol, Miostat

Func. class.: Miotic, cholinergic

Action: Contracts sphincter muscle of iris; causes spasms of ciliary muscle, deepening of anterior chamber

Uses: Miosis in ocular surgery, glaucoma (open-angle, narrow-angle)

Dosage and routes:

Ocular surgery

• *Adult:* INSTILL 0.5 ml (intraocular) 0.01% sol in anterior chamber of eye (done by physician) for miosis during surgery

Glaucoma

• *Adult:* INSTILL 1-2 gtt (topical) 0.75%-3% sol in eye bid-tid

Available forms: 0.75%, 1.5%, 2.25%, 3% sol for topical use; oph sol 0.01%,

Side effects/adverse reactions:

CV: ***Marked hypotension,*** bradycardia, headache

GI: Nausea, vomiting, abdominal discomfort, diarrhea, salivation

EENT: Blurred vision, varying degrees of myopia, decreased visual acuity in dim light, slight conjunctival hyperemia, altered distance vision, decreased night vision, eye ache

RESP: Asthma attacks

Contraindications: Hypersensitivity; when miosis is undesirable; corneal abrasions

Precautions: Bradycardia, CAD, hyperthyroidism, asthma, pregnancy, obstruction of GI or urinary tract, peptic ulcer, parkinsonism, epilepsy, peritonitis

Pharmacokinetics:

Instill/Oint: Miosis onset 10-20 min, duration 4-8 hr; decreased intraocular pressure onset 4 hr; duration 8 hr

NURSING CONSIDERATIONS

Assess:

• Heart, respiratory rate, B/P

Perform/provide:

• Use of reconstituted sol immediately; discard unused portion

Evaluate:

• Therapeutic response: decreasing intraocular pressure, miosis during ocular surgery

Teach patient/family:

• To report change in vision, blurring or loss of sight, trouble breathing, sweating, flushing
• Method of instillation, including pressure on lacrimal sac for 1 min, and not to touch dropper to eye, use demonstration, return demonstration
• That long-term therapy may be required in glaucoma
• That blurred vision will decrease with repeated use of drug

* Available in Canada only

• Not to drive during 1st few days of treatment

carbamazepine (℞)

(kar-ba-maz′e-peen)

Apo-Carbamazepine*, Epitol, Mazepine*, Novo Carbamaz*, Tegretol

Func. class.: Anticonvulsant

Chem. class.: Iminostilbene derivative

Action: Inhibits nerve impulses by limiting influx of sodium ions across cell membrane in motor cortex

Uses: Tonic-clonic, complex-partial, mixed seizures; trigeminal neuralgia

Investigational uses: Diabetes insipidus, bipolar disorder, neurogenic pain

Dosage and routes:

Seizures

• *Adult and child >12 yr:* PO 200 mg bid, may be increased by 200 mg/day in divided doses q6-8h; maintenance 800-1200 mg/day maximum 1200 mg/day; adjustment is needed to minimum dose to control seizures

• *Child <12 yr:* PO 10-20 mg/kg/day in 2-3 divided doses

Trigeminal neuralgia

• *Adult:* PO 100 mg bid with meals; may increase 100 mg q12h until pain subsides, not to exceed 1.2 g/day; maintenance is 200-400 mg bid

Available forms: Tabs, chewable 100 mg; tabs 200 mg; ext-rel tabs 200, 400 mg; oral susp 100 mg/5 ml

Side effects/adverse reactions:

HEMA: ***Thrombocytopenia, agranulocytosis, leukocytosis, neutropenia, aplastic anemia, eosinophilia,*** increased pro-time

CNS: Drowsiness, dizziness, confusion, fatigue, ***paralysis,*** headache, hallucinations, worsening of seizures

GI: Nausea, constipation, diarrhea, anorexia, vomiting, abdominal pain, stomatitis, glossitis, increased liver enzymes, ***hepatitis***

INTEG: Rash, ***Stevens-Johnson syndrome,*** urticaria

EENT: Tinnitus, dry mouth, blurred vision, diplopia, nystagmus, conjunctivitis

CV: ***Hypertension, CHF,*** hypotension, aggravation of cardiac artery disease

RESP: Pulmonary hypersensitivity (fever, dyspnea, pneumonitis)

GU: Frequency, retention, albuminuria, glycosuria, impotence, increased BUN

Contraindications: Hypersensitivity to carbamazepine or tricyclic antidepressants, bone marrow depression, concomitant use of MAOIs

Precautions: Glaucoma, hepatic disease, renal disease, cardiac disease, psychosis, pregnancy (C), lactation, child <6 yr

Pharmacokinetics:

PO: Onset slow, peak 4-8 hr; metabolized by liver; excreted in urine, feces; crosses placenta; excreted in breast milk; half-life 14-16 hr

Interactions:

• Toxicity: troleandomycin, erythromycin, cimetidine, isoniazid, propoxyphene, lithium

• Decreased effects of phenobarbital, phenytoin, primidone

• Increased effects of vasopressin, lypressin, desmopressin

Lab test interferences:

Decrease: Thyroid function tests

NURSING CONSIDERATIONS

Assess:

• Renal studies: urinalysis, BUN, urine creatinine q3mo

• Blood studies: RBC, Hct, Hgb, reticulocyte counts qwk for 4 wk

then qmo; if myelosuppression occurs, drug should be discontinued
• Hepatic studies: ALT, AST, bilirubin
• Drug levels during initial treatment; should remain at 3-9 µg/ml; anorexia may indicate increased blood levels
• Description of seizures
• Mental status: mood, sensorium, affect, behavioral changes; if mental status changes, notify prescriber
• Eye problems: need for ophthalmic examinations before, during, after treatment (slit lamp, fundoscopy, tonometry)
• Allergic reaction: purpura, red raised rash; if these occur, drug should be discontinued
• Blood dyscrasias: fever, sore throat, bruising, rash, jaundice
• Toxicity: bone marrow depression, nausea, vomiting, ataxia, diplopia, cardiovascular collapse, Stevens-Johnson syndrome

Administer:
• With food, milk to decrease GI symptoms
• Chewable tablets; tell patient to chew tablet, not swallow it whole

Perform/provide:
• Storage at room temperature
• Hard candy, frequent rinsing of mouth, gum for dry mouth
• Assistance with ambulation during early part of treatment; dizziness occurs

Evaluate:
• Therapeutic response: decreased seizure activity, document on patient's chart

Teach patient/family:
• To carry Medic Alert ID stating patient's name, drugs taken, condition, physician's name, phone number
• To avoid driving, other activities that require alertness
• To avoid alcohol ingestion; convulsions may result
• Not to discontinue medication quickly after long-term use
• That urine may turn pink to brown

Treatment of overdose: Lavage, VS

carbidopa-levodopa (℞)

(kar-bi-doe'pa) (lee-voe-doe'pa)
carbidopa/levodopa, Sinemet, Sinemet CR

Func. class.: Antiparkinson agent
Chem. class.: Catecholamine

Action: Decarboxylation of levodopa to periphery is inhibited by carbidopa; more levodopa is made available for transport to brain and conversion to dopamine in the brain

Uses: Parkinson's disease, parkinsonism resulting from carbon monoxide, chronic manganese intoxication, cerebral arteriosclerosis

Dosage and routes:
• *Adult:* PO 3-6 tabs of 25 mg carbidopa/250 mg levodopa qd in divided doses, not to exceed 8 tabs/day; SUS REL 1 tablet bid at intervals of not less than 6 hr usual: 2-8 tabs/day at intervals of 4-8 hr

Available forms: Tabs 10/100, 25/100, 25 mg carbidopa/250 mg levodopa sus rel tab: 50 mg/200 mg carbidopa/levodopa

Side effects/adverse reactions:

HEMA: ***Hemolytic anemia, leukopenia, agranulocytosis***

CNS: Involuntary choreiform movements, hand tremors, fatigue, headache, anxiety, twitching, numbness, weakness, confusion, agitation, insomnia, nightmares, psychosis, hallucination, hypomania, severe depression, dizziness

GI: Nausea, vomiting, anorexia, abdominal distress, dry mouth flatulence, dysphagia, bitter taste, diarrhea, constipation
INTEG: Rash, sweating, alopecia
CV: Orthostatic hypotension, tachycardia, hypertension, palpitation
EENT: Blurred vision, diplopia, dilated pupils
MISC: Urinary retention, incontinence, weight change, dark urine
Contraindications: Hypersensitivity, narrow-angle glaucoma, undiagnosed skin lesions
Precautions: Renal disease, cardiac disease, hepatic disease, respiratory disease, MI with dysrhythmias, convulsions, peptic ulcer, pregnancy (C), lactation
Pharmacokinetics:
PO: Peak 1-3 hr, exceted in urine (metabolites)
Interactions:
- Hypertensive crisis: MAOIs, furazolidone
- Decreased effects of levodopa: anticholinergics, hydantoins, methionine, papaverine, pyridoxine, tricyclics, benzodiazepines
- Increased effects of levodopa: antacids, metoclopramide

Lab test interferences:
False positive: Urine ketones
False negative: Urine glucose
False increase: Uric acid, urine protein
Decrease: VMA, BUN, creatinine
NURSING CONSIDERATIONS
Assess:
- B/P, respiration
- Mental status: affect, mood, behavioral changes, depression, complete suicide assessment

Administer:
- Drug until NPO before surgery
- Adjust dosage to response
- With meals; limit protein taken with drug
- Only after MAOIs have been discontinued for 2 wk; if previously on levodopa, discontinue for at least 8 hr before change to carbidopa-levodopa

Perform/provide:
- Assistance with ambulation during beginning therapy
- Testing for diabetes mellitus, acromegaly if on long-term therapy

Evaluate:
- Therapeutic response: decrease in akathisia, improved mood

Teach patient/family:
- To change positions slowly to prevent orthostatic hypotension
- To report side effects: twitching, eye spasms; indicate overdose
- To use drug exactly as prescribed; if discontinued abruptly, parkinsonian crisis may occur; physician may recommend drug-free holidays
- That urine, sweat may darken
- To use physical activities to maintain mobility, lessen spasms
- That improvement may not occur for 3-4 months

carboplatin (℞)
(kar-boe-pla'-tin)
Paraplatin
Func. class.: Antineoplastic alkylating agent
Chem. class.: Platinum coordination compound

Action: Produces interstrand DNA cross-links and to a lesser extent DNA-protein cross-links; activity is not cell cycle phase specific
Uses: Palliative treatment of ovarian carcinoma recurrent after treatment with other antineoplastic agents, including cisplatin
Dosage and routes: (single agent):
- *Adult:* IV INF 360 mg/m^2 given over >15 min on day 1 q4wk; do not

repeat single intermittent courses until neutrophil count is >2,000/mm^3 and platelet count is >100,000/mm^3

Available forms: Inj 50, 150, 450 mg/vial

Side effects/adverse reactions:

EENT: Tinnitus, hearing loss, *vestibular toxicity*

HEMA: ***Thrombocytopenia, leukopenia, pancytopenia, neutropenia,*** anemia, bleeding

CV: Cardiac abnormalities

GI: Severe nausea, vomiting, diarrhea, weight loss

GU: ***Renal tubular damage,*** renal insufficiency, impotence, sterility, amenorrhea, gynecomastia

INTEG: Alopecia, dermatitis, rash, erythema, pruritus, urticaria

CNS: ***Convulsions, central neurotoxicity,*** peripheral neuropathy

RESP: Mucositis

META: Hypomagnesemia, hypocalcemia, hypokalemia, hyponatremia, hyperuremia

Contraindications: Hypersensitivity to this drug, platinum products, mannitol; severe bone marrow depression, significant bleeding, pregnancy (D)

Precautions: Radiation therapy within 1 mo, chemotherapy within 1 mo, lactation, liver disease

Pharmacokinetics: Initial half-life 1-2 hr, postdistribution half-life 2½-6 hr, not bound to plasma proteins, excreted by the kidneys

Interactions:

• Increased nephrotoxicity or ototoxicity: aminoglycosides

Y-site compatibilities: Fludarabine, melphalan, ondansetron, paclitaxel, sargramostim, vinorelbine

Additive compatibilities: Ifosfamide, ifosfamide with etoposide

Solution compatibilities: D_5/0.2% NaCl, D_5/0.45% NaCl, D_5/0.9% NaCl, 0.9% NaCl, sterile water for inj

NURSING CONSIDERATIONS

Assess:

• CBC, differential, platelet count weekly; withhold drug if WBC count is <4000/mm^3 or platelet count is <100,000/mm^3; notify prescriber of results

• Renal function studies: BUN, creatinine, serum uric acid, urine CrCL before and during therapy

• I&O ratio; report fall in urine output to <30 ml/hr

• Monitor temperature q4h (may indicate beginning of infection)

• Liver function tests before and during therapy (bilirubin, AST [SGOT], ALT [SGPT], LDH) as needed or monthly

• Bleeding; hematuria, stool guaiac, bruising or petechiae, mucosa or orifices q8h

• Dyspnea, rales, unproductive cough, chest pain, tachypnea

• Food preferences; list likes, dislikes

• Effects of alopecia on body image; discuss feelings about body changes

• Yellowing of skin, sclera, dark urine, clay-colored stools, itchy skin, abdominal pain, fever, diarrhea

• Edema in feet, joint pain, stomach pain, shaking

• Inflammation of mucosa, breaks in skin

Administer:

• IV after diluting 10 mg/ml of sterile water for inj, D_5W, NS (10 mg/ml); then further dilute with the same sol 1-4 mg/ml; give over 15 min or more (INT INF)

• IV INF over 5-6 hr; do not use needles or IV administration sets containing aluminum; may cause precipitate

• Antiemetic 30-60 min before giving drug and PRN for vomiting

* Available in Canada only

- Allopurinol or sodium bicarbonate to maintain uric acid levels, alkalinization of urine
- Antibiotics for prophylaxis of infection
- Diuretic (furosemide 40 mg IV) after infusion

Perform/provide:

- Storage protected from light at room temperature; reconstituted sol stable for 8 hr at room temp
- Deep-breathing exercises with patient tid-qid; place in semi-Fowler's position
- Increase fluid intake to 2-3 L/day to prevent urate deposits and calculi formation and to speed elimination of drug
- Diet low in purines: organ meats (kidney, liver), dried beans, peas to maintain alkaline urine

Evaluate:

- Therapeutic response: decreasing size of tumor, spread of malignancy

Teach patient/family:

- To report any complaints or side effects to nurse or prescriber
- That impotence or amenorrhea can occur; reversible after treatment is discontinued
- To report any changes in breathing or coughing
- That hair may be lost during treatment; a wig or hairpiece may make patient feel better; new hair may be different in color, texture

carboprost (℞)

(kar'boe-prost)

Hemabate, Prostin/15M*

Func. class.: Oxytocic

Chem. class.: Prostaglandin

Action: Stimulates uterine contractions, causing complete abortion in approximately 16 hr

Uses: Abortion at 13-20 wk gestation

Dosage and routes:

- *Adult:* IM 250 µg, then 250 µg q1½-3½ hr, may increase to 500 µg if no response, not to exceed 12 mg total dose

Available forms: Inj IM 250 µg/ml carboprost, 83 µg/ml tromethamine

Side effects/adverse reactions:

CNS: *Fever, chills,* headache

GI: *Nausea, vomiting, diarrhea*

Contraindications: Hypersensitivity, severe hepatic disease, severe renal disease, PID, respiratory disease, cardiac disease

Precautions: Asthma, anemia, jaundice, diabetes mellitus, convulsive disorders, past uterine surgery, pregnancy (C)

Pharmacokinetics: Onset: 15 min, peak 2 hr; metabolized in lungs, liver; excreted in urine (metabolites)

NURSING CONSIDERATIONS

Assess:

- B/P, pulse; watch for change that may indicate hemorrhage
- Respiratory rate, rhythm, depth; notify prescriber of abnormalities
- For length, duration of contraction; notify prescriber of contractions lasting over 1 min or absence of contractions
- For incomplete abortion, pregnancy must be terminated by another method; drug is teratogenic

Administer:

- IM in deep muscle mass; rotate injection sites if additional doses are given
- With crash cart on unit

Perform/provide:

- Emotional support before and after the abortion

Evaluate:

- Therapeutic response: expulsion of fetus

Teach patient/family:
• To report increased blood loss, abdominal cramps, increased temperature, foul-smelling lochia
• Methods of comfort control and pain control

carisoprodol (℞)

(kar-eye-soe-proe′dole)
carisoprodol, Rela, Soma, Soprodol, Soridol
Func. class.: Skeletal muscle relaxant, central acting
Chem. class.: Meprobamate congener

Combination products: Soma Compound: carisoprodol 200 mg, aspirin 325 mg

Action: Depresses CNS by blocking interneuronal activity in descending reticular formation, spinal cord, producing sedation
Uses: Relieving pain, stiffness in musculoskeletal disorders
Dosage and routes:
• *Adult and child >12 yr:* PO 350 mg tid, hs
Available forms: Tabs 350 mg
Side effects/adverse reactions:
CNS: Dizziness, weakness, drowsiness, headache, tremor, depression, insomnia, ataxia, irritability
EENT: Diplopia, temporary loss of vision
CV: Postural hypotension, tachycardia
GI: Nausea, vomiting, hiccups, epigastric discomfort
INTEG: Rash, pruritus, fever, facial flushing
Contraindications: Hypersensitivity, child <12 yr, intermittent porphyria
Precautions: Renal disease, hepatic disease, addictive personality, pregnancy (C), elderly, lactation

Pharmacokinetics:
PO: Onset ½ hr, duration 4-6 hr; metabolized by liver; excreted in urine; crosses placenta; excreted in breast milk (large amounts); half-life 8 hr
Interactions:
• Increased CNS depression: alcohol, tricyclic antidepressants, narcotics, barbiturates, sedatives, hypnotics

NURSING CONSIDERATIONS
Assess:
• Blood studies: CBC, WBC, differential; blood dyscrasias may occur
• Liver function studies: AST, ALT, alk phosphatase; hepatitis may occur
• ECG in epileptic patients; poor seizure control has occurred with patients taking this drug
• Idiosyncratic reaction, anaphylaxis within a few min or hr of 1st to 4th dose
• Allergic reactions: rash, fever, respiratory distress
• Severe weakness, numbness in extremities
• Psychologic dependency: increased need for medication, more frequent requests for medication, increased pain
• CNS depression: dizziness, drowsiness, psychiatric symptoms
Administer:
• With meals for GI symptoms
Perform/provide:
• Storage in tight container at room temperature
• Assistance with ambulation if dizziness, drowsiness occurs, especially elderly
Evaluate:
• Therapeutic response: decreased pain, spasticity
Teach patient/family:
• Not to discontinue medication quickly; insomnia, nausea, head-

ache, spasticity, tachycardia will occur; drug should be tapered off over 1-2 wk
• Not to take with alcohol, other CNS depressants
• To avoid hazardous activities if drowsiness, dizziness occur
• To avoid using OTC medication: cough preparations, antihistamines, unless directed by physician

Treatment of overdose: Induce emesis of conscious patient, lavage, dialysis

carmustine (℞)

(kar-mus′teen)

BiCNU BCNU

Func. class.: Antineoplastic alkylating agent

Chem. class.: Nitrosourea

Action: Alkylates DNA, RNA; is able to inhibit enzymes that allow synthesis of amino acids in proteins; activity is not cell cycle phase specific

Uses: Brain tumors such as glioblastoma, medulloblastoma, astrocytoma; multiple myeloma, Hodgkin's disease, other lymphomas, GI, breast, bronchogenic, renal carcinomas

Dosage and routes:
• *Adult:* IV 75-100 mg/m^2 over 1-2 hr × 2 days or 200 mg/m^2 × 1 dose q6-8wk; if leukocytes fall below 2000 or platelets below 75,000, only 50% of dose should be given

Available forms: Inj IV 100 mg; powder

Side effects/adverse reactions:
HEMA: ***Thrombocytopenia, leukopenia, myelosuppression, anemia***
GI: Nausea, vomiting, anorexia, stomatitis, ***hepatotoxicity***
GU: Azotemia, ***renal failure***
INTEG: Burning, hyperpigmentation at injection site
RESP: ***Fibrosis, pulmonary infiltrate***

Contraindications: Hypersensitivity, leukopenia, thrombocytopenia

Precautions: Pregnancy (D), lactation

Pharmacokinetics: Degraded within 15 min; crosses blood-brain barrier; 70% excreted in urine within 96 hr; 10% excreted as CO_2; fate of 20% is unknown

Interactions:
• Increased toxicity: other antineoplastics, radiation
• Enhanced action: vit A, caffeine
• Increased toxicity: cimetidine, other antineoplastics, radiation

Y-site compatibilities: Fludarabine, melphalan, ondansetron, sargramostim, vinorelbine

NURSING CONSIDERATIONS

Assess:
• CBC, differential, platelet count weekly; withhold drug if WBC is <4000 or platelet count is <75,000; notify prescriber of results
• Liver function tests: AST, ALT, bilirubin
• Pulmonary function tests, chest x-ray films before, during therapy; chest film should be obtained q2wk during treatment
• Renal function studies: BUN, serum uric acid, urine CrCl before, during therapy
• I&O ratio; report fall in urine output of 30 ml/hr
• Monitor for cold, cough, fever (may indicate beginning infection)
• Bleeding: hematuria, guaiac, bruising, petechiae, mucosa, orifices q8h
• Dyspnea, rales, unproductive cough, chest pain, tachypnea
• Food preferences; list likes, dislikes
• Inflammation of mucosa, breaks in skin

Administer:

- IV after diluting 100 mg drug/3 ml ethyl alcohol (provided); then further dilute 27 ml sterile H_2O for inj; then dilute with 100-500 ml 0.9% NaCl or D_5W, give over 1 hr or more, reduce rate if discomfort is felt
- Antiemetic 30-60 min before giving drug to prevent vomiting
- Antibiotics for prophylaxis of infection

Perform/provide:

- Storage in refrigerator
- Strict medical asepsis, protective isolation if WBC levels are low
- Special skin care
- Deep-breathing exercises with patient tid-qid; place in semi-Fowler's position
- Increase fluid intake to 2-3 L/day to prevent urate deposits, calculi formation
- Rinsing of mouth tid-qid with water or club soda; brushing of teeth bid-tid with soft brush or cotton-tipped applicators for stomatitis; use unwaxed dental floss, use viscous lidocaine (Xylocaine)
- Warm compresses at injection site for inflammation; reduce flow rate if patient complains of burning at injection site

Evaluate:

- Therapeutic response: decreasing size of tumor, spread of malignancy

Teach patient/family:

- Protective isolation precautions
- To report any changes in breathing or coughing
- To avoid foods with citric acid, hot or rough texture
- To report any bleeding, white spots, ulceration in mouth to prescriber; tell patient to examine mouth qd
- To avoid use of aspirin, ibuprofen, razors, commercial mouthwash
- To report signs of anemia (fatigue, irritability, shortness of breath, faintness)
- To report signs of infection (sore throat, fever)

---

carteolol (℞)

(kar-tee'oh-lole)

Cartrol, Ocupress

Func. class.: Antihypertensive

Chem. class.: Nonselective β-blocker

Action: Produces fall in B/P without reflex tachycardia or significant reduction in heart rate through mixture of α-blocking, β-blocking effects and intrinsic sympathomimetic activity; elevated plasma renins are reduced

Uses: Mild to moderate hypertension, ophthalmic, intraocular, open-angle glaucoma

Dosage and routes:

- *Adult:* PO 2.5 mg tid initially, may gradually increase to desired response; OPH i gtt bid

Available forms: Tabs 2.5, 5 mg; oph sol 1%

Side effects/adverse reactions:

CV: Orthostatic hypotension, ***bradycardia, CHF, chest pain, ventricular dysrhythmias, AV block, peripheral vascular insufficiency,*** palpitations

CNS: Dizziness, mental changes, drowsiness, fatigue, headache, catatonia, depression, anxiety, nightmares, paresthesia, lethargy, insomnia, decreased concentration

GI: Nausea, vomiting, diarrhea, dry mouth, flatulence, constipation, anorexia

INTEG: Rash, alopecia, urticaria, pruritus, fever

HEMA: ***Agranulocytosis, thrombocytopenic purpura (rare)***

---

* Available in Canada only

EENT: Tinnitus, visual changes, sore throat, double vision, dry burning eyes
GU: Impotence, dysuria, ejaculatory failure, urinary retention
RESP: ***Bronchospasm,*** dyspnea, wheezing, nasal stuffiness, pharyngitis
MS: Joint pain, arthralgia, muscle cramps, pain
OTHER: Facial swelling, decreased exercise tolerance, weight change, Raynaud's disease

Contraindications: Hypersensitivity to β-blockers, cardiogenic shock, heart block (2nd or 3rd degree), sinus bradycardia, CHF, bronchial asthma

Precautions: Major surgery, pregnancy (C), lactation, diabetes mellitus, renal disease, thyroid disease, COPD, well-compensated heart failure, nonallergic bronchospasm

Pharmacokinetics:
PO: Onset 1-2 hr, peak 2-4 hr, duration 8-12 hr, half-life 6-8 hr; metabolized by liver (metabolites inactive); excreted in urine, bile; crosses placenta; excreted in breast milk

Interactions:
- Increased hypotension: diuretics, other antihypertensives, halothane, nitroglycerin, prazosin
- Decreased β-blocker effects: sympathomimetics, nonsteroidal antiinflammatory agents, salicylates
- Increased hypoglycemic effect: insulin
- Increased effects of lidocaine
- Decreased bronchodilating effects of theophylline β-agonists

Lab test interferences:
False increase: Urinary catecholamines
Interference: Glucose, insulin tolerance tests

NURSING CONSIDERATIONS

Assess:
- I&O, weight daily
- B/P, pulse q4h; note rate, rhythm, quality
- Apical/radial pulse before administration; notify physician of any significant changes
- Baselines in renal, liver function tests before therapy begins
- Edema in feet, legs daily
- Skin turgor, dryness of mucous membranes for hydration status

Administer:
- PO: ac, hs; tablet may be crushed or swallowed whole
- Reduced dosage in renal dysfunction

Perform/provide:
- Storage in dry area at room temperature; do not freeze

Evaluate:
- Therapeutic response: decreased B/P after 1-2 wk

Teach patient/family:
- Not to discontinue drug abruptly; taper over 2 wk, or may precipitate angina
- Not to use OTC products containing α-adrenergic stimulants (nasal decongestants, OTC cold preparations) unless directed by prescriber
- To report bradycardia, dizziness, confusion, depression, fever
- To take pulse at home, advise when to notify prescriber
- To avoid alcohol, smoking, sodium intake
- To comply with weight control, dietary adjustments, modified exercise program
- To carry Medic Alert ID to identify drug being taken, allergies
- To avoid hazardous activities if dizziness is present
- To report symptoms of CHF: difficult breathing, especially on exertion or when lying down, night cough, swelling of extremities

• To take medication hs to minimize orthostatic hypotension
• To wear support hose to minimize effects of orthostatic hypotension
• Method of instillation if using ophthalmic

Treatment of overdose: Lavage, IV atropine for bradycardia, IV theophylline for bronchospasm, digitalis, O_2, diuretic for cardiac failure; hemodialysis is useful for removal; administer vasopressor (norepinephrine) for hypotension, isoproterenol for heart block

cascara sagrada/ cascara sagrada aromatic fluid extract/ cascara sagrada fluid extract (OTC)

(kas-kar′a)

Func. class.: Laxative
Chem. class.: Anthraquinone

Action: Direct chemical irritation in colon; increases propulsion of stool

Uses: Constipation; bowel or rectal preparation for surgery or examination

Dosage and routes:
• *Adult:* PO 325 mg hs; FLUID 1 ml qd; AROMATIC FLUID 5 ml qd
• *Child 2-12 yr:* PO/FLUID/AROMATIC FLUID ½ adult dose
• *Child <2 yr:* PO/FLUID/AROMATIC FLUID ¼ adult dose

Available forms: Powder, tabs 325 mg; oral sol

Side effects/adverse reactions:
GI: Nausea, vomiting, anorexia, cramps, diarrhea
META: Hypocalcemia, enteropathy, alkalosis, hypokalemia, ***tetany***

Contraindications: Hypersensitivity, GI bleeding, obstruction, CHF, lactation, abdominal pain, nausea/vomiting, appendicitis, acute surgical abdomen, alcoholics (aromatic form)

Precautions: Pregnancy (C)

Pharmacokinetics:
PO: Peak 6-12 hr; metabolized by liver; excreted by kidneys, in feces

Interactions:
• Decreased absorption of these drugs: antibiotics, digitalis, nitrofurantoin, salicylates, tetracyclines, oral anticoagulants

NURSING CONSIDERATIONS

Assess:
• Blood, urine electrolytes if drug is used often by patient
• I&O ratio to identify fluid loss
• Cause of constipation; identify whether fluids, bulk, or exercise missing from lifestyle
• Cramping, rectal bleeding, nausea, vomiting; if these symptoms occur, drug should be discontinued

Administer:
• Alone for better absorption; do not take within 1 hr of other drugs or within 1 hr of antacids, milk
• In morning or evening (oral dose)

Evaluate:
• Therapeutic response: decrease in constipation

Teach patient/family:
• To swallow tabs whole; do not chew
• Not to use laxatives for long-term therapy; bowel tone will be lost
• That normal bowel movements do not always occur daily
• Not to use in presence of abdominal pain, nausea, vomiting
• To notify physician if constipation unrelieved or of symptoms of electrolyte imbalance: muscle cramps, pain, weakness, dizziness

cefaclor (℞)

(sef'a-klor)

Ceclor

Func. class.: Antibiotic

Chem. class.: Cephalosporin (2nd generation)

Action: Inhibits bacterial cell wall synthesis, which renders cell wall osmotically unstable, leading to cell death

Uses: Gram-negative bacilli: *H. influenzae, E. coli, P. mirabilis, Klebsiella;* gram-positive organisms: *S. pneumoniae, S. pyogenes, S. aureus;* upper and lower respiratory tract, urinary tract, skin infections, otitis media

Dosage and routes:

- *Adult:* PO 250-500 mg q8h, not to exceed 4 g/day
- *Child >1 mo:* PO 20-40 mg/kg qd in divided doses q8h, or total daily dose may be divided and given q12h, not to exceed 1 g/day

Available forms: Caps 250, 500 mg; oral susp 125, 187, 250, 375 mg/5 ml

Side effects/adverse reactions:

CNS: Headache, dizziness, weakness, paresthesia, fever, chills

GI: Nausea, vomiting, *diarrhea, anorexia,* pain, glossitis, bleeding, increased AST (SGOT), ALT (SGPT), bilirubin, LDH, alk phosphatase, abdominal pain

GU: Proteinuria, vaginitis, pruritus, candidiasis, increased BUN, ***nephrotoxicity, renal failure***

HEMA: ***Leukopenia, thrombocytopenia, agranulocytosis,*** anemia, ***neutropenia, lymphocytosis, eosinophilia, pancytopenia, hemolytic anemia***

INTEG: Rash, urticaria, dermatitis, ***anaphylaxis***

RESP: Dyspnea

Contraindications: Hypersensitivity to cephalosporins, infants <1 mo

Precautions: Hypersensitivity to penicillins, pregnancy (B), lactation, renal disease

Pharmacokinetics: Peak ½-1 hr, half-life 36-54 min; 25% bound by plasma proteins; 60%-85% eliminated unchanged in urine in 8 hr; crosses placenta; excreted in breast milk

Interactions:

- Decreased effects: tetracyclines, erythromycins
- Increased toxicity: aminoglycosides, furosemide, probenecid, sulfinpyrazone, colistin, ethacrynic acid, vancomycin

Lab test interferences:

Increase (false): Creatinine (serum urine), urinary 17-KS

False positive: Urinary protein, direct Coombs' test, urine glucose

Interference: Cross-matching

NURSING CONSIDERATIONS

Assess:

- Sensitivity to penicillins and other cephalosporins
- Nephrotoxicity: increased BUN, creatinine
- I&O daily
- Blood studies: AST, ALT, CBC, Hct, bilirubin, LDH, alk phosphatase, Coombs' test monthly if patient is on long-term therapy
- Electrolytes: K, Na, Cl monthly if patient is on long-term therapy
- Bowel pattern qd; if severe diarrhea occurs, drug should be discontinued; may indicate pseudomembranous colitis
- Urine output; if decreasing, notify prescriber (may indicate nephrotoxicity)
- Allergic reactions: rash, urticaria, pruritus, chills, fever, joint pain; angioedema may occur a few days after therapy begins

• Bleeding: ecchymosis, bleeding gums, hematuria, stool guaiac daily
• Overgrowth of infection: perineal itching, fever, malaise, redness, pain, swelling, drainage, rash, diarrhea, change in cough, sputum

Administer:
• For 10-14 days to ensure organism death, prevent superinfection
• With food if needed for GI symptoms
• After C&S completed

Evaluate:
• Therapeutic response: decreased symptoms of infection

Teach patient/family:
• If diabetic, to use Clinistix or Ketodiastix, blood glucose level
• Not to drink alcohol or meds with alcohol: reaction may occur
• To use yogurt or buttermilk to maintain intestinal flora, decrease diarrhea
• To take all medication prescribed for length of time ordered
• To report sore throat, bruising, bleeding, joint pain; may indicate blood dyscrasias (rare)

Treatment of anaphylaxis: Epinephrine, antihistamines, resuscitate if needed

cefadroxil (℞)

(sef-a-drox'ill)
cefadroxil, Duricef
Func. class.: Antibiotic
Chem. class.: Cephalosporin (1st generation)

Action: Inhibits bacterial cell wall synthesis, rendering cell wall osmotically unstable, leading to cell death

Uses: Gram-negative bacilli: *E. coli, P. mirabilis, Klebsiella (UTI only);* gram-positive organisms: *S. pneumoniae, S. pyogenes, S. aureus;* upper, lower respiratory tract, urinary tract, skin infections, otitis media; tonsillitis; particularly UTIs

Dosage and routes:
• *Adult:* PO 1-2 g qd or q12h, give a loading dose of 1 g initially; dosage reduction indicated in renal impairment (CrCl <50 ml/min)
• *Child:* 30 mg/kg/day

Available forms: Caps 500 mg; tabs 1 g; oral susp 125, 250, 500 mg/5 ml

Side effects/adverse reactions:
CNS: Headache, dizziness, weakness, paresthesia, fever, chills
GI: Nausea, vomiting, *diarrhea, anorexia,* pain, glossitis, bleeding, increased AST (SGOT), ALT (SGPT), bilirubin, LDH, alk phosphatase, abdominal pain, ***pseudomembranous colitis***
GU: Proteinuria, vaginitis, pruritus, candidiasis, increased BUN, ***nephrotoxicity, renal failure***
HEMA: ***Leukopenia, thrombocytopenia, agranulocytosis,*** anemia, ***neutropenia, lymphocytosis, eosinophilia, pancytopenia, hemolytic anemia***
INTEG: Rash, urticaria, dermatitis, ***anaphylaxis***
RESP: Dyspnea

Contraindications: Hypersensitivity to cephalosporins, infants <1 mo

Precautions: Hypersensitivity to penicillins, pregnancy (B), lactation, renal disease

Pharmacokinetics: Peak 1-1½ hr, half-life 1-2 hr; 20% bound by plasma proteins; crosses placenta; excreted in breast milk

Interactions:
• Decreased effects: tetracyclines, erythromycins
• Increased toxicity: aminoglycosides, furosemide, probenecid, sulfinpyrazone, colistin, ethacrynic acid, vancomycin

* Available in Canada only

Lab test interferences:
Increase (false): Creatinine (serum urine), urinary 17-KS
False positive: Urinary protein, direct Coombs' test, urine glucose
Interference: Cross-matching

NURSING CONSIDERATIONS

Assess:
- Sensitivity to penicillin and other cephalosporins
- Nephrotoxicity: increased BUN, creatinine
- I&O daily
- Blood studies: AST (SGOT), ALT (SGPT), CBC, Hct, bilirubin, LDH, alk phosphatase, Coombs' test monthly if patient is on long-term therapy
- Electrolytes: K, Na, Cl monthly if patient is on long-term therapy
- Bowel pattern qd; if severe diarrhea occurs, drug should be discontinued; may indicate pseudomembranous colitis
- Urine output: if decreasing, notify prescriber; may indicate nephrotoxicity
- Allergic reactions: rash, urticaria, pruritus, chills, fever, joint pain; angioedema; may occur few days after therapy begins
- Bleeding: ecchymosis, bleeding gums, hematuria, stool guaiac daily
- Overgrowth of infection: perineal itching, fever, malaise, redness, pain, swelling, drainage, rash, diarrhea, change in cough, sputum

Administer:
- For 10-14 days to ensure organism death, prevent superinfection
- With food if needed for GI symptoms
- After C&S completed

Evaluate:
- Therapeutic response: decreased symptoms of infection

Teach patient/family:
- If diabetic to use Clinistix or Ketodiastix, blood glucose level
- Not to drink alcohol or use meds with alcohol: reaction may occur
- To use yogurt or buttermilk to maintain intestinal flora, decrease diarrhea
- To take all medication prescribed for length of time ordered
- To report sore throat, bruising, bleeding, joint pain; may indicate blood dyscrasias (rare)

Treatment of anaphylaxis: Epinephrine, antihistamines; resuscitate if needed

---

cefamandole (℞)
(sef-a-man'dole)
Mandol
Func. class.: Antibiotic
Chem. class.: Cephalosporin (2nd generation)

Action: Inhibits bacterial cell wall synthesis, rendering cell wall osmotically unstable, leading to cell death

Uses: Gram-negative bacilli: *H. influenzae, E. coli, P. mirabilis, Klebsiella;* gram-positive organisms: *S. pneumoniae, S. pyogenes, S. aureus;* upper, lower respiratory tract, urinary tract, skin infections, peritonitis, septicemia, surgical prophylaxis

Dosage and routes:
- *Adult:* IM/IV 500 mg-1 g q4-8h; may give up to 2 g q4h for severe infections
- *Child >1 mo:* IM/IV 50-100 mg/kg/day in divided doses q4-8h, not to exceed adult dose
- Dosage reduction indicated in renal impairment (CrCl <5 ml/min)

Available forms: Inj IM, IV 1, 2, 10 g

Side effects/adverse reactions:
CNS: Headache, dizziness, weakness, paresthesia, fever, chills

GI: Nausea, vomiting, diarrhea, anorexia, pain, glossitis, bleeding, increased AST (SGOT), ALT (SGPT), bilirubin, LDH, alk phosphatase, abdominal pain

GU: Proteinuria, vaginitis, pruritus, candidiasis, increased BUN, ***nephrotoxicity, renal failure***

HEMA: ***Leukopenia, thrombocytopenia, agranulocytosis,*** anemia, ***neutropenia, lymphocytosis, eosinophilia, pancytopenia, hemolytic anemia,*** bleeding, ***hypoprothrombinemia***

INTEG: Rash, urticaria, dermatitis, ***anaphylaxis***

RESP: Dyspnea

Contraindications: Hypersensitivity to cephalosporins, infants <1 mo

Precautions: Hypersensitivity to penicillins, pregnancy (B), lactation, renal disease

Pharmacokinetics: Peak 1-1½ hr, half-life ½-1 hr; 60%-75% bound by plasma proteins; crosses placenta; excreted in breast milk

Interactions:

- Decreased effects: tetracyclines, erythromycins
- Increased toxicity: aminoglycosides, furosemide, probenecid, sulfinpyrazone, colistin, ethacrynic acid, vancomycin
- Disulfiram reaction: disulfiram

Y-site compatibilities: Acyclovir, cyclophosphamide, hydromorphone, magnesium sulfate, meperidine, morphine, perphenazine

Syringe compatibility: Heparin

Additive compatibilities: Clindamycin, floxacillin, furosemide, metronidazole, or verapamil

Lab test interferences:

Increase (false): Urinary 17-KS

False positive: Urinary protein, direct Coombs', urine glucose

Interference: Cross-matching

NURSING CONSIDERATIONS

Assess:

- Sensitivity to penicillin or other cephalosporins
- Nephrotoxicity: increased BUN, creatinine
- Blood studies: AST (SGOT), ALT (SGPT), CBC, Hct, bilirubin, LDH, alk phosphatase, Coombs' test, protime monthly if patient is on long-term therapy
- Electrolytes: K, Na, Cl monthly if patient is on long-term therapy
- Bowel pattern qd; if severe diarrhea occurs, drug should be discontinued; may indicate pseudomembranous colitis
- IV site for extravasation or phlebitis, change site q72h
- Urine output: if decreasing, notify prescriber; may indicate nephrotoxicity
- Allergic reactions: rash, urticaria, pruritus, chills, fever, joint pain, angioedema; may occur few days after therapy begins
- Bleeding: ecchymosis, bleeding gums, hematuria, stool guaiac
- Overgrowth of infection: perineal itching, fever, malaise, redness, pain, swelling, drainage, rash, diarrhea, change in cough, sputum

Administer:

- IV; check often for irritation, extravasation; dilute 1 g or less of drug/10 ml or more normal saline or sterile H_2O for inj; run over 3-5 min; may be further diluted with 100 ml of compatible sol and run over 15-30 min via Y-tube or 3-way stopcock; may also be diluted in 1 L compatible sol, run over prescribed rate
- For 10-14 days to ensure organism death, prevent superimposed infection
- After C&S completed

Evaluate:
• Therapeutic response: decreased symptoms of infection

Teach patient/family:
• If diabetic, to use Clinistix or Ketodiastix, blood glucose level
• Not to drink alcohol or meds with alcohol: reaction may occur
• To report sore throat, bruising, bleeding, joint pain; may indicate blood dyscrasias (rare)

Treatment of anaphylaxis: Epinephrine, antihistamines, resuscitate if needed

cefazolin (℞)

(sef-a'zoe-lin)

Ancef, cefazolin sodium, Kefzol, Zolicef

Func. class.: Antibiotic

Chem. class.: Cephalosporin (1st generation)

Action: Inhibits bacterial cell wall synthesis, rendering cell wall osmotically unstable, leading to cell death

Uses: Gram-negative bacilli: *H. influenzae, E. coli, P. mirabilis, Klebsiella;* gram-positive organisms: *S. pneumoniae, S. pyogenes, S. aureus;* upper, lower respiratory tract, urinary tract, skin infections, bone, joint, biliary, genital infections, endocarditis, surgical prophylaxis, septicemia

Dosage and routes:

Life-threatening infections
• *Adult:* IM/IV 1-1.5 g q6h
• *Child >1 mo:* IM/IV 100 mg/kg in 3-4 equal doses

Mild/moderate infections
• *Adult:* IM/IV 250-500 mg q8h
• *Child >1 mo:* IM/IV 25-50 mg/kg in 3-4 equal doses
• Dosage reduction indicated in renal impairment (CrCl <54 ml/min)

Available forms: Inj IM, IV, 500 mg, 1, 5, 10, 20 g

Side effects/adverse reactions:

CNS: Headache, dizziness, weakness, paresthesia, fever, chills

GI: Nausea, vomiting, *diarrhea, anorexia,* pain, glossitis, bleeding, increased AST (SGOT), ALT (SGPT), bilirubin, LDH, alk phosphatase, abdominal pain, oral candidiasis

GU: Proteinuria, vaginitis, pruritus, candidiasis, increased BUN, ***nephrotoxicity, renal failure***

HEMA: ***Leukopenia, thrombocytopenia, agranulocytosis,*** anemia, ***neutropenia, lymphocytosis, eosinophilia, pancytopenia, hemolytic anemia (rare)***

INTEG: Rash, urticaria, dermatitis, ***anaphylaxis***

Contraindications: Hypersensitivity to cephalosporins, infants <1 mo

Precautions: Hypersensitivity to penicillins, pregnancy (B), lactation, renal disease

Pharmacokinetics:

IM: Peak ½-2 hr, half-life 1½-2¼ hr

IV: Peak 10 min; eliminated unchanged in urine; 70% to 86% protein bound

Interactions:
• Increased toxicity: aminoglycosides, furosemide, colistin, ethacrynic acid

Y-site compatibilities: Acyclovir, atracurium, calcium gluconate, cyclophosphamide, enalaprilat, esmolol, famotidine, fluconazole, fludarabine, foscarnet, labetalol, lidocaine, magnesium sulfate, melphalan, meperidine, morphine, multivitamins, ondansetron, perphenazine, pancuronium, regular insulin, sargramostim, vecuronium, vitamin B complex with C

Syringe compatibilities: Heparin, vitamin B complex

Additive compatibilities: Aztreonam, cimetidine, clindamycin, metronidazole, verapamil
Lab test interferences:
Increase (false): Urinary 17-KS
False positive: Urinary protein, direct Coombs' test, urine glucose
Interference: Cross-matching
NURSING CONSIDERATIONS
Assess:
• Sensitivity to penicillin or other cephalosporins
• Nephrotoxicity: increased BUN, creatinine
• I&O daily
• Blood studies: AST (SGOT), ALT (SGPT), CBC, Hct, alk phosphatase, bilirubin, LDH, Coombs' test monthly if patient is on long-term therapy
• Electrolytes: K, Na, Cl monthly if patient is on long-term therapy
• Bowel pattern qd; if severe diarrhea occurs, drug should be discontinued; may indicate pseudomembranous colitis
• IV site for extravasation or phlebitis, change site q72h
• Urine output: if decreasing, notify physician; may indicate nephrotoxicity
• Allergic reactions: rash, urticaria, pruritus, chills, fever, joint pain, angioedema; may occur few days after therapy begins
• Overgrowth of infection: perineal itching, fever, malaise, redness, pain, swelling, drainage, rash, diarrhea, change in cough, sputum
Administer:
• IV; check for irritation, extravasation often; dilute in 10 ml sterile H_2O for inj and run over 3-5 min; may be further diluted with 50-100 ml of NS, D_5W sol and run over ½-1 hr by Y-tube or 3-way stopcock
• For 10-14 days to ensure organism death, prevent superinfection
• After C&S completed
Evaluate:
• Therapeutic response: decreased fever, malaise, chills
Teach patient/family:
• If diabetic, check blood glucose level
Treatment of anaphylaxis: Epinephrine, antihistamines, resuscitate if needed

cefixime (℞)

(se-fix' eem)
Suprax
Func. class.: Broad-spectrum antibiotic
Chem. class.: Cephalosporin (3rd generation)

Action: Inhibits bacterial cell wall synthesis, rendering cell wall osmotically unstable, leading to cell death
Uses: Uncomplicated UTI *(E. coli, P. mirabilis),* pharyngitis and tonsillitis *(S. pyogenes),* otitis media *(H. influenzae), M. catarrhalis,* acute bronchitis, and acute exacerbations of chronic bronchitis *(S. pneumoniae, H. influenzae)*
Dosage and routes:
• *Adult:* PO 400 mg qd as a single dose or 200 mg q12h
• Child >50 kg or >12 yrs: PO use adult dosage
• Child: <50 kg or <12 years: PO 8 mg/kg/day as a single dose or 4 mg/kg q12h
Available forms: Tabs 200, 400 g; powder for oral susp 100 mg/5 ml
Side effects/adverse reactions:
CNS: Headache, dizziness, paresthesia, fever, chills, lethargy, fatigue, confusion
GI: Nausea, vomiting, diarrhea, anorexia, pain, glossitis, bleeding, increased AST (SGOT), ALT (SGPT),

bilirubin, LDH, alk phosphatase, heartburn, dysgeusia, flatulence
GU: ***Proteinuria,*** vaginitis, pruritis, increased BUN, ***nephrotoxicity, renal failure,*** pyuria, dysuria
HEMA: ***Leukopenia, thrombocytopenia, agranulocytosis,*** anemia, ***neutropenia, lymphocytosis, eosinophilia, pancytopenia, hemolytic anemia (rare)***
INTEG: Rash, urticaria, ***exfoliative dermatitis, anaphylaxis***
RESP: ***Bronchospasm,*** dyspnea, tight chest

Contraindications: Hypersensitivity to cephalosporins, infants <6 mo

Precautions: Hypersensitivity to penicillins, pregnancy (B), lactation, renal disease

Pharmacokinetics:
PO: Peak 1 hr, half-life 3-4 hr, 65% bound by plasma proteins, 50% eliminated unchanged in urine; crosses placenta; excreted in breast milk

Interactions:
- Increased renal toxicity: aminoglycosides, furosemide, colistin, ethacrynic acid, vancomycin

Lab test interferences:
Increase (false): Urinary 17-KS
False positive: Urinary protein, direct Coombs', urine glucose
Interference: Cross-matching

NURSING CONSIDERATIONS

Assess:
- Sensitivity to penicillin or other cephalosporins
- Nephrotoxicity: increased BUN, creatinine
- Blood studies: AST (SGOT), ALT (SGPT), CBC, Hct, bilirubin, LDH, alk phosphatase; Coombs' test monthly if patient is on long-term therapy
- Bowel pattern qd; if severe diarrhea occurs, drug should be discontinued (may indicate pseudomembranous colitis)
- Urine output: if decreasing, notify physician (may indicate nephrotoxicity)
- Allergic reactions: rash, urticaria, pruritus, chills, fever, joint pain, angioedema; may occur a few days after therapy begins
- Bleeding: ecchymosis, bleeding, itching, fever, malaise, redness, pain, swelling, drainage, rash, diarrhea, change in cough, sputum

Administer:
- For 10-14 days to ensure organism death, prevent superinfection
- After C&S completed

Evaluate:
- Therapeutic response: decreased fever, malaise, chills

Teach patient/family:
- To report sore throat, bruising, bleeding, joint pain (may indicate blood dyscrasias [rare])
- If diabetic, check blood glucose level

Treatment of anaphylaxis: Epinephrine, antihistamines, resuscitate if needed

cefmetazole (℞)
(sef-met′a-zole)
Zefazone
Func. class.: Broad-spectrum antibiotic
Chem. class.: Cephalosporin (2nd generation)

Action: Inhibits bacterial cell wall synthesis, rendering cell wall osmotically unstable, leading to cell death

Uses: Gram-negative bacilli: *H. influenzae, E. coli, Proteus, Klebsiella, B. fragilis;* gram-positive organisms: *S. pneumoniae, S. pyogenes, S. aureus;* anaerobes, including *Clostridium;* infections of lower respiratory tract, urinary tract, skin, bone; septicemia; intraabdominal infections

Dosage and routes:

• *Adult:* IV 1-8 g divided q6-12h × 5-14 days

Available forms: Powder for inj 1, 2 gm/vial

Side effects/adverse reactions:

CNS: Headache, sizziness, paresthesia, fever, chills, lethargy, fatigue, confusion

GI: Nausea, vomiting, diarrhea, anorexia, pain, glossitis, bleeding, increased AST (SGOT), ALT (SGPT), bilirubin, LDH, alk phosphatase, heartburn, flatulence

GU: ***Proteinuria,*** vaginitis, pruritus, candidiasis, increased BUN, ***nephrotoxicity, renal failure***

HEMA: ***Leukopenia, thrombocytopenia, agranulocytosis, eosinophilia, pancytopenia, hemolytic anemia (rare)***

INTEG: Rash, urticaria, ***exfoliative dermatitis,*** thrombophlebitis ***angioedema,*** erythema, pruitus

SYST: ***Anaphylaxis***

Contraindications: Hypersensitivity to cephalosporins, infants <1 mo

Precautions: Hypersensitivity to penicillins, pregnancy (B), lactation, renal disease

Pharmacokinetics:

IM: Peak 30-45 min; 68% bound by plasma proteins, excreted by kidneys; half-life 1-3 hr

Interactions:

• Incompatible in sol with aminoglycosides

• Increased renal toxicity and ototoxicity: aminoglycosides, furosemide, colistin, ethacrynic acid, vancomycin

• Increased plasma level of cefmetazole

Lab test interferences:

Increase (false): Creatinine (serum urine), urinary 17-KS

False positive: Urinary protein, direct Coombs' test, urine glucose

Interference: Cross-matching

NURSING CONSIDERATIONS

Assess:

• Sensitivity to penicillin and other cephalosporins

• Nephrotoxicity: increased BUN, creatinine

• Blood studies: AST (SGOT), ALT (SGPT), CBC, Hct, bilirubin, LDH, alk phosphatase, Coombs' test monthly if patient is on long-term therapy

• Electrolytes: K, Na, Cl monthly if patient is on long-term therapy

• Bowel pattern qd; if severe diarrhea occurs, drug should be discontinued (may indicate pseudomembranous colitis)

• IV site for extravasation or phlebitis; change site q72h

• Urine output: if decreasing, notify prescriber (may indicate nephrotoxicity)

• Allergic reactions: rash, urticaria, pruritis, chills, fever, joint pain, 7-10 days after therapy begins

• Overgrowth of infection: perineal itching, fever, malaise, redness, pain, swelling, drainage, rash, diarrhea, change in cough, sputum

Administer:

• IV after diluting 3.7 or 10 ml sterile H_2O for inj, 2 gm/7 or 15 ml, shake, let stand until clear, run over 3-5 min; may be further diluted in 50-100 ml of D_5W, NS, LR to 1-20 mg/ml and run over ½-1 hr by Y-tube or 3-way stopcock

• For 10-14 days to ensure organism death, prevent superinfection

• After C&S completed

Evaluate:

• Therapeutic response: decreased fever, malaise, chills

Teach patient/family:

• If diabetic, check blood glucose level

* Available in Canada only

• To report sore throat, bruising, bleeding, joint pain (may indicate blood dyscrasias [rare])

Treatment of anaphylaxis: Epinephrine, antihistamines, resuscitate if needed

cefonicid (℞)

(se-fon′i-sid)

Monocid

Func. class.: Antibiotic

Chem. class.: Cephalosporin (2nd generation)

Action: Inhibits bacterial cell wall synthesis, rendering cell wall osmotically unstable, leading to cell death

Uses: Gram-negative bacilli: *H. influenzae, E. coli, P. mirabilis, Klebsiella;* gram-positive organisms: *S. pneumoniae, S. pyogenes, S. aureus;* lower respiratory tract, urinary tract, skin infections, otitis media, peritonitis, septicemia

Dosage and routes:

Life-threatening infections

• *Adult:* IM/IV BOL or INF 1-2 g/24 hr; divide in two doses if giving 2 g

• Dosage reduction indicated in renal impairment

Available forms: Inj IM, IV, 500 mg, 1, 10 g

Side effects/adverse reactions:

CNS: Headache, dizziness, weakness, paresthesia, fever, chills

GI: Nausea, vomiting, diarrhea, anorexia, pain, glossitis, bleeding, increased AST (SGOT), ALT (SGPT), bilirubin, LDH, alk phosphatase, abdominal pain

GU: Proteinuria, vaginitis, pruritus, candidiasis, increased BUN, ***nephrotoxicity, renal failure***

HEMA: ***Leukopenia, thrombocytopenia, agranulocytosis,*** anemia, ***neutropenia, lymphocytosis, eosinophilia, pancytopenia, hemolytic anemia (rare)***

INTEG: Rash, urticaria, dermatitis, ***anaphylaxis***

Contraindications: Hypersensitivity to cephalosporins, infants <1 mo

Precautions: Hypersensitivity to penicillins, pregnancy (B), lactation, renal disease

Pharmacokinetics:

IV: Onset 5 min

IM: Peak 1 hr

Half-life 4½ hr; excreted in breast milk; 98% protein bound

Interactions:

• Decreased effects: tetracyclines, erythromycins

• Increased toxicity: aminoglycosides, furosemide, colistin, ethacrynic acid, vancomycin, other cephalosporins

Y-site compatibility: Acyclovir

Additive compatibility: Clindamycin

Lab test interferences:

Increase (false): Urinary 17-KS

False positive: Urinary protein, direct Coombs' test, urine glucose

Interference: Cross-matching

NURSING CONSIDERATIONS

Assess:

• Sensitivity to penicillin and other cephalosporins

• Nephrotoxicity: increased BUN, creatinine

• Blood studies: AST (SGOT), ALT (SGPT), CBC, Hct, bilirubin, LDH, alk phosphatase, Coombs' test monthly if patient on long-term therapy

• Electrolytes: K, Na, Cl monthly if patient is on long-term therapy

• Bowel pattern qd; if severe diarrhea occurs, drug should be discontinued; may indicate pseudomembranous colitis

• Urine output: if decreasing, notify prescriber; may indicate nephrotoxicity

C

• Allergic reactions: rash, urticaria, pruritus, chills, fever, joint pain, angioedema; may occur few days after therapy begins
• Overgrowth of infection: perineal itching, fever, malaise, redness, pain, swelling, drainage, rash, diarrhea, change in cough, sputum

Administer:

• IV direct dilute 0.5 g/2 ml or 1 g/2.5 ml sterile H_2O for inj and give by Y-tube or 3-way stopcock over 3-5 min
• IV INT INF may be further diluted in 50-100 ml D_5W, NS and given over 30 min; slight yellowing of sol does not affect potency
• IV; check for irritation, extravasation often
• For 10-14 days to ensure organism death, prevent superimposed infection
• After C&S completed

Evaluate:

• Therapeutic response: decreased symptoms of infection

Teach patient/family:

• If diabetic, check blood glucose level
• To report sore throat, bruising, bleeding, joint pain; may indicate blood dyscrasias (rare)

Treatment of anaphylaxis: Epinephrine, antihistamines, resuscitate if needed

cefoperazone (℞)

(sef-oh-per′a-zone)
Cefobid
Func. class.: Antibiotic, broad-spectrum
Chem. class.: Cephalosporin (3rd generation)

Action: Inhibits bacterial cell wall synthesis, rendering cell wall osmotically unstable, leading to cell death

Uses: Gram-negative bacilli: *H. influenzae, E. coli, P. mirabilis, Klebsiella, Enterobacter, Serratia, Citrobacter, Providencia, P. aeruginosa;* lower respiratory tract, urinary tract, skin, bone infections, bacterial septicemia, peritonitis, PID

Dosage and routes:

Mild/moderate infections
• *Adult:* IM/IV 1-2 g q12h

Severe infections
• *Adult:* IM/IV 6-12 g/day divided in 2-4 equal doses

Available forms: Inj IM, IV, 1, 2 g

Side effects/adverse reactions:

CNS: Headache, dizziness, weakness, paresthesia, fever, chills
GI: Nausea, vomiting, diarrhea, anorexia, pain, glossitis, bleeding, increased AST (SGOT), ALT (SGPT), bilirubin, LDH, alk phosphatase, abdominal pain, pseudomembranous colitis
GU: Proteinuria, vaginitis, pruritus, candidiasis, increased BUN, ***nephrotoxicity, renal failure***
HEMA: ***Leukopenia, thrombocytopenia, agranulocytosis,*** anemia, ***neutropenia, lymphocytosis, eosinophilia, pancytopenia, hemolytic anemia, bleeding, hypoprothrombinemia (rare)***
INTEG: Rash, urticaria, dermatitis, ***anaphylaxis***
RESP: Dyspnea

Contraindications: Hypersensitivity to cephalosporins, infants <1 mo

Precautions: Hypersensitivity to penicillins, pregnancy (B), lactation, renal disease

Pharmacokinetics:

IV: Onset 5 min, peak 5-20 min, duration 6-8 hr
IM: Peak 1-2 hr, duration 6-8 hr
Half-life 2 hr; 70%-75% is eliminated unchanged in bile; 20%-30%

unchanged in urine; excreted in breast milk (small amounts)

Interactions:

• Increased toxicity: aminoglycosides, furosemide, probenecid, colistin, ethacrynic acid, vancomycin

• Disulfiram-like reactions if alcohol ingested within 24-72 hr of cefoperazone administration

Y-site compatibilities: Acyclovir, cyclophosphamide, enalaprilat, esmolol, famotidine, foscarnet, fludarabine, hydromorphone, magnesium sulfate, melphalan, morphine

Syringe compatibility: Heparin

Additive compatibilities: Cimetidine, clindamycin, furosemide

Lab test interferences:

Increase (false): Urinary 17-KS

False positive: Urinary protein, direct Coombs' test, urine glucose

Interference: Cross-matching

NURSING CONSIDERATIONS

Assess:

• Sensitivity to penicillin, other cephalosporins

• Nephrotoxicity: increased BUN, creatinine

• Blood studies: AST (SGOT), ALT (SGPT), CBC, Hct, bilirubin, LDH, alk phosphatase, Coombs' test, protime monthly if patient on long-term therapy

• Electrolytes: K, Na, Cl monthly if patient is on long-term therapy

• Bowel pattern qd; if severe diarrhea occurs, drug should be discontinued; may indicate pseudomembranous colitis

• IV site for extravasation or phlebitis; change site q72h

• Urine output: if decreasing, notify prescriber; may indicate nephrotoxicity

• Allergic reactions: rash, urticaria, pruritus, chills, fever, joint pain, angioedema; may occur few days after therapy begins

• Bleeding: ecchymosis, bleeding gums, hematuria, stool guaiac

• Overgrowth of infection: perineal itching, fever, malaise, redness, pain, swelling, drainage, rash, diarrhea, change in cough, sputum

Administer:

• IV after diluting 1 g/ml sterile H_2O for inj, or 0.9% NaCl; shake, give over 3-5 min; each g may be further diluted with 20-40 ml D_5W, NS given over 30 min or as a cont inf over 6-24 hr to a concentration no greater than 25 mg/ml

• IM for concentration >250 mg/ml, dilute in sterile water, then lidocaine, inject deeply

• For 10-14 days to ensure organism death, prevent superinfection

• After C&S completed

Evaluate:

• Therapeutic response: decreased symptoms of infection

Teach patient/family:

• Not to drink alcohol during or for 3 days after use

• To report sore throat, bruising, bleeding, joint pain; may indicate blood dyscrasias (rare)

Treatment of anaphylaxis: Epinephrine, antihistamines, resuscitate if needed

ceforanide (℞)

(sef-or'a-nide)

Precef

Func. class.: Antibiotic, broad spectrum

Chem. class.: Cephalosporin (2nd generation)

Action: Inhibits bacterial cell wall synthesis, rendering cell wall osmotically unstable and leading to cell death

Uses: Gram-negative bacilli: *H. influenzae, E. coli, P. mirabilis, Kleb-*

siella; gram-positive organisms: *S. pneumoniae, S. aureus;* lower respiratory tract, urinary tract, skin, bone infections, septicemia, endocarditis

Dosage and routes:

- *Adult:* IM/IV 0.5-1 g q12h
- *Child:* IM/IV 20-40 mg/kg/day in 2 equal doses q12h
- Dosage reduction indicated in renal impairment (CrCl <59 ml/min)

Available forms: Powder for inj IM, IV 500 mg, 1, 10 g

Side effects/adverse reactions:

CNS: Headache, dizziness, weakness, paresthesia, fever, chills

GI: Nausea, vomiting, diarrhea, anorexia, pain, glossitis, bleeding, increased AST (SGOT), ALT (SGPT), bilirubin, LDH, alk phosphatase, abdominal pain

GU: Proteinuria, vaginitis, pruritus, increased BUN, ***nephrotoxicity, renal failure***

HEMA: ***Leukopenia, thrombocytopenia, agranulocytosis,*** anemia, ***neutropenia, lymphocytosis, eosinophilia, pancytopenia, hemolytic anemia (rare)***

INTEG: Rash, urticaria, dermatitis, ***anaphylaxis***

RESP: Dyspnea

Contraindications: Hypersensitivity to cephalosporins, infants <1 mo

Precautions: Hypersensitivity to penicillins, pregnancy (B), lactation, renal disease

Pharmacokinetics:

IV: Peak 2 hr

IM: Peak 1 hr

Half-life 2½-3 hr; 80% is bound by plasma proteins; 90% is eliminated unchanged in urine; crosses placenta; excreted in breast milk

Interactions:

- Increased toxicity: aminoglycosides, furosemide, probenecid, colistin, ethacrynic acid, vancomycin

Y-site compatibilities: Acyclovir, cyclophosphamide, fludarabine, hydromorphone, magnesium sulfate, melphalan, meperidine, morphine, paclitaxel, ondansetron, perphanazine, sargramostim

Lab test interferences:

Increase (false): Urinary 17-KS

False positive: Urinary protein, direct Coombs' test, urine glucose

Interference: Cross-matching

NURSING CONSIDERATIONS

Assess:

- Sensitivity to penicillin, other cephalosporins
- Nephrotoxicity: increased BUN, creatinine
- Blood studies: AST (SGOT), ALT (SGPT), CBC, Hct, bilirubin, LDH, alk phosphatase, Coombs' test monthly if patient on long-term therapy
- Electrolytes: K, Na, Cl monthly if patient is on long-term therapy
- Urine output: if decreasing, notify prescriber; may indicate nephrotoxicity
- Allergic reactions: rash, urticaria, pruritus, chills, fever, joint pain, angioedema; may occur few days after therapy begins
- Overgrowth of infection: perineal itching, fever, malaise, redness, pain, swelling, drainage, rash, diarrhea, change in cough, sputum
- Bowel pattern qd; if severe diarrhea occurs, drug should be discontinued; may indicate pseudomembranous colitis
- IV site for extravasation or phlebitis; change site q72h

Administer:

- IV direct after diluting 0.5 g/5 ml NS or sterile H_2O for inj; give over 3-5 min
- IV INF may be further diluted in 50-100 ml D_5W, NS and given over 30 min

• For 10-14 days to ensure organism death, prevent superinfection
• After C&S completed

Evaluate:
• Therapeutic response: decreased symptoms of infection

Teach patient/family:
• If diabetic, check blood glucose level
• Not to drink alcohol or meds with alcohol, as reaction may occur
• To report sore throat, bruising, bleeding, joint pain; may indicate blood dyscrasias (rare)

Treatment of anaphylaxis: Epinephrine, antihistamines; resuscitate if needed

cefotaxime (℞)

(sef-oh-tax′eem)
Claforan

Func. class.: Antibiotic, broad-spectrum
Chem. class.: Cephalosporin (3rd generation)

Action: Inhibits bacterial cell wall synthesis, rendering cell wall osmotically unstable, leading to cell death

Uses: Gram-negative organisms: *H. influenzae, E. coli, N. gonorrhoeae, N. meningitidis, P. mirabilis, Klebsiella, Citrobacter, Serratia, Salmonella, Shigella;* gram-positive organisms: *S. pneumoniae, S. pyogenes, S. aureus,* lower serious respiratory tract, urinary tract, skin, bone, gonococcal infections, bacteremia, septicemia, meningitis

Dosage and routes:
• *Adult:* IM/IV 1 g q8-12h

Severe infections
• *Adult:* IM/IV 2 g q4h, not to exceed 12 g/day
• Uncomplicated gonorrhea, 1 g IM
• Dosage reduction indicated for severe renal impairment (CrCl <20 ml/min)

Available forms: Powder for inj IM, IV, 1, 2, 10 g; frozen inj/IV 20, 40 mg/ml

Side effects/adverse reactions:
CNS: Headache, dizziness, weakness, paresthesia, fever, chills
GI: Nausea, vomiting, diarrhea, anorexia, pain, glossitis, bleeding, increased AST (SGOT), ALT (SGPT), bilirubin, LDH, alk phosphatase, abdominal pain
GU: Proteinuria, vaginitis, pruritus, candidiasis, increased BUN, ***nephrotoxicity, renal failure***
HEMA: ***Leukopenia, thrombocytopenia, agranulocytosis,*** anemia, ***neutropenia, lymphocytosis, eosinophilia, pancytopenia, hemolytic anemia (rare)***
INTEG: Rash, urticaria, dermatitis, ***anaphylaxis,*** pain, induration (IM), inflammation (IV)

Contraindications: Hypersensitivity to cephalosporins, infants <1 mo

Precautions: Hypersensitivity to penicillins, pregnancy (B), lactation, renal disease

Pharmacokinetics:
IV: Onset 5 min
IM: Onset 30 min
Half-life 1 hr; 35%-65% is bound by plasma proteins; 40%-65% is eliminated unchanged in urine in 24 hr; 25% metabolized to active metabolites; excreted in breast milk (small amounts)

Interactions:
• Incompatible with aminoglycosides, aminophylline, HCO_3, erythromycins
• Increased toxicity: aminoglycosides, furosemide, colistin, ethacrynic acid, vancomycin

Lab test interferences:
Increase (false): Urinary 17-KS

False positive: Urinary protein, direct Coombs' test, urine glucose
Interference: Cross-matching

NURSING CONSIDERATIONS

Assess:

• Sensitivity to penicillin, other cephalosporins
• Nephrotoxicity: increased BUN, creatinine
• Blood studies: AST (SGOT), ALT (SGPT), CBC, Hct, bilirubin, LDH, alk phosphatase, Coombs' test monthly if patient is on long-term therapy
• Electrolytes: K, Na, Cl monthly if patient on long-term therapy
• Bowel pattern qd; if severe diarrhea occurs, drug should be discontinued; may indicate pseudomembranous colitis
• IV site for extravasation or phlebitis; change site q72h
• Urine output: if decreasing, notify prescriber; may indicate nephrotoxicity
• Allergic reactions: rash, urticaria, pruritis, chills, fever, joint pain, angioedema; may occur few days after therapy begins
• Bleeding: ecchymosis, bleeding gums, hematuria, stool guaiac
• Overgrowth of infection: perineal itching, fever, malaise, redness, pain, swelling, drainage, rash, diarrhea, change in cough, sputum

Administer:

• IV after diluting 1g/10 ml D_5W, NS, sterile H_2O for inj and give over 3-5 min by Y-tube or 3-way stopcock; may be diluted further with 50-100 ml of normal saline or D_5W; run over ½-1 hr; discontinue primary inf during administration; or may be diluted in larger vol of sol and given as a cont inf over 6-24 hr
• For 10-14 days to ensure organism death, prevent superinfection
• After C&S completed

Evaluate:

• Therapeutic response: decreased symptoms of infection

Teach patient/family:

• To report sore throat, bruising, bleeding, joint pain; may indicate blood dyscrasias (rare)
• If diabetic, check blood glucose level

Treatment of anaphylaxis: Epinephrine, antihistamines; resuscitate if needed

cefotetan (℞)

(sef'oh-tee-tan)
Cefotan
Func. class.: Antibiotic, broad spectrum
Chem. class.: Cephalosporin (2nd generation)

Action: Inhibits bacterial cell wall synthesis, which renders cell osmotically unstable, leading to cell death

Uses: Gram-negative organisms: *H. influenzae, E. coli, E. aerogenes, P. mirabilis, Klebsiella, Citrobacter, Enterobacter, Salmonella, Shigella, Acinetobacter, B. fragilis, Neisseria, Serratia;* gram-positive organisms: *S. pneumoniae, S. pyogenes, S. aureus;* upper, lower, serious respiratory tract, urinary tract, skin, gonococcal, intraabdominal infections, septicemia, meningitis

Dosages and routes:

• *Adult:* IV/IM 1-2g q12h × 5-10 days

Perioperative prophylaxis

• *Adult:* IV 1-2 g ½-1 hr before surgery

Available forms: Inj (IV, IM) 1, 2, 10 g

Side effects/adverse reactions:

CNS: Headache, dizziness, weakness, paresthesia, fever, chills

* Available in Canada only

GI: Nausea, vomiting, diarrhea, anorexia, pain, glossitis, bleeding, increased AST (SGOT), ALT (SGPT), bilirubin, LDH, alk phosphatase, ***pseudomembranous colitis***
GU: Proteinuria, vaginitis, pruritus, candidiasis, increased BUN, ***nephrotoxicity, renal failure***
HEMA: ***Leukopenia, thrombocytopenia, agranulocytosis,*** anemia, ***neutropenia, lymphocytosis, eosinophilia, pancytopenia, hemolytic anemia (rare)***
INTEG: Rash, urticaria, dermatitis
RESP: Dyspnea, ***anaphylaxis***

Contraindications: Hypersensitivity to cephalosporins; children

Precautions: Hypersensitivity to penicillins, pregnancy (B), lactation, renal disease

Pharmacokinetics:
IV/IM: Peak 1½-3 hr; half-life 3-5 hr, 70%-90% bound by plasma proteins, 50%-80% eliminated unchanged in urine, crosses placenta, excreted in milk

Interactions:
- Increased toxicity: aminoglycosides

Y-site compatibilities: Famotidine, fluconazole, fludarabine, regular insulin, meperidine, morphine, sargramostim

Lab test interferences:
Increase (false): Urinary 17-KS
False positive: Urinary protein, direct Coombs' test, urine glucose
Interference: Cross-matching

NURSING CONSIDERATIONS

Assess:
- Sensitivity to penicillin or other cephalosporins
- Nephrotoxicity: increased BUN, creatinine
- Blood studies: AST (SGOT), ALT (SGPT), CBC, Hct, bilirubin, LDH, alk phosphatase, Coombs' test monthly if patient is on long-term therapy
- Electrolytes: K, Na, Cl monthly if patient on long-term therapy
- Bowel pattern qd; if severe diarrhea occurs, drug should be discontinued; may indicate pseudomembranous colitis
- IV site for extravasation, phlebitis, change site q72h
- Urine output: if decreasing, notify prescriber; may indicate nephrotoxicity
- Allergic reactions: rash, urticaria, pruritus, chills, fever; may occur a few days after therapy begins
- Bleeding: ecchymosis, bleeding gums, hematuria, stool guaiac
- Overgrowth of infection: perineal itching, fever, malaise, redness, swelling, drainage, rash, diarrhea, change in cough, sputum

Administer:
- IV direct after diluting 1 g/10 ml sterile H_2O for inj and give over 3-5 min; may be diluted further with 50-100 ml of normal saline or D_5W, shake; run over ½-1 hr by Y-tube or 3-way stopcock; discontinue primary inf during administration
- For 5-10 days to ensure organism death, prevent superinfection
- After C&S

Evaluate:
- Therapeutic response: decreased symptoms of infection

Teach patient/family:
- To report sore throat, bruising, bleeding, joint pain; may indicate blood dyscrasias (rare)
- To report severe diarrhea; may indicate pseudomembranous colitis

Treatment of anaphylaxis: Epinephrine, antihistamines; resuscitate if needed

cefoxitin (℞)

(se-fox'i-tin)
Mefoxin
Func. class.: Antibiotic, broad-spectrum
Chem. class.: Cephamycin (2nd generation)

Action: Inhibits bacterial cell wall synthesis, rendering cell wall osmotically unstable, leading to cell death

Uses: Gram-negative bacilli: *H. influenzae, E. coli, Proteus, Klebsiella, B. fragilis, N. gonorrhoeae;* gram-positive organisms: *S. pneumoniae, S. pyogenes, S. aureus;* anaerobes including *Clostridium,* lower respiratory tract, urinary tract, skin, bone, gonococcal infections, septicemia, peritonitis

Dosage and routes:
- *Adult:* IM/IV 1-2 g q6-8h
- Dosage reduction indicated in renal impairment (CrCl <50 ml/min)
- Uncomplicated gonorrhea 2 g IM as single dose with 1 g PO probenecid at same time

Severe infections
- *Adult:* IM/IV 2 g q4h

Available forms: Powder for inj IM, IV 1, 2, 10 g

Side effects/adverse reactions:
CNS: Headache, dizziness, weakness, paresthesia, fever, chills
GI: Nausea, vomiting, diarrhea, anorexia, pain, glossitis, bleeding, increased AST (SGOT), ALT (SGPT), bilirubin, LDH, alk phosphatase, abdominal pain
GU: Proteinuria, vaginitis, pruritus, candidiasis, increased BUN, ***nephrotoxicity, renal failure***
HEMA: ***Leukopenia, thrombocytopenia, agranulocytosis,*** anemia, ***neutropenia, lymphocytosis, eosinophilia, pancytopenia, hemolytic anemia (rare)***
INTEG: Rash, urticaria, dermatitis, thrombophlebitis
SYST: ***Anaphylaxis***

Contraindications: Hypersensitivity to cephalosporins; infants <1 mo

Precautions: Hypersensitivity to penicillins, pregnancy (B), lactation, renal disease

Pharmacokinetics:
IV: Peak 3 min
IM: Peak 15-60 min
Half-life 1 hr, 55%-75% bound by plasma proteins, 90%-100% eliminated unchanged in urine; crosses placenta, blood-brain barrier, eliminated in breast milk, not metabolized

Interactions:
- Increased toxicity: aminoglycosides, furosemide, colistin, ethacrynic acid, vancomycin

Y-site compatibilities: Acyclovir, cyclophosphamide, famotidine, fluconazole, foscarnet, hydromorphone, magnesium sulfate, meperidine, morphine, ondansetron, perphenazine

Additive compatibilities: Amikacin, cimetidine, clindamycin, gentamicin, kanamycin, multivitamins, sodium bicarbonate, tobramycin, verapamil, vitamin B complex with C

Syringe compatibility: Heparin

Lab test interferences:
Increase (false): Creatinine (serum urine), urinary 17-KS
False positive: Urinary protein, direct Coombs' test, urine glucose
Interference: Cross-matching

NURSING CONSIDERATIONS

Assess:
- Sensitivity to penicillin, other cephalosporins
- Nephrotoxicity: increased BUN, creatinine
- Blood studies: AST (SGOT), ALT (SGPT), CBC, Hct, bilirubin, LDH,

* Available in Canada only

alk phosphatase, Coombs' test monthly if patient is on long-term therapy
- Electrolytes: K, Na, Cl monthly if patient is on long-term therapy
- Bowel pattern qd; if severe diarrhea occurs, drug should be discontinued (may indicate pseudomembranous colitis)
- IV site for extravasation or phlebitis; change site q72h
- Urine output: if decreasing, notify prescriber; may indicate nephrotoxicity
- Allergic reactions: rash, urticaria, pruritis, chills, fever, joint pain, angioedema; may occur few days after therapy begins
- Bleeding: ecchymosis, bleeding gums, hematuria, stool guaiac
- Overgrowth of infection: perineal itching, fever, malaise, redness, pain, swelling, drainage, rash, diarrhea, change in cough, sputum

Administer:
- IV after diluting 1 g or less/10 ml or more D_5W, NS and give over 3-5 min; may be diluted further with 50-100 ml of normal saline or D_5W; run over ½-1 hr by Y-tube or 3-way stopcock; discontinue primary inf during administration; by cont inf at prescribed rate
- For 10-14 days to ensure organism death, prevent superimposed infection
- After C&S completed

Evaluate:
- Therapeutic response: decreased symptoms of infection

Teach patient/family:
- If diabetic, check blood glucose level
- To report severe diarrhea; may indicate pseudomembranous colitis
- To report sore throat, bruising, bleeding, joint pain; may indicate blood dyscrasias (rare)

Treatment of anaphylaxis: Epinephrine, antihistamines; resuscitate if needed

cefpodoxime (℞)
(sef-poe-dox'eem)
Vantin
Func. class.: Antibiotic
Chem. class.: Cephalosporin (2nd generation)

Action: Inhibits bacterial cell synthesis, which renders cell wall osmotically unstable

Uses: Gram-negative bacilli: *N. gonorrhoeae, H. influenzae, E. coli, P. mirabilis, Klebsiella;* gram-positive organisms: *S. pneumoniae, S. pyogenes, S. aureus;* upper and lower respiratory tract, urinary tract, skin infections, otitis media, sexually transmitted diseases

Dosage and routes:
- *Adult (>13 years of age):* pneumonia: 200 mg q12h for 14 days; uncomplicated gonorrhea: 200 mg single dose; skin and skin structure: 400 mg q12h for 7-14 days; pharyngitis and tonsillitis: 100 mg q12h for 10 days; uncomplicated UTI: 100 mg q12h for 7 days; dosing interval increased in presence of severe renal impairment
- *Child (5 mo-12 yrs):* acute otitis media: 5 mg/kg q12h for 14 days; pharyngitis/tonsillitis: 5 mg/kg q12h (max 100 mg/dose or 200 mg/day) for 10 days

Available forms: Tabs 100, 200 mg; granules for suspension 50 mg/5 ml and 100 mg/5 ml

Side effects/adverse reactions:
CNS: Headache, dizziness, lethargy, fatigue, paresthesia, fever, chills
GI: Nausea, vomiting, diarrhea, anorexia, pain, glossitis, bleeding, in-

creased AST (SGOT), ALT (SGPT), bilirubin, LDH, alk phosphatase
GU: ***Proteinuria, vaginitis, pruritus, candidiasis, increased BUN, nephrotoxicity, renal failure***
HEMA: ***Leukopenia, thrombocytopenia, agranulocytosis, anemia, neutropenia, lymphocytosis, eosinophilia, pancytopenia, hemolytic anemia (rare)***
INTEG: Rash, urticaria, dermatitis
RESP: Dyspnea
SYST: ***Anaphylaxis***

Contraindications: Hypersensitivity to cephalosporins; infants

Precautions: Hypersensitivity to penicillins, pregnancy (B), lactation, renal disease

Pharmacokinetics:

Half-life 2-3 min; 25% bound by plasma proteins; 30% eliminated unchanged in urine in 8 hr; crosses placenta; excreted in breast milk

Interactions:

- Increased toxicity: aminoglycosides, probenecid, colistin, vancomycin

Y-site compatibilities: Famotidine, fluconazole, fludarabine, regular insulin, meperidine, morphine, sargramostim

Lab test interferences:

False increase: Creatinine (serum urine), urinary 17-KS
False positive: Urinary protein, direct Coombs' test, urine glucose
Interference: Cross-matching

NURSING CONSIDERATIONS

Assess:

- Sensitivity to penicillins and other cephalosporins
- Nephrotoxicity: increased BUN, creatinine
- Blood studies: AST (SGOT), ALT (SGPT), CBC, Hct, bilirubin, LDH, alk phosphatase, Coombs' test monthly if patient on long-term therapy
- Electrolytes: K, Na, Cl monthly if patient on long-term therapy
- Bowel pattern qd; if severe diarrhea occurs, drug should be discontinued; may indicate pseudomembranous colitis
- Urine output: if decreasing, notify physician (may indicate nephrotoxicity)
- Allergic reactions: rash, urticaria, pruritus, chills, fever, joint pain; angioedema may occur a few days after therapy begins
- Bleeding: ecchymosis, bleeding gums, hematuria, stool guaiac
- Overgrowth of infection: perineal itching, fever, malaise, redness, pain, swelling, drainage, rash, diarrhea, change in cough, sputum

Administer:

- For 10-14 days to ensure organism death, prevent superinfection
- With food to enhance absorption
- After C&S completed

Evaluate:

- Therapeutic response: decreased symptoms of infection

Teach patient/family:

- If diabetic, monitor blood glucose level
- To use yogurt or buttermilk to maintain intestinal flora, decrease diarrhea
- To take all med prescribed for length of time ordered
- To report sore throat, bruising, bleeding, joint pain; may indicate blood dyscrasias (rare)

Treatment of anaphylaxis: Epinephrine, antihistamines; resuscitate if needed

* Available in Canada only

cefprozil (℞)

(sef-proe'zill)

Cefzil

Func. class.: Antibiotic, broad spectrum

Chem. class.: 2nd generation cephalosporin

Action: Inhibits bacterial cell wall synthesis, which renders cell wall osmotically unstable, leading to cell death

Uses: Pharyngitis/tonsillitis, otitis media, secondary bacterial infection of acute bronchitis, and acute bacterial exacerbation of chronic bronchitis and uncomplicated skin and skin structure infections

Dosage and routes:

Upper respiratory infections

• *Adult:* PO 500 mg qd × 10 days

Otitis media

• *Child:* (6 mo-12 yr) PO 15 mg/kg q12h × 10 days

Lower respiratory infections

• *Adult:* PO 500 mg bid × 10 days

Skin/skin structure infections

• *Adult:* PO 250-500 mg q12h × 10 days

Available forms: Tabs 250, 500 mg; susp 125, 250 mg/5ml

Side effects/adverse reactions:

CNS: Dizziness, headache, weakness, paresthesia, fever, chills

GU: ***Nephrotoxicity, proteinuria, increased BUN, renal failure, hematuria,*** vaginitis, genitoanal pruritus, candidiasis

GI: Diarrhea, nausea, vomiting, pain, glossitis, anorexia, bleeding, increased AST (SGOT), ALT (SGPT), bilirubin, LDH, alk phosphatase, abdominal pain, ***pseudomembranous colitis,*** flatulence

HEMA: ***Leukopenia, thrombocytopenia, agranulocytosis, anemia, neutropenia, lymphocytosis, eosinophilia, pancytopenia, hemolytic anemia (rare)***

INTEG: Rash, urticaria, dermatitis

RESP: Dyspnea

SYST: ***Anaphylaxis***

Contraindications: Hypersensitivity to cephalosporins

Precautions: Pregnancy (B), lactation, elderly, hypersensitivity to penicillins, renal disease

Pharmacokinetics:

PO: Peak 6-10 hr; plasma protein binding 99%; elimination half-life 25 hr; extensively metabolized to an active metabolite

Interactions:

• Decreased effects of: tetracyclines, erythromycins, chloramphenicol

• Increased toxicity of aminoglycosides, colistin

Y-site compatibilities: Famotidine, fluconazole, fludarabine, regular insulin, meperidine, morphine, sargramostim

Lab test interferences:

Increase (false): Urinary 17-KS

False positive: Urinary protein, direct Coombs' test, urine glucose

Interference: Cross-matching

NURSING CONSIDERATIONS

Assess:

• Sensitivity to penicillin, other cephalosporins

• Nephrotoxicity: increased BUN, creatinine

• Blood studies: AST (SGOT), ALT (SGPT), CBC, Hct, bilirubin, LDH, alk phosphatase, Coombs' test monthly

• Bowel pattern qd; if severe diarrhea occurs, drug should be discontinued; may indicate pseudomembranous colitis

• Urine output: if decreasing, notify prescriber; may indicate nephrotoxicity

• Allergic reactions: rash, urticaria, pruritus, chills, fever, joint pain, an-

gioedema; may occur few days after therapy begins
• Bleeding: ecchymosis, bleeding gums, hematuria, stool guaiac
• Overgrowth of infection: perineal itching, fever, malaise, redness, pain, swelling, drainage, rash, diarrhea, change in cough, sputum

Administer:
• For 10-14 days to ensure organism death, prevent superimposed infection
• After C&S

Evaluate:
• Therapeutic response: negative C&S

Teach patient/family:
• To report severe diarrhea; may indicate pseudomembranous colitis
• To report sore throat, bruising, bleeding, joint pain; may indicate blood dyscrasias (rare)

Treatment of anaphylaxis: Epinephrine, antihistamines; resuscitate if needed

ceftazidime (℞)

(sef'tay-zi-deem)

Ceptaz, Fortaz, Magnacef*, Pentacef, Tazicef, Tazidime

Func. class.: Antibiotic, broad-spectrum

Chem. class.: Cephalosporin (3rd generation)

Action: Inhibits bacterial cell wall synthesis, which renders cell osmotically unstable

Uses: Gram-negative organisms: *H. influenzae, E. coli, E. aerogenes, P. aeruginosa, P. mirabilis, Klebsiella, Citrobacter, Enterobacter, Salmonella, Shigella, Acinetobacter, B. fragilis, Neisseria, Serratia;* gram-positive organisms: *S. pneumoniae, S. pyogenes, S. aureus;* upper, lower, serious respiratory tract, urinary tract, skin, gonococcal, intraabdominal infections; septicemia, meningitis

Dosage and routes:
• *Adult:* IV/IM 1 g q8-12h × 5-10 days
• *Children:* IV 30-50 mg/kg q8h not to exceed 6 g/day
• *Neonates:* IV 30-50 mg/kg q12h

Available forms: Inj (IV, IM), 500 mg, 1, 2, 6 g

Side effects/adverse reactions:
CNS: Headache, dizziness, weakness, paresthesia, fever, chills
GI: Nausea, vomiting, diarrhea, anorexia, pain, glossitis, bleeding, increased AST (SGOT), ALT (SGPT), bilirubin, LDH, alk phosphatase
GU: Proteinuria, vaginitis, pruritus, candidiasis, increased BUN, ***nephrotoxicity, renal failure***
HEMA: ***Leukopenia, thrombocytopenia, agranulocytosis,*** anemia, ***neutropenia, lymphocytosis, eosinophilia, pancytopenia, hemolytic anemia (rare)***
INTEG: Rash, urticaria, dermatitis
SYST: ***Anaphylaxis***
RESP: Dyspnea

Contraindications: Hypersensitivity to cephalosporins, children

Precautions: Hypersensitivity to penicillins, pregnancy (B), lactation, renal disease

Pharmacokinetics:
IV/IM: Peak 1 hr, half-life ½-1 hr, 90% bound by plasma proteins, 80% eliminated unchanged in urine, crosses placenta, excreted in breast milk

Interactions:
• Increased toxicity: aminoglycosides

Y-site compatibilities: Acyclovir, ciprofloxacin, enalaprilat, esmolol, fludarabine, foscarnet, hydromorphone, labetalol, meperidine, melphalan, morphine, ondansetron, pa-

* Available in Canada only

clitaxel, vinorelbine tartrate, zidovudine

Additive compatibilities: Ciprofloxacin, clindamycin, metronidazole

Lab test interferences:

Increase (false): Urinary 17-KS

False positive: Urinary protein, direct Coombs' test, urine glucose

Interference: Cross-matching

NURSING CONSIDERATIONS

Assess:

• Sensitivity to penicillin, other cephalosporins

• Nephrotoxicity: increased BUN, creatinine

• Blood studies: AST (SGOT), ALT (SGPT), CBC, Hct, bilirubin, LDH, alk phosphatase, Coombs' test monthly if patient on long-term therapy

• Electrolytes: K, Na, Cl monthly if patient on long-term therapy

• Bowel pattern qd; if severe diarrhea occurs, drug should be discontinued; may indicate pseudomembranous colitis

• IV site for extravasation, phlebitis, change site q72h

• Urine output: if decreasing, notify prescriber; may indicate nephrotoxicity

• Allergic reactions: rash, urticaria, pruritus, chills, fever; may occur a few days after therapy begins

• Bleeding: ecchymosis, bleeding gums, hematuria, stool guaiac

• Overgrowth of infection: perineal itching, fever, malaise, redness, swelling, drainage, rash, diarrhea, change in cough, sputum

Administer:

• IV after diluting 1 g/10 ml sterile H_2O for inj, shake, invert needle, push plunger, insert needle through stopper and keep in sol, expel bubbles and give over 3-5 min; may be diluted further with 50-100 ml of normal saline or D_5W; run over ½-1 hr, give through Y-tube or 3-way stopcock, discontinue primary inf during administration

• For 5-10 days to ensure organism death, prevent superinfection

• After C&S is taken

Evaluate:

• Therapeutic response: decreased symptoms of infection

Teach patient/family:

• To report sore throat, bruising, bleeding, joint pain; may indicate blood dyscrasias

• To report severe diarrhea; may indicate pseudomembranous colitis

• If diabetic, check blood glucose level

Treatment of anaphylaxis: Epinephrine, antihistamines; resuscitate if needed

ceftizoxime (℞)

(sef-ti-zox'eem)

Cefizox

Func. class.: Antibiotic, broad-spectrum

Chem. class.: Cephalosporin (3rd generation)

Action: Inhibits bacterial cell wall synthesis, which renders cell wall osmotically unstable, leading to cell death

Uses: Gram-negative organisms: *H. influenzae, E. coli, E. aerogenes, P. mirabilis, Klebsiella, Enterobacter;* gram-positive organisms: *S. pneumoniae, S. pyogenes, S. aureus;* lower serious respiratory tract, urinary tract, skin, intraabdominal infections, septicemia, meningitis, bone, joint infections, PID caused by *N. gonorrhoeae*

Dosage and routes:

• *Adult:* IM/IV 1-2 g q8-12h, may give up to 4g q8h in life-threatening infections

PID

• *Adult:* IV 2 g q8h, may increase to 4 g q8h in severe infections

Available forms: Inj 1, 2, 10 g/100 ml piggyback, 50 ml/5% D

Side effects/adverse reactions:

CNS: Headache, dizziness, paresthesia, fever

GI: Nausea, vomiting, diarrhea, anorexia, pain, glossitis, bleeding, increased AST (SGOT), ALT (SGPT), bilirubin, LDH, alk phosphatase, abdominal pain, ***pseudomembranous colitis***

GU: Proteinuria, vaginitis, pruritus, candidiasis

HEMA: ***Leukopenia, thrombocytopenia, agranulocytosis,*** anemia, ***neutropenia, eosinophilia, hemolytic anemia (rare)***

INTEG: Rash, urticaria, dermatitis

RESP: Dyspnea

SYST: ***Anaphylaxis***

Contraindications: Hypersensitivity to cephalosporins, infants <1 mo

Precautions: Hypersensitivity to penicillins, pregnancy (B), lactation, renal disease

Pharmacokinetics:

IV: Onset 5 min

IM: Peak 1 hr

Half-life 5-8 hr; 90% bound by plasma proteins; 36%-60% eliminated unchanged in urine; crosses placenta; excreted in breast milk

Interactions:

• Increased toxicity: aminoglycosides, furosemide, colistin, ethacrynic acid

Y-site compatibilities: Acyclovir, enalaprilat, esmolol, famotidine, fludarabine, foscarnet, hydromorphone, labetalol, melphalan, meperidine, morphine, ondansetron, sargramostim, vinorelbine tartrate

Additive compatibility: Clindamycin

Lab test interferences:

Increase (false): Urinary 17-KS

False positive: Urinary protein, direct Coombs' test, urine glucose

Interference: Cross-matching

NURSING CONSIDERATIONS

Assess:

• Sensitivity to penicillin, other cephalosporins

• Nephrotoxicity: increased BUN, creatinine

• Blood studies: AST (SGOT), ALT (SGPT), CBC, Hct, bilirubin, LDH, alk phosphatase, Coombs' test monthly if patient on long-term therapy

• Electrolytes: K, Na, Cl monthly if patient on long-term therapy

• Bowel pattern qd; if severe diarrhea occurs, drug should be discontinued; may indicate pseudomembranous colitis

• IV site for extravasation, phlebitis; change site q72h

• Allergic reactions: rash, urticaria, pruritus, chills, fever, joint pain, angioedema; may occur few days after therapy begins

• Bleeding: ecchymosis, bleeding gums, hematuria, stool guaiac

• Overgrowth of infection: perineal itching, fever, malaise, redness, pain, swelling, drainage, rash, diarrhea, change in cough, sputum

Administer:

• IV after diluting 1 g/10 ml sterile water, shake and give over 3-5 min; may be diluted further with 50-100 ml NS or D_5W give through Y-tube or 3-way stopcock; run over ½-1 hr

• For 10-14 days to ensure organism death, prevent superinfection

• After C&S

Evaluate:

• Therapeutic response: decreased symptoms of infection

Teach patient/family:

• If diabetic, check blood glucose level

---

* Available in Canada only

• To report sore throat, bruising, bleeding, joint pain; may indicate blood dyscrasias (rare)

Treatment of anaphylaxis: Epinephrine, antihistamines; resuscitate if needed

---

ceftriaxone (℞)

(sef-try-ax′one)

Rocephin

Func. class.: Antibiotic, broad spectrum

Chem. class.: Cephalosporin (3rd generation)

Action: Inhibits bacterial cell wall synthesis, which renders cell wall osmotically unstable, leading to cell death

Uses: Gram-negative organisms: *H. influenzae, E. coli, E. aerogenes, P. mirabilis, Klebsiella, Citrobacter, Enterobacter, Salmonella, Shigella, Acinetobacter, B. fragilis, Neisseria, Serratia;* gram-positive organisms: *S. pneumoniae, S. pyogenes, S. aureus;* lower serious respiratory tract, urinary tract, skin, gonococcal, intraabdominal infections, septicemia, meningitis, bone, joint infections

Dosage and routes:

• *Adult:* IM/IV 1-2 g qd or in two equal doses

• *Child:* IM/IV 50-75 mg/kg/day in equal doses q12h

Uncomplicated gonorrhea

• 250 mg IM as single dose

• Dosage reduction may be indicated in severe renal impairment (CrCl <10 ml/min)

Meningitis

• *Adult and child:* IM/IV 100 mg/kg/day in equal doses q12h

Surgical prophylaxis

• Adult: IV 1 g ½-2 hr preop

Available forms: Inj IM, IV 500 mg, 1, 2, 10 g

Side effects/adverse reactions:

CNS: Headache, dizziness, weakness, paresthesia, fever, chills

GI: Nausea, vomiting, diarrhea, anorexia, pain, glossitis, bleeding, increased AST (SGOT), ALT (SGPT), bilirubin, LDH, alk phosphatase, abdominal pain, ***pseudomembranous colitis***

GU: Proteinuria, vaginitis, pruritus, candidiasis, increased BUN, ***nephrotoxicity, renal failure***

HEMA: ***Leukopenia, thrombocytopenia, agranulocytosis,*** anemia, ***neutropenia, lymphocytosis, eosinophilia, pancytopenia, hemolytic anemia***

INTEG: Rash, urticaria, dermatitis

RESP: Dyspnea

SYST: ***Anaphylaxis***

Contraindications: Hypersensitivity to cephalosporins, infants <1 mo

Precautions: Hypersensitivity to penicillins, pregnancy (B), lactation, renal disease

Pharmacokinetics:

IV: Onset 5 min

IM: Peak 1 hr

Half-life 5-8 hr, 90% bound by plasma proteins; 35%-60% eliminated unchanged in urine; crosses placenta; excreted in breast milk

Interactions:

• Increased toxicity: aminoglycosides, furosemide, probenecid, sulfinpyrazone, colistin, ethacrynic acid

Y-site compatibilities: Acyclovir, fludarabine, foscarnet, melphalan, meperidine, morphine, paclitaxel, sargramostim, vinorelbine tartrate

Additive compatibilities: Amino acids or sodium bicarbonate

Lab test interferences:

Increase (false): Urinary 17-KS

False positive: Urinary protein, direct Coombs' test, urine glucose

Interference: Cross-matching

NURSING CONSIDERATIONS

Assess:

- Sensitivity to penicillin, other cephalosporins
- Nephrotoxicity: increased BUN, creatinine
- Blood studies: AST (SGOT), ALT (SGPT), CBC, Hct, bilirubin, LDH, alk phosphatase, Coombs' test monthly if patient is on long-term therapy
- Electrolytes: K, Na, Cl monthly if patient is on long-term therapy
- Bowel pattern qd; if severe diarrhea occurs, drug should be discontinued; may indicate pseudomembranous colitis
- IV site for extravasation, phlebitis; change site q72h
- Urine output: if decreasing, notify prescriber; may indicate nephrotoxicity
- Allergic reactions: rash, urticaria, pruritus, chills, fever, joint pain, angioedema; may occur few days after therapy begins
- Bleeding: ecchymosis, bleeding gums, hematuria, stool guaiac
- Overgrowth of infection: perineal itching, fever, malaise, redness, pain, swelling, drainage, rash, diarrhea, change in cough, sputum

Administer:

- For 10-14 days to ensure organism death, prevent superinfection
- IV after diluting 250 mg/2.4 ml D_5W, H_2O for inj, 0.9% NaCl; may be further diluted with 50-100 ml NS, D_5W, $D_{10}W$ shake; run over ½-1 hr
- After C&S

Evaluate:

- Therapeutic response: decreased symptoms of infection

Teach patient/family:

- If diabetic, check blood glucose level
- To report severe diarrhea; may indicate pseudomembranous colitis
- To report sore throat, bruising, bleeding, joint pain; may indicate blood dyscrasias (rare)

Treatment of anaphylaxis: Epinephrine, antihistamines; resuscitate if needed

---

cefuroxime (℞)

(sef-fyoor-ox'eem)

Ceftin, Kefurox, Zihacef

Func. class.: Antibiotic, broad-spectrum

Chem. class.: Cephalosporin (2nd generation)

Action: Inhibits bacterial cell wall synthesis, rendering cell wall osmotically unstable

Uses: Gram-negative bacilli *(H. influenzae, E. coli, Neisseria, P. mirabilis, Klebsiella);* gram-positive organisms *(S. pneumoniae, S. pyogenes, S. aureus);* serious lower respiratory tract, urinary tract, skin, gonococcal infections; septicemia; meningitis

Dosage and routes:

- *Adult and child:* PO 250 mg q12h; may increase to 500 mg q12h in serious infections
- *Adult:* IM/IV 750 mg-1.5 g q8h for 5-10 days

Urinary tract infections

- *Adult:* PO 125 mg q12h; may increase to 250 mg q12h if needed

Otitis media

- Child <2 yr: PO 125 mg bid
- Child >2 yr: PO 250 mg bid

Surgical prophylaxis

- *Adult:* IV 1.5 g ½-1 hr preop

Severe infections

- *Adult:* IM/IV 1.5 g q6h; may give up to 3 g q8h for bacterial meningitis

---

* Available in Canada only

• *Child >3 mo:* IM/IV 50-100 mg/kg/day; may give up to 200-240 mg/kg/day IV in divided doses for bacterial meningitis
• Dosage reduction indicated in severe renal impairment (CrCl < 20 ml/min)
Uncomplicated gonorrhea
• 1.5 g IM as single dose with oral probenecid in 2 separate sites
Available forms: Tabs 125, 250, 500 mg, inj 150 mg, 1.5, 7.5 g; Inj IM, IV 750 mg, 1.5 g, pwd
Side effects/adverse reactions:
CNS: Headache, dizziness, weakness, paresthesia, fever, chills
GI: Nausea, vomiting, diarrhea, anorexia, pain, glossitis, bleeding, increased AST (SGOT), ALT (SGPT), bilirubin, LDH, alk phosphatase, abdominal pain, ***pseudomembranous colitis***
GU: Proteinuria, vaginitis, pruritus, candidiasis, increased BUN, ***nephrotoxicity, renal failure***
HEMA: ***Leukopenia, thrombocytopenia, agranulocytosis,*** anemia, ***neutropenia, lymphocytosis, eosinophilia, pancytopenia, hemolytic anemia (rare)***
INTEG: Rash, urticaria, dermatitis
SYST: ***Anaphylaxis***
Contraindications: Hypersensitivity to cephalosporins, infants <1 mo
Precautions: Hypersensitivity to penicillins, pregnancy (B), lactation, renal disease
Pharmacokinetics:
65% excreted unchanged in urine, half-life 1-2 hr in normal renal function
Interactions:
• Increased side effects: aminoglycosides, furosemide, colistin, ethacrynic acid
Lab test interferences:
Increase (false): Creatinine (serum urine), urinary 17-KS
False positive: Urinary protein, direct Coombs' test, urine glucose
Interferences: Cross-matching

NURSING CONSIDERATIONS

Assess:
• Sensitivity to penicillin or other cephalosporins
• Nephrotoxicity: increased BUN, creatinine
• Blood studies: AST (SGOT), ALT (SGPT), CBC, Hct, bilirubin, LDH, alk phosphatase, Coombs' test monthly if patient is on long-term therapy
• Electrolytes: K, Na, Cl monthly if patient is on long-term therapy
• Bowel pattern qd; if severe diarrhea occurs, drug should be discontinued; may indicate pseudomembranous colitis
• Urine output: if decreasing, notify prescriber; may indicate nephrotoxicity
• Allergic reactions: rash, urticaria, pruritus, chills, fever, joint pain, angioedema; may occur a few days after therapy begins
• Bleeding: ecchymosis, bleeding gums, hematuria, stool guaiac
• Overgrowth of infection: perineal itching, fever, malaise, redness, pain, swelling, drainage, rash, diarrhea, change in cough, sputum
Administer:
• For 10-14 days to ensure organism death, prevent superinfection
• With food if needed for GI symptoms
• After C&S
Evaluate:
• Therapeutic response: decreased symptoms of infection
Teach patient/family:
• To use yogurt or buttermilk to maintain intestinal flora, decrease diarrhea
• To take all medication prescribed for length of time ordered

• To report sore throat, bruising, bleeding, joint pain; may indicate blood dyscrasias (rare)
• If diabetic, check blood glucose level

Treatment of anaphylaxis: Epinephrine, antihistamine; resuscitate if needed

cephalexin (℞)

(sef-a-lex'in)

Biocef, cephalexin, Ceporex*, Keflex, Keftab, Novolexin*, Nu-Cephalex*

Func. class.: Antibiotic

Chem. class.: Cephalosporin (1st generation)

Action: Inhibits bacterial cell wall synthesis, rendering cell wall osmotically unstable, leading to cell death

Uses: Gram-negative bacilli: *H. influenzae, E. coli, P. mirabilis, Klebsiella;* gram-positive organisms: *S. pneumoniae, S. pyogenes, S. aureus;* upper, lower respiratory tract, urinary tract, skin, bone infections, otitis media

Dosage and routes:
• *Adult:* PO 250-500 mg q6h
• *Child:* PO 25-50 mg/kg/day in 4 equal doses

Moderate skin infections
500 mg q12h

Severe infections
• *Adult:* PO 500 mg-1 g q6h
• *Child:* PO 50-100 mg/kg/day in 4 equal doses
• Dosage reduction indicated in renal impairment (CrCl <50 ml/min)

Available forms: Caps 250, 500 mg; tabs 250, 500, 1 g; oral susp 125, 250 mg/5 ml

Side effects/adverse reactions:
CNS: Headache, dizziness, weakness, paresthesia, fever, chills
GI: Nausea, vomiting, diarrhea, anorexia, pain, glossitis, bleeding, increased AST (SGOT), ALT (SGPT), bilirubin, LDH, alk phosphatase, abdominal pain, ***pseudomembranous colitis***
GU: Proteinuria, vaginitis, pruritus, candidiasis, increased BUN, ***nephrotoxicity, renal failure***
HEMA: ***Leukopenia, thrombocytopenia, agranulocytosis,*** anemia, ***neutropenia, lymphocytosis, eosinophilia, pancytopenia, hemolytic anemia (rare)***
INTEG: Rash, urticaria, dermatitis
RESP: Dyspnea
SYST: ***Anaphylaxis***

Contraindications: Hypersensitivity to cephalosporins, infants <1 mo.

Precautions: Hypersensitivity to penicillins, pregnancy (B), lactation, renal disease

Pharmacokinetics:
PO: Peak 1 hr, duration 6-8 hr, half-life 30-72 min; 5%-15% bound by plasma proteins; 90%-100% eliminated unchanged in urine; crosses placenta; excreted in breast milk

Interactions:
• Increased toxicity: aminoglycosides, furosemide, colistin, ethacrynic acid, vancomycin

Lab test interferences:
Increase (false): Creatinine (serum urine), urinary 17-KS
False positive: Urinary protein, direct Coombs' test, urine glucose
Interference: Cross-matching

NURSING CONSIDERATIONS

Assess:
• Sensitivity to penicillin, other cephalosporins
• Nephrotoxicity: increased BUN, creatinine
• Blood studies: AST (SGOT), ALT (SGPT), CBC, Hct, bilirubin, LDH, alk phosphatase, Coombs' test monthly if patient is on long-term therapy

* Available in Canada only

• Electrolytes: K, Na, Cl monthly if patient is on long-term therapy
• Bowel pattern qd; if severe diarrhea occurs, drug should be discontinued; may indicate pseudomembranous colitis
• Urine output: if decreasing, notify prescriber; may indicate nephrotoxicity
• Allergic reactions: rash, urticaria, pruritus, chills, fever, joint pain, angioedema; may occur few days after therapy begins
• Bleeding: ecchymosis, bleeding gums, hematuria, stool guaiac
• Overgrowth of infection: perineal itching, fever, malaise, redness, pain, swelling, drainage, rash, diarrhea, change in cough, sputum

Administer:
• For 10-14 days to ensure organism death, prevent superinfection
• With food if needed for GI symptoms
• After C&S

Evaluate:
• Therapeutic response: decreased symptoms of infection

Teach patient/family:
• If diabetic, check blood glucose level
• To use yogurt or buttermilk to maintain intestinal flora, decrease diarrhea
• To take all medication prescribed for length of time ordered
• To report sore throat, bruising, bleeding, joint pain; may indicate blood dyscrasias (rare)
• To report severe diarrhea; may indicate pseudomembranous colitis

Treatment of anaphylaxis: Epinephrine, antihistamines, resuscitate if needed

cephalothin (℞)

(sef-a-loe'thin)
cephalothin sodium, Ceporacin*, Keflin, Keflin Neutral, Seffin Neutral

Func. class.: Broad-spectrum antibiotic

Chem. class.: Cephalosporin (1st generation)

Action: Inhibits bacterial cell wall synthesis, rendering cell wall osmotically unstable and leading to cell death by binding to the cell wall membrane

Uses: Gram-negative bacilli: *H. influenzae, E. coli, P. mirabilis, Klebsiella, Salmonella, Shigella;* gram-positive organisms: *S. pneumoniae, S. pyogenes, S. aureus;* lower respiratory tract, urinary tract, skin and bone infections; septicemia, endocarditis, bacterial peritonitis

Dosage and routes:
• *Adult:* IM/IV 500 mg-1 g q4-6h
• *Child:* IM/IV 14-27 mg/kg q4h or 20-40 mg/kg q6h
• Dosage reduction indicated in renal impairment (CrCl 50 ml/min)

Uncomplicated gonorrhea
• 2 g IM as single dose

Severe infections
• *Adult:* IM/IV 1-2 g q4h

Available forms: Powder for inj IM, IV 1, 2, 20 g; frozen IV 20, 30, 40 mg/ml

Side effects/adverse reactions:
CNS: Headache, dizziness, weakness, paresthesia, fever, chills
GI: Nausea, vomiting, diarrhea, anorexia, pain, glossitis, bleeding; increased AST (SGOT), ALT (SGPT), bilirubin, LDH, alk phosphatase; abdominal pain, ***pseudomembranous colitis***
GU: ***Proteinuria,*** vaginitis, pruri-

tus, candidiasis, increased BUN, ***nephrotoxicity, renal failure***

HEMA: ***Leukopenia, thrombocytopenia, agranulocytosis,*** anemia, ***neutropenia, lymphocytosis, eosinophilia, pancytopenia, hemolytic anemia (rare)***

INTEG: Rash, urticaria, dermatitis

RESP: Dyspnea

SYST: ***Anaphylaxis***

Contraindications: Hypersensitivity to cephalosporins

Precautions: Hypersensitivity to penicillins, pregnancy (B), lactation, renal disease

Pharmacokinetics: Well absorbed (IM)

IV: Peak 15 min

IM: Peak 30 min

Half-life ½-1 hr, 65%-80% bound by plasma proteins, 50%-75% eliminated unchanged in urine in 8 hr; crosses placenta, excreted in breast milk, deacetylated in kidneys, liver

Interactions:

- Decreased effects: Tetracyclines, erythromycins
- Increased toxicity: Aminoglycosides, furosemide, colistin, ethacrynic acid, vancomycin

Y-site compatibilities: Cyclophosphamide, famotidine, heparin, hydromorphone, magnesium sulfate, meperidine, morphine, multivitamins, perphenazine, potassium chloride, vitamin B complex with C

Syringe compatibility: Cimetidine

Additive compatibilities: Ascorbic acid, chloramphenicol, clindamycin, fluorouracil, hydrocortisone sodium succinate, isoproterenol, magnesium sulfate, metaraminol bitartrate, methicillin, methotrexate, potassium chloride, prednisolone sodium phosphate, procaine, sodium bicarbonate

Lab test interferences:

False increase: Creatinine (serum, urine), urinary 17-KS

False positive: Urinary protein, direct Coombs', urine glucose, Clinitest

Interference: Cross-matching

NURSING CONSIDERATIONS

Assess:

- Infection: fever, wound drainage, sputum, malaise
- Nephrotoxicity: increased BUN, creatinine I&O daily and weight; if output is decreasing, notify prescriber
- Sensitivity to penicillin, other cephalosporins
- Blood studies: AST (SGOT), ALT (SGPT), CBC
- Hct, bilirubin, LDH, alk phosphatase, Coombs' test monthly if patient is on long-term therapy
- Electrolytes: K, Na, Cl monthly if patient is on long-term therapy
- Bowel pattern qd; if severe diarrhea occurs, drug should be discontinued; may indicate pseudomembranous colitis
- IV site for extravasation, phlebitis; change site q72h
- Allergic reactions: rash, urticaria, pruritus, chills, fever, wheezing, joint pain, angioedema; may occur few days after therapy begins; keep resuscitation equipment and epinephrine on unit
- Bleeding: ecchymosis, bleeding gums, hematuria, stool guaiac
- Overgrowth of infection: perineal itching, fever, malaise, redness, pain, swelling, drainage, rash, diarrhea, change in cough, sputum

Administer:

- Clear solution; do not give cloudy sol
- IV after diluting 1 g or less/10 ml or more of sterile H_2O for inj; give over 3-5 min; may be further diluted with 50 ml D_5W, NS by Y-tube or 3-way stopcock; run over 15-30 min;

* Available in Canada only

discontinue primary IV during administration; may also be given by continuous infusion
• IM after reconstituting with 4 ml sterile H_2O for inj/1 g vial
• For 10-14 days to ensure organism death, prevent superinfection after C&S
• Insert IM in deep muscle mass, massage

Evaluate:
• Therapeutic response: decreased symptoms of infection

Teach patient/family:
• If diabetic, check blood glucose level
• To report sore throat, bruising, bleeding, joint pain; may indicate blood dyscrasias (rare)
• To report severe diarrhea; may indicate pseudomembranous colitis
• To report furry tongue, loose, foul-smelling stools; vaginal itching may indicate superinfection

Treatment of anaphylaxis: Epinephrine, antihistamines; resuscitate if needed

cephapirin (℞)

(sef-a-pye'rin)
Cefadyl, cephaprin sodium
Func. class.: Antibiotic, broad spectrum
Chem. class.: Cephalosporin (1st generation)

Action: Inhibits bacterial cell wall synthesis, rendering cell wall osmotically unstable, leading to cell death

Uses: Gram-negative bacilli: *H. influenzae, E. coli, P. mirabilis, Klebsiella;* gram-positive organisms: *S. pneumoniae, S. viridans, S. aureus;* lower respiratory tract, urinary tract, skin infections, septicemia, endocarditis, bacterial peritonitis

Dosage and routes:
• *Adult:* IM/IV 500 mg-1 g q4-6h
• *Child:* IM/IV 40-80 mg/kg/day given in divided doses q6h or 10-20 mg/kg q6h
• Dosage reduction indicated in renal impairment (CrCl <50 ml/min)

Available forms: Powder for inj IM, IV 500 mg, 1, 2, 20 g; IV only 1, 2, 4 g

Side effects/adverse reactions:
CNS: Headache, dizziness, weakness, paresthesia, fever, chills
GI: Nausea, vomiting, diarrhea, anorexia, pain, glossitis, bleeding, increased AST (SGOT), ALT (SGPT), bilirubin, LDH, alk phosphatase, abdominal pain, ***pseudomembranous colitis***
GU: Proteinuria, vaginitis, pruritus, candidiasis, increased BUN, ***nephrotoxicity, renal failure***
HEMA: ***Leukopenia, thrombocytopenia, agranulocytosis,*** anemia, ***neutropenia, lymphocytosis, eosinophilia, pancytopenia, hemolytic anemia (rare)***
INTEG: Rash, urticaria, dermatitis
RESP: Dyspnea
SYST: ***Anaphylaxis***

Contraindications: Hypersensitivity to cephalosporins, infants <1 mo

Precautions: Hypersensitivity to penicillins, pregnancy (B), lactation, renal disease

Pharmacokinetics:
IV: Peak 5 min
IM: Peak 30 min
Half-life 21-47 min; 44%-50% bound by plasma proteins; 40%-70% eliminated unchanged in urine; crosses placenta; excreted in breast milk; metabolized in liver

Interactions:
• Tetracyclines, aminoglycosides, aminophylline, epinephrine, lev-

arterenol, mannitol, phenytoin, thiopental
• Increased toxicity: aminoglycosides, furosemide, colistin, ethacrynic acid
Y-site compatibilities: Acyclovir, cyclophosphamide, famotidine, heparin, hydrocortisone sodium succinate, hydromorphone, magnesium sulfate, meperidine, morphine, multivitamins, perphenazine, potassium chloride, vitamin B complex with C
Additive compatibilities: Bleomycin, calcium chloride, calcium gluconate, chloramphenicol, diphenhydramine, ergonovine maleate, heparin, hydrocortisone sodium phosphate, hydrocortisone sodium succinate, metaraminol bitartrate, oxacillin, penicillin G potassium, pentobarbital, phenobarbital, phytonadione, potassium chloride, sodium bicarbonate, succinylcholine, verapamil, warfarin, vitamin B complex
Lab test interferences:
Increase (false:) Creatinine (serum urine), urinary 17-KS
False positive: Urinary protein, direct Coombs' test, urine glucose
Interference: Cross-matching

NURSING CONSIDERATIONS

Assess:
• Sensitivity to penicillin, other cephalosporins
• Nephrotoxicity: increased BUN, creatinine
• Blood studies: AST (SGOT), ALT (SGPT), CBC, Hct, bilirubin, LDH, alk phosphatase, Coombs' test monthly if patient is on long-term therapy
• Electrolytes: K, Na, Cl monthly if patient is on long-term therapy
• Bowel pattern qd; if severe diarrhea occurs, drug should be discontinued; may indicate pseudomembranous colitis
• IV site for extravasation, phlebitis; change site q72h
• Urine output: if decreasing, notify prescriber; may indicate nephrotoxicity
• Allergic reactions: rash, urticaria, pruritus, chills, fever, joint pain, angioedema; may occur few days after therapy begins
• Bleeding: ecchymosis, bleeding gums, hematuria, stool guaiac
• Overgrowth of infection: perineal itching, fever, malaise, redness, pain, swelling, drainage, rash, diarrhea, change in cough, sputum

Administer:
• IV after diluting 1 g or less/10 ml or more NS, D_5W, or bacteriostatic H_2O for inj; give 1 g or less/5 min or more; may be further diluted in 50-100 ml of D_5W, NS; run over 15 min; discontinue primary inf during administration; may also be given by continuous infusion
• For 10-14 days to ensure organism death, prevent superinfection
• After C&S

Evaluate:
• Therapeutic response: decreased symptoms of infection

Teach patient/family:
• If diabetic, check blood glucose level
• To report severe diarrhea; may indicate pseudomembranous colitis
• To report sore throat, bruising, bleeding, joint pain; may indicate blood dyscrasias (rare)

Treatment of anaphylaxis: Epinephrine, antihistamines; resuscitate if needed

cephradine (℞)

(sef'ra-deen)

cephradine, Velosef

Func. class.: Antibiotic

Chem. class.: Cephalosporin (1st generation)

Action: Inhibits bacterial cell wall synthesis, rendering cell wall osmotically unstable, leading to cell death

Uses: Gram-negative bacilli: *H. influenzae, E. coli, P. mirabilis, Klebsiella;* gram-positive organisms: *S. pneumoniae, S. pyogenes, S. aureus;* serious respiratory tract, urinary tract, skin infections, otitis media

Dosage and routes:

- *Adult:* IM/IV 500 mg-1 g q4-6h not to exceed 8 g/day; PO 250 mg-1 g q6-12h
- *Child >1 yr.:* IM/IV 12-25 mg/kg q6h; max 4 g/day PO 6-12 mg/kg q6h

Available forms: Powder for inj IM, IV 250, 500 mg, 1, 2 g; caps 250, 500 mg; oral susp 125, 250 mg/5 ml

Side effects/adverse reactions:

CNS: Headache, dizziness, weakness, paresthesia, fever, chills

GI: Nausea, vomiting, diarrhea, anorexia, pain, glossitis, bleeding, increased AST (SGOT), ALT (SGPT), bilirubin, LDH, alk phosphatase, abdominal pain, ***pseudomembranous colitis***

GU: Proteinuria, vaginitis, pruritus, candidiasis, increased BUN, ***nephrotoxicity, renal failure***

HEMA: ***Leukopenia, thrombocytopenia, agranulocytosis,*** anemia, ***neutropenia, lymphocytosis, eosinophilia, pancytopenia, hemolytic anemia (rare)***

INTEG: Rash, urticaria, dermatitis

RESP: Dyspnea

SYST: ***Anaphylaxis***

Contraindications: Hypersensitivity to cephalosporins, infants <1 mo

Precautions: Hypersensitivity to penicillins, pregnancy (B), lactation, renal disease

Pharmacokinetics:

PO: Peak 1 hr

IV: Peak 5 min

IM: Peak 1 hr

Half-life 0.75-1.5 h; 20% bound by plasma proteins; 80%-90% eliminated unchanged in urine; crosses placenta; excreted in breast milk

Interactions:

- Incompatible in sol with tetracyclines, erythromycins, calcium salts, magnesium salts, aminoglycosides, epinephrine, lidocaine, all antibiotics, Ringer's sol
- Increased toxicity: aminoglycosides, furosemide, colistin, ethacrynic acid, vancomycin

Lab test interferences:

Increase (false): Creatinine (serum urine), urinary 17-KS

False positive: Urinary protein, direct Coombs' test, urine glucose

Interference: Cross-matching

NURSING CONSIDERATIONS

Assess:

- Sensitivity to penicillin or other cephalosporins
- Nephrotoxicity: increased BUN, creatinine
- Blood studies: AST (SGOT), ALT (SGPT), CBC, Hct, bilirubin, LDH, alk phosphatase, Coombs' test monthly if patient is on long-term therapy
- Electrolytes: K, Na, Cl monthly if patient is on long-term therapy
- Bowel pattern qd; if severe diarrhea occurs, drug should be discontinued; may indicate pseudomembranous colitis
- IV site for extravasation, phlebitis; change site q72h

• Urine output: if decreasing, notify prescriber; may indicate nephrotoxicity
• Allergic reactions: rash, urticaria, pruritus, chills, fever, joint pain, angioedema; may occur few days after therapy begins
• Bleeding: ecchymosis, bleeding gums, hematuria, stool guaiac
• Overgrowth of infection: perineal itching, fever, malaise, redness, pain, swelling, drainage, rash, diarrhea, change in cough, sputum

Administer:
• IV after diluting 500 mg or less/5 ml or more sterile H_2O for inj; give over 3-5 min; may be further diluted 500 mg or less/10-20 ml D_5W, NS; give through Y-tube or 3-way stopcock, run over ½-1 hr
• For 10-14 days to ensure organism death, prevent superinfection
• With food if needed for GI symptoms
• After C&S

Evaluate:
• Therapeutic response: decreased symptoms of infection

Teach patient/family:
• If diabetic, check blood glucose level
• To use yogurt or buttermilk to maintain intestinal flora, decrease diarrhea
• To take all medication prescribed for length of time ordered
• To report sore throat, bruising, bleeding, joint pain; may indicate blood dyscrasias (rare)

Treatment of anaphylaxis: Epinephrine, antihistamines, resuscitate if needed

chenodiol (℞)

(kee-noe-dye'ole)
Chenix
Func. class.: Antilithic
Chem. class.: Chenodeoxycholic acid

Action: Suppresses synthesis of cholesterol, cholic acid, replacing cholic acid with drug metabolite, which leads to the degradation of gallstones

Uses: Dissolving gallstones instead of surgery; drug has no effect on radiopaque, calcified gallstones or bile pigment stones

Dosage and routes:
• *Adult:* PO 250 mg bid × 2 wk, then increased by 250 mg/day, not to exceed 16 mg/kg/day × 24 mo

Available forms: Tabs 250 mg

Side effects/adverse reactions:
HEMA: ***Leukopenia***
GI: Diarrhea, fecal urgency, heartburn, nausea, cramps, increased ALT, AST, LDH, vomiting, dysphagia, absence of taste, ***hepatotoxicity,*** flatulence, dyspepsia

Contraindications: Hypersensitivity, hepatic disease, bile duct obstruction, biliary GI fistula, pregnancy (X)

Precautions: Lactation, children, atherosclerosis, elderly

Pharmacokinetics: Metabolized by liver; excreted in feces (metabolite/unchanged drug); crosses placenta

Interactions:
• Decreased action of chenodiol: cholestyramine, colestipol, aluminum antacids, estrogens, clofibrate

NURSING CONSIDERATIONS

Assess:
• Vital signs, cardiac status: checking for dysrhythmias, increased rate, palpitations
• I&O ratio; check for urinary re-

tention or hesitancy, especially elderly
• Oral cholecystogram or ultrasonogram q6-9mo
• GI complaints: nausea, vomiting, anorexia, diarrhea; if diarrhea is severe, dosage may have to be decreased

Administer:
• With meals for better absorption
• Antidiarrheals if diarrhea occurs

Perform/provide:
• Storage at room temperature
• Increased fluids, bulk, exercise to patient's lifestyle to decrease constipation

Evaluate:
• Therapeutic response: absence of pain (epigastric), gallstones on diagnostic testing

Teach patient/family:
• That stone dissolution may take 6-24 mo; therapy is discontinued in 18 mo if gallstones are still intact
• To notify prescriber if pregnancy is suspected; birth defects may occur

chloral hydrate (℞)

(klor al hye'drate)
Aquachloral Supprettes, chloral hydrate, Noctec, Novochlorhydrate*
Func. class.: Sedative-hypnotic
Chem. class.: Chloral derivative

Controlled Substance Schedule IV (USA), Schedule F (Canada)

Action: Reduction product trichloroethanol produces mild cerebral depression, which causes sleep

Uses: Sedation, insomnia

Dosage and routes:

Sedation
• *Adult:* PO/REC 250 mg tid pc
• *Child:* PO 8 mg/kg tid, not to exceed 500 mg tid

Insomnia
• *Adult:* PO/REC 500 mg-1 g ½ hr before hs
• *Child:* PO/REC 50 mg/kg in one dose

Available forms: Caps 250, 500 mg; syr 250, 500 mg/5 ml; supp 325, 500, 650 mg

Side effects/adverse reactions:
HEMA: ***Eosinophilia, leukopenia***
CNS: Drowsiness, dizziness, stimulation, nightmares, ataxia, hangover (rare), light-headedness, headache, paranoia
GI: Nausea, vomiting, flatulence, diarrhea, unpleasant taste, ***gastric necrosis***
INTEG: Rash, urticaria, angioedema, fever, purpura, eczema
CV: Hypotension, dysrhythmias
RESP: ***Depression***

Contraindications: Hypersensitivity to this drug or triclofos, severe renal disease, severe hepatic disease, GI disorders (oral forms), gastritis

Precautions: Severe cardiac disease, depression, suicidal individuals, asthma, intermittent porphyria, pregnancy (C), lactation, elderly

Pharmacokinetics:
PO: Onset 30 min-1 hr, duration 4-8 hr
REC: Onset slow, duration 4-6 hr; metabolized by liver; excreted by kidneys (inactive metabolite) and feces; crosses placenta; excreted in breast milk; metabolite is highly protein bound

Interactions:
• Increased action: oral anticoagulants, furosemide
• Increased action of both drugs: alcohol, CNS depressants

Lab test interferences:
Interferences: Urine catecholamines, urinary 17-OHCS

False positive: Urine glucose (copper sulfate test)

NURSING CONSIDERATIONS

Assess:

• Blood studies: Hct, Hgb, RBCs, serum folate (if on long-term therapy), pro-time in patients receiving anticoagulants
• Mental status: mood, sensorium, affect, memory (long, short)
• Physical dependency: more frequent requests for medication, shakes, anxiety, pinpoint pupils
• Respiratory dysfunction: respiratory depression, character, rate, rhythm; hold drug if respirations <10/min or if pupils dilated (rare)
• Blood dyscrasias: fever, sore throat, bruising, rash, jaundice, epistaxis (rare)
• History of substance abuse, cardiac disease, gastritis

Administer:

• After removal of cigarettes, to prevent fires
• After trying conservative measures for insomnia
• ½-1 hr before hs for sleeplessness
• On empty stomach with full glass of water or juice for best absorption and to decrease corrosion (do not chew); after meals to decrease GI symptoms if using for sedation

Perform/provide:

• Assistance with ambulation after receiving dose, especially elderly
• Safety measure: side rails, nightlight, call bell within easy reach
• Checking to see PO medication swallowed
• Storage in dark container, suppositories in refrigerator

Evaluate:

• Therapeutic response: ability to sleep at night, decreased amount of early morning awakening if taking drug for insomnia

Teach patient/family:

• To avoid driving, other activities requiring alertness
• To avoid alcohol ingestion, CNS depressants; serious CNS depression may result
• Not to discontinue medication quickly after long-term use; drug should be tapered over 1-2 wk
• That effects may take 2 nights for benefits to be noticed
• Alternative measures to improve sleep (reading, exercise several hours before hs, warm bath, warm milk, TV, self-hypnosis, deep breathing)

Treatment of overdose: Lavage, activated charcoal; monitor electrolytes, vital signs

chlorambucil (℞)

(klor-am′byoo-sil)

Leukeran

Func. class.: Antineoplastic alkylating agent

Chem. class.: Nitrogen mustard

Action: Alkylates DNA, RNA; inhibits enzymes that allow synthesis of amino acids in proteins; activity is not cell cycle phase specific

Uses: Chronic lymphocytic leukemia, Hodgkin's disease, other lymphomas, macroglobulinemia, nephrotic syndrome, breast carcinoma, choreocarcinoma, ovarian carcinoma

Dosage and routes:

• *Adult:* PO 0.1-0.2 mg/kg/day for 3-6 wk initially, then 2-6 mg/day; maintenance 0.2 mg/kg for 2-4 wk; course may be repeated at 2-4 wk intervals
• *Child:* PO 0.1-0.2 mg/kg/day in divided doses or 4.5 mg/m^2/day as 1 dose or in divided doses

Available forms: Tabs 2 mg

Side effects/adverse reactions:

CNS: ***Convulsions in children***

* Available in Canada only

HEMA: ***Thrombocytopenia, leukopenia, pancytopenia*** (prolonged use), ***permanent bone marrow depression***
GI: Nausea, vomiting, diarrhea, weight loss, hepatoxicity, jaundice
GU: Hyperuremia
INTEG: Alopecia (rare), dermatitis, rash
RESP: ***Fibrosis, pneumonitis***
Contraindications: Radiation therapy within 1 mo, chemotherapy within 1 mo, thrombocytopenia, smallpox vaccination, pregnancy (1st trimester) (D), lactation
Precautions: ***Pneumococcus*** vaccination
Pharmacokinetics: Well absorbed orally; metabolized in liver; excreted in urine; half-life 2 hr
Interactions:
• Increased toxicity: other antineoplastics, radiation

NURSING CONSIDERATIONS
Assess:
• Bleeding: hematuria, guaiac, bruising or petechiae, mucosa or orifices q8h
• Food preferences; list likes, dislikes
• Yellowing of skin, sclera, dark urine, clay-colored stools, itchy skin, abdominal pain, fever, diarrhea
• Dyspnea, rales, unproductive cough, chest pain, tachypnea
• Effects of alopecia on body image; discuss feelings about body changes (rare)
• CBC, differential, platelet count weekly; withhold drug if WBC is <4000 or platelet count is <75,000; notify prescriber of results
• Pulmonary functions test, chest x-ray films before, during therapy; chest film should be obtained q2wk during treatment
• Renal function studies: BUN, serum uric acid, urine CrCl before, during therapy
• I&O ratio; report fall in urine output of <30 ml/hr
• Monitor temperature q4h (may indicate beginning infection)
• Liver function tests before, during therapy (bilirubin, AST, ALT, LDH) as needed or monthly
Administer:
• Antacid before oral agent; give drug 2 hr after evening meal, before bedtime
• Antiemetic 30-60 min before giving drug to prevent vomiting
• Allopurinol or sodium bicarbonate to maintain uric acid levels, alkalinization of urine
• Antibiotics for prophylaxis of infection
Perform/provide:
• Storage in tight container
• Strict medical asepsis, protective isolation if WBC levels are low
• Increase fluid intake to 2-3 L/day to prevent urate deposits, calculi formation
• Diet low in purines: organ meats (kidney, liver), dried beans, peas to maintain alkaline urine
Evaluate:
• Therapeutic response: decreased size of tumor, spread of malignancy
Teach patient/family:
• To report signs of infection: increased temperature, sore throat, flu symptoms
• To report signs of anemia: fatigue, headache, faintness, shortness of breath, irritability
• To report bleeding; avoid use of razors, commercial mouthwash
• To avoid use of aspirin products, ibuprofen
• About protective isolation precautions
• To report any changes in breathing or coughing
• That hair may be lost during treatment; a wig or hairpiece may make

patient feel better; new hair may be different in color, texture (rare)

chloramphenicol/chloramphenicol palmitate/chloramphenicol sodium succinate (℞)

(klor-am-fen′i-kole)

chloramphenicol, chloramphenicol sodium succinate, Chloromycetin Kapseals, Chloromycetin Sodium Succinate, Chloromycetin Palmitate, Novochlorocap*

Func. class.: Antibacterial/antirickettsial

Chem. class.: Dichloroacetic acid derivative

Action: Binds to 50S ribosomal subunit, which interferes with or inhibits protein synthesis

Uses: Infections caused by *H. influenzae, S. typhi, Rickettsia, Neisseria,* mycoplasma

Dosage and routes:

• *Adult and child:* PO/IV 50-75 mg/kg/day in divided doses q6h, 100 mg/kg/day (for meningitis only)

• *Premature infants and neonates:* IV/PO 25 mg/kg/day in divided doses q6h

Available forms: Inj (IV) 1 g; caps 250, 500 mg; oral susp 150 mg/5 ml

Side effects/adverse reactions:

HEMA: ***Anemia, thrombocytopenia, aplastic anemia, granulocytopenia, leukopenia*** (rare)

EENT: Optic neuritis, blindness

GI: Nausea, vomiting, diarrhea, abdominal pain, xerostomia, glossitis, colitis, pruritus ani

INTEG: Itching, urticaria, contact dermatitis, rash

CV: ***Gray syndrome in newborns: failure to feed, pallor, cyanosis, abdominal distention, irregular respiration, vasomotor collapse***

CNS: Headache, *depression,* confusion

Contraindications: Hypersensitivity, severe renal disease, severe hepatic disease, minor infections

Precautions: Hepatic disease, renal disease, infants, children, bone marrow depression (drug-induced), pregnancy (C), lactation

Pharmacokinetics:

PO/IV: Peak 1-2 hr, duration 8 hr, half-life 1½-4 hr; conjugated in liver; excreted in urine (up to 15% as free drug), breast milk, feces; crosses placenta

Interactions:

• Increased action of phenytoin, tolbutamide, chlorpropamide, phenobarbital

• Increased prothrombin time: anticoagulants

• Decreased action of iron, Vit B_{12}, folic acid, penicillins

• Avoid use with myelosuppressive drugs

Y-site compatibilities: Acyclovir, cyclophosphamide, enalaprilat, esmolol, foscarnet, hydromorphone, labetalol, magnesium sulfate, meperidine, morphine, perphenazine

Syringe compatibility: Heparin

NURSING CONSIDERATIONS

Assess:

• Signs of infection, anemia

• Any patient with compromised renal system; drug is excreted slowly in poor renal system function; toxicity may occur rapidly

• Liver studies: AST (SGOT), ALT (SGPT)

• Blood studies: WBC, RBC, Hct, Hgb, platelets, serum iron, reticulocytes; drug should be discontinued if bone marrow is depressed

• Renal studies: urinalysis, protein, blood, BUN, creatinine

• C&S before drug therapy; may be given as soon as culture is taken

* Available in Canada only

• Drug level in impaired hepatic, renal systems
• Bowel pattern before, during treatment
• Skin eruptions, itching, dermatitis after administration
• Respiratory status: rate, character, wheezing, tightness in chest
• Allergies before treatment, reaction of each medication; place allergies on chart, bright red letters; notify all people giving drugs
• Neonates for beginning Gray syndrome: cyanosis, abdominal distention, irregular respiration, failure to feed; drug should be discontinued immediately

Administer:
• IV after diluting 1 g/10 ml of sterile H_2O for inj or D_5W (10% sol); give over >1 min; may be further diluted in 50-100 ml of D_5W; give through Y-tube, 3-way stopcock, or additive inf set; run over ½-1 hr
• Oral form on empty stomach with full glass of water
• IM route not recommended

Perform/provide:
• Storage of capsules in tight container at room temperature, reconstituted sol at room temp 30 days
• Adrenalin, suction, tracheostomy set, endotracheal intubation equipment on unit
• Adequate intake of fluids (2 L) during diarrhea episodes

Evaluate:
• Therapeutic response: decreased symptoms of infection

Teach patient/family:
• Aspects of drug therapy: need to complete entire course to ensure organism death (10-14 days); culture may be taken after complete course of medication
• To report sore throat, fever, fatigue, unusual bleeding, bruising; could indicate bone marrow depression (may occur weeks or months after termination of drug)
• That drug must be taken in equal intervals around clock to maintain blood levels

Treatment of hypersensitivity: Withdraw drug, maintain airway, administer epinephrine, aminophylline, O_2, IV corticosteroids

chloramphenicol (ophthalmic) (℞)

(klor-am-fen′i-kole)

AK-Chlor, Chloramphenicol, Chloramphenicol Ophthalmic, Chloromycetin Ophthalmic, Chloroptic, Chloroptic S.O.P., Fenicol*, Isopto Fenical*, Pentamycin*

Func. class.: Antiinfective

Action: Inhibits bacterial protein synthesis

Uses: Infection of eye

Dosage and routes:
• *Adult and child:* INSTILL 2 gtt in eye qd-qid until desired response; TOP apply oint to conjunctival sac q3-6h as needed or hs if using gtt also

Available forms: Oint 1%; sol 0.25, 0.5%, 25 mg; pwd for sol 25 mg/vial

Side effects/adverse reactions:
EENT: Poor corneal wound healing, temporary visual haze, overgrowth of nonsusceptible organisms

Contraindications: Hypersensitivity

Precautions: Antibiotic hypersensitivity, pregnancy (C)

NURSING CONSIDERATIONS

Assess:
• Allergy: itching, lacrimation, redness, swelling

Administer:
• After washing hands, cleanse

crusts or discharge from eye before application
• Apply pressure to lacrimal sac for 1 min to prevent systemic absorption

Perform/provide:
• Storage at room temperature; protect from light

Evaluate:
• Therapeutic response: absence of redness, inflammation, tearing

Teach patient/family:
• To use drug exactly as prescribed
• Not to use eye makeup, towels, washcloths, eye medication of others; reinfection may occur
• That drug container tip should not touch eye
• To report itching, increased redness, burning, stinging, swelling; drug should be discontinued
• That drug may cause blurred vision when ointment is applied
• That prolonged or frequent use may lead to serious reactions: hypersensitivity, bone marrow depression

chloramphenicol (otic) (℞)

(klor-am-fen'i-kole)
Chloromycetin Otic, Sopamycetin*
Func. class.: Broad-spectrum otic antibiotic
Chem. class: Antibacterial

Action: Inhibits protein synthesis in susceptible gram-positive, gram-negative microorganisms
Uses: Ear infection (external)
Dosage and routes:
• *Adult and child:* INSTILL 2-3 gtts tid
Available forms: Sol 0.5%
Side effects/adverse reactions:
EENT: Itching, irritation in ear
INTEG: Rash, urticaria, contact dermatitis, burning, ***angioedema***
HEMA: ***Bone marrow hypoplasia, aplastic anemia***
Contraindications: Hypersensitivity, perforated eardrum
Precautions: Inner ear infections

NURSING CONSIDERATIONS

Assess:
• For redness, swelling, pain in ear, which indicates superinfection

Administer:
• After removing impacted cerumen by irrigation
• After cleaning stopper with alcohol
• After restraining child if necessary
• Warming solution to body temp; do not warm above body temp; loss of potency will occur

Perform/provide:
• Storage at room temperature, protection from light

Evaluate:
• Therapeutic response: decreased ear pain

Teach patient/family:
• Method of instillation, using aseptic technique, including not touching dropper to ear; by demonstration, return demonstration
• That dizziness may occur after instillation

chloramphenicol (topical) (℞)

(klor-am-fen'i-kole)
Chloromycetin
Func. class.: Local antiinfective
Chem. class.: Antibacterial

Action: Interferes with bacterial protein synthesis
Uses: Skin infections (bacterial)
Dosage and routes:
• *Adult and child:* TOP apply to affected area bid-qid

* Available in Canada only

Available forms: Cream 1%
Side effects/adverse reactions:
HEMA: ***Blood dyscrasias***
INTEG: Rash, urticaria, stinging, burning, vesicular, maculopapular dermatitis, ***angioedema***
Contraindications: Hypersensitivity
Precautions: Pregnancy (C), lactation

NURSING CONSIDERATIONS
Assess:
- Allergic reaction: burning, stinging, swelling, redness
- Signs and symptoms of blood dyscrasias

Administer:
- Enough medication to cover lesions completely
- After cleansing with soap, water before each application; dry well

Perform/provide:
- Storage at room temperature in dry place; protect from light

Evaluate:
- Therapeutic response: decrease in size, number of lesions

Teach patient/family:
- To use medical asepsis (hand washing) before, after each application to prevent further infection
- To apply with glove to prevent further infection
- To avoid use of OTC creams, ointments, lotions unless directed by prescriber
- To notify prescriber if conditions worsen or of rash or irritation
- To watch for superinfections with diarrhea

chlordiazepoxide (℞)

(klor-dye-az-e-pox′ide)
Apo-Chlordiazepoxide*, chlordiazepoxide HCl, Libritabs, Librium, Medilium*, Mitran, Novopoxide*, Resposans-10, Solium*, Sereen
Func. class.: Antianxiety
Chem. class.: Benzodiazepine

Combination products: Clindex, Clinoxide, Clipoxide, Librax, Lidox: chlordiazepoxide HCl 5 mg with clidinium bromide 2.5 mg; Librax: chlordiazepoxide HCl 5 mg, clidinium bromide 2.5 mg; Limbitrol 5-12.5: chlordiazepoxide 5 mg, amitriptyline HCl 12.5 mg; Limbitrol 10-25: chlordiazepoxide 10 mg, amitriptyline HCl 25 mg; Menrium 5-2: chlordiazepoxide 5 mg with esterified estrogens 0.2 mg; Menrium 5-4: chlordiazepoxide 5 mg with esterified estrogens 0.4 mg; Menrium 10-4: chlordiazepoxide 10 mg with esterified estrogens 0.4 mg

Controlled Substance Schedule IV
Action: Potentiates the actions of GABA, especially in the limbic system, reticular formation
Uses: Short-term management of anxiety, acute alcohol withdrawal, preoperatively for relaxation
Dosage and routes:
Mild anxiety
- *Adult:* PO 5-10 mg tid-qid
- *Child >6 yr:* 5 mg bid-qid, not to exceed 10 mg bid-tid

Severe anxiety
- *Adult:* PO 20-25 mg tid-qid

Preoperatively
- *Adult:* PO 5-10 mg tid-qid on day before surgery; IM 50-100 mg 1 hr before surgery

Alcohol withdrawal
- *Adult:* PO/IM/IV 50-100 mg, not to exceed 300 mg/day

Available forms: Caps 5, 10, 25 mg; tabs 5, 10, 25 mg; powder for IM inj 100 mg ampule

Side effects/adverse reactions:

CNS: Dizziness, drowsiness, confusion, headache, anxiety, tremors, stimulation, fatigue, depression, insomnia, hallucinations

GI: Constipation, dry mouth, nausea, vomiting, anorexia, diarrhea

INTEG: Rash, dermatitis, itching

CV: Orthostatic hypotension, ***ECG changes, tachycardia,*** hypotension

EENT: Blurred vision, tinnitus, mydriasis

Contraindications: Hypersensitivity to benzodiazepines, narrow-angle glaucoma, psychosis, pregnancy (D), lactation, child <18 yr

Precautions: Elderly, debilitated, hepatic disease, renal disease

Pharmacokinetics:

PO: Onset 30 min, peak ½ hr, duration 4-6 hr; metabolized by liver, excreted by kidneys; crosses placenta, excreted in breast milk; half-life 5-30 hr

Interactions:

• Decreased effects of chlordiazepoxide: oral contraceptives, rifampin, valproic acid

• Increased effects of chlordiazepoxide: CNS depressants, alcohol, cimetidine, disulfiram, oral contraceptives

Syringe incompatibility: Benzquinamide

Y-site compatibilities: Heparin, hydrocortisone sodium succinate, potassium chloride, Vitamin B with C

Solution compatibilities: D_5W, Ringer's, 0.9% NaCl

Lab test interferences:

Increase: AST/ALT, serum bilirubin

False increase: 17-OHCS

Decrease: RAIU

NURSING CONSIDERATIONS

Assess:

• B/P (lying, standing), pulse; if systolic B/P drops 20 mm Hg, hold drug, notify prescriber

• Blood studies: CBC during long-term therapy; blood dyscrasias have occurred rarely

• Hepatic studies: AST (SGOT), ALT (SGPT), bilirubin, creatinine, LDH, alk phosphatase

• I&O; may indicate renal dysfunction

• For ataxia, oversedation in elderly, debilitated patients

• Mental status: mood, sensorium, affect, sleeping pattern, drowsiness, dizziness

• Physical dependency, withdrawal symptoms: headache, nausea, vomiting, muscle pain, weakness after long-term use

• Suicidal tendencies, paradoxic reactions such as excitement, stimulation, acute rage

Administer:

• By IV 5 ml NS/100 mg powder; agitate ampule gently; give through Y-tube or 3-way stopcock; give 100 mg or less over ≥1 min; do not use IM diluent for IV use

• With food or milk for GI symptoms

• Crushed if patient is unable to swallow medication whole

• Sugarless gum, hard candy, frequent sips of water for dry mouth

Perform/provide:

• Assistance with ambulation during beginning therapy, since drowsiness/dizziness occurs

• Safety measures, including side rails

• Check to see PO medication has been swallowed

Evaluate:

• Therapeutic response: decreased anxiety, restlessness, sleeplessness

* Available in Canada only

Teach patient/family:
• That drug may be taken with food
• Not to be used for everyday stress or used longer than 4 mo, unless directed by prescriber
• Not to take more than prescribed amount; may be habit-forming
• To avoid OTC preparations unless approved by prescriber
• To avoid driving, activities that require alertness; drowsiness may occur
• To avoid alcohol ingestion, other psychotropic medications, unless directed by prescriber
• Not to discontinue medication abruptly after long-term use; may precipitate convulsions
• To rise slowly or fainting may occur, especially elderly
• That drowsiness may worsen at beginning of treatment

Treatment of overdose: Lavage, VS, supportive care, give flumazenil

chloroprocaine (℞)

(klor′-oh-pro-kane)
Nesacaine, Nesacaine MPF
Func. class.: Local anesthetic
Chem. class.: Ester

Action: Competes with calcium for sites in nerve membrane that control sodium transport across cell membrane; decreases rise of depolarization phase of action potential
Uses: Epidural anesthesia, peripheral nerve block, caudal anesthesia, infiltration block
Dosage and routes:
Varies by route of anesthesia
Available forms: Inj 1%, 2%, 3%
Side effects/adverse reactions:
CNS: Anxiety, restlessness, ***convulsions, loss of consciousness,*** drowsiness, disorientation, tremors, shivering
CV: ***Myocardial depression, cardiac arrest, dysrhythmias,*** bradycardia, hypotension, hypertension, fetal bradycardia
GI: Nausea, vomiting
EENT: Blurred vision, tinnitus, pupil constriction
INTEG: Rash, urticaria, allergic reactions, edema, burning, skin discoloration at injection site, tissue necrosis
RESP: ***Status asthmaticus, respiratory arrest, anaphylaxis***
Contraindications: Hypersensitivity, child <12 yr, elderly, severe liver disease
Precautions: Elderly, severe drug allergies, pregnancy (C), lactation
Pharmacokinetics: Duration ½-1 hr; metabolized by liver; excreted in urine (metabolites)
Interactions:
• Dysrhythmias: epinephrine, halothane, enflurane
• Hypertension: MAOIs, tricyclic antidepressants, phenothiazines

NURSING CONSIDERATIONS
Assess:
• B/P, pulse, respiration during treatment
• Fetal heart tones if used during labor
• Allergic reactions: rash, urticaria, itching
• Cardiac status: ECG for dysrhythmias, pulse, B/P during anesthesia
Administer:
• Only with crash cart, resuscitative equipment nearby
• Only drugs without preservatives for epidural or caudal anesthesia
Perform/provide:
• Use of new solution; discard unused portions
Evaluate:
• Therapeutic response: anesthesia necessary for procedure

Treatment of overdose: Airway, O_2, vasopressor, IV fluids, anticonvulsants for seizures

chloroquine (℞)

(klor'oh-kwin)

Aralen HCl, Aralen Phosphate, chloroquine phosphate, Novo-chloroquine*

Func. class.: Antimalarial

Chem. class.: Synthetic 4-aminoquinoline derivative

Action: Inhibits parasite replications, transcription of DNA to RNA by forming complexes with DNA of parasite

Uses: Malaria of *Plasmodium vivax, P. malariae, P. ovale, P. falciparum* (some strains), amebiasis

Dosage and routes:

Malaria suppression

• *Adult and child:* PO 5 mg/kg/wk on same day of week, not to exceed 500 mg; treatment should begin 1-2 wk before exposure and for 8 wk after; if treatment begins after exposure, 600 mg for adult and 10 mg/kg for children in 2 divided doses 6 hr apart

Extraintestinal amebiasis

• *Adult:* IM 200-250 mg qd (HCl) up to 12 days, then 1 g (phosphate) qd × 2 days, then 500 mg qd × 2-3 wk

• *Child:* IM/PO 10 mg/kg qd (HCl) × 2-3 wk, not to exceed 300 mg/day

Available forms: Tabs 250, 500 mg; inj IM 50 mg/ml

Side effects/adverse reactions:

CV: Hypotension, heart block, asystole with syncope, ECG changes

INTEG: Pruritus, pigmentary changes, skin eruptions, lichen planus-like eruptions, eczema, ***exfoliative dermatitis***

CNS: Headache, stimulation, fatigue, ***convulsion,*** psychosis

EENT: Blurred vision, corneal changes, retinal changes, difficulty focusing, tinnitus, vertigo, deafness, photophobia, corneal edema

GI: Nausea, vomiting, anorexia, diarrhea, cramps

HEMA: ***Thrombocytopenia, agranulocytosis, hemolytic anemia, leukopenia***

Contraindications: Hypersensitivity, retinal field changes, porphyria

Precautions: Pregnancy (C), children, blood dyscrasias, severe GI disease, neurologic disease, alcoholism, hepatic disease, G6PD deficiency, psoriasis, eczema, lactation, porphyria

Pharmacokinetics:

PO: Peak 1-6 hr, half-life 3-5 days; metabolized in the liver; excreted in urine, feces, breast milk; crosses placenta

Interactions:

• Decreased action of chloroquine: magnesium aluminum compounds, kaolin

• Reduced oral clearance and metabolism of chloroquine: cimetidine

NURSING CONSIDERATIONS

Assess:

• Ophthalmic test if long-term treatment or dosage >150 mg/day

• Liver studies qwk: AST (SGOT), ALT (SGPT), bilirubin

• Blood studies: CBC, since blood dyscrasias occur

• ECG during therapy

• Watch for depression of T waves, widening of QRS complex

• Allergic reactions: pruritus, rash, urticaria

• Blood dyscrasias: malaise, fever, bruising, bleeding (rare)

• For ototoxicity (tinnitus, vertigo, change in hearing); audiometric testing should be done before, after treatment

• For toxicity: blurring vision; difficulty focusing; headache; dizzi-

* Available in Canada only

ness; decreased knee, ankle reflexes; drug should be discontinued immediately

Administer:

• Before or after meals at same time each day to maintain drug level

• IM after aspirating to avoid injection into blood system, which may cause hypotension, asystole, heart block; rotate injection sites

Perform/provide:

• Storage in tight, light-resistant container at room temp; keep injection in cool environment

Evaluate:

• Therapeutic response: decreased symptoms of infection

Teach patient/family:

• To use sunglasses in bright sunlight to decrease photophobia

• That urine may turn rust or brown color

• To report hearing, visual problems, fever, fatigue, bruising, bleeding, which may indicate blood dyscrasias

Treatment of overdose: Induce vomiting, gastric lavage, administer barbiturate (ultrashort-acting), vasopressin; tracheostomy may be necessary

chlorothiazide (℞)

(klor-oh-thye'a-zide)

Diachlor, Diuril, Diuril Sodium

Func. class.: Diuretic

Chem. class.: Thiazide; sulfonamide derivative

Combination products: Diupres-250: chlorothiazide 250 mg, reserpine 0.125 mg; Diupres-500: chlorothiazide 500 mg, reserpine 0.125 mg

Action: Acts on distal tubule by increasing excretion of water, sodium, chloride, potassium, magnesium

Uses: Edema, hypertension, diuresis

Dosage and routes:

Edema, hypertension

• *Adult:* PO/IV 500 mg-2 g qd in 2 divided doses

Diuresis

• *Child >6 mo:* PO 20 mg/kg/day in 2 divided doses

Available forms: Tabs 250, 500 mg; oral susp 250 mg/5 ml; inj 500 mg

Side effects/adverse reactions:

CNS: Drowsiness, paresthesia, anxiety, depression, headache, *dizziness, fatigue, weakness*

CV: Irregular pulse, orthostatic hypotension, palpitations, volume depletion

EENT: Blurred vision

ELECT: *Hypokalemia,* hypercalcemia, hyponatremia, hypochloremia, hypophosphatemia, hypomagnesemia

GI: *Nausea, vomiting, anorexia,* constipation, diarrhea, cramps, pancreatitis, GI irritation, ***hepatitis***

GU: *Frequency,* polyuria, ***uremia,*** glucosuria

HEMA: ***Aplastic anemia, hemolytic anemia, leukopenia, agranulocytosis, thrombocytopenia, neutropenia***

INTEG: *Rash,* urticaria, purpura, photosensitivity, fever

META: Hyperglycemia, *hyperuricemia,* hypomagnesemia, increased creatinine, BUN

Contraindications: Hypersensitivity to thiazides or sulfonamides, anuria, renal decompensation, pregnancy (D), lactation

Precautions: Hypokalemia, renal disease, hepatic disease, gout, COPD, lupus erythematosus, diabetes mellitus, elderly

Pharmacokinetics: Not well absorbed PO

PO: Onset 2 hr, peak 4 hr, duration 6-12 hr; crosses placenta, excreted in breast milk, excreted unchanged by the kidneys; half-life 2 hr

Interactions:

• Increased toxicity: lithium, nondepolarizing skeletal muscle relaxants, digitalis
• Increased hypotension: other antihypertensives, alcohol
• Decreased effects of: antidiabetics, sulfonylureas
• Decreased absorption of thiazides: cholestyramine, colestipol
• Decreased hypotensive response: indomethacin
• Hypokalemia: ticarcillin, glucocorticoids, amphotericin, mezlocillin, piperacillin
• Hyperglycemia, hyperuricemia, hypotension: diazoxide

Additive compatibilities: Cimetidine, lidocaine, nafcillin, sodium bicarbonate

Lab test interferences:

False negative: Phentolamine and tyramine tests
Interference: Urine steroid tests
Increase: BSP retention, Ca, amylase, parathyroid test
Decrease: PBI, PSP

NURSING CONSIDERATIONS

Assess:

• Weight, I&O daily to determine fluid loss; effect of drug may be decreased if used qd
• Rate, depth, rhythm of respirations; effect of exertion
• B/P lying, standing; postural hypotension may occur, especially in elderly
• Electrolytes: K, Na, Cl; include BUN, blood glucose, CBC, serum creatinine, blood pH, ABGs, uric acid, Ca, Mg
• Glucose in urine if patient is diabetic
• Improvement in CVP q8h
• Signs of metabolic alkalosis: drowsiness, restlessness
• Rashes, temperature elevation qd
• Confusion, especially in elderly; take safety precautions if needed

Administer:

• IV after diluting 0.5 g/18 ml or more of sterile water for inj; may be diluted further with Ringer's, LR, 0.45% NaCl, 0.9% NaCl, D_5W, $D_{10}W$, check for extravasation; give over 5 min (0.5 g/5 m)
• In AM to avoid interference with sleep if using drug as a diuretic
• K replacement if K less than 3 mg/dl
• With food if nausea occurs; absorption may be decreased slightly; tablets may be crushed
• After shaking suspension

Evaluate:

• Therapeutic response: improvement in edema of feet, legs, sacral area daily if medication is being used for CHF

Teach patient/family:

• To rise slowly from lying or sitting position; orthostatic hypotension may occur
• To notify prescriber of muscle weakness, cramps, nausea, dizziness
• That drug may be taken with food or milk; to take at same time each day; not to double dose; dehydration may occur
• That blood sugar may be increased in diabetics
• To take early in day to avoid nocturia
• To use sunscreen (not with PABA); use protective clothing to prevent photosensitivity
• To weigh weekly and notify prescriber of change of >3 lb
• To eat diet high in K
• Not to take OTC medications without consulting prescriber

Treatment of overdose: Lavage if taken orally; monitor electrolytes; administer dextrose in saline; monitor hydration, CV, renal status

chlorpheniramine (OTC, ℞)

(klor-fen-eer'a-meen)

Aller-Chlor, Chlo-Amine, Chlor-Pro, Chlorate, chlorpheniramine maleate, Chlor-Pro 10, Chlorspan 12, Chlortab-B, Chlortab-4, ChlorTrimeton, Chlor-Trimeton Repetabs, Pedia Care Allergy Formula, Pfeiffer's Allergy, Phenetron, Telachlor, Teldrin, Trimegen

Func. class.: Antihistamine

Chem. class.: Alkylamine, H_1-receptor antagonist

Action: Acts on blood vessels, GI system, respiratory system, by competing with histamine for H_1-receptor site; decreases allergic response by blocking histamine

Uses: Allergy symptoms, rhinitis

Dosage and routes:

• *Adult:* PO 2-4 mg tid-qid, not to exceed 36 mg/day; TIME-REL 8-12 mg bid-tid, not to exceed 36 mg/day; IM/IV/SC 5-40 mg/day

• *Child 6-12 yr:* PO 2 mg q4-6h, not to exceed 12 mg/day; SUS REL 8 mg hs or qd, SUS REL not recommended for child <6 yr

• *Child 2-5 yr:* PO 1 mg q4-6h, not to exceed 4 mg/day

Available forms: Tabs, chewable 2 mg; tabs 4, 8, 12 mg; tabs, time-rel 8, 12 mg; caps, time-rel 8, 12 mg; syr 2 mg/5 ml; inj IM, SC, IV 10, 100 mg/ml

Side effects/adverse reactions:

CNS: *Dizziness, drowsiness,* poor coordination, fatigue, anxiety, euphoria, confusion, paresthesia, neuritis

RESP: Increased thick secretions, wheezing, chest tightness

HEMA: ***Thrombocytopenia, agranulocytosis, hemolytic anemia***

GI: Dry mouth, nausea, anorexia, diarrhea

INTEG: Photosensitivity

GU: *Retention,* dysuria, frequency

EENT: Blurred vision, dilated pupils, tinnitus, nasal stuffiness, dry nose, throat, mouth

Contraindications: Hypersensitivity to H_1-receptor antagonists, acute asthma attack, lower respiratory tract disease

Precautions: Increased intraocular pressure, renal disease, cardiac disease, hypertension, bronchial asthma, seizure disorder, stenosed peptic ulcers, hyperthyroidism, prostatic hypertrophy, bladder neck obstruction, pregnancy (B), lactation, elderly

Pharmacokinetics:

PO: Onset 20-60 min, duration 8-12 hr; detoxified in liver; excreted by kidneys; (metabolites/free drug); half-life 20-24 hr

Interactions:

• Increased CNS depression: barbiturates, narcotics, hypnotics, tricyclic antidepressants, alcohol

• Decreased effect of oral anticoagulants, heparin

• Increased effect of chlorpheniramine: MAOIs

Additive compatibility: Amikacin

Lab test interferences:

False negative: Skin allergy tests

NURSING CONSIDERATIONS

Assess:

• I&O ratio; be alert for urinary retention, frequency, dysuria; drug should be discontinued

• CBC during long-term therapy

• Blood dyscrasias: thrombocytopenia, agranulocytosis (rare)

• Respiratory status: rate, rhythm, increase in bronchial secretions, wheezing, chest tightness

Administer:

• IV undiluted at ≥10 mg/1 min

• With meals for GI symptoms; absorption may slightly decrease

Perform/provide:

• Hard candy, gum, frequent rinsing of mouth for dryness

• Storage in tight container at room temp

Evaluate:

• Therapeutic response: absence of running, congested nose, rashes

Teach patient/family:

• Not to chew or crush sustained-release forms

• All aspects of drug use; to notify prescriber of confusion/sedation/hypotension

• That this drug decreases anticoagulant (oral) effect

• To avoid driving, other hazardous activity if drowsiness occurs, especially elderly

• To avoid concurrent use of alcohol, other CNS depressants

Treatment of overdose: Administer ipecac syrup or lavage, diazepam, vasopressors, barbiturates (short-acting)

chlorpromazine (℞)

(klor-proe′ma-zeen)

chlorpromazine HCl, Chlorpromanyl*, Largactil*, Novo-Chlorpromazine*, Ormazine, Thor-prom, Thorazine, Thorazine Spansules

Func. class.: Antipsychotic/neuroleptic

Chem. class.: Phenothiazine-aliphatic

Action: Depresses cerebral cortex, hypothalamus, limbic system, which control activity aggression; blocks neurotransmission produced by dopamine at synapse; exhibits a strong α-adrenergic, anticholinergic blocking action; mechanism for antipsychotic effects is unclear

Uses: Psychotic disorders, mania, schizophrenia, anxiety, intractable hiccups, nausea, vomiting; preoperatively for relaxation; acute intermittent porphyria, behavioral problems in children

Dosage and routes:

Psychiatry

• *Adult:* PO 10-50 mg q1-4h initially, then increase up to 2 g/day if necessary

• *Adult:* IM 10-50 mg q1-4h

• *Child:* PO 0.25 mg/lb q4-6h or 0.5 mg/kg

• *Child:* IM 0.25 mg/lb q6-8h or 0.5 mg/kg

• *Child:* REC 0.5 mg/lb q6-8h or 1 mg/kg

Nausea and vomiting

• *Adult:* PO 10-25 mg q4-6h prn; IM 25-50 mg q3h prn; REC 50-100 mg q6-8h prn, not to exceed 400 mg/day

• *Child:* PO 0.25 mg/lb q4-6h prn, IM 0.25 mg/lb q6-8h prn not to exceed 40 mg/day (<5 yr) or 75 mg/day (5-12 yr); REC 0.5 mg/lb: q6-8h prn

• *Adult:* IV 25-50 mg qd-qid

• *Child:* IV 0.55 mg/kg q6-8h

Intractable hiccups

• *Adult:* PO 25-50 mg tid-qid; IM 25-50 mg (only if PO dose does not work); IV 25-50 mg in 500-1000 ml NS (only for severe hiccups)

Available forms: Tabs 10, 25, 50, 100, 200 mg; time-rel caps 30, 75, 150, 200, 300 mg; syr 10 mg/5ml; conc 30, 100 mg/ml; supp 25, 100 mg; inj IM, IV 25 mg/ml

Side effects/adverse reactions:

CV: Orthostatic hypotension, hy-

* Available in Canada only

pertension, ***cardiac arrest,*** ECG changes, ***tachycardia***
EENT: Blurred vision, glaucoma, dry eyes
GI: Dry mouth, nausea, vomiting, anorexia, constipation, diarrhea, jaundice, weight gain
GU: Urinary retention, urinary frequency, enuresis, impotence, amenorrhea, gynecomastia, breast engorgement
HEMA: Anemia, ***leukopenia, leukocytosis, agranulocytosis***
INTEG: Rash, photosensitivity, dermatitis
RESP: ***Laryngospasm,*** dyspnea, ***respiratory depression***
CNS: EPS: pseudoparkinsonism, akathisia, dystonia, tardive dyskinesia, seizures, *headache,* ***neuroleptic malignant syndrome*** *(rare)*
Contraindications: Hypersensitivity, circulatory collapse, liver damage, cerebral arteriosclerosis, coronary disease, severe hypertension/hypotension, blood dyscrasias, coma, child <2 years, brain damage, bone marrow depression, alcohol and barbiturate withdrawal
Precautions: Pregnancy (C), lactation, seizure disorders, hypertension, hepatic disease, cardiac disease, elderly
Pharmacokinetics:
PO: Absorption variable, widely distributed; onset erratic 30-60 min, duration 4-6 hr
IM: Well absorbed; peak 15-20 min, duration 4 to 8 hr
IV: Onset 5 min, peak 10 min, duration unknown
PO-ER: Onset 30-60 min, peak unknown, duration 10-12 hr
REC: Onset erratic, duration 3 hr; metabolized by liver, excreted in urine (metabolites), crosses placenta, enters breast milk; 95% bound to plasma proteins; elimination half-life 10-30 hr

Interactions:
- Oversedation: other CNS depressants, alcohol, barbiturate anesthetics, antihistamines, sedatives /hypnotics, antidepressants
- Toxicity: epinephrine
- Decreased absorption: aluminum hydroxide, magnesium hydroxide antacids
- Decreased antiparkinson activity: levodopa, bromocriptine
- Decreased serum chlorpromazine: lithium
- Increased effects of both drugs: β-adrenergic blockers, alcohol
- Increased anticholinergic effects: anticholinergics
- Agranulocystosis: antithyroid agents

Syringe compatibilities: Atropine, butorphanol, diphenhydramine, doxapram, droperidol, fentanyl, glycopyrrolate, hydromorphone, hydroxyzine, meperidine, metoclopramide, midazolam, morphine, pentozocine, perphenazine, prochlorperazine, promazine, promethazine, scopolamine
Y-site compatibilities: Heparin, hydrocortisone sodium succinate, ondansetron, potassium chloride methohexital, penicillin G, phenobarbital
Additive compatibilities: Ascorbic acid, ethacrynate, netilmicin
Lab test interferences:
Increase: Liver function tests, cardiac enzymes, cholesterol, blood glucose, prolactin, bilirubin, PBI, cholinesterase, ^{131}I, alk phosphatase, leukocytes, granulocytes, platelets
Decrease: Hormones (blood and urine)
False positive: Pregnancy tests, PKU
False negative: Urinary steroids, 17-OHCS

NURSING CONSIDERATIONS

Assess:
- Mental status: orientation, mood, behavior, presence of hallucinations

and type before initial administration and monthly
• Swallowing of PO medication; check for hoarding or giving of medication to other patients
• I&O ratio; palpate bladder if low urinary output occurs, especially in elderly
• Bilirubin, CBC, liver function studies monthly
• Urinalysis recommended before, during prolonged therapy
• Affect, orientation, LOC, reflexes, gait, coordination, sleep pattern disturbances
• B/P sitting, standing, lying; take pulse and respirations q4h during initial treatment; establish baseline before starting treatment; report drops of 30 mm Hg; obtain baseline ECG, Q-wave and T-wave changes
• Dizziness, faintness, palpitations, tachycardia on rising
• For neuroleptic malignant syndrome: hyperpyrexia, muscle rigidity, increased CPK, altered mental status, for acute dystonia (check chewing, swallowing, eyes, pin rolling)
• EPS including akathisia (inability to sit still, no pattern to movements), tardive dyskinesia (bizarre movements of the jaw, mouth, tongue, extremities), pseudoparkinsonism (rigidity, tremors, pill rolling, shuffling gait)
• Skin turgor daily
• Constipation, urinary retention daily; increase bulk, H_2O in diet

Administer:
• IM, inject in deep muscle mass, do not give SC
• IV after diluting 1 mg/1 ml with NS, give 1 mg or less/2 min or more; may be further diluted in 500-1000 ml of NS
• Antiparkinsonian agent for EPS
• Rectal after placing in refrigerator for ½ hour if too soft to insert
• Drug in liquid form mixed in glass of juice or cola if hoarding is suspected
• Decreased dose in elderly
• PO with full glass of water, milk; or with food to decrease GI upset

Perform/provide:
• Decreased stimuli by dimming lights, avoiding loud noises
• Supervised ambulation until stabilized on medication; do not involve in strenuous exercise program because fainting is possible; patient should not stand still for long periods
• Increased fluids to prevent constipation
• Sips of water, candy, gum for dry mouth
• Storage in tight, light-resistant container, oral sol in amber bottle

Evaluate:
• Therapeutic response: decrease in emotional excitement, hallucinations, delusions, paranoia, reorganization of patterns of thought, speech

Teach patient/family:
• To use good oral hygiene; frequent rinsing of mouth, sugarless gum for dry mouth
• To avoid hazardous activities until drug response is determined
• That orthostatic hypotension occurs often and to rise from sitting or lying position gradually
• To remain lying down after IM injection for at least 30 min
• To avoid hot tubs, hot showers, tub baths, since hypotension may occur
• To avoid abrupt withdrawal of this drug, or EPS may result; drug should be withdrawn slowly
• To avoid OTC preparations (cough, hay fever, cold) unless approved by

prescriber, since serious drug interactions may occur; avoid use with alcohol, CNS depressants; increased drowsiness may occur
• To use a sunscreen and sunglasses to prevent burns
• About EPS and necessity of meticulous oral hygiene, since oral candidiasis may occur
• To take antacids 2 hr before or after this drug
• To report sore throat, malaise, fever, bleeding, mouth sores; CBC should be drawn and drug discontinued
• That in hot weather, heat stroke may occur; take extra precautions to stay cool
• That urine may turn pink or red

Treatment of overdose: Lavage if orally ingested; provide airway; *do not induce vomiting or use epinephrine*

chlorpropamide (℞)

(klor-proe'pa-mide)
Chloronase*, Chlorpropamide, Diabinese, Novopropamide*
Func. class.: Antidiabetic
Chem. class.: Sulfonylurea (1st generation)

Action: Causes functioning β-cells in pancreas to release insulin, leading to drop in blood glucose levels; may improve insulin binding to insulin receptors or increase the number of insulin receptors with prolonged administration. May also reduce basal hepatic glucose secretion; not effective if patient lacks functioning β-cells

Uses: Stable adult-onset diabetes mellitus (type II) NIDDM

Dosage and routes:
• *Adult:* PO 100-250 mg qd, initially, then 100-500 mg maintenance according to response; not to exceed 750 mg/day

Available forms: Tabs 100, 250 mg scored

Side effects/adverse reactions:
CNS: Headache, weakness, dizziness, drowsiness, tinnitus, fatigue, vertigo
*GI: **Hepatotoxicity, cholestatic jaundice,*** nausea, vomiting, diarrhea, heartburn
*HEMA: **Leukopenia, thrombocytopenia, agranulocytosis, aplastic anemia, pancytopenia, hemolytic anemia***
INTEG: Rash, allergic reactions, pruritus, urticaria, eczema, photosensitivity, erythema
*ENDO: **Hypoglycemia,*** hyponatremia

Contraindications: Hypersensitivity to sulfonylureas, juvenile or brittle diabetes, pregnancy (D), lactation, renal failure

Precautions: Elderly, cardiac disease, thyroid disease, renal disease, hepatic disease, severe hypoglycemic reactions

Pharmacokinetics:
PO: Completely absorbed by GI route, onset 1 hr, peak 3-6 hr, duration 60 hr, half-life 36 hr; metabolized in liver; excreted in urine (metabolites and unchanged drug), breast milk; 90%-95% plasma protein bound

Interactions:
• Increased hypoglycemic effects: oral anticoagulants, salicylates, sulfonamides, NSAIDS, chloramphenicol, cimetidine, MAOIs, insulin, guanethidine, methyldopa, probenecid, ranitidine
• Increased effects of chlorpropamide: insulin, MAOIs
• Decreased digoxin levels: digoxin
• Decreased effect of both drugs: diazoxide

• Disulfiram-like reaction: alcohol
• Decreased action of chlorpropamide: calcium channel blockers, corticosteroids, oral contraceptives, thiazide diuretics, thyroid preparations, estrogens, phenobarbital, phenytoin, rifampin, sympathomimetics

NURSING CONSIDERATIONS

Assess:

• Hypoglycemic/hyperglycemic reaction soon after meals

Administer:

• Drug 30 min before meals

Perform/provide:

• Storage in tight container in cool environment

Evaluate:

• Therapeutic response: decrease in polyuria, polydipsia, polyphagia, clear sensorium, absence of dizziness, stable gait

Teach patient/family:

• To check for symptoms of cholestatic jaundice: dark urine, pruritus, yellow sclera; prescriber should be notified
• To use capillary blood glucose test or Chemstrip tid
• Symptoms of hypo/hyperglycemia, what to do about each
• That this drug must be taken daily; explain consequence of discontinuing drug abruptly
• To take drug in morning to prevent hypoglycemic reactions at night; have glucagon emergency kit available
• To avoid OTC medications unless directed by prescriber
• That diabetes is lifelong illness; drug will not cure disease
• That all food in diet plan must be eaten to prevent hypoglycemia
• To carry Medic Alert ID for emergency purposes
• Not to drink alcohol

Treatment of overdose: glucose 25 g IV, via dextrose 50% sol, 50 ml or 1 mg glucagon

chlorthalidone (℞)

(klor-thal'i-done)

Apo-Chlorthalidone*, chlorthalidone, Hygroton, Hylidone, Novothalidone*, Thalitone, Uridon*

Func. class.: Diuretic

Chem. class.: Thiazide-like phthalimidine derivative

Action: Acts on distal tubule by increasing excretion of water, sodium, chloride, potassium, magnesium, bicarbonate

Uses: Edema, hypertension, diuresis, CHF, nephrotic syndrome

Dosage and routes:

• *Adult:* PO 25-100 mg/day or 100 mg every other day
• *Child:* PO 2 mg/kg 3 ×/wk

Available forms: Tabs 25, 50, 100 mg

Side effects/adverse reactions:

GU: Frequency, polyuria, ***uremia,*** glucosuria, impotence

CNS: Drowsiness, paresthesia, anxiety, depression, headache, *dizziness, fatigue, weakness*

GI: Nausea, vomiting, anorexia, constipation, diarrhea, cramps, pancreatitis, GI irritation, ***hepatitis***

EENT: Blurred vision

INTEG: Rash, urticaria, purpura, photosensitivity, fever

META: Hyperglycemia, hyperuremia, increased creatinine, BUN, gout

HEMA: ***Aplastic anemia, hemolytic anemia, leukopenia, agranulocytosis, thrombocytopenia, neutropenia***

CV: Irregular pulse, orthostatic hypotension, palpitations, volume depletion

ELECT: Hypokalemia, hypomagnesemia, hypercalcemia, hyponatremia, hypochloremia

* Available in Canada only

Contraindications: Hypersensitivity to thiazides or sulfonamides, anuria, renal decompensation, lactation

Precautions: Hypokalemia, renal disease, pregnancy (C), lactation, hepatic disease, gout, diabetes mellitus, elderly

Pharmacokinetics:

PO: Onset 2 hr, peak 6 hr, duration 24-72 hr; excreted unchanged by kidneys; crosses placenta; enters breast milk; half-life 40 hr

Interactions:

- Increased toxicity: lithium, nondepolarizing skeletal muscle relaxants
- Decreased effects of antidiabetics
- Decreased absorption of thiazides: cholestyramine, colestipol
- Decreased hypotensive response: indomethacin, NSAIDs
- Hyperglycemia, hyperuricemia, hypotension: diazoxide

Lab test interferences:

Increase: BSP retention, Ca, cholesterol, triglycerides, amylase

Decrease: PBI, PSP, parathyroid test

NURSING CONSIDERATIONS

Assess:

- Weight, I&O daily to determine fluid loss; effect of drug may be decreased if used qd
- Rate, depth, rhythm of respiration, effect of exertion
- B/P lying, standing; postural hypotension may occur
- Electrolytes: K, Mg, Na, Cl; include BUN, blood sugar, CBC, serum creatinine, blood pH, ABGs, uric acid, Ca
- Glucose in urine if patient is diabetic
- Signs of metabolic alkalosis: drowsiness, restlessness
- Signs of hypokalemia: postural hypotension, malaise, fatigue, tachycardia, leg cramps, weakness
- Rashes, temperature elevation qd
- Confusion, especially in elderly; take safety precautions if needed

Administer:

- In AM to avoid interference with sleep if using drug as a diuretic
- K replacement if K less than 3 mg/dl
- With food if nausea occurs; absorption may be decreased slightly

Evaluate:

- Therapeutic response: improvement in edema of feet, legs, sacral area daily if medication used in CHF

Teach patient/family:

- To increase fluid intake to 2-3 L/day unless contraindicated, to rise slowly from lying or sitting position
- To notify prescriber of muscle weakness, cramps, nausea, dizziness
- That drug may be taken with food or milk
- That blood sugar may be increased in diabetics
- To use sunscreen to protect against photosensitivity
- To take early in day to avoid nocturia

Treatment of overdose: Lavage if taken orally, monitor electrolytes, administer dextrose in NS, monitor hydration, CV, renal status

chlorzoxazone (℞)

(klor-zox′a-zone)

chlorzoxazone, Paraflex, Parafon Forte DSC, Remular-S

Func. class.: Skeletal muscle relaxant

Chem. class.: Benzoxazole derivative

Combination products: Blanex: chlorzoxazone 250 mg, acetaminophen 300 mg; Chlorofon-F, Chlorzone Forte, Paracet Forte, Parafon Forte, Zoxaphen: chlorzoxazone 250 mg with acetaminophen 300 mg;

Lobac: chloroxazone 250 mg, acetaminophen 300 mg; Mus-Lax: chlorzoxazone 250 mg, acetaminophen 300 mg; Polyflex: chlorzoxazone 250 mg, acetaminophen 300 mg; Skelez: chlorzoxazone 250 mg, acetaminophen 300 mg; Zoxaphen: chlorzoxazone 250 mg, acetaminophen 300 mg

---

Action: Inhibits multisynaptic reflex arcs
Uses: Relieving pain, spasm in musculoskeletal conditions
Dosage and routes:
- *Adult:* PO 250-750 mg tid-qid
- *Child:* PO 20 mg/kg/day in divided doses bid-tid

Available forms: Tabs 250 mg
Side effects/adverse reactions:
GU: Urine discoloration
HEMA: ***Granulocytopenia, anemia***
CNS: *Dizziness, drowsiness,* headache, insomnia, stimulation, malaise
GI: *Nausea,* vomiting, anorexia, diarrhea, constipation, ***hepatotoxicity, jaundice***
INTEG: Rash, pruritus, petechiae, ecchymoses, ***angioedema***
SYST: ***Anaphylaxis***
Contraindications: Hypersensitivity, impaired hepatic function
Precautions: Pregnancy (C), lactation, hepatic disease, elderly
Pharmacokinetics:
PO: Onset 1 hr, peak 3-4 hr, duration 6 hr, half-life 1 hr; metabolized in liver; excreted in urine (metabolites)
Interactions:
- Increased CNS depression: alcohol, tricyclic antidepressants, narcotics, barbiturates, sedatives, hypnotics

NURSING CONSIDERATIONS
Assess:
- Blood studies: CBC, WBC, differential for blood dyscrasias
- Liver function studies: AST, ALT, alk phosphatase; hepatitis may occur; hold dose and notify prescriber of signs of hepatotoxicity
- EEG in epileptic patients; poor seizure control has occurred
- Allergic reactions: rash, fever, respiratory distress
- Severe weakness, numbness in extremities
- Psychologic dependency: increased need for medication, more frequent requests for medication, increased pain
- CNS depression: dizziness, drowsiness, psychiatric symptoms

Administer:
- With meals for GI symptoms

Perform/provide:
- Storage in tight container at room temperature
- Assistance with ambulation if dizziness or drowsiness occurs, especially elderly

Evaluate:
- Therapeutic response: decreased pain, spasticity

Teach patient/family:
- Not to discontinue quickly; insomnia, nausea, headache, spasticity, tachycardia will occur; drug should be tapered over 1-2 wk
- Not to take with alcohol, other CNS depressants
- To avoid hazardous activities if drowsiness, dizziness occurs
- To avoid using OTC medication: cough preparations, antihistamines, unless directed by prescriber
- That urine may be orange or purple

Treatment of overdose: Gastric lavage or induce emesis, then administer activated charcoal; use other supportive treatment as necessary; monitor cardiac function

---

* Available in Canada only

cholestyramine (℞)

(koe-less-tir'a-meen)

Cholybar, Questran, Questran Light

Func. class.: Antilipemic

Chem. class.: Bile acid sequestrant

Action: Absorbs, combines with bile acids to form insoluble complex that is excreted through feces; loss of bile acids lowers cholesterol levels

Uses: Primary hypercholesterolemia, pruritus associated with biliary obstruction, diarrhea caused by excess bile acid, digitalis toxicity, xanthomas

Dosage and routes:

• *Adult:* PO 4 g ac, and hs, not to exceed 32 g/day

• *Child:* PO 240 mg/kg/day in 3 divided doses with food or drink

Available forms: Powder 9 g/4 g cholestyramine

Side effects/adverse reactions:

CNS: Headache, dizziness, drowsiness, vertigo, tinnitus

MS: Muscle, joint pain

GI: Constipation, abdominal pain, nausea, fecal impaction, hemorrhoids, flatulence, vomiting, steatorrhea, peptic ulcer

INTEG: Rash, irritation of perianal area, tongue, skin

HEMA: Decreased vit A, D, K, red cell folate content, ***hyperchloremic acidosis, bleeding,*** decreased protime

Contraindications: Hypersensitivity, biliary obstruction

Precautions: Pregnancy (C), lactation, children

Pharmacokinetics:

PO: Excreted in feces, maximum effect in 2 wk

Interactions:

• Decreased absorption of phenylbutazone, warfarin, thiazides, digitalis, penicillin G, tetracyclines, cephalexin, phenobarbital, folic acid, corticosteroids, iron, thyroid, clindamycin, trimethoprim, chenodiol, fat-soluble vitamins

Lab test interferences:

Increase: Liver function studies, Cl, PO_4

NURSING CONSIDERATIONS

Assess:

• Cardiac glycoside level, if both drugs are being administered

• For signs of vit A, D, K deficiency

• Serum cholesterol, triglyceride levels, electrolytes if on extended therapy

• Bowel pattern daily; increase bulk, H_2O in diet for constipation

Administer:

• Drug ac, hs; give all other medications 1 hr before cholestyramine or 4 hr after cholestyramine to avoid poor absorption

• Drug mixed/applesauce or stirred into beverage (2-6 oz), do not take dry, let stand for 2 min

• Supplemental doses of vit A, D, K, if levels are low

Evaluate:

• Therapeutic response: decreased cholesterol level (hyperlipidemia); diarrhea, pruritus (excess bile acids)

Teach patient/family:

• Symptoms of hypoprothrombinemia: bleeding mucous membranes, dark tarry stools, hematuria, petechiae; report immediately

• Importance of compliance; toxicity may result if doses missed

• That risk factors should be decreased: high-fat diet, smoking, alcohol consumption, absence of exercise

• Not to discontinue suddenly

choline salicylate (℞)

(koe'leen)

Arthropan

Func. class.: Nonnarcotic analgesic

Chem. class.: Salicylate

Action: Blocks pain impulses in CNS that occur in response to inhibition of prostaglandin synthesis; antipyretic action results from inhibition of hypothalamic heat-regulating center to produce vasodilation to allow heat dissipation

Uses: Mild to moderate pain or fever including arthritis, juvenile rheumatoid arthritis

Dosage and routes:

Arthritis

• *Adult and child >12 yr:* PO 870-1740 mg qid; max 6 × /day

Pain/fever

• *Adult:* PO 870 mg q3-4h prn

• *Child 3-6 yr:* PO 105-210 mg q4h prn

Available forms: Liq 870 mg/5 ml

Side effects/adverse reactions:

HEMA: ***Thrombocytopenia, agranulocytosis, leukopenia, neutropenia, hemolytic anemia,*** increased pro-time

CNS: Stimulation, drowsiness, dizziness, confusion, ***convulsion,*** headache, flushing, hallucinations, ***coma***

GI: Nausea, vomiting, GI bleeding, diarrhea, heartburn, anorexia, ***hepatitis***

INTEG: Rash, urticaria, bruising

EENT: Tinnitus, hearing loss

CV: Rapid pulse, pulmonary edema

RESP: Wheezing, hyperpnea

ENDO: Hypoglycemia, hyponatremia, hypokalemia

Contraindications: Hypersensitivity to salicylates, GI bleeding, bleeding disorders, children <3 yr, Vit K deficiency, children with flulike symptoms

Precautions: Anemia, hepatic disease, renal disease, Hodgkin's disease, pregnancy (C), lactation

Pharmacokinetics:

PO: Onset 15-30 min; metabolized by liver; crosses placenta; excreted in breast milk, by kidneys

Interactions:

• Decreased effects of choline: antacids, steroids, urinary alkalizers

• Increased blood loss: alcohol, heparin

• Increased effects of anticoagulants, insulin, methotrexate

• Decreased effects of probenecid, spironolactone, sulfinpyrazone, sulfonylamides

• Toxic effects: PABA, furosemide, carbonic anhydrase inhibitors

• Decreased blood sugar levels: salicylates

• GI bleeding: steroids, antiinflammatories

Lab test interferences:

Increase: Coagulation studies, liver function studies, serum uric acid, amylase, CO_2, urinary protein

Decrease: Serum K, PBI, cholesterol

Interference: Urine catecholamines, pregnancy test

NURSING CONSIDERATIONS

Assess:

• Liver function studies: AST, ALT, bilirubin, creatinine (long-term therapy)

• Renal function studies: BUN, urine creatinine (long-term therapy)

• Blood studies: CBC, Hct, Hgb, pro-time (long-term therapy)

• I&O ratio; decreasing output may indicate renal failure (long-term therapy)

• Hepatotoxicity: dark urine; clay-colored stools; yellowing of skin, sclera; itching; abdominal pain; fever; diarrhea (long-term therapy)

* Available in Canada only

• Allergic reactions: rash, urticaria; drug may have to be discontinued
• Renal dysfunction: decreased urine output
• Ototoxicity: tinnitus, ringing, roaring in ears; audiometric testing needed before, after long-term therapy
• Visual changes: blurring, halos, corneal, retinal damage
• Edema in feet, ankles, legs
• Drug history; many interactions

Administer:
• Mixed with fruit juice, carbonated beverage, water

Evaluate:
• Therapeutic response: decreased pain, fever, stiffness of joints

Teach patient/family:
• To report any symptoms of hepatotoxicity, renal toxicity, visual changes, ototoxicity, allergic reactions, bleeding (long-term therapy)
• Not to exceed recommended dosage; acute poisoning may result
• To read label on other OTC drugs; many contain aspirin
• That therapeutic response takes 2 wk (arthritis)
• To avoid alcohol ingestion; GI bleeding may occur
• That if anticoagulants are given with this drug, this drug should be decreased 2 wk before surgery

Treatment of overdose: Lavage, activated charcoal, monitor electrolytes, VS

chorionic gonadotropin, human (℞)

(go-nad'oh-troe-pin)
APL, Chorex-5, Chorex-10, Choron 10, Gonic, Pregnyl, Profasi

Func. class.: Human chorionic gonadotropin
Chem. class.: Polypeptide hormone

Action: Stimulates production of gonadal steroids, androgens; stimulates corpus luteum to produce progesterone

Uses: Infertility, anovulation, hypogonadism, nonobstructive cryptorchidism

Dosage and routes:
• Dosage regimens vary widely

Infertility/anovulation
• *Adult:* IM 10,000 U 1 day after last dose of menotropins

Hypogonadism
• *Adult:* IM 500-1000 U 3 × wk × 3 wk, then 2 × wk × 3 wk, or 4000 U 3 × wk × 6-9 mo, then 2000 U 3 × wk × 3 mo

Cryptorchidism
• *Child (boy 4-9 yr):* IM 5000 U qod × 4 doses

Available forms: Powder for inj 500, 1000, 2000 U/ml

Side effects/adverse reactions:
CNS: Headache, depression, fatigue, anxiety, irritability
GU: Gynecomastia, early puberty, edema, ***ectopic pregnancy***
INTEG: *Pain at injection site*

Contraindications: Hypersensitivity, pituitary hypertrophy/tumor, early puberty, prostatic cancer, pregnancy (X)

Precautions: Asthma, migraine headache, convulsive disorders, cardiac disease, renal disease, lactation, children <4 yr

Pharmacokinetics:

IM: Peak 6 hr, half-life 11-24 hr, excreted by kidneys

NURSING CONSIDERATIONS

Assess:

• Weight weekly; notify prescriber if weekly weight gain is >5 lb

• B/P before, during treatment

• Be alert for decreasing urinary output, increasing edema

• Edema, hypertension

Administer:

• Only after clomiphene citrate has been tried on anovulatory patient

• After reconstitution with diluent enclosed in package

Perform/provide:

• Refrigeration for up to 2 mo

Evaluate:

• Therapeutic response: ovulation, fertility

Teach patient/family:

• To report facial, axillary, pubic hair, change in voice, penile enlargement, acne in male, abdominal pain, distention, vaginal bleeding in women

• To report symptoms of ectopic pregnancy: dizziness, pain on one side or in shoulder, pallor, weak thready pulse, hemorrhage; shock may proceed rapidly

chymopapain (℞)

(kye'moe-pa-pane)

Chymodiactin

Func. class.: Enzyme

Chem. class.: Proteolytic

Action: Hydrolyzes noncollagenous polypeptides that maintain structure of chondromucoprotein; activity decreases pressure on disk

Uses: Herniated lumbar intervertebral disk

Dosage and routes:

• *Adult:* INJ 2-4 mKat U/disk injected intradiskally, not to exceed 10 mKat U in a multiple herniation

Available forms: Powder for inj 4, 10 mKat U/vial

Side effects/adverse reactions:

CNS: ***Paraplegia, cerebral hemorrhage,*** headache, dizziness, paresthesia, numbness of extremities

INTEG: Rash, urticaria, itching

GI: Nausea, paralytic ileus

MS: Back pain, stiffness, spasm, acute transverse myelitis, weakness, leg pain

SYSTEM: ***Anaphylaxis***

GU: Urinary retention

Contraindications: Hypersensitivity to this drug, papaya, meat tenderizer; severe spondylolisthesis; severe progressing paralysis; spinal cord tumor; cauda equina lesion, previous use

Precautions: Pregnancy (C), lactation, children

Pharmacokinetics: Onset 30 min, duration 24 hr

Interactions:

• Dysrhythmias: halothane anesthetics plus epinephrine

NURSING CONSIDERATIONS

Assess:

• RBCs, ESR before treatment

• Respiratory rate, rhythm, depth; notify physician of abnormalities

• Anaphylaxis for several days after injection

• Neuro status after surgery; elimination status for paralytic ileus

• For allergies: iodine, papaya, meat tenderizer; if allergies are identified, drug should not be used

Administer:

• Only with epinephrine available for anaphylaxis

• Only in lumbar spine by physician

• After diluting with sterile water for injection, use within 60 min

• After completing allergy test (ChymoFAST)

Evaluate:

• Therapeutic response: absence of back pain, increased mobility

Teach patient/family

• To report allergic reactions up to 2 wk after injection

• To be aware of possible infection; redness, swelling, pain

ciclopirox (℞)

(sye-kloe-peer′ox)

Loprox

Func. class.: Local antiinfective

Chem. class.: Antifungal

Action: Interferes with fungal cell membrane, which increases permeability, leaking of cell nutrients

Uses: Tinea cruris, tinea corporis, tinea pedis, tinea versicolor, cutaneous candidiasis

Dosage and routes:

• *Adult and child >10 yr:* TOP rub into affected area bid

Available forms: Cream 1%, lotion 1%

Side effects/adverse reactions:

INTEG: Rash, urticaria, stinging, burning, pruritus, pain

Contraindications: Hypersensitivity

Precautions: Pregnancy (B), lactation, child <10 yr

NURSING CONSIDERATIONS

Assess:

• Allergic reaction: burning, stinging, swelling, redness

Administer:

• Enough medication to cover lesions completely

• After cleansing with soap, water before each application; dry well

Perform/provide:

• Storage at room temperature in dry place

Evaluate:

• Therapeutic response: decrease in size, number of lesions

Teach patient/family:

• To apply with glove to prevent further infection

• To avoid use of OTC creams, ointments, lotions unless directed by prescriber

• To continue even though condition improves

• To wash hands before, after each application

• Not to cover with occlusive dressing

• To change shoes and socks once a day during treatment of tinea pedis

• To report blisters, burning, oozing, swelling

cimetidine (OTC, ℞)

(sye-met′i-deen)

Apo-Cimetidine*, Tagamet, Peptol*, Novocimetine*

Func. class.: H_2 histamine receptor antagonist

Chem. class.: Imidazole derivative

Action: Inhibits histamine at H_2 receptor site in the gastric parietal cells, which inhibits gastric acid secretion

Uses: Short-term treatment of duodenal and gastric ulcers and maintenance; management of GERD and Zollinger-Ellison syndrome

Investigational uses: Prevention of aspiration pneumonitis, stress ulcers, upper GI bleeding

Dosage and routes:

Treatment of active ulcers

• *Adult and child:* PO 300 mg qid with meals, hs × 8 wk or 400 mg bid, 800 mg hs; after 8 wk give hs dose only; IV BOL 300 mg/20 ml 0.9% NaCl over 1-2 min q6h; IV INF 300 mg/50 ml D_5W over 15-20

C

min; IM 300 mg q6h, not to exceed 2400 mg

Prophylaxis of duodenal ulcer

• *Adult and child >16 yr:* 400 mg hs

GERD

Adult: PO 800-1600 mg/day in divided doses

Hypersecretory conditions (Zollinger-Ellison syndrome)

Adult: PO/IM/IV 300-600 mg q6h; may increase to 12 g/day if needed

Upper GI bleeding prophylaxis

Adult: IV 50 mg/hr; lowered in renal disease

Aspiration pneumonitis prophylaxis

Adult: IM/IV 300 mg IM 1 hr before anesthesia, then 300 mg IV q4h until patient is alert

Available forms: Tabs 100, 200, 300, 400, 800 mg; liq 300 mg/5 ml; inj IV 300 mg/2 ml, 300 mg/50 ml 0.9% NaCl

Side effects/adverse reactions:

CNS: Confusion, headache, depression, dizziness, anxiety, weakness, psychosis, tremors, ***convulsions***

CV: Bradycardia, tachycardia

GI: Diarrhea, abdominal cramps, ***paralytic ileus, jaundice***

GU: Gynecomastia, galactorrhea, impotence, increase in BUN, creatinine

HEMA: ***Agranulocytosis, thrombocytopenia, neutropenia, aplastic anemia, increase in pro-time***

INTEG: Urticaria, rash, alopecia, sweating, flushing, ***exfoliative dermatitis***

Contraindications: Hypersensitivity

Precautions: Pregnancy (B), lactation, child <16 yr, organic brain syndrome, hepatic disease, renal disease, elderly

Pharmacokinetics: Well absorbed (PO, IM)

IM/IV: Onset 10 min, peak ½ hour, duration 4-5 hours

PO: Peak 1-1½ hr, half-life 1½-2 hrs; 30%-40% metabolized by liver, excreted in urine unchanged, crosses placenta, enters breast milk

Interactions:

• Increased toxicity: oral anticoagulants, benzodiazepines, metoprolol, propranolol, phenytoin, quinidine, theophylline, tricyclic antidepressants, lidocaine, procainamide, carmustine, flecainide, narcotic analgesics, succinylcholine

• Decreased absorption of cimetidine: antacids, anticholinergics, metoclopramide

• Decreased effectiveness: smoking

• Decreased absorption: ketoconazole, iron salts, tetracyclines, indomethacin

• Decreased absorption of tocainide

Syringe compatibilities: Atropine, butorphanol, cephalothin, diazepam, diphenhydramine, doxapram, droperidol, fentanyl, glycopyrrolate, heparin, hydromorphone, hydroxyzine, lorazepam, meperidine, midazolam, morphine, nafcillin, nalbuphine, penicillin GT sodium, pentazocine, perphenazine, prochlorperazine, promazine, promethazine, scopolamine, sodium acetate, NaCl, sodium lactate, sterile water

Y-site compatibilities: Acyclovir, aminophylline, amrinone, atracurium, enalaprilat, esmolol, foscarnet, haloperidol heparin, hetastarch, idarubicin, labetalol, melphalan, ondansetron, paclitaxel, pancuronium, tolazoline, vecuronium, vinorelbine, zidovudine

Additive compatibilities: Acetazolamide, amikacin, aminophylline, cefoxitin, chlorothiazide, clindamycin, colistimethate, dexamethasone, digoxin, epinephrine, erythromycin, ethacrynate, furosemide, gen-

* Available in Canada only

tamicin, insulin, isoproterenol, lidocaine, lincomycin, metaraminol bitartrate, methylprednisolone, norepinephrine, penicillin G potassium, phytonadione, polymyxin B, potassium chloride, protamine sulfate, quinidine, sodium nitroprusside, tetracycline, verapamil, vitamin B complex

Lab test interferences:
Increase: Alk phosphatase, AST, creatinine
False positive: Gastric bleeding test, Hemocult

NURSING CONSIDERATIONS

Assess:
• Gastric pH (5 should be maintained), also epigastric pain and duration, intensity; aggravating, ameliorating factors
• I&O ratio, BUN, creatinine, CBC with differential monthly

Administer:
• IV after diluting 300 mg/20 ml of NS for inj; give over ≥2 min; may be diluted 300 mg/50 ml of D_5W; run over 15-20 min; or total daily dose (900 mg) diluted in 100-1000 ml D_5W given over 24 hr
• With meals for prolonged drug effect; antacids 1 hr before or 1 hr after cimetidine

Perform/provide:
• Storage of diluted sol at room temp up to 48 hr

Evaluate:
• Therapeutic response: decreased pain in abdomen; healing of ulcers, absence of gastroesophageal reflex

Teach patient/family:
• That gynecomastia, impotence may occur, are reversible
• To avoid driving, other hazardous activities until patient is stabilized on this medication; drowsiness or dizziness may occur
• To avoid black pepper, caffeine, alcohol, harsh spices, extremes in temp of food
• To avoid OTC preparations: aspirin, cough, cold preparations; condition may worsen
• That smoking decreases the effectiveness of the drug
• That drug must be continued for prescribed time to be effective and taken exactly as prescribed; doses not to be doubled
• To report bruising, fatigue, malaise; blood dyscrasias may occur
• To report to prescriber diarrhea, black tarry stools, sore throat, rash

ciprofloxacin (℞)

(sip-ro-floks'a-sin)
Ciloxan, Cipro, Cipro IV
Func. class.: Broad-spectrum antibiotic
Chem. class.: Fluoroquinolone antibacterial

Action: Interferes with conversion of intermediate DNA fragments into high-molecular-weight DNA in bacteria; DNA gyrase inhibitor

Uses: Infection caused by susceptible *E. coli, E. cloacae, P. mirabilis, K. pneumoniae, P. vulgaris, C. freundi, S. marcescens, P. aeruginosa, S. aureus, Enterobacter*

Dosage and routes:

Uncomplicated urinary tract infections
• *Adult:* PO 250 mg q12h; IV 200 mg q12h

Complicated/severe urinary tract infections
• *Adult:* PO 500 mg q12h; IV 400 mg q12h

Respiratory, bone, skin, joint infections
• *Adult:* PO 500-750 mg q12h; IV 400 mg q12h

Corneal ulcers, conjunctivitis
• *Adult:* OPHTL 1-2 drops q15-30 min, then 1-2 drops 4-6 times daily

Available forms: Tabs 250, 500, 750 mg; IV 200 mg/100 ml D_5, 400 mg/200 ml D_5; 200, 400 mg vial; oph sol

Side effects/adverse reactions:

CNS: Headache, dizziness, fatigue, insomnia, depression, restlessness, seizures, confusion

GI: Nausea, diarrhea, increased ALT (SGPT), AST (SGOT), flatulence, heartburn, vomiting, oral candidiasis, dysphagia

INTEG: Rash, pruritus, urticaria, photosensitivity, flushing, fever, chills

MS: Blurred vision, tinnitus

Contraindications: Hypersensitivity to quinolones

Precautions: Pregnancy (C), lactation, children, renal disease, epilepsy

Pharmacokinetics:

PO: Peak 1 hr, half-life 3-4 hr; excreted in urine as active drug, metabolites

Interactions:

- Decreased absorption of ciproflaxin: magnesium antacids, aluminum hydroxide, zinc, iron, sucralfate, calcium
- Increased serum levels of ciprofloxacin: probenecid
- Increased theophylline levels when used with ciprofloxacin

Y-site compatibilities: Aztreonam, ceftazidime, heparin, piperacillin, tobramycin

Additive compatibilities: Amikacin, aztreonam, ceftazidime, gentamicin, metronidazole, piperacillin, tobramycin

Syringe compatibility: Heparin

NURSING CONSIDERATIONS

Assess:

- CNS symptoms: headache, dizziness, fatigue, insomnia, depression
- Kidney, liver function studies: BUN, creatinine, AST (SGOT), ALT (SGPT)
- I&O ratio, urine pH <5.5 is ideal
- Allergic reactions: fever, flushing, rash, urticaria, pruritus

Administer:

- IV over 1 hr as an INF, comes in premixed plastic INF container or diluted 20 or 40 ml vial to a final conc of 0.5-2 mg/ml of NS or D_5W; give through Y-tube or 3-way stopcock
- After clean-catch urine for C&S

Perform/provide:

- Limited intake of alkaline foods, drugs: milk, dairy products, alkaline antacids, sodium bicarbonate

Evaluate:

- Therapeutic response: decreased pain, frequency, urgency, C&S—absence of infection

Teach patient/family:

- Not to take any products containing magnesium or calcium (such as antacids), iron, or aluminum with this drug or within 2 hr of drug
- That photosensitivity may occur; patient should avoid sunlight or use sunscreen to prevent burns
- That fluids must be increased to 3 L/day to avoid crystallization in kidneys
- If dizziness occurs, to ambulate, perform activities with assistance
- To complete full course of drug therapy
- To contact physician if adverse reaction occurs
- To take with food to decrease GI irritation

---

cisapride (℞)

(siss'a-pride)

Propulsid

Func. class.: Cholinergic

Action: Enhances response to acetylcholine at the myenteric plexus

Uses: Treatment of heartburn

Dosage and routes:
• *Adult:* PO 10 mg qid at least 15 min ac and hs; may increase to 20 mg; elderly may need higher dosage
Available forms: Tabs 10, 20 mg
Side effects/adverse reactions:
RESP: Rhinitis, sinusitis, coughing
CNS: Headache, sleeplessness, anxiety, nervousness, pain, fever
GI: Diarrhea, constipation, nausea, anorexia, abdominal pain, flatulence, dyspepsia
GU: UTI, frequency
INTEG: Pruritus, rash
Contraindications: Hypersensitivity; GI hemorrhage, obstruction, perforation
Precautions: Pregnancy (C), lactation, children, elderly, electrolyte disturbances, congenital prolonged QT syndrome
Pharmacokinetics:
PO: Rapidly absorbed; onset ½-1 hr, peak 1-1½ hr; extensively metabolized by liver, excreted in urine, (metabolite); 98% bound to plasma proteins; terminal half-life 6-12 hr
Interactions:
• Inhibition of metabolism of cisapride: ketoconazole, itraconazole, miconazole, troleandomycin; do not use together
• Decreased action of cisapride: anticholinergics
• Increased peak plasma levels: cimetidine, H_2 antagonists
• Increased coagulation time: anticoagulants

NURSING CONSIDERATIONS
Assess:
• GI complaints: nausea, vomiting, anorexia, constipation
Administer:
• ½-1 hr before meals for better absorption
Evaluate:
• Therapeutic response: absence of heartburn
Teach patient/family:
• To avoid alcohol, other CNS depressants that will enhance sedating properties of this drug
• To increase fluids, bulk in diet for constipation
Treatment of overdose: Gastric lavage or activated charcoal, general support

cisplatin (℞)
(sis′pla-tin)
CDDP Platinol, Platinol-AQ
Func. class.: Antineoplastic alkylating agent
Chem. class.: Inorganic heavy metal

Action: Alkylates DNA, RNA; inhibits enzymes that allow synthesis of amino acids in proteins; activity is not cell cycle phase specific
Uses: Advanced bladder cancer, adjunctive in metastatic testicular cancer, adjunctive in metastatic ovarian cancer, head, neck cancer, esophagus, prostate, lung and cervical cancer, lymphoma
Dosage and routes:
Testicular cancer
• *Adult:* IV 20 mg/m² qd × 5 days, repeat q3wk for 3 cycles or more, depending on response
Bladder cancer
• *Adult:* IV 50-70 mg/m² q3-4wk
Ovarian cancer
• *Adult:* IV 100 mg/m² q4wk or 50 mg/m² q3wk with doxorubicin therapy; mix with 2 L NaCl and 37.5 g mannitol over 6 hr
Available forms: Inj IV 10, 50, 100 mg
Side effects/adverse reactions:
EENT: Tinnitus, hearing loss, vestibular toxicity
HEMA: ***Thrombocytopenia, leukopenia, pancytopenia***

CV: Cardiac abnormalities
GI: Severe nausea, vomiting, diarrhea, weight loss
GU: ***Renal tubular damage,*** renal insufficiency, impotence, sterility, amenorrhea, gynecomastia, hyperuremia
INTEG: Alopecia, dermatitis
CNS: ***Convulsions,*** peripheral neuropathy
RESP: ***Fibrosis***
META: Hypomagnesemia, hypocalcemia, hypokalemia, hypophosphatemia
SYST: ***Hypersensitivity reaction***

Contraindications: Radiation therapy or chemotherapy within 1 mo, thrombocytopenia, smallpox vaccination

Precautions: Pneumococcus vaccination, pregnancy (D), lactation

Pharmacokinetics: Well absorbed orally, metabolized in liver, excreted in urine; half-life 2 hr

Interactions:
- Increased nephrotoxicity: aminoglycosides
- Decreased effects of phenytoin

Y-site compatibilities: Bleomycin, cyclophosphamide, doxapram, doxorubicin, droperidol, fludarabine, fluorouracil, furosemide, heparin, leucovorin, melphalan, methotrexate, metoclopramide, mitomycin, ondansetron, paclitaxel, sargramostim, vinblastine, vincristine, vinorelbine

Syringe compatibilities: Bleomycin, cyclophosphamide, doxapram, doxorubicin, droperidol, fluorouracil, furosemide, heparin, leucovorin, methotrexate, metoclopramide, mitomycin, vinblastine, vincristine

Additive compatibilities: Cyclophosphamide with etoposide, etoposide, etoposide with floxuridine, floxuridine, floxuridine with leucovorin calcium, hydroxyzine, ifosfamide, ifosfamide with etoposide, leucovorin, magnesium sulfate, mannitol

Solution compatibilities: D_5/0.225% NaCl, D_5/0.45% NaCl, D_5/0.9% NaCl, D_5/0.45% NaCl with mannitol 1.875%, D_5/0.33% NaCl with KCl 20 mEq and mannitol 1.875%, 0.9% NaCl, 0.45% NaCl, 0.3% NaCl, 0.225% NaCl, water

NURSING CONSIDERATIONS

Assess:
- CBC, differential, platelet count weekly; withhold drug if WBC is <4000 or platelet count is <75,000; notify prescriber of results
- Renal function studies: BUN, creatinine, serum uric acid, urine CrCl before, electrolytes during therapy
- I&O ratio; report fall in urine output of <30 ml/hr
- Monitor temperature q4h (may indicate beginning infection)
- Liver function tests before, during therapy (bilirubin, AST [SGOT], ALT [SGPT], LDH) as needed or monthly
- Bleeding: hematuria, guaiac, bruising or petechiae, mucosa or orifices q8h, obtain prescription for viscous lidocaine (Xylocaine)
- Dyspnea, rales, unproductive cough, chest pain, tachypnea
- Food preferences; list likes, dislikes
- Effects of alopecia on body image; discuss feelings about body changes
- Yellowing of skin, sclera; dark urine; clay-colored stools; itchy skin; abdominal pain; fever; diarrhea
- Edema in feet, joint pain, stomach pain, shaking
- Inflammation of mucosa, breaks in skin

Administer:
- IV after diluting 10 mg/10 ml or

* Available in Canada only

50 mg/50 ml sterile H_2O for inj; withdraw prescribed dose, dilute ½ dose with 1000 ml D_5 O.2 NaCl or D_5 O.45 NaCl with 37.5 g mannitol; IV INF is given over 3-4 hr; use a 0.45 μm filter; total dose 2 L over 6-8 hr; check site for irritation, phlebitis; do not use equipment containing aluminum

- Hydrate patient with 1-2 L fluids over 8-12 hr before treatment
- Epinephrine for hypersensitivity reaction
- Antiemetic 30-60 min before giving drug and prn
- Allopurinol or sodium bicarbonate to maintain uric acid levels, alkalinization of urine
- Antibiotics for prophylaxis of infection
- Diuretic (furosemide 40 mg IV) or mannitol after infusion

Perform/provide:

- Strict medical asepsis, protective isolation if WBC levels are low
- Comprehensive oral hygiene
- Storage protected from light in refrigerator (dry powder)
- Deep breathing exercises with patient tid-qid; place in semi-Fowler's position
- Increase fluid intake to 2-3 L/day to prevent urate deposits, calculi formation, elimination of drug
- Diet low in purines: organ meats (kidney, liver), dried beans, peas to maintain alkaline urine

Evaluate:

- Therapeutic response: decreased tumor size, spread of malignancy

Teach patient/family:

- To report signs of infection: increased temperature, sore throat, flu symptoms
- To report signs of anemia: fatigue, headache, faintness, shortness of breath, irritability
- To report bleeding: avoid use of razors, commercial mouthwash
- To avoid aspirin, ibuprofen
- About protective isolation
- To report any complaints or side effects to nurse or physician
- That impotence or amenorrhea can occur; reversible after discontinuing treatment
- To report any changes in breathing, coughing
- That hair may be lost during treatment; a wig or hairpiece may make patient feel better; new hair may be different in color, texture

cladribine (CdA) (℞)

(clay-dry'bine)

Leustatin

Func. class.: Antineoplastic antibiotic

Chem. class.: Purine nucleoside analog

Action: Phosphylated while passively crossing the cell membrane, causing cell death by not properly repairing single-strand DNA

Uses: Treatment of active hairy cell leukemia; may be useful in chronic lymphocytic leukemia, non-Hodgkin's lymphomas, acute myeloid leukemia, autoimmune hemolytic anemia

Dosage and routes:

Single daily dose

- *Adult:* IV 1 day × 0.09 mg/kg diluted with 0.9% NaCl 500 ml; give over 24 hr × 7 days

Seven-day infusion

- *Adult:* IV 7 days × 0.09 mg/kg diluted with 0.9% NaCl qs to 100 ml; pass through 0.22 microfilter

Available forms: Sol 1 mg/ml

Side effects/adverse reactions:

CNS: Headache, dizziness, insomnia

CV: Edema, tachycardia

GI: Nausea, vomiting, anorexia, diarrhea, constipation, abdominal pain
HEMA: ***Neutropenia, anemia, thrombocytopenia, bone marrow hypocellularity,*** purpura, epistaxis, petechia
INTEG: Rash, inj site reactions, pruritus
MS: Myalgia, arthralgia
RESP: Cough, upper respiratory infection, dyspnea, shortness of breath, abnormal chest sounds, pneumonia
SYST: Fever, infection, fatigue, pain, allergic reaction, chills, ***death, sepsis***

Contraindications: Hypersensitivity

Precautions: Renal disease, pregnancy (D), lactation, children, bone marrow depression, hepatic disease, neurologic disease

Pharmacokinetics:
IV: Terminal half-life 5.4 hr

NURSING CONSIDERATIONS

Assess:

- CBC, differential, platelet count weekly; withhold drug if WBC $<4000/mm^3$ or platelet count $<75{,}000/mm^3$; notify prescriber
- Renal function studies: BUN, serum uric acid, urine CrCl, electrolytes before, during therapy
- I&O ratio; report urine output <30 ml/hr
- Monitor temperature q4h; fever may indicate beginning infection
- Liver function tests before, during therapy: bilirubin, AST, ALT, alk phosphatase as needed or monthly
- Local irritation, pain, burning at injection site
- Symptoms indicating severe allergic reaction: rash, pruritus, urticaria, purpuric skin lesions, itching, flushing
- GI symptoms: frequency of stools, cramping

Administer:

- Antiemetic 30-60 min before giving drug to prevent vomiting
- Use gloves, gown to mix IV sol
- Use bacteriostatic (0.9% NaCl, 0.9% benzyl alcohol preserved) to prepare 7-day inf; pass both cladribine and diluent through sterile 0.22 μm hydrophilic syr filter as each sol is introduced into inf reservoir; add dose of cladribine to inf reservoir using filter, then bacteriostatic 0.9% NaCl to bring sol total to 100 ml; after preparation, clamp line, disconnect filter, discard; aspirate air bubbles (reservoir) using syr, dry filter or sterile vat filter assembly; reclamp line, discard filter and syr; infuse continuously × 7 days
- Add dose for single daily dose to inf bag (500 ml 0.9% NaCl); infuse continuously over 24 hr; repeat daily dose × 7 days
- Do not admix with other IV drugs or sol

Perform/provide:

- Hydrocortisone, sodium thiosulfate to infiltration area, ice compress after stopping inf
- Strict hand-washing technique, gloves, protective covering
- Liquid diet: carbonated beverages; gelatin may be added if patient is not nauseated or vomiting
- Storage in refrigerator; protect from light; reconstituted or diluted sol may be stored at room temp no longer than 8 hr; discard single-use vials of unused sol

Evaluate:

- Therapeutic response: decrease in symptoms of hairy cell leukemia

Teach patient/family:

- To report any complaints, side effects to nurse or prescriber
- To avoid crowds, sources of infection when granulocyte count low

clarithromycin (℞)

(klare-ith'row-my-sin)
Biaxin
Func. class.: Antibacterial
Chem. class.: Macrolide antibiotic

Action: Binds to 50S ribosomal subunits of susceptible bacteria and suppresses protein synthesis
Uses: Mild to moderate infections of the upper respiratory tract, lower respiratory tract, uncomplicated skin and skin structure infections caused by *S. pneumoniae, M. pneumoniae, L. pneumophilia, M. catarrhalis, N. gonorrhoeae, C. diphtheriae, L. monocytogenes, H. influenzae, S. pyogenes, S. aureus, M. avium* (mac), complex infection in AIDS patients
Dosage and routes:
• *Adult:* PO 250-500 mg bid for 7-14 days; 500 mg bid continues for *M. avium* (mac)
Available forms: Tabs 250, 500 mg
Side effects/adverse reactions:
INTEG: Rash, urticaria, pruritus
GI: Nausea, vomiting, diarrhea, ***hepatotoxicity,*** abdominal pain, stomatitis, heartburn, anorexia, abnormal taste
GU: Vaginitis, moniliasis
MISC: Headache
Contraindications: Hypersensitivity
Precautions: Pregnancy (C), lactation, hepatic, renal disease, elderly
Pharmacokinetics: Peak 2 hr, duration 12 hr, half-life 4-6 hr; metabolized by the liver; excreted in bile, feces
Interactions:
• Arrhythmias: terfenadine, astemizole
• Increased effects of oral anticoagulants, digoxin, theophylline, methylprednisolone, cyclosporine, bromocriptine, disopyramide, carbamazepine
• Decreased action: clindamycin
• Increased or decreased action: penicillins
Lab test interferences:
False increase: 17-OHCS/17-KS, AST, ALT
Decrease: Folate assay
NURSING CONSIDERATIONS
Assess:
• I&O ratio; report hematuria, oliguria in renal disease
• Liver studies: AST, ALT
• Renal studies: urinalysis, protein, blood
• C&S before drug therapy; drug may be given as soon as culture is taken; C&S may be repeated after treatment
• Bowel pattern before, during treatment
• Skin eruptions, itching
• Respiratory status: rate, character, wheezing, tightness in chest; discontinue drug
• Allergies before treatment, reaction of each medication; place allergies on chart in bright red, notify all people giving drugs
Administer:
• Adequate intake of fluids (2 L) during diarrhea episodes
Perform/provide:
• Storage at room temp
Evaluate:
• Therapeutic response: C&S negative for infection
Teach patient/family:
• To take with full glass H_2O; may give with food for GI symptoms
• To report sore throat, fever, fatigue; may indicate superinfection
• To notify nurse of diarrhea stools, dark urine, pale stools, yellow discoloration of eyes or skin, severe abdominal pain
• To take at evenly spaced intervals; complete dosage regimen

Treatment of hypersensitivity: Withdraw drug, maintain airway, administer epinephrine, aminophylline, O_2, IV corticosteroids

clemastine (℞)

(klem'as-teen)

Tavist, Tavist-1

Func. class.: Antihistamine

Chem. class.: Ethanolamine derivative, H_1-receptor antagonist

Action: Acts on blood vessels, GI, respiratory system by competing with histamine for H_1-receptor site; decreases allergic response by blocking histamine

Uses: Allergy symptoms, rhinitis, angioedema, urticaria

Dosage and routes:

• *Adult and child >12 yr:* PO 1.34-2.68 mg bid-tid, not to exceed 8.04 mg/day

Available forms: Tabs 1.34, 2.68 mg; syr 0.67 mg/ml

Side effects/adverse reactions:

CNS: *Dizziness, drowsiness,* poor coordination, fatigue, anxiety, euphoria, confusion, paresthesia, neuritis

CV: Hypotension, palpitations, tachycardia

RESP: Increased thick secretions, wheezing, chest tightness

HEMA: ***Thrombocytopenia, agranulocytosis, hemolytic anemia***

GI: *Constipation,* dry mouth, nausea, vomiting, anorexia, diarrhea

INTEG: Rash, urticaria, photosensitivity

GU: *Retention,* dysuria, frequency

EENT: Blurred vision, dilated pupils, tinnitus, nasal stuffiness, dry nose, throat, mouth

Contraindications: Hypersensitivity to H_1-receptor antagonists, acute asthma attack, lower respiratory tract disease

Precautions: Increased intraocular pressure, renal disease, cardiac disease, hypertension, bronchial asthma, seizure disorder, stenosed peptic ulcers, hyperthyroidism, prostatic hypertrophy, bladder neck obstruction, pregnancy (B), lactation, elderly

Pharmacokinetics:

PO: Peak 5-7 hr, duration 10-12 hr or more; metabolized in liver, excreted by kidneys

Interactions:

• Increased CNS depression: barbiturates, narcotics, hypnotics, tricyclic antidepressants, alcohol

• Decreased effect of oral anticoagulants, heparin

• Increased effect of clemastine: MAOIs

Lab test interferences:

False negative: Skin allergy tests

NURSING CONSIDERATIONS

Assess:

• I&O ratio; be alert for urinary retention, frequency, dysuria; drug should be discontinued

• CBC during long-term therapy

• Blood dyscrasias: thrombocytopenia, agranulocytosis (rare)

• Respiratory status: rate, rhythm, increase in bronchial secretions, wheezing, chest tightness

• Cardiac status: palpitations, increased pulse, hypotension

Administer:

• With meals for GI symptoms; absorption may slightly decrease

Perform/provide:

• Hard candy, gum, frequent rinsing of mouth for dryness

• Storage in tight container at room temp

Evaluate:

• Therapeutic response: absence of running or congested nose or rashes

Teach patient/family:
- All aspects of drug use; to notify prescriber of confusion, sedation, hypotension
- To avoid driving, other hazardous activity if drowsiness occurs
- To avoid concurrent use of alcohol, other CNS depressants
- That drug decreases anticoagulant (oral) effect
- To change position slowly, as drug may cause dizziness, hypotension (elderly)

Treatment of overdose: Administer ipecac syrup or lavage, diazepam, vasopressors, barbiturates (short-acting)

clidinium (℞)

(kli-di'nee-um)

Quarzan

Func. class.: GI anticholinergic

Chem. class.: Synthetic quaternary ammonium antimuscarinic

Combination products: Clindex, Clinoxide, Clipoxide, Librax, Lidox, Lidoxide: clidinium bromide 2.5 mg with chlordiazepoxide HCl 5 mg

Action: Inhibits muscarinic actions of acetylcholine at postganglionic parasympathetic neuroeffector sites

Uses: Treatment of peptic ulcer disease in combination with other drugs

Dosage and routes:
- *Adult:* PO 2.5-5 mg tid-qid ac, hs
- *Elderly:* PO 2.5 mg tid ac

Available forms: Caps 2.5, 5 mg

Side effects/adverse reactions:

CNS: Confusion, stimulation in elderly, headache, insomnia, dizziness, drowsiness, anxiety, weakness, hallucination

GI: Dry mouth, constipation, ***paralytic ileus,*** heartburn, nausea, vomiting, dysphagia, absence of taste

GU: Hesitancy, retention, impotence

CV: Palpitations, tachycardia

EENT: Blurred vision, photophobia, mydriasis, cycloplegia, increased ocular tension

INTEG: Urticaria, rash, pruritus, anhidrosis, fever, allergic reactions

Contraindications: Hypersensitivity to anticholinergics, narrow-angle glaucoma, GI obstruction, myasthenia gravis, paralytic ileus, GI atony, toxic megacolon

Precautions: Hyperthyroidism, coronary artery disease, dysrhythmias, CHF, ulcerative colitis, hypertension, hiatal hernia, hepatic disease, renal disease, pregnancy (C), lactation, urinary retention, prostatic hypertrophy, elderly

Pharmacokinetics:

PO: Onset 1 hr, duration 3 hr; ionized, excreted in urine

Interactions:
- Increased anticholinergic effect: amantadine, tricyclic antidepressants, MAOIs
- Decreased effect of phenothiazines, levodopa, ketoconazole

NURSING CONSIDERATIONS

Assess:
- VS, cardiac status: dysrhythmias, increased rate, palpitations
- I&O ratio; urinary retention or hesitancy, especially elderly
- GI complaints: pain, bleeding (frank or occult), nausea, vomiting, anorexia

Administer:
- ½-1 hr ac for better absorption
- Decreased dose to elderly patients, since their metabolism may be slowed
- Gum, hard candy, frequent rinsing of mouth for dryness of oral cavity

Perform/provide:
- Storage in tight container protected from light
- Increased fluids, bulk, exercise to decrease constipation

Evaluate:
• Therapeutic response: absence of epigastric pain, bleeding, nausea, vomiting

Teach patient/family:
• To avoid driving, other hazardous activities until stabilized on medication
• To avoid alcohol, other CNS depressants; will enhance sedating properties of this drug
• To avoid hot environments; stroke may occur, drug suppresses perspiration
• To use sunglasses when outside to prevent photophobia, may cause blurred vision
• To drink plenty of fluids
• To report dysphagia

---

clindamycin (℞)

(klin-da-mye'sin)
Cleocin HCl, Clindamycin HCl, Dalacin C*/Cleocin Pediatric/ Cleocin Phosphate, Clindamycin Phosphate

Func. class.: Antibacterial

Chem. class.: Lincomycin derivative

Action: Binds to 50S subunit of bacterial ribosomes, suppresses protein synthesis

Uses: Infections caused by staphylococci, streptococci, pneumococci, *Rickettsia, Fusobacterium, Actinomyces, Peptococcus, Bacteroides*

Dosage and routes:
• *Adults:* PO 150-450 mg q6h; IM/IV 300-900 mg q6-12h, not to exceed 4800 mg/day
• *Child >1 mo:* PO 8-25 mg/kg/day in divided doses q6-8h; IM/IV 15-40 mg/kg/day in divided doses q6-8h (3-4 equal doses)
• *PID:* Adult IV 600 mg qid plus gentamicin

Available forms: Inj 150-300 mg/ml; caps 75, 150-300 mg; oral sol 75 mg/ml

Side effects/adverse reactions:
HEMA: ***Leukopenia, eosinophilia, agranulocytosis, thrombocytopenia, polyarthritis***
GI: Nausea, vomiting, abdominal pain, diarrhea, ***pseudomembranous colitis,*** anorexia, weight loss
GU: Increased AST, ALT, bilirubin, alk phosphatase, jaundice, *vaginitis,* urinary frequency
EENT: Rash, urticaria, pruritus, erythema, pain, abscess at injection site

Contraindications: Hypersensitivity to this drug or lincomycin, ulcerative colitis/enteritis, infants <1 mo

Precautions: Renal disease, liver disease, GI disease, elderly, pregnancy (B), lactation, tartrazine sensitivity

Pharmacokinetics:
PO: Peak 45 min, duration 6 hr
IM: Peak 3 hr, duration 8-12 hr
Half-life 2½ hr; metabolized in liver; excreted in urine, bile, feces as active/inactive metabolites; crosses placenta; excreted in breast milk

Interactions:
• Increased neuromuscular blockade: nondepolarizing muscle relaxants

Syringe compatibilities: Amikacin, aztreonam, gentamicin, heparin

Y-site compatibilities: Cyclophosphamide, enalaprilat, esmolol, foscarnet, hydromorphone, labetolol, magnesium sulfate, melphalan, meperidine, morphine, multivitamins, odansetron, perphenazine, vinorelbine, zidovudine

Lab test interferences:
Increase: Alk phosphatase, bilirubin, CPK, AST (SGOT), ALT (SGPT)

---

* Available in Canada only

NURSING CONSIDERATIONS

Assess:

- Liver studies: AST (SGOT), ALT (SGPT)
- Blood studies: WBC, RBC, Hct, Hgb, platelets, serum iron, reticulocytes; drug should be discontinued if bone marrow depression occurs
- Renal studies: urinalysis, protein, blood, BUN, creatinine
- C&S before drug therapy; drug may be given as soon as culture is taken
- B/P, pulse in patient receiving drug parenterally
- Bowel pattern before, during treatment; if severe diarrhea occurs, drug should be discontinued; may indicate pseudomembranous colitis
- Skin eruptions, itching, dermatitis after administration
- Respiratory status: rate, character, wheezing, tightness in chest
- Allergies before treatment, reaction of each medication; place allergies on chart in bright red letters; notify all people giving drugs

Administer:

- IV by infusion only; do not administer bolus dose; dilute 300 mg or less/50 ml or more of D_5W, NS; may be further diluted in greater amounts of D_5W, NS and given as a cont inf in acute PID; give first dose 10 mg/min over ½ hr, then 0.75 mg/min; increased rates may be used to keep serum blood levels higher; run over >10 min; no more than 1200 mg in a single 1-hr inf
- IM deep injection; rotate sites
- Orally with at least 8 oz H_2O

Perform/provide:

- Storage at room temp (caps) up to 2 wk (reconstituted)
- Epinephrine, suction, tracheostomy set, endotracheal intubation equipment on unit
- Adequate intake of fluids (2 L) during diarrhea episodes

Evaluate:

- Therapeutic response: decreased temperature, negative C&S

Teach patient/family:

- To take oral drug with full glass H_2O; may give with food for GI symptoms; antiperistaltic drugs may worsen diarrhea
- Aspects of drug therapy: need to complete entire course of medication to ensure organism death (10-14 days); culture may be taken after completed medication course
- To report sore throat, fever, fatigue; may indicate superinfection
- That drug must be taken in equal intervals around clock to maintain blood levels
- To notify nurse or prescriber of diarrhea

Treatment of hypersensitivity: Withdraw drug; maintain airway; administer epinephrine, aminophylline, O_2, IV corticosteroids

clioquinol (OTC)

(klee-oh-kwee'nole)

Vioform

Func. class.: Local antifungal

Chem. class.: Halogenated hydroxyquinoline

Action: Increases cell membrane permeability in susceptible organisms by binding sterols; decreases potassium, sodium, and nutrients in cell

Uses: Cutaneous infections: athlete's foot, eczema, ringworm, other fungal infections

Dosage and routes:

TOP: apply to affected area bid or tid × 7 days only

Available forms: cream, oint 3%

Side effects/adverse reactions:

INTEG: Rash, urticaria, stinging,

burning, dry skin, pruritus, contact dermatitis, erythema, redness, staining of hair and skin

Contraindications: Hypersensitivity to iodine, chloroxine

Precautions: Pregnancy (C), varicella, viral skin conditions, deep or puncture wounds, serious burns, children

Pharmacokinetics: Some absorbed through the skin, excreted in urine (conjugated form), the rest excreted slowly

Lab test interference:

Interference: Thyroid function tests

NURSING CONSIDERATIONS

Assess:

- Allergic reaction: burning, stinging, swelling, redness

Administer:

- Enough medication to cover lesions completely
- After cleansing with soap and water before application; dry well

Perform/provide:

- Storage at room temperature in dry place

Evaluate:

- Therapeutic response: decrease in size, number of lesions

Teach patient/family:

- To avoid use of OTC creams, ointments, lotions unless directed by prescriber
- To use medical asepsis (hand washing) before, after each application to prevent further infection
- Not to cover with occlusive dressing
- To continue even if condition improves
- That drug may stain clothing, skin, hair

clobetasol (℞)

(klo-bet′a-sol)

Temovate

Func. class.: Topical corticosteroid

Chem. class.: Synthetic fluorinated agent, group I potency

Action: Antipruritic, antiinflammatory

Uses: Psoriasis, eczema, contact dermatitis, pruritus; usually reserved for severe dermatoses that have not responded to less potent formulation

Dosage and routes:

- *Adult and child:* Apply to affected area bid

Available forms: Oint 0.05%; cream 0.05%

Side effects/adverse reactions:

INTEG: Burning, dryness, itching, irritation, acne, folliculitis, hypertrichosis, perioral dermatitis, hypopigmentation, atrophy, striae, miliaria, allergic contact dermatitis, secondary infection

Contraindications: Hypersensitivity to corticosteroids, fungal infections

Precautions: Pregnancy (C), lactation, viral, bacterial infections

NURSING CONSIDERATIONS

Assess:

- Temp; if fever develops, drug should be discontinued
- For systemic absorption: increased temp, inflammation, irritation

Administer:

- Only to affected areas; do not get in eyes
- Leaving uncovered or lightly covered; occlusive dressing not recommended; systemic absorption may occur
- Only to dermatoses; do not use on weeping, denuded, or infected area

* Available in Canada only

Perform/provide:
- Cleansing before application
- Treatment for a few days after area has cleared
- Storage at room temperature

Evaluate:
- Therapeutic response: absence of severe itching, patches on skin, flaking

Teach patient/family:
- To avoid sunlight on affected area; burns may occur
- To limit treatment to 14 days using <50 g/wk

clocortolone (℞)

(klo-kort′o-lone)

Cloderm

Func. class.: Topical corticosteroid

Chem. class.: Synthetic fluorinated agent, group IV potency

Action: Antipruritic, antiinflammatory

Uses: Psoriasis, eczema, contact dermatitis, pruritus

Dosage and routes:
- *Adult and child:* Apply to affected area tid or qid

Available forms: Cream 0.1%

Side effects/adverse reactions:

INTEG: Burning, dryness, itching, irritation, acne, folliculitis, hypertrichosis, perioral dermatitis, hypopigmentation, atrophy, striae, miliaria, allergic contact dermatitis, secondary infection

Contraindications: Hypersensitivity to corticosteroids, fungal infections

Precautions: Pregnancy (C), lactation, viral, bacterial infections

NURSING CONSIDERATIONS

Assess:
- Temp; if fever develops, drug should be discontinued
- For systemic absorption: increased temp, inflammation, irritation

Administer:
- Only to affected areas; do not get in eyes
- Medication, then cover with occlusive dressing (only if prescribed), seal to normal skin, change q12h; systemic absorption may occur
- Only to dermatoses; do not use on weeping, denuded, or infected area

Perform/provide:
- Cleansing before application of drug
- Treatment for a few days after area has cleared
- Storage at room temperature

Evaluate:
- Therapeutic response: absence of severe itching, patches on skin, flaking

Teach patient/family:
- To avoid sunlight on affected area; burns may occur

clofazimine (℞)

(kloe-fa′zi-meen)

Lamprene

Func. class.: Leprostatic

Action: Inhibits mycobacterial growth, binds to mycobacterial DNA; exerts antiinflammatory properties in controlling leprosy reactions

Uses: Lepromatous leprosy, dapsone-resistant leprosy, lepromatous leprosy complicated by erythema nodosum leprosum

Dosage and routes:

Erythema nodosum leprosum
- *Adult:* PO: 100-200 mg qd × 3 mo, then taper dosage to 100 mg when disease is controlled; do not exceed 200 mg/day

Dapsone-resistant leprosy
- *Adult:* PO: 100 mg/day in combination with at least one other an-

tileprosy drug × 3 yr, then 100 mg qd clofazimine (only)
Available forms: Caps 50, 100 mg
Side effects/adverse reactions:
GI: Diarrhea, nausea, vomiting, abdominal pain, intolerance, ***GI bleeding, obstruction,*** anorexia, constipation, ***hepatitis,*** jaundice
EENT: Pigmentation of cornea, conjunctiva, drying, burning, itching, irritation
INTEG: Pink or brown discoloration, dryness, pruritus, rash, photosensitivity, acne, monilial cheilosis
CNS: Dizziness, headache, fatigue, drowsiness
MISC: Discolored urine, feces, sputum, sweat
Precautions: Pregnancy (C), lactation, children, abdominal pain, diarrhea, depression
Pharmacokinetics: Deposited in fatty tissue, reticuloendothelial system; half-life 70 days; small amount excreted in feces, sputum, sweat
Lab test interferences:
Increase: Albumin, bilirubin, AST (SGPT), eosinophilia, hypokalemia
NURSING CONSIDERATIONS
Assess:
• Liver studies qwk: ALT (SGOT), AST (SGPT), bilirubin
• Renal studies: BUN, creatinine, I&O, specific gravity, urinalysis before; qmo
• Blood level of drug
• Mental status often: affect, mood, behavioral changes; psychosis may occur
• Hepatic status: decreased appetite, jaundice, dark urine, fatigue
Administer:
• With meals to decrease GI symptoms
• Antiemetic if vomiting occurs
• After C&S is completed; qmo to detect resistance
Perform/provide:
• Infants to be kept with mother infected with leprosy; breastfeeding during drug therapy is encouraged
Evaluate:
• Therapeutic response: decreased symptoms of infection
Teach patient/family:
• That therapeutic effects may occur after 3-6 mo of drug therapy
• That compliance with dosage schedule, length is necessary
• That scheduled appointments must be kept or relapse may occur
• That drug must be taken with meals
• Skin, sweat, sputum, urine, feces discoloration, although reversible, may take several months or years to disappear

---

clofibrate (℞)

(kloe-fye'brate)
Atromid-S, Claripen*, Claripex*, Clofibrate
Func. class.: Antilipemic
Chem. class.: Aryloxisobutyric acid derivative

Action: Inhibits biosynthesis of VLDL, LDL, which are responsible for triglyceride development, mobilizes triglycerides from tissue, increases excretion of neutral sterols
Uses: Hyperlipidemia; xanthoma tuberosum; types III, IV, V hyperlipidemia
Dosage and routes:
• *Adult:* PO 2 g/day in 4 divided doses
Available forms: Caps 500 mg
Side effects/adverse reactions:
GI: Nausea, vomiting, dyspepsia, increased liver enzymes, stomatitis, flatulence, hepatomegaly, gastritis, increased cholelithiasis, weight gain
INTEG: Rash, urticaria, pruritus, dry hair and skin, alopecia

---

* Available in Canada only

HEMA: ***Leukopenia,*** anemia, ***eosinophilia,*** bleeding
CNS: Fatigue, weakness, drowsiness, dizziness
GU: Decreased libido, impotence, dysuria, proteinuria, oliguria, ***hematuria***
MS: Myalgias, arthralgias
CV: Angina, dysrhythmias, thrombophlebitis, ***pulmonary emboli***
MISC: Polyphagia, weight gain
Contraindications: Severe hepatic disease, severe renal disease, primary biliary cirrhosis
Precautions: Peptic ulcer, pregnancy (C), lactation
Pharmacokinetics:
PO: Peak 2-6 hr, plasma protein binding >90%; half-life 6-25 hr, excreted in urine, metabolized in liver
Interactions:
- Increased effects of sulfonylureas, insulin
- Increased toxicity of clofibrate: probenecid
- Increased anticoagulant effects: oral anticoagulants
- Decreased effects of clofibrate: rifampin

Lab test interferences:
Increase: Liver function studies, CPK, BSP, thymol turbidity

NURSING CONSIDERATIONS
Assess:
- Renal and hepatic levels (long-term therapy)
- Bowel pattern daily; increase bulk, water in diet for constipation

Administer:
- Drug with meals if GI symptoms occur

Evaluate:
- Therapeutic response: decreased triglycerides, diarrhea, pruritus (excess bile acids)

Teach patient/family:
- That compliance is needed, since toxicity may result if doses are missed
- That risk factors should be decreased: high-fat diet, smoking, alcohol consumption, absence of exercise
- That birth control should be practiced while on this drug
- To report GU symptoms: decreased libido, impotence, dysuria, proteinuria, oliguria, hematuria

clomiphene (℞)

(kloe'mi-feen)
Clomid, clomiphene citrate, Milophene, Serophene
Func. class.: Ovulation stimulant
Chem. class.: Nonsteroidal antiestrogenic

Action: Increases LH, FSH release from the pituitary, which increase maturation of ovarian follicle, ovulation, development of corpus luteum
Uses: Female infertility (ovulatory failure)
Dosage and routes:
- *Adult:* PO 50-100 mg qd × 5 days or 50-100 mg qd beginning on day 5 of cycle; may be repeated until conception occurs or 3 cycles of therapy have been completed

Available forms: Tabs 50 mg
Side effects/adverse reactions:
CV: Vasomotor flushing, phlebitis, deep-vein thrombosis
EENT: Blurred vision, diplopia, photophobia
CNS: Headache, depression, restlessness, anxiety, nervousness, fatigue, insomnia, dizziness, flushing
GI: Nausea, vomiting, constipation, abdominal pain, bloating
INTEG: Rash, dermatitis, urticaria, alopecia
GU: Polyuria, frequency, birth defects, spontaneous abortions, mul-

tiple ovulation, breast pain, oliguria, abnormal uterine bleeding
Contraindications: Hypersensitivity, pregnancy (X), hepatic disease, undiagnosed uterine bleeding, uncontrolled thyroid or adrenal dysfunction, intracranial lesion, ovarian cysts
Precautions: Hypertension, depression, convulsions, diabetes mellitus
Pharmacokinetics: Metabolized in liver, excreted in feces
Lab test interferences:
Increase: FSH/LH, BSP, thyroxine, TBG

NURSING CONSIDERATIONS

Administer:
• After discontinuing estrogen therapy
• At same time qd to maintain drug level

Evaluate:
• Therapeutic response: fertility

Teach patient/family:
• That multiple births are common
• To notify prescriber if low abdominal pain occurs; may indicate ovarian cyst, cyst rupture
• If dose is missed, double at next time; if more than one dose is missed, call prescriber
• That response usually occurs 4-10 days after last day of treatment
• Method for taking, recording basal body temp to determine whether ovulation has occurred
• If ovulation can be determined (there is a slight decrease in temp, then a sharp increase for ovulation), to attempt coitus 3 days before and qod until after ovulation
• If pregnancy is suspected, to notify prescriber immediately

clomipramine (℞)
(kloe-mip′ra-meen)
Anafranil
Func. class.: Antipsychotic
Chem. class.: Tertiary amine

Action: Not known. Potent inhibitor of serotonin uptake; also increases dopamine metabolism
Uses: Depression, dysphoria, phobias, anxiety, agoraphobia, obsessive-compulsive disorder
Dosage and routes:
Obsessive-compulsive disorder
• *Adult:* PO 25 mg hs and increase gradually over 4 wk to 75-300 mg/day in divided doses
• *Child (10-18 yr):* PO 25-50 mg/day gradually increased; not to exceed 200 mg/day
Depression
• *Adult:* PO 50-150 mg/day in a single or divided dose
Anxiety/agoraphobia
• *Adult:* PO 25-75 mg/day
Available forms: Caps 25, 50, 75 mg
Side effects/adverse reactions:
HEMA: ***Agranulocytosis, neutropenia, pancytopenia***
CV: Hypotension, tachycardia, ***cardiac arrest***
CNS: Dizziness, tremors, mania, ***seizures,*** aggressiveness, EPS
ENDO: Galactorrhea, hyperprolactinemia
META: Hyponatremia
GI: Constipation, dry mouth, nausea, dyspepsia
GU: Delayed ejaculation, anorgasmy, retention
INTEG: Diaphoresis, photosensitivity
Contraindications: Hypersensitivity
Precautions: Seizures, suicidal patients, elderly, pregnancy (C), lactation

Pharmacokinetics: Extensively bound to tissue and plasma proteins; demethylated in liver; active metabolites excreted in urine; half-life: 21 hr parent compound, 36 hr metabolite

Interactions:
• Hypotensive antagonism: bethanidine
• Toxicity: phenothiazines, cimetidine
• Ethanol reaction: disulfiram, guanadrel increased or decreased effects
• Increased or decreased effects of clomipramine: estrogens
• Delirium: ethchlorvynol
• Hypertensive crisis, convulsions, hypertensive episode: MAOIs
• Decreased seizure threshold: phenytoin, phenobarbital

Lab test interferences:
Increase: Prolactin, TBG
Decrease: Serum thyroid hormone

NURSING CONSIDERATIONS

Assess:
• B/P (lying, standing), pulse q4h; if systolic B/P drops 20 mm Hg, withhold drug, notify prescriber; take vital signs q4h in patients with cardiovascular disease
• Blood studies: CBC, leukocytes, differential, cardiac enzymes if patient is receiving long-term therapy
• Hepatic studies: AST (SGOT), ALT (SGPT), bilirubin
• Mental status: mood, sensorium, affect, suicidal tendencies; increase in psychiatric symptoms: depression, panic
• Urinary retention, constipation; constipation more likely in children
• Withdrawal symptoms: headache, nausea, vomiting, muscle pain, weakness; not usual unless drug discontinued abruptly
• Alcohol consumption; if alcohol consumed, withhold dose until AM

Administer:
• Increased fluids, bulk in diet for constipation, especially elderly
• With food or milk for GI symptoms
• Gum, hard candy, or frequent sips of water for dry mouth

Perform/provide:
• Storage in tight container at room temp; do not freeze
• Assistance with ambulation during beginning therapy, since drowsiness/dizziness occurs
• Safety measures, including side rails, primarily in elderly
• Checking to see PO medication swallowed

Evaluate:
• Therapeutic response: decreased anxiety, depression

Teach patient/family:
• That the effects may take 2-3 wk
• To use caution in driving, other activities requiring alertness because of drowsiness, dizziness, blurred vision
• To avoid alcohol ingestion, other CNS depressants
• Not to discontinue medication quickly after long-term use; may cause nausea, headache, malaise
• To wear sunscreen, protective clothing to prevent photosensitivity

Treatment of overdose: ECG monitoring; induce emesis; lavage, activated charcoal; anticonvulsant

clonazepam (℞)

(kloe-na'zi-pam)
Klonopin, Rivoiril
Func. class.: Anticonvulsant
Chem. class.: Benzodiazepine derivative

Controlled Substance Schedule IV

Action: Inhibits spike, wave formation in absence seizures (petit mal), decreases amplitude, frequency, duration, spread of discharge in minor motor seizures

Uses: Absence, atypical absence, akinetic, myoclonic seizures

Dosage and routes:

• *Adult:* PO Not to exceed 1.5 mg/day in 3 divided doses; may be increased 0.5-1 mg q3 days until desired response, not to exceed 20 mg/day

• *Child <10 yr or 30 kg:* PO 0.01-0.03 mg/kg/day in divided doses q8h, not to exceed 0.05 mg/kg/day; may be increased 0.25-0.5 mg q3d until desired response, not to exceed 0.1-0.2 mg/kg/day

Available forms: Tabs 0.5, 1, 2 mg

Side effects/adverse reactions:

HEMA: ***Thrombocytopenia, leukocytosis, eosinophilia***

CNS: Drowsiness, dizziness, confusion, behavioral changes, tremors, insomnia, headache, suicidal tendencies, slurred speech

GI: Nausea, constipation, polyphagia, anorexia, xerostomia, diarrhea, gastritis, sore gums

INTEG: Rash, alopecia, hirsutism

EENT: Increased salivation, nystagmus, diplopia, abnormal eye movements

RESP: ***Respiratory depression,*** dyspnea, congestion

CV: Palpitations, bradycardia

GU: Dysuria, enuresis, nocturia, retention

Contraindications: Hypersensitivity to benzodiazepines, acute narrow-angle glaucoma

Precautions: Open-angle glaucoma, chronic respiratory disease, pregnancy (C), lactation, renal, hepatic disease, elderly

Pharmacokinetics:

PO: Peak 1-2 hr; metabolized by liver; excreted in urine; half-life 18-50 hr

Interactions:

• Increased CNS depression: alcohol, barbiturates, narcotics, antidepressants, other anticonvulsants, general anesthetics, hypnotics, sedatives

• Decreased effect of carbamazepine

• Seizures: valproic acid

Lab test interferences:

Increase: AST (SGPT), alk phosphatase

NURSING CONSIDERATIONS

Assess:

• Renal studies: urinalysis, BUN, urine creatinine

• Blood studies: RBC, Hct, Hgb, reticulocyte counts qwk for 4 wk, then qmo

• Hepatic studies: ALT (SGOT), AST (SGPT), bilirubin, creatinine

• Drug levels during initial treatment (therapeutic 20-80 mg/ml)

• Signs of physical withdrawal if medication suddenly discontinued

• Mental status: mood, sensorium, affect, oversedation, behavioral changes; if mental status changes, notify prescriber

• Eye problems: need for ophthalmic exam before, during, after treatment (slit lamp, fundoscopy, tonometry)

• Allergic reaction: red raised rash; drug should be discontinued

• Blood dyscrasias: fever, sore throat, bruising, rash, jaundice

• Toxicity: bone marrow depression, nausea, vomiting, ataxia, diplopia, cardiovascular collapse

Administer:

• With food, milk for GI symptoms

Perform/provide:

• Storage at room temperature

• Assistance with ambulation during early part of treatment; dizziness occurs, especially elderly

Evaluate:

• Therapeutic response: decreased seizure activity, document on patient's chart

Teach patient/family:
• To carry ID card or Medic Alert bracelet stating name, drugs taken, condition, prescriber's name, phone number
• To avoid driving, other activities that require alertness
• To avoid alcohol ingestion, CNS depressants; increased sedation may occur
• Not to discontinue medication quickly after long-term use; taper off over several weeks

Treatment of overdose: Lavage, activated charcoal, monitor electrolytes, VS, administer vasopressors

clonidine (℞)

(klon'i-deen)

Catapres, Catapress-TTS, clonidine HCl, Dixarit*

Func. class.: Antihypertensive

Chem. class.: Central α-adrenergic agonist

Combination products: Combipres 0.1 mg: clonidine HCl 0.1 mg with chlorthalidone 15 mg; Combipres 0.2 mg: clonidine HCl 0.2 mg with chlorthalidone 15 mg

Action: Inhibits sympathetic vasomotor center in CNS, which reduces impulses in sympathetic nervous system; blood pressure, pulse rate, cardiac output decrease

Uses: Mild to moderate hypertension, used alone or in combination

Investigational uses: Narcotic withdrawal, prevention of vascular headaches, treatment of menopausal symptoms, dysmenorrhea, attention deficit disorder

Dosage and routes:

Hypertension
• *Adult:* PO/TRANS 0.1 mg bid, then increase by 0.1 mg/day or 0.2 mg/day until desired response; range 0.2-0.8 mg/day in divided doses

Opioid withdrawal
Adult: PO 0.3-1.2 mg/day; decreased dosage given over several days

Available forms: Tabs 0.1, 0.2, 0.3 mg; trans sys 2.5, 5, 7.5 mg delivering 0.1, 0.2, 0.3 mg/24 hr, respectively

Side effects/adverse reactions:
CNS: Drowsiness, sedation, headache, fatigue, nightmares, insomnia, mental changes, anxiety, depression, hallucinations, delirium
CV: Orthostatic hypotension, palpitations, ***CHF;*** ECG abnormalities
EENT: Taste change, parotid pain
ENDO: Hyperglycemia
GI: Nausea, vomiting, malaise, constipation, dry mouth
GU: Impotence, dysuria, *nocturia,* gynecomastia
INTEG: Rash, alopecia, facial pallor, pruritus, hives, edema, burning papules, excoriation (transdermal patches)
MS: Muscle, joint pain; leg cramps

Contraindications: Hypersensitivity

Precautions: MI (recent), diabetes mellitus, chronic renal failure, Raynaud's disease, thyroid disease, depression, COPD, child <12 (patches), asthma, pregnancy (C), lactation, elderly

Pharmacokinetics: Absorbed well
PO: Onset ½ to 1 hr, peak 2-4 hr, duration 8 hr; half-life 12-16 hr
TOP: Onset 3 days, duration 1 wk; metabolized by liver (metabolites), excreted in urine (30% unchanged, inactive metabolites, feces), crosses blood-brain barrier, excreted in breast milk

Interactions:
• Increased CNS depression: narcotics, sedatives, hypnotics, anesthetics, alcohol

• Decreased hypotensive effects: tricyclic antidepressants, MAOIs, appetite suppressants, amphetamines
• Increased hypotensive effects: diuretics, other antihypertensive nitrates
• Increased bradycardia: β-blockers, cardiac glycosides

Lab test interferences:
Increase: Blood glucose
Decrease: VMA, catecholamines aldosterone

NURSING CONSIDERATIONS

Assess:
• Blood studies: neutrophils, decreased platelets
• Renal studies: protein, BUN, creatinine; increased levels may indicate nephrotic syndrome
• Baselines in renal, liver function tests before therapy begins; K levels, although hyperkalemia rare
• Dipstick of urine for protein qd in first morning specimen; if protein is increased, a 24-hr urinary protein should be collected
• B/P, pulse if used for hypertension
• For narcotic withdrawal including fever, diarrhea, nausea, vomiting, cramps, insomnia, shivering, dilated pupils
• Edema in feet, legs daily; monitor I&O; check for falling output
• Allergic reaction: rash, fever, pruritus, urticaria; drug should be discontinued if antihistamines fail to help
• Allergic reaction from patches: rash, urticaria, angioedema; should not continue to use
• Symptoms of CHF: edema, dyspnea, wet rales, B/P
• Renal symptoms: polyuria, oliguria, frequency
• For retinal degeneration: periodic eye exam

Administer:
• IV infusion of 0.9% NaCl (as ordered) to expand fluid volume if severe hypotension occurs
• SL if patient is unable to swallow
• PO: give last dose at hs
• Topical patch q/wk; apply to site without hair; best absorption over chest or upper arm; rotate sides with each application; clean site before application; apply firmly, especially around edges

Perform/provide:
• Storage of patches in cool environment, tablets in tight container

Evaluate:
• Therapeutic response: decrease in B/P in hypertension, decrease in withdrawal symptoms (narcotic)

Teach patient/family:
• To avoid hazardous activities, since drug may cause drowsiness
• To administer 1 hr before meals
• Not to discontinue drug abruptly, or withdrawal symptoms may occur: anxiety, increased B/P, headache, insomnia, increased pulse, tremors, nausea, sweating
• Not to use OTC (cough, cold, or allergy) products unless directed by prescriber
• To avoid sunlight, wear sunscreen; photosensitivity may occur
• To comply with dosage schedule even if feeling better
• To rise slowly to sitting or standing position to minimize orthostatic hypotension, especially elderly
• To notify prescriber of mouth sores, sore throat, fever, swelling of hands, feet, irregular heartbeat, chest pain, signs of angioedema
• About excessive perspiration, dehydration, vomiting; diarrhea may lead to fall in blood pressure; consult prescriber if these occur
• That drug may cause dizziness, fainting; light-headedness may occur during 1st few days of therapy
• That drug may cause dry mouth;

use hard candy, saliva product, or frequent rinsing of mouth
• That compliance is necessary; not to skip or stop drug unless directed by prescriber
• That drug may cause skin rash or impaired perspiration
• That response may take 2-3 days if drug is given transdermally; instruct on administration of patch
Treatment of overdose: Supportive treatment; administer tolazoline, atropine, dopamine prn

clorazepate (℞)

(klor-az'e-pate)
clorazepate dipotassium, Gen-Xene, Novoclopate*, Tranxene, Tranxene-SD, Tranxene-SD Half Strength
Func. class.: Antianxiety
Chem. class.: Benzodiazepine

Controlled Substance Schedule IV
Action: Potentiates the actions of GABA, especially in limbic system, reticular formation
Uses: Anxiety, acute alcohol withdrawal, adjunct in seizure disorders
Dosage and routes:
Anxiety
• *Adult:* PO 15-60 mg/day
Alcohol withdrawal
• *Adult:* PO 30 mg then 30-60 mg in divided doses; day 2, 45-90 mg in divided doses; day 3, 22.5-45 mg in divided doses; day 4, 15-30 mg in divided doses; then reduce daily dose to 7.5-15 mg
Seizure disorders
• *Adult and child >12 yr:* PO 7.5 mg tid; may increase by 7.5 mg/wk or less, not to exceed 90 mg/day
• *Child 9-12 yr:* PO 7.5 mg bid; may increase by 7.5 mg/wk or less, not to exceed 60 mg/day

Available forms: Caps 3.75, 7.5, 15 mg; tabs 3.75, 7.5, 15 mg, single-dose tab 11.25, 22.5 mg
Side effects/adverse reactions:
CNS: Dizziness, drowsiness, confusion, headache, anxiety, tremors, stimulation, fatigue, depression, insomnia, hallucinations, lethargy
GI: Constipation, dry mouth, nausea, vomiting, anorexia, diarrhea
INTEG: Rash, dermatitis, itching
CV: Orthostatic hypotension, ***ECG changes, tachycardia,*** hypotension
EENT: Blurred vision, tinnitus, mydriasis
Contraindications: Hypersensitivity to benzodiazepines, narrow-angle glaucoma, psychosis, pregnancy (D), lactation, child <18 yr
Precautions: Elderly, debilitated, hepatic disease, renal disease
Pharmacokinetics:
PO: Onset 15 min, peak 1-2 hr, duration 4-6 hr; metabolized by liver, excreted by kidneys; crosses placenta, breast milk; half-life 30-100 hr
Interactions:
• Decreased effects of clorazepate: valproic acid
• Increased effects of clorazepate: CNS depressants, alcohol, disulfiram, oral contraceptives, antidepressants, MAOIs, cimetidine
Lab test interferences:
Increase: AST (SGOT), ALT (SGPT), serum bilirubin
Decrease: RAIU
False increase: 17-OHCS
NURSING CONSIDERATIONS
Assess:
• B/P (lying, standing), pulse; if systolic B/P drops 20 mm Hg, hold drug, notify prescriber
• Blood studies: CBC during long-term therapy; blood dyscrasias have occurred rarely

• Hepatic studies: AST (SGOT), ALT (SGPT), bilirubin, creatinine, LDH, alk phosphatase
• I&O; may indicate renal dysfunction
• Mental status: mood, sensorium, affect, sleeping pattern, drowsiness, dizziness
• Physical dependency, withdrawal symptoms: headache, nausea, vomiting, muscle pain, weakness after long-term use
• Suicidal tendencies

Administer:
• With food, milk for GI symptoms
• Crushed if patient cannot swallow whole
• Sugarless gum, hard candy, frequent sips of water for dry mouth

Perform/provide:
• Assistance with ambulation during beginning therapy, for drowsiness/dizziness, especially elderly
• Safety measures, including side rails
• Check to see PO medication has been swallowed

Evaluate:
• Therapeutic response: decreased anxiety, restlessness, insomnia

Teach patient/family:
• That drug may be taken with food
• Not to be used for everyday stress or used longer than 4 mo, unless directed by prescriber; not to take more than prescribed amount; may be habit forming
• To avoid OTC preparations unless approved by prescriber
• To avoid driving, activities that require alertness; drowsiness may occur, especially elderly
• To avoid alcohol ingestion, other psychotropic medications, unless directed by prescriber
• Not to discontinue medication abruptly after long-term use
• To rise slowly or fainting may occur
• That drowsiness may worsen at beginning of treatment

Treatment of overdose: Lavage, VS, supportive care, flumazenil

clotrimazole (OTC, ℞)

(kloe-trim'a-zole)

Mycelex Troches, Lotrimin, Lotrimin AF, Mycelex, Mycelex OTC, Canesten*, FemCare, Gyne-Lotrimin, Mycelex-G, Mycelex-7, Mycelex Twin Pack

Func. class.: Local antifungal

Chem. class.: Imidazole derivative

Action: Interferes with fungal DNA replication; binds sterols in fungal cell membrane, which increases permeability, leaking of cell nutrients; fungicidal

Uses: Tinea pedis, tinea cruris, tinea corporis, tinea versicolor, *C. albicans* infection of the vagina, vulva, throat, mouth

Dosage and routes:
• *Adult and child:* TOP rub into affected area bid × 1-8 wk; LOZ dissolve in mouth 5 ×/day × 2 wk; INTRA VAG 1 applicator/1 tab × 1-2 wk hs

Available forms: Cream, sol, lotion 1%; vag tabs 100, 500 mg; vag cream 1%, troches 10 mg

Side effects/adverse reactions:
INTEG: Rash, urticaria, stinging, burning, peeling, blistering, skin fissures
OTHER: Abdominal cramps, bloating, urinary frequency, dyspareunia

Contraindications: Hypersensitivity

Precautions: Pregnancy (B), lactation

* Available in Canada only

NURSING CONSIDERATIONS
Assess:
• Allergic reaction: burning, stinging, swelling, redness
Administer:
• 1 applicator or 1 tab intravaginally each night
• Enough medication to cover lesions completely
• After cleansing with soap, water before each application; dry well
Perform/provide:
• Storage at room temp in dry place
Evaluate:
• Therapeutic response: decrease in size, number of lesions, decrease in itching, white patches around vulva
Teach patient/family:
• To apply with glove to prevent further infection
• To avoid use of OTC creams, ointments, lotions unless directed by prescriber
• To wash hands before, after each application
• To abstain from sexual intercourse during vaginal/vulvular treatment
• To use continuously even during menstrual period
• To report to prescriber if infection persists or returns in 2 mo; pregnancy or a serious medical condition may be the cause

cloxacillin (℞)

(klox-a-sill′in)

Apo Cloxi*, cloxacillin sodium, Cloxapen, Novocloxin*, Nu-Clox*, Orbenin*, Tegopen

Func. class.: Broad-spectrum antibiotic

Chem. class.: Penicillinase-resistant penicillin

Action: Interferes with cell wall replication of susceptible organisms; the cell wall, rendered osmotically unstable, swells, bursts from osmotic pressure
Uses: Gram-positive cocci *(S. aureus, S. pyogenes, E. pyogenes, S. pneumoniae),* penicillinase-producing staphylococci
Dosage and routes:
• *Adult:* PO 1-4 g/day in divided doses q6h
• *Child:* PO 50-100 mg/kg in divided doses q6h
Available forms: Caps 250, 500 mg; powder for oral susp 125 mg/5 ml
Side effects/adverse reactions:
HEMA: Anemia, increased bleeding time, ***bone marrow depression, granulocytopenia***
GI: Nausea, vomiting, diarrhea, increased AST (SGOT), ALT (SGPT), abdominal pain, glossitis, colitis
GU: Oliguria, proteinuria, hematuria, *vaginitis, moniliasis,* ***glomerulonephritis***
CNS: Lethargy, hallucinations, anxiety, depression, twitching, ***coma, convulsions***
Contraindications: Hypersensitivity to penicillins; neonates
Precautions: Pregnancy (B), lactation, hypersensitivity to cephalosporins
Pharmacokinetics:
PO: Peak 1 hr, duration 6 hr; half-life 30-60 min; metabolized in liver; excreted in urine, bile, breast milk; crosses placenta
Interactions:
• Decreased antimicrobial effectiveness of cloxacillin: tetracyclines, erythromycins
• Increased cloxacillin concentrations: aspirin, probenecid
Lab test interferences:
False positive: Urine glucose, urine protein
Decreased: Uric acid
NURSING CONSIDERATIONS
Assess:
• I&O ratio; report hematuria, olig-

uria, since penicillin in high doses is nephrotoxic
• Any patient with compromised renal system, since drug is excreted slowly in poor renal system function; toxicity may occur rapidly
• Liver studies: AST (SGOT), ALT (SGPT)
• Blood studies: WBC, RBC, H&H, bleeding time
• Renal studies: urinalysis, protein, blood
• Culture, sensitivity before drug therapy; drug may be taken as soon as culture is taken
• Bowel pattern before, during treatment
• Skin eruptions after administration of penicillin to 1 wk after discontinuing drug
• Respiratory status: rate, character, wheezing, tightness in chest
• Allergies before initiation of treatment; reaction of each medication; place allergies on chart in bright red

Administer:
• After C&S completed

Perform/provide:
• Adrenaline, suction, tracheostomy set, endotracheal intubation equipment on unit
• Adequate intake of fluids (2 L) during diarrhea episodes
• Scratch test to assess allergy after securing order from prescriber; usually done when penicillin is only drug of choice
• Storage in tight container; after reconstituting, store in refrigerator for 2 wk, room temperature 1 wk

Evaluate:
• Therapeutic response: absence of fever, draining wounds

Teach patient/family:
• Aspects of drug therapy including need to complete entire course of medication to ensure organism death (10-14 days); culture may be taken after completed course of medication
• To report sore throat, fever, fatigue (may indicate superinfection)
• To wear or carry a Medic Alert ID if allergic to penicillins
• To notify nurse of diarrhea
• To take on an empty stomach with a full glass of water

Treatment of overdose: Withdraw drug; maintain airway; administer epinephrine, aminophylline, O_2, IV corticosteroids for anaphylaxis

clozapine (℞)

(clo'za-pin)
Clozaril
Func. class.: Antipsychotic
Chem. class.: Tricyclic dibenzodiazepine derivative

Action: Interferes with dopamine receptor binding with lack of extrapyramidal symptoms; also acts as an adrenergic, cholinergic, histaminergic, serotonergic antagonist

Uses: Management of psychotic symptoms in schizophrenic patients for whom other antipsychotics have failed

Dosage and routes:
• *Adult:* PO 25 mg qd or bid; may increase by 25-50 mg/day; normal range 300-450 mg/day after 2 wk; do not increase dose more than 2 × per wk; do not exceed 900 mg/day; use lowest dose to control symptoms

Available forms: Tabs 25, 100 mg

Side effects/adverse reactions:
CNS: Sedation, salivation, dizziness, headache, tremors, sleep problems, akinesia, fever, ***seizures,*** *sweating, akathisia, confusion, fatigue, insomnia,* depression, slurred speech, anxiety
GI: Drooling or excessive salivation, constipation, nausea, abdomi-

* Available in Canada only

nal discomfort, vomiting, diarrhea, anorexia
MS: Weakness; pain in back, neck, legs; spasm
CV: Tachycardia, hypotension, hypertension, chest pain, ECG changes
GU: Urinary abnormalities, incontinence, ejaculation dysfunction, frequency, urgency, retention
RESP: Dyspnea, nasal congestion, throat discomfort
HEMA: ***Leukopenia, neutropenia, agranulocytosis, eosinophilia***
Contraindications: Hypersensitivity, myeloproliferative disorders, severe granulocytopenia, CNS depression, coma, narrow-angle glaucoma
Precautions: Pregnancy (B); lactation; children <16; hepatic, renal, cardiac disease; seizures; prostatic enlargement; elderly

Pharmacokinetics:
Steady state 2.5 hr; 95% protein bound; completely metabolized by liver; excreted in urine and feces (metabolites); half-life 8-12 hr

Interactions:
- Increased anticholinergic effects: anticholinergics
- Increased hypotension: antihypertensives
- Increased CNS depression: CNS drugs
- Increased bone marrow suppression: antineoplastics, other drugs suppressing bone marrow
- Increased plasma concentrations: warfarin, digoxin, other highly protein-bound drugs

Lab test interferences:
Increase: Liver function tests, cardiac enzymes, cholesterol, blood glucose, bilirubin, PBI, cholinesterase, ^{131}I
False positive: Pregnancy tests, PKU
False negative: Urinary steroids, 17-OHCS

NURSING CONSIDERATIONS
Assess:
- Swallowing of PO medication; check for hoarding or giving of medication to other patients
- I&O ratio; obtain baseline before treatment begins; palpate bladder if low urinary output occurs
- Bilirubin, CBC, liver function studies monthly; discontinue treatment if WBC <3000/mm^3 or a granulocyte <1500/mm^3
- Urinalysis is recommended before, during prolonged therapy
- Affect, orientation, LOC, reflexes, gait, coordination, sleep pattern disturbances
- B/P standing and lying; take pulse and respirations q4h during initial treatment; establish baseline before starting treatment; report drops of 30 mm Hg
- Dizziness, faintness, palpitations, tachycardia on rising
- EPS including akathisia (inability to sit still, no pattern to movements), tardive dyskinesia (bizarre movements of the jaw, mouth, tongue, extremities), pseudoparkinsonism (rigidity, tremors, pill rolling, shuffling gait)
- Skin turgor daily
- Constipation, urinary retention daily; if these occur, increase bulk, water in diet, especially elderly

Administer:
- Antiparkinsonian agent for EPS

Perform/provide:
- Decreased noise input by dimming lights, avoiding loud noises
- Supervised ambulation until stabilized on medication; do not involve in strenuous exercise program because fainting is possible; patient should not stand still for long periods
- Increased fluids to prevent constipation

• Storage in tight, light-resistant container

Evaluate:

• Therapeutic response: decrease in emotional excitement, hallucinations, delusions, paranoia, reorganization of patterns of thought, speech

Teach patient/family:

• That orthostatic hypotension occurs often, and to rise from sitting or lying position gradually

• To avoid hot tubs, hot showers, tub baths; hypotension may occur

• To avoid abrupt withdrawal of this drug, or EPS may result; drug should be withdrawn slowly

• To avoid OTC preparations (cough, hay fever, cold) unless approved by prescriber, since serious drug interactions may occur; avoid use with alcohol or CNS depressants; increased drowsiness may occur

• Regarding compliance with drug regimen

• About EPS and necessity for meticulous oral hygiene, since oral candidiasis may occur

• To report sore throat, malaise, fever, bleeding, mouth sores; if these occur, CBC should be drawn and drug discontinued

• In hot weather, heat stroke may occur; take extra precautions to stay cool

• To avoid driving, other hazardous activities; seizures may occur

• To notify physician if pregnant or if pregnancy is intended

Treatment of overdose: Lavage, activated charcoal; provide an airway; do not induce vomiting

codeine (℞)

(koe'deen)

Paveral*

Func. class.: Narcotic analgesics

Chem. class.: Opiate, phenathrene derivative

Combination products: Caladryl: diphenhydramine HCl 1% with calamine 8%, camphor 0.1%; Calcidrine: codeine 8.4 mg/5 ml with calcium iodide anhydrous 152 mg/5 ml; Capital and Codeine: codeine 30 mg with acetaminophen 325 mg; Copavin Pulvules: codeine sulfate 15 mg with papaverine HCl; Penntuss: codeine polistirex equivalent to codeine 10 mg/5 ml with chlorpheniramine polistirex equivalent to chlorpheniramine maleate 4 mg/5 ml; Soma Compound with Codeine: codeine 16 mg, aspirin 325 mg, carisoprodol 200 mg

Controlled Substance Schedule II, III, IV, V (depends on route)

Action: Depresses pain impulse transmission at the spinal cord level by interacting with opioid receptors

Uses: Moderate to severe pain, nonproductive cough

Investigational uses: Diarrhea

Dosage and routes:

Pain

• *Adult:* PO 15-60 mg q4h prn; IM/SC 15-60 mg q4h prn

• *Child:* PO 3 mg/kg/day in divided doses q4h prn

Cough

• *Adult:* PO 10-20 mg q4-6h, not to exceed 120 mg/day

• *Child:* PO 1-1.5 mg/kg/day in 4 divided doses, not to exceed 60 mg/day

Diarrhea

• *Adult:* PO 30 mg; may repeat qid prn

* Available in Canada only

Available forms: Inj 15, 30, 60 mg/ml; tabs 15, 30, 60 mg; oral sol 10 mg/5 ml*, 15 mg/5 ml

Side effects/adverse reactions:

CNS: Drowsiness, sedation, dizziness, agitation, dependency, lethargy, restlessness

GI: Nausea, vomiting, anorexia, constipation

RESP: ***Respiratory depression, respiratory paralysis***

CV: Bradycardia, palpitations, orthostatic hypotension, tachycardia

GU: Urinary retention

INTEG: Flushing, rash, urticaria

Contraindications: Hypersensitivity to opiates, respiratory depression, increased intracranial pressure, seizure disorders, severe respiratory disorders

Precautions: Elderly, cardiac dysrhythmias, pregnancy (C), lactation

Pharmacokinetics: Onset 15-30 min, peak 1-2 hr, duration 4-6 hr; metabolized by liver; excreted by kidneys, in breast milk; crosses placenta; half-life 2½-4 hr

Interactions:

- Effects may be increased with other CNS depressants: alcohol, narcotics, sedative/hypnotics, antipsychotics, skeletal muscle relaxants

NURSING CONSIDERATIONS

Assess:

- I&O ratio; check for decreasing output; may indicate urinary retention, especially elderly
- By using pain-scoring method
- For productive cough
- Cough: type, duration, ability to raise secretion
- CNS changes, dizziness, drowsiness, hallucinations, euphoria, LOC, pupil reaction
- Allergic reactions: rash, urticaria
- Respiratory dysfunction: respiratory depression, character, rate rhythm; notify prescriber if respirations are <10/min, shallow
- Need for pain medication, tolerance

Administer:

- With antiemetic for nausea, vomiting
- When pain is beginning to return; determine dosage interval by patient response

Perform/provide:

- Storage in light-resistant container at room temp
- Assistance with ambulation if needed
- Safety measures: top side rails, night-light, call bell

Evaluate:

- Therapeutic response: decrease in pain, absence of grimacing, decreased cough

Teach patient/family:

- To report any symptoms of CNS changes, allergic reactions
- That physical dependency may result after extended periods
- To change position slowly; orthostatic hypotension may occur
- To avoid hazardous activities if drowsiness, dizziness occurs
- To avoid alcohol, other CNS depressants unless directed by prescriber

colchicine (℞)

(kol′chi-seen)

Func. class.: Antigout agent

Chem. class.: Colchicum autumnale alkaloid

Action: Inhibits microtubule formation of lactic acid in leukocytes, which decreases phagocytosis and inflammation in joints

Uses: Gout, gouty arthritis (prevention, treatment); to arrest progression of neurologic disability in multiple sclerosis

Dosage and routes:

Prevention

• *Adult:* PO 0.5-1.8 mg qd depending on severity; IV 0.5-1 mg 1-2 × day

Treatment

• *Adult:* PO 0.5-1.2 mg, then 0.5-1.2 mg q1h, until pain decreases or side effects occur

Available forms: Tabs 0.5, 0.6, 1 mg*

Side effects/adverse reactions:

MISC: Myopathy, alopecia, reversible azoospermia, peripheral neuritis

GU: Hematuria, oliguria, renal damage

HEMA: ***Agranulocytosis, thrombocytopenia, aplastic anemia, pancytopenia***

GI: Nausea, vomiting, anorexia, malaise, metallic taste, cramps, peptic ulcer, diarrhea

INTEG: Chills, dermatitis, pruritus, purpura, erythema

Contraindications: Hypersensitivity; serious GI, renal, hepatic, cardiac disorders; blood dyscrasias

Precautions: Severe renal disease, blood dyscrasias, pregnancy (C), hepatic disease, elderly, lactation, children

Pharmacokinetics:

PO: Peak ½-2 hr, half-life 20 min; deacetylates in liver; excreted in feces (metabolites/active drug)

Interactions:

• Decreased action of colchicine: acidifying agents

• Decreased action of Vit B_{12}

• Increased action of CNS depressants, sympathomimetics

• Increased action of colchicine: alkalinizers

• Considered incompatible in syringe with other drugs

Lab test interferences:

Increase: Alk phosphatase, AST/ALT

False positive: RBC, Hgb

NURSING CONSIDERATIONS

Assess:

• I&O ratio; observe for decrease in urinary output

• CBC, platelets, reticulocytes before, during therapy (q3mo)

• Coombs' test for Coombs' negative hemolytic anemia

Administer:

• Oral: on empty stomach only, to facilitate absorption

Evaluate:

• Therapeutic response: decreased stone formation on x-ray, decreased pain in kidney region, absence of hematuria, decreased pain in joints

Teach patient/family:

• To increase fluid intake to 3-4 L/day

• To avoid alcohol, OTC preparations that contain alcohol; skin rashes have occurred

• To report any pain, redness, or hard area, usually in legs

• Importance of complying with medical regimen; the possibility of bone marrow depression occurring

colestipol (℞)

(koe-les'ti-pole)

Colestid

Func. class.: Antilipemic

Chem. class.: Bile sequestrant, resin exchange agent

Action: Absorbs, combines with bile acids to form insoluble complex excreted through feces; loss of bile acids lowers cholesterol levels

Uses: Primary hypercholesterolemia, xanthomas, digitalis toxicity, pruritus due to biliary obstruction, diarrhea due to bile acids

Dosage and routes:

• *Adult:* PO 15-30 g/day in 2-4 divided doses

* Available in Canada only

Available forms: Granules
Side effects/adverse reactions:
GI: Constipation, abdominal pain, nausea, fecal impaction, hemorrhoids, flatulence, vomiting, steatorrhea, peptic ulcer
INTEG: Rash, irritation of perianal area, tongue, skin
HEMA: Decreased Vit A, D, K, red folate content, ***hyperchloremic acidosis,*** bleeding, decreased pro-time
Contraindications: Hypersensitivity, biliary obstruction
Precautions: Pregnancy (B), lactation, children, bleeding disorders
Pharmacokinetics:
PO: Excreted in feces
Interactions:
- May reduce action of thiazide, digitalis, warfarin, penicillin G, folic acid, phenylbutazone, tetracycline, corticosteroids, iron, thyroid agents, clindamycin, trimethoprim, chenodiol, fat-soluble vitamins, cephalexin, phenobarbital

Lab test interferences:
Increase: Liver function studies, chloride, PO_4
NURSING CONSIDERATIONS
Assess:
- Cardiac glycoside levels, if both drugs are being administered
- For signs of Vit A, D, K deficiency
- Serum cholesterol, triglyceride levels, electrolytes (extended therapy)
- Bowel pattern daily; increase bulk, water in diet if constipation develops

Administer:
- Drug ac, hs; give all other medications 1 hr before colestipol or 4 hr after colestipol to avoid poor absorption
- Drug mixed in applesauce or stirred into beverage (2-6 oz); do not take dry; let stand for 2 min
- Supplemental doses of Vit A, D, K if levels are low

Evaluate:
- Therapeutic response: decreased triglycerides, diarrhea, pruritus (excess bile acids)

Teach patient/family:
- Symptoms of hypoprothrombinemia: bleeding mucous membranes, dark tarry stools, hematuria, petechiae; report immediately
- That compliance is needed; toxicity may result if doses are missed
- That risk factors should be decreased: high-fat diet, smoking, alcohol consumption, absence of exercise

colfosceril (℞)
(kohl-foss'sir-ill)
Exosurf Neonatal
Func. class.: Synthetic lung surfactant
Chem. class.: Dipalmitoylphosphatidylcholine (DPPC)

Action: Surfactant maintains lung inflation and prevents collapse by lowering surface tension
Uses: Treatment of respiratory distress syndrome (RDS) in premature infants
Dosage and routes:
Prophylactic treatment
Endotracheally: 5 ml/kg as soon as possible after birth and repeat doses 12 and 24 hr later to infants remaining on mechanical ventilation
Rescue treatment
Endotracheally: administer in two 2.5 ml/kg doses; give initial dose after treatment of RDS, then second dose in 12 hr
Available forms: 108 mg/10 ml/vial with sterile H_2O for inj and 5 endotracheal tube adapters
Side effects/adverse reactions:
RESP: ***Apnea, pulmonary hemorrhage, pulmonary air leak, congenital pneumonia***

SYST: ***Nonpulmonary fatal infections***

Precautions: Congenital anomalies, prophylactic treatment

Pharmacokinetics: Distributed to all lobes, alveolar spaces, distal airways; alveolar half-life 12 hr; 90% of alveolar phospholipids recycled

NURSING CONSIDERATIONS

Assess:

- Respiratory rate, rhythm, character, chest expansion, color, transcutaneous saturation, ABGs
- Endotracheal tube placement before dosing
- For apnea after endotracheal administration
- Reflux of drug into the endotracheal tube during administration; stop drug if this occurs; if needed, increase peak inspiratory pressure on ventilator by 4-5 cm H_2O until tube is cleared

Administer:

- Suction before administration
- After selecting adapter that corresponds to diameter of endotracheal tube, insert adapter into tube by twisting, connect breathing circuit to adapter, remove cap from adapter sideport, attach syringe to sideport; after dose is completed, remove syringe, recap sideport
- After reconstituting each vial with 8 ml preservative-free sterile water for injection, fill 10-12 ml syringe with 8 ml preservative-free sterile water for injection, using an 18-19G needle; allow vacuum in vial to draw liquid into vial; aspirate 8 ml out of vial into syringe while maintaining vacuum; release syringe plunger; repeat aspiration, release until adequately mixed; draw dose into syringe from below froth in vial; do not use if large particles are present
- By endotracheal administration only by persons trained in neonatal intubation and ventilation, after first 2.5 ml dose is given while infant is in midline position, turn head/torso 45° to right for 30 sec, then give 2nd dose; turn to left for 30 sec; do not suction for 2 hr unless needed

Perform/provide:

- Reduction in peak ventilator inspiratory pressures immediately if chest expansion improves substantially after dose
- Reduction in FiO_2 in small, repeated steps when infant becomes pink and transcutaneous oxygen saturation is in excess of 95%; oxygen saturation should remain between 90% and 95%
- Suction all infants before administration to prevent mucus plugging; if endotracheal tube obstruction is suspected, remove obstruction, replace tube immediately
- Storage at room temp in dry place

Evaluate:

- Therapeutic response: decreased respiratory distress

---

corticotropin (ACTH) (℞)

(kor-ti-koe-troe′pin)

ACTH, Acthar, corticotropin, ACTH-40, ACTH-80, H.P. Acthar Gel

Func. class.: Pituitary hormone

Chem. class.: Adrenocorticotropic hormone

Action: Stimulates adrenal cortex to produce, secrete corticosterone, cortisol

Uses: Testing adrenocortical function, treatment of adrenal insufficiency caused by administration of corticosteroids (long term), multiple sclerosis

Dosage and routes:

Testing of adrenocortical function

* Available in Canada only

• *Adult:* IM/SC up to 80 U in divided doses; IV 10-25 U in 500 ml D_5W given over 8 hr

Inflammation

• *Adult:* SC/IM 40 U in 4 divided doses (aqueous) or 40 U q12-24h (gel/repository form)

Available forms: Inj IM, IV, SC 40, 80 U/vial, repository inj IM, SC 40, 80/ml

Side effects/adverse reactions:

INTEG: Impaired wound healing, rash, urticaria, hirsutism, petechiae, ecchymoses, sweating, acne, hyperpigmentation

CNS: ***Convulsions,*** dizziness, euphoria, insomnia, headache, mood swings, behavioral changes, depression, psychosis

GI: Nausea, vomiting, ***peptic ulcer perforation,*** pancreatitis, distention, ulcerative esophagitis

GU: Water, sodium retention, hypokalemia

EENT: Cataracts, glaucoma

MS: Weakness, osteoporosis, compression fractures, muscle atrophy, steroid myopathy, myalgia, arthralgia

ENDO: Cushingoid symptoms, diabetes mellitus, antibody formation, growth retardation in children, menstrual irregularities

Contraindications: Hypersensitivity, scleroderma, osteoporosis, CHF, peptic ulcer disease, hypertension, systemic fungal infections, smallpox vaccination, recent surgery, ocular herpes simplex, primary adrenocortical insufficiency/hyperfunction

Precautions: Pregnancy (C), lactation, latent TB, hepatic disease, hypothyroiditis, childbearing age, psychiatric diagnosis, myasthenia gravis, acute gouty arthritis

Pharmacokinetics:

IV/IM/SC: Onset <6 hr, duration 2-4 hr, repository duration up to 3 days, half-life <20 min, excreted in urine

Interactions:

• Possible ulceration: salicylates, alcohol, corticosteroids

• Hypokalemia: diuretics (K-depleting), amphotericin B

• Hyperglycemia: insulin, oral hypoglycemic agents

Additive compatibilities: Calcium gluconate, chloramphenicol, cytarabine, dimenhydrinate, erythromycin gluceptate, heparin, hydrocortisone sodium succinate, methicillin, norepinephrine, oxytetracycline, penicillin G potassium, potassium chloride, tetracycline, vancomycin

NURSING CONSIDERATIONS

Assess:

• Baseline ECG, B/P, chest x-ray, GTT

• Pulse, B/P

• I&O ratio; weight qwk, report gain over 5 lb/wk

• 2 hr postprandial, chest x-ray, serum K, 17 KS, 17-OHCS, cortisol, during long-term treatment

• Dependent edema, moon face, pulmonary edema, cerebral edema

• Infection; drug may mask

• Increased stress in patient's life that may require increased corticosteroids

• Mental status: affect, mood, increased aggressiveness, irritability; change may require decreased steroids

• Growth rate of child

• Hypoadrenalism in neonates if drug was given during pregnancy

• Allergic reaction: rash, urticaria, fever, nausea, vomiting, dyspnea; drug should be discontinued immediately, administer epinephrine 1:1000

Administer:

• Test for hypersensitivity for individuals allergic to pork products

• Decreased Na, increase K for dependent edema
• Increase protein diet for N loss
• Gel at room temp, give deep IM using 21G needle
• May be used to treat edema
• IV; give over 2 min; dilute 25 U/1 ml sterile H_2O or NS or 40 U/2 ml; may dilute 10-25 U/500 ml compatible sol; give over 8 hr

Perform/provide:
• Storage in refrigerator of unused portion; use within 24 hr

Evaluate:
• Therapeutic response: absence of inflammation, pain, increased muscle strength in myasthenia gravis

Teach patient/family:
• To avoid vaccinations during drug treatment
• To maintain hydration up to 2 L/day unless contraindicated
• To avoid OTC products: salicylates, products with alcohol
• Not to discontinue medication abruptly; adrenal crisis may occur; should be tapered over several wk
• To wear Medic Alert ID specifying steroid therapy
• That drug does not cure condition, only decreases symptoms
• To notify prescriber of infection: fever, sore throat, muscular pain
• To tell patient to notify anyone involved in medical or dental care that this drug is being taken

cortisone (℞)

(kor′ti-sone)
Cortone
Func. class.: Corticosteroid, synthetic
Chem. class.: Glucocorticoid, short-acting

Action: Decreases inflammation by suppression of migration of polymorphonuclear leukocytes, fibroblasts, reversal of increased capillary permeability and lysosomal stabilization

Uses: Inflammation, severe allergy, adrenal insufficiency, collagen disorders, respiratory, dermatologic disorders

Dosage and routes:
• *Adult:* PO/IM 25-300 mg qd or q2 days, titrated to response

Available forms: Tabs 5, 10, 25 mg; inj 50 mg/ml

Side effects/adverse reactions:
INTEG: Acne, poor wound healing, ecchymosis, bruising, petechiae
CNS: Depression, flushing, sweating, headache, mood changes
CV: Hypertension, ***circulatory collapse, thrombophlebitis, embolism,*** tachycardia, ***necrotizing angiitis, CHF,*** edema
HEMA: ***Thrombocytopenia***
MS: Fractures, osteoporosis, weakness
GI: Diarrhea, nausea, abdominal distention, ***GI hemorrhage,*** increased appetite, ***pancreatitis***
EENT: Fungal infections, increased intraocular pressure, blurred vision

Contraindications: Psychosis, hypersensitivity, idiopathic thrombocytopenia, acute glomerulonephritis, amebiasis, fungal infections, nonasthmatic bronchial disease, child <2 yr, AIDS, TB

Precautions: Pregnancy (C), lactation, diabetes mellitus, glaucoma, osteoporosis, seizure disorders, ulcerative colitis, CHF, myasthenia gravis, renal disease, esophagitis, peptic ulcer

Pharmacokinetics:
PO: Peak 2 hr, duration 1½ days
IM: Peak 20-48 hr, duration 1½ days

Interactions:
• Decreased action of cortisone: cholestyramine, colestipol, barbiturates,

* Available in Canada only

rifampin, ephedrine, phenytoin, theophylline
• Decreased effects of anticoagulants, anticonvulsants, antidiabetics, ambenonium, neostigmine, isoniazid, toxoids, vaccines, anticholinesterases, salicylates, somatrem
• Increased side effects: alcohol, salicylates, indomethacin, amphotericin B, digitalis, cyclosporine, diuretics
• Increased action of cortisone: salicylates, estrogens, indomethacin, oral contraceptives, ketoconazole, macrolide antibiotics

Lab test interferences:
Increase: Cholesterol, Na, blood glucose, uric acid, Ca, urine glucose
Decrease: Ca, K, T_4, T_3, thyroid ^{131}I uptake test, urine 17-OHCS, 17-KS, PBI
False negative: Skin allergy tests

NURSING CONSIDERATIONS

Assess:
• K, blood sugar, urine glucose while on long-term therapy; hypokalemia and hyperglycemia
• Weight daily; notify prescriber of weekly gain >5 lb
• B/P q4h, pulse; notify prescriber if chest pain occurs
• I&O ratio; be alert for decreasing urinary output and increasing edema
• Plasma cortisol levels during long-term therapy (normal level: 138-635 nmol/L SI units if drawn at 8 AM)
• Infection: fever, WBC even after withdrawal of medication; drug masks infection
• K depletion: paresthesias, fatigue, nausea, vomiting, depression, polyuria, dysrhythmias, weakness
• Edema, hypertension, cardiac symptoms
• Mental status: affect, mood, behavioral changes, aggression

Administer:
• After shaking suspension (parenteral)
• Titrated dose; use lowest effective dose
• IM inj deeply in large mass; rotate sites; avoid deltoid; use a 21G needle
• In one dose in AM to prevent adrenal suppression; avoid SC administration; tissue may be damaged
• With food or milk to decrease GI symptoms

Perform/provide:
• Assistance with ambulation in patient with bone tissue disease to prevent fractures

Evaluate:
• Therapeutic response: ease of respirations, decreased inflammation

Teach patient/family:
• That ID as steroid user should be carried at all times
• To notify physician if therapeutic response decreases; dosage adjustment may be needed
• Not to discontinue abruptly or adrenal crisis can result
• To avoid OTC products: salicylates, alcohol in cough products, cold preparations unless directed by prescriber
• All aspects of drug usage, including cushingoid symptoms
• Symptoms of adrenal insufficiency: nausea, anorexia, fatigue, dizziness, dyspnea, weakness, joint pain

cosyntropin (℞)

(koe-sin-troe′pin)
Cortrosyn, Synacthen, Tetracosactrin
Func. class.: Pituitary hormone
Chem. class.: Synthetic polypeptide

Action: Stimulates adrenal cortex

to produce, secrete corticosterone, cortisol

Uses: Testing adrenocortical function

Dosage and routes:

• *Adult and child >2 yr:* IM/IV 0.25-1 mg between blood sampling

• *Child <2 yr:* IM/IV 0.125 mg

Available forms: Inj IM, IV 0.25 mg/vial

Side effects/adverse reactions:

INTEG: Rash, urticaria, pruritus, flushing

Contraindications: Hypersensitivity

Precautions: Pregnancy (C)

Pharmacokinetics:

IV/IM: Onset 5 min, peak 1 hr, duration 2-4 hr

Interactions:

• Considered incompatible with any drug in syringe or sol

• Incompatible with blood, blood products

NURSING CONSIDERATIONS

Assess:

• Plasma cortisol levels at ½-1 hr after drug administered (>5 μg/dl is normal), at end of 1 hr, levels should have doubled

• Dependent edema, moon face, pulmonary edema, cerebral edema

• Infection; drug may mask

• Increased stress in patient's life that may require increased corticosteroids

• Mental status: affect, mood, increased aggressiveness, irritability; change may require decreased steroids

• Growth rate of child

• Hypoadrenalism in neonates if drug was given during pregnancy

• Allergic reaction: rash, urticaria, fever, nausea, vomiting, dyspnea; drug should be discontinued immediately; administer epinephrine 1:1000

Administer:

• After reconstitution with 1 ml 0.9% NaCl/0.25 mg by direct IV over 2 min; may be further diluted in D_5 or NS; run 40 mg/hr over 4-8 hr as an inf

Perform/provide:

• Storage at room temp 24 hr or refrigerated 3 wk

Evaluate:

• Therapeutic response: absence of inflammation, pain, increased muscle strength in myasthenia gravis

Teach patient/family:

• To avoid vaccinations during drug treatment

• To maintain hydration up to 2 L/day unless contraindicated

• To avoid OTC products: salicylates, products with alcohol

• Not to discontinue abruptly; thyroid crisis may occur; drug should be tapered over several wk

• To wear Medic Alert ID specifying steroid therapy

• That drug does not cure condition, only decreases symptoms

• To notify prescriber of infection: fever, sore throat, muscular pain

• To tell patient to notify anyone involved in medical or dental care that this drug is being taken

cromolyn (℞)

(kroe'moe-lin)

Intal, Intal p*, Nasalcrom, Rynacrom*, Gastrocrom

Func. class.: Antiasthmatic

Chem. class.: Mast cell stabilizer

Action: Stabilizes the membrane of the sensitized mast cell, preventing release of chemical mediators after an antigen-IgE interaction

Uses: Allergic rhinitis, severe perennial bronchial asthma, prevention of exercise-induced broncho-

* Available in Canada only

spasm, acute bronchospasm induced by environmental pollutants, mastocytosis

Dosage and routes:

Allergic rhinitis

• *Adult and child >6 yr:* NASAL SOL 1 spray in each nostril tid-qid, not to exceed 6 doses/day

Bronchospasm

• *Adult and child >6 yr:* INH 20 mg <1 hr before exercise

Bronchial asthma

• *Adult and child >6 yr:* INH 20 mg qid; NEB 20 mg qid by nebulization

Available forms: Sol 40 mg/ml; inh, caps for inh, 20 mg; oral caps 100 mg; neb sol 20 mg; aerosol 800 μg/actuation

Side effects/adverse reactions:

EENT: Throat irritation, cough, nasal congestion, burning eyes

CNS: Headache, dizziness, neuritis

GU: Frequency, dysuria

GI: Nausea, vomiting, anorexia, dry mouth, bitter taste

INTEG: Rash, urticaria, angioedema

MS: Joint pain/swelling

Contraindications: Hypersensitivity to this drug or lactose, status asthmaticus

Precautions: Pregnancy (B), lactation, renal disease, hepatic disease, child <5 yr

Pharmacokinetics:

INH: Peak 15 min, duration 4-6 hr; excreted unchanged in feces; half-life 80 min

NURSING CONSIDERATIONS

Assess:

• Eosinophil count during treatment

• Respiratory status: rate, rhythm, characteristics, cough, wheezing, dyspnea

Administer:

• By inhalation/nebulizer only

• Gargle, sip of water to decrease irritation in throat

Evaluate:

• Therapeutic response: decrease in asthmatic symptoms, congested, runny nose

Teach patient/family:

• To clear mucus before using

• Proper inhalation technique: exhale; using inhaler, inhale deeply with head tipped back to open airway; remove; hold breath; exhale; repeat until all of drug is inhaled, use demonstration; return demonstration

• That therapeutic effect may take up to 4 wk

• Not to swallow capsule

• That drug is preventive only, not restorative

---

crotamiton (℞)

(kroe-tam′i-ton)

Eurax

Func. class.: Scabicide

Chem. class.: Synthetic chloroformate salt

Action: Unknown; toxic to *Sarcoptes scabiei*

Uses: Scabies, pruritus

Dosage and routes:

Scabies

• *Adult and child:* CREAM wash area with soap, water; remove visible crusts, apply cream, apply another coat in 24 hr, remove with soap, water in 48 hr

Pruritus

Massage into affected area, repeat as necessary

Available forms: Cream 10%; lotion 10%

Side effects/adverse reactions:

INTEG: Itching, rash, irritation, contact dermatitis

Contraindications: Hypersensitivity, skin inflammation, abrasions, breaks in skin, mucous membranes

Precautions: Children, pregnancy (C)

NURSING CONSIDERATIONS

Assess:

- Area of body involved, including crusts, brownish trails on skin, itching papules in skin folds

Administer:

- After patient bathes with soap, water; remove all crusts
- From chin down; do not apply to face, lips, mouth, eyes, any mucous membrane, anus, or meatus
- Topical corticosteroids as ordered to decrease contact dermatitis; antihistamines for pruritus
- Lotions of menthol or phenol to control itching
- Topical antibiotics for infection

Perform/provide:

- Storage in tight, light-resistant container
- Isolation until skin, scalp have cleared, treatment complete

Evaluate:

- Therapeutic response: decreased itching after several wk, decreased redness

Teach patient/family:

- To change clothing and bed linen the morning after treatment; affected person should have separate towels and linens
- To shake well before using
- To wash all inhabitants' clothing, using hot water, dry in hot dryer for >20 min; preventive treatment may be required for all persons living in same house to decrease spread of infection
- That itching may continue for 4-6 wk
- That drug must be reapplied if accidentally washed off, or treatment will be ineffective
- To avoid contact with eyes, face, meatus, mucous membranes, or irritation may occur
- To discontinue use and notify prescriber of irritation, sensitization

cyanocobalamin (vit B_{12})/hydroxocobalamin (vit $B_{12}a$) (OTC, ℞)

(sye-an-oh-koe-bal'a-min)

Bedoz*, B_{12} Resin, Cobex, Crystamine, Crysti-12, Cyanabin*, Cyanoject, Cyomin, Ener-B, Pernavite, Redisol, Rubesol-1000, Rubion*, Rubramin PC, Sytobex, Vitamin B_{12}

Func. class.: Vit B_{12}, water-soluble vitamin

Action: Needed for adequate nerve functioning, protein and carbohydrate metabolism, normal growth, RBC development, cell reproduction

Uses: Vit B_{12} deficiency, pernicious anemia, vit B_{12} malabsorption syndrome, Schilling test, increased requirements with pregnancy, thyrotoxicosis, hemolytic anemia, hemorrhage, renal and hepatic disease

Dosage and routes:

- *Adult:* PO 25 μg qd × 5-10 days, maintenance 100-200 mg IM qmo; IM/SC 30-100 μg qd × 5-10 days, maintenance 100-200 μg IM qmo
- *Child:* PO 1 μg qd × 5-10 days, maintenance 60 μg IM qmo or more; IM/SC 1-30 μg qd × 5-10 days, maintenance 60 μg IM qmo or more

Pernicious anemia/malabsorption syndrome

- *Adult:* IM 100-1000 μg qd × 2 wk, then 100-1000 μg IM qmo
- *Child:* IM 100-500 μg over 2 wk or more given in 100-500 μg doses, then 60 μg IM/SC monthly

Schilling test

- *Adult and child:* IM 1000 μg in one dose

Available forms: Tabs 25, 50, 100, 250, 500, 1000 μg; inj IM 100, 120, 1000 μg/ml

* Available in Canada only

Side effects/adverse reactions:
CNS: Flushing, optic nerve atrophy
GI: Diarrhea
CV: ***CHF,*** peripheral vascular thrombosis, ***pulmonary edema***
INTEG: Itching, rash, pain at site
META: Hypokalemia
SYST: ***Anaphylactic shock***
Contraindications: Hypersensitivity, optic nerve atrophy
Precautions: Pregnancy (A), lactation, children
Pharmacokinetics: Stored in liver, kidneys, stomach; 50%-90% excreted in urine; crosses placenta, excreted in breast milk
Interactions:
• Decreased absorption: aminoglycosides, anticonvulsants, colchicine, chloramphenicol, aminosalicylic acid, K preparation, cimetidine
• Increased absorption: prednisone
Y-site compatibilities: Heparin, hydrocortisone sodium succinate, potassium chloride
Solution compatibilities: Dextrose/Ringer's or lactated Ringer's combinations, dextrose/saline combinations, D_5W, $D_{10}W$, 0.45% NaCl, Ringer's or lactated Ringer's sol, ascorbic acid
Lab test interferences:
False positive: Intrinsic factor
NURSING CONSIDERATIONS
Assess:
• GI function: diarrhea, constipation
• K levels during beginning treatment
• CBC for increase in reticulocyte count during 1st week of therapy, then increase in RBC and hemoglobin
• Nutritional status: egg yolks, fish, organ meats, dairy products, clams, oysters: good sources of vit B_{12}
• For pulmonary edema, worsening of CHF in cardiac patients
Administer:
• With fruit juice to disguise taste; immediately after mixing
• With meals if possible for better absorption
• By IM inj for pernicious anemia for life unless contraindicated
• IV route not recommended but may be admixed in TPN solution
Perform/provide:
• Protection from light and heat
Evaluate:
• Therapeutic response: decreased anorexia, dyspnea on exertion, palpitations, paresthesias, psychosis, visual disturbances
Teach patient/family
• That treatment must continue for life for pernicious anemia
• To eat well-balanced diet
• To avoid contact with persons with infection; infections common
Treatment of overdose: Discontinue drug

cyclandelate (℞)
(sye-klan′da-late)
Cyclan, Cyclandelate, Cyclospasmol
Func. class.: Peripheral vasodilator
Chem. class.: Nonnitrate

Action: Relaxes vascular smooth muscle, dilates peripheral vascular smooth muscle by direct action
Uses: Intermittent claudication, thrombophlebitis, Raynaud's phenomenon, ischemic cerebrovascular disease, arteriosclerosis obliterans, nocturnal leg cramps
Dosage and routes:
• *Adult:* PO 200 mg qid, not to exceed 400 mg qid; maintenance dose 400-800 mg/day in 2-4 divided doses
Available forms: Tabs 200, 400 mg; caps 200, 400 mg

Side effects/adverse reactions:
HEMA: Increased bleeding time (rare)
CV: ***Tachycardia***
CNS: Headache, paresthesias, dizziness, weakness
GI: Heartburn, eructation, nausea, pyrosis
INTEG: Sweating, flushing
Contraindications: Hypersensitivity
Precautions: Glaucoma, pregnancy (C), lactation, recent MI, hypertension, severe obliterative coronary artery or cerebrovascular disease
Pharmacokinetics:
PO: Onset 15 min, peak 1½ hr, duration 4 hr

NURSING CONSIDERATIONS
Assess:
- Bleeding time in individuals with bleeding disorders
- Cardiac status: B/P, pulse, rate, rhythm, character; watch for increasing pulse

Administer:
- With meals for GI symptoms

Perform/provide:
- Storage in air-tight container at room temp

Evaluate:
- Therapeutic response: ability to walk without pain, increased temperature in extremities, increased pulse volume

Teach patient/family:
- That medication is not cure; may have to be taken for life
- That it is necessary to quit smoking to prevent excessive vasoconstriction
- That improvement may be sudden but usually occurs gradually over several weeks
- To report headache, weakness, increased pulse, as drug may have to be decreased or discontinued
- To avoid hazardous activities until stabilized on medication; dizziness may occur

cyclizine (OTC, ℞)

(sye'kli-zeen)
Marezine
Func. class.: Antiemetic, antihistamine, anticholinergic
Chem. class.: H_2-receptor antagonist, piperazine derivative

Action: Acts centrally by blocking chemoreceptor trigger zone, which in turn acts on vomiting center
Uses: Motion sickness, prevention of postoperative vomiting
Dosage and routes:
Vomiting
- *Adult:* IM 50 mg ½ hr before termination of surgery, then q4-6h prn (lactate)
- *Child:* IM 3 mg/kg divided in 3 equal doses

Motion sickness
- *Adult:* PO 50 mg then q4-6h prn, not to exceed 200 mg/day (HCl)
- *Child:* PO 25 mg q4-6h prn

Available forms: Tabs 50 mg; inj 50 mg/ml
Side effects/adverse reactions:
CNS: Drowsiness, dizziness, vertigo, fatigue, restlessness, headache, insomnia, hallucinations (auditory/visual), hallucinations and ***convulsions*** in children
GI: Nausea, anorexia
EENT: Dry mouth, blurred vision, tinnitus
Contraindications: Hypersensitivity to cyclizines, shock
Precautions: Children, narrow-angle glaucoma, urinary retention, lactation, prostatic hypertrophy, elderly, pregnancy (B), lactation
Pharmacokinetics:
PO: Duration 4-6 hr; other pharmacokinetics not known

* Available in Canada only

Interactions:

- May increase effect: alcohol, tranquilizers, narcotics

Lab test interferences:

False negative: Allergy skin testing

NURSING CONSIDERATIONS

Assess:

- VS, B/P
- Signs of toxicity of other drugs or masking of symptoms of disease: brain tumor, intestinal obstruction
- Observe for drowsiness/dizziness

Administer:

- IM injection in large muscle mass; aspirate to avoid IV administration
- Tablets may be swallowed whole, chewed, or allowed to dissolve

Evaluate:

- Therapeutic response: absence of motion sickness, vomiting

Teach patient/family:

- That a false-negative result may occur with skin testing; skin testing procedures should not be scheduled for 4 days after discontinuing use
- To avoid hazardous activities or activities requiring alertness; dizziness may occur; instruct patient to request assistance with ambulation
- To avoid alcohol, other depressants

cyclobenzaprine (℞)

(sye-kloe-ben'za-preen)

cyclobenzaprine HCl, Cycloflex, Flexeril

Func. class.: Skeletal muscle relaxant, central acting

Chem. class.: Tricyclic amine salt

Action: Unknown; may be related to antidepressant effects

Uses: Adjunct for relief of muscle spasm and pain in musculoskeletal conditions

Dosage and routes:

- *Adult:* PO 10 mg tid × 1 wk, not to exceed 60 mg/day × 3 wk

Available forms: Tabs 10 mg

Side effects/adverse reactions:

CNS: Dizziness, weakness, drowsiness, headache, tremor, depression, insomnia, confusion, paresthesia

EENT: Diplopia, temporary loss of vision

CV: Postural hypotension, tachycardia, dysrhythmias

GI: Nausea, vomiting, hiccups, dry mouth

INTEG: Rash, pruritus, fever, facial flushing, sweating

GU: Urinary retention, frequency, change in libido

Contraindications: Acute recovery phase of myocardial infarction, dysrhythmias, heart block, CHF, hypersensitivity, child <12 yr, intermittent porphyria, thyroid disease

Precautions: Renal disease, hepatic disease, addictive personality, pregnancy (B), lactation, elderly

Pharmacokinetics:

PO: Onset 1 hr, peak 3-8 hr, duration 12-24 hr, half-life 1-3 days; metabolized by liver; excreted in urine; crosses placenta; excreted in breast milk

Interactions:

- Decreased effects of guanethidine
- Increased CNS depression: alcohol, tricyclic antidepressants, narcotics, barbiturates, sedatives, hypnotics
- Do not use within 14 days of MAOI

NURSING CONSIDERATIONS

Assess:

- Blood studies: CBC, WBC, differential for blood dyscrasias
- Liver function studies: AST, ALT, alk phosphatase; hepatitis may occur
- ECG in epileptic patients; poor seizure control has occurred

• Allergic reactions: rash, fever, respiratory distress
• Severe weakness, numbness in extremities
• Psychologic dependency: increased need for medication, more frequent requests for medication, increased pain
• CNS depression: dizziness, drowsiness, psychiatric symptoms

Administer:
• With meals for GI symptoms

Perform/provide:
• Storage in tight container at room temperature
• Assistance with ambulation if dizziness, drowsiness occur, especially elderly

Evaluate:
• Therapeutic response: decreased pain, spasticity; muscle spasms of acute, painful musculoskeletal conditions generally short term; long-term therapy seldom warranted

Teach patient/family:
• Not to discontinue medication quickly; insomnia, nausea, headache, spasticity, tachycardia will occur; drug should be tapered off over 1-2 wk
• Not to take with alcohol, other CNS depressants
• To avoid hazardous activities if drowsiness/dizziness occurs
• To avoid using OTC medication: cough preparations, antihistamines, unless directed by prescriber
• To use gum, frequent sips of water for dry mouth

Treatment of overdose: Empty stomach with emesis, gastric lavage, then administer activated charcoal; use anticonvulsants if indicated; monitor cardiac function

cyclopentolate (℞)

(sye-kloe-pen'toe-late)
AK-Pentolate, Cyclogyl, cyclopentolate, Pentolair

Func. class.: Mydriatic, cycloplegic, anticholinergic

Combination products: Cyclomydril Ophthalmic: cyclopentolate HCl 0.2%, phenylephrine HCl 1%

Action: Blocks response of iris sphincter muscle, ciliary muscle of the lens to cholinergic stimulation, resulting in dilation, paralysis of accommodation

Uses: Cycloplegic refraction, mydriasis

Dosage and routes:
• *Adult:* INSTILL SOL 1 gtt of a 1-2% sol, then 1 gtt in 5 min
• *Child >6 yr:* INSTILL SOL 1 gtt of a 0.5%-2% sol, then 1 gtt in 5 min of a 0.5%-1% sol

Available forms: Sol 0.5%, 1%, 2%

Side effects/adverse reactions:

SYST: Tachycardia, confusion, fever, flushing, dry skin, dry mouth, abdominal discomfort (infants: bladder distention, irregular pulse, ***respiratory depression***)

EENT: Blurred vision, temporary burning sensation on instillation, eye dryness, photophobia, conjunctivitis, increased intraocular pressure

CNS: Psychotic reaction, behavior disturbances, ataxia, restlessness, hallucinations, somnolence, disorientation, failure to recognize people, ***grand mal seizures,*** irritability

GI: Abdominal distention, vomiting

Contraindications: Hypersensitivity, infants <3 mo, open- or narrow-angle glaucoma, conjunctivitis

Precautions: Pregnancy (C), elderly, lactation, children, Down syndrome

Pharmacokinetics:
Instill: Peak 30-60 min (mydriasis), 25-75 min (cycloplegia), duration ¼-1 day

NURSING CONSIDERATIONS

Administer:
- After shaking vial to mix drug to clear sol, push stopper to mix sterile H_2O with powder
- After cleaning stopper with rubbing alcohol
- Immediately after reconstituting, discard unused portion

Evaluate:
- Therapeutic response: mydriasis

Teach patient/family:
- To report change in vision, blurring, loss of sight, trouble breathing, sweating, flushing
- Method of instillation: pressure on lacrimal sac for 1 min; do not touch dropper to eye
- That blurred vision will decrease with repeated use of drug
- That drug will burn when instilled
- To wear dark sunglasses for photophobia
- Not to do hazardous activities until able to see

cyclophosphamide (℞)

(sye-kloe-foss'fa-mide)

Cytoxan, Neosar, Procytox*

Func. class.: Antineoplastic alkylating agent

Chem. class.: Nitrogen mustard

Action: Alkylates DNA, RNA; inhibits enzymes that allow synthesis of amino acids in proteins; is also responsible for cross-linking DNA strands; activity is not cell cycle phase specific

Uses: Hodgkin's disease; lymphomas; leukemia; cancer of female reproductive tract, lung, prostate; multiple myeloma; neuroblastoma; retinoblastoma; Ewing's sarcoma

Dosage and routes:
- *Adult:* PO initially 1-5 mg/kg over 2-5 days, maintenance is 1-5 mg/kg; IV initially 40-50 mg/kg in divided doses over 2-5 days, maintenance 10-15 mg/kg q7-10 days, or 3-5 mg/kg q3 days
- *Child:* PO/IV 2-8 mg/kg or 60-250 mg/m^2 in divided doses for 6 or more days; maintenance 10-15 mg/kg q7-10 days or 30 mg/kg q3-4 wk; dose should be reduced by half when bone marrow depression occurs

Available forms: Powder for inj IV 100, 200, 500 mg, 1, 2 g; tabs 25, 50 mg

Side effects/adverse reactions:

CV: ***Cardiotoxicity*** (high doses)

HEMA: ***Thrombocytopenia, leukopenia, pancytopenia; myelosuppression***

GI: Nausea, vomiting, diarrhea, weight loss, colitis, ***hepatotoxicity***

GU: ***Hemorrhagic cystitis,*** *hematuria, neoplasms, amenorrhea, azoospermia, sterility, ovarian fibrosis*

INTEG: Alopecia, dermatitis

RESP: ***Fibrosis***

ENDO: Syndrome of inappropriate antidiuretic hormone (SIADH)

CNS: Headache, dizziness

Contraindications: Lactation, pregnancy (D)

Precautions: Radiation therapy

Pharmacokinetics:
Metabolized by liver; excreted in urine; half-life 4-6½ hr; 50% bound to plasma proteins

Interactions:
- Increased toxicity: aminoglycosides
- Increased metabolism of cyclophosphamide: phenobarbital
- Potentiation of cyclophosphamide: succinylcholine

• Increased bone marrow depression: allopurinol, thiazides
• Decreased digoxin levels: digoxin

Y-site compatibilities: Amikacin, ampicillin, azlocillin bleomycin, cefamandole, cefazolin, cefoperazone, ceforanide, cefotaxime, cefoxitin, cefuroxime, cephalothin, cephapirin, chloramphenicol sodium succinate, cisplatin, clindamycin, doxorubicin, doxycycline, droperidol, erythromycin lactobionate, fludarabine, fluorouracil, furosemide, gentamicin, heparin, idarubicin, kanamycin, leucovorin, melphalan, methotrexate, metoclopramide, metronidazole, mezlocillin, mihocycline, mitomycin, moxalactam, nafcillin, ondansetron, oxacillin, paclitaxel, penicillin G potassium, piperacillin, sargramostim, tetracycline, ticarcillin, ticarcillin-clavulanic, tobramycin, trimethoprim-sulfamethoxazole, vancomycin, vinblastine, vincristine, vinorelbine

Syringe compatibilities: Bleomycin, cisplatin, doxapram, doxorubicin, droperidol, fluorouracil, furosemide, heparin, leucovorin, metoclopramide, methotrexate, mitomycin, mitoxantrone, vinblastine, vincristine

Additive compatibilities: Cisplatin with etoposide, hydroxyzine, methotrexate, methotrexate with fluorouracil

Solution compatibilities: Amino acids 4.25%/D_{25}, D_5/0.9% NaCl, D_5W, 0.9% NaCl

Lab test interferences:
Increase: Uric acid
False positive: Pap test
False negative: PPD, mumps, trichophytin, *Candida*
Decrease: Pseudocholinesterase

NURSING CONSIDERATIONS

Assess:

• CBC, differential, platelet count weekly; withhold drug if WBC is <4000 or platelet count is <75,000; notify prescriber of results
• Pulmonary function tests, chest x-ray films before, during therapy; chest film should be obtained q2 wk during treatment
• Renal function studies: BUN, serum uric acid, urine CrCl before, during therapy
• I&O ratio; report fall in urine output of <30 ml/hr
• Monitor temperature q4h (may indicate beginning infection)
• Liver function tests before, during therapy (bilirubin, AST [SGOT], ALT [SGPT], LDH) as needed or monthly
• Bleeding: hematuria, guaiac, bruising or petechiae, mucosa or orifices q8h
• Dyspnea, rales, unproductive cough, chest pain, tachypnea
• Food preferences; list likes, dislikes
• Effects of alopecia on body image, discuss feelings about body changes
• Yellowing of skin, sclera; dark urine; clay-colored stools; itchy skin; abdominal pain; fever; diarrhea
• Edema in feet, joint pain, stomach pain, shaking
• Inflammation of mucosa, breaks in skin
• Buccal cavity q8h for dryness, sores or ulceration, white patches, oral pain, bleeding, dysphagia; obtain prescription for viscous lidocaine (Xylocaine)
• Symptoms indicating severe allergic reaction: rash, pruritus, urticaria, purpuric skin lesions, itching, flushing
• Tachypnea, ECG changes, dyspnea, edema, fatigue

Administer:

• Fluids IV or PO before chemotherapy to hydrate patient

* Available in Canada only

• Antacid before oral agent, give after evening meal, before bedtime
• Antiemetic 30-60 min before giving drug and prn
• Allopurinol or sodium bicarbonate to maintain uric acid levels, alkalinization of urine
• Prevent hyperuricemia
• Antibiotics for prophylaxis of infection
• IV after diluting 100 mg/5 ml of sterile H_2O or bacteriostatic H_2O; shake; let stand until clear; may be further diluted in up to 250 ml D_5 or NS; give 100 mg or less/min through 3-way stopcock of glucose or saline inf
• Using 21, 23, 25G needle; check site for irritation, phlebitis
• Topical or systemic analgesics for pain
• Local or systemic drugs for infection
• In AM so drug can be eliminated before hs

Perform/provide:
• Storage in tight container at room temperature
• Strict medical asepsis, protective isolation if WBC levels are low
• Special skin care
• Deep-breathing exercises with patient tid-qid; place in semi-Fowler's position
• Increase fluid intake to 2-3 L/day to prevent urate deposits, calculi formation, reduce incidence of hemorrhagic cystitis
• Diet low in purines: organ meats (kidney, liver), dried beans, peas to maintain alkaline urine
• Rinsing of mouth tid-qid with water, club soda; brushing of teeth bid-tid with soft brush or cotton-tipped applicators for stomatitis; use unwaxed dental floss
• Warm compresses at injection site for inflammation

Evaluate:
• Therapeutic response: decreased tumor size, spread of malignancy

Teach patient/family:
• About protective isolation
• That amenorrhea can occur; reversible after stopping treatment
• To report any changes in breathing or coughing
• That hair may be lost during treatment; a wig or hairpiece may make patient feel better; new hair may be different in color, texture
• To avoid foods with citric acid, hot or rough texture
• To report any bleeding, white spots, ulcerations in mouth to prescriber; tell patient to examine mouth qd
• To report signs of infection: increased temperature, sore throat, flu symptoms
• To report signs of anemia: fatigue, headache, faintness, shortness of breath, irritability
• To report bleeding: avoid use of razors, commercial mouthwash
• To avoid use of aspirin products, ibuprofen

cycloserine (℞)

(sye-kloe-ser′een)
Seromycin Pulvules
Func. class.: Antitubercular
Chem. class.: S. orchidaceus, antibiotic

Action: Inhibits cell wall synthesis, analog of D-alanine
Uses: Pulmonary tuberculosis, extrapulmonary as adjunctive
Dosage and routes:
• *Adult:* PO 250 mg q12h × 14 days, then 250 mg q8h × 2 wk if no signs of toxicity, then 250 mg q6h if no signs of toxicity, not to exceed 1 g/day

• *Child:* PO 10-20 mg/kg/day (max 0.75-1 g) individual doses
Available forms: Caps 250 mg
Side effects/adverse reactions:
INTEG: Dermatitis, photosensitivity
CV: ***CHF***
CNS: Headache, anxiety, drowsiness, tremors, ***convulsions,*** lethargy, depression, confusion, psychosis, aggression
HEMA: ***Megaloblastic anemia,*** Vit B_{12}, folic acid deficiency, leukocytosis
Contraindications: Hypersensitivity, seizure disorders, renal disease, alcoholism (chronic), depression, severe anxiety, lactation, anemia
Precautions: Pregnancy (C), children
Pharmacokinetics:
PO: Peak 3-8 hr; excreted unchanged in urine; crosses placenta; excreted in breast milk
Interactions:
• Seizures: alcohol
• May increase CNS toxicity: isoniazid, ethionamide
Lab test interferences:
Increase: AST/ALT
NURSING CONSIDERATIONS
Assess:
• Liver studies qwk: ALT, AST, bilirubin
• Blood levels of drug; keep <30 µg/ml or toxicity may occur
• Mental status often: affect, mood, behavioral changes, psychosis may occur
Administer:
• Using pipette provided; use glass container to prevent adherence to sides
• After C&S is completed, qmo to detect resistance
• Pyridoxine (200-300 mg/day) if ordered to prevent neurotoxicity
Perform/provide:
• Storage in air-tight container at room temp
Evaluate:
• Therapeutic response: decreased symptoms of TB
Teach patient/family:
• To avoid alcohol while taking drug
• That compliance with dosage schedule, length is necessary
• To report neurotoxicity: confusion, headache, drowsiness, tremors, paresthesias, mental changes
• To avoid hazardous activities if drowsiness or dizziness occurs
Treatment of overdose: Administer Vit B_6, anticonvulsants, lavage, O_2, assisted respiration

cyclosporine (℞)

(sye'kloe-spor-een)
Ciclosporine, Cyclosporin A, Sandimmune
Func. class.: Immunosuppressant
Chem. class.: Fungus-derived peptide

Action: Produces immunosuppression by inhibiting lymphocytes (T)
Uses: Organ transplants to prevent rejection
Dosage and routes:
• *Adult and child:* PO 15 mg/kg several hours before surgery, daily for 2 wk, reduce dosage by 2.5 mg/kg/wk to 5-10 mg/kg/day; IV 5-6 mg/kg several hours before surgery, daily, switch to PO form as soon as possible
Available forms: Oral sol 100 mg/ml; inj IV 50 mg/ml; soft gelatin caps 25, 100 mg
Side effects/adverse reactions:
GI: Nausea, vomiting, diarrhea, *oral Candida, gum hyperplasia,* ***hepatotoxicity,*** pancreatitis
INTEG: Rash, acne, *hirsutism*
CNS: Tremors, headache

* Available in Canada only

GU: ***Albuminuria, hematuria, proteinuria, renal failure***

Contraindications: Hypersensitivity

Precautions: Severe renal disease, severe hepatic disease, pregnancy (C)

Pharmacokinetics: Peak 4 hr, highly protein bound, half-life (biphasic) 1.2 hr, 25 hr; metabolized in liver; excreted in feces; crosses placenta; excreted in breast milk

Interactions:

- Increased action of cyclosporine: amphotericin B, cimetidine, ketoconazole
- Decreased action of cyclosporine: phenytoin, rifampin
- Compatibility information unknown; give separately

NURSING CONSIDERATIONS

Assess:

- Renal studies: BUN, creatinine at least monthly during treatment, 3 mo after treatment
- Liver function studies: alk phosphatase, AST, ALT, bilirubin
- Drug blood level during treatment
- Hepatotoxicity: dark urine, jaundice, itching, light-colored stools; drug should be discontinued

Administer:

- IV after diluting each 50 mg/20-100 ml of NS or D_5W; run over 2-6 hr; use an infusion pump, glass inf bottles only
- For several days before transplant surgery
- With corticosteroids
- With meals for GI upset or in chocolate milk
- With oral antifungal for *Candida* infections

Evaluate:

- Therapeutic response: absence of rejection

Teach patient/family:

- To report fever, chills, sore throat, fatigue, since serious infections may occur
- To use contraceptive measures during treatment, for 12 wk after ending therapy

cyproheptadine (℞)

(si-proe-hep'ta-deen)

cyproheptadine HCl, Periactin

Func. class.: Antihistamine, H_1-receptor antagonist

Chem. class.: Piperidine

Action: Acts on blood vessels, GI, respiratory system by competing with histamine for H_1-receptor site; decreases allergic response by blocking histamine

Uses: Allergy symptoms, rhinitis, pruritus, cold urticaria

Investigational uses: Appetite stimulant, management of vascular headache

Dosage and routes:

- *Adult:* PO 4 mg tid-qid, not to exceed 0.5 mg/kg/day
- *Child 7-14 yr:* PO 4 mg bid-tid, not to exceed 16 mg/day
- *Child 2-6 yr:* PO 2 mg bid-tid, not to exceed 12 mg/day

Available forms: Tabs 4 mg; syr 2 mg/5 ml

Side effects/adverse reactions:

CNS: *Dizziness, drowsiness,* poor coordination, fatigue, anxiety, euphoria, confusion, paresthesia, neuritis

CV: Hypotension, palpitations, tachycardia

RESP: Increased thick secretions, wheezing, chest tightness

GI: *Constipation,* dry mouth, nausea, vomiting, anorexia, diarrhea, weight gain

INTEG: Rash, urticaria, photosensitivity

GU: Retention, dysuria, frequency, increased appetite
EENT: Blurred vision, dilated pupils; tinnitus; nasal stuffiness; dry nose, throat, mouth
Contraindications: Hypersensitivity to H_1-receptor antagonist, acute asthma attack, lower respiratory tract disease
Precautions: Increased intraocular pressure, renal disease, cardiac disease, hypertension, bronchial asthma, seizure disorder, stenosed peptic ulcers, hyperthyroidism, prostatic hypertrophy, bladder neck obstruction, pregnancy (B), lactation, elderly
Pharmacokinetics:
PO: Duration 4-6 hr; metabolized in liver; excreted by kidneys; excreted in breast milk
Interactions:
- Increased CNS depression: barbiturates, narcotics, hypnotics, tricyclic antidepressants, alcohol
- Decreased effect of oral anticoagulants, heparin
- Increased effect of cyproheptadine: MAOIs

Lab test interferences:
False negative: Skin allergy tests
NURSING CONSIDERATIONS
Assess:
- I&O ratio; be alert for urinary retention, frequency, dysuria; drug should be discontinued
- CBC during long-term therapy
- Respiratory status: rate, rhythm, increase in bronchial secretions, wheezing, chest tightness
- Cardiac status: palpitations, increased pulse, hypotension

Administer:
- With meals for GI symptoms; absorption may slightly decrease

Perform/provide:
- Hard candy, gum, frequent rinsing of mouth for dryness
- Storage in air-tight container at room temp

Evaluate:
- Therapeutic response: absence of running or congested nose, rashes

Teach patient/family:
- All aspects of drug use; to notify prescriber of confusion, sedation, hypotension
- That this drug decreases anticoagulant (oral) effect
- To avoid driving, other hazardous activity if drowsiness occurs, especially elderly
- To avoid concurrent use of alcohol, other CNS depressants

Treatment of overdose: Ipecac syrup or lavage, diazepam, vasopressors, barbiturates (short-acting)

---

cytarabine (℞)

(sye-tare'a-been)
cytarabine, Cytosar*, Cytosar-U, Tarabine PFS
Func. class.: Antineoplastic, antimetabolite
Chem. class.: Pyrimidine nucleoside

Action: Competes with physiologic substrate of DNA synthesis, thus interfering with cell replication in the S phase of the cell cycle (before mitosis)
Uses: Acute myelocytic leukemia, acute lymphocytic leukemia, chronic myelocytic leukemia, and in combination for non-Hodgkin's lymphomas in children
Dosage and routes:
Acute myelocytic leukemia
- *Adult:* IV INF 200 mg/m^2/day × 5 days; INTRATHECAL 5-50 mg/m^2/day × 3 days/wk or 30 mg/m^2/day q4d

In combination
- *Child:* IV INF 100 mg/m^2/day × 5-10 days

---

* Available in Canada only

Available forms: Inj IV, intrathecal 100, 500 mg, 1, 2 g

Side effects/adverse reactions:

HEMA: Thrombophlebitis, bleeding, ***thrombocytopenia, leukopenia, myelosuppression, anemia***

GI: Nausea, vomiting, anorexia, diarrhea, stomatitis, ***hepatotoxicity,*** abdominal pain, hematemesis, ***GI hemorrhage***

EENT: Sore throat, conjunctivitis

GU: Urinary retention, ***renal failure, hyperuricemia***

INTEG: Rash, fever, freckling, cellulitis

RESP: ***Pneumonia,*** dyspnea

CV: Chest pain, ***cardiopathy***

CNS: Neuritis, dizziness, headache, personality changes, ataxia, mechanical dysphasia, ***coma***

CYTARABINE SYNDROME: Fever, myalgia, bone pain, chest pain, rash, conjunctivitis, malaise (6-12 hr after administration)

Contraindications: Hypersensitivity, infants, pregnancy (1st trimester)

Precautions: Renal disease, hepatic disease, pregnancy (C), lactation

Pharmacokinetics:

INTRATHECAL: Half-life 2 hr; metabolized in liver; excreted in urine (primarily inactive metabolite); crosses blood-brain barrier, placenta

IV: Distribution half-life 10 min, elimination half-life 1-3 hr

Interactions:

- Increased toxicity: radiation or other antineoplastics
- Decreased effects of oral digoxin

Syringe compatibility: Metoclopramide

Y-site compatibilities: Amsacrine, fludarabine, ondansetron, sargramostim

Additive compatibilities: Corticotropin, daunorubicin with etoposide, hydroxyzine, lincomycin, methotrexate, potassium chloride, prednisolone, sodium bicarbonate, vincristine

Solution compatibilities: Amino acids, 4.25%/D_{25}, D_5/LR, D_5/0.2% NaCl, D_5/0.9% NaCl, D_{10}/0.9% NaCl, D_5W, invert sugar 10% in electrolyte #1, Ringer's LR, 0.9% NaCl, sodium lactate 1/6 mol/L, TPN #57

NURSING CONSIDERATIONS

Assess:

- CBC (RBC, Hct, Hgb), differential, platelet count weekly; withhold drug if WBC is <4000/mm^3, platelet count is <75,000/mm^3, or RBC, Hct, Hgb low; notify prescriber of these results
- Renal function studies: BUN, serum uric acid, urine creatinine clearance, electrolytes before and during therapy
- I&O ratio; report fall in urine output to <30 ml/hr
- Monitor temperature q4h; fever may indicate beginning infection; no rectal temperatures
- Liver function tests before and during therapy: bilirubin, ALT (SGOT), AST (SGPT), alk phosphatase, as needed or monthly
- Blood uric acid during therapy
- Cytarabine syndrome: fever, myalgia, bone pain, chest pain, rash, conjunctivitis, malaise; corticosteroids may be ordered
- Bleeding: hematuria, guaiac, bruising or petechiae, mucosa or orifices q8h
- Dyspnea, rales, unproductive cough, chest pain, tachypnea, fatigue, increased pulse, pallor, lethargy, personality changes, with high doses
- Food preferences; list likes, dislikes
- Edema in feet, joint pain, stomach pain, shaking

• Inflammation of mucosa, breaks in skin
• Yellowing of skin, sclera; dark urine; clay-colored stools; itchy skin; abdominal pain; fever; diarrhea
• Buccal cavity q8h for dryness, sores or ulceration, white patches, oral pain, bleeding, dysphagia
• Local irritation, pain, burning, discoloration at injection site
• GI symptoms: frequency of stools, cramping
• Acidosis, signs of dehydration: rapid respirations, poor skin turgor, decreased urine output, dry skin, restlessness, weakness

Administer:
• IV after diluting 100 mg/5 ml of sterile H_2O for inj; given by direct IV over 1-3 min through free-flowing tubing (IV); may be further diluted in 50-100 ml NS or D_5W, given over 30 min to 24 hr depending on dose
• Antiemetic 30-60 min before giving drug and prn
• Allopurinol or sodium bicarbonate to maintain uric acid levels and alkalinization of the urine
• Prevent hyperuricemia
• Topical or systemic analgesics for pain
• Transfusion for anemia
• Antispasmodic for GI symptoms

Perform/provide:
• Strict medical asepsis and protective isolation if WBC levels are low
• Increase fluid intake to 2-3 L/day to prevent urate deposits and calculi formation, unless contraindicated
• Diet low in purines: absence of organ meats (kidney, liver), dried beans, peas to prevent increased urate deposits
• Rinsing of mouth tid-qid with water, club soda; brushing of teeth bid-tid with soft brush or cotton-tipped applicators for stomatitis; use unwaxed dental floss
• HOB raised to facilitate breathing if dyspnea or pneumonia

Evaluate:
• Therapeutic response: decreased tumor size, spread of malignancy

Teach patient/family:
• Why protective isolation necessary
• To report any coughing, chest pain, changes in breathing; may indicate beginning pneumonia
• To avoid foods with citric acid, hot or rough texture if stomatitis is present
• To report stomatitis: any bleeding, white spots, ulcerations in mouth; tell patient to examine mouth qd, report any symptoms
• To report signs of infection: increased temperature, sore throat, flu symptoms
• To report signs of anemia: fatigue, headache, faintness, shortness of breath, irritability
• To report bleeding; avoid use of razors, commercial mouthwash
• To avoid use of aspirin products or ibuprofen

dacarbazine (DTIC) (℞)

(da-kar′ba-zeen)
DTIC-Dome, DTIC
Func. class.: Antineoplastic alkylating agent
Chem. class.: Cytotoxic triazine

Action: Alkylates DNA, RNA; inhibits enzymes that allow synthesis of amino acids in proteins; also responsible for cross-linking DNA strands; activity is not cell cycle phase specific

Uses: Hodgkin's disease, sarcomas,

neuroblastoma, malignant melanoma

Dosage and routes:

• *Adult:* IV 2-4.5 mg/kg or 70-160 mg/m^2 qd × 10 days; repeat q4wk depending on response or 250 mg/m^2 qd × 5 days; repeat q3wk

Available forms: Inj IV 100, 200 mg

Side effects/adverse reactions:

HEMA: ***Thrombocytopenia, leukopenia,*** anemia

GI: Nausea, anorexia, vomiting, ***hepatotoxicity***

CNS: Facial paresthesia, flushing, fever, malaise

INTEG: Alopecia, dermatitis, pain at injection site

Contraindications: Lactation

Precautions: Radiation therapy, pregnancy (1st trimester) (C)

Pharmacokinetics:

Metabolized by liver; excreted in urine; half-life 35 min, terminal 5 hr, 5% protein bound

Interactions:

• Decreased effectiveness of dacarbazine: phenytoin, phenobarbital

Y-site compatibilities: Fludarabine, melphalan, ondansetron, sargramostim, paclitaxel, vinorelbine

Additive incompatibilities: Hydrocortisone sodium succinate, cysteine

Additive compatibilities: Bleomycin, carmustine, cyclophosphamide, cytarabine, dactinomycin, doxorubicin, fluorouracil, mercaptopurine, methotrexate, vinblastine

NURSING CONSIDERATIONS

Assess:

• CBC, differential, platelet count weekly; withhold drug if WBC <4000 or platelet count <75,000; notify prescriber of results

• Monitor temp q4h (may indicate beginning infection)

• Liver function tests before, during therapy (bilirubin, AST, ALT, LDH) as needed or monthly

• Bleeding: hematuria, guaiac, bruising or petechiae, mucosa or orifices q8h

• Food preferences; list likes, dislikes

• Effects of alopecia on body image, discuss feelings about body changes

• Yellowing of skin, sclera; dark urine; clay-colored stools; itchy skin; abdominal pain; fever; diarrhea

• Inflammation of mucosa, breaks in skin

Administer:

• Antiemetic 30-60 min before giving drug to prevent vomiting

• Antibiotics for prophylaxis of infection

• After diluting 100 mg/9.9 ml of sterile H_2O for inj (10 mg/ml), give by direct IV over 1 min through Y-tube or 3-way stopcock; may be further diluted in 50-250 ml D_5W or NS for inj, given as an inf over ½ hr

• Watch for extravasation; give Na thiosulfate 10% 4 ml plus sterile H_2O 5 ml, 3-5 ml SC if needed

Perform/provide:

• Storage in light-resistant container, dry area

• Strict medical asepsis, protective isolation if WBC levels are low

• Increase fluid intake to 2-3 L/day to prevent urate deposits, calculi formation

• Warm compresses at injection site for inflammation

Evaluate:

• Therapeutic response: decreased tumor size, spread of malignancy

Teach patient/family:

• About protective isolation

• Advise patient to avoid prolonged exposure to sun

• That hair may be lost during treatment; a wig or hairpiece may make the patient feel better; new hair may be different in color, texture
• To report signs of infection: fever, sore throat, flu symptoms
• To report signs of anemia: fatigue, headache, faintness, shortness of breath, irritability
• To report bleeding; avoid use of razors, commercial mouthwash
• To avoid use of aspirin products or ibuprofen

dactinomycin (℞)

(dak-ti-noe-mye'sin)
Cosmegen
Func. class.: Antineoplastic, antibiotic

Action: Inhibits DNA, RNA, protein synthesis; derived from *S. parrullus;* replication is decreased by binding to DNA, which causes strand splitting; cell cycle nonspecific; a vesicant
Uses: Sarcomas, melanomas, trophoblastic tumors in women, testicular cancer, Wilms' tumor, rhabdomyosarcoma
Dosage and routes:
• *Adult:* IV 500 μg/m^2/day × 5 days; stop drug for 2-4 wk; then repeat cycle
• *Child:* IV 15 μg/kg/day × 5 days, not to exceed 500 μg/day; stop drug until bone marrow recovery, then repeat cycle
Available forms: Inj IV 0.5 mg/vial
Side effects/adverse reactions:
HEMA: ***Thrombocytopenia, leukopenia, aplastic anemia***
GI: Nausea, vomiting, anorexia, stomatitis, ***hepatotoxicity,*** abdominal pain, diarrhea
INTEG: Rash, alopecia, pain at injection site, folliculitis, acne, desquamation, ***extravasation***
EENT: Chelitis, dysphagia, esophagitis
CNS: Malaise, fatigue, lethargy, fever
MS: Myalgia
Contraindications: Hypersensitivity, herpes infection, child <6 mo
Precautions: Renal disease, hepatic disease, pregnancy (C), lactation, bone marrow depression
Pharmacokinetics: Half-life 36 hr
IV: onset 2-5 min; concentrates in kidneys, liver, spleen; does not cross blood-brain barrier; excreted in feces and urine
Interactions:
• Increased toxicity: other antineoplastics, radiation
Y-site compatibilities: Fludarabine, ondansetron, sargramostim
Lab test interferences:
Increase: Uric acid

NURSING CONSIDERATIONS

Assess:
• CBC, differential, platelet count weekly; withhold drug if WBC is <4000/mm^3 or platelet count is <75,000/mm^3; notify prescriber
• Renal function studies: BUN, serum uric acid, urine CrCl, electrolytes before, during therapy
• I&O ratio; report fall in urine output to <30 ml/hr
• Monitor temp q4h; fever may indicate beginning infection
• Liver function tests before, during therapy: bilirubin, AST, ALT, alk phosphatase, as needed or monthly
• Bleeding: hematuria, guaiac stools, bruising, petechiae, mucosa or orifices q8h
• Food preferences; list likes, dislikes
• Effects of alopecia on body image; discuss feelings about body changes
• Inflammation of mucosa, breaks in skin
• Yellowing of skin, sclera; dark

* Available in Canada only

urine; clay-colored stools; itchy skin; abdominal pain; fever; diarrhea

• Buccal cavity q8h for dryness, sores, ulceration, white patches, oral pain, bleeding, dysphagia

• Local irritation, pain, burning at injection site

• Symptoms indicating severe allergic reaction: rash, pruritus, urticaria, purpuric skin lesions, itching, flushing

• GI symptoms: frequency of stools, cramping, nausea, vomiting, anorexia

• Acidosis, signs of dehydration: rapid respirations, poor skin turgor, decreased urine output, dry skin, restlessness, weakness, sunken eyeball in children

Administer:

• After diluting 0.5 mg/1.1 ml of sterile H_2O for inj without preservative; use 2.2 ml (0.25 mg/ml), give by direct IV at 0.5 mg or less/min through Y-tube or 3-way stopcock of inf in progress; may be further diluted if required in 50 ml D_5W or NS for infusion; run over 10-15 min

• Antiemetic 30-60 min before giving drug to prevent vomiting

• Check for extravasation at inj site

• Topical or systemic analgesics for pain

• Local or systemic drugs for infection

• Hydrocortisone, sodium thiosulfate to infiltration area, and ice compress after stopping infusion

• Antispasmodic for GI symptoms: cramping, diarrhea, nausea, vomiting

Perform/provide:

• Strict hand-washing technique, gloves and protective covering

• Liquid diet: carbonated beverages; gelatin may be added if patient is not nauseated or vomiting

• Rinsing of mouth tid-qid with water, club soda; brushing of teeth bid-qid with soft brush or cotton-tipped applicators for stomatitis; use unwaxed dental floss to prevent injury

• Storage in cool, dark environment; do not expose to bright light or freeze

Evaluate:

• Therapeutic response: decreased tumor size, spread of malignancy

Teach patient/family:

• To avoid alcohol while taking this drug

• That contraception is needed during treatment and for 4-6 months after discontinuing therapy

• To avoid vaccinations without order by prescriber

• To report any complaints, side effects to nurse or prescriber

• That hair may be lost during treatment after 1-2 wks and that wig or hairpiece may make patient feel better; tell patient that new hair may be different in color, texture

• To avoid foods with citric acid, hot or rough texture when stomatitis is present

• To report any bleeding, white spots, ulcerations in mouth to prescriber; tell patient to examine mouth qd

• To avoid crowds, person with known infection when granulocyte count is low

dalteparin (℞)

(dal-tep'a-rin)

Fragmin

Func. class.: Anticoagulant

Chem. class.: Low molecular weight heparin

Action: Prevents conversion of fibrinogen to fibrin and prothrombin to thrombin by enhancing inhibitory effects of antithrombin III

Uses: Prevention of deep vein thrombosis in abdominal surgery patients

Dosage and routes:

• *Adult:* SC 2500 IU each day starting 1-2 hr prior to surgery and repeat qd × 5-10 days post operatively

• To be used SC only

Available forms:

Prefilled syringes, 2500 antifactor-Xa IU/0.2 ml

Side effects/adverse reactions:

CNS: ***Intracranial bleeding***

SYST: Hypersensitivity, ***hemorrhage, anaphylaxis*** possible

HEMA: ***Thrombocytopenia***

INTEG: Pruritus, superficial wound infection

Contraindications: Hypersensitivity to this drug, heparin, or other anticoagulants; hemophilia, leukemia with bleeding, thrombocytopenic purpura, cerebrovascular hemorrhage, cerebral aneurysm, severe hypertension, other severe cardiac disease

Precautions: Elderly, pregnancy (B), hepatic disease, severe renal disease, blood dyscrasias, subacute bacterial endocarditis, acute nephritis, lactation, child, recent childbirth, peptic ulcer disease, pericarditis, pericardial effusion, recent lumbar puncture, vasculitis, other diseases where bleeding is possible

Pharmacokinetics: Excreted by kidneys, half-life 2 hr, peak 4 hr onset and duration unknown

Interactions:

• Increased risk of bleeding: aspirin, oral anticoagulants, platelet inhibitors

NURSING CONSIDERATIONS

Assess:

• For blood studies (Hct, occult blood in stools) during treatment since bleeding can occur

• For bleeding gums, petechiae, ecchymosis, black tarry stools, hematuria, epistaxis, decrease in Hct, B/P; may indicate bleeding, possible hemorrhage; notify prescriber immediately, drug should be discontinued

• For hypersensitivity: fever, skin rash, urticaria; notify prescriber immediately

• For needed dosage change q1-2wk; dose may need to be decreased if bleeding occurs

Administer:

• Do not give IM or IV drug route; approved is SC only

• By SC only; have patient sit or lie down; SC inj may be around the navel in a U-shape, upper outer side of thigh or upper outer quadrangle of the buttocks; rotate inj sites

• Changing needles is not recommended

Evaluate:

• Therapeutic response: absence of deep-vein thrombosis

Teach patient/family:

• To avoid OTC preparations that may cause serious drug interactions unless directed by prescriber; may contain aspirin; other anticoagulants

• To use soft-bristle toothbrush to avoid bleeding gums, avoid contact sports, use electric razor, avoid IM injection

• To report any signs of bleeding: gums, under skin, urine, stools; unusual bruising

Treatment of overdose:

Protamine sulfate 1% given IV; 1 mg protamine/100 anti-Xa IU of Fragmin given

danazol (℞)

(da'na-zole)

Cyclomen*, danazol, Danocrine

Func. class.: Androgen

Chem. class.: α-Ethinyl testosterone derivative

Action: Atrophy of endometrial tissue; decreases FSH, LH, which are controlled by pituitary; this leads to amenorrhea/anovulation

Uses: Endometriosis, prevention of hereditary angioedema, fibrocystic breast disease

Dosage and routes:

Endometriosis

• *Adult:* PO initial dose 500 mg bid, then decreased to 400 mg bid × 3-9 mo

Fibrocystic breast disease

• *Adult:* PO 100-400 mg qd in 2 divided doses × 2-6 mo

Hereditary angioedema

• *Adult:* PO 200 mg bid-tid until desired response, then decrease dose to 100 mg at 1-3 mo intervals

Available forms: Caps 50, 100, 200 mg

Side effects/adverse reactions:

INTEG: Rash, acneiform lesions, oily hair, skin, flushing, sweating, acne vulgaris, alopecia, hirsutism, pruritis

CNS: Dizziness, headache, fatigue, tremors, paresthesias, flushing, sweating, anxiety, lability, insomnia, carpal tunnel syndrome

MS: Cramps, spasms

CV: Increased B/P

GU: Hematuria, amenorrhea, atrophic vaginitis, decreased libido, decreased breast size, clitoral hypertrophy, testicular atrophy

GI: Nausea, vomiting, constipation, weight gain, ***cholestatic jaundice***

EENT: Conjunctional edema, nasal congestion

ENDO: Abnormal GTT

Contraindications: Severe renal, severe cardiac, severe hepatic disease, hypersensitivity, genital bleeding (abnormal)

Precautions: Migraine headaches, seizure disorders, pregnancy (C)

Interactions:

• Increased effects of oral antidiabetics, oxyphenbutazone

• Increased prothrombin time: anticoagulants

• Increased edema: ACTH, adrenal steroids

• Decreased effects of: insulin

Lab test interferences:

Increase: Cholesterol

Decrease: Cholesterol, T_4, T_3, thyroid ^{131}I uptake test, 17-KS, PBI

Interferences: GTT

NURSING CONSIDERATIONS

Assess:

• K, blood sugar, urine glucose while on long-term therapy

• Weight daily; notify prescriber if weekly weight gain is >5 lb; drug should be decreased or discontinued

• I&O ratio; be alert for decreasing urinary output, increasing edema

• Edema, hypertension, cardiac symptoms, jaundice

• Mental status: affect, mood, behavioral changes, aggression, sleep disorders, depression anxiety, lability

• Signs of virilization: deepening of voice, decreased libido, facial hair that may not be reversible

• Hypercalcemia: GI symptoms, polydipsia, polyuria, increased calcium levels above 11 mg/dl, loss of muscle tone

Administer:

• With food or milk to decrease GI symptoms (i.e., nausea, vomiting, anorexia, dyspepsia)

Perform/provide:
• Storage in air-tight container at room temperature; do not freeze
• ROM exercise for patients who are immobile to relieve cramps and spasms

Evaluate:
• Therapeutic response: decreased pain in endometriosis; decreased size, pain in fibrocystic breast disease

Teach patient/family:
• To notify prescriber if therapeutic response decreases
• Not to discontinue medication abruptly; to taper over several wk
• To report menstrual irregularities; that amenorrhea usually occurs but menstruation resumes 2-3 mo after termination of therapy without medical intervention
• About routine breast self-exam and to report any increase in nodule size
• That drug should induce anovulation; reversible within 60-90 days after drug is discontinued and treatment will need to be resumed
• That endometriosis tends to recur after drug is discontinued

---

dantrolene (℞)

(dan'troe-leen)

Dantrium, Dantrium Intravenous

Func. class.: Skeletal muscle relaxant, direct acting

Chem. class.: Hydantoin

Action: Interferes with intracellular release of calcium from the sarcoplasmic reticulium necessary to initiate contraction; slow catabolism in malignant hyperthermia

Uses: Spasticity in multiple sclerosis, stroke, spinal cord injury, cerebral palsy, malignant hyperthermia

Dosage and routes:

Spasticity
• *Adult:* PO 25 mg/day; may increase by 25-100 mg bid-qid, not to exceed 400 mg/day × 1 wk
• *Child:* PO 1 mg/kg/day given in divided doses bid-tid; dosage may increase gradually, not to exceed 100 mg qid

Prevention of malignant hyperthermia
• *Adult and Child:* PO 4-8 mg/kg/day in 3-4 divided doses × 1-2 days prior to procedures, give last dose 4 hr preop

Malignant hyperthermia
• *Adult and child:* IV 1 mg/kg, may repeat to total dose of 10 mg/kg; PO 4-8 mg/kg/day in 4 divided doses × 3 days to prevent further hyperthermia

Available forms: Caps 25, 50, 100 mg; powder for inj IV 20 mg/vial

Side effects/adverse reactions:

CNS: *Dizziness, weakness, fatigue, drowsiness,* headache, disorientation, insomnia, paresthesias, tremors

EENT: Nasal congestion, blurred vision, mydriasis

HEMA: ***Eosinophilia***

CV: Hypotension, chest pain, palpitations

GI: *Nausea,* constipation, vomiting, increased AST (SGOT), alk phosphatase, abdominal pain, dry mouth, anorexia, hepatitis dyspepsia

GU: Urinary frequency, nocturia, impotence, crystalluria

INTEG: Rash, pruritus, photosensitivity

Contraindications: Hypersensitivity, compromised pulmonary function, active hepatic disease, impaired myocardial function

Precautions: Peptic ulcer disease, renal disease, hepatic disease, stroke,

---

* Available in Canada only

seizure disorder, diabetes mellitus, pregnancy (C), lactation, elderly

Pharmacokinetics:

PO: Peak 5 hr; highly protein bound; half-life 8 hr; metabolized in liver; excreted in urine (metabolites)

Interactions:

• Dysrhythmias: verapamil
• Increased CNS depression: alcohol, tricyclic antidepressants, narcotics, barbiturates, sedatives, hypnotics, magnessium sulfate, antihistamines
• Hepatotoxicity: estrogens
• Considered incompatible in sol or syringe; compatibility unknown

NURSING CONSIDERATIONS

Assess:

• For increased seizure activity, ECG in epilepsy patient; poor seizure control has occurred
• I&O ratio; check for urinary retention, frequency, hesitancy, especially elderly
• Hepatic function by frequent determination of AST (SGOT), ALT (SGPT), renal function studies, BUN, creatinine, CBC
• Allergic reactions: rash, fever, respiratory distress
• Severe weakness, numbness in extremities, prescriber should be notified and drug discontinued
• Tolerance: increased need for medication, more frequent requests for medication, increased pain
• CNS depression: dizziness, drowsiness, insomnia, psychiatric symptoms
• Signs of hepatotoxicity: jaundice, yellow sclera, pain in abdomen, nausea, fever, prescriber should be notified, drug should be discontinued

Administer:

• With meals for GI symptoms, caps may be opened and mixed with food/liquid
• IV after diluting 20 mg/60 ml sterile H_2O for inj without bacteriostatic agent (333 μg/ml); shake until clear; give by rapid IV push through Y-tube or 3-way stopcock; follow by prescribed doses immediately

Perform/provide:

• Storage in tight container at room temperature; protect diluted sol from light, use within 6 hr
• Gum, frequent sips of water for dry mouth
• Assistance with ambulation if dizziness/drowsiness occurs

Evaluate:

• Therapeutic response: decreased pain, spasticity

Teach patient/family:

• Not to discontinue medication quickly; hallucinations, spasticity, tachycardia will occur; drug should be tapered off over 1-2 wk; notify prescriber of abdominal pain, jaundiced sclera, clay-colored stools, change in color of urine
• Not to take with alcohol, other CNS depressants
• That if improvement does not occur within 6 wk, prescriber may discontinue
• To avoid altering activities while taking this drug
• To avoid hazardous activities if drowsiness, dizziness occurs
• To avoid using OTC medication: cough preparations, antihistamines, unless directed by prescriber

Treatment of overdose: Induce emesis of conscious patient; lavage, dialysis

dapiprazole (℞)

(da-pip′ra-zole)

Rev-Eyes

Func. class.: Ophthalmic α-adrenergic blocking agents

Action: Blocks α-adrenergic receptors in smooth muscle in the eye;

miosis occurs through effect on the iris dilator muscle
Uses: Iatrogenically induces mydriasis produced by adrenergic or parasympatholytic agents
Dosage and routes:
• *Adult:* INSTILL 2 gtt, then 2 gtt 5 min later applied to the conjunctiva; do not use more than qwk
Available forms: Pwd for lyophilized 25 mg (0.5% sol reconstituted)
Side effects/adverse reactions:
EENT: Burning, ptosis, lid erythema, lid edema, itching, keratitis, corneal edema; brow ache, photophobia, headaches, eye dryness, tearing, blurring vision
Contraindications: Hypersensitivity, acute iritis
Precautions: Pregnancy (B), lactation, children, severe cardiovascular disease

NURSING CONSIDERATIONS

Assess:
• Cardiac status; watch for bradycardia, palpitations, especially in cardiac disease (including hypertension)

Administer:
• By instillation after tearing off aluminum seals; remove and discard rubber plugs from drugs and diluent; remove dropper and attach to vial; shake

Perform/provide:
• Storage at room temp after reconstituting × 21 days

Teach patient/family:
• That drug may cause burning, itching, blurring, dryness of eye
• Method for instillation
• Discard unused solution or solution that is not clear and colorless

dapsone (DDS) (℞)

(dap'sone)
Avlosulfon*, Dapsone
Func. class.: Leprostatic
Chem. class.: Sulfone

Action: Bactericidal and bacteriostatic against *M. leprae*
Uses: Hansen's disease, PCP (*Pneumocystitis carinii* pneumonia)
Dosage and routes:
Hansen's disease
• *Adult:* PO 100 mg qd with rifampin 600 mg qd × 6 mo
PCP
• *Adult:* PO 50-100 mg/day usually given with trimethoprin 20 mg/kg/day in 4 divided doses
Available forms: Tabs 25, 100 mg
Side effects/adverse reactions:
INTEG: ***Exfoliative dermatitis,*** photosensitivity
CNS: Peripheral neuropathy, headache, anxiety, drowsiness, tremors, ***convulsions,*** lethargy, depression, confusion, psychosis, aggression
GI: Nausea, vomiting, abdominal pain, anorexia
GU: Proteinuria, nephrotic syndrome, renal papillary necrosis
EENT: Blurred vision, optic neuritis, photophobia
HEMA: ***Megaloblastic anemia***
Contraindications: Hypersensitivity to sulfones, severe anemia
Precautions: Renal disease, hepatic disease, G6PD deficiency, pregnancy (A), lactation
Pharmacokinetics:
Rapid complete absorption; half-life 25-31 hr; highly bound to plasma protein; metabolized in liver; excreted in urine
Interactions:
• Increased side effects: hemolytic agents

* Available in Canada only

• Increased action of dapsone: probenecid, folic acid antagonists
• Decreased blood levels of dapsone: rifampin
• Decreased bactericidal action: PABA
• Decreased GI absorption of dapsone: activated charcoal

NURSING CONSIDERATIONS

Assess:
• Temp; if >101° F (38.3° C), drug should be reduced
• Liver studies qwk: ALT (SGPT), AST (SGOT), bilirubin
• Renal status: BUN, creatinine, output, specific gravity, urinalysis before; qmo
• Blood levels of drug
• For anemia: Hct, Hgb, fatigue; for peripheral neuritis; or exfoliative dermatitis
• Mental status often: affect, mood, behavioral changes; psychosis may occur
• Hepatic status: decreased appetite, jaundice, dark urine, fatigue

Administer:
• With meals for GI symptoms
• Antiemetic if vomiting occurs
• After C&S is completed; qmo to detect resistance

Perform/provide:
• Infants kept with mothers infected with leprosy; breastfeeding during drug therapy encouraged

Evaluate:
• Therapeutic response: decreased symptoms of Hansen's disease

Teach patient/family:
• That therapeutic effects may occur after 3-6 mo of drug therapy
• That compliance with dosage schedule, duration is necessary
• To avoid hazardous machinery if drowsiness occurs

daunorubicin (℞)

(daw-noe-roo'bi-sin)

Cerubidine

Func. class.: Antineoplastic, antibiotic

Chem. class.: Anthracycline glycoside

Action: Inhibits DNA synthesis, primarily; derived from *S. verticillus;* replication is decreased by binding to DNA, which causes strand splitting; cell cycle specific (S phase); a vesicant

Uses: Myelogenous, monocytic leukemia, acute nonlymphocytic leukemia, Ewing's sarcoma, Wilms' tumor, neuroblastoma, rhabdomyosarcoma

Dosage and routes:

Single agent
• *Adult:* IV 60 mg/m^2/day × 3-5 day q4wk

In combination
• *Adult:* IV 45 mg/m^2/day × 3 days, then 2 days of subsequent courses with cytosine arabinoside

Available forms: Inj IV 20 mg powder/vial

Side effects/adverse reactions:

HEMA: ***Thrombocytopenia, leukopenia, anemia***

GI: Nausea, vomiting, anorexia, mucositis, ***hepatotoxicity***

GU: Impotence, sterility, amenorrhea, gynecomastia, hyperuricemia

INTEG: Rash, ***extravasation,*** dermatitis, reversible alopecia, cellulitis, thrombophlebitis at injection site

CV: ***Dysrhythmias, CHF, pericarditis, myocarditis,*** peripheral edema

CNS: Fever, chills

Contraindications: Hypersensitivity, pregnancy (1st trimester) (D), lactation, systemic infections, cardiac disease

Precautions: Renal, hepatic disease; gout; bone marrow depression

Pharmacokinetics: Half-life 18½ hr; metabolized by liver; crosses placenta; excreted in breast milk, urine, bile

Interactions:

• Increased toxicity: other antineoplastics, radiation

• Incompatible with dexamethasone, heparin

Y-site compatibilities: Ondansetron, melphalan, vinorelbine

Additive compatibilities: Cytarabine with etoposide, hydrocortisone sodium succinate; not recommended for admixing

Solution compatibilities: $D_{3.3}$/0.3% NaCl, D_5W, Normosol R, Ringer's, 0.9% NaCl

Lab test interferences:

Increase: Uric acid

NURSING CONSIDERATIONS

Assess:

• CBC, differential, platelet count weekly; withhold drug if WBC is $<4000/mm^3$ or platelet count is $<75,000/mm^3$; notify prescriber

• Blood, urine uric acid levels

• Renal function studies: BUN, serum uric acid, urine CrCl, electrolytes before, during therapy

• I&O ratio; report fall in urine output to <30 ml/hr

• Monitor temperature q4h; fever may indicate beginning infection

• Liver function tests before, during therapy: bilirubin, AST (SGOT), ALT (SGPT), alk phosphatase as needed or monthly

• ECG; watch for ST-T wave changes, low QRS and T, possible dysrhythmias (sinus tachycardia, heart block, PVCs)

• Bleeding: hematuria, guaiac stools, bruising or petechiae, mucosa or orifices q8h

• Food preferences; list likes, dislikes

• Effects of alopecia on body image; discuss feelings about body changes

• Inflammation of mucosa, breaks in skin

• Yellowing of skin, sclera; dark urine; clay-colored stools; itchy skin; abdominal pain; fever; diarrhea

• Buccal cavity q8h for dryness, sores or ulceration, white patches, oral pain, bleeding, dysphagia

• Local irritation, pain, burning at injection site

• GI symptoms: frequency of stools, cramping

• Acidosis, signs of dehydration: rapid respirations, poor skin turgor, decreased urine output, dry skin, restlessness, weakness

• Cardiac status: B/P, pulse, character, rhythm, rate

Administer:

• IV after diluting 20 mg/4 ml sterile H_2O for inj (5 mg/ml), rotate, further dilute in 10-15 ml NS; give over 3-5 min by direct IV through Y-tube or 3-way stopcock of inf of D_5 or NS

• Antiemetic 30-60 min before giving drug and 6-10 hr after treatment to prevent vomiting

• Allopurinol or sodium bicarbonate to reduce uric acid levels, alkalinization of urine

• Transfusion for anemia

• Antispasmodic for GI symptoms

• Hydrocortisone for extravasation; apply ice compress after stopping infusion

Perform/provide:

• Strict hand-washing technique, gloves, protective clothing

• Liquid diet: carbonated beverages, gelatin may be added if patient is not nauseated or vomiting

• Increased fluid intake to 2-3 L/day to prevent urate and calculi formation

• Diet low in purines: absence of organ meats (kidney, liver), dried beans, peas to reduce uric acid level
• Rinsing of mouth tid-qid with water, club soda; brushing of teeth bid-qid with soft brush or cotton-tipped applicators for stomatitis; use unwaxed dental floss
• Storage at room temp 24 hr after reconstituting or 48 hr refrigerated

Evaluate:
• Therapeutic response: decreased tumor size, spread of malignancy

Teach patient/family:
• To report any complaints, side effects to nurse or prescriber
• That hair may be lost during treatment and wig or hairpiece may make patient feel better; tell patient that new hair may be different in color, texture
• To avoid foods with citric acid, hot or rough texture
• To report any bleeding, white spots, ulcerations in mouth; tell patient to examine mouth qd
• That urine and other body fluids may be red-orange for 48 hr

deferoxamine (℞)

(de-fer-ox′a-meen)
Desferal
Func. class.: Heavy metal antagonist
Chem. class.: Chelating agent

Action: Binds iron ions (ferric ions) to form water-soluble complex that is removed by kidneys
Uses: Acute, chronic iron intoxication, hemochromatosis, hemosiderosis
Dosage and routes:
Acute iron toxicity
• *Adult and child:* IM/IV 1 g, then 500 mg q4h × 2 doses, then 500 mg q4-12h × 2 doses, not to exceed 15 mg/kg/hr or 6 g/24 hr
Chronic iron toxicity
• *Adult and child:* IM 500 mg-1 g/day plus IV INF 2 g given by separate line with each blood transfusion, not to exceed 15 mg/kg/hr or 6 g/24 hr; SC 1-2 g over 8-24 hr by SC infusion pump
Available forms: Powder for inj IV, IM, SC 500 mg/vial
Side effects/adverse reactions:
CNS: Flushing, shock following rapid IV
INTEG: Urticaria, erythema, pruritus, pain at injection site, fever
CV: Hypotension, tachycardia
GI: Diarrhea, abdominal cramps
EENT: Blurred vision, cataracts, decreased healing, ***ototoxicity***
MS: Leg cramps
GU: Dysuria, pyelonephritis
SYST: ***Anaphylaxis***
Contraindications: Hypersensitivity, anuria, severe renal disease, child <3 yr
Precautions: Pregnancy (C), lactation
Pharmacokinetics:
Primarily forms a complex excreted by kidneys as complex, unchanged drug
Interactions:
• Incompatible with other drugs in sol or syringe

NURSING CONSIDERATIONS
Assess:
• Poisoning; type of agent, time, amount ingested
• Acute, early iron toxicity: nausea, vomiting, abdominal cramping, bloody diarrhea
• Acute later iron toxicity: loss of consciousness, shock, metabolic acidosis
• Inj site for redness, inflammation, pain
• For blood in stools
• Vision and hearing periodically

- VS
- I&O, kidney function studies: BUN, creatinine, CrCl, serum iron levels
- Allergic reactions: rash, urticaria; drug should be discontinued

Administer:

- IV (used for shock) after diluting 500 mg/2 ml H_2O for inj; when dissolved, must be further diluted with D_5W or LR or NS; run at <15 mg/kg/hr; 2 g/1000 ml usually given over 24 hr; to be used only for short time; IM is preferred route
- IM after diluting with 2 ml sterile water for injection per 500 mg of drug; rotate injection sites
- SC route use abdominal SC tissue by infusion pump × 8-24 hrs/treatment
- Only when epinephrine 1:1000 is on unit for anaphylaxis

Evaluate:

- Therapeutic response: decreased symptoms of heavy metal intoxication

Teach patient/family:

- That urine may turn red
- To avoid Vit C preparations

demeclocycline (℞)

(dem-e-kloe-sye′kleen)

Declomycin

Func. class.: Broad-spectrum antibiotic/antiinfective

Chem. class.: Tetracycline

Action: Inhibits protein synthesis, phosphorylation in microorganisms by binding to 30S ribosomal subunits, reversibly binding to 50S ribosomal subunits; bacteriostatic

Uses: Uncommon gram-positive/gram-negative bacteria, protozoa, *Rickettsia, Mycoplasma*

Dosage and routes:

- *Adult:* PO 150 mg q6h or 300 mg q12h
- *Child >8 yr:* PO 6-12 mg/kg/day in divided doses q6-12h

Gonorrhea

- *Adult:* PO 600 mg, then 300 mg q12h × 4 days, total 3 g

SIADH

- *Adult:* PO 600-1200 mg/day in divided doses

Available forms: Tabs 150, 300 mg; caps 150 mg

Side effects/adverse reactions:

CNS: Fever, headache, paresthesia

HEMA: ***Eosinophilia, neutropenia, thrombocytopenia, leukocytosis, hemolytic anemia***

EENT: Dysphagia, glossitis, decreased calcification of deciduous teeth, abdominal pain, oral candidiasis

GI: Nausea, vomiting, diarrhea, anorexia, enterocolitis, ***hepatotoxicity,*** flatulence, abdominal cramps, epigastric burning, stomatitis, ***psuedomembranous colitis***

CV: Pericarditis

GU: Increased BUN, polyuria, polydipsia, ***renal failure, nephrotoxicity***

INTEG: Rash, urticaria, photosenitivity, increased pigmentation, ***exfoliative dermatitis,*** pruritus, angioedema

Contraindications: Hypersensitivity to tetracyclines, children <8 yr, pregnancy (D)

Precautions: Renal disease, hepatic disease, lactation, nephrogenic diabetes insipidus

Pharmacokinetics:

PO: Peak 3-6 hr, duration 48-72 hr, half-life 10-17 hr; excreted in urine; crosses placenta; excreted in breast milk; 36%-91% bound to serum protein

Interactions:

- Decreased effect of demeclocycline: antacids, $NaHCO_3$, dairy, alkali products, iron, kaolin, pectin, cimetidine

• Increased effect: anticoagulants
• Decreased effect: penicillins, oral contraceptives
• Nephrotoxicity: methoxyflurane

Lab test interferences:

False negative: Urine glucose with Clinistix or Tes-Tape

False increase: Urinary catecholamines, AST (SGOT), ALT (SGPT), BUN

NURSING CONSIDERATIONS

Assess:

• I&O ratio
• Blood studies: PT, CBC, AST, ALT, BUN, creatinine
• Urine specific gravity, Na
• Signs of infection
• Allergic reactions: rash, itching, pruritus, angioedema
• Nausea, vomiting, diarrhea; administer antiemetic, antacids as ordered
• Overgrowth of infection: increased temperature, malaise, redness, pain, swelling, drainage, perineal itching, diarrhea, changes in cough, sputum

Administer:

• On empty stomach 1 hr ac or 2 hr pc with 8 oz H_2O
• After C&S
• 2 hr before or after laxative or ferrous products; 3 hr after antacid or kaolin-pectin products

Perform/provide:

• Storage in tight, light-resistant container at room temp

Evaluate:

• Therapeutic response: decreased temperature, absence of lesions, negative C&S

Teach patient/family:

• To avoid sun exposure; sunscreen does not seem to decrease photosensitivity
• If diabetic, to avoid use of Clinistix, Diastix, or Tes-Tape for urine glucose testing
• That all prescribed medication must be taken to prevent superinfection
• To avoid milk products; take with full glass of water

desipramine (℞)

(dess-ip′ra-meen)

Desipramine HCl, Norpramin, Pertofrane

Func. class.: Antidepressant—tricyclic

Chem. class.: Dibenzazepine, secondary amine

Action: Blocks reuptake of norepinephrine, serotonin into nerve endings, increasing action of norepinephrine, serotonin in nerve cells

Uses: Depression

Dosage and routes:

• *Adult:* PO 75-150 mg/day in divided doses; may increase to 300 mg/day or may give daily dose hs
• *Adolescent/geriatric:* PO 25-50 mg/day, may increase to 100 mg/day

Available forms: Tabs 10, 25, 50, 75, 100, 150 mg; caps 25, 50 mg

Side effects/adverse reactions:

HEMA: ***Agranulocytosis, thrombocytopenia, eosinophilia, leukopenia***

CNS: Dizziness, drowsiness, confusion, headache, anxiety, tremors, stimulation, weakness, insomnia, nightmares, EPS (elderly), increased psychiatric symptoms, paresthesia

GI: Diarrhea, dry mouth, nausea, vomiting, ***paralytic ileus,*** increased appetite, cramps, epigastric distress, jaundice, ***hepatitis,*** stomatitis, constipation

GU: Retention, ***acute renal failure***

INTEG: Rash, urticaria, sweating, pruritus, photosensitivity

CV: Orthostatic hypotension, ECG changes, tachycardia, ***hypertension,*** palpitations
EENT: Blurred vision, tinnitus, mydriasis, ophthalmoplegia
Contraindications: Hypersensitivity to tricyclic antidepressants, recovery phase of myocardial infarction, narrow-angle glaucoma, convulsive disorders, prostatic hypertrophy, child <12 yr
Precautions: Suicidal patients, severe depression, increased intraocular pressure, elderly, pregnancy (C), lactation
Pharmacokinetics:
PO: Steady state 2-11 days; metabolized by liver; excreted by kidneys; crosses placenta; half-life 14-62 hr
Interactions:
• Decreased effects of guanethidine, clonidine, indirect acting sympathomimetics (ephedrine)
• Increased effects of direct-acting sympathomimetics (epinephrine) alcohol, barbiturates, benzodiazepines, CNS depressants
• Hyperpyretic crisis, convulsions, hypertensive episode: MAOI (pargyline [Eutonyl])
Lab test interferences:
Increase: Serum bilirubin, blood glucose, alk phosphatase
False increase: Urinary catecholamines
Decrease: VMA, 5-HIAA

NURSING CONSIDERATIONS
Assess:
• B/P (lying, standing), pulse q4h; if systolic B/P drops 20 mm Hg, hold drug, notify prescriber; take vital signs q4h in patients with cardiovascular disease
• Blood studies: CBC, leukocytes, differential, cardiac enzymes if patient is receiving long-term therapy
• Hepatic studies: AST, ALT, bilirubin
• Weight qwk, appetite may increase with drug
• ECG for flattening of T wave, bundle branch block, AV block, dysrhythmias in cardiac patients
• EPS primarily in elderly: rigidity, dystonia, akathisia
• Mental status: mood, sensorium, affect, suicidal tendencies, increase in psychiatric symptoms: depression, panic
• Urinary retention, constipation; constipation most likely in children
• Withdrawal symptoms: headache, nausea, vomiting, muscle pain, weakness; not usual unless drug discontinued abruptly
• Alcohol consumption; if consumed, hold dose until morning
Administer:
• Increased fluids, bulk in diet for constipation, especially in elderly
• With food, milk for GI symptoms
• Crushed if patient is unable to swallow medication whole
• Dosage hs if oversedation occurs during day; may take entire dose hs; elderly may not tolerate once/day dosing
• Gum, hard candy, frequent sips of water for dry mouth
Perform/provide:
• Storage at room temp
• Assistance with ambulation during beginning therapy for drowsiness/dizziness
• Safety measures, including side rails, primarily in elderly
• Checking to see PO medication swallowed
Evaluate:
• Therapeutic response: decreased depression
Teach patient/family:
• That therapeutic effects may take 2-3 wk

* Available in Canada only

• To use caution in driving, other activities requiring alertness because of drowsiness, dizziness, blurred vision
• To avoid alcohol ingestion, other CNS depressants
• Not to discontinue medication quickly after long-term use; may cause nausea, headache, malaise
• To wear sunscreen or large hat, since photosensitivity occurs

Treatment of overdose: ECG monitoring; induce emesis; lavage, activated charcoal; administer anticonvulsant

---

desmopressin (℞)

(des-moe-press'in)

Concentraid, DDAVP

Func. class.: Pituitary hormone

Chem. class.: Synthetic antidiuretic hormone

Action: Promotes reabsorption of water by action on renal tubular epithelium; causes smooth muscle constriction, increase in plasma factor VIII levels, which increases platelet aggregation resulting in vasopressor effect, similar to vasopressin

Uses: Hemophilia A, von Willebrand's disease type 1, nonnephrogenic diabetes insipidus, symptoms of polyuria/polydipsia caused by pituitary dysfunction, nocturnal enuresis

Dosage and routes:

Diabetes insipidus

• *Adult:* INTRANASAL 0.1-0.4 mg qd in divided doses (1-4 sprays with pump); IV/SC 0.2-0.4 mg qd in divided doses
• *Child 3 mo to 12 yr:* INTRANASAL 0.05-0.3 mg qd in divided doses

Hemophilia/von Willebrand's disease

• *Adult and child:* IV 0.3 μg/kg in NaCl over 15-30 min; may repeat if needed

Available forms: Intranasal pipets 0.01 mg/ml, inj IV, SC 4 μg/ml, Rhihal Tube del 2.5 mg/vial

Side effects/adverse reactions:

EENT: Nasal irritation, congestion, rhinitis

CNS: Drowsiness, headache, lethargy, flushing

GU: Vulval pain

GI: Nausea, heartburn, cramps

CV: Increased B/P

Contraindications: Hypersensitivity, nephrogenic diabetes insipidus

Precautions: Pregnancy (B), CAD, lactation, hypertension

Pharmacokinetics:

Nasal: Onset 1 hr, peak 1-2 hr, duration 8-20 hr, half-life 8 min, 76 min (terminal)

Interactions:

• Increased response: carbamazepine, chlorpropamide, clofibrate
• Decreased response; lithium, alcohol, demeclocyclines, heparin, large doses of epinephrine
• Compatibility not known

NURSING CONSIDERATIONS

Assess:

• Pulse, B/P when giving IV or SC
• I&O ratio, weight daily; check for edema in extremities; if water retention is severe, diuretic may be prescribed
• Water intoxication: lethargy, behavioral changes, disorientation, neuromuscular excitability
• Intranasal use: nausea, congestion, cramps, headache; usually decreased with decreased dose

Administer:

• Undiluted over 1 min in diabetes insipidus
• Diluted, one single dose/50 ml of NS (adult & child >10 kg), a single dose/10 ml as an IV inf over 15-30 min in von Willebrand's disease or hemophilia A

Perform/provide:
• Storage in refrigerator or cool environment

Evaluate:
• Therapeutic response: absence of severe thirst, decreased urine output, osmolality

Teach patient/family:
• Technique for nasal instillation: to insert tube into nostril to instill drug
• To avoid OTC products: cough, hay fever products, since these preparations may contain epinephrine, decrease drug response; do not use with alcohol
• To wear Medic Alert ID specifying therapy
• If dose is missed, take when remembered up to 1 hr before next dose; do not double dose

desonide (℞)

(dess'oh-nide)
DesOwen, Tridesilon
Func. class.: Topical corticosteroid
Chem. class.: Synthetic nonfluorinated agent, group IV potency

Action: Antipruritic, antiinflammatory

Uses: Psoriasis, eczema, contact dermatitis, pruritus

Dosage and routes:
• *Adult and child:* Apply to affected area bid-tid

Available forms: Cream 0.05%; oint 0.05%

Side effects/adverse reactions:
INTEG: Burning, dryness, itching, irritation, acne, folliculitis, hypertrichosis, perioral dermatitis, hypopigmentation, atrophy, striae, miliaria, allergic contact dermatitis, secondary infection

Contraindications: Hypersensitivity to corticosteroids, fungal infections

Precautions: Pregnancy (C), lactation, viral infections, bacterial infections

NURSING CONSIDERATIONS

Assess:
• Temperature; if fever develops, drug should be discontinued
• For systemic absorption: increased temperature, inflammation, irritation

Administer:
• Only to affected areas; do not get in eyes
• Medication; then cover with occlusive dressing if prescribed; seal to normal skin; change q12h; systemic absorption may occur
• Only to dermatoses; do not use on weeping, denuded, infected area

Perform/provide:
• Cleansing before application
• Treatment for a few days after area has cleared
• Storage at room temp

Evaluate:
• Therapeutic response: absence of severe itching, patches on skin, flaking

Teach patient/family:
• To avoid sunlight on affected area; burns may occur

desoximetasone (℞)

(des-ox-i-met'a-sone)
Desoximetasone, Topicort, Topicort LP
Func. class.: Topical corticosteroid
Chem. class.: Synthetic fluorinated agent, group II potency (0.25%), group III potency (0.05%)

Action: Antipruritic, antiinflammatory

* Available in Canada only

Uses: Psoriasis, eczema, contact dermatitis, pruritus
Dosage and routes:
• *Adult and child:* TOP apply to affected area bid-tid
Available forms: Cream 0.05% (LP), 0.25%; oint 0.25%; gel 0.05%
Side effects/adverse reactions:
INTEG: Burning, dryness, itching, irritation, acne, folliculitis, hypertrichosis, perioral dermatitis, hypopigmentation, atrophy, striae, miliaria, allergic contact dermatitis, secondary infection
Contraindications: Hypersensitivity to corticosteroids, fungal infections
Precautions: Pregnancy (C), lactation, viral infections, bacterial infections
NURSING CONSIDERATIONS
Assess:
• Temp; if fever develops, drug should be discontinued
• For systemic absorption: fever, inflammation, irritation
Administer:
• Only to affected areas; do not get in eyes
• Medication; cover with occlusive dressing if prescribed; seal to normal skin; change q12h; use occlusive dressing with extreme caution (group II potency); systemic absorption may occur
• Only to dermatoses; do not use on weeping, denuded, infected area
Perform/provide:
• Cleansing before application
• Treatment for a few days after area has cleared
• Storage at room temp
Evaluate:
• Therapeutic response: absence of severe itching, patches on skin, flaking
Teach patient/family:
• To avoid sunlight on affected area; burns may occur

dexamethasone (℞)

(dex-a-meth'a-sone)
Aeroseb-Dex, Decaderm, Decaspray
Func. class.: Topical corticosteroid
Chem. class.: Synthetic fluorinated agent

Action: Antipruritic, antiinflammatory
Uses: Corticosteroid-responsive dermatoses
Dosage and routes:
• *Adult and child:* TOP apply to affected area bid-qid
Available forms: Gel 0.1%; aerosol 0.01%, 0.04%
Side effects/adverse reactions:
INTEG: Burning, dryness, itching, irritation, acne, folliculitis, hypertrichosis, perioral dermatitis, hypopigmentation, atrophy of the epidermis, striae, miliaria, allergic contact dermatitis, secondary infection
Contraindications: Hypersensitivity to corticosteroids, fungal infections, viral infections
Precautions: Pregnancy (C), lactation, viral, bacterial infections
NURSING CONSIDERATIONS
Assess:
• Temp; if fever develops, drug should be discontinued
• Systemic absorption: fever, infection, irritation
Administer:
• Only to affected areas; do not get in eyes
• Then cover with occlusive dressing if ordered; seal to normal skin; change q12h; systemic absorption may occur
• Only to dermatoses; do not use on weeping, denuded, infected area
Perform/provide:
• Cleansing before application

• Treatment for a few days after area has cleared
• Storage at room temp

Evaluate:
• Therapeutic response: absence of severe itching, patches on skin, flaking

Teach patient/family:
• To avoid sunlight on affected area; burns may occur

dexamethasone/ dexamethasone acetate/dexamethasone sodium phosphate (℞)

(dex-a-meth′a-sone)

Aeroseb-Dex, Decaderm, Decaspray, Dalalone D.P., Dalalone L.A., Decadron-LA, Decaject-L.A., Dexacen LA-8, Dexamethasone Acetate, Dexasone L.A., Dexone LA, Solurex LA, Dalalone, Decadron Phosphate, Decaject, Dexacen-4, Dexamethasone Sodium Phosphate, Dexasone, Dexone, Hexadrol Phosphate, Solurex, Decadron Phosphate Respihaler

Func. class.: Corticosteroid

Chem. class.: Glucocorticoid, long-acting

Combination products: Decadron with Xylocaine: dexamethasone PO_4 4 mg, lidocaine HCl 10 mg/ml

Action: Decreases inflammation by suppression of migration of polymorphonuclear leukocytes, fibroblasts, reversal of increased capillary permeability and lysosomal stabilization

Uses: Inflammation, allergies, neoplasms, cerebral edema, septic shock, collagen disorders

Dosage and routes:

Inflammation
• *Adult:* PO 0.25-4 mg bid-qid IM 4-16 mg q1-3 wk (acetate)

Shock
• *Adult:* IV 1-6 mg/kg or 40 mg q2-6h (phosphate)

Cerebral edema
• *Adult:* IV 10 mg, then 4-6 mg IM q6h × 2-4 days, then taper over 1 wk
• *Child:* PO 0.2 mg/kg/day in divided doses

Available forms: Tabs 0.25, 0.5, 0.75, 1, 1.5, 3, 4, 6 mg; inj IM acetate 8, 16 mg/ml; inj IV phosphate 4, 10 mg/ml; elix 0.5 mg/5 ml; oral sol 0.5 mg/5 ml, 0.5 mg/1 ml

Side effects/adverse reactions:
INTEG: Acne, poor wound healing, ecchymosis, petechiae
CNS: *Depression, flushing, sweating,* headache, mood changes
CV: *Hypertension,* ***circulatory collapse, thrombophlebitis, embolism,*** tachycardia, edema
HEMA: ***Thrombocytopenia***
MS: Fractures, osteoporosis, weakness
GI: *Diarrhea, nausea, abdominal distention,* ***GI hemorrhage,*** *increased appetite,* ***pancreatitis***
EENT: Fungal infections, increased intraocular pressure, blurred vision

Contraindications: Psychosis, hypersensitivity, idiopathic thrombocytopenia, acute glomerulonephritis, amebiasis, fungal infections, nonasthmatic bronchial disease, child <2 yr, AIDS, TB

Precautions: Pregnancy (C), lactation, diabetes mellitus, glaucoma, osteoporosis, seizure disorders, ulcerative colitis, CHF, myasthenia gravis, renal disease, peptic ulcer, esophagitis

Pharmacokinetics:
PO: Peak 1-2 h, duration 2⅓ days
IM: Peak 8 h, duration 6 days
Half-life 3-4½ hr

Interactions:

- Decreased action of dexamethasone: cholestyramine, colestipol, barbiturates, rifampin, ephedrine, phenytoin, theophylline, antacids
- Decreased effects of anticoagulants, anticonvulsants, antidiabetics, ambenonium, neostigmine, isoniazid, toxoids, vaccines, anticholinesterases, salicylates, somatrem
- Increased side effects: alcohol, salicylates, indomethacin, amphotericin B, digitalis, cyclosporine, diuretics
- Increased action of dexamethasone: salicylates, estrogens, indomethacin, oral contraceptives, ketoconazole, macrolide antibiotics
- Incompatible with amikacin, daunorubicin, doxorubicin, metaraminol, prochlorperazine, vancomycin

Lab test interferences:

Increase: Cholesterol, Na, blood glucose, uric acid, Ca, urine glucose
Decrease: Ca, K, T_4, T_3, thyroid ^{131}I uptake test, urine 17-OHCS, 17-KS, PBI
False negative: Skin allergy tests

NURSING CONSIDERATIONS

Assess:

- K, blood sugar, urine glucose while on long-term therapy; hypokalemia and hyperglycemia
- Weight daily; notify prescriber of weekly gain >5 lb
- B/P q4h, pulse; notify prescriber of chest pain
- I&O ratio; be alert for decreasing urinary output, increasing edema
- Plasma cortisol levels during long-term therapy (normal: 138-635 nmol/L SI units when drawn at 8 AM)
- Infection: fever, WBC even after withdrawal of medication; drug masks infection
- Potassium depletion: paresthesias, fatigue, nausea, vomiting, depression, polyuria, dysrhythmias, weakness
- Edema, hypertension, cardiac symptoms
- Mental status: affect, mood, behavioral changes, aggression

Administer:

- IV undiluted direct over 1 min or less or diluted with NS or D_5W and give as an IV inf at prescribed rate
- After shaking suspension (parenteral); do not give suspension IV
- Titrated dose; use lowest effective dose
- IM inj deeply in large muscle mass; rotate sites; avoid deltoid; use 21G needle
- In one dose in AM to prevent adrenal suppression; avoid SC administration; may damage tissue
- With food or milk to decrease GI symptoms

Perform/provide:

- Assistance with ambulation in patient with bone tissue disease to prevent fractures

Evaluate:

- Therapeutic response: ease of respirations, decreased inflammation

Teach patient/family:

- That ID as steroid user should be carried
- To notify prescriber if therapeutic response decreases; dosage adjustment may be needed
- Not to discontinue abruptly or adrenal crisis can result
- To avoid OTC products: salicylates, alcohol in cough products, cold preparations unless directed by prescriber
- To teach patient all aspects of drug usage, including cushingoid symptoms
- Symptoms of adrenal insufficiency: nausea, anorexia, fatigue, dizziness, dyspnea, weakness, joint pain

dexamethasone/ dexamethasone sodium phosphate (℞)

(dex-a-meth'a-sone)

AK-Dex, Dexamethasone Ophthalmic Suspension, Decadron Phosphate, Maxidex

Func. class.: Ophthalmic anti-inflammatory

Action: Reduces inflammation, resulting in decreased pain, photophobia, hyperemia, cellular infiltration

Uses: Inflammation of eye, lids, conjunctiva, cornea; uveitis; iridocyclitis; allergic condition; burns; foreign bodies

Dosage and routes:

• *Adult and child:* INSTILL 1-2 gtt into conjunctival sac q1-4h depending on condition

Available forms: Oint 0.05%; ophthalmic sol 0.1%; oph susp 0.1%

Side effects/adverse reactions:

EENT: ***Increased intraocular pressure,*** poor corneal wound healing, increased possibility of corneal infection, glaucoma exacerbation, ***optic nerve damage,*** decreased acuity, visual field, cataracts

Contraindications: Hypersensitivity, acute superficial herpes simplex, fungal/viral diseases of eye or conjunctiva, active diabetes mellitus, ocular TB, eye infection

Precautions: Corneal abrasion, glaucoma, pregnancy (C)

NURSING CONSIDERATIONS

Perform/provide:

• Storage in light-resistant container

Evaluate:

• Therapeutic response: absence of swelling, redness, exudate

Teach patient/family:

• Instillation method: pressure on lacrimal duct for 1 min

• Not to share eye medications

• Not to use if purulent drainage is present

• To shake before using

• Not to discontinue abruptly; taper over 1-2 wk

dexamethasone sodium phosphate (℞)

(dex-a-meth'a-sone)

Decadron Phosphate

Func. class.: Topical corticosteroid

Chem. class.: Synthetic fluorinated agent, group VI potency

Action: Antipruritic, antiinflammatory

Uses: Psoriasis, eczema, contact dermatitis, pruritus

Dosage and routes:

• *Adult and child:* Apply to affected area tid-qid

Available forms: Cream 0.1%

Side effects/adverse reactions:

INTEG: Burning, dryness, itching, irritation, acne, folliculitis, hypertrichosis, perioral dermatitis, hypopigmentation, atrophy, striae, miliaria, allergic contact dermatitis, secondary infection

Contraindications: Hypersensitivity to corticosteroids, fungal infections

Precautions: Pregnancy (C), lactation, viral infections, bacterial infections

NURSING CONSIDERATIONS

Assess:

• For systemic absorption: fever, inflammation, irritation

• Temp; if fever develops, drug should be discontinued

Administer:

• Only to affected areas; do not get in eyes

• Medication; then cover with occlusive dressing if prescribed; seal to normal skin; change q12h; systemic absorption may occur
• Only to dermatoses; do not use on weeping, denuded, or infected area

Perform/provide:
• Cleansing before application
• Treatment for a few days after area has cleared
• Storage at room temp

Evaluate:
• Therapeutic response: absence of severe itching, patches on skin, flaking

Teach patient/family:
• To avoid sunlight on affected area; burns may occur

dexamethasone sodium phosphate (nasal) (℞)

(dex-a-meth'a-sone)

Decadron Phosphate Turbinaire

Func. class.: Steroid, intranasal

Chem. class.: Glucocorticoid

Action: Long-acting synthetic adrenocorticoid with antiinflammatory activity, minimal mineralocorticoid properties

Uses: Inflammation (not within sinuses), nasal polyps, allergic conditions of nose

Dosage and routes:
• *Adult:* SPRAY 1-2 sprays bid-tid, not to exceed 12/day
• *Child 6-12 yr:* SPRAY 1-2 sprays bid, not to exceed 8/day

Available forms: 84 μg/metered spray

Side effects/adverse reactions:
EENT: Nasal irritation, dryness, rebound congestion, epistaxis, sneezing, ***infarction of nasal mucosa***
INTEG: Urticaria
CNS: Headache, dizziness
SYST: ***CHF, convulsions,*** increased sodium, hypertension

Contraindications: Hypersensitivity, child <12 yr, localized infection of nose, acute status asthmaticus

Precautions: Lactation, nasal trauma, pregnancy (C)

NURSING CONSIDERATIONS

Assess:
• Adrenal suppression: 17-KS, plasma cortisol for decreased levels
• Nasal passages during long-term treatment for changes in mucus
• For edema, increased B/P, increase in K^+ during treatment; indicates systemic absorption

Administer:
• After cleaning spray container daily with warm water; dry thoroughly

Perform/provide:
• Storage in cool environment; do not puncture or incinerate container

Evaluate:
• Therapeutic response: decreased inflammation, redness

Teach patient/family:
• To clear nasal passages if sneezing attack occurs, repeat dose
• To continue using product even if mild nasal bleeding occurs; is usually transient
• Method of instillation after providing written instructions from manufacturer
• To clear nasal passages before administration; use decongestant if needed; shake inhaler; invert; tilt head backward; insert nozzle into nostril away from septum; hold other nostril closed; depress activator; inhale through nose; exhale through mouth
• To decrease gradually if drug has been used consistently
• That only 1 person should use a single-container drug

• For irritation, dryness, epistaxis, drug may be discontinued
• That benefit requires regular use, takes several days

dexchlorpheniramine (℞)

(dex-klor-fen-eer'a-meen)
Dexchlor, Dexchlorpheniramine Maleate, Poladex, Polaramine

Func. class.: Antihistamine
Chem. class.: Alkylamine derivative, H_1-receptor antagonist

Action: Acts on blood vessels, GI, respiratory system by competing with histamine for H_1-receptor site; decreases allergic response by blocking histamine

Uses: Allergy symptoms, rhinitis, pruritus, contact dermatitis

Dosage and routes:
• *Adult:* PO 1-2 mg tid-qid; REPEAT ACTION 4-6 mg bid-tid
• *Child 6-11 yr:* PO 1 mg q4-6h, or TIME REL 4 mg hs
• *Child 2-5 yr:* PO 0.5 mg q4-6h; do not use repeat action form

Available forms: Tabs 2 mg; repeat-action tab 4, 6 mg; syr 2 mg/5 ml

Side effects/adverse reactions:
CNS: *Dizziness, drowsiness,* poor coordination, fatigue, anxiety, euphoria, confusion, paresthesia, neuritis
CV: Hypotension, palpitations, tachycardia
RESP: Increased thick secretions, wheezing, chest tightness
GI: *Constipation,* dry mouth, nausea, vomiting, anorexia, diarrhea
INTEG: Rash, urticaria, photosensitivity
GU: *Retention,* dysuria, frequency
EENT: Blurred vision, dilated pupils, tinnitus, nasal stuffiness, dry nose, throat, mouth

Contraindications: Hypersensitivity to H_1-receptor antagonist; acute asthma attack, lower respiratory tract disease

Precautions: Increased intraocular pressure, renal disease, cardiac disease, hypertension, bronchial asthma, seizure disorder, stenosed peptic ulcers, hyperthyroidism, prostatic hypertrophy, bladder neck obstruction, pregnancy (B), lactation, elderly

Pharmacokinetics:
PO: Onset 15 min, peak 3 hr, duration 3-6 hr; metabolized in liver; excreted by kidneys (inactive metabolites); excreted in breast milk (small amounts)

Interactions:
• Increased CNS depression: barbiturates, narcotics, hypnotics, tricyclic antidepressants, alcohol
• Decreased effect: oral anticoagulants, heparin
• Increased effect of dexchlorpheniramine: MAOIs

Lab test interferences:
False negative: Skin allergy tests

NURSING CONSIDERATIONS

Assess:
• I&O ratio; be alert for urinary retention, frequency, dysuria; drug should be discontinued
• CBC during long-term therapy
• Respiratory status: rate, rhythm, increase in bronchial secretions, wheezing, chest tightness
• Cardiac status: palpitations, increased pulse, hypotension

Administer:
• With meals for GI symptoms; absorption may slightly decrease

Perform/provide:
• Hard candy, gum, frequent rinsing of mouth for dryness
• Storage in tight container at room temp

* Available in Canada only

Evaluate:
- Therapeutic response: absence of running or congested nose or rashes

Teach patient/family:
- All aspects of drug use; to notify prescriber of confusion/sedation/hypotension
- To avoid driving, other hazardous activity if drowsiness occurs, especially elderly
- That this drug decreases anticoagulant (oral) effect
- To avoid concurrent use of alcohol, other CNS depressants

Treatment of overdose: Ipecac syrup or lavage, diazepam, vasopressors, barbiturates (short-acting)

dextran 40 (℞)

Dextran 40, Gentran 40, LMD 10%, Rheomacrodex

Func. class.: Plasma volume expander

Chem. class.: Low molecular weight polysaccharide

Action: Similar to human albumin, which expands plasma volume by drawing fluid from interstitial space to intravascular space

Uses: Expand plasma volume, prophylaxis of embolism, thrombosis

Dosage and routes:

Shock
- *Adult:* IV INF 500 ml over 15-30 min, total dose in 24 hr not to exceed 20 ml/kg; subsequent doses given slowly; if given >24 hr, not to exceed 10 ml/kg/day; not to exceed therapy >5 days

Thrombosis/embolism
- *Adult:* IV INF 500-1000 ml, then 500 ml/day × 3 days, then 500 ml q2-3 days × 2 wk if needed

Available forms: 10% dextran 40/5% dextrose, 10% dextran 40/0.9% NaCl

Side effects/adverse reactions:

HEMA: Decreased hematocrit, platelet function, increased bleeding/coagulation times

INTEG: Rash, urticaria, pruritus, angioedema, chills, fever, flushing

RESP: Wheezing, dyspnea, ***bronchospasm, pulmonary edema***

CV: Hypotension, ***cardiac arrest***

GU: ***Osmotic nephrosis, renal failure, stasis,*** hyponatremia

GI: Nausea, vomiting, increased AST, ALT

SYST: ***Anaphylaxis***

Contraindications: Hypersensitivity, renal failure, CHF (severe), extreme dehydration

Precautions: Active hemorrhage, pregnancy (C)

Pharmacokinetics:

IV: Expands blood vol 1-2 × amount infused; excreted in urine and feces

Interactions:
- Incompatible with chlortetracycline, phytonadione, promethazine
- Incompatible with any drug in sol

Lab test interferences:

False increase: Blood glucose, urinary protein, bilirubin, total protein

Interference: Rh test, blood typing/crossmatching

NURSING CONSIDERATIONS

Assess:
- VS q5min × 30 min
- CVP during infusion (5-10 cm H_2O—normal range)
- Urine output q1h; watch for increase in urinary output, which is common; if output does not increase, infusion should be decreased or discontinued
- I&O ratio and specific gravity, urine osmolarity; if specific gravity is very low, renal clearance is low; drug should be discontinued
- Allergy: rash, urticaria, pruritus, wheezing, dyspnea, bronchospasm, drug should be discontinued immediately

• Circulatory overload: increased pulse, respirations, SOB, wheezing, chest tightness, chest pain
• Dehydration after infusion: decreased output, decreased specific gravity of urine, increased temp, poor skin turgor, increased specific gravity, dry skin

Administer:
• After prescribed dilution; may give inital 500 mg at 15-30 min; distribute remainder of daily dose over 8-24 hr
• After crossmatch is drawn, if blood is to be given also
• Dextran 1 (Promit) to prevent anaphylaxis if ordered

Perform/provide:
• Storage at constant temperature 15°-30° C (59°-86° F); discard unused portions, protect from freezing

Evaluate:
• Therapeutic response: increased plasma volume

dextran 70/75 (℞)

Dextran 70, Dextran 75, Gentran 75, Macrodex

Func. class.: Plasma volume expander

Chem. class.: High molecular weight polysaccharide

Action: Similar to human albumin, which expands plasma volume by drawing fluid from interstitial spaces to intravascular space

Uses: Expand plasma volume in hypovolemic shock or impending shock

Dosage and routes:
• *Adult:* IV INF 500-1000 ml not to exceed 20-40 ml/min, not to exceed 10 ml/kg/24 hr if therapy >24 hr

Available forms: 70/75 dextran in 0.9% NaCl, D_5%

Side effects/adverse reactions:
HEMA: Decreased hematocrit, platelet function; increased bleeding/coagulation times
INTEG: Rash, urticaria, pruritus, angioedema, chills, fever, flushing
RESP: Wheezing, dyspnea, ***bronchospasm, pulmonary edema***
CV: Hypotension, ***cardiac arrest***
GU: ***Osmotic nephrosis, renal failure, stasis,*** hypernatremia
GI: Nausea, vomiting, increased AST, ALT
SYST: ***Anaphylaxis***

Contraindications: Hypersensitivity, renal failure, CHF (severe), extreme dehydration

Precautions: Active hemorrhage, pregnancy (C)

Pharmacokinetics:
IV: Expands blood vol 1-2 × amount infused; excreted in urine, feces

Lab test interferences:
False increase: Blood glucose, urinary protein, bilirubin, total protein
Interferences: Rh test, blood typing/crossmatching

NURSING CONSIDERATIONS

Assess:
• VS q5min × 30 min
• CVP during infusion (5-10 cm H_2O—normal range)
• Urine output q1h; watch for increase in urinary output, which is common; if output does not increase, infusion should be decreased or discontinued
• I&O ratio and specific gravity, urine osmolarity; if specific gravity is very low, renal clearance is low; drug should be discontinued
• Allergy: rash, urticaria, pruritus, wheezing, dyspnea, bronchospasm; drug should be discontinued immediately
• Circulatory overload: increased pulse, respirations, SOB, wheezing, chest tightness, chest pain

* Available in Canada only

• Dehydration after infusion: decreased output, increased temp, poor skin turgor, increased specific gravity, dry skin

Administer:

• After prescribed dilution, may give inital 500 mg at 20-40 ml/min, reduce flow to lowest rate

• After crossmatch is drawn, if blood is to be given also

• Dextran 1 (Promit) to prevent anaphylaxis

Perform/provide:

• Storage at constant temperature <25° C (77° F); discard unused portions; do not use unless clear

Evaluate:

• Therapeutic response: increased plasma volume

dextroamphetamine (℞)

(dex-troe-am-fet'a-meen)

Dexedrine, Dexedrine Spansules, dextroamphetamine sulfate, Ferndex, Oxydess II, Spancap #1

Func. class.: Cerebral stimulant

Chem. class.: Amphetamine

Combination products: Biphetamine 12½: dextroamphetamine 6.25 mg, amphetamine 6.25 mg; Biphetamine 20: dextroamphetamine 10 mg, amphetamine 10 mg

Controlled Substance Schedule II

Action: Increases release of norepinephrine, dopamine in cerebral cortex to reticular activating system

Uses: Narcolepsy, attention deficit disorder with hyperactivity

Dosage and routes:

Narcolepsy

• *Adult:* PO 5-60 mg qd in divided doses

• *Child >12 yr:* PO 10 mg qd increasing by 10 mg/day at weekly intervals

• *Child 6-12 yr:* PO 5 mg qd increasing by 5 mg/wk (max 60 mg/day)

Attention deficit disorder

• *Child >6 yr:* PO 5 mg qd-bid increasing by 5 mg/day at weekly intervals

• *Child 3-6 yr:* PO 2.5 mg qd increasing by 2.5 mg/day at weekly intervals

Available forms: Tabs 5, 10 mg; caps sus rel 5, 10, 15 mg; elix 5 mg/5 ml

Side effects/adverse reactions:

CNS: Hyperactivity, insomnia, restlessness, talkativeness, dizziness, headache, chills, stimulation, dysphoria, irritability, aggressiveness, tremor, dependence, addiction

GI: Anorexia, dry mouth, diarrhea, constipation, weight loss, metallic taste

GU: Impotence, change in libido

CV: Palpitations, tachycardia, hypertension, decrease in heart rate, dysrhythmias

INTEG: Urticaria

Contraindications: Hypersensitivity to sympathomimetic amines, hyperthyroidism, hypertension, glaucoma, severe arteriosclerosis, drug abuse, cardiovascular disease, anxiety

Precautions: Gilles de la Tourette's disorder, pregnancy (C), lactation, child <3 yr

Pharmacokinetics:

PO: Onset 30 min, peak 1-3 hr, duration 4-20 hr; metabolized by liver; urine excretion pH dependent; crosses placenta, breast milk; half-life 10-30 hr

Interactions:

• Hypertensive crisis: MAOIs or within 14 days of MAOIs, furazolidine

• Increased effect of dextroamphetamine: acetazolamide, antacids, sodium bicarbonate, phenothiazines, haloperidol
• Decreased effect of dextroamphetamine: barbiturates, ascorbic acid, ammonium chloride, tricyclics
• Decreased effect: guanethidine

NURSING CONSIDERATIONS

Assess:
• VS, B/P; this drug may reverse antihypertensives; check patients with cardiac disease often
• CBC, urinalysis; in diabetes: blood sugar, urine sugar; insulin changes may be required, since eating will decrease
• Height, growth rate in children; growth rate may be decreased
• Mental status: mood, sensorium, affect, stimulation, insomnia, irritability
• Tolerance or dependency: an increased amount may be used to get same effect; will develop after long-term use
• Overdose: pain, fever, dehydration, insomnia, hyperactivity

Administer:
• At least 6 hr before hs to avoid sleeplessness
• Gum, hard candy, frequent sips of water for dry mouth

Evaluate:
• Therapeutic response: increased CNS stimulation, decreased drowsiness

Teach patient/family:
• Not to crush or chew sus rel forms
• To decrease caffeine consumption (coffee, tea, cola, chocolate); may increase irritability, stimulation
• To avoid OTC preparations unless approved by prescriber
• To taper drug over several weeks; depression, increased sleeping, lethargy
• To avoid alcohol ingestion
• To avoid hazardous activities until stabilized on medication
• To get needed rest; patient will feel more tired at end of day

Treatment of overdose: Administer fluids, hemodialysis or peritoneal dialysis; antihypertensive for increased B/P, ammonium Cl for increased excretion

dextromethorphan (OTC)

(dex-troe-meth-or′fan)

Balminil DM*, Benylin DM, Broncho-Grippol-DM*, Children's Hold, Delsym, Dextromethorphan, Hold DM, Koffex*, Neo-DM*, Orex DM*, Pertussin, Pertussin ES, Robidex*, Robitussin Cough Calmers, Robitussin Pediatric, Sedatuss*, St. Joseph Cough Suppressant, Sucrets Cough Control, Suppress, Trocal, Vicks Formula 44

Func. class.: Antitussive, nonnarcotic

Chem. class.: Levorphanol derivative

Combination products: Benylin DM: dextromethorphan hydrobromide 5 mg/5 ml with guaifenesin 100 mg/5 ml; Children's Hold 4 Hour: dextromethorphan hydrobromide 3.75 mg with phenylpropanolamine HCl 6.25 mg; Comtrex: dextromethorphan hydrobromide 10 mg with acetaminophen 325 mg, chlorpheniramine maleate 2 mg, phenylpropanolamine hydrochloride 12.5 mg; Comtrex: dextromethorphan hydrobromide 3.3 mg/5 ml with acetaminophen 108.3 mg/5 ml, chlorpheniramine maleate 0.67 mg/5 ml, phenylpropanolamine HCl 4.2 mg/5 ml; Conar: dextromethorphan hy-

* Available in Canada only

drobromide 15 mg with acetaminophen 300 mg, guaifenesin 100 mg, phenylephrine HCl 10 mg; Conar Expectorant: dextromethorphan hydrobromide 15 mg/5 ml with guaifenesin 100 mg/5 ml, phenylephrine HCl 10 mg/5 ml; Conar Syrup: dextromethorphan hydrobromide 15 mg/5 ml with phenylephrine HCl 10 mg/5 ml; Contac Jr.: dextromethorphan hydrobromide 5 mg/5 ml with acetaminophen 160 mg/5 ml, pseudoephedrine HCl 15 mg/5 ml; Contac Severe Cold Formula, Nyquil Nighttime Cold Medicine, Nytime Cold Medicine, Quiet Nite: dextromethorphan hydrobromide 5 mg/ 5 ml with acetaminophen 167 mg/5 ml, doxylamine succinate 1.25 mg/5 ml, pseudoephedrine HCl 10 mg/5 ml; CoTylenol Cold Medication Tablets: dextromethorphan hydrobromide 15 mg with acetaminophen 325 mg, chlorpheniramine maleate 2 mg, pseudoephedrine HCl 30 mg; CoTylenol: dextromethorphan hydrobromide 5 mg/5 ml with acetaminophen 108.3 mg/5 ml, chlorpheniramine maleate 0.67 mg/5ml, pseudoephedrine HCl 10 mg/5 ml; Cremacoat 3: dextromethorphan hydrobromide 6.7 mg/5 ml with guaifenesin 66.7 mg/5 ml, phenylpropanolamine HCl 12.5 mg/5 ml; Cremacoat 4: dextromethorphan hydrobromide 6.7 mg/5 ml with doxylamine succinate 2.5 mg/5 ml, phenylpropanolamine HCl 12.5 mg/5 ml; Dimetane-DX Cough Syrup: dextromethorphan hydrobromide 10 mg/5 ml with brompheniramine maleate 2 mg/5 ml, pseudoephedrine HCl 30 mg/5 ml; Dorcol Children's Cough Syrup: dextromethorphan hydrobromide 5 mg/ 5 ml with guaifenesin 50 mg/5 ml, pseudoephedrine HCl 15 mg/5 ml; Iophen DM, Tussi-Organidin DM: dextromethorphan hydrobromide 10 mg/5 ml with iodinated glycerol 30 mg/5 ml; Mediqueall: dextromethorphan hydrobromide 15 mg with pseudoephedrine HCl 30 mg; Naldecon-DX Adult: dextromethorphan hydrobromide 15 mg/5 ml with guaifenesin 200 mg/ 5 ml, phenylpropanolamine HCl 18 mg/5 ml; Naldecon-DX Children's Syrup: dextromethorphan hydrobromide 7.5 mg/5 ml with guaifenesin 100 mg/5 ml, phenylpropanolamine HCl 9 mg/5 ml; Novahistine Cough and Cold Formula: dextromethorphanhydrobromide 10 mg/5 ml with chlorpheniramine maleate 2 mg/5 ml, pseudoephedrine HCl 30 mg/5 ml; Orthoxicol Cough Syrup: dextromethorphan hydrobromide 10 mg/5 ml with methoxyphenamine HCl 17 mg/5 ml; Phenergan with Dextromethorphan: dextromethorphan hydrobromide 15 mg/5 ml with promethazine HCl 6.35 mg/5ml; Robitussin-DM: dextromethorphan hydrobromide 15 mg/5 ml, guaifenesin 100 mg/5 ml; Spec-T Sore Throat Cough Suppressant: dextromethorphan hydrobromide 10 mg with benzocaine 10 mg; Sudafed Cough Syrup: dextromethorphan hydrobromide 5 mg/5 ml with guaifenesin 100 mg/5 ml, pseudoephedrine HCl 15 mg/5 ml; Triaminic-DM Cough Formula: dextromethorphan hydrobromide 10 mg/5 ml with phenylpropanolamine HCl 12.5 mg/5 ml; Triaminicol: dextromethorphan hydrobromide 10 mg/5 ml with chlorpheniramine maleate 2 mg/5 ml, phenylpropanolamine HCl 12.5 mg/5 ml; Vicks Childrens Cough Syrup: dextromethorphan hydrobromide 3.5 mg/5 ml with guaifenesin 25 mg/5 ml; Vicks Cough Silencers: dextromethorphan hydrobromide 2.5 mg with benzocaine 1 mg; Vicks Daycare: dextromethorphan hydrobromide 10 mg with acetaminophen 325 mg, guaifenesin 100 mg, pseudoephedrine HCl 30 mg; Vicks Daycare: dextromethorphan hydrobromide 3.3 mg/5 ml with acetaminophen 108.3 mg/5 ml, guaifenesin 33.3 mg/5 ml, pseudoephedrine HCl 10 mg/5 ml; Vicks Formula 44 Cough Control Discs: dextromethorphan hydrobromide 5 mg with benzocaine 1.25 mg; Vicks Formula 44 Cough Mixture: dextromethorphan hydrobromide 15 mg/5 ml with doxylamine succinate 3.75 mg/5 ml; Vicks Formula 44D: dextromethorphan hydrobromide 10 mg/5 ml with guaifenesin 66.7 mg/5 ml, pseudoephedrine HCl 20 mg/5 ml; Vicks Formula 44M: dextromethorphan hydrobromide 7.4 mg/5 ml with acetaminophen 125 mg/5 ml, guaifenesin 50 mg/5 ml, pseudoephedrine HCl 15 mg/5 ml

---

Action: Depresses cough center in medulla by direct effect

Uses: Nonproductive cough

Dosage and routes:

• *Adult:* PO 10-20 mg q4h, or 30 mg q6-8h, not to exceed 120 mg/day; SUS-REL LIQ 60 mg bid, not to exceed 120 mg/day

• *Child 6-12 yr:* PO 5-10 mg q4h; SUS-REL LIQ 30 mg bid, not to exceed 60 mg/day

• *Child 2-6 yr:* PO 2.5-5 mg q4h, or 7.5 mg q6-8h, not to exceed 30 mg/day

Available forms: Loz 2.5, 5 mg; sol 3.5, 5, 7.5, 10, 15 mg/5 ml; syrup 15 mg/15 ml, 10 mg/5 ml; sus-action Liq 30 mg/5 ml

Side effects/adverse reactions:

CNS: Dizziness

GI: Nausea

Contraindications: Hypersensitivity, asthma/emphysema, productive cough

Precautions: Nausea/vomiting, fever, persistent headache, pregnancy (C)

Pharmacokinetics:

PO: Onset 15-30 min, duration 3-6 hr

SUS: Duration 12 hr

Interactions:

• Do not give with MAOIs or within 2 wk of MAOIs, penicillins, salicylates, tetracyclines, phenobarbital, iodines (high doses)

NURSING CONSIDERATIONS

Assess:

• Cough: type, frequency, character including sputum

Administer:

• Decreased dose to elderly patients; metabolism may be slowed

Perform/provide:

• Increased fluids to liquefy secretions

• Humidification of patient's room

Evaluate:

• Therapeutic response: absence of cough

Teach patient/family:

• To avoid driving, other hazardous activities until patient is stabilized on this medication

• To avoid smoking, smoke-filled rooms, perfumes, dust, environmental pollutants, cleaners that increase cough

• To avoid alcohol, other CNS depressants

• To notify prescriber if cough persists over a few days

---

dextrose (D-glucose) (℞)

Glucose, Glutose, Insta-Glucose, Insulin Reaction

Func. class.: Caloric

Action: Needed for adequate utilization of amino acids; decreases protein, nitrogen loss; prevents ketosis

---

* Available in Canada only

Uses: Increases intake of calories; increases fluids in patients unable to take adequate fluids, calories orally
Investigational uses: Varicose veins, acute alcohol intoxication
Dosage and routes:
• *Adult and child:* IV depends on individual requirements
Available forms: Inj IV 2.5%, 5%, 10%, 20%, 40%, 50%, 60%, 70%; oral gel 40%; chew tab 5 g
Side effects/adverse reactions:
CNS: Confusion, ***loss of consciousness,*** dizziness
CV: Hypertension, ***CHF, pulmonary edema***
GU: ***Glycosuria, osmotic diuresis***
ENDO: Hyperglycemia, rebound hypoglycemia, hyperosmolar syndrome, hyperglycemic nonketotic syndrome
INTEG: Chills, flushing, warm feeling, rash, urticaria, extravasation necrosis
Contraindications: Hyperglycemia, delirium tremens, hemorrhage (cranial/spinal), CHF
Precautions: Renal, liver, cardiac disease, diabetes mellitus

NURSING CONSIDERATIONS
Assess:
• Electrolytes (K, Na, Ca, Cl, Mg), blood glucose, ammonia, phosphate
• Injection site for extravasation: redness along vein, edema at site, necrosis, pain, hard tender area; site should be changed immediately
• Monitor temperature q4h for increased fever, indicating infection; if infection suspected, infusion is discontinued, tubing, bottle, catheter tip cultured
• Serum glucose in patients receiving hypotonic glucose 50% and over
• Nutritional status: calorie count by dietitian
Administer:
• Only (4%) protein and dextrose (up to 12.5%) via peripheral vein; stronger sol: central IV administration
• May be given undiluted via prepared sol give 10% sol, 5 ml/15 sec, 10% sol, 1000 ml/3 hr or more 20% sol, 500 ml/½-1 hr 50% sol, 10 ml/min
• Oral glucose preparations (gel, chew tabs) are to be used in conscious patients only; check serum blood glucose after first dose
• After changing IV catheter, dressing q24h with aseptic technique
Evaluate:
• Therapeutic response: increased weight
Teach patient/family
• Reason for dextrose infusion
• Review hypo/hyperglycemia symptoms
• Review blood glucose monitoring procedure

dezocine (℞)
(dez′oh-seen)
Dalgan
Func. class.: Narcotic agonist-antagonist analgesic
Chem. class.: Opioid, synthetic

Action: Depresses pain impulse transmission at the spinal cord level by interacting with opioid receptors
Uses: Severe pain
Dosage and routes:
Adult: IM 5-20 mg q3-6h, not to exceed 120 mg/day; IV 2.5-10 mg q2-4h
Available forms: IM, IV inj 5, 10, 15 mg single-dose vials, multiple dose 10 mg/ml
Side effects/adverse reactions:
CV: Hypotension, pulse irregularity, hypertension, chest pain, pallor, edema, thrombophlebitis
CNS: Drowsiness, dizziness, confusion, sedation, anxiety, headache, de-

pression, delirium, sleep disturbances, dependency
GI: Nausea, vomiting, anorexia, constipation, cramps, abdominal pain, dry mouth, diarrhea
INTEG: Injection site reactions, pruritus, rash, sweating, chills
RESP: ***Respiratory depression,*** hiccups
GU: Urinary frequency, hesitancy, retention
EENT: Blurred vision, slurred speech, diplopia

Contraindications: Hypersensitivity

Precautions: Addictive personality, pregnancy (C), lactation, increased intracranial pressure, respiratory depression, hepatic disease, renal disease, child <18 yr, elderly, biliary surgery, COPD, sulfite sensitivity

Pharmacokinetics:
IM: Onset 30 min, peak 50-90 min, duration 2-4 hr
IV: onset 10 min, peak 30 min, duration 2-4 hr
Metabolized by liver; excreted by kidneys; may cross placenta

Interactions:
- Incompatibility: not known
- Increased CNS depression: alcohol, narcotics, sedative/hypnotics, antipsychotics, skeletal muscle relaxants, general anesthetics, tranquilizers

NURSING CONSIDERATIONS
Assess:
- I&O ratio; decreasing output may indicate urinary retention
- CNS changes: dizziness, drowsiness, hallucinations, euphoria, LOC, pupil reaction
- Allergic reactions: rash, urticaria
- Respiratory dysfunction: respiratory depression, character, rate, rhythm of respirations; notify prescriber if <10/min, shallow
- Need for pain medication, physical dependence

Administer:
- Undiluted 5 mg or less over 2-3 min
- With antiemetic if nausea, vomiting occur
- When pain is beginning to return; determine dosage interval by patient response

Perform/provide:
- Storage in light-resistant area at room temp
- Assistance with ambulation
- Safety measures: top side rails, night-light, call bell in easy reach

Evaluate:
- Therapeutic response: decrease in pain

Teach patient/family:
- To report any symptoms of CNS changes, allergic reactions
- That physical dependency may result after extended use
- That withdrawal symptoms may occur: nausea, vomiting, cramps, fever, faintness, anorexia

Treatment of overdose: Naloxone 0.2-0.8 IV, O_2, IV fluids, vasopressors

diazepam (℞)

(dye-az′-e-pam)
Diazepam, Diazepam Intensol, D-Tran*, E-Pam*, Meval*, Novodipam*, Stress-Pam*, Valium, Valrelease, Vivol*, Vazepam, Zetran
Func. class.: Antianxiety
Chem. class.: Benzodiazepine

Controlled Substance Schedule IV

Action: Potentiates the actions of GABA, especially in limbic system, reticular formation; enhances presympathetic inhibition, inhibits spinal polysynaptic afferent paths

* Available in Canada only

Uses: Anxiety, acute alcohol withdrawal, adjunct in seizure disorders; preoperatively, skeletal muscle relaxation

Dosage and routes:

Anxiety/convulsive disorders

• *Adult:* PO 2-10 mg tid-qid; EXT REL 15-30 mg qd

• *Child >6 mo:* PO 1-2.5 mg tid-qid

Tetanic muscle spasms

• *Child <5 yr:* IM/IV 5-10 mg q3-4h prn

• *Infants >30 days:* IM/IV 1-2 mg q3-4h prn

Status epilepticus

• *Adult:* IV BOL 5-20 mg, 2 mg/min, may repeat q5-10m, not to exceed 60 mg; may repeat in 30 min if seizures reappear

• *Child:* IV BOL 0.1-0.3 mg/kg (1 mg/min over 3 min); may repeat q15m × 2 doses

Available forms: Tabs 2, 5, 10 mg; caps ext rel 15 mg, IM/IV inj

Side effects/adverse reactions:

CNS: Dizziness, drowsiness, confusion, headache, anxiety, tremors, stimulation, fatigue, depression, insomnia, hallucinations

CV: Orthostatic hypotension, ***ECG changes, tachycardia,*** hypotension

EENT: Blurred vision, tinnitus, mydriasis

GI: Constipation, dry mouth, nausea, vomiting, anorexia, diarrhea

INTEG: Rash, dermatitis, itching

Contraindications: Hypersensitivity to benzodiazepines, narrow-angle glaucoma, psychosis, pregnancy (D), lactation

Precautions: Elderly, debilitated, hepatic disease, renal disease

Pharmacokinetics:

PO: Rapidly absorbed; onset ½ hr, duration 2-3 hr

IM: Onset 15-30 min, duration 1-1½ hr; absorption slow and erratic

IV: Onset 1-5 min, duration 15 min

• Metabolized by liver, excreted by kidneys, crosses placenta, excreted in breast milk, crosses the blood-brain barrier; half-life 20-50 hr, more effective by mouth

Interactions:

• Decreased effects of diazepam: oral contraceptives, rifampin, valproic acid, cimetidine, disulfiram, narcotic analgesics

• Increased CNS depression: CNS depressants, alcohol

Y-site compatibilities: Dobutamine, nafcillin, quinidine

Syringe compatibility: Cimetidine

Lab test interferences:

Increase: AST (SGOT)/ALT (SGPT), serum bilirubin

False increase: 17-OHCS

Decrease: RAIU

NURSING CONSIDERATIONS

Assess:

• B/P (lying, standing), pulse; respiratory rate; if systolic B/P drops 20 mm Hg, hold drug, notify physician; respirations q5-15 min if given IV

• Blood studies: CBC during long-term therapy; blood dyscrasias (rare)

• Degree of anxiety; what precipitates anxiety and whether drug controls symptoms

• For alcohol withdrawal symptoms, including hallucinations (visual, auditory), delirium, irritability, agitation, fine to coarse tremors

• For seizure control and type, duration, intensity of convulsions

• Hepatic studies: AST (SGOT), ALT (SGPT), bilirubin, creatinine, LDH alk phosphatase

• IV site for thrombosis or phlebitis, which may occur rapidly

• Mental status: mood, sensorium, affect, sleeping pattern, drowsiness, dizziness

• Physical dependency, withdrawal symptoms: headache, nausea, vomiting, muscle pain, weakness after long-term use

• Suicidal tendencies

Administer:

• IV into large vein; do not dilute or mix with any other drug; give IV 5 mg or less/1 min or total dose over 3 min or more (children, infants); continuous infusion is not recommended

• With food or milk for GI symptoms; crushed if patient is unable to swallow medication whole; do not crush ext rel capsules

• Sugarless gum, hard candy, frequent sips of water for dry mouth

• Reduced narcotic dose by ⅓ if given concomitantly with diazepam

Perform/provide:

• Assistance with ambulation during beginning therapy, for drowsiness, dizziness

• Safety measures, including side rails

• Check to see PO medication has been swallowed

Evaluate:

• Therapeutic response: decreased anxiety, restlessness, insomnia

Teach patient/family:

• That drug may be taken with food

• Not to be used for everyday stress or used longer than 4 mo unless directed by prescriber; no more than prescribed amount; may be habit forming

• To avoid OTC preparations unless approved by prescriber

• To avoid driving, activities that require alertness; drowsiness may occur

• To avoid alcohol, other psychotropic medications unless directed by prescriber

• Not to discontinue medication abruptly after long-term use

• To rise slowly or fainting may occur, especially in elderly

• That drowsiness may worsen at beginning of treatment

Treatment of overdose: Lavage, VS, supportive care

diazoxide (℞)

(dye-az-ox'ide)

diazoxide, parenteral, Hyperstat IV

Func. class.: Antihypertensive

Chem. class.: Vasodilator

Action: Vasodilates arteriolar smooth muscle by direct relaxation; a reduction in blood pressure with concomitant increases in heart rate, cardiac output

Uses: Hypertensive crisis when urgent decrease of diastolic pressure required; increase blood glucose levels in hyperinsulinism

Dosage and routes:

• *Adult:* IV BOL 1-3 mg/kg rapidly up to a max of 150 mg in a single injection; dose may be repeated at 5-15 min intervals until desired response is achieved; give IV in 30 sec or less

• *Child:* IV BOL 1-2 mg/kg rapidly; administration same as adult, not to exceed 150 mg

Available forms: Inj IV 15 mg/ml

Side effects/adverse reactions:

CV: ***Hypotension,*** T-wave changes, angina pectoris, palpitations, ***supraventricular tachycardia, edema,*** rebound hypertension

CNS: Headache, sleepiness, euphoria, anxiety, EPS, confusion, tinnitus, blurred vision, dizziness, weakness

GI: Nausea, vomiting, dry mouth

INTEG: Rash

HEMA: Decreased hemoglobin, hematocrit, ***thrombocytopenia***

GU: Breast tenderness; increased BUN, fluid, electrolyte imbalances; Na, water retention

* Available in Canada only

ENDO: Hyperglycemia in diabetics, transient hyperglycemia in nondiabetics

Contraindications: Hypersensitivity to thiazides, sulfonamides, hypertension of aortic coarctation or AV shunt, pheochromocytoma, dissecting aortic aneurysm

Precautions: Tachycardia, fluid, electrolyte imbalances, pregnancy (C), lactation, impaired cerebral or cardiac circulation, children

Pharmacokinetics:

IV: Onset 1-2 min, peak 5 min, duration 3-12 hr; half-life 20-36 hr, excreted slowly in urine, crosses blood-brain barrier, placenta

Interactions:

- Increased hyperuricemic, antihypertensive effects of diazoxide: thiazide diuretics
- Hyperglycemia: sulfonylurens
- Decreased anticonvulsant effect: hydantoins

Syringe compatibility: Heparin

NURSING CONSIDERATIONS

Assess:

- B/P q5min until stabilized, then q1h × 2 hr, then q4h
- Pulse, jugular venous distention q4h
- Electrolytes, blood studies: K, Na, Cl, CO_2, CBC, serum glucose
- Weight daily, I&O
- Edema in feet, legs daily
- Skin turgor, dryness of mucous membranes for hydration status
- Rales, dyspnea, orthopnea
- IV site for extravasation, rate
- Signs of CHF: dyspnea, edema, wet rales
- Postural hypotension, take B/P sitting, standing

Administer:

- Undiluted; give over ½ min or less
- To patient in recumbent position; keep in that position for 1 hr after administration

Perform/provide:

- Protection from light

Evaluate:

- Therapeutic response: decreased B/P, primarily diastolic pressure

Treatment of overdose: Dopamine, or norepinephrine for hypotension, dialysis, Trendelenburg maneuver

D

diazoxide (oral) (℞)

(dye-az-ox′ide)

Proglycem

Func. class.: Hyperglycemic

Chem. class.: Benzothiadiazine

Action: Decreases release of insulin from β-cells in pancreas, increasing blood glucose

Uses: Hypoglycemia caused by hyperinsulinism

Dosage and routes:

- *Adult and child:* PO 3-8 mg/kg/day in 2-3 divided doses q8-12h
- *Infants and neonates:* PO 8-15 mg/kg/day in 2-3 divided doses q8-12h

Available forms: Caps 50 mg; oral susp 50 mg/ml

Side effects/adverse reactions:

GU: Reversible nephrotic syndrome, decreased urinary output, hematuria

CNS: Headache, weakness, malaise, anxiety, dizziness, insomnia, paresthesia

EENT: Diplopia, cataracts, ring scotoma, subconjunctival hemorrhage, lacrimation

HEMA: ***Thrombocytopenia, leukopenia,*** eosinophilia, decreased Hgb, Hct

INTEG: Increased hair growth or loss of scalp hair, rash, dermatitis, herpes

GI: Nausea, vomiting, anorexia, abdominal pain, transient loss of taste, diarrhea

CV: Tachycardia, palpitations, hypotension, transient hypertension

META: Hyperuricemia, sodium/fluid retention, ketoacidosis, hyperglycemia, azotemia
Contraindications: Hypersensitivity to this drug or thiazides, functional hypoglycemia
Precautions: Pregnancy (C), lactation, renal disease, diabetes mellitus, CV disease, gout
Pharmacokinetics:
PO: Onset 1 hr, duration 8 hr, half-life 28 hr; excreted unchanged by kidneys; crosses blood-brain barrier, placenta
Interactions:
- Increased effects of diazoxide: phenothiazines, thiazide diuretics
- Decreased effects of phenytoin
- Increased effects of antihypertensives, oral anticoagulants
- Decreased effects of diazoxide: α-adrenergic blockers, sulfonylureas, insulin

Lab test interferences:
Increase: Bilirubin, uric acid, blood glucose
Decrease: Creatinine, Hgb, Hct, plasma-free fatty acids
NURSING CONSIDERATIONS
Assess:
- I&O ratio, weight weekly
- Electrolytes (K, Na, Cl), glucose, Hct, Hgb, platelets, differential
- Urine for glucose, ketones qd

Administer:
- Shake susp before using

Perform/provide:
- Susp storage: protect from light

Evaluate:
- Therapeutic response: adequate blood, urine glucose, absence of ketones in urine

Teach patient/family:
- That if not effective within 2-3 wk, drug may be discontinued
- That any hirsutism is reversible after discontinuing treatment

dibucaine HCl (topical) (OTC)
(dye'byoo-kane)
dibucaine, Nupercainal
Func. class.: Topical anesthetic
Chem. class.: Amide

Action: Inhibits nerve impulses from sensory nerves, which produces anesthesia
Uses: Pruritus, sunburn, toothache, sore throat, cold sores, oral pain, rectal pain and irritation
Dosage and routes:
- *Adult and child:* TOP apply qid as needed; REC insert tid and after each BM

Available forms: Cream 0.5%; oint 1%
Side effects/adverse reactions:
INTEG: Rash, irritation, sensitization
Contraindications: Hypersensitivity, infants <1 yr, application to large areas, ophthalmic use
Precautions: Child <6 yr, sepsis, pregnancy (C), denuded skin
Pharmacokinetics: Peak <5 mins, duration 15-45 mins
NURSING CONSIDERATIONS
Assess:
- Allergy: rash, irritation, reddening, swelling
- Infection: if affected area is infected, do not apply

Administer:
- After cleansing and drying of affected area

Evaluate:
- Therapeutic response: absence of pain, itching of affected area

Teach patient/family:
- To report rash, irritation, redness, swelling
- How to apply cream, ointment

diclofenac (℞)

(dye-kloe'fen-ak)

Cataflam, Voltaren, Voltaren SR

Func. class.: Nonsteroidal antiinflammatory

Chem. class.: Phenylacetic acid

Action: Inhibits prostaglandin synthesis by decreasing enzyme needed for biosynthesis; analgesic, antiinflammatory, antipyretic

Uses: Acute, chronic rheumatoid arthritis, osteoarthritis, ankylosing spondylitis, analgesia, primary dysmenorrhea; ophthl postoperative inflammation after cataract extraction

Dosage and routes:

Osteoarthritis

• *Adult:* PO 100-150 mg/day in 2-3 divided doses

Rheumatoid arthritis

• *Adult:* PO 150-200 mg/day in divided doses

Ankylosing spondylitis

• *Adult:* PO 100-125 mg/day in 4-5 divided doses give 25 mg qid and 25 mg hs if needed

Postcataract surgery

• *Adult:* OPHTH i gtt of 0.1% sol qid × 2 wk 24 hr post surgery

Analgesia/primary dysmenorrhea

Adult: PO 50 mg tid, max 150 mg/day (potassium tab only)

Available forms: Tabs enteric coated 25, 50, 75 mg; tabs 50 mg (potassium); ophth sol 1%

Side effects/adverse reactions:

GI: Nausea, anorexia, vomiting, diarrhea, ***jaundice, cholestatic hepatitis,*** constipation, flatulence, cramps, dry mouth, peptic ulcer, GI bleeding

CNS: Dizziness, drowsiness, fatigue, tremors, confusion, insomnia, anxiety, depression, nervousness, paresthesia, muscle weakness

CV: ***CHF,*** tachycardia, peripheral edema, palpitations, ***dysrhythmias,*** hypotension, hypertension, fluid retention

INTEG: Purpura, rash, pruritus, sweating, erythema, petechiae, photosensitivity, alopecia

GU: ***Nephrotoxicity: dysuria, hematuria, oliguria, azotemia, cystitis, UTI***

HEMA: ***Blood dyscrasias,*** epistaxis, bruising

EENT: Tinnitus, hearing loss, blurred vision

RESP: Dyspnea, hemoptysis, pharyngitis, ***bronchospasm, laryngeal edema,*** rhinitis, shortness of breath

Contraindications: Hypersensitivity to aspirin, iodides, other nonsteroidal antiinflammatory agents, asthma

Precautions: Pregnancy (B) 1st, 2nd trimester, lactation, children, bleeding disorders, GI disorders, cardiac disorders, hypersensitivity to other antiinflammatory agents

Pharmacokinetics:

PO: Peak 2-3 hr, elimination half-life 1-2 hr, 90% bound to plasma proteins, metabolized in liver to metabolite, excreted in urine

Interactions:

• Decreased antihypertensive effect: β-blockers, diuretics

• Increased anticoagulant effect: coumarin

• Increased toxicity: phenytoin, sulfonamides, sulfonylurea, digoxin, lithium

• Increased plasma levels of diclofenac: probenecid, K-sparing diuretics

NURSING CONSIDERATIONS

Assess:

• Blood counts during therapy; watch for decreasing platelets; if low, therapy may need to be discontinued, restarted after hematologic recovery

• Blood dyscrasias (thrombocytopenia): bruising, fatigue, bleeding, poor healing
Evaluate:
• Therapeutic response: decreased inflammation in joints
Teach patient/family:
• That drug must be continued for prescribed time to be effective
• To report bleeding, bruising, fatigue, malaise; blood dyscrasias do occur
• To avoid aspirin, alcoholic beverages
• To take with food, milk, or antacids to avoid GI upset, to swallow whole
• To use caution when driving; drowsiness, dizziness may occur
• To take with a full glass of water to enhance absorption; do not crush, break, or chew

dicloxacillin (℞)

(dye-klox-a-sill′-in)
Dicloxacillin sodium, Dycill, Dynapen, Pathocil
Func. class.: Broad-spectrum antibiotic
Chem. class.: Penicillinase-resistant penicillin

Action: Interferes with cell wall replication of susceptible organisms; osmotically unstable cell wall swells, bursts from osmotic pressure
Uses: Effective for gram-positive cocci *(S. aureus, S. pyogenes, S. viridans, S. faecalis, S. bovis, S. pneumoniae)*, infections caused by penicillinase-producing *Staphylococcus*
Dosage and routes:
• *Adult:* PO 0.5-4 g/day in divided doses q6h
• *Child:* PO 12.5-25 mg/kg in divided doses q6h, max 4 g/d
Available forms: Caps 125, 250, 500 mg; powder for oral susp 62.5 mg/5 ml
Side effects/adverse reactions:
HEMA: Anemia, increased bleeding time, ***bone marrow depression, granulocytopenia***
GI: Nausea, vomiting, diarrhea, increased AST (SGOT), ALT (SGPT), abdominal pain, glossitis, pseudomembranous colitis
GU: ***Oliguria, proteinuria, hematuria,*** *vaginitis, moniliasis,* ***glomerulonephritis***
CNS: Lethargy, hallucinations, anxiety, depression, twitching, ***coma, convulsions***
SYST: ***Anaphylaxis***
Contraindications: Hypersensitivity to penicillins; neonates
Precautions: Hypersensitivity to cephalosporins, pregnancy (B), lactation
Pharmacokinetics:
PO: Peak 1 hr, duration 4-6 hr, half-life 30-60 min; metabolized in liver; excreted in urine, bile, breast milk; crosses placenta
Interactions:
• Decreased antimicrobial effectiveness of dicloxacillin: tetracyclines, erythromycins
• Increased dicloxacillin concentrations: aspirin, probenecid
Lab test interferences:
False positive: Urine glucose, urine protein

NURSING CONSIDERATIONS
Assess:
• I&O ratio; report hematuria, oliguria, since penicillin in high doses is nephrotoxic
• Any patient with compromised renal system, since drug is excreted slowly in poor renal system function; toxicity may occur rapidly
• Blood studies: WBC, RBC, Hgb, Hct, bleeding time
• Renal studies: urinalysis, protein, blood

* Available in Canada only

• C&S before drug therapy; drug may be given as soon as culture is taken
• WBC and diff, ALT (SGOT), AST (SGPT), BUN, creatinine for patients on long-term therapy
• Bowel pattern before, during treatment
• Skin eruptions after administration of penicillin to 1 wk after discontinuing drug
• Respiratory status: rate, character, wheezing, tightness in chest
• Allergies before initiation of treatment, reaction of each medication; highlight allergies on chart in red

Administer:
• Drug after C&S
• On an empty stomach with a full glass of water

Perform/provide:
• Adrenalin, suction, tracheostomy set, endotracheal intubation equipment
• Adequate fluid intake (2 L) during diarrhea episodes
• Scratch test to assess allergy after securing order from prescriber; usually done when penicillin is only drug of choice
• Storage in tight container; after reconstituting, store in refrigerator up to 2 wk

Evaluate:
• Therapeutic response: absence of fever, draining wounds

Teach patient/family:
• Aspects of drug therapy, including need to complete course of medication to ensure organism death (10-14 days); culture may be taken after completed course
• To report sore throat, fever, fatigue; may indicate superinfection
• To wear or carry Medic Alert ID if allergic to penicillins
• To notify nurse of diarrhea

Treatment of anaphylaxis: Withdraw drug; maintain airway; administer epinephrine, aminophylline, O_2, IV corticosteroids

dicyclomine (℞)

(dye-sye'kloe-meen)

Antispas, Bentyl, Bentylol*, Byclomine, Dibent, Dicyclomine HCL, Di-Spaz, Formulex*, Neoquess, OR-Tyl, Spasmoject, Viserol

Func. class.: Gastrointestinal anticholinergic

Chem. class.: Synthetic tertiary amine

Action: Inhibits muscarinic actions of acetylcholine at postganglionic parasympathetic neuroeffector sites

Uses: Treatment of peptic ulcer disease in combination with other drugs; infant colic

Dosage and routes:
• *Adult:* PO 10-20 mg tid-qid; IM 20 mg q4-6h
• *Child >2 yr:* PO 10 mg tid-qid
• *Child 6 mo-2 yr:* PO 5 mg tid-qid

Available forms: Caps 10, 20 mg; tabs 20 mg; syr 10 mg/5 ml; inj IM 10 mg/ml

Side effects/adverse reactions:

CNS: Confusion, stimulation in elderly, headache, insomnia, dizziness, drowsiness, anxiety, weakness, hallucination; ***seizures, coma*** (child <3 mo)

GI: Dry mouth, constipation, ***paralytic ileus,*** heartburn, nausea, vomiting, dysphagia, absence of taste

GU: Hesitancy, retention, impotence

CV: Palpitations, tachycardia

EENT: Blurred vision, photophobia, mydriasis, cycloplegia, increased ocular tension

INTEG: Urticaria, rash, pruritus, anhidrosis, fever, allergic reactions

Contraindications: Hypersensitivity to anticholinergics, narrow-angle glaucoma, GI obstruction, myasthenia gravis, paralytic ileus, GI atony, toxic megacolon

Precautions: Hyperthyroidism, coronary artery disease, dysrhythmias, CHF, ulcerative colitis, hypertension, hiatal hernia, hepatic disease, renal disease, pregnancy (B), lactation, urinary retention, prostatic hypertrophy

Pharmacokinetics:

PO: Onset 1-2 hr, duration 3-4 hr; metabolized by liver; excreted in urine

Interactions:

- Increased anticholinergic effect: amantadine, tricylic antidepressants, MAOIs, H_1 antihistamines
- Decreased effect of phenothiazines, levodopa, ketoconazole

NURSING CONSIDERATIONS

Assess:

- VS, cardiac status: checking for dysrhythmias, increased rate, palpitations
- I&O ratio; check for urinary retention or hesitancy
- GI complaints: pain, bleeding (frank or occult), nausea, vomiting, anorexia

Administer:

- ½-1 hr ac for better absorption
- Decreased dose to elderly patients; metabolism may be slowed
- Gum, hard candy, frequent rinsing of mouth for dry oral cavity

Perform/provide:

- Storage in tight container protected from light
- Increased fluids, bulk, exercise to decrease constipation

Evaluate:

- Therapeutic response: absence of epigastric pain, bleeding, nausea, vomiting

Teach patient/family:

- To avoid driving, other hazardous activities until stabilized on medication; may cause blurred vision
- To avoid alcohol, other CNS depressants; will enhance sedating properties of this drug
- To avoid hot environments; stroke may occur; drug suppresses perspiration
- To use sunglasses when outside to prevent photophobia
- To drink plenty of fluids
- To report dysphagia

didanosine (ddI, dideoxyinosine) (℞)

(dye-dan'o-seen)

Videx, ddI, Dideoxyinosine

Func. class.: Antiviral

Chem. class.: Synthetic purine nucleoside of deoxyadenosine

Action: Nucleoside analog incorporating into cellular DNA by viral reverse transcriptase, thereby terminating the cellular DNA chain

Uses: Advanced HIV, AIDS infections in adults and children who have been unable to use zidovudine or who have not responded to treatment

Dosage and routes:

- *Adult:* PO >75 kg, 300 mg bid tabs, or 375 mg bid buffered pwd; 50-74 kg, 200 mg bid tabs, or 250 mg bid buffered pwd; 35-49 kg, 125 mg bid tabs, or 167 mg bid buffered pwd
- *Child:* PO 1.1-1.4 m^2, 100 mg bid tabs, or 125 mg bid pedi pwd; 0.8-1 m^2, 75 mg bid tabs, or 94 mg bid pedi pwd; 0.5-0.7 m^2, 50 mg bid tabs, or 62 mg bid pedi pwd; <0.4 m^2, 25 mg bid tabs, or 31 mg bid pedi pwd

Available forms: Tabs, buffered, chewable/dispersible 25, 50, 100, 150 mg; pwd for oral sol, buffered

100, 167, 250, 375 mg; pwd for oral sol, pedi 2, 4 g

Side effects/adverse reactions:

GI: ***Pancreatitis,*** diarrhea, nausea, vomiting, abdominal pain, constipation, stomatitis, dyspepsia, liver abnormalities, flatulence, taste perversion, dry mouth, oral thrush, melena, increased ALT, AST, alk phosphatase, amylase

GU: Increased bilirubin, uric acid

CNS: ***Peripheral neuropathy, seizures,*** confusion, anxiety, hypertonia, abnormal thinking, asthenia, insomnia, ***CNS depression,*** pain, dizziness, chills, fever

RESP: Cough, pneumonia, dyspnea, asthma, epistaxis, hypoventilation, sinusitis

INTEG: Rash, pruritus, alopecia, ecchymosis, hemorrhage, petechiae, sweating

MS: Myalgia, arthritis, myopathy, muscular atrophy

CV: Hypertension, vasodilation, dysrhythmia, syncope, CHF, palpitation

EENT: Ear pain, otitis, photophobia, visual impairment

HEMA: ***Leukopenia, granulocytopenia, thrombocytopenia, anemia***

Contraindications: Hypersensitivity

Precautions: Renal, hepatic disease, pregnancy (B), lactation, children, sodium-restricted diets, elevated amylase, preexistant peripheral neuropathy

Pharmacokinetics:

PO: Elimination half-life 1.62 hr, extensive metabolism is thought to occur; administration within 5 min of food will decrease absorption

Interactions:

• Decreased absorption: ketoconazole, dapsone, food

• Do not give with tetracyclines

• Decreased concentrations of fluoroquinolone antibiotics

NURSING CONSIDERATIONS

Assess:

• Peripheral neuropathy: tingling or pain in hands and feet, distal numbness

• Pancreatitis: Abdominal pain, nausea, vomiting, elevated liver enzymes; drug should be discontinued, since condition can be fatal

• Children by dilated retinal examination q6mo to rule out retinal depigmentation

• CBC, differential, platelet count qmo; withhold drug if WBC is <4000 or platelet count is <75,000; notify prescriber of results; alk phosphatase, monitor amylase

• Renal function studies: BUN, serum uric acid, urine CrCl before, during therapy

• Temperature q4h, may indicate beginning infection

• Liver function tests before, during therapy (bilirubin, AST [SGOT], ALT [SGPT]) as needed or qmo

Administer:

• Antibiotics for prophylaxis of infection

Perform/provide:

• Strict medical asepsis, protective isolation if WBC levels are low

• Cleanup of powdered products; use wet mop or damp sponge

Evaluate:

• Therapeutic response: absence of infection; symptoms of HIV

Teach patient/family:

• To take on an empty stomach; not to take dapsone at same time as ddi

• To report signs of infection: increased temperature, sore throat, flu symptoms

• To report signs of anemia: fatigue, headache, faintness, shortness of breath, irritability

• To report bleeding; avoid use of razors, commercial mouthwash

D

• That hair may be lost during therapy (rare); a wig or hairpiece may make patient feel better

dienestrol (℞)

(dye-en-ess′trole)

DV, Ortho Dienestrol

Func. class.: Estrogen

Chem. class.: Nonsteroidal synthetic estrogen

Action: Needed for adequate functioning of female reproductive system, it affects release of pituitary gonadotropins, inhibits ovulation, adequate calcium use in bone structures

Uses: Atrophic vaginitis, kraurosis vulvae

Dosage and routes:

• *Adult:* VAG CREAM 1-2 applications qd × 2 wk, then ½ dose × 2 wk, then 1 application

Available forms: Vag cream 0.01%

Side effects/adverse reactions:

CNS: Dizziness, headache, migraines, depression

CV: Hypotension, thrombophlebitis, edema, ***thromboembolism, stroke, pulmonary embolism, myocardial infarction***

GI: Nausea, vomiting, diarrhea, anorexia, pancreatitis, cramps, constipation, increased appetite, increased weight, ***cholestatic jaundice***

EENT: Contact lens intolerance, increased myopia, astigmatism

GU: Amenorrhea, cervical erosion, breakthrough bleeding, dysmenorrhea, vaginal candidiasis, breast changes, gynecomastia, testicular atrophy, impotence

INTEG: Rash, urticaria, acne, hirsutism, alopecia, oily skin, seborrhea, purpura, melasma

META: Folic acid deficiency, hypercalcemia, hyperglycemia

Contraindications: Breast cancer, thromboembolic disorders, reproductive cancer, genital bleeding (abnormal, undiagnosed), pregnancy (X), lactation

Precautions: Hypertension, asthma, blood dyscrasias, gallbladder disease, CHF, diabetes mellitus, bone disease, depression, migraine headache, convulsive disorders, hepatic disease, renal disease, family history of cancer of the breast or reproductive tract

Pharmacokinetics:

TOP: Degraded in liver; excreted in urine; crosses placenta; excreted in breast milk

Interactions:

• Decreased action of anticoagulants, oral hypoglycemics

• Toxicity: tricyclic antidepressants

• Decreased action of dienestrol: anticonvulsants, barbiturates, phenylbutazone, rifampin

• Increased action of: corticosteroids

NURSING CONSIDERATIONS

Assess:

• Weight daily; notify prescriber of weekly weight gain >5 lb

• B/P q4h

• I&O ratio; be alert for decreasing urinary output and increasing edema

• Liver function studies including ALT (SGOT), AST (SGPT), bilirubin

• Edema, hypertension, cardiac symptoms, jaundice

• Mental status: affect, mood, behavioral changes, aggression

• Hypercalcemia

Administer:

• At hs for better absorption

• Titrated dose; use lowest effective dose to prevent adverse reactions

• Dosage reduction should continue at 3-6 month intervals

* Available in Canada only

Perform/provide:
• Storage in tight, light-resistant container in refrigerator
Evaluate:
• Therapeutic response: decreased symptoms of vaginitis, kraurosis
Teach patient/family:
• How to fill applicator and insert cream
• To check with prescriber before using any OTC drugs
• To report breast lumps, vaginal bleeding, edema, jaundice, dark urine, clay-colored stools, dyspnea, headache, blurred vision, abdominal pain, numbness or stiffness in legs, chest pain
• To stop using product and report to prescriber if pregnancy is suspected

diethylstilbestrol/diethylstilbestrol diphosphate (℞)

(dye-eth-il-stil-bess'trole)
DES, diethylstilbestrol, Honvol*, Stilphostrol
Func. class.: Estrogen
Chem. class.: Nonsteroidal synthetic estrogen

Action: Needed for adequate functioning of female reproductive system, it affects release of pituitary gonadotropins, inhibits ovulation, adequate calcium use in bone structures

Uses: Breast cancer, prostatic cancer

Dosage and routes:
Prostatic cancer
• *Adult:* PO 1-3 mg qd, then 1 mg qd; PO 50-200 mg tid (diphosphate); IM 5 mg 2×/wk, then 4 mg 2×/wk; IV 0.25-1 g qd × 5 days, then 1-2×/wk
Breast cancer (postmenopausal)
• *Adult:* PO 15 mg qd
Available forms: Tabs 1, 5 mg; diethylstilbestrol diphosphate tab 50 mg; inj 0.25 gm

Side effects/adverse reactions:
CNS: Dizziness, headache, migraines, depression
CV: Hypotension, thrombophlebitis, edema, ***thromboembolism, stroke, pulmonary embolism, myocardial infarction***
GI: Nausea, vomiting, diarrhea, anorexia, pancreatitis, cramps, constipation, increased appetite, increased weight, ***cholestatic jaundice***
EENT: Contact lens intolerance, increased myopia, astigmatism
GU: Amenorrhea, cervical erosion, breakthrough bleeding, dysmenorrhea, vaginal candidiasis, breast changes, *gynecomastia, testicular atrophy, impotence*
INTEG: Rash, urticaria, acne, hirsutism, alopecia, oily skin, seborrhea, purpura, melasma
META: Folic acid deficiency, hypercalcemia, hyperglycemia

Contraindications: Premenopausal breast cancer, thromboembolic disorders, reproductive cancer, genital bleeding (abnormal, undiagnosed), pregnancy (X), lactation

Precautions: Hypertension, asthma, blood dyscrasias, gallbladder disease, CHF, diabetes mellitus, bone disease blocking agents

Interactions:
• Decreased action of anticoagulants, oral hypoglycemics
• Toxicity: tricyclic antidepressants
• Decreased action of diethylstilbestrol: anticonvulsants, barbiturates, phenylbutazone, rifampin
• Increased action of corticosteroids
• Incompatibility: not known

Lab test interferences:
Increase: BSP retention test, PBI, T_4, serum Na, platelet aggressabil-

ity, thyroxine-binding globulin (TBG), prothrombin, factors VII, VIII, IX, X, triglycerides
Decrease: Serum folate, serum triglyceride, T_3 resin uptake test, glucose tolerance test, antithrombin III, pregnanediol, metyraponetest
False positive: LE prep, antinuclear antibodies

NURSING CONSIDERATIONS

Assess:

• Urine glucose in patient with diabetes; urine glucose may rise
• Weight daily, notify prescriber of weekly weight gain >5 lb; if increase, diuretic may be ordered
• B/P q4h, watch for increase caused by H_2O and Na retention
• I&O ratio; be alert for decreasing urinary output and increasing edema
• Liver function studies, including AST (SGOT), ALT (SGPT), bilirubin, alk phosphatase
• Edema, hypertension, cardiac symptoms, jaundice
• Mental status: affect, mood, behavioral changes, aggression

Administer:

• IV after diluting in 300 ml dextrose or NS sol; give at 1-2 ml/min × 15 min; may increase rate to complete infusion 1 hr after starting
• Titrated dose; use lowest effective dose
• In one dose in AM for prostatic cancer
• With food, milk for GI symptoms

Evaluate:

• Therapeutic response: absence of breast engorgement, reversal of menopause or decrease in tumor size in prostatic cancer

Teach patient/family:

• To weigh weekly, report gain >5 lb
• To report breast lumps, vaginal bleeding, edema, jaundice, dark urine, clay-colored stools, dyspnea, headache, blurred vision, abdominal pain, numbness or stiffness in legs, chest pain; male to report impotence or gynecomastia
• To check with prescriber before taking any OTC drugs

difenoxin HCl/atropine sulfate diphenoxylate/atropine (℞)

(dye-fen-ox'in)
Diphenatol, Lofene, Logene, Lomotil, Lomanate, Lo-Trol, Motofen, Nor-Mil
Func. class.: Antidiarrheal
Chem. class.: Phenylpiperidine derivative, opiate agonist

Controlled Substance Schedule IV (difenoxin); V diphenoxylate
Action: Inhibits gastric motility by acting on mucosal receptors responsible for peristalsis
Uses: Acute nonspecific and acute exacerbations of chronic functional diarrhea

Dosage and routes:

• *Adult:* PO 2 mg, then 1 mg after each loose stool or 1 mg q3-4h as needed, not to exceed 8 mg/24 hr

Available forms: Tab 1 mg difenoxin HCl, 0.025 mg atropine; tabs 2.5 mg diphenoxylate/0.025 mg atropine; liq 2.5 mg diphenoxylate/0.025 mg atropine/5 ml

Side effects/adverse reactions:

CNS: Dizziness, drowsiness, lightheadedness, headache, fatigue, nervousness, insomnia, confusion
GI: Nausea, vomiting, dry mouth, epigastric distress, constipation
EENT: Burning eyes, blurred vision

Contraindications: Hypersensitivity, pseudomembranous enterocolitis, jaundice, glaucoma, child <2 yr, severe electrolyte imbalances, diar-

* Available in Canada only

rhea associated with organisms that penetrate intestinal mucosa
Precautions: Hepatic disease, renal disease, ulcerative colitis, pregnancy (C), lactation, severe liver disease
Pharmacokinetics:
PO: Onset 40-60 min, peak 2 hr, duration 3-4 hr, terminal half-life 12-14 hr; metabolized in liver to inactive metabolite; excreted in urine, feces
Interactions:
• Do not use with MAOIs; hypertensive crisis may occur
• Increased action of alcohol, narcotics, barbiturates, other CNS depressants, anticholinergics
NURSING CONSIDERATIONS
Assess:
• Electrolytes (K, Na, Cl) if on long-term therapy
• Bowel pattern before; for rebound constipation after termination of medication; bowel sounds
• Response after 48 hr; if none, drug should be discontinued
• Abdominal distention, toxic megacolon, which may occur in ulcerative colitis
Administer:
• For 48 hr only; if no response, drug should be discontinued
Evaluate:
• Therapeutic response: decreased diarrhea
Teach patient/family:
• To avoid OTC products unless directed by prescriber; may contain alcohol
• Not to exceed recommended dose
• That drug may be habit forming
• Not to engage in hazardous activities; drowsiness may occur

diflorasone (℞)
(die-floor′a-sone)
Florone, Florone E, Maxiflor, Psorcon
Func. class.: Topical corticosteroid
Chem. class.: Synthetic fluorinated agent, group II potency

D

Action: Antipruritic, antiinflammatory
Uses: Psoriasis, eczema, contact dermatitis, pruritus
Dosage and routes:
• *Adult and child:* Apply to affected area qd-tid
Available forms: Cream 0.05%; oint 0.05%
Side effects/adverse reactions:
INTEG: Burning, dryness, itching, irritation, acne, folliculitis, hypertrichosis, perioral dermatitis, hypopigmentation, atrophy, striae, miliaria, allergic contact dermatitis, secondary infection
Contraindications: Hypersensitivity to corticosteroids, fungal infections
Precautions: Pregnancy (C), lactation, viral, bacterial infections
NURSING CONSIDERATIONS
Assess:
• Temp; if fever develops, drug should be discontinued
• For systemic absorption: fever, inflammation, irritation
Administer:
• Only to affected areas; do not get in eyes
• Medication; then cover with occlusive dressing if prescribed; seal to normal skin; change q12h; use occlusive dressing with extreme caution; systemic absorption may occur
• Only to dermatoses; do not use on weeping, denuded, infected area

Perform/provide:
• Cleansing before application
• Treatment for a few days after area has cleared
• Storage at room temperature

Evaluate:
• Therapeutic response: absence of severe itching, patches on skin, flaking

Teach patient/family:
• To avoid sunlight on affected area; burns may occur

---

diflunisal (℞)

(dye-floo′ni-sal)
Diflunisal, Dolobid
Func. class.: Nonsteroidal anti-inflammatory
Chem. class.: Salicylate derivative

Action: May block pain impulses in CNS that occur in response to inhibition of prostaglandin synthesis; antipyretic action results from inhibition of hypothalamic heat-regulating center to produce vasodilation to allow heat dissipation

Uses: Mild to moderate pain or fever including arthritis; 3-4 times more potent than aspirin

Dosage and routes:
Pain/fever
• *Adult:* PO loading dose 1 g; then 500-1000 mg/day in 2 divided doses, q12h, not to exceed 1500 mg/day

Available forms: Tabs 250, 500 mg

Side effects/adverse reactions:
HEMA: ***Thrombocytopenia, agranulocytosis, leukopenia, neutropenia, hemolytic anemia,*** increased pro-time
CNS: Stimulation, drowsiness, dizziness, confusion, ***convulsions,*** headache, flushing, hallucinations, coma
GI: Nausea, vomiting, GI bleeding, diarrhea, heartburn, anorexia, ***hepatitis***
INTEG: Rash, urticaria, bruising
EENT: Blurred vision, decreased acuity, corneal deposits
CV: Rapid pulse, ***pulmonary edema***
RESP: Wheezing, hyperpnea
ENDO: Hypoglycemia, hyponatremia, hypokalemia

Contraindications: Hypersensitivity to salicylates, GI bleeding, bleeding disorders, children <12 yr, Vit K deficiency

Precautions: Anemia, hepatic disease, renal disease, Hodgkin's disease, pregnancy (C), lactation

Pharmacokinetics:
PO: Onset 15-30 min, peak 2-3 hr, half-life 10-12 hr; metabolized by liver; excreted by kidneys; crosses placenta; 99% protein bound; excreted in breast milk

Interactions:
• Decreased effects of diflunisal: antacids, steroids, urinary alkalizers
• Increased blood loss: alcohol, heparin
• Increased effects of anticoagulants, insulin, methotrexate, hydrochlorothiazide, acetaminophen
• Decreased effects of probenecid, spironolactone, sulfinpyrazone, sulfa drugs
• Toxic effects: PABA
• Decreased blood sugar levels: salicylates

Lab test interferences:
Increase: Coagulation, liver function studies, serum uric acid, amylase, CO_2, urinary protein
Decrease: Serum K, PBI, cholesterol
Interfere: Urine catecholamines, pregnancy test

NURSING CONSIDERATIONS

Assess:
• Liver function studies: AST (SGOT), ALT (SGPT), bilirubin, creatinine (long-term therapy)

---

* Available in Canada only

- Renal function studies: BUN, urine creatinine (long-term therapy)
- Blood studies: CBC, Hct, Hgb, pro-time (long-term therapy)
- I&O ratio; decreasing output may indicate renal failure (long-term therapy)
- Hepatotoxicity: dark urine; clay-colored stools; yellowing of skin, sclera; itching; abdominal pain; fever; diarrhea (long-term therapy)
- Allergic reactions: rash, urticaria; drug may have to be discontinued
- Renal dysfunction: decreased urine output
- Ototoxicity: tinnitus, ringing, roaring in ears; audiometric testing is needed before, after long-term therapy
- Visual changes: blurring, halos, corneal, retinal damage
- Edema in feet, ankles, legs
- Drug history; many interactions

Administer:

- To patient whole
- With food, milk for gastric symptoms

Evaluate:

- Therapeutic response: decreased pain, stiffness of joints

Teach patient/family:

- To report any symptoms of hepatotoxicity, renal toxicity, visual changes, ototoxicity, allergic reactions (long-term therapy)
- Not to exceed recommended dosage; acute poisoning may result
- To read label on other OTC drugs; many contain aspirin
- That therapeutic response takes 2 wk (arthritis)
- To avoid alcohol ingestion; GI bleeding may occur

Treatment of overdose: Lavage, activated charcoal, monitor electrolytes, VS

digitoxin (℞)

(di-ji-tox'in)

Crystodign, digitoxin

Func. class.: Antidysrhythmic, cardiac glycoside cardiotonic

Chem. class.: Digitalis preparation

Action: Acts by increased influx of calcium ions from extracellular to intracellular cytoplasm, increasing force of contraction and cardiac output; decreases conduction velocity through AV node; prolongs effective refractory period

Uses: CHF, atrial fibrillation, atrial flutter, atrial tachycardia, rapid digitalization in these disorders

Dosage and routes:

- *Adult and child >12 yr:* PO 1.2-1.6 initially; give in divided doses over 24 hr; 150 μg qd; maintenance 10% initial dose

Available forms: Tabs 50, 100, 150, 200 μg

Side effects/adverse reactions:

CNS: Headache, drowsiness, apathy, confusion, disorientation, fatigue, depression, hallucinations

CV: ***Dysrhythmias,*** *hypotension, bradycardia,* AV block

GI: Nausea, vomiting, anorexia, abdominal pain, diarrhea

EENT: Blurred vision, yellow-green halos, photophobia, diplopia

MS: Muscular weakness

Contraindications: Hypersensitivity to digitalis, ventricular fibrillation, ventricular tachycardia, carotid sinus syndrome, 2nd or 3rd degree heart block

Precautions: Hepatic disease, acute MI, AV block, hypokalemia, hypomagnesemia, sinus node disease, lactation, severe respiratory disease, hypothyroidism, elderly, pregnancy (C), lactation

Pharmacokinetics:
PO: Onset ½-2 hr, peak 4-12 hr; duration 2-3 wk, half-life 4-20 days; metabolized in liver; excreted in urine
Interactions:
• Hypokalemia: thiazides
• Increased blood levels: spironolactone
• Decreased effects: hydantoins, aminoglutethimide, rifampin, phenylbutazone, barbiturates, cholestyramine, colestipol
• Toxicity: adrenergics, diuretics, succinylcholine, quinidine, thioamines
• Decreased level of digitoxin: thyroid agents
Lab test interferences:
Increase: CPK
NURSING CONSIDERATIONS
Assess:
• Apical pulse for 1 min before giving drug; if pulse <60, take again in 1 hr; if <60, call prescriber
• Electrolytes: K, Na, Cl, Ca; renal function studies: BUN, creatinine; blood studies: ALT (SGOT), AST (SGPT), bilirubin
• Monitor drug levels (therapeutic level 25-35 ng/ml)
• Cardiac status: apical pulse, character, rate, rhythm
Administer:
• K supplements if ordered for K levels <3.0 mg/dl
Evaluate:
• Therapeutic response: decreased weight, edema, pulse, respiration and increased urine output
Teach patient/family:
• Not to stop drug abruptly; teach all aspects of drug, digitalis toxicity; to keep tabs in container protected from light
• To avoid OTC medications; many adverse interactions
Treatment of overdose: Discontinue drug, administer K, digoxin immune FAB, monitor ECG

digoxin (℞)

(di-jox'in)
digoxin, Lanoxicaps, Lanoxin
Func. class.: Antidysrhythmic, cardiac glycoside
Chem. class.: Digitalis preparation

Action: Inhibits the sodium-potassium ATPase, which makes more calcium available for contractile proteins, resulting in increased cardiac output
Uses: CHF, atrial fibrillation, atrial flutter, atrial tachycardia, cardiogenic shock, paroxysmal atrial tachycardia, rapid digitalization in these disorders
Dosage and routes:
• *Adult:* IV 0.5 mg given over >5 min, then PO 0.125-0.5 mg qd in divided doses q4-6hr as needed
• *Elderly:* PO 0.125 mg qd maintenance
• *Child >2 yr:* PO 0.02-0.04 mg/kg divided q8h over 24 hr; maintenance 0.006-0.012 mg/kg qd in divided doses q12hr; IV loading dose 0.015-0.035 mg/kg over >5 min
• *Child 1 mo-2 yr:* IV 0.03-0.05 mg/kg in divided doses over >5 min q48h; change to PO as soon as possible; PO 0.035-0.060 mg/kg divided in 3 doses over 24 hr; maintenance 0.01-0.02 mg/kg in divided doses q12h
• *Neonates:* IV loading dose 0.02-0.03 mg/kg over >5 min in divided doses q4-8h; change to PO as soon as possible; PO loading dose 0.035 mg/kg divided q8h over 24h; maintenance 0.01 mg/kg in divided doses q12h

• *Premature infants:* IV 0.015-0.025 mg/kg divided in 3 doses over 24 hr, given over >5 min; maintenance 0.003-0.009 mg/kg in divided doses q12h

Available forms: Caps 50, 100, 200 μg; elix 50 μg/ml; tabs 125, 250, 500 μg; inj 100, 250 μg/ml: pediatric inj 10 μg/ml

Side effects/adverse reactions:

CNS: Headache, drowsiness, apathy, confusion, disorientation, fatigue, depression, hallucinations

CV: ***Dysrhythmias,*** *hypotension,* bradycardia, ***AV block***

EENT: Blurred vision, yellow-green halos, photophobia, diplopia

GI: Nausea, vomiting, anorexia, abdominal pain, diarrhea

Contraindications: Hypersensitivity to digitalis, ventricular fibrillation, ventricular tachycardia, carotid sinus syndrome, 2nd or 3rd degree heart block

Precautions: Renal disease, acute MI, AV block, severe respiratory disease, hypothyroidism, elderly, pregnancy (C), sinus nodal disease, lactation, hypokalemia

Pharmacokinetics:

PO: Onset ½-2 hr, peak 6-8 hr, duration 3-4 days

IV: Onset 5-30 min, peak 1-5 hr, duration variable, half-life 1.5 days; excreted in urine

Interactions:

• Hypokalemia: diuretics, amphotericin B, carbenicillin, ticarcillin, corticosteroids, piperacillin

• Decreased digoxin level: thyroid agents

• Increased blood levels: propantheline bromide, spironolactone quinidine, verapamil, aminoglycosides PO, amiodarone, anticholinergics, quinine

• Increased bradycardia: β-adrenergic blockers, antidysrythmics

• Toxicity: adrenergics, amphotericin, corticosteroids, diuretics, glucose, insulin, reserpine, succinylcholine, quinidine, thioamines

Syringe compatibility: Heparin, milrinone

Y-site compatibilities: Amrinone, famotidine, meperidine, milrinone, morphine, potassium chloride, vitamin B with C

Additive compatibilities: Bretylium, cimetidine, floxacillin, furosemide, lidocaine, verapamil

Lab test interferences:

Increase: CPK

NURSING CONSIDERATIONS

Assess:

• Apical pulse for 1 min before giving drug; if pulse <60 in adult or <90 in an infant, take again in 1 hr; if <60 in adult, call prescriber; note rate, rhythm, character; monitor ECG continuously during parenteral loading dose

• Electrolytes: K, Na, Cl, Mg, Ca; renal function studies: BUN, creatinine; blood studies: ALT (SGOT), AST (SGPT), bilirubin, Hct, Hgb before initiating treatment and periodically thereafter

• I&O ratio, daily weights; monitor turgor, lung sounds, edema

• Monitor drug levels (therapeutic level 0.5-2 ng/ml)

• Cardiac status: apical pulse, character, rate, rhythm

Administer:

• PO with or without food; may crush tabs, mix with food/fluids

• K supplements if ordered for K levels <3, or foods high in K: bananas, orange juice

• IV undiluted or 1 ml of drug/4 ml sterile H_2O, D_5, or NS; give over >5 min through Y-tube or 3-way stopcock; during digitalization close monitoring is necessary

Perform/provide:

• Storage protected from light

Evaluate:
Therapeutic response: decreased weight, edema, pulse, respiration, rales; increased urine output; serum digoxin level (0.5-2 ng/ml)

Teach patient/family:
• Not to stop drug abruptly; teach all aspects of drug, to take exactly as ordered
• To avoid OTC medications, since many adverse drug interactions may occur; do not take antacid at same time
• To notify prescriber of any loss of appetite, lower stomach pain, diarrhea, weakness, drowsiness, headache, blurred or yellow vision, rash, depression, toxicity
• Toxic symptoms of this drug and when to notify prescriber
• To maintain a sodium-restricted diet as ordered
• To report shortness of breath, difficulty breathing, weight gain, edema, persistent cough

Treatment of overdose: Discontinue drug; give K; monitor ECG, give adrenergic blocking agent, digoxin immune FAB

digoxin immune FAB (ovine) (℞)

(di-jox′in)
Digibind
Func. class.: Antidote—digoxin specific

Action: Antibody fragments bind to free digoxin to reverse digoxin toxicity by not allowing digoxin to bind to sites of action

Uses: Life-threatening digoxin or digitoxin toxicity

Dosage and routes:
Digoxin toxicity
• *Adult:* IV dose (mg) = dose ingested (mg) × 0.8 × 66.7; if ingested amount is unknown, give 800 mg IV; if digoxin liquid caps or digitoxin used, do not multiply ingested dose by 0.8

Available forms: Inj 40 mg/vial (binds 0.6 mg digoxin or digitoxin)

Side effects/adverse reactions:
CV: ***CHF,*** ventricular rate increase, ***atrial fibrillation,*** low cardiac output
RESP: ***Impaired respiratory function, rapid respiratory rate***
META: ***Hypokalemia***
INTEG: Hypersensitivity, allergic reactions, facial swelling, redness

Contraindications: Mild digoxin toxicity, hypersensitivity

Precautions: Children, lactation, cardiac disease, renal disease, pregnancy (C)

Pharmacokinetics:
IV: Peaks after completion of infusion, onset 30 min (variable); not known if crosses placenta, breast milk; half-life biphasic—14-20 hr; prolonged in renal disease; excreted by kidneys

Interactions:
• Considered incompatible with all drugs in syringe or sol

Lab test interferences:
Interfere: Immunoassay digoxin

NURSING CONSIDERATIONS

Assess:
• Hypokalemia: ST depression, flat T waves, presence of U wave, ventricular dysrhythmia; K levels may decrease rapidly

Administer:
• After diluting 40 mg/4 ml of sterile H_2O for inj 10 mg/ml mix; may be further diluted with normal saline, sol should be clear, colorless
• By bolus if cardiac arrest is imminent or IV over 30 min using a 0.22 µm filter

Perform/provide:
• Storage of reconstituted sol for up to 4 hr in refrigerator

* Available in Canada only

Teach patient/family:
• The purpose of medication; to report fever, chills, itching, swelling, dyspnea
• To advise dentists, doctors that this drug has been used

Evaluate:
• Therapeutic response: correction of digoxin toxicity; check digoxin levels

---

dihydroergotamine (℞)

(dye-hye-droe-er-got'a-meen)
D.H.E. 45
Func. class.: α-Adrenergic blocker
Chem. class.: Ergot alkaloid (dihydrogenated)

Action: Constricts smooth muscle in periphery, cranial blood vessels; inhibits norepinephrine uptake

Uses: Vascular headache (migraine or histamine)

Dosage and routes:
• *Adult:* IM/IV 1 mg; may repeat q1-2h if needed, not to exceed 3 mg/day or 6 mg/wk

Available forms: Inj 1 mg/ml

Side effects/adverse reactions:
CNS: Numbness in fingers, toes, weakness
CV: Transient tachycardia, chest pain, bradycardia, increase or decrease in B/P, *gangrene*
GI: Nausea, vomiting
MS: Muscle pain

Contraindications: Hypersensitivity to ergot preparations, occlusion (peripheral, vascular), CAD, hepatic disease, pregnancy (X), renal disease, peptic ulcer, hypertension, lactation, children, uremia

Pharmacokinetics:
IM: Onset 15-30 min, peak 2 hr, duration 3-4 hr
IV: Onset 5 min, peak 45 min, duration 3-4 hr
Half-life 1.3-4 hr

Interactions:
• Increased effects: troleandomycin
• Increased vasoconstriction: β-blockers
• Incompatible with any drug in syringe or sol

NURSING CONSIDERATIONS

Assess:
• Weight daily, check for peripheral edema in feet, legs
• For stress level, activity, recreation, coping mechanisms
• Neurologic status: LOC, blurring vision, nausea, vomiting, tingling in extremities that precede headache
• Ingestion of tyramine (pickled products, beer, wine, aged cheese), food additives, preservatives, colorings, artificial sweeteners, chocolate, caffeine; may precipitate these headaches

Administer:
• IV undiluted; give 1 mg or less/min
• IM dose, which takes 20 min for effect, or IV for immediate effect
• At beginning of headache; dose must be titrated to patient response
• Only to women who are not pregnant; harm to fetus may occur

Perform/provide:
• Storage in dark area; do not use discolored solutions
• Quiet, calm environment with decreased stimulation for noise, bright light, excessive talking

Evaluate:
• Therapeutic response: decrease in frequency, severity of headache

Teach patient/family:
• Not to use OTC medications; serious drug interactions may occur
• To report side effects: increased vasoconstriction starting with cold extremities, then paresthesia, weakness

• That an increase in headaches may occur when this drug is discontinued after long-term use
• To keep drug out of reach of children; death may occur

dihydrotachysterol (℞)

(dye-hye-droe-tak-iss′ter-ole)
DHT Intensol, DHT, Hytakerol
Func. class.: Parathyroid agent (calcium regulator)
Chem. class.: Vitamin D analog

Action: Increases intestinal absorption of calcium for bones, increases renal tubular absorption of phosphate; regulates calcium levels by regulating calcitonin, parathyroid hormone
Uses: Renal osteodystrophy, hypoparathyroidism, pseudohypoparathyroidism, familial hypophosphatemia, postoperative tetany
Dosage and routes:
Hypophosphatemia
• *Adult and child:* PO 0.5-2 mg qd, maintenance 0.3-1.5 mg qd
Hypoparathyroidism/pseudohypoparathyroidism
• *Adult:* PO 0.8-2.4 mg qd × 4 days, maintenance 0.2-2 mg qd regulated by serum calcium levels
• *Child:* PO 1-5 mg qd × 1 wk, maintenance 0.2-1 mg qd regulated by serum Ca levels
Renal osteodystrophy
• *Adult:* PO 0.1-0.25 mg qd, then 0.2-1 mg/day
Available forms: Tabs 0.125, 0.2, 0.4 mg; caps 0.125 mg; oral sol 0.2, 0.25 mg/5 ml
Side effects/adverse reactions:
EENT: Tinnitus
CNS: Drowsiness, headache, vertigo, fever, lethargy
GI: Nausea, diarrhea, vomiting, jaundice, anorexia, dry mouth, constipation, cramps, metallic taste
MS: Myalgia, arthralgia, decreased bone development
GU: ***Polyuria,*** hypercalciuria, hyperphosphatemia, ***hematuria***
Contraindications: Hypersensitivity, renal disease, hyperphosphatemia, hypercalcemia
Precautions: Pregnancy (C), renal calculi, lactation, CV disease
Pharmacokinetics:
PO: Onset 2 wk; metabolized by liver, excreted in feces (active/inactive)
Interactions:
• Decreased absorption of dihydrotachysterol: cholestyramine, colestipol, HCl, mineral oil
• Hypercalcemia: thiazide diuretics, calcium supplements
• Cardiac dysrhythmias: cardiac glycosides, verapamil
• Decreased effect of dihydrotachysterol: corticosteroids, phenytoin, barbiturates
Lab test interferences:
False increase: Cholesterol
NURSING CONSIDERATIONS
Assess:
• BUN, urinary Ca, AST (SGOT), ALT (SGPT), cholesterol, creatinine, alk phosphatase, uric acid, chlorine, magnesium, electrolytes, urine pH, phosphate; may increase calcium, should be kept at 9-10 mg/dl, vit D 50-135 IU/dl, phosphate 70 mg/dl
• Alk phosphatase; may be decreased
• For increased blood level, since toxic reactions may occur rapidly
• For dry mouth, metallic taste, polyuria, bone pain, muscle weakness, headache, fatigue, tinnitus, change in LOC, irregular pulse, dysrhythmias, increased respirations, anorexia, nausea, vomiting, cramps, diarrhea, constipation; may indicate hypercalcemia

* Available in Canada only

• Renal status: decreased urinary output (oliguria, anuria), edema in extremities, weight gain >5 lb, periorbital edema
• Nutritional status, diet for sources of vit D (milk, some seafood), Ca (dairy products, dark green vegetables), phosphates (dairy products) must be avoided

Administer:
• PO, may be increased q4wk depending on blood level

Perform/provide:
• Storage in tight, light-resistant containers at room temperature
• Restriction of Na, K if required
• Restriction of fluids if required for chronic renal failure

Evaluate:
• Therapeutic response: prevention of bone deficiencies

Teach patient/family:
• Symptoms of hypercalcemia
• About foods rich in calcium, vit D

dihydroxyaluminum sodium carbonate (OTC)

(dye hye drox'ee-a-loom-a-nim)
Rolaids Antacid
Func. class.: Antacid
Chem. class.: Aluminum product

Action: Neutralizes gastric acidity, reduces pepsin
Uses: Antacid
Dosage and routes:
• *Adult:* PO 1-2 as needed; may give up to 2-4 tabs
Available forms: Chewable tab 334 mg
Side effects/adverse reactions:
GI: Constipation, ***obstruction***
Contraindications: Hypersensitivity to aluminum products
Precautions: Elderly, sodium/fluid restriction, decreased GI motility, GI obstruction, dehydration, severe renal disease, CHF, pregnancy (C)
Pharmacokinetics:
PO: Onset 20-40 min, excreted in feces
Interactions:
• Decreased effectiveness of: tetracyclines, ketoconazole, isoniazid, phenothiazines, iron salts, digitalis
• Constipation; increase bulk in the diet if needed

NURSING CONSIDERATIONS

Administer:
• Laxatives or stool softeners if constipation occurs

Evaluate:
• Therapeutic response: absence of pain, decreased acidity

Teach patient/family:
• To increase fluids to 2 L/day unless contraindicated
• To avoid long-term use; high sodium content

diltiazem (℞)

(dil-tye'a-zem)
Apo-Diltiaz*, Cardizem, Cardizem SR, Cardizem CD, diltiazem, Dilacor-XR
Func. class.: Calcium channel blocker
Chem. class.: Benzothiazepine

Action: Inhibits calcium ion influx across cell membrane during cardiac depolarization; produces relaxation of coronary vascular smooth muscle, dilates coronary arteries, slows SA/AV node conduction times, dilates peripheral arteries
Uses: Oral: angina pectoris due to coronary insufficiency, hypertension, vasospasm; parenteral: atrial fibrillation, flutter, paroxysmal supraventricular tachycardia

Dosage and routes:
- *Adult:* PO 30 mg qid, increasing dose gradually to 180-360 mg/day in divided doses or 60-120 mg bid; may increase to 240-360 mg/day
- *Adult IV:* 0.25 mg/kg over BOL 2 min initially, then 0.35 mg/kg may be given after 15 min; if no response, may give CONT INF 5-15 mg/hr for up to 24 hrs
- *Adult:* PO (Cardizem CD) qd

Available forms: Tabs 30, 60, 90, 120 mg; caps sus rel 60, 90, 120, 180, 240, 300 mg; inj (IV) 5 mg/ml (5, 10 ml)

Side effects/adverse reactions:
CV: Dysrhythmia, edema, ***CHF,*** bradycardia, hypotension, palpitations, heart block, peripheral edema, angina
GI: Nausea, vomiting, diarrhea, gastric upset, constipation, increased liver function studies
GU: Nocturia, polyuria, ***acute renal failure***
INTEG: Rash, pruritus, flushing, photosensitivity
CNS: Headache, fatigue, drowsiness, dizziness, depression, weakness, insomnia, tremor, paresthesia

Contraindications: Sick sinus syndrome, 2nd or 3rd degree heart block, hypotension less than 90 mm Hg systolic, acute MI, pulmonary congestion

Precautions: CHF, hypotension, hepatic injury, pregnancy (C), lactation, children, renal disease

Pharmacokinetics: Onset 30-60 min, peak 2-3 hr, immediate rel, 6-11 sus rel, half-life 3½-9 hr; metabolized by liver; excreted in urine (96% as metabolites)

Interactions:
- Increased effects of β-blockers, digitalis, lithium, carbamazepine, cyclosporine
- Increased effects of diltiazem: cimetidine

NURSING CONSIDERATIONS

Assess:
- Blood levels (therapeutic levels: 0.025-0.1 μg/ml)
- Cardiac status: B/P, pulse, respiration, ECG and intervals PR, QRS, QT

Administer:
- Before meals, hs (PO)
- IV undiluted over 2 min or diluted 125 mg/100 ml, 250 mg/250 ml, of D_5W, 0.9% NaCl, D_5/0.45% NaCl, give 10 mg/hr may increase by 5 mg/hr to 15 mg/hr, continue infusion up to 24 hr

Perform/provide:
- Storage in tight container at room temperature

Evaluate:
- Therapeutic response: decreased anginal pain, decreased B/P

Teach patient/family:
- How to take pulse before taking drug; record or graph should be kept
- To avoid hazardous activities until stabilized on drug, dizziness is no longer a problem
- To limit caffeine consumption
- To avoid OTC drugs unless directed by prescriber
- Importance of complying with all areas of medical regimen: diet, exercise, stress reduction, drug therapy; sit on side of bed for 5-10 min prior to OOB; do not lift heavy items
- Not to crush sus rel caps
- To report dizziness, shortness of breath, palpitations
- Not to discontinue abruptly
- To take with a full glass of water

Treatment of overdose: Defibrillation, atropine for AV block, vasopressor for hypotension

---

dimenhydrinate (OTC, ℞)

(dye-men-hye'dri-nate)

Calm-X, dimenhydrinate, Dimetabs, Dinate, Dommanate, Dramamine, Dramanate, Dramocen, Dramoject, Dymenate, Gravol*, Hydrate, Marmine, Nauseal*, Nauseatol*, Nico-Vert, Novodimenate*, Travamine*, Triptone Caplets, Wehamine

Func. class.: Antiemetic, antihistamine, anticholinergic

Chem. class.: H_1-receptor antagonist, ethanolamine derivative

Action: Vestibular stimulation is decreased

Uses: Motion sickness, nausea, vomiting

Dosage and routes:

- *Adult:* PO 50-100 mg q4h; REC 100 mg qd or bid; IM/IV 50 mg as needed
- *Child:* IM/PO 5 mg/kg divided in 4 equal doses

Available forms: Tabs 50 mg; inj 50 mg/ml; liq 12.5 mg/4 ml; supp 50, 100 mg; chew tabs 50 mg; caps 50 mg

Side effects/adverse reactions:

CNS: Drowsiness, restlessness, headache, dizziness, insomnia, confusion, nervousness, tingling, vertigo; hallucinations and ***convulsions*** in young children

GI: Nausea, anorexia, diarrhea, vomiting, constipation

CV: Hypertension, hypotension, palpitation

INTEG: Rash, urticaria, fever, chills, flushing

EENT: Dry mouth, blurred vision, diplopia, nasal congestion, photosensitivity

Contraindications: Hypersensitivity to narcotics, shock

Precautions: Children, cardiac dysrhythmias, elderly, asthma, pregnancy (B), lactation, prostatic hypertrophy, bladder-neck obstruction, narrow-angle glaucoma, stenosing peptic ulcer, pyloroduodenal obstruction

Pharmacokinetics:

IM/PO: Duration 4-6 hr

Interactions:

- Increased effect: alcohol, other CNS depressants
- May mask ototoxic symptoms associated with aminoglycosides

Syringe compatibilities: Atropine, diphenhydramine, droperidol, fentanyl, heparin, meperidine, metoclopramide, morphine, pentazocine, perphenazine, ranitidine, scopolamine

Additive compatibilities: Amikacin, calcium gluconate, chloramphenicol, corticotropin, erythromycin, heparin, hydroxyzine, methicillin, norepinephrine, oxytetracycline, penicillin G potassium, pentobarbital, phenobarbital, potassium chloride, prochlorperazine, vancomycin, vitamin B with C

Lab test interferences:

False negative: Allergy skin testing

NURSING CONSIDERATIONS

Assess:

- VS, B/P; check patients with cardiac disease more often
- Signs of toxicity of other drugs or masking of symptoms of disease: brain tumor, intestinal obstruction
- Observe for drowsiness, dizziness

Administer:

- IV after diluting 50 mg/10 ml of NaCl inj; give 50 mg or less over 2 min
- IM injection in large muscle mass; aspirate to avoid IV administration
- Tablets may be swallowed whole, chewed, or allowed to dissolve

Evaluate:
• Therapeutic response: absence of nausea, vomiting

Teach patient/family:
• That a false-negative result may occur with skin testing; these procedures should not be scheduled for 4 days after discontinuing use
• To avoid hazardous activities, activities requiring alertness; dizziness may occur; instruct patient to request assistance with ambulation
• To avoid alcohol, other depressants

dimercaprol (℞)

(dye-mer-cap'role)

BAL in Oil, British Anti-Lewisite*, dimercaptopropanol

Func. class.: Heavy metal antagonist

Chem. class.: Chelating agent (dithiol compound)

Action: Binds ions from arsenic, gold, mercury, lead, copper to form water-soluble complex removed by kidneys

Uses: Arsenic, gold, mercury, lead poisoning

Dosage and routes:

Severe gold/arsenic poisoning
• *Adult:* IM 3 mg/kg q4h × 2 days then qid × 1 day, then bid × 10 days

Mild gold/arsenic poisoning
• *Adult:* IM 2.5 mg/kg qid × 2 days, then bid × 1 day, then qd × 10 days

Acute lead poisoning
• *Adult:* IM 4 mg/kg, then q4h with edetate calcium disodium 12.5 mg/kg IM, not to exceed 5 mg/kg/dose

Mercury poisoning
• *Adult:* IM 5 mg/kg, then 2.5 mg/kg/day or bid × 10 days

Available forms: Inj IM 100 mg/ml

Side effects/adverse reactions:
CNS: Headache, paresthesia, anxiety, tremors, ***convulsions, shock***
INTEG: Urticaria, erythema, pruritus, pain at injection site, fever, burning of lips, mouth, throat
CV: Hypertension, tachycardia
GI: Nausea, vomiting, salivation
EENT: Rhinorrhea, throat pain or constriction, lacrimation
GU: Burning sensation in penis, ***nephrotoxicity***
SYST: ***Anaphylaxis,*** metabolic acidosis

Contraindications: Hypersensitivity, anuria, hepatic insufficiency, poisoning of other metals, severe renal disease, child <3 yr, pregnancy (D)

Precautions: Hypertension, lactation, G6PD deficiency

Pharmacokinetics:
Metabolized by plasma enzymes, excreted by kidneys as complex, unchanged drug within 4 hr

Interactions:
• Increased toxicity: iron, selenium, uranium, cadmium

Lab test interferences:
Decrease: RAIU test

NURSING CONSIDERATIONS

Assess:
• B/P, increasing B/P or tachycardia, respirations, pulse, check temp q4hr; drug may cause fever in children, burning sensation of mouth, lips, eyes, throat
• Monitor I&O, kidney function studies: BUN, creatinine, CrCl; report decreases in output
• Urine: pH, albumin, casts, blood; metal levels daily
• Allergic reactions (rash, urticaria); if these occur, drug should be discontinued

Administer:
• IM in deep muscle mass; rotate injection sites; if giving EDTA also, give in separate site; observe for sterile abscesses

* Available in Canada only

- Only when epinephrine 1:1000 is on unit for anaphylaxis
- Being careful not to allow drug to touch skin; contact dermatitis can occur
- Acetazolamide or sodium citrate to decrease pH of urine, which decreases renal damage
- Give within 2 hr of ingestion; have antihistamine available for allergic reaction

Evaluate:

- Therapeutic response: decreasing level of metal in the blood

Teach patient/family:

- That breath may be odorous
- Explain all aspects of drug administration

dinoprostone (℞)

(dye-noe-prost'one)

Cervidil, Prepidil, Prostin E_2

Func. class.: Oxytocic, abortifacient

Chem. class.: Prostaglandin E_2

Action: Stimulates uterine contractions, causing abortion; acts within 30 hr for complete abortion

Uses: Abortion during 2nd trimester, benign hydatidiform mole, expulsion of uterine contents in fetal deaths to 28 wk, missed abortion, to efface and dilate the cervix in pregnancy at term

Dosage and routes:

- *Adult:* VAG SUPP 20 mg, repeat q3-5h until abortion occurs, max dose is 240 mg
- *Adult:* GEL; warm up to room temperature, choose correct length shielded catheter (10 or 20 mm), fill catheter by pushing plunger; patient should remain recumbent for 15-30 min
- *Adult:* INSERT 10 mg, remove upon onset of active labor or 12 hrs of insertion

Available forms: Vag supp 20 mg, gel 0.5 mg/3 gm (prefilled syringe); vaginal insert 10 mg; gel 0.5 mg

Side effects/adverse reactions:

CNS: Headache, dizziness, chills, fever

CV: Hypotension

GI: Nausea, vomiting, diarrhea

GU: Vaginitis, vaginal pain, vulvitis, vaginismus

INTEG: Rash, skin color changes

MS: Leg cramps, joint swelling, weakness

EENT: Blurred vision

INSERT: Uterine hyperstimulation, fever, nausea, vomiting, diarrhea, abdominal pain

GEL: Uterine contractile abnormality, GI side effects, back pain, fever

FETAL: Bradycardia (i.e., deceleration)

Contraindications: Hypersensitivity, uterine fibrosis, cervical stenosis, pelvic surgery, pelvic inflammatory disease, respiratory disease

Precautions: Hepatic disease, renal disease, cardiac disease, asthma, anemia, jaundice, diabetes mellitus, convulsive disorders, hypertension, hypotension

Pharmacokinetics:

SUPP: Onset 10 min, duration 2-3 hr; metabolized in spleen, kidney, lungs; excreted in urine

NURSING CONSIDERATIONS

Assess:

- Dilatation, effacement of cervix and uterine contraction, fetal heart tones, check for contractions over 1 min
- For fever that occurs ½ hr after suppository insertion (abortion)
- Respiratory rate, rhythm, depth; notify prescriber of abnormalities, pulse, B/P, temperature
- Vaginal discharge: check for itching, irritation; indicates vaginal infection

• For fever, chills: increase fluids or give tepid sponge bath or blanket
Administer:
• By insert: transversely in the posterior fornix of the vagina immediately after removal from foil package; do not insert without retrieval system
• By gel: after warming to room temperature, remove seal from end of syringe, and remove the protective end cap and insert into plunger stopper assembly; make sure patient is in dorsal position
• Antiemetic/antidiarrheal before administration of this drug
Evaluate:
• Therapeutic response: expulsion of fetus
Teach patient/family:
• To remain supine for 10-15 min after insertion
• To report excessive cramping, bleeding, chills, fever
• Methods of pain, comfort control

diphenhydramine (OTC, ℞)

(dye-fen-hye'dra-meen)

Allerdryl*, AllerMax, Banophen, Belix, Bena-D 10, Bena-D 50, Benadryl, Benadryl 25, Benadryl Kapseals, Benahist 10, Benahist 50, Ben-Allergin-50, Benoject, Benoject-10, Benoject-50, Benylin Cough, Bydramine, Compōz, Dermamycin, Diahist, Diphenacen-50, Diphen Cough, Diphenhist, Diphenhydramine HCl, Dormarex 2, Dormin, Dyrexin, Genahist, Hydramine, Hydramyn, Hyrexin-50, Insomnal*, Nidryl, Nordryl, Nordryl Cough, Nytol, Phendry, Scot-Tussin Allergy, Silphen Cough, Sleep-Eze 3, Sleepinal, Sominex 2, Sominex Caplets, Tusstat, Twilite, Uni-Bent Cough, Wehdryl

Func. class.: Antihistamine

Chem. class.: Ethanolamine derivative, H_1-receptor antagonist

Combination products: Benadryl: diphenhydramine HCl 25 mg with pseudoephedrine HCl 60 mg; Benylin: diphenhydramine HCl 12.5 mg/5 ml with pseudoephedrine HCl 30 mg/5 ml; Ziradyl: diphenhydramine HCl 2% with zinc oxide 2%

Action: Acts on blood vessels, GI, respiratory system by competing with histamine for H_1-receptor site; decreases allergic response by blocking histamine
Uses: Allergy symptoms, rhinitis, motion sickness, antiparkinsonism, nighttime sedation, infant colic, nonproductive cough
Dosage and routes:
• *Adult:* PO 25-50 mg q4-6h, not to

* Available in Canada only

exceed 400 mg/day; IM/IV 10-50 mg, not to exceed 400 mg/day
• *Child >12 kg:* PO/IM/IV 5 mg/kg/day in 4 divided doses, not to exceed 300 mg/day
Available forms: Caps 25, 50 mg; tabs 25, 50 mg; elix 12.5 mg/5 ml; syr 12.5 mg/5 ml; inj IM, IV 50 mg/ml; cream 1, 2%; lotion 1%
Side effects/adverse reactions:
CNS: Dizziness, drowsiness, poor coordination, fatigue, anxiety, euphoria, confusion, paresthesia, neuritis
RESP: Increased thick secretions, wheezing, chest tightness
HEMA: ***Thrombocytopenia, agranulocytosis, hemolytic anemia***
GI: Dry mouth, nausea, anorexia, diarrhea
INTEG: Photosensitivity
GU: Retention, dysuria, frequency
EENT: Blurred vision, dilated pupils, tinnitus, nasal stuffiness, dry nose, throat, mouth
Contraindications: Hypersensitivity to H_1-receptor antagonist, acute asthma attack, lower respiratory tract disease
Precautions: Increased intraocular pressure, renal disease, cardiac disease, hypertension, bronchial asthma, seizure disorder, stenosed peptic ulcers, hyperthyroidism, prostatic hypertrophy, bladder neck obstruction, pregnancy (C), lacation
Pharmacokinetics:
PO: Peak 1-3 hr, duration 4-7 hr; *IM:* Onset ½ hr, peak 1-4 hr, duration 4-7 hr; *IV:* Onset immediate, duration 4-7 hr; metabolized in liver, excreted by kidneys; crosses placenta, excreted in breast milk; half-life 2-7 hr
Interactions:
• Increased CNS depression: barbiturates, narcotics, hypnotics, tricyclic antidepressants, alcohol
• Decreased effect of: oral anticoagulants, heparin
• Increased effect of: diphenhydramine: MAOIs
Syringe compatibilities: Atropine, butorphanol, chlorpromazine, cimetidine, dimenhydrinate, droperidol, fentanyl, glycopyrrolate, hydromorphone, hydroxyzine, meperidine, metoclopromide, midazolam, morphine, nalbuphine, pentazocine, perphenazine, prochlorperazine, promazine, promethazine, ranitidine, scopolamine
Y-site compatibilities: Acyclovir, amsacrine, fluconazole, fludarabine, heparin, meperidine, ondansetron, sargramostim, idarubicin, melphalan, paclitaxel, vinorelbine
Additive compatibilities: Amikacin, aminophylline, bleomycin, cephaparin, erythromycin, methyldopate, nafcillin, netilmicin, methicillin, penicillin G potassium, polymyxin B, tetracycline, vitamin B with C
Lab test interferences:
False negative: Skin allergy tests

NURSING CONSIDERATIONS

Assess:
• I&O ratio; be alert for urinary retention, frequency, dysuria; drug should be discontinued
• CBC during long-term therapy; blood dyscrasias
• Respiratory status: rate, rhythm, increase in bronchial secretions, wheezing, chest tightness
Administer:
• With meals for GI symptoms; absorption may slightly decrease
• IV undiluted; give 25 mg/1 min
• Deep IM in large muscle; rotate site
• Hs only if using for sleep aid
Perform/provide:
• Hard candy, gum, frequent rinsing of mouth for dryness

• Storage in tight container at room temperature

Evaluate:

• Therapeutic response: absence of running or congested nose or rashes, improved sleep

Teach patient/family:

• All aspects of drug use; to notify prescriber of confusion, sedation, hypotension

• To avoid driving, other hazardous activity if drowsiness occurs

• That this drug may decrease anticoagulant (oral)

• To avoid concurrent use of alcohol, other CNS depressants

Treatment of overdose: Administer ipecac syrup or lavage, diazepam, vasopressors, barbiturates (short-acting)

diphenidol (℞)

(dye-fen'i-dole)

Vontrol

Func. class.: Antiemetic

Chem. class.: Trihexyphenidyl derivative

Action: May act as dopamine antagonist at chemoreceptor trigger zone to inhibit vomiting

Uses: Nausea, vomiting, peripheral dizziness

Dosage and routes:

• *Adult:* PO 25-50 mg q4h

• *Children >23 kg:* PO 25 mg q4h prn; do not exceed 5.5 mg/kg/ 24 hr

Available forms: Tabs 25 mg

Side effects/adverse reactions:

CNS: *Drowsiness,* fatigue, restlessness, tremor, headache, stimulation, dizziness, insomnia, twitching, disorientation, confusion, sleep disturbance, auditory, visual hallucination, depression

GI: Nausea, indigestion

CV: Hypotension

INTEG: Rash

EENT: Dry mouth, blurred vision

Contraindications: Hypersensitivity, psychosis, anuria

Precautions: Children, prostatic hypertrophy, glaucoma, pyloric and duodenal stenosis, elderly, pregnancy (C), lactation

Pharmacokinetics:

PO: Onset 30-45 min, duration 3-6 hr, metabolized by liver, excreted by kidneys

NURSING CONSIDERATIONS

Assess:

• VS, B/P; check patients with cardiac disease more often

• Observe for CNS adverse effects: confusion, hallucination

• Monitor I&O (90% excreted in urine)

• Signs of toxicity of other drugs or masking of symptoms of disease: brain tumor, intestinal obstruction

• Drowsiness, dizziness

Administer:

• Tabs may be swallowed whole, chewed, or allowed to dissolve

Evaluate:

• Therapeutic response: absence of nausea, vomiting

Teach patient/family:

• To avoid alcohol, other depressants

• That drug should be used only under close supervision

diphtheria and tetanus toxoids and pertussis vaccine (DPT) (℞)

Diphtheria and Tetanus Toxoids and Pertussis Vaccine, Tri-Immunol

Func. class.: Vaccine/toxoid

Action: Provide immunity to diphtheria, tetanus, pertussis by stimu-

* Available in Canada only

lating antibody/antitoxin production

Uses: Prevention of diphtheria, tetanus, pertussis

Dosage and routes:

• *Child >6 wk-6 yr:* IM 0.5 ml at 2, 4, 6 mos, 1½ yr; booster needed 0.5 ml at age 6

Available forms: Inj IM diphtheria 12.5 LfU, tetanus 5 LfU, pertussis 4 U/0.5 ml

Side effects/adverse reactions:

GI: Nausea, vomiting, anorexia

INTEG: Skin abscess, urticaria, itching, swelling, erythema, edema at site

CV: Tachycardia, hypotension

SYST: Lymphadenitis, ***anaphylaxis,*** fever, chills, malaise

CNS: Crying, fretfulness, fever, drowsiness, ***seizures***

MS: Osteomyelitis

Contraindications: Hypersensitivity, active infection, poliomyelitis outbreak, immunosuppression, febrile illness

Precautions: Pregnancy

Interactions:

• Decreased response to toxoid: immunosuppressive agents: antineoplastics, corticosteroids, radiation therapy; alkylating agents

NURSING CONSIDERATIONS

Assess:

• For skin reactions: swelling, rash, urticaria

• For anaphylaxis: inability to breathe, bronchospasm

Administer:

• At least 4 wk apart × 3 doses

• Only with epinephrine 1:1000 on unit to treat laryngospasm

• IM only; not to be given SC (vastus lateralis in infants)

Perform/provide:

• Storage in refrigerator, do not freeze

• Written record of immunization

Evaluate:

• For history of allergies, skin conditions (eczema, psoriasis, dermatitis), reactions to vaccinations

Teach patient/family:

• That doses are given at least 4 wk apart × 3 doses; booster needed at 10 yr intervals, diphtheria/tetanus

D

dipivefrin (℞)

(dye-pi've-frin)

dipivefrin, Propine

Func. class.: Adrenergic agonist

Chem. class.: Diesterified epinephrine

Action: Converted to epinephrine, which decreases aqueous production and increases outflow

Uses: Open-angle glaucoma

Dosage and routes:

• *Adult:* INSTILL 1 gtt q12h

Available forms: Sol 0.1%

Side effects/adverse reactions:

CV: Hypertension, tachycardia, dysrhythmias

EENT: Burning, stinging, mydriasis, photophobia

Contraindications: Hypersensitivity, narrow-angle glaucoma

Precautions: Pregnancy (B), lactation, children, aphakia

Pharmacokinetics:

Instill: Onset 30 min, peak 1 hr, duration 12 hr

NURSING CONSIDERATIONS

Perform/provide:

• Storage at room temperature

Evaluate:

• Therapeutic response: decrease in aqueous humor of eye

Teach patient/family:

• To report stinging, burning, itching, lacrimation, puffiness

• Method of instillation, including pressure on lacrimal sac for 1 min and not to touch dropper to eye

• Not to catch up missed doses

dipyridamole (℞)

(dye-peer-id'a-mole)

Apo-Dipyridamole*, dipyridamole, Persantine, Persantine IV

Func. class.: Coronary vasodilator, antiplatelet

Chem. class.: Nonnitrate

Action: Inhibits adenosine uptake, which produces coronary vasodilation; increases oxygen saturation in coronary tissues, coronary blood flow; acts on small resistance vessels with little effect on vascular resistance; may increase development of collateral circulation; decreases platelet aggregation by the inhibition of phosphodiesterase (an enzyme)

Uses: Prevention of transient ischemic attacks, inhibition of platelet adhesion to prevent myocardial reinfarction, thromboembolism, with warfarin in prosthetic heart valves, prevention of coronary bypass graft occlusion with aspirin; possibly effective for long-term therapy of chronic angina pectoris

Dosage and routes:

TIA

- *Adult:* PO 50 mg tid, 1 hr ac, not to exceed 400 mg qd

Inhibition of platelet adhesion

- *Adult:* PO 50-75 mg qid in combination with aspirin or warfarin; IV 570 μg/Kg

Available forms: Tabs 25, 50, 75 mg, IV 10 mg/2 ml

Side effects/adverse reactions:

CV: Postural hypotension

CNS: Headache, dizziness, weakness, fainting, syncope

GI: Nausea, vomiting, anorexia, diarrhea

INTEG: Rash, flushing

Contraindications: Hypersensitivity, hypotension

Precautions: Pregnancy (C), lactation

Pharmacokinetics:

PO: Peak 2-2½ hr, duration 6 hr; therapeutic response may take several months; metabolized in liver; excreted in bile; undergoes enterohepatic recirculation

Interactions:

- Incompatibility not known
- Additive antiplatelet effects: ASA, NSAID
- Increased bleeding: Coumadin

NURSING CONSIDERATIONS

Assess:

- B/P, pulse during treatment until stable; take B/P lying, standing; orthostatic hypotension is common
- Cardiac status: chest pain, what aggravates or ameliorates condition

Administer:

- IV after diluting each 5 mg/2 ml or more D_5W, 0.45% NaCl, or 0.9% NaCl to a total vol of 20-50 ml; give over 4 min; do not give undiluted
- On an empty stomach: 1 hr before meals or 2 hr after; give with 8 oz water for better absorption

Perform/provide:

- Storage at room temperature

Evaluate:

- Therapeutic response: decreased chest pain (angina), decreased platelet adhesion

Teach patient/family:

- That medication is not cure; may have to be taken continuously in evenly spaced doses only as directed
- That it is necessary to quit smoking to prevent excessive vasoconstriction
- To avoid hazardous activities until stabilized on medication; dizziness may occur
- To rise slowly from sitting or lying to prevent orthostatic hypotension
- Not to use alcohol or OTC medi-

* Available in Canada only

cations unless approved by prescriber

Treatment of overdose: Administer IV phenylephrine

disopyramide (℞)

(dye-soe-peer'a-mide)

disopyramide, Napamide, Norpace, Norpace CR, Rhythmodan

Func. class.: Antidysrhythmic (Class IA)

Chem. class.: Nonnitrate

Action: Prolongs duration of action potential and effective refractory period; reduces disparity in refractory between normal and infarcted myocardium; prevents increased myocardial excitability and conduction contractility

Uses: PVCs, ventricular tachycardia, supraventricular tachycardia, atrial flutter, fibrillation

Investigational uses: Supraventricular tachycardia (prevention, treatment)

Dosage and routes:

• *Adult:* PO 100-200 mg q6h, in renal dysfunction 100 mg q6h; SUS REL CAPS 200 mg q12h

• *Child 12-18 yr:* PO 6-15 mg/kg/day, in divided doses q6h

• *Child 4-12 yr:* PO 10-15 mg/kg/day in divided doses q6h

• *Child 1-4 yr:* PO 10-20 mg/kg/day in divided doses q6h

• *Child <1 yr:* PO 10-30 mg/kg/day, in divided doses q6h

Available forms: Caps 100, 150 mg (as phosphate); sus rel caps, 100, 150 mg

Side effects/adverse reactions:

GU: Retention, hesitancy, impotence, urinary frequency, urgency

CNS: Headache, dizziness, psychosis, fatigue, depression, paresthesias, anxiety, insomnia

GI: Dry mouth, constipation, nausea, anorexia, flatulence, diarrhea, vomiting

CV: Hypotension, bradycardia, angina, PVCs, tachycardia, increases QRS, QT segments, ***cardiac arrest,*** edema, weight gain, AV block, ***CHF,*** syncope, chest pain

META: Hypoglycemia

INTEG: Rash, pruritus, urticaria

MS: Weakness, pain in extremities

EENT: Blurred vision, dry nose, throat, eyes, narrow-angle glaucoma

HEMA: ***Thrombocytopenia, agranulocytosis,*** anemia (rare), decreased Hgb, Hct

Contraindications: Hypersensitivity, 2nd or 3rd degree block, cardiogenic shock, CHF (uncompensated), sick sinus syndrome, QT prolongation

Precautions: Pregnancy (C), lactation, diabetes mellitus, renal disease, children, hepatic disease, myasthenia gravis, narrow-angle glaucoma, cardiomyopathy, conduction abnormalities

Pharmacokinetics:

PO: Peak 30 min-3 hr, duration 6-12 hr; half-life 4-10 hr; metabolized in liver; excreted in feces, urine, breast milk; crosses placenta

Interactions:

• Increased effects of disopyramide: quinidine, procainamide, propranolol, lidocaine, atenolol, other antidysrhythmics

• Do not administer within 48 hr of verapamil

• Increased side effects of disopyramide: anticholinergics

• Decreased effects of disopyramide: phenytoin, rifampin

Lab test interferences:

Increase: Liver enzymes, lipids, BUN, creatinine

Decrease: Hgb/Hct, blood glucose

NURSING CONSIDERATIONS

Assess:

• Apical pulse for 1 min; if less than 60, check again in 1 hr; if still less than 60, notify prescriber
• ECG; check for increased QT, widening QRS; drug should be discontinued
• Blood level during treatment (therapeutic level 2-8 μg/ml); ANA titer
• Weight daily; a rapid weight gain should be reported
• For dehydration or hypovolemia, I&O ratio, electrolytes (Na, K, Cl)
• Liver, kidney function studies (AST [SGOT], ALT [SGPT], bilirubin, BUN, creatinine) during treatment
• Diabetics for signs of hypoglycemia
• B/P continuously for hypotension, hypertension
• Increase in QRS, QT; drug should be discontinued
• For rebound hypertension after 1-2 hr
• Constipation: increased bulk in diet, water, stool softeners, or laxatives needed
• Cardiac rate, respiration: rate, rhythm, character
• Urinary hesitancy, frequency or a change in I&O ratio; check for edema daily; check for toxicity

Administer:

• Do not crush or break sus rel cap; give 1 hr before or 2 hr after meals
• Sugar-free gum, frequent sips of water for dry mouth
• Reduced dosage slowly with ECG monitoring

Evaluate:

• Therapeutic response: decreased dysrhythmias

Teach patient/family:

• To take drug exactly as prescribed; if dose is missed take within 3-4 hr of next dose, do not double dose
• To avoid alcohol, or severe hypotension may occur; to avoid OTC drugs, or serious drug interactions may occur
• To make position change slowly during early therapy to prevent orthostatic hypotension
• To avoid hazardous activities if dizziness or blurred vision occurs
• Importance of complying with drug regimen; tell patient that this drug does not cure condition

Treatment of overdose: O_2, artificial ventilation, ECG, dopamine for circulatory depression, diazepam or thiopental for convulsions, gastric lavage

disulfiram (℞)

(dye-sul'fram)

Antabuse, disulfiram

Func. class.: Alcohol deterrent

Chem. class.: Aldehyde dehydrogenase inhibitor

Action: Blocks oxidation of alcohol at acetaldehyde stage; accumulation of acetaldehyde produces the disulfiram-alcohol reaction

Uses: Chronic alcoholism (as adjunct)

Dosage and routes:

• *Adult:* PO 250-500 mg qd × 1-2 wk, then 125-500 mg qd until fully socially recovered

Available forms: Tabs 250, 500 mg

Side effects/adverse reactions:

CNS: Headache, drowsiness, restlessness, dizziness, fatigue, tremors, psychosis, neuritis, sweating, ***convulsions, death,*** peripheral neuropathy

GI: Nausea, vomiting, anorexia, severe thirst, ***hepatotoxicity,*** metallic, garliclike aftertaste

INTEG: Rash, dermatitis, urticaria

Disulfiram reaction: Alcohol reaction: flushing, throbbing, head-

ache, respiratory difficulty, nausea, vomiting, sweating, thirst, chest pain, palpitations, dyspnea, hyperventilation, tachycardia, confusion, CV collapse, MI, CHF, convulsions, death
Contraindications: Hypersensitivity, alcohol intoxication, psychoses, CV disease, pregnancy (X), lactation
Precautions: Hypothyroidism, hepatic disease, diabetes mellitus, seizure disorders, nephritis, cerebral damage
Pharmacokinetics:
PO: Onset 12 hr; oxidized by liver; excreted unchanged in feces
Interactions:
• Increased effects of tricyclic antidepressants, diazepam, oral anticoagulants, paraldehyde, phenytoin, chlordiazepoxide, isoniazid, caffeine
• Disulfiram reaction: alcohol
• Psychosis: metronidazole
Lab test interferences:
Increase: Cholesterol
Decrease: ^{131}I uptake, PBI, VMA
NURSING CONSIDERATIONS
Assess:
• Liver function studies q2wk during therapy; AST (SGOT), ALT (SGPT)
• CBC, SMA q3-6 mo to detect any abnormality, including increased cholesterol q6mo
• Mental status: affect, mood, drug history, ability to follow treatment, abstain from alcohol
• For signs of hepatotoxicity: jaundice, dark urine, clay-colored stools, abdominal pain
Administer:
• Only with patient's knowledge; do not give to intoxicated person
• Once per day in the AM or hs if drowsiness occurs
• Only after patient has not been drinking for >12 hr
• Tabs may be crushed and mixed with liquid
Evaluate:
• Therapeutic response: prevention of alcohol intake
Teach patient/family:
• Effect of this drug if alcohol is taken; written consent for disulfiram therapy should be obtained
• That shaving lotions, creams, lotions, cough preparations, skin products must be checked for alcohol content; even in small amount, alcohol can produce a reaction
• That tolerance will not develop if treatment is prolonged
• That reaction may occur for 2 wk after last dose
• That tablets can be crushed, mixed with beverage
• To carry ID listing disulfiram therapy
• To avoid driving, hazardous tasks if drowsiness occurs
• That disulfiram reaction can be fatal; occurs 15 min after drinking and may last several hours
• Give written instructions and symptoms of alcohol—disulfiram reaction
Treatment of overdose: IV Vit C, ephedrine sulfate, antihistamines, O_2

DNase (recombinant human deoxyribonuclease I) (℞)

Pulmozyme

Func. class.: Cystic fibrosis agent (orphan drug)

Action: May break down molecules in large amounts of infected sputum; improves air flow, lessens chance of bacterial infection
Uses: Management of cystic fibrosis
Dosage and routes:
Child 5-20 yr: INH 2.5 mg qd

Available forms: Neb 2.5 mg
Side effects/adverse reactions:
RESP: Possibly laryngitis, hoarseness, hemoptysis, transient decrease in pulmonary function
Contraindications: Hypersensitivity
NURSING CONSIDERATIONS
Assess:
• Resp function: B/P, pulse, lung sounds
Administer:
• By nebulization only
Evaluate:
• Therapeutic response: decreased thick tenacious secretions, ease of respirations
Teach patient/family:
• To rinse mouth after use
• About all aspects of drug; avoid smoking, smoke-filled rooms, persons with respiratory infections

dobutamine (℞)

(doe-byoo'ta-meen)
Dobutrex
Func. class.: Adrenergic direct-acting β_1-agonist
Chem. class.: Catecholamine

Action: Causes increased contractility, increased coronary blood flow and heart rate by acting on β-1 receptors in heart
Uses: Cardiac surgery, refractory heart failure
Investigational uses: Cardiogenic shock in children
Dosage and routes:
• *Adult:* IV INF 2.5-10 μg/kg/min; may increase to 40 μg/kg/min if needed
Available forms: Inj 250 mg vial IV
Side effects/adverse reactions:
CNS: Anxiety, headache, dizziness
CV: Palpitations, tachycardia, hypertension, PVCs, angina
GI: Heartburn, nausea, vomiting
MS: Muscle cramps (leg)
Contraindications: Hypersensitivity, idiopathic hypertrophic subaortic stenosis
Precautions: Pregnancy (C), lactation, children, hypertension
Pharmacokinetics:
IV: Onset 1-5 min, peak 10 min, half-life 2 min; metabolized in liver (inactive metabolites); excreted in urine
Interactions:
• Dysrhythmias: general anesthetics
• Decreased action of dobutamine: other β-blockers
• Increased B/P: oxytocics
• Increased pressor effect and dysrhythmias: tricyclic antidepressant, MAOIs
Syringe compatibilities: Heparin, ranitidine
Y-site compatibilities: Amrinone, atracurium, bretylium, calcium chloride, calcium gluconate, diazepam, diltiazem, dopamine, enalaprilat, famotidine, haloperidol, insulin, lidocaine, magnesium sulfate, nitroglycerin, pancuronium, potassium chloride, ranitidine, sodium nitroprusside, streptokinase, tolazoline, vecuronium, verapamil, zidovudine
Additive compatibilities: Atropine, dopamine, epinephrine, hydralazine, indomethacin, isoproterenol, lidocaine, meperidine, metaraminol bitartrate, morphine, nitroglycerin, norepinephrine, phenotolamine, phenylephrine, procainamide, propranolol, ranitidine
NURSING CONSIDERATIONS
Assess:
• Hypovolemia; if present correct first
• Oxygenation/perfusion deficit (check B/P, chest pain, dizziness, loss of consciousness)
• Heart failure: S_3 gallop, dyspnea, neck vein distention, bibasilar crack-

les in patients with CHF, cardiomyopathy
- I&O ratio
- ECG during administration continuously; if B/P increases, drug is decreased CVP or PWP during infusion if possible
- B/P and pulse q5min after parenteral route

Administer:
- IV diluting each 250 mg/10 ml of sterile H_2O or D_5 for inj; may be further diluted to 50 ml or more given at prescribed rate; should be gradually increased to desired rate
- Plasma expanders for hypovolemia
- Parenteral (IV) dose slowly, after reconstituting, then diluting with at least 50 ml of D_5W, 0.9% NS, or Na lactate

Perform/provide:
- Storage of reconstituted solution if refrigerated for <24 hr

Evaluate:
- Therapeutic response: increased B/P with stabilization

Teach patient/family:
- Reason for drug administration

Treatment of overdose: Administer a β_1 adrenergic blocker

docusate calcium/docusate potassium/docusate sodium (℞)

(dok'yoo-sate)

DC Softgels, Docusate Calcium, Pro-Cal-Sof, Sulfalax Calcium, Surfak/Dialose, Diocto-K, Kasof/Colace, Correctol Extra Gentle, Diocto, Dioeze, Disonate, Docusate Sodium, DOK, DOS Softgel, Doxinate, D-S-S, Modane Soft, Regulex SS, Regutol,

Func. class.: Laxative, emollient

Chem. class.: Anionic surfactant

Combination products: Peri-Colace: docusate sodium 100 mg with cusanthranol 30 mg; Persistin: salsalate 487.5 mg with aspirin 162.5 mg

Action: Increases water, fat penetration in intestine; allows for easier passage of stool

Uses: To soften stools

Dosage and routes:
- *Adult:* PO 50-300 mg qd (sodium) or 240 mg (calcium or potassium) prn; ENEMA 5 ml (sodium)
- *Child >12 yr:* ENEMA 2 ml (sodium)
- *Child 6-12 yr:* PO 40-120 mg qd (sodium)
- *Child 3-6 yr:* PO 20-60 mg qd (sodium)
- *Child <3 yr:* PO 10-40 mg qd (sodium)

Available forms: *Calcium:* cap 50, 240 mg; *potassium:* cap 100, 240 mg; *sodium:* cap 50, 100, 240, 250 mg; tab 100 mg; syrup 50, 60 mg/15 ml; liquid 150 mg/15 ml; Sol 50 mg/ml; enema 283 mg/3.9 cap

Side effects/adverse reactions:
GI: Nausea, anorexia, cramps, diarrhea
INTEG: Rash
EENT: Bitter taste, throat irritation
Contraindications: Hypersensitivity, obstruction, fecal impaction, nausea/vomiting
Precautions: Pregnancy (C), lactation
Pharmacokinetics: Onset 24-72 hr

NURSING CONSIDERATIONS

Assess:
- Cause of constipation; identify whether fluids, bulk, or exercise are missing from lifestyle
- Cramping, rectal bleeding, nausea, vomiting; if these symptoms occur, drug should be discontinued

Administer:
- Alone with 8 oz H_2O only for better absorption; do not take within 1 hr of other drugs or within 1 hr of antacids, milk, or H_2 blockers
- In morning or evening (oral dose)

Perform/provide:
- Storage in cool environment; do not freeze

Evaluate:
- Therapeutic response: decrease in constipation

Teach patient/family:
- To swallow tabs whole; do not chew
- That normal bowel movements do not always occur daily
- Not to use in presence of abdominal pain, nausea, vomiting
- To notify prescriber if constipation unrelieved or if symptoms of electrolyte imbalance occur: muscle cramps, pain, weakness, dizziness, excessive thirst
- To keep out of children's reach

dopamine (℞)

(doe'pa-meen)
Dopastat, dopamine HCl, Intropin, Revimine*
Func. class.: Agonist
Chem. class.: Catecholamine

Action: Causes increased cardiac output; acts on α-receptors, causing vasoconstriction in blood vessels; low dose causes renal and mesenteric vasodilation
Uses: Shock; increased perfusion; hypotension
Dosage and routes:
- *Adult:* IV INF 2-5 μg/kg/min, not to exceed 50 μg/kg/min, titrate to patient's response

Available forms: Inj 0.8, 1.6, 40, 80, 160 mg/ml
Side effects/adverse reactions:
CNS: Headache
CV: Palpitations, tachycardia, hypertension, ectopic beats, angina, wide QRS complex, peripheral vasoconstriction
GI: Nausea, vomiting, diarrhea
INTEG: Necrosis, tissue sloughing with extravasation, ***gangrene***
RESP: Dyspnea
Contraindications: Hypersensitivity, ventricular fibrillation, tachydysrhythmias, pheochromocytoma
Precautions: Pregnancy (C), lactation, arterial embolism, peripheral vascular disease
Pharmacokinetics:
IV: Onset 5 min, duration <10 min; metabolized in liver; excreted in urine (metabolites)
Interactions:
- Do not use within 2 wk of MAOIs, phenytoin, barbiturates; or hypertensive crisis may result
- Dysrhythmias: general anesthetics

* Available in Canada only

• Decreased action of dopamine: other β-blockers
• Increased B/P: oxytocics
• Increased pressor effect: tricyclic antidepressant, MAOIs
• Additive effect: diuretics

Y-site compatibilities: Amrinone, atracurium, diltiazem, dobutamine, esmolol, famotidine, foscarnet, haloperidol, heparin, hydrocortisone sodium succinate, labetalol, lidocaine, meperidine, morphine, nitroglycerin, pancuronium, potassium chloride, ranitidine, sodium nitroprusside, streptokinase, tolazoline, vecuronium, verapamil, vitamin B with C, zidovudine

NURSING CONSIDERATIONS

Assess:

• Hypovolemia; if present, correct first
• Oxygenation/perfusion deficit (check B/P, chest pain, dizziness, loss of consciousness)
• Heart failure: S_3 gallop, dyspnea, neck vein distention, bibasilar crackles in patients with CHF, cardiomyopathy
• I&O ratio
• ECG during administration continuously; if B/P increases, drug is decreased
• B/P and pulse q5min after parenteral route
• CVP or PWP during infusion if possible
• Paresthesias and coldness of extremities; peripheral blood flow may decrease
• Injection site: tissue sloughing; if this occurs, administer phentolamine mixed with NS

Administer:

• Plasma expanders for hypovolemia
• IV after diluting 200 mg/250-500 ml of D_5W, D_5 0.45% NaCl, D_5 0.9% NaCl, D_5LR, LR
• Parenteral IV dose slowly; after reconstituting, use infusion pump; flush line before infusing; infuse as secondary IV line

Perform/provide:

• Storage of reconstituted sol if refrigerated no longer than 24 hr
• Do not use discolored sol

Evaluate:

• Therapeutic response: increased B/P with stabilization

Teach patient/family:

• Reason for drug administration

Treatment of overdose: Administer a β_1-adrenergic blocker

dorzolamide (℞)

(dor-zol'a-mide)
Truscopt
Func. class.: Carbonic anhydrase inhibitor

Action: The enzyme carbonic anhydrase is inhibited in the eye causing decreased aqueous humor secretion

Uses: Open-angle glaucoma, ocular hypertension

Dosage and routes:

• *Adult:* INSTILL 1 gtt tid in each eye

Available forms: Sol 2%

Side effects/adverse reactions:

CNS: Headache
CV: Hypertension, tachycardia, dysrhythmias
GI: Bitter taste
EENT: Burning, stinging

Contraindications: Hypersensitivity

Precautions: Pregnancy (C), lactation, child, aphakia, hypersensitivity to carbonic anhydrase inhibitors, sulfonamides, thiazide diuretics, ocular inhibitors, hepatic, renal insufficiency

Pharmacokinetics: Peak 2 hr, duration 8-12 hr

NURSING CONSIDERATIONS

Assess:

- Ophth exams, intraocular pressure
- Blood counts, liver, renal function tests, serum electrolytes (long-term treatment)

Perform/provide:

- Dark storage at room temp

Evaluate:

- Therapeutic response: Absence of increased intraocular pressure

Teach patient/family:

- How to instill drops
- Drug may cause burning, itching, blurring, dryness of eye area

doxacurium (℞)

(dox'a-cure-ee-um)

Nuromax

Func. class.: Neuromuscular blocker (nondepolarizing)

Action: Inhibits transmission of nerve impulses by binding with cholinergic receptor sites, antagonizing action of acetylcholine

Uses: Facilitation of endotracheal intubation, skeletal muscle relaxation during mechanical ventilation, surgery, or general anesthesia

Dosage and routes:

- *Adult:* IV 0.05 mg/kg; 0.08 mg/kg is used for prolonged neuromuscular blockade; maintenance 0.025 mg/kg
- *Child 2-12 yr:* IV 0.03-0.05 mg/kg; may increase for maintenance dose

Available forms: Inj 1 mg/ml

Side effects/adverse reactions:

CV: ***Decreased B/P, ventricular fibrillation, myocardial infarction, cardiovascular accident***

RESP: ***Prolonged apnea, bronchospasm, wheezing, respiratory depression***

EENT: Diplopia

MS: *Weakness,* prolonged skeletal muscle relaxation, ***paralysis***

INTEG: Rash, urticaria

Contraindications: Hypersensitivity

Precautions: Pregnancy (C), renal, hepatic disease, lactation, children <3 mo, fluid and electrolyte imbalances, neuromuscular disease, respiratory disease, obesity, elderly, severe burns

Pharmacokinetics: Not metabolized; excretion of unchanged drug in urine and bile

Interactions:

- Increased neuromuscular blockade: Aminoglycosides, quinidine, local anesthetics, polymyxin antibiotics, enflurane, isoflurane, tetracyclines, halothane, magnesium, colistin, procainamide, bacitracin, lincomycin, clindamycin, lithium
- Longer onset and shorter duration of doxacurium: phenytoin, carbamazepine

Solution compatibilities: LR, D_5/LR, D_5/0.9% NaCl

NURSING CONSIDERATIONS

Assess:

- For electrolyte imblances (K, Mg); may lead to increased action of this drug
- Vital signs (B/P, pulse, respirations, airway) until fully recovered; rate, depth, pattern of respirations, strength of hand grip
- I&O ratio; check for urinary retention, frequency, hesitancy
- Recovery: decreased paralysis of face, diaphragm, leg, arm, rest of body
- Allergic reactions: rash, fever, respiratory distress, pruritus; drug should be discontinued

Administer:

- Using nerve stimulator by anesthesiologist to determine neuromuscular blockade

* Available in Canada only

• After succinylcholine effects subside
• Anticholinesterase to reverse neuromuscular blockade
• By slow IV over 1-2 min (only by qualified persons, usually an anesthesiologist)
• Only fresh sol

Perform/provide:
• Storage at room temp; do not freeze
• Reassurance if communication is difficult during recovery from neuromuscular blockade
• Use reconstituted sol within 24 hr
• Frequent (q2h) instillation of artificial tears and covering eyes to prevent drying of cornea

Evaluate:
• Therapeutic response: paralysis of jaw, eyelid, head, neck, rest of body

Treatment of overdose: Neostigmine; monitor VS; may require mechanical ventilation

---

doxapram (℞)
(dox'a-pram)
Dopram
Func. class.: Analeptic

Action: Respiratory stimulation through activation of peripheral carotid chemoreceptor; with higher doses medullary respiratory centers are stimulated; general CNS stimulation

Uses: Chronic obstructive pulmonary disease (COPD), postanesthesia respiratory stimulation, prevention of acute hypercapnia, drug-induced CNS depression

Dosage and routes:

Postanesthesia
• *Adult:* IV inj 0.5-1 mg/kg, not to exceed 1.5 mg/kg total as a single injection; IV inf 250 mg in 250 ml sol, not to exceed 4 mg/kg; run at 1-3 mg/min

Drug-induced CNS depression
Adult: IV priming dose of 2 mg/kg, repeated in 5 min; repeat q1-2h till patient awakes; IV inf priming dose 2 mg/kg at 1-3 mg/min, not to exceed 3 g/d

COPD (Hypercapnia)
• *Adult:* IV inf 1-2 mg/min, not to exceed 3 mg/min for no longer than 2 hr

Available forms: Inj IV 20 mg/ml

Side effects/adverse reactions:
CNS: ***Convulsions,*** (clonus/generalized), *headache,* restlessness, dizziness, confusion, paresthesias, flushing, sweating, bilateral Babinski's sign, rigidity, depression
GI: Nausea, vomiting, diarrhea, hiccups
GU: Retention, incontinence
CV: Chest pain, hypertension, change in heart rate, lowered T waves, tachycardia, arrhythmias
INTEG: Pruritus, irritation at injection site
EENT: Pupil dilation, sneezing
RESP: ***Laryngospasm, bronchospasm,*** rebound hypoventilation, dyspnea, cough, tachypnea, hiccoughs

Contraindications: Hypersensitivity, seizure disorders, severe hyper tension, severe bronchial asthma, severe dyspnea, severe cardiac disorders, pneumothorax, pulmonary embolism, severe respiratory disease, newborns

Precautions: Bronchial asthma, pheochromocytoma, severe tachycardia, dysrhythmias, pregnancy (B), hypertension, lactation, children

Pharmacokinetics:
IV: Onset 20-40 sec, peak 1-2 min, duration 5-10 min; metabolized by liver; excreted by kidneys (metabolites); half-life 2.5-4 hr

Interactions:
• Synergistic pressor effect: MAOIs, sympathomimetics

• Cardiac dysrhythmias: halothane, cyclopropane, enflurane

Syringe compatibilities: Amikacin, bumetadine, chlorpromazine, cimetidine, cisplatin, cyclophosphamide, deslanoside, dopamine, doxycycline, epinephrine, hydroxyzine, imipramine, isoniazid, lincomycin, methotrexate, netilmicin, phytonadione, pyridoxine, terbutaline, thiamine, tobramycin, vincristine

NURSING CONSIDERATIONS

Assess:

• BP, heart rate, deep tendon reflexes, ABGs, LOC before administration, q30min

• PO_2, Pco_2, O_2 saturation during treatment

• Hypertension, dysrhythmias, tachycardia, dyspnea, skeletal muscle hyperactivity; may indicate overdosage; discontinue drug

• Respiratory stimulation: increased rate, abnormal rhythm

• Extravasation; change IV site q48h

Administer:

• IV undiluted or diluted with equal parts of sterile H_2O for inj; may be diluted 250 mg/250 ml of D_5W, $D_{10}W$ and run as infusion

• IV undiluted over 5 min; IV inf at 1-3 mg/min; adjust for desired respiratory response, using infusion pump IV; if an inf is used after initial dose, start at 1-3 mg/min depending on patient response; D/C after 2 hr; wait 1-2 hr and repeat

• Only after adequate airway is established

• After O_2, IV barbiturates, resuscitative equipment available

Perform/provide:

• Placing patient in Sims' position to prevent aspiration of vomitus

• Discontinue infusion if side effects occur; narrow margin of safety

Teach patient/family:

• Purpose of medication

Evaluate:

• Therapeutic response: increased breathing capacity

Treatment of overdose: Lavage, activated charcoal; monitor electrolytes, vital signs

doxazosin (℞)

dox-ay'zoe-sin)

Cardura

Func. class.: Peripheral α_1-adrenergic blocker

Chem. class.: Quinozoline

Action: Peripheral blood vessels are dilated, peripheral resistance lowered; reduction in blood pressure results from α_1-adrenergic receptors being blocked

Uses: Hypertension, urinary outflow obstruction, symptoms of benign prostatic hyperplasia

Investigational uses: CHF with digoxin and diuretics

Dosage and routes:

Adult: PO 1 mg qd, increasing up to 16 mg qd if required; usual range 4-16 mg/day

Available forms: Tabs 1, 2, 4, 8 mg

Side effects/adverse reactions:

CV: Palpitations, orthostatic hypotension, tachycardia, edema, dysrhythmias, chest pain

CNS: Dizziness, headache, drowsiness, anxiety, depression, vertigo, weakness, fatigue, asthenia

GI: Nausea, vomiting, diarrhea, constipation, abdominal pain

GU: Incontinence, polyuria

EENT: Epistaxis, tinnitus, dry mouth, red sclera, pharyngitis, rhinitis

Contraindications: Hypersensitivity to quinazolines

Precautions: Pregnancy (C), children, lactation, hepatic disease

Pharmacokinetics:

PO: Onset 2 hr, peak 2-6 hr, duration 6-12 hr; half-life 22 hr; metabolized in liver; excreted via bile/feces (<63%) and in urine (9%); extensively protein bound (98%)

Interaction:

- Increased hypotensive effects: β-blockers, verapamil
- Decreased hypotensive effects: indomethacin
- Decreased effects of clonidine

NURSING CONSIDERATIONS

Assess:

- B/P 2-6 hr after each dose and with each increase; postural effects may occur
- Pulse, jugular venous distention q4h
- BUN, uric acid if on long-term therapy
- I&O, weight daily
- Edema in feet, legs daily
- Skin turgor, dryness of mucous membranes for hydration status
- Rales, dyspnea, orthopnea q30min

Administer:

- Whole; do not chew or crush tablets; may be given with food

Perform/provide:

- Storage in tight container in cool environment

Evaluate:

- Therapeutic response: decreased B/P

Teach patient/family:

- That fainting occasionally occurs after 1st dose; do not drive or operate machinery for 4 hr after 1st dose or after dosage increase or take 1st dose hs

Treatment of overdose: Administer volume expanders or vasopressors; discontinue drug; place in supine position

doxepin (℞)

(dox'e-pin)

doxepin HCl, Sinequan, Sinequan Concentrate, Triadapin*

Func. class.: Antidepressant, tricyclic

Chem. class.: Dibenzoxepin, tertiary amine

Action: Blocks reuptake of norepinephrine, serotonin into nerve endings, increasing action of norepinephrine, serotonin in nerve cells

Uses: Major depression, anxiety

Investigational uses: Chronic pain management

Dosage and routes:

- *Adult:* PO 50-75 mg/day in divided doses; may increase to 300 mg/day or may give daily dose hs

Available forms: Caps 10, 25, 50, 75, 100, 150 mg; oral conc 10 mg/ml

Side effects/adverse reactions:

HEMA: ***Agranulocytosis, thrombocytopenia, eosinophilia, leukopenia***

CNS: Dizziness, drowsiness, confusion, headache, anxiety, tremors, stimulation, weakness, insomnia, nightmares, EPS (elderly), increased psychiatric symptoms, paresthesia

GI: Diarrhea, dry mouth, nausea, vomiting, ***paralytic ileus,*** increased appetite, cramps, epigastric distress, jaundice, ***hepatitis,*** stomatitis, constipation

GU: Retention, ***acute renal failure***

INTEG: Rash, urticaria, sweating, pruritus, photosensitivity

CV: Orthostatic hypotension, ECG changes, tachycardia, ***hypertension,*** palpitations

EENT: Blurred vision, tinnitus, mydriasis, ophthalmoplegia, glossitis

Contraindications: Hypersensitivity to tricyclic antidepressants, uri-

nary retention, narrow-angle glaucoma, prostatic hypertrophy
Precautions: Suicidal patients, elderly, pregnancy (C), lactation
Pharmacokinetics:
PO: Steady state 2-8 days; metabolized by liver; excreted by kidneys; crosses placenta; excreted in breast milk; half-life 8-24 hr
Interactions:
- Decreased effects of guanethidine, clonidine, indirect-acting sympathomimetics (ephedrine)
- Increased effects of direct-acting sympathomimetics (epinephrine), alcohol, barbiturates, benzodiazepines, CNS depressants
- Hyperpyretic crisis, convulsions, hypertensive episode: MAOI (pargyline [Eutonyl])

Lab test interferences:
Increase: Serum bilirubin, blood glucose, alk phosphatase
False increase: Urinary catecholamines
Decrease: VMA, 5-HIAA

NURSING CONSIDERATIONS

Assess:
- B/P (lying, standing), pulse q4h; if systolic B/P drops 20 mm Hg, hold drug, notify prescriber; take vital signs q4h in patients with cardiovascular disease
- Blood studies: CBC, leukocytes, differential, cardiac enzymes if patient is receiving long-term therapy
- Hepatic studies: AST (SGOT), ALT (SGPT), bilirubin
- Weight qwk; appetite may increase with drug
- ECG for flattening of T wave, bundle branch block, AV block, dysrhythmias in cardiac patients
- EPS primarily in elderly: rigidity, dystonia, akathisia
- Mental status: mood, sensorium, affect, suicidal tendencies, an increase in psychiatric symptoms: depression, panic
- Urinary retention, constipation; constipation most likely in children
- Withdrawal symptoms: headache, nausea, vomiting, muscle pain, weakness; not usual unless drug is discontinued abruptly
- Alcohol consumption; if alcohol is consumed, hold dose until morning

Administer:
- Increased fluids, bulk in diet for constipation, urinary retention
- With food, milk for GI symptoms
- Dosage hs for oversedation during day; may take entire dose hs; elderly may not tolerate qd dosing
- Gum, hard candy, or frequent sips of water for dry mouth
- Concentrate with fruit juice, water, or milk to disguise taste

Perform/provide:
- Storage in tight container protected from direct sunlight
- Assistance with ambulation during beginning therapy, since drowsiness/dizziness occurs
- Safety measures, including side rails, primarily for elderly
- Checking to see PO medication swallowed

Evaluate:
- Therapeutic response: decreased anxiety, depression

Teach patient/family:
- That therapeutic effects may take 2-3 wk
- To use caution in driving, other activities requiring alertness, because of drowsiness, dizziness, blurred vision
- To avoid alcohol ingestion, other CNS depressants
- Not to discontinue medication quickly after long-term use; may cause nausea, headache, malaise
- To wear sunscreen or large hat, since photosensitivity occurs

Treatment of overdose: ECG monitoring; induce emesis; lavage, acti-

* Available in Canada only

vated charcoal; administer anticonvulsant

doxorubicin (℞)

(dox-oh-roo'bi-sin)

Adriamycin, Adriamycin PFS, Adriamycin RDF, Doxorubicin HCl, Rubex

Func. class.: Antineoplastic, antibiotic

Chem. class.: Anthracycline glycoside

Action: Inhibits DNA synthesis primarily; derived from *Streptomyces peucetius;* replication is decreased by binding to DNA, which causes strand splitting; active throughout entire cell cycle; a vesicant

Uses: Wilms' tumor; bladder, breast, cervical, head, neck, liver, lung, ovarian, prostatic, stomach, testicular, thyroid cancer; Hodgkin's disease; acute lymphoblastic leukemia; myeloblastic leukemia; neuroblastomas; lymphomas; sarcomas

Dosage and routes:

• *Adult:* 60-75 mg/m^2 q3wk, or 30 mg/m^2 on days 1-3 of 4-wk cycle, not to exceed 550 mg/m^2 cumulative dose

Available forms: Inj IV 10, 20, 50 mg

Side effects/adverse reactions:

HEMA: ***Thrombocytopenia, leukopenia, anemia***

GI: Nausea, vomiting, anorexia, mucositis, ***hepatotoxicity***

GU: Impotence, sterility, amenorrhea, gynecomastia, hyperuricemia

INTEG: Rash, necrosis at injection site, dermatitis, reversible alopecia, cellulitis, thrombophlebitis at injection site

CV: Increased B/P, ***sinus tachycardia, PVCs,*** chest pain, ***bradycardia, extra systoles***

Contraindications: Hypersensitivity, pregnancy (1st trimester) (D), lactation, systemic infections

Precautions: Renal, hepatic, cardiac disease, gout, bone marrow depression (severe)

Pharmacokinetics: Triphasic pattern of elimination; half-life 12 min, 3⅓ hr, 29⅔ hr; metabolized by liver; crosses placenta; excreted in urine, bile, breast milk

Interactions:

• Increased toxicity: other antineoplastics or radiation

• Decreased serum digoxin levels: digoxin

• Decreased antibody response: live virus vaccine

Syringe compatibilities: Bleomycin, cisplatin, cyclophosphamide, droperidol, fluorouracil, leucovorin calcium, methotrexate, metoclopramide, mitomycin, vincristine

Y-site compatibilities: Bleomycin, cisplatin, cyclophosphamide, droperidol, fluorouracil, leucovorin calcium, methotrexate, metoclopramide, mitomycin, vinblastine, vincristine

Lab test interferences:

Increase: Uric acid

NURSING CONSIDERATIONS

Assess:

• CBC, differential, platelet count weekly; withhold drug if WBC is <4000/mm^3 or platelet count is <75,000/mm^3; notify prescriber of these results

• Blood, urine uric acid levels

• Renal function studies: BUN, serum uric acid, urine CrCl, electrolytes before, during therapy

• I&O ratio; report fall in urine output to <30 ml/hr

• Monitor temperature q4h; fever may indicate beginning infection

• Liver function tests before, during therapy: bilirubin, AST, ALT, alk phosphatase as needed or monthly

• ECG; watch for ST-T wave changes, low QRS and T, possible dysrhythmias (sinus tachycardia, heart block, PVCs)
• Bleeding: hematuria, guaiac, bruising or petechiae, mucosa or orifices q8h
• Food preferences; list likes, dislikes
• Effects of alopecia on body image; discuss feelings about body changes
• Inflammation of mucosa, breaks in skin
• Yellowing of skin and sclera, dark urine, clay-colored stools, itchy skin, abdominal pain, fever, diarrhea
• Buccal cavity q8h for dryness, sores, ulceration, white patches, oral pain, bleeding, dysphagia
• Alkalosis if severe vomiting is present
• Local irritation, pain, burning at injection site
• GI symptoms: frequency of stools, cramping
• Acidosis, signs of dehydration: rapid respirations, poor skin turgor, decreased urine output, dry skin, restlessness, weakness
• Cardiac status: B/P, pulse, character, rhythm, rate, ABGs, ECG

Administer:
• Hydrocortisone, dexamethasone or sodium bicarbonate (1 mEq/1 ml) for extravasation; apply ice compresses
• Antiemetic 30-60 min before giving drug to prevent vomiting
• Allopurinol or sodium bicarbonate to maintain uric acid levels, alkalinization of urine
• IV after diluting 10 mg/5 ml of NaCl for inj; another 5 ml of diluent/10 mg is recommended; shake; give over 3-5 min; give through Y-tube or 3-way stopcock through free-flowing 5% dextrose inf or NS
• Topical or systemic analgesics for pain
• Transfusion for anemia
• Antispasmodic for GI symptoms

Perform/provide:
• Strict hand-washing technique, gloves, protective clothing
• Liquid diet: carbonated beverages, Jell-O may be added if patient is not nauseated or vomiting
• Increased fluid intake to 2-3 L/day to prevent urate, calculi formation
• Diet low in purines: absence of organ meats (kidney, liver), dried beans, peas to maintain alkaline urine
• Rinsing of mouth tid-qid with water, club soda; brushing of teeth bid-tid with soft brush or cotton-tipped applicators for stomatitis; use unwaxed dental floss
• Storage at room temperature for 24 hr after reconstituting or 48 hr refrigerated

Evaluate:
• Therapeutic response: decreased tumor size, spread of malignancy

Teach patient/family:
• To report any complaints, side effects to nurse or prescriber
• That hair may be lost during treatment and wig or hairpiece may make the patient feel better; tell patient that new hair may be different in color, texture
• To avoid foods with citric acid, hot or rough texture
• To report any bleeding, white spots, ulcerations in mouth to prescriber; tell patient to examine mouth qd
• That urine and other body fluids may be red-orange for 48 hr
• To avoid crowds and persons with infections when granulocyte count is low
• That contraceptive measures are recommended during therapy

• To avoid vaccinations; reactions may occur

doxycycline (℞)

(dox-i-sye'kleen)

Apo-Doxy*, Doryx, Doxy 100, Doxy 200, Doxy-Caps, Doxychel Hyclate, Doxycin*, Doxycycline, Monodox, Novodoxyclin*, Vibramycin, Vibramycin IV, Vibra-Tabs, Vovox

Func. class.: Broad-spectrum antibiotic/antiinfective

Chem. class.: Tetracycline

Action: Inhibits protein synthesis, prosphorylation in microorganisms by binding to 30S ribosomal subunits, reversibly binding to 50S ribosomal subunits; bacteriostatic

Uses: Syphilis, *C. trachomatis,* gonorrhea, lymphogranuloma venereum, uncommon gram-negative/positive organisms, malaria prophylaxis

Investigational uses: Traveler's diarrhea, Lyme disease, prevention of chronic bronchitis

Dosage and routes:

• *Adult:* PO 100 mg q12h on day 1, then 100 mg/d; IV 200 mg in 1-2 inf on day 1, then 100-200 mg/d

• *Child >8 yr:* PO/IV 4.4 mg/kg/d in divided doses q12h on day 1, then 2.2-4.4 mg/kg/d

Gonorrhea (uncomplicated)

• *Adult:* PO 200 mg, then 100 mg hs and 100 mg bid × 3d or 300 mg, then 300 mg in 1 hr; disseminated; 100 mg PO bid × at least 7d

Malaria prophylaxis

• *Adult:* 100 mg qd 1-2 days prior to travel and daily during travel

C. trachomatis

• *Adult:* PO 100 mg bid × 7d

Syphilis

• *Adult:* PO 300 mg/day in divided doses × 10d

Available forms: Tabs 50, 100 mg; caps 50, 100 mg; syr 50 mg/ml; powder for inj IV 100, 200 mg; powder for oral susp 25 mg/5 ml

Side effects/adverse reactions:

CNS: Fever

HEMA: ***Eosinophilia, neutropenia, thrombocytopenia, hemolytic anemia***

EENT: Dysphagia, glossitis, decreased calcification of deciduous teeth, oral candidiasis

GI: Nausea, abdominal pain, vomiting, diarrhea, anorexia, enterocolitis, ***hepatotoxicity,*** flatulence, abdominal cramps, gastric burning, stomatitis

CV: Pericarditis

GU: Increased BUN

INTEG: Rash, urticaria, photosensitivity, increased pigmentation, ***exfoliative dermatitis,*** pruritus, ***angioedema***

Contraindications: Hypersensitivity to tetracyclines, children <8 yr, pregnancy (D)

Precautions: Hepatic disease, lactation

Pharmacokinetics:

PO: Peak 1½-4 hr, half-life 15-22 hr; excreted in bile, 25%-93% protein bound

Interactions:

• Decreased effects of doxycycline: antacids, $NaHCO_3$, dairy products, alkali products, iron, kaolin/pectin, barbiturates, carbemazine, phenytoin, cimetidine

• Increased effect: anticoagulants

• Decreased effects: penicillins, oral contraceptives

Y-site compatibilities: Acyclovir, amiodarone, cyclophosphamide, hydromorphone, magnesium sulfate, melphalan, meperidine, morphine, ondansetron, perphenazine, sargramostim, vinorelbine

Additive compatibility: Ranitidine
Syringe compatibility: Doxapram
Lab test interferences:
False negative: Urine glucose with Clinistix or Tes-Tape
False increase: Urinary catecholamines; ALT, AST

NURSING CONSIDERATIONS
Assess:
- I&O ratio
- Blood studies: PT, CBC, AST, ALT, BUN, creatinine
- Signs of infection
- Allergic reactions: rash, itching, pruritus, angioedema
- Nausea, vomiting, diarrhea; administer antiemetic, antacids as ordered
- Overgrowth of infection: fever, malaise, redness, pain, swelling, drainage, perineal itching, diarrhea, changes in cough or sputum
- IV site for phlebitis/thrombosis; drug is highly irritating

Administer:
- IV after diluting 100 mg or less/10 ml of sterile H_2O or NS for inj; further dilute with 100-1000 ml of NaCl, D_5, Ringer's 10% invert sugar in water, LR D_5LR, Normosol-M, Normosol-R in D_5W; run 100 mg or less over 1-4 hr; do not give IM/SC; inf must be completed in 6 hr, when diluted in LR sol, or 12 hr in other sol
- After C&S
- 2 hr before or after laxative or ferrous products; 3 hr after antacid or kaolin-pectin products

Perform/provide:
- Storage in tight, light-resistant container at room temp

Evaluate:
- Therapeutic response: decreased temperature, absence of lesions, negative C&S

Teach patient/family:
- To avoid sun, since burns may occur; sunscreen does not seem to decrease photosensitivity
- That all prescribed medication must be taken to prevent superinfection
- To take with a full glass of water; may take with food or milk

---

D-penicillamine (℞)

(pen-i-sill'a-meen)
Cuprimine, Depen
Func. class.: Heavy metal antagonist
Chem. class.: Chelating agent (thiol compound)

Action: Binds with ions of lead, mercury, copper, iron, zinc to form a water-soluble complex excreted by kidneys
Uses: Wilson's disease, rheumatoid arthritis, cystinuria, lead poisoning
Dosage and routes:
Cystinuria
- *Adult:* PO 250 mg qid ac, not to exceed 5 g/day
- *Child:* PO 30 mg/kg/day in divided doses qid ac

Wilson's disease
- *Adult:* PO 250 mg qid ac
- *Child:* PO 20 mg/kg/day in divided doses ac

Rheumatoid arthritis
- *Adult:* PO 125-250 mg/day, then increased 250 mg q2-3mo if needed, not to exceed 1 g/day

Available forms: Caps 125, 250 mg; tabs 250 mg
Side effects/adverse reactions:
HEMA: ***Thrombocytopenia, granulocytopenia, leukopenia, hemolytic anemia, aplastic anemia, eosinophilia,*** lupus syndrome, increased sedimentation rate
INTEG: Urticaria, erythema, pruritus, fever, ecchymosis, alopecia

CV: Hypotension, tachycardia
GI: Diarrhea, abdominal cramping, nausea, vomiting, ***hepatotoxicity***, anorexia, pain, peptic ulcer
EENT: Tinnitus, optic neuritis
MS: Arthralgia
GU: ***Proteinuria, nephrotic syndrome, glomerulonephritis***
SYST: ***Anaphylaxis***
RESP: Pneumonitis, ***asthma, pulmonary fibrosis***

Contraindications: Hypersensitivity to penicillins, anuria, agranulocytosis, severe renal disease, pregnancy (D), lactation

Pharmacokinetics:
PO: Peak 1 hr, metabolized in liver, excreted in urine

Interactions:
- Increased side effects: oxyphenbutazone, phenylbutazone, gold salts, antimalarials, cytotoxics
- Decreased absorption of D-penicillamine: oral iron, antacids, food

NURSING CONSIDERATIONS

Assess:
- Monitor hepatic, renal studies: AST/ALT, alk phosphatase, BUN, creatinine
- Monitor I&O, temperature
- Monitor platelet, neutropenia, WBC, H&H; if WBC <3500/mm^3 or if platelets <100,000/mm^3, drug should be discontinued
- Allergic reactions (rash, urticaria); if these occur, drug should be discontinued

Administer:
- On an empty stomach, ½-1 hr before meals; at least 2 hr after meals
- Vit B_6 daily, depleted when this drug is used
- Only when epinephrine 1:1000 is on unit for anaphylaxis
- Fluids to 3 L/day to prevent renal failure

Evaluate:
- Therapeutic response: absence of pain, rigidity in joints (rheumatoid arthritis)

Teach patient/family:
- That urine may be red
- That therapeutic effect may take 1-3 mo
- To report sore throat, easy bruising, bleeding from mucous membranes; may indicate bone marrow depression

D

droperidol (℞)

(droe-per'i-dole)
Droperidol, Inapsine
Func. class.: Neuroleptic
Chem. class.: Butyrophenone derivative

Action: Acts on CNS at subcortical levels, produces tranquilization, sleep; antiemetic

Uses: Premedication for surgery; induction, maintenance in general anesthesia; postoperatively for nausea, vomiting

Dosage and routes:

Induction
- *Adult:* IV/IM 0.22-0.275 mg/kg given with analgesic or general anesthetic; may give 1.25-2.5 mg additionally
- *Child 2-12 yr:* IV 88-165 μg/kg, titrated to response needed

Premedication
- *Adult:* IM 2.5-10 mg ½-1 hr before surgery
- *Child 2-12 yr:* IM 1-1.5 mg/20-25 lb

Maintaining general anesthesia
- *Adult:* IV 1.25-2.5 mg

Regional anesthesia adjunct
- *Adult:* IV/IM 2.5-5 mg

Diagnostic procedures without general anesthesia
- *Adult:* IM 2.5-10 mg ½-1 hr prior to procedure; 1.25-2.5 mg may be needed

Available forms: Inj IM, IV 2.5 mg/ml

Side effects/adverse reactions:

RESP: ***Laryngospasm, bronchospasm***

CNS: Dystonia, akathisia, flexion of arms, fine tremors, dizziness, anxiety, drowsiness, restlessness, hallucination, depression

CV: Tachycardia, hypotension

EENT: Upward rotation of eyes, oculogyric crisis

INTEG: Chills, facial sweating, shivering

Contraindications: Hypersensitivity, child <2 yr, pregnancy (C), lactation

Precautions: Elderly, cardiovascular disease (hypotension, bradydysrhythmias), renal disease, liver disease, Parkinson's disease

Pharmacokinetics:

IM/IV: Onset 3-10 min, peak ½ hr, duration 3-6 hr; metabolized in liver; excreted in urine as metabolites; crosses placenta

Interactions:

- Increased CNS depression: alcohol, narcotics, barbiturates, antipsychotics or other CNS depressants
- Decreased effects of amphetamines, anticonvulsants, anticoagulants, when given with this drug
- Increased intraocular pressure: anticholinergics, antiparkinson drugs
- Increased side effects of lithium

Syringe compatibilities: Atropine, bleomycin, butorphanol, chlorpromazine, cimetidine, cisplatin, cyclophosphamide, dimenhydrinate, diphenhydramine, doxorubicin, fentanyl, glycopyrrolate, hydroxyzine, meperidine, metoclopramide, midazolam, mitomycin, morphine, nalbuphine, pentazocine, perphenazine, prochlorperazine, promazine, promethazine, scopolamine, vinblastine, vincristine

Y-site compatibilities: Bleomycin, buprenorphine, cisplatin, cyclophosphamide, doxorubicin, hydrocortisone sodium succinate, metoclopramide, mitomycin, ondansetron, potassium chloride, vinblastine, vincristine, vitamin B with C

NURSING CONSIDERATIONS

Assess:

- VS q10m during IV administration, q30m after IM dose
- EPS: dystonia, akathisia
- For increasing heart rate or decreasing B/P, notify prescriber at once; do not place patient in Trendelenburg position, or sympathetic blockade may occur, causing respiratory arrest

Administer:

- IV undiluted; give through Y-tube or 3-way stopcock at 10 mg or less/min; titrate to patient response; may be given as an infusion by adding dose to 250 ml LR, D_5W, 0.9% NaCl
- Anticholinergics (benztropine, diphenhydramine) for EPS
- Only with crash cart, resuscitative equipment nearby
- IM deep in large muscle mass

Perform/provide:

- Slow movement of patient to avoid orthostatic hypotension

Evaluate:

- Therapeutic response: decreased anxiety, absence of vomiting during and after surgery
- To rise slowly from sitting or standing to minimize orthostatic hypotension

dyphylline (℞)

(dye'fi-lin)

Dilor, Dyflex-200, Dyflex-400, Dylline, Dyphylline, Lufyllin, Lufyllin-400, Neothylline, Protophylline*

Func. class.: Bronchodilator

Chem. class.: Xanthine, ethylenediamide

Combination products: Lufyllin-EPG Tablets: dyphylline 100 mg, ephedrine 16 mg, guaifenesin 200 mg, phenobarbital 16 mg; Lufyllin-EPG Elixir: dyphylline 150 mg, ephedrine 24 mg, guaifenesin 300 mg, phenobarbital 24 mg, alcohol

Action: Relaxes smooth muscle of respiratory system by blocking phosphodiesterase, which increases cyclic AMP; cyclic AMP results in positive inotropic, chronotropic effects, bronchodilation, stimulation of CNS

Uses: Bronchial asthma, bronchospasm in chronic bronchitis, COPD

Dosage and routes:

- *Adult:* PO 200-800 mg q6h; IM 250-500 mg q6h injected slowly
- *Child >6 yr:* PO 4-7 mg/kg/day in 4 divided doses

Available forms: Tabs 200, 400 mg; elix 100, 160 mg/15 ml; inj IM 250 mg/ml

Side effects/adverse reactions:

CNS: Anxiety, restlessness, insomnia, dizziness, ***convulsions,*** headache, light-headedness, muscle twitching

CV: Palpitations, sinus tachycardia, hypotension, flushing, dysrhythmias

GI: Nausea, vomiting, anorexia, dyspepsia, epigastric pain

INTEG: Flushing, urticaria

RESP: Tachypnea

OTHER: Fever, dehydration, ***albuminuria,*** hyperglycemia

Contraindications: Hypersensitivity to xanthines, tachydysrhythmias

Precautions: Elderly, CHF, cor pulmonale, hepatic disease, active peptic ulcer disease, diabetes mellitus, hyperthyroidism, hypertension, children, renal disease, pregnancy (C), lactation, glaucoma

Pharmacokinetics: Peak 1 hr, half-life 2 hr, excreted in urine unchanged

Interactions:

- Do not mix in syringe with other drugs
- Increased action of dyphylline: cimetidine, propranolol, erythromycin, troleandomycin
- May increase effects of anticoagulants
- Cardiotoxicity: β-blockers
- Increased metabolism: barbiturates, phenytoin
- Decreased elimination of dyphylline: uricosurics

NURSING CONSIDERATIONS

Assess:

- Dyphylline blood levels; toxicity may occur with small increase above 20 μg/ml
- Monitor I&O; diuresis occurs; dehydration may result in elderly or children
- Whether theophylline was given recently
- Auscultate lung fields bilaterally; notify prescriber of abnormalities
- Allergic reactions: rash, urticaria; drug should be discontinued

Administer:

- PO after meals to decrease GI symptoms; absorption may be affected
- Avoid IM injection; pain occurs

Perform/provide

- Storage protected from light, at room temperature

Evaluate:

- Therapeutic response: decreased dyspnea, respiratory rate, rhythm

Teach patient/family

- To check OTC medications, current prescription medications for ephedrine; will increase stimulation; not to drink alcohol or caffeine
- To avoid hazardous activities; dizziness, drowsiness, blurred vision may occur
- For GI upset, to take drug with 8 oz water; avoid taking with food, since absorption may be decreased

echothiophate (℞)

(ek-oh-thye′oh-fate)

Ecostigmine Iodide, Phospholine Iodide

Func. class.: Miotic

Chem. class.: Cholinesterase inhibitor, irreversible

Action: Prevents breakdown of neurotransmitter acetylcholine, which then accumulates, causing enhancement, prolongation of its physiologic effects

Uses: Glaucoma (open-angle), accommodative esotropia, treatment of obstructed aqueous outflow; extremely effective in control of chronic wide-angle glaucoma, aphakic glaucoma, congenital glaucoma

Dosage and routes:

- *Adult and child:* INSTILL 1 gtt of 0.03%, or 0.125% sol qd in conjunctival sac, not to exceed 1 gtt bid

Available forms: Powder for reconstitution, 1.5 mg (0.03%), 3 mg (0.06%), 6.25 mg (0.125%), 12.5 mg (0.25%) with 5 ml diluent

Side effects/adverse reactions:

GU: Frequency

CV: Hypotension, bradycardia, ***cardiac arrest***

INTEG: Sweating, pallor, cyanosis

RESP: ***Bronchospasm***

GI: Nausea, vomiting, abdominal cramps, diarrhea

EENT: Blurred vision, stinging, burning, lacrimation, lid muscle twitching; conjunctival, ciliary redness; brow ache; headache; induced myopia; iris cysts; hyperemia; hyphema

Contraindications: Hypersensitivity, ureitis

Precautions: Asthma, bradycardia, parkinsonism, peptic ulcer, pregnancy (C)

Interactions:

- Decreased effect of echothiophate: pilocarpine
- Increased effect of both drugs: ambenonium, edrophonium, neostigmine, physostigmine, pyridostigmine
- Increased effects of general anesthetics

NURSING CONSIDERATIONS

Assess:

- Specific condition being treated
- History (e.g., asthma, cardiac disease), possible sensitivity, contraindications, drug interactions

Administer:

- After checking vial for concentration
- Immediately after reconstituting; discard unused portion
- After reconstituting powder with diluent provided

Evaluate:

- Therapeutic response: decreased aqueous humor in eye

Teach patient/family:

- Why patient is receiving medication; patient, family should have a clear regimen as well as name of medication
- To report change in vision, blurring or loss of sight, trouble breathing, sweating, flushing
- Method of instillation, including pressure on lacrimal sac for 1 min, not to touch dropper to eye
- That long-term therapy may be required

- That blurred vision will decrease with repeated use of drug
- That patient may experience stinging, dull ache or tearing, which should subside in a few minutes; if it persists, contact prescriber
- That patient may experience decreased visual ability at night; instruct not to drive
- To use drops at night to eliminate hazardous transient blurring

econazole (℞)

(e-kone′a-zole)

Spectazole

Func. class.: Local antiinfective

Chem. class.: Imidazole derivative, antifungal

Action: Interferes with fungal cell membrane, which increases permeability, leaking of cell nutrients

Uses: Tinea pedis, tinea cruris, tinea corporis, tinea versicolor, cutaneous candidiasis

Dosage and routes:

- *Adult and child:* TOP apply to affected area bid-qid depending on condition

Available forms: Cream 1%

Side effects/adverse reactions:

INTEG: Rash, urticaria, stinging, burning, pruritus

Contraindications: Hypersensitivity

Precautions: Pregnancy (C), lactation

NURSING CONSIDERATIONS

Assess:

- Allergic reaction: burning, stinging, swelling, redness

Administer:

- After cleansing with soap, water before each application, dry well
- Enough medication to cover lesions completely
- For 2 wk in tinea cruris, tinea corporis, *Candida* infections; 1 mo tinea pedis

Perform/provide:

- Storage at room temp in dry place

Evaluate:

- Therapeutic response: decrease in size, number of lesions

Teach patient/family:

- To use asepsis (hand washing) before, after each application
- To apply with glove to prevent further infection
- To avoid use of OTC creams, ointments, lotions unless directed by prescriber
- Not to cover with occlusive dressing
- To continue even though condition improves
- To notify prescriber if condition worsens

edetate calcium disodium (℞)

(ed′e-tate)

calcium disodium versenate, calcium EDTA, edathamil calcium disodium, sodium calcium edetate

Func. class.: Heavy metal antagonist (antidote)

Chem. class.: Chelating agent

Action: Binds ions of lead to form a water-soluble complex that is removed by kidneys

Uses: Lead poisoning, acute lead encephalopathy

Dosage and routes:

Acute lead encephalopathy

- *Adult and child:* 1.5 g/m^2/day × 3-5 days, with dimercaprol, may be given again after 4 days off drug

Lead poisoning

- *Adult:* IV 1 g/250-500 ml D_5W or 0.9% NaCl over 1-2 hr or q12h ×

3-5 days; may repeat after 2 days; not to exceed 50 mg/kg/day; may be given as CONT INF over 8-24 hr

- *Adult:* IM 35 mg/kg bid
- *Child:* IM 35 mg/kg/day in divided doses q8-12h, not to exceed 50 mg/kg/day; may give for 3-5 days, off 4 days before next course

Available forms: Inj 200 mg/ml

Side effects/adverse reactions:

CNS: Headache, paresthesia, numbness

INTEG: Urticaria, erythema, pruritus, pain at injection site, fever, cheilosis

CV: Hypotension, dysrhythmias, thrombophlebitis

GI: Vomiting, *diarrhea, abdominal cramps, anorexia,* cheilosis, histamine-like reaction with GI distress

EENT: Nasal congestion, sneezing

MS: Leg cramps, myalgia, arthralgia, weakness

GU: ***Hematuria, renal tubular necrosis, proteinuria***

Contraindications: Hypersensitivity, anuria, poisoning of other metals, severe renal disease, child <3 yr

Precautions: Hypertension, pregnancy (C), lactation, gout, active TB

Pharmacokinetics:

Not metabolized; excreted in urine; half-life 20-60 min (IV), 90 min (IM)

Interactions:

Increased toxicity: cardiac glycosides, glucocorticoids

Additive compatibility: Netilmicin

Lab test interferences:

Decrease: Cholesterol/triglycerides, K, blood glucose

NURSING CONSIDERATIONS

Assess:

- VS, B/P, pulse, respirations, weigh daily
- Monitor I&O, kidney function studies: BUN, creatinine, CrCl; watch for decreasing urine output
- Neuro status: watch for paresthesias, beginning convulsions
- Urine: pH, albumin, casts, blood, coproporphyrins, calcium
- For febrile reactions that may occur 4-8 hr following drug therapy
- Cardiac abnormalities: dysrhythmias, hypotension, tachycardia
- Allergic reactions (rash, urticaria); drug should be discontinued

Administer:

- EDTA, BAL separately
- IV 5 ml EDTA/250-500 ml of D_5W, 0.9% NaCl give over 1 hr in less severe lead toxicity; over 2 hr in severe lead toxicity also may be given over 8-24 hr, IM is preferred route
- IM in large muscle mass; rotate injection sites; procaine HCl should be added to IM injection (1 ml procaine 1% to each ml concentrated drug) to minimize pain at injection site
- Only when epinephrine 1:1000 is on unit for anaphylaxis
- IV fluids to ensure adequate hydration before administration

Evaluate:

- Therapeutic response: decreased symptoms of lead poisoning

edetate disodium (℞)

(ed'e-tate)

Chealamide, Disodium EDTA, Disotate, Endrate

Func. class.: Metal antagonist

Chem. class.: Chelating agent

Action: Binds with ions of calcium, zinc, magnesium to form a water-soluble complex excreted from kidneys

* Available in Canada only

Uses: Hypercalcemic crisis, control of ventricular arrhythmias associated with digitalis toxicity

Dosage and routes:

• *Adult and child:* IV INF 15-50 mg/kg/day, diluted in 500 ml D_5W or 0.9% NaCl, given over 3-4 hr, not to exceed 3 g/day (adult) or 70 mg/kg/day (child); allow 5 days between courses (child), 2 days (adult)

Available forms: Inj conc 150 mg/ml

Side effects/adverse reactions:

CNS: Headache, paresthesia, ***numbness***

INTEG: Urticaria, ***exfoliative dermatitis,*** erythema, pain at injection site

CV: Hypotension, thrombophlebitis

GI: Nausea, vomiting, diarrhea

GU: Dysuria, pyelonephritis, ***nephrotoxicity,*** hyperuricemia, hypomagnesemia, polyuria, ***proteinuria, renal tubular necrosis, hypocalcemia***

Contraindications: Hypersensitivity, anuria, hepatic insufficiency, poisoning of other metals, severe renal disease, child <3 yr, seizure disorders, active/inactive TB

Precautions: Hypertension, pregnancy (C), lactation

Pharmacokinetics:

Excreted in urine as calcium chelate

Interactions:

• Incompatible in 5% alcohol

Lab test interferences:

False decrease: Calcium

Decrease: Magnesium, alk phosphatase

NURSING CONSIDERATIONS

Assess:

• VS, B/P, pulse; if hypotension occurs, drug should be discontinued

• Monitor I&O, kidney function studies: BUN, creatinine, CrCl, Ca (must be done following each administration)

• Hypocalcemia: numbness of feet, hands, tongue, lips; positive Chvostek's, Trousseau's signs; convulsions; stupor

• Cardiac abnormalities: dysrhythmias, hypotension, tachycardia

• Allergic reactions (rash, urticaria); if these occur, drug should be discontinued

Administer:

• IV inf after diluting in 500 ml dextrose, or isotonic saline sol, not to exceed 15 mg of actual medication/min, total dose is usually given over 3-4 hr

• Only when IV Ca preparation is on unit for emergency use

• EDTA, BAL separately

• IV use infusion pump, rotate infusion sites, observe site for redness, inflammation

• IV fluids to ensure adequate hydration before administration of drug

Perform/provide:

• Assistance with ambulation

Evaluate:

• Therapeutic response: Ca levels 9-10 mg/dl; absence of hypercalcemic symptoms

Teach patient/family:

• To remain recumbent for ½ hr to prevent postural hypotension

• To make position changes slowly to prevent fainting

• That dosage schedule must be followed

• That breath may be odorous

edrophonium (℞)

(ed-roe-fone'yum)

Enlon, Reversol, Tensilon

Func. class.: Cholinergics, anticholinesterase

Chem. class.: Quaternary ammonium compound

Action: Inhibits destruction of acetylcholine, which increases concentration at sites where acetylcholine is released; this facilitates transmission of impulses across myoneural junction

Uses: To diagnose myasthenia gravis; curare antagonist; differentiation of myasthenic crisis from cholinergic crisis

Dosage and routes:

Tensilon test (myasthenia gravis diagnosis)

• *Adult:* IV 1-2 mg over 15-30 sec, then 8 mg if no response; IM: 10 mg; if cholinergic reaction occurs, retest after ½ hr with 2 mg IM

• *Child >34 kg:* IV 2 mg; if no response in 45 sec, then 1 mg q45 sec, not to exceed 10 mg; IM 5 mg

• *Child <34 kg:* IV 1 mg; if no response in 45 sec, then 1 mg q45 sec, not to exceed 5 mg; IM 5 mg

• *Infant:* IV 0.5 mg

Reversal of nondepolarizing neuromuscular blockers

• *Adult:* IV 10 mg over 30-45 sec, may repeat, not to exceed 40 mg

Differentiation of myasthenic crisis from cholinergic crisis

• *Adult:* IV 1 mg, if no response in 1 min, may repeat

Available forms: Inj 10 mg/ml

Side effects/adverse reactions:

INTEG: Rash, urticaria

CNS: Dizziness, headache, sweating, weakness, ***convulsions,*** incoordination, ***paralysis,*** drowsiness, ***loss of consciousness***

GI: Nausea, diarrhea, vomiting, cramps, increased salivary and gastric secretions, dysphagia, increased peristalsis

CV: Tachycardia, dysrhythmias, bradycardia, hypotension, AV block, ECG changes, ***cardiac arrest,*** syncope

GU: Frequency, incontinence, urgency

RESP: ***Respiratory depression, bronchospasm, constriction, laryngospasm, respiratory arrest,*** dyspnea

EENT: Miosis, blurred vision, lacrimation, visual changes

Contraindications: Obstruction of intestine, renal system, hypersensitivity

Precautions: Seizure disorders, bronchial asthma, coronary occlusion, hyperthyroidism, dysrhythmias, peptic ulcer, megacolon, poor GI motility, pregnancy (C), bradycardia, hypotension

Pharmacokinetics:

IV: Onset 30-60 sec, duration 6-15 min

IM: Onset 2-10 min, duration 12-45 min

Interactions:

• Decreased action of edrophonium: procainamide, quinidine, aminoglycosides, anesthetics, mecamylamine, polymyxin, magnesium, corticosteroids, antidysrythmics

• Bradycardia: digitalis

Y-site compatibilities: Heparin, hydrocortisone, potassium chloride, vitamin B with C

NURSING CONSIDERATIONS

Assess:

• VS, respiration during test; muscle strength

• Diabetic patient carefully, since this drug lowers blood glucose

Administer:

• IV undiluted 2 mg or less over 15-30 sec; as a curare antagonist, over 30-45 sec; or given as continuous infusion in myasthenia crisis

• Only with atropine sulfate available for cholinergic crisis

• Only after all other cholinergics have been discontinued

Perform/provide:

• Storage at room temperature

Evaluate:

• Therapeutic response: increased muscle strength, hand grasp; improved gait; absence of labored breathing (if severe)

Teach patient/family:
• To wear Medic Alert ID specifying myasthenia gravis, drugs taken
Treatment of overdose:
Respiratory support, atropine 1-4 mg (IV)

enalapril/ enalaprilat (℞)

(e-nal'a-pril)/(e-nal'a-pril-at)
Vasotec, Vasotec IV

Func. class.: Antihypertensive
Chem. class.: Angiotensin-converting enzyme inhibitor

Combination products: Vaseretic: enalapril maleate 10 mg with hydrochlorothiazide 25 mg

Action: Selectively suppresses renin-angiotensin-aldosterone system; inhibits ACE; prevents conversion of angiotensin I to angiotensin II, dilation of arterial, venous vessels
Uses: Hypertension, CHF
Dosage and routes:
• *Adult:* PO 5 mg/day, may increase or decrease to desired response range 10-40 mg/day
Hypertension
• *Adult:* IV 1.25 mg q6h over 5 min
Patients on diuretics
• *Adult:* IV 0.625 mg over 5 min, may give additional doses of 1.25 mg q6h
Renal impairment
• *Adult:* IV 1.25 mg q6h with CrCl <3 mg/dl or 0.625 mg if CrCl >3 mg/dl
Available forms: Tabs 2.5, 5, 10, 20 mg; inj 1.25 mg/ml
Side effects/adverse reactions:
CV: Hypotension, chest pain, tachycardia, dysrhythmias
CNS: Insomnia, dizziness, paresthesias, headache, fatigue, anxiety
GI: Nausea, vomiting, colitis, cramps, diarrhea, constipation, flatulence, dry mouth, loss of taste
INTEG: Rash, purpura, alopecia, hyperhidrosis
HEMA: ***Agranulocytosis, neutropenia***
EENT: Tinnitus, visual changes, sore throat, double vision, dry burning eyes
GU: ***Proteinuria, renal failure,*** increased frequency of polyuria or oliguria
RESP: Dyspnea, cough, rales, angioedema
META: Hyperkalemia
Contraindications: Hypersensitivity
Precautions: Renal disease, hyperkalemia, pregnancy (C), lactation
Pharmacokinetics:
PO: Peak 4-6 hr; half-life 1½ hr; metabolized by liver to active metabolite, excreted in urine
IV: Onset 5-15 min, peak up to 4 hr
Interactions:
• Hypersensitivity: allopurinol
• Severe hypotension: diuretics, other antihypertensives
• Decreased effects of enalapril: aspirin, antacids
• Increased K levels: salt substitutes, K-sparing diuretics, K supplements
• May increase effects of ergots, neuromuscular blocking agents, antihypertensives, hypoglycemics, barbiturates, reserpine, levodopa
• Effects may be increased by phenothiazines, diuretics, phenytoin, quinidine, nifedipine
Y-site compatibilities: Amikacin, aminophylline, ampicillin, ampicillin/sulbactam, aztreonam, butorphanol, calcium gluconate, cefazolin, cefoperazone, ceftazidime, ceftizoxime, chloramphenicol, cimetidine, clindamycin, erythromycin lactobionate, esmolol, famotidine,

fentanyl, ganciclovir, gentamicin, heparin, hetastarch, hydrocortisone sodium succinate, labetalol, lidocaine, magnesium sulfate, melphalan, methylprednisolone sodium succinate, metronidazole, morphine, nafcillin, penicillin G, potassium, phenobarbital, piperacillin, potassium chloride, potassium phosphate, ranitidine, sodium acetate, tobramycin, trimethoprim/sulfamethoxazole, vancomycin, vinorelbine

Lab test interferences:

Interference: Glucose/insulin tolerance tests

NURSING CONSIDERATIONS

Assess:

- B/P, pulse q4h; note rate, rhythm, quality
- Electrolytes: K, Na, Cl
- Baselines in renal, liver function tests before therapy begins
- Edema in feet, legs daily
- Skin turgor, dryness of mucous membranes for hydration status
- Symptoms of CHF: edema, dyspnea, wet rales

Administer:

- IV, undiluted over 5 min, use diluent provided or 50 ml D_5W, 0.9% NaCl, 0.9% NaCl in D_5W or LR, Isolyte E, give through Y-tube of free-flowing inf of 0.9% NaCl, D_5W, LR, Isolyte E

Evaluate:

- Therapeutic response: decreased B/P

Teach patient/family:

- Not to use OTC (cough, cold, or allergy) products unless directed by prescriber
- To avoid sunlight or wear sunscreen for photosensitivity
- To comply with dosage schedule, even if feeling better
- To notify prescriber of mouth sores, sore throat, fever, swelling of hands or feet, irregular heartbeat, chest pain, signs of angioedema
- Excessive perspiration, dehydration, vomiting, diarrhea; may lead to fall in blood pressure—consult prescriber if these occur
- That drug may cause dizziness, fainting; light-headedness may occur during 1st few days of therapy
- That drug may cause skin rash or impaired perspiration
- Not to discontinue drug abruptly
- Not to use OTC products unless directed by prescriber
- To rise slowly to sitting or standing position to minimize orthostatic hypotension

Treatment of overdose: Lavage, IV atropine for bradycardia, IV theophylline for bronchospasm, digitalis, O_2, diuretic for cardiac failure, hemodialysis

enoxacin (℞)

(e-nox'a-sin)

Penetrex

Func. class.: Antiinfective

Chem. class.: Fluoroquinolone

Action: Inhibits the enzyme that repairs bacterial DNA, thereby preventing bacterial replication; DNA-gyrase inhibitor

Uses: Uncomplicated urethral or cervical gonorrhea, uncomplicated and complicated UTI. Effective against staphylococci, *Aeromonas* sp., *Citrobacter* sp., *Enterobacter* sp., *Escherichia coli, Hemophilus ducreyi, Klebsiella* sp., *Moranella morganii, Neisseria gonorrhea, Proteus vulgaris, Proteus mirabilis, Providencia* sp., *Pseudomonas aeruginosa, Serratia*

Dosage and routes:

Gonorrhea

- *Adult:* PO 400 mg as a single dose

Uncomplicated UTI

* Available in Canada only

• *Adult:* PO 200 mg bid × 7 days
Complicated UTI
• *Adult:* PO 400 mg bid × 14 days
Available forms: Tabs 200, 400 mg
Side effects/adverse reactions:
CNS: Dizziness, headache, fatigue, somnolence, depression, insomnia, anxiety
GI: Diarrhea, nausea, vomiting, anorexia, flatulence, heartburn, abdominal pain, dry mouth, increased AST (SGOT), ALT (SGPT)
INTEG: Rash, pruritus, photosensitivity
EENT: Visual disturbances, dizziness
Contraindications: Hypersensitivity to quinolones
Precautions: Pregnancy (C), lactation, children, elderly, renal disease, seizure disorders
Pharmacokinetics:
PO: Peak 1 hr, half-life 3-6 hr, steady state 2 days; excreted in urine as unchanged drug, metabolites
Interactions:
• Decreased effects of enoxacin: antacids, nitrofurantoin, iron salts, sucralfate, antineoplastics
• Increased enoxacin levels: probenecid, cimetidine
• Increased toxicity: theophylline, cyclosporin, caffeine
NURSING CONSIDERATIONS
Assess:
• Kidney, liver function studies: BUN, creatinine, AST (SGOT), ALT (SGPT)
• I&O ratio, urine pH; <5.5 is ideal
• CNS symptoms: insomnia, vertigo, headache, agitation, confusion
• Allergic reactions: rash, flushing, urticaria, pruritus
Administer:
• After clean-catch urine for C&S
Perform/provide:
• Limited intake of alkaline foods, drugs; milk, dairy products, peanuts, vegetables, alkaline actacids, sodium bicarbonate
Evaluate:
• Therapeutic response: negative C&S, absence of symptoms of infection
Teach patient/family:
• Fluids must be increased to 3L/day to avoid crystallization in kidneys
• If dizziness occurs, to ambulate, perform activities with assistance
• Not to take within 2 hr of antacids, calcium, iron, milk, sucralfate
• To use sunscreen, protective clothing for photosensitivity
• To complete full course of drug therapy, take 1 hr ac or 2 hr pc
• To contact prescriber if adverse reactions occur

enoxaparin (℞)

(ee-nox'a-par-in)
Lovenox
Func. class.: Antithrombotic
Chem. class.: Unfractionated porcine heparin

Action: Prevents conversion of fibrinogen to fibrin and prothrombin to thrombin by enhancing inhibitory effects of antithrombin III; produces higher ratio of anti-factor X_a to antifactor IIa
Uses: Prevention of deep-vein thrombosis, pulmonary emboli in hip and knee replacement
Dosage and routes:
• *Adult:* SC 30 mg bid immediately after surgery; continue to administer until deep-vein thrombosis no longer a threat (7-14 days)
Available forms: Inj 30 mg/0.3 ml, prefilled syringes
Side effects/adverse reactions:
CNS: Fever, confusion
GI: Nausea

GU: Edema, peripheral edema
HEMA: ***Hypochromic anemia, thrombocytopenia,*** bleeding
INTEG: Ecchymosis
Contraindications: Hypersensitivity to this drug, heparin, or pork; hemophilia, leukemia with bleeding, peptic ulcer disease, thrombocytopenic purpura
Precautions: Alcoholism, elderly, pregnancy (C), hepatic disease (severe), renal disease (severe), blood dyscrasias, severe hypertension, subacute bacterial endocarditis, acute nephritis, lactation, children
Pharmacokinetics:
SC: Maximum antithrombin activity (3-5 hr)
Elimination half-life 4½ hr
Interactions:
- Increased action of enoxaprin: oral anticoagulants, salicylates
- Do not mix with other drugs or infusion fluids

NURSING CONSIDERATIONS
Assess:
- Blood studies (Hct, platelets, occult blood in stools); thrombocytopenia may occur
- Bleeding gums, petechiae, ecchymosis, black tarry stools, hematuria
- Partial prothrombin time, which should be 1½-2 × control, PTT often done qd, APTT, ACT

Administer:
- Only after screening patient for bleeding disorders
- SC only; do not give IM
- To recumbent patient; give SC; rotate inj sites (left/right anterolateral, left/right posterolateral abdominal wall)
- Insert whole length of needle into skin fold held with thumb and forefinger
- Only this drug when ordered; not interchangeable with heparin
- At same time each day to maintain steady blood levels
- Do not massage area or aspirate when giving SC injection
- Avoiding all IM injections that may cause bleeding

Perform/provide:
- Storage at 77° F (25° C); do not freeze

Evaluate:
- Therapeutic response: prevention of deep vein thrombosis

Teach patient/family:
- To use soft-bristle toothbrush to avoid bleeding gums, to use electric razor
- To report any signs of bleeding: gums, under skin, urine, stools

Treatment of overdose:
Protamine SO_4 10% sol; dose should equal dose of enoxaparin

ephedrine (nasal) (OTC)

(e-fed′rin)
Vatronol Nose Drops
Func. class.: Nasal decongestant
Chem. class.: Indirect/direct sympathomimetic amine

Action: Relaxes bronchial smooth muscle, increases diameter of nasal passage by action on β_2-adrenergic receptors
Uses: Nasal congestion associated with colds, hay fever, sinusitis, other allergic conditions, adjunct in middle ear infections
Dosage and routes:
- *Adult and child:* INSTILL 3-4 gtts, q4h or small amount of gel in each nostril q4h

Available forms: Sol 0.5% sulfate; gel 0.6% HCl
Side effects/adverse reactions:
GI: Nausea, vomiting, anorexia
EENT: Irritation, burning, sneezing,

* Available in Canada only

stinging, dryness, rebound congestion
INTEG: Contact dermatitis
CNS: Anxiety, restlessness, tremors, weakness, insomnia, dizziness, fever, headache
Contraindications: Hypersensitivity to sympathomimetic amines
Precautions: Child <6 yr, elderly, diabetes, cardiovascular disease, hypertension, hyperthyroidism, increased ICP, prostatic hypertrophy, pregnancy (C)
Interactions:
- Hypertension: MAOIs, β-adrenergic blockers
- Hypotension: methyldopa, mecamylamine, reserpine

NURSING CONSIDERATIONS
Assess:
- Redness, swelling, pain in nasal passages

Administer:
- No more than q4h; for <4 consecutive days

Perform/provide:
- Environmental humidification to decrease nasal congestion, dryness
- Storage in light-resistant containers; do not expose to high temperatures

Evaluate:
- Therapeutic response: decreased congestion, runny nose

Teach patient/family:
- That stinging may occur for a few applications; drying of mucosa may be decreased by environmental humidification
- To notify prescriber if irregular pulse, insomnia, dizziness, or tremors occur
- Proper administration to avoid systemic absorption

ephedrine (℞)
(e-fed′rin)
Ephedrine, Ephedrine sulfate, Neorespin
Func. class.: Adrenergic, mixed direct and indirect effects
Chem. class.: Phenylisopropylamine

Action: Causes increased contractility and heart rate by acting on β-receptors in the heart; also acts on α-receptors, causing vasoconstriction in blood vessels
Uses: Shock; increased perfusion; hypotension, bronchodilation
Dosage and routes:
Vasopressor
- *Adult:* IM/SC 25-50 mg, not to exceed 150 mg/24 hr; IV 10-25 mg, not to exceed 150 mg/24 hr
- *Child:* SC/IV 3 mg/kg/day or 25-100 mg/m^2/day in divided doses q4-6h

Bronchodilator
- *Adult:* PO 25-50 mg bid-qid, not to exceed 400 mg/day; IM/SC 12.5-25 mg
- *Child:* PO 2-3 mg/kg/day or 100 mg/m^2/day in 4-6 divided doses

Orthostatic hypotension
- *Adult:* PO 25 mg qd-qid
- *Child:* PO 3 mg/kg/day in 4-6 divided doses

Stimulation
- *Adult:* PO 25-50 mg q3-4 hr prn
- *Child:* PO 3 mg/kg/day or 100 mg/m^2/day in divided doses

Available forms: Inj 25, 50 mg/ml; caps 25, 50 mg; syr 11, 20 mg/5 ml
Side effects/adverse reactions:
CNS: Tremors, anxiety, insomnia, headache, dizziness, confusion, hallucinations, ***convulsions, CNS depression***
GU: Dysuria, urinary retention

CV: Palpitations, tachycardia, hypertension, chest pain, ***dysrhythmias***
GI: Anorexia, nausea, vomiting
RESP: ***Dyspnea***
Contraindications: Hypersensitivity to sympathomimetics, narrow-angle glaucoma
Precautions: Pregnancy (C), lactation, cardiac disorders, hyperthyroidism, diabetes mellitus, prostatic hypertrophy
Pharmacokinetics:
PO: Onset 15-60 min, duration 2-4 hr
IV: Onset 5 min, duration 2 hr
Metabolized in liver; excreted in urine (unchanged), breast milk; crosses blood-brain barrier, placenta
Interactions:
• Do not use with MAOIs or tricyclic antidepressants; hypertensive crisis may occur
• Decreased effect of ephedrine: methyldopa, urinary acidifiers, rauwolfia alkaloids
• Increased effect of this drug: urinary alkalizers
• Dysrhythmia: halothane, anesthetics, digitalis
• Decreased effect of guanethidine
Solution compatibilities: 0.9% NaCl, 0.45% NaCl, D_5W, $D_{10}W$, Ringers, LR, ionosol
NURSING CONSIDERATIONS
Assess:
• I&O ratio
• ECG during administration continuously; if B/P increases, drug is decreased
• B/P and pulse q5min after parenteral route
• CVP or PWP during infusion if possible
• For paresthesias and coldness of extremities; peripheral blood flow may decrease
• Injection site: tissue sloughing; if this occurs, administer phentolamine mixed with 0.9% NaCl
Administer:
• IV undiluted through Y-tube or 3-way stopcock; give 10 mg or less over 1 min
• Plasma expanders for hypovolemia
Perform/provide:
• Storage of reconstituted sol refrigerated no longer than 24 hr
• Do not use discolored sol
Evaluate:
• Therapeutic response: increased B/P with stabilization
Teach patient/family:
• Reason for drug administration
Treatment of overdose: Administer phentolamine for hypertension, diazepam for convulsions

epinephrine/epinephrine bitartrate/epinephrine HCl (℞)

(ep-i-nef′rin)

Adrenalin Chloride, Adrenalin Chloride Solution, Asthma Haler, Asthma Nefrin, Bronitin Mist, Bronkaid Mist, Epinal, Epinephrine, Epinephrine HCl, Epinephrine Pediatric, Epipen Jr., Epitrate, Eppy/N, Glaucon, Medihaler-Epi, Micro-Nefrin, Nephron Inhalant, Primatene Mist, S-2 Inhalant, Sus-Phrine, Vaponefrin

Func. class.: Adrenergic
Chem. class.: Catecholamine

Combination products: E-Pilo: epinephrine bitartrate 1%, pilocarpine HCl 1%, 2%, 3%, 4%, 6%

Action: β_1- and β_2-agonist causing increased levels of cyclic AMP producing bronchodilation, cardiac, and CNS stimulation; large doses cause vasoconstriction; small doses can cause vasodilation via β_2-vascular receptors

Uses: Acute asthmatic attacks, hemostasis, bronchospasm, anaphylaxis, allergic reactions, cardiac arrest, adjunct in anesthesia

Dosage and routes:

Asthma

- *Adult and child:* INH 1-2 puffs of 1:100 or 2.25% racemic q15min

Bronchodilator

- *Adult:* SC 0.2-0.5 mg q20min-4 hr max 1 mg/dose

Anaphylatic Shock/Vasopressor

- *Adult:*SC/IM 0.5 mg, repeat q5min if needed, then IV; IV 0.1-0.25 mg, repeat q5-15min or inf 1 μg/min, increase to 4 μg/min if needed
- *Child:* SC/IM/IV 10 μg/kg, repeat q5-15min up to 0.3 mg

Anaphylatic Reaction

- *Adult:* SC/IM 0.2-0.5 mg, repeat q10-15min, do not exceed 1 mg/dose
- *Child:* SC 0.01 mg/kg, repeat q15min, ×2 doses, then q4hr, max 0.5 mg/dose

Cardiac arrest

- *Adult:* IC, IV, endotracheal 0.1-1 mg repeat q5min prn
- *Child:* IC, IV, endotracheal 5-10 μg q5min, may use 0.1 μ/kg/min IV inf after inital dose

Available forms: Aerosol 0.16 mg/spray, 0.2 mg/spray, 0.25 mg/spray; inj 1:1000 (1 mg/ml), 1:200 (5 mg/ml), 0.01 mg/ml (1:100,000), 0.1 mg/ml (1:10,000), 0.5 mg/ml (1:2,000); sol for nebulization 1:100, 1.25%, 2.25% (base)

Side effects/adverse reactions:

GU: Urinary retention

CNS: Tremors, anxiety, insomnia, headache, dizziness, confusion, hallucinations, ***cerebral hemorrhage***

CV: Palpitations, tachycardia, hypertension, *dysrhythmias,* increased T wave

GI: Anorexia, nausea, vomiting

RESP: Dyspnea

Contraindications: Hypersensitivity to sympathomimetics, narrow-angle glaucoma

Precautions: Pregnancy (C), lactation, cardiac disorders, hyperthyroidism, diabetes mellitus, prostatic hypertrophy

Pharmacokinetics:

SC: Onset 3-5 min, duration 20 min

PO, INH: Onset 1 min

Interactions:

- Do not use with MAOIs or tricyclic antidepressants; hypertensive crisis may occur
- Decreased effect of epinephrine: methyldopa, urinary acidifiers, rauwolfia alkaloids and β-blockers
- Increased effect of epinephrine: urinary alkalizers

Y-site compatibilities: Amrinone, atracurium, calcium chloride, calcium gluconate, famotidine, heparin, hydrocortisone sodium succinate, pancuronium, phytonadione, potassium chloride, vecuronium, vitamin B with C

Syringe compatibilities: Doxapram, heparin, milrinone

Additive compatibilities: Amikacin, cimetidine, dobutamide, floxacillin, furosemide, metaraminol, verapamil

NURSING CONSIDERATIONS

Assess:

- ECG during administration continuously; if B/P increases, drug is decreased
- B/P and pulse q5min after parenteral route
- CVP or PCWP during infusion if possible
- Injection site: tissue sloughing; administer phentolamine with NS

Administer:

- Parenteral IV dose slowly, after reconstituting 1 mg (1:1000 sol)/10 ml or more NS; to prepare a 1:10,000 sol for maintenance, may be further diluted in 500 ml D_5W; give 1 mg or less over 1 min or more through Y-tube or 3-way stopcock; 1 mg = 1 ml of 1:1000 or 10 ml of 1:10,000

Perform/provide:

- Storage of reconstituted sol refrigerated no longer than 24 hr
- Do not use discolored sol

Evaluate:

- Therapeutic response: increased B/P with stabilization or ease of breathing

Teach patient/family:

- Reason for drug administration
- To rinse mouth after use to prevent dryness after inhalation
- Not to take OTC preparations

Treatment of overdose: Administer an α-blocker and a β-blocker

epinephrine bitartrate/epinephrine HCl/epinephryl borate (optic) (℞)

(ep-i-nef′rin)

Epitrate, Mytrate/Epifrin, Glaucon/Epinal, Eppy*

Func. class.: Mydriatic, adrenergic agonist

Chem. class.: Sympathomimetic amine

Action: Contracts radial muscle of the iris, lowers intraocular pressure by enhancing aqueous humor outflow

Uses: Open-angle glaucoma

Dosage and routes:

- *Adult and child:* INSTILL SOL 1-2 gtt 1%-2% sol, determined by tonometric reading (bitartrate); 1 gtt of a 0.5%-2% sol (HCl) or 0.5%-1% (borate)

Available forms: Sol 0.1%, 0.5%, 1%, 2% (HCl), borate 0.5%, 1%

Side effects/adverse reactions:

CV: Palpitations, tachycardia, headache, hypertension, faintness, trembling

EENT: Blurred vision, eye pain, ocular irritation, tearing

Contraindications: Hypersensitivity to sympathomimetic amines, narrow-angle glaucoma, dysrhythmias, cardiogenic shock, cerebral arteriosclerosis

Precautions: Elderly, hyperthyroidism, heart disease, diabetes mellitus, hypertension, pregnancy (C), asthma, lactation, children

Pharmacokinetics:

Instill: Onset 1 hr, peak 4-8 hr, duration 12-24 hr

Interactions:

- Dysrhythmias: cyclopropane, halogenated hydrocarbons
- Increased pressor effects: tricyclic antidepressants, antihistamines, β-blockers, MAOIs

NURSING CONSIDERATIONS

Assess:

- Allergic reaction: itching, edema of eyelids, eye discharge; drug should be discontinued
- Tonometer readings during long-term treatment
- B/P, pulse, respirations

Evaluate:

- Therapeutic response: mydriasis

Teach patient/family:

- To report change in vision, blurring or loss of sight, trouble breathing, sweating, pallor
- Method of instillation: pressure on lacrimal sac for 1 min; do not touch dropper to eye
- That long-term therapy may be required for glaucoma
- To check OTC drugs for other sympathetic nervous system stimulants (e.g., phenylephrine)
- Not to use sol if brown or contains a precipitate

* Available in Canada only

• Not to use while wearing soft contact lenses

epinephrine (nasal) (OTC)

(ep-i-nef′rin)

Adrenalin Chloride

Func. class.: Nasal decongestant

Chem. class.: Sympathomimetic amine

Action: Relaxes bronchial smooth muscle, increases diameter of nasal passage by action on β-adrenergics

Uses: Nasal congestion, superficial bleeding

Dosage and routes:

• *Adult and child >6 yr old:* TOP apply to affected area with sterile swab

Available forms: Sol 0.1%

Side effects/adverse reactions:

GI: Nausea, vomiting, anorexia

EENT: Irritation, burning, sneezing, stinging, dryness, rebound congestion

INTEG: Contact dermatitis

CNS: Anxiety, restlessness, tremors, weakness, insomnia, dizziness, fever, headache

Contraindications: Hypersensitivity to sympathomimetic amines

Precautions: Child <6 yr, elderly, diabetes, cardiovascular disease, hypertension, hyperthyroidism, increased ICP, prostatic hypertrophy, pregnancy (C)

Interactions:

• Hypertension: MAOIs, β-adrenergic blockers

• Hypotension: methyldopa, mecamylamine, reserpine

NURSING CONSIDERATIONS

Assess:

• For redness, swelling, pain in nasal passages

Administer:

• No more than q4h; for <4 consecutive days

Perform/provide:

• Environmental humidification to decrease nasal congestion, dryness

• Storage in light-resistant container; do not expose to high temp

Evaluate:

• Therapeutic response: decreased congestion, bleeding

Teach patient/family:

• That stinging may occur for a few applications; drying of mucosa may be decreased by environmental humidification

• To notify prescriber of irregular pulse, insomnia, dizziness, tremors

• Proper administration to avoid systemic absorption

epoetin alpha (℞)

(ee-poe′e-tin al′fa)

Epogen, EPO, Procrit

Func. class.: Hormone

Chem. class.: Amino acid polypeptide

Action: Erythropoietin is one factor controlling rate of red cell production; drug is developed by recombinant DNA technology

Uses: Anemia caused by reduced endogenous erythropoietin production, primarily end-stage renal disease; to correct hemostatic defect in uremia; anemia due to AZT treatment in HIV patients; anemia due to chemotherapy

Dosage and routes:

• *Adult:* IV 5-500 U/kg 3 ×/wk

Anemia secondary to chemotherapy

• *Adult:* SC 150 U/kg 3 ×/wk, may increase after 2 mo up to 300 U/kg 3 × wk

Anemia in chronic renal failure

• *Adult:* SC/IV 50-100 U/kg 3 ×/wk,

then adjust dose by 25 U/kg/dose to maintain HCT

Anemia secondary to zidovudine treatment

• *Adult:* SC/IV 100 U/kg 3 ×/wk × 2 mo, may increase by 50-100 U/kg q1-2 mo, up to 300 U/kg 3 ×/wk

Available forms: 2000, 3000, 4000, 10,000 U/ml

Side effects/adverse reactions:

CV: *Hypertension,* ***hypertensive encephalopathy***

CNS: ***Seizures,*** coldness, sweating

MS: Bone pain

Contraindications: Hypersensitivity

Pharmacokinetics:

IV: Metabolized in body; extent of metabolism unknown; onset of increased reticulocyte count 1-2 wk

NURSING CONSIDERATIONS

Assess:

• Renal studies: urinalysis, protein, blood, BUN, creatinine

• Blood studies: reticulocyte count weekly

• I&O; report drop in output to <50 ml/hr

• CNS symptoms: coldness, sweating

• CV status: B/P; hypertension may occur rapidly leading to hypertension encephalopathy

Evaluate:

• Therapeutic response: increase in reticulocyte count in 1-2 wk, increased appetite, enhanced sense of well-being

ergoloid (℞)

(er'goe-loid)

Ergoloid Mesylates, Gerimal, Hydergine, Hydergine LC

Func. class.: Migraine agent

Chem. class.: Ergot alkaloid–amino acid

Action: May increase cerebral metabolism and blood flow

Uses: Dementias: senile, Alzheimer's, multiinfarct, primary progressive

Dosage and routes:

• *Adult:* PO/SL 1 mg tid, may increase to 4.5-12 mg/day

Available forms: Tabs SL 0.5, 1 mg; tabs 1 mg; cap 1 mg; liquid 1 mg/ml

Side effects/adverse reactions:

GI: Nausea, vomiting, sublingual irritation

Contraindications: Hypersensitivity to ergot preparations; psychosis

Precautions: Acute intermittent porphyria, pregnancy (C), lactation

Pharmacokinetics:

PO: Peak 1 hr; metabolized in liver; excreted as metabolites in feces; crosses blood-brain barrier; half-life 3½ hr

NURSING CONSIDERATIONS

Assess:

• Weight daily; check for peripheral edema in feet, legs

• B/P and pulse, check regularly

• Neurologic status: LOC, blurring vision, nausea, vomiting, tingling in extremities before headache

• Toxicity: dyspnea; hypotension or hypertension; rapid, weak pulse; delirium; nausea; vomiting; bradycardia

Administer:

• With or after meals to avoid GI symptoms; do not crush or chew SL tab

Perform/provide:
• Storage in well-closed container at room temp
Evaluate:
• Therapeutic response: decreased forgetfulness, increased mental alertness and ability for self-care
Teach patient/family:
• To change positions slowly and to move extremities before walking
• To maintain dosage at approved level; not to increase drug
• To report side effects, including increased vasoconstriction starting with cold extremities, then paresthesia, weakness
• That 6 mo treatment may be required; some improvement occurs in 1 mo
• To keep drug out of reach of children; death may occur
Treatment of overdose: Induce emesis if orally ingested, or gastric lavage; administer saline cathartic, keep warm

ergonovine (℞)
(er-goe-noe'veen)
Ergotrate Maleate, ergonovine maleate
Func. class.: Oxytocic
Chem. class.: Ergot alkaloid

Action: Stimulates uterine contractions and vascular smooth muscle, decreases bleeding
Uses: Postpartum or postabortion hemorrhage
Investigational uses: To induce a coronary artery spasm
Dosage and routes:
Oxytoxic:
• *Adult:* IM 0.2 mg q2-4h, not to exceed 5 doses; IV 0.2 mg given over 1 min
Induced coronary artery spasm
• *Adult:* IV 50 μg q5min up to 400 μg or when chest pain occurs

Available forms: Inj 0.2 mg/ml
Side effects/adverse reactions:
CNS: Headache, dizziness, fainting
CV: Hypertension, chest pain
GI: Nausea, vomiting
INTEG: Sweating
RESP: Dyspnea
EENT: Tinnitus
GU: Cramping
Contraindications: Hypersensitivity to ergot medication, augmentation of labor, before delivery of placenta, spontaneous abortion (threatened), pelvic inflammatory disease
Precautions: Hepatic disease, renal disease, cardiac disease, asthma, anemia, convulsive disorders, hypertension, glaucoma, obliterative vascular disease
Pharmacokinetics:
IM: Onset 2-5 min, duration 3 hr
IV: Onset immediate, duration 45 min
Metabolized in liver, excreted in urine
Interactions:
• Hypertension: sympathomimetics, ergots
NURSING CONSIDERATIONS
Assess:
• Ergotism: nausea, vomiting, weakness, muscular pain, insensitivity to cold, paresthesias of extremities; drug should be discontinued
• B/P, pulse; watch for change that may indicate hemorrhage
• Respiratory rate, rhythm, depth; notify prescriber of abnormalities
• Fundal tone, nonphasic contractions; check for relaxation
Administer:
• IV undiluted through Y-tube or 3-way stopcock
• IM in deep muscle mass; rotate injection sites if additional doses are given
• With emergency equipment available

Evaluate:

• Therapeutic response: decreased blood loss, severe cramping

Teach patient/family:

• To report increased blood loss, increased temp, or foul-smelling lochia; that cramping is normal

Treatment of overdose:
Stop drug, give vasodilators, heparin, dextran

---

ergotamine (℞)

(er-got′a-meen)

Ergostat Ergomar*, Gynergen*, Medihaler Ergotamine*

Func. class.: α-Adrenergic blocker

Chem. class.: Ergot alkaloid-amino acid

Combination products: Bellergal-S: ergotamine tartrate 0.6 mg with levorotatory belladonna alkaloids, malates 0.2 mg (of lavorotatory belladonna alkaloids 40 mg); Cafergot: ergotamine tartrate 1 mg with caffeine 100 mg; Cafergot suppositories: ergotamine tartrate 2 mg, caffeine 100 mg; Ergocaff: ergotamine tartrate 1 mg, caffeine 100 mg; Migral: ergotamine tartrate 1 mg, caffeine 50 mg, cyclizine HCl 25 mg; Wigraine: ergotamine tartrate 1 mg, caffeine 100 mg, levorotatory belladonna alkaloids 0.1 mg, phenacetin 130 mg; Wigraine Suppositories: ergotamine tartrate 2 mg, caffeine 100 mg, tartaric acid 21.5 mg

---

Action: Constricts smooth muscle in peripheral, cranial blood vessels, relaxes uterine muscle; blocks serotonin release

Uses: Vascular headache (migraine, cluster histamine)

Dosage and routes:

• *Adult:* 2 mg, then 1-2 mg qh or q ½ hr for SL, not to exceed 6 mg/day or 10 mg/wk; INH 1 puff, may repeat in 5 min, not to exceed 6/24 hr or 15 sprays/wk

Available forms: SL tabs 2 mg; tabs 1 mg; oral inh 360 μg/dose

Side effects/adverse reactions:

CNS: Numbness in fingers, toes, headache, weakness

CV: Transient tachycardia, chest pain, bradycardia, edema, claudication, increase or decrease in B/P

GI: Nausea, vomiting, diarrhea, abdominal cramps

MS: Muscle pain

Contraindications: Hypersensitivity to ergot preparations, occlusion (peripheral, vascular), CAD, hepatic disease, renal disease, peptic ulcer, hypertension, pregnancy (X)

Precautions: Lactation, children, anemia

Pharmacokinetics:

PO: Peak 30 min-3 hr; metabolized in liver; excreted as metabolites in feces; crosses blood-brain barrier; excreted in breast milk

Interactions:

• Increased effects: troleandomycin

• Increased vasoconstriction: β-blockers

NURSING CONSIDERATIONS

Assess:

• Ergotism: nausea, vomiting, weakness, muscular pain, insensitivity to cold, paresthesia of extremities; drug should be discontinued

• Weight daily, check for peripheral edema in feet, legs

• For stress level, activity, recreation, coping mechanisms

• Neurologic status: LOC, blurring vision, nausea, vomiting, tingling in extremities that occur preceding the headache

• Ingestion of tyramine foods (pickled products, beer, wine, aged cheese), food additives, preservatives, colorings, artificial sweeten-

---

* Available in Canada only

ers, chocolate, caffeine; may precipitate headaches
• Toxicity: dyspnea, hypotension or hypertension, rapid, weak pulse, delirium, nausea, vomiting

Administer:
• At beginning of headache; dose must be titrated to patient response
• By SL route if possible for better, faster absorption
• With or after meals to avoid GI symptoms (PO route only)
• Not to pregnant women; harm to fetus may occur

Perform/provide:
• Quiet, calm environment with decreased stimulation for noise, bright light, or excessive talking

Evaluate:
• Therapeutic response: decrease in frequency, severity of headache

Teach patient/family:
• Not to use OTC medications; serious drug interactions may occur
• To maintain dose at approved level; not to increase even if drug does not relieve headache
• To report side effects including increased vasoconstriction starting with cold extremities, then paresthesia, weakness
• That an increase in headaches may occur when this drug is discontinued after long-term use
• To keep drug out of reach of children; death may occur
• How to use inhaler

Treatment of overdose: Induce emesis or gastric lavage if orally ingested; administer saline cathartic; keep warm

erythrityl (℞)
(e-ri′thri-till)
Cardilate
Func. class.: Vasodilator, coronary
Chem. class.: Nitrate

Action: Decreases preload, afterload, which is responsible for decreasing left ventricular end diastolic pressure, systemic vascular resistance; improves exercise tolerance

Uses: Chronic stable angina pectoris, prophylaxis of angina pain, pulmonary arteriolar dilation

Dosage and routes:
• *Adult:* PO 10-30 mg tid; SL 5-15 mg before stressful activity

Available forms: Chew tabs 10 mg; tabs 5, 10 mg

Side effects/adverse reactions:
CV: Postural hypotension, tachycardia, ***collapse,*** syncope, edema
GI: Nausea, vomiting
INTEG: Pallor, sweating, rash
CNS: Headache, flushing, dizziness ***weakness, fainting***
MISC: Twitching, hemolytic anemia, ***methemoglobinemia***

Contraindications: Hypersensitivity to this drug or nitrites, severe anemia, increased intracranial pressure, cerebral hemorrhage, acute MI, head trauma

Precautions: Postural hypotension, pregnancy (C), lactation, children, hypertropic cardiomyopathy, glaucoma

Pharmacokinetics:
PO: Onset 30 min, peak 1-1½ hr, duration 6 hr
SL: Onset 5-10 min, peak 30-45 min, duration 3 hr; metabolized by liver, excreted in urine

Interactions:
• Increased effects: β-blockers, di-

uretics, antihypertensives, alcohol products

Lab test interferences:
Decrease: Cholesterol

NURSING CONSIDERATIONS

Assess:
- For orthostatic B/P, pulse during beginning therapy
- Pain: duration, time started, activity being performed, character
- Tolerance if taken over long period
- Headache, light-headedness, decreased B/P; may need decreased dosage

Administer:
- With 8 oz of water on empty stomach (oral tablet)
- After checking expiration date

Evaluate:
- Therapeutic response: decrease or prevention of anginal pain

Teach patient/family:
- To keep tabs in original container
- If 3 SL tabs do not relieve pain, patient may have MI
- To avoid alcohol products
- That drug may cause headache; tolerance occurs over time
- That drug may be taken before stressful activity: exercise, sexual activity
- Not to chew or swallow SL tabs
- That SL may sting when drug comes in contact with mucous membranes
- To avoid hazardous activities if dizziness occurs
- Importance of complying with complete medical regimen
- To make position changes slowly to prevent fainting

erythromycin (ophthalmic) (℞)

(er-ith-roe-mye'sin)

AK-Mycin, Erythromycin, Ilotycin

Func. class.: Antiinfective

Action: Inhibits bacterial protein synthesis

Uses: Infection of external eye, prophylaxis of ophthalmia neonatorium due to *N. gonorrhoeae, C. trachomatis*

Dosage and routes:
- *Adult and child:* Apply OINT qd-qid as needed

Ophthalmia neonatorum
- *Neonates:* Apply to conjunctival sacs immediately after delivery

Available forms: Oint 0.5%

Side effects/adverse reactions:
EENT: Poor corneal wound healing, temporary visual haze, overgrowth of nonsusceptible organisms

Contraindications: Hypersensitivity, epitheleal herpes, varicella, mycobacterial, fungal infections, simplex keratitis

Precautions: Antibiotic hypersensitivity

NURSING CONSIDERATIONS

Assess:
- Allergy: itching, lacrimation, redness, swelling

Administer:
- After washing hands; cleanse crusts or discharge from eye before application

Perform/provide:
- Storage at room temp in air-tight container

Evaluate:
- Therapeutic response: absence of redness, inflammation, tearing

Teach patient/family:
- To use drug exactly as prescribed
- Not to use eye makeup, towels,

washcloths, eye medication of others; reinfection may occur
• That drug container tip should not be touched to eye
• To report itching, increased redness, burning, stinging, swelling; drug should be discontinued
• That vision may blur when ointment is applied

erythromycin (topical) (OTC)

(er-ith-roe-mye'sin)

A/T/S, Akne-Mycin, C-Solve 2, Erycette, Eryderm, Erygel, Erymax, Erythromycin, E-Solve 2, ETS-2%, Staticin, Theramycin Z, T-Stat

Func. class.: Local antiinfective

Chem. class.: Macrolide antibacterial

Action: Interferes with bacterial protein synthesis

Uses: Pyoderma, acne vulgaris

Dosage and routes:
• *Adult and child:* TOP apply to affected area tid-qid

Available forms: Top sol, ointment 1.5%, 2%; gel 2%

Side effects/adverse reactions:
INTEG: Rash, urticaria, stinging, burning, pruritus, dry, scaly, oily skin

Contraindications: Hypersensitivity

Precautions: Pregnancy (C), lactation, child <12 yr

Interactions:
Avoid use with clindamycin, abrasive agents, acids, alkaline media

NURSING CONSIDERATIONS

Assess:
• Allergic reaction: burning, stinging, swelling, redness

Administer:
• After cleansing with soap, water before each application; dry well
• Enough medication to cover lesions completely

Perform/provide:
• Storage at room temp in dry place; after reconstitution, store in refrigerator

Evaluate:
• Therapeutic response: decrease in size, number of lesions

Teach patient/family:
• To use asepsis (hand washing) before, after each application
• To apply with glove to prevent further infection
• To avoid use of OTC creams, ointments, lotions unless directed by prescriber
• To avoid use near eyes, nose, mouth
• To monitor for superinfection
• To report skin irritation to prescriber

erythromycin base, erythromycin estolate, erythromycin ethylsuccinate, erythromycin gluceptate, erythromycin lactobionate, erythromycin stearate (℞)

(eh-rith-roe-mye'sin)

Apo-Erythro-EC*, E-Base, E-Mycin, Erybid*, Eryc, Ery-Tab, erythromycin, erythromycin base, Erthromycin Filmtabs, Novorythro*, PCE Dispertab, Robimycin Robitabs/Erythromid*, erythromycin estolate, Ilosone, Ilosone Pulvules/E.E.S. 200, E.E.S. 400, Eryped, Ery Ped Drops, Eryped 200, Eryped 400, erythromycin ethylsuccinate/erythromycin lactobionate, Ilotycin Gluceptate

Func. class.: Antibacterial

Chem. class.: Macrolide antibiotic

Combination products: Pediazole: erythromycin ethlysuccinate 200 mg (of erythromycin) per 5 ml with sulfisoxazole acetyl 600 mg (of sulfisoxazole) per 5 ml

Action: Binds to 50S ribosomal subunits of susceptible bacteria and suppresses protein synthesis

Uses: Infections caused by *N. gonorrhoeae;* mild to moderate respiratory tract, skin, soft tissue infections caused by *S. pneumoniae, M. pneumoniae, C. diphtheriae, B. pertussis, T. pallidum, B. burgdorferi, L. monocytogenes;* syphilis; Legionnaire's disease, *L. pneumophila, C. trachomatis; H. influenzae* (when used with sulfonamides)

Dosage and routes:

Soft tissue infections

• *Adult:* PO 250-500 mg q6h (base, estolate, stearate); PO 400-800 mg q6h (ethylsuccinate); IV INF 15-20 mg/kg/day (lactobionate)

• *Child:* PO 30-50 mg/kg/day in divided doses q6h (salts); IV 15-20 mg/kg/day in divided doses q4-6h (lactobionate)

N. gonorrhoeae/PID

• *Adult:* IV 500 mg q6h × 3 days (gluceptate, lactobionate), then PO 250 mg (base, estolate, stearate) or 400 mg (ethylsuccinate) q6h × 1 wk

Syphilis

Adult: PO 30 g in divided doses over 15 days (base, estolate, stearate)

Chlamydia

• *Adult:* PO 500 mg q6h × 1 wk or 250 mg qid × 2 wk

• *Infant:* PO 50 mg/kg/day in 4 divided doses × 3 wk or more

• *Newborn:* PO 50 mg/kg/day in 4 divided doses × 2 wk or more

Intestinal amebiasis

• *Adult:* PO 250 mg q6h × 10-14 days (base, estolate, stearate)

• *Child:* PO 30-50 mg/kg/day in divided doses q6h × 10-14 days (base, estolate, stearate)

Available forms: Base: tabs, enteric-coated 250, 333, 500 mg; tabs film-coated 250, 500 mg; caps, enteric-coated 125, 250 mg; estolate: tabs chewable 125, 250 mg; tabs 500 mg; caps 125, 250 mg; drops 100 mg/ml; susp 125, 250 mg/5ml; stearate: tabs, film-coated 250, 500 mg; ethylsuccinate: tabs, chewable 200, 400 mg; 100 mg/2.5 ml, 200, 400 mg/5 ml; susp 200, 400 mg powder for suspension 100 mg/2.5 ml, 200 and 400 mg/5 ml powder for inj; 500 mg and 1 g (lactobionate), 250 mg, 500 mg, 1 g (as gluceptate)

* Available in Canada only

Side effects/adverse reactions:
INTEG: Rash, urticaria, pruritus, thrombophlebitis (IV site)
GI: Nausea, vomiting, diarrhea, ***hepatotoxicity,*** abdominal pain, stomatitis, heartburn, anorexia, pruritus ani
GU: Vaginitis, moniliasis
EENT: Hearing loss, tinnitus
Contraindications: Hypersensitivity, preexisting liver disease (estolate)
Precautions: Pregnancy (C), hepatic disease, lactation
Pharmacokinetics: Peak 4 hr, duration 6 hr, half-life 1-2 hr; metabolized in liver; excreted in bile, feces
Interactions:
• Arrhythmias: astemizole, terfenadine
• Increased action of oral anticoagulants, digitalis, theophylline, methylprednisolone, cyclosporine, bromocriptine, disopyramide, ergots, triazolam
Additive compatibilities: Calcium gluconate, corticotropin, dimenhydrinate, heparin, hydrocortisone sodium succinate, methicillin, penicillin G potassium, potassium chloride, sodium bicarbonate
Erythromycin lactobionate:
Aminophylline, ampicillin, cimetidine, diphenhydramine, hydrocortisone sodium succinate, lidocaine, methicillin, penicillin G potassium, penicillin G sodium, pentobarbital, polymyxin B, potassium chloride, prednisolone sodium phosphate, prochlorperazine, promazine, sodium bicarbonate, sodium iodide, verapamil
Syringe compatibility: Methicillin
Y-site compatibilities: Acyclovir, amiodarone, cyclophosphamide, enalaprilat, esmolol, famotidine, foscarnet, hydromorphone, idarubicin, labetol, magnesium sulfate, meperidine, morphine, multivitamins, perphenazine, vitamin B with C, zidovudine
Lab test interferences:
False increase: 17-OHCS/17-KS, AST (SGOT)/ALT (SGPT)
Decrease: Folate assay

NURSING CONSIDERATIONS

Assess:
• I&O ratio; report hematuria, oliguria in renal disease
• Liver studies: AST (SGOT), ALT (SGPT)
• Renal studies: urinalysis, protein, blood
• C&S before drug therapy; drug may be given as soon as culture is taken; C&S may be repeated after treatment
• Bowel pattern before, during treatment
• Skin eruptions, itching
• Respiratory status: rate, character, wheezing, tightness in chest; discontinue drug if these occur
• Allergies before treatment, reaction of each medication; place allergies on chart in bright red; notify all people giving drugs
Administer:
• IV after diluting 500 mg or less/10 ml sterile H_2O without preservatives; dilute further in 80-250 ml of 0.9% NaCl, LR, Normosol-R; may be further diluted to 1 mg/ml and given as continuous infusion; run 1 g or less/100 ml over ½-1 hr; continuous infusion over 6 hr, may require buffers to neutralize pH if dilution is < 250 ml, use infusion pump
• Do not give by IM or IV push
• Enteric-coated tablets may be given with food
Perform/provide:
• Storage at room temp
• Adequate intake of fluids (2 L) during diarrhea episodes

Evaluate:
• Therapeutic response: decreased symptoms of infection
Teach patient/family:
• To take oral drug with full glass of water; with food for GI symptoms
• Do not take with fruit juice
• To report sore throat, fever, fatigue; could indicate superinfection
• To notify nurse of diarrhea stools, dark urine, pale stools, yellow discoloration of eyes or skin, and severe abdominal pain
• To take at evenly spaced intervals; complete dosage regimen
Treatment of hypersensitivity: Withdraw drug; maintain airway; administer epinephrine, aminophylline, O_2, IV corticosteroids

esmolol (℞)
(ess'moe-lol)
Brevibloc
Func. class.: β-Adrenergic blocker (antidysrhythmic II)

Action: Competitively blocks stimulation of β_1-adrenergic receptors in the myocardium; produces negative chronotropic, inotropic activity (decreases rate of SA node discharge, increases recovery time), slows conduction of AV node, decreases heart rate, decreases O_2 consumption in myocardium; also decreases renin-aldosterone-angiotensin system at high doses; inhibits β_2-receptors in bronchial system slightly
Uses: Supraventricular tachycardia, noncompensatory tachycardia, hypertensive crisis
Dosage and routes:
• *Adult:* IV loading dose—500 μg/kg/min over 1 min; maintenance—50 μg/kg/min for 4 min; may repeat q5min, increasing maintenance inf by 50 μg/kg/min (max of 200 μg/kg/min), titrate to patient response

Available forms: Inj 10 mg, 250 mg/ml
Side effects/adverse reactions:
INTEG: Induration, inflammation at site, discoloration, edema, erythema, burning pallor, flushing, rash, pruritus, dry skin, alopecia
CNS: Confusion, light-headedness, paresthesia, somnolence, fever, dizziness, fatigue, headache, depression, anxiety
GI: Nausea, vomiting, anorexia, gastric pain, flatulence, constipation, heartburn, bloating
CV: Hypotension, bradycardia, chest pain, peripheral ischemia, shortness of breath, ***CHF,*** conduction disturbances
GU: Urinary retention, impotence, dysuria
RESP: ***Bronchospasm,*** dyspnea, cough, wheeziness, nasal stuffiness
Contraindications: 2nd or 3rd degree heart block, cardiogenic shock, CHF, cardiac failure, hypersensitivity
Precautions: Hypotension, pregnancy (C), peripheral vascular disease, diabetes, hypoglycemia, thyrotoxicosis, renal disease, lactation
Pharmacokinetics: Onset very rapid, duration short, half-life 9 min; metabolized by hydrolysis of the ester linkage; excreted via kidneys
Interactions:
• Increased digoxin levels: digoxin
• Increased esmolol levels: morphine
• Reversal of esmolol effects: isoproterenol, norepinephrine, dopamine, dobutamine
• Increased effects of both drugs: disopyramide
• Increased effects of lidocaine
Y-site compatibilities: Amikacin, aminophylline, ampicillin, atracurium, butorphanol, calcium chloride, cefazolin, cefoperazone,

ceftazidime, ceftizoxime, chloramphenicol, cimetidine, clindamycin, co-trimoxazole, dopamine, enalaprilat, erythromycin, lactobionate, famotidine, fentanyl, furosemide, gentamicin, heparin, hydrocortisone sodium succinate, magnesium sulfate, methyldopate, metronidazole, morphine sulfate, nafcillin, pancuronium, penicillin G potassium, phenytoin, piperacillin, polymyxin B, potassium chloride, potassium phosphate, ranitidine, sodium acetate, streptomycin, tobramycin, vancomycin, vecuronium

Additive compatibilities: Aminophylline, bretyllium, heparin

Lab test interferences:

Interference: Glucose/insulin tolerance test

NURSING CONSIDERATIONS

Assess:

- I&O ratio, weight daily
- B/P, pulse q4h; note rate, rhythm, quality; rapid changes can cause shock; if systolic <100 or diastolic <60, notify prescriber before giving drug
- Apical/radial pulse before administration; notify prescriber if <60 bpm
- Baselines in renal, liver function tests before therapy begins
- Breath sounds and respiratory pattern
- Respiratory pattern: wheezing from bronchospasm
- Edema in feet, legs daily
- Skin turgor, dryness of mucous membranes for hydration status

Administer:

- Reduced dosage in cool environment
- IV diluted 5 g/20 ml of D_5W, D_5R, D_5 0.9% NaCl, 0.45% NaCl, LR D_5 0.45% NaCl 0.9% NaCl further dilute in the remaining 480 ml (10 mg/ml) and give as infusion; give loading dose over 1 min, then maintenance over 4 min; may repeat loading dose q5min with increased maintenance dose; maintenance dose should not be >200 μg/kg/min and be given up to 48 hr; dose should be tapered at 25 μg/kg/min; use infusion pump

Perform/provide:

- Storage protected from light, moisture; in cool environment

Evaluate:

- Therapeutic response: lower B/P immediately, lower heart rate

Treatment of overdose: Discontinue drug

---

estazolam (℞)

(ess-taz'oh-lam)

ProSom

Func. class.: Sedative-hypnotic

Chem. class.: Benzodiazepine derivative

Controlled Substance Schedule IV (US)

Action: Produces CNS depression at the limbic, thalamic, hypothalamic levels of the CNS; may be mediated by neurotransmitter γ-aminobutyric acid (GABA); results are sedation, hypnosis, skeletal muscle relaxation, anticonvulsant activity, anxiolytic action

Uses: Insomnia

Dosage and routes:

- *Adult:* PO 1-2 mg hs
- *Geriatric:* PO 0.5 mg hs

Available forms: Tabs 1, 2 mg

Side effects/adverse reactions:

INTEG: Dermatitis, allergy, sweating, flushing, pruritus

HEMA: ***Leukopenia, granulocytopenia (rare)***

CNS: Lethargy, drowsiness, daytime sedation, dizziness, confusion, lightheadedness, headache, anxiety, irritability, weakness, tremors, depression, lack of coordination

GI: Nausea, vomiting, diarrhea, heartburn, abdominal pain, constipation, anorexia, taste alteration
CV: Chest pain, pulse changes, palpitations, tachycardia
MISC: Joint pain, congestion
Contraindications: Hypersensitivity to benzodiazepines, pregnancy (X), sleep apnea
Precautions: Hepatic disease, renal disease, suicidal individuals, drug abuse, elderly, psychosis, child <18, lactation, depression, pulmonary insufficiency
Pharmacokinetics: Onset 15-45 min, peak 1½-2 hr, duration 7-8 hr; metabolized by liver; excreted by kidneys (inactive/active metabolites); crosses placenta; excreted in breast milk
Interactions:
- Increased effects of estazolam: cimetidine, disulfiram, isoniazid, probenecid, oral contraceptives
- Increased CNS depression: alcohol, CNS depressants
- Decreased effect of estazolam: theophylline, rifampin, smoking, caffeine

NURSING CONSIDERATIONS
Assess:
- Blood studies: Hct, Hgb, RBCs (if on long-term therapy)
- For REM rebound if abruptly discontinued after 3 wk of use
- Hepatic studies: AST (SGOT), ALT (SGPT), bilirubin
- Mental status: mood, sensorium, affect, memory (long, short)
- Blood dyscrasias: fever, sore throat, bruising, rash, jaundice, epistaxis (rare)
- Type of sleep problem: falling asleep, staying asleep

Administer:
- After removal of cigarettes to prevent fire
- After trying conservative measures for insomnia
- ½-1 hr before hs for sleeplessness
- On empty stomach for fast onset; with food for GI symptoms

Perform/provide:
- Assistance with ambulation after receiving dose
- Safety measures: side rails, nightlight, call bell within easy reach
- Checking to see PO medication has been swallowed
- Storage in tight container in cool environment

Evaluate:
- Therapeutic response: ability to sleep at night, fewer early AM awakenings

Teach patient/family:
- To avoid driving, other activities requiring alertness until drug is stabilized

---

esterified estrogens (℞)

Climestrone*, Estratab, Menest, Neo-Estrone*
Func. class.: Estrogen
Chem. class.: Nonsteroidal synthetic estrogen

Combination products: Estratest: esterified estrogens 1.25 mg, methyltestosterone 2.5 mg; Estratest HS: esterified estrogens 0.625 mg, methyltestosterone 1.25 mg

Action: Needed for adequate functioning of female reproductive system; affects release of pituitary gonadotropins, inhibits ovulation, adequate calcium use in bone
Uses: Menopause, prostatic cancer, hypogonadism, castration, primary ovarian failure
Dosage and routes:
Menopause
- *Adult:* PO 0.3-3.75 mg qd 3wk on, 1 wk off

Hypogonadism/castration/ovarian failure
• *Adult:* PO 2.5 mg qd-tid 3wk on, 1 wk off
Prostatic cancer
• *Adult:* PO 1.25-2.5 mg tid
Breast cancer
• *Adult:* PO 10 mg tid × 3 mo or longer
Available forms: Tabs 0.3, 0.625, 1.25, 2.5 mg
Side effects/adverse reactions:
CNS: Dizziness, headache, migraines, depression
CV: Hypotension, thrombophlebitis, edema, ***thromboembolism, stroke, pulmonary embolism, myocardial infarction***
GI: Nausea, vomiting, diarrhea, anorexia, pancreatitis, cramps, constipation, increased appetite, increased weight, ***cholestatic jaundice***
EENT: Contact lens intolerance, increased myopia, astigmatism
GU: Amenorrhea, cervical erosion, breakthrough bleeding, dysmenorrhea, vaginal candidiasis, breast changes, *gynecomastia, testicular atrophy, impotence*
INTEG: Rash, urticaria, acne, hirsutism, alopecia, oily skin, seborrhea, purpura, melasma
META: Folic acid deficiency, hypercalcemia, hyperglycemia
Contraindications: Breast cancer, thromboembolic disorders, reproductive cancer, genital bleeding (abnormal, undiagnosed), pregnancy (X)
Precautions: Hypertension, asthma, blood dyscrasias, gallbladder disease, CHF, diabetes mellitus, bone disease, depression, migraine headache, convulsive disorders, hepatic disease, renal disease, family history of cancer of breast or reproductive tract

Pharmacokinetics:
PO: Degraded in liver; excreted in urine; crosses placenta; excreted in breast milk
Interactions:
• Decreased action of anticoagulants, oral hypoglycemics
• Toxicity: tricyclic antidepressants
• Decreased action of estrogens: anticonvulsants, barbiturates, phenylbutazone, rifampin
• Increased action of corticosteroids

NURSING CONSIDERATIONS

Assess:
• Blood glucose in patient with diabetes
• Weight daily; notify prescriber of weekly weight gain >5 lb; if increase, diuretic may be ordered
• B/P q4h; watch for increase caused by H_2O and Na retention
• I&O ratio; be alert for decreasing urinary output and increasing edema
• Liver function studies, including AST (SGOT), ALT (SGPT), bilirubin, alk phosphatase
• Edema, hypertension, cardiac symptoms, jaundice
• Mental status: affect, mood, behavioral changes, aggression
• Hypercalcemia
Administer:
• Titrated dose; use lowest effective dose
• With food or milk to decrease GI symptoms
Evaluate:
• Therapeutic response: reversal of menopause or decrease in tumor size in prostatic cancer
Teach patient/family:
• To weigh weekly, report gain >5 lb
• To check with prescriber before using OTC drugs
• To report breast lumps, vaginal bleeding, edema, jaundice, dark urine, clay-colored stools, dyspnea,

headache, blurred vision, abdominal pain, numbness or stiffness in legs, chest pain; male to report impotence or gynecomastia

estradiol/estradiol cypionate/estradiol valerate/estradiol transdermal system (℞)

(ess-tra-dye'ole)

Cypionate, depGynogen, Depo Estadiol, Depogen, Dura-Estrin, Estra-D, Estradiol Cypionate, Estro-Cyp, Estroject-LA, Estronol-LA/Estrace, Estraderm/Deladiol-40, Delestrogen, Dioval 40, Dioval XX, Duragen-10, Duragen-20, Duragen-40, Estradiol Valerate, Estra-L 20, Estra-L 40, Gynogen L.A. "10," Gynogen L.A. "20," Gynogen L.A. "40," L.A.E. 20, Valergen 10, Valergen 20, Valergen 40/Estace, Estraderm TTS

Func. class.: Estrogen

Chem. class.: Nonsteroidal synthetic estrogen

Action: Needed for adequate functioning of female reproductive system; affects release of pituitary gonadotropins, inhibits ovulation, adequate calcium use in bone

Uses: Menopause, inoperable breast cancer, prostatic cancer, atrophic vaginitis, kraurosis vulvae, hypogonadism, castration, primary ovarian failure, prevention of osteoporosis

Dosage and routes:

Hormone replacement

• *Adult:* TD 0.05-0.1 mg/24 hrs, apply 2 ×/wk

Menopause/hypogonadism/castration/ovarian failure

• *Adult:* PO 1-2 mg qd 3wk on, 1 wk off or 5 days on, 2 days off; IM 0.2-1 mg qwk

Prostatic cancer

• *Adult:* IM 30 mg q1-2wk (valerate); PO 1-2 mg tid (oral estradiol)

Breast cancer

• *Adult:* PO 10 mg tid × 3 mo or longer

Atropic vaginitis

• *Adult:* VAG CREAM 2-4 g qd × 1-2 wk, then 1 g 1-3 ×/wk

Kraurosis vulvae

• *Adult:* IM 1-1.5 mg 1-2 ×/wk

Available forms: Estradiol tabs 1, 2 mg; cypionate injection 5 mg/ml; valerate injection 10, 20, 40 mg/ml; transderm 0.05, 0.1 mg/24 hr release rate; vag cream 100 µg/gm

Side effects/adverse reactions:

CNS: Dizziness, headache, migraines, depression

CV: Hypotension, thrombophlebitis, edema, ***thromboembolism, stroke, pulmonary embolism, myocardial infarction***

GI: Nausea, vomiting, diarrhea, anorexia, pancreatitis, cramps, constipation, increased appetite, increased weight, ***cholestatic jaundice***

EENT: Contact lens intolerance, increased myopia, astigmatism

GU: Amenorrhea, cervical erosion, breakthrough bleeding, dysmenorrhea, vaginal candidiasis, breast changes, *gynecomastia, testicular atrophy, impotence*

INTEG: Rash, urticaria, acne, hirsutism, alopecia, oily skin, seborrhea, purpura, melasma

META: Folic acid deficiency, hypercalcemia, hyperglycemia

Contraindications: Breast cancer, thromboembolic disorders, reproductive cancer, genital bleeding (abnormal, undiagnosed), pregnancy (X)

Precautions: Hypertension, asthma, blood dyscrasias, gallbladder dis-

* Available in Canada only

ease, CHF, diabetes mellitus, bone disease, depression, migraine headache, convulsive disorders, hepatic disease, renal disease, family history of cancer of breast or reproductive tract

Pharmacokinetics:

PO/IH/TOP: Degraded in liver; excreted in urine; crosses placenta; excreted in breast milk

Interactions:

• Decreased action of anticoagulants, oral hypoglycemics
• Toxicity: tricyclic antidepressants
• Decreased action of estradiol: anticonvulsants, barbiturates, phenylbutazone, rifampin, milk products, calcium
• Increased action of: corticosteroids

Lab test interferences:

Increase: BSP retention test, PBI, T_4, serum sodium, platelet aggregation, thyroxine-binding globulin (TBG), prothrombin, factors VII, VIII, IX, X, triglycerides
Decrease: Serum folate, serum triglyceride, T_3 resin uptake test, glucose tolerance test, antithrombin III, pregnanediol, metyrapone test
False positive: LE prep, antinuclear antibodies

NURSING CONSIDERATIONS

Assess:

• Blood glucose of diabetic patient
• Weight daily, notify prescriber of weekly weight gain >5 lb; if increase, diuretic may be ordered
• B/P q4h, watch for increase caused by H_2O and Na retention
• I&O ratio; decreasing urinary output, increasing edema
• Liver function studies, including AST (SGOT), ALT (SGPT), bilirubin, alk phosphatase
• Hypertension, cardiac symptoms, jaundice, hypercalcemia
• Mental status: affect, mood, behavioral changes, aggression

Administer:

• Titrated dose; use lowest effective dose
• IM injection deeply in large muscle mass
• With food or milk to decrease GI symptoms (oral)
• Apply to trunk of body 2 ×/wk (transdermal)
• On intermittent cycle schedule: 3 wk on, then 1 wk off; if patch falls off reapply (transdermal)

Evaluate:

• Therapeutic response: reversal of menopause or decrease in tumor size in prostatic cancer

Teach patient/family:

• To weigh weekly, report gain >5 lb
• To report breast lumps, vaginal bleeding, edema, jaundice, dark urine, clay-colored stools, dyspnea, headache, blurred vision, abdominal pain, numbness or stiffness in legs, chest pain; male to report impotence or gynecomastia

estramustine (℞)

(ess-tra-muss'teen)
Emcyt
Func. class.: Antineoplastic
Chem. class.: Hormone: estrogen

Action: Combination drug consisting of nitrogen mustard/estrogen; estrogen is a carrier for the nitrogen mustard into estrogen-dependent tissue; acts like a weak alkylating agent

Uses: Metastatic prostate cancer

Dosage and routes:

• *Adult:* PO 10-16 mg/kg in 3-4 divided doses/day; treatment may continue for ≥3 mo or 600 mg/m^2/day in 3 divided doses

Available forms: Caps 140 mg

Side effects/adverse reactions:
GI: Nausea, vomiting, anorexia, ***hepatotoxicity***
GU: ***Renal failure,*** impotence, gynecomastia
INTEG: Rash, urticaria, pruritus, flushing, alopecia
RESP: Dyspnea, ***emboli,*** hoarseness
CV: ***Myocardial infarction,*** hypertension, ***CHF, CVA***
CNS: Headache, anxiety, seizures, insomnia, mood swings
Contraindications: Hypersensitivity to estradiol, thromboembolic disorders, pregnancy (D)
Precautions: Edema, hepatic disease, CVA, MI, seizures, hypertension, diabetes mellitus
Pharmacokinetics:
PO: Peak 1-2 hr, executed via biliary tract; excreted in bile; half-life 20 hr (terminal)

NURSING CONSIDERATIONS
Assess:
- Renal function studies: BUN, serum uric acid, urine CrCl, electrolytes before, during therapy
- I&O ratio; report fall in urine output to <30 ml/hr
- Liver function tests before, during therapy (bilirubin, AST [SGOT], ALT [SGPT], LDH) as needed or monthly
- Dyspnea, chest pain, tachypnea, fatigue, increased pulse, pallor, lethargy
- Food preferences; list likes, dislikes
- Edema in feet, joint, stomach pain, shaking
- Inflammation of mucosa, breaks in skin
- Yellowing of skin, sclera, dark urine, clay-colored stools, itchy skin, abdominal pain, fever, diarrhea
- Symptoms indicating severe allergic reaction: rash, pruritus, urticaria, purpuric skin lesions, itching, flushing
- Tachycardia, ECG changes, dyspnea, edema, fatigue, leg cramps; may indicate cardiac toxicity

Administer:
- In divided doses over 1-3 mo; give antiemetic if nausea, vomiting, or anorexia become severe

Evaluate:
- Therapeutic response: decreased tumor size, spread of malignancy

Teach patient/family:
- To report any complaints, side effects to nurse or prescriber
- That gynecomastia, impotence can occur and are reversible after discontinuing treatment
- To report any changes in breathing, coughing
- Importance of immediately reporting GI bleeding
- To use contraception during use; positive mutagenic effects

---

estrogenic substances, conjugated (℞)

C.E.S,* conjugated estrogens, Conjugated Estrogens C.S.D*, Premarin, Premarin Intravenous

Func. class.: Estrogen

Chem. class.: Nonsteroidal synthetic estrogen

Action: Needed for adequate functioning of female reproductive system; it affects release of pituitary gonadotropins, inhibits ovulation, adequate calcium use in bone
Uses: Menopause, inoperable breast cancer, prostatic cancer, abnormal uterine bleeding, hypogonadism, castration, primary ovarian failure, osteoporosis
Dosage and routes:
Menopause
- *Adult:* PO 0.3-1.25 mg qd 3wk on, 1 wk off

* Available in Canada only

Osteoporosis
• *Adult:* PO 0.625 mg qd or in cycle
Atrophic Vaginitis
• *Adult:* VAG CREAM 2-4 g ml qd × 21 days, off 7 days, repeat
Prostatic cancer
• *Adult:* PO 1.25-2.5 mg tid
Breast cancer
• *Adult:* PO 10 mg tid × 3 mo or longer
Abnormal uterine bleeding
• *Adult:* IV/IM 25 mg, repeat in 6-12 hr
Castration/primary ovarian failure
• *Adult:* PO 1.25 mg qd 3wk on, 1 wk off
Hypogonadism
• *Adult:* PO 2.5 mg bid-tid × 20 days/mo

Available forms: Tabs 0.3, 0.625, 0.9, 1.25, 2.5 mg; inj 25 mg/vial; vag cream 0.625 mg/g

Side effects/adverse reactions:
CNS: Dizziness, headache, migraine, depression
CV: Hypotension, thrombophlebitis, edema, ***thromboembolism, stroke, pulmonary embolism, myocardial infarction***
GI: Nausea, vomiting, diarrhea, anorexia, pancreatitis, cramps, constipation, increased appetite, increased weight, ***cholestatic jaundice***
EENT: Contact lens intolerance, increased myopia, astigmatism
GU: Amenorrhea, cervical erosion, breakthrough bleeding, dysmenorrhea, vaginal candidiasis, breast changes, *gynecomastia, testicular atrophy, impotence*
INTEG: Rash, urticaria, acne, hirsutism, alopecia, oily skin, seborrhea, purpura, melasma
META: Folic acid deficiency, hypercalcemia, hyperglycemia

Contraindications: Breast cancer, thromboembolic disorders, reproductive cancer, genital bleeding (abnormal, undiagnosed), pregnancy (X), lactation

Precautions: Hypertension, asthma, blood dyscrasias, gallbladder disease, CHF, diabetes mellitus, bone disease, depression, migraine headache, convulsive disorders, hepatic disease, renal disease, family history of cancer of breast or reproductive tract

Pharmacokinetics:
PO/IV/IM: Degraded in liver, excreted in urine, crosses placenta, excreted in breast milk

Interactions:
• Decreased action of anticoagulants, oral hypoglycemics
• Toxicity: tricyclic antidepressants
• Decreased action of estrogens: anticonvulsants, barbiturates, phenylbutazone, rifampin
• Increased action of corticosteroids

NURSING CONSIDERATIONS

Assess:
• Blood glucose if diabetic patient
• Weight daily; notify prescriber of weekly weight gain >5 lb; if increase, diuretic may be ordered
• B/P q4h; watch for increase caused by H_2O and Na retention
• I&O ratio; be alert for decreasing urinary output, increasing edema
• Liver function studies; AST (SGOT), ALT (SGPT), bilirubin, alk phosphatase
• Hypertension, cardiac symptoms, jaundice, hypercalcemia
• Mental status: affect, mood, behavioral changes, aggression

Administer:
• Titrated dose, use lowest effective dose
• IM reconstitute after withdrawing >5 ml of air from container and inject sterile diluent on vial side rotate to dissolve; give injection deep in large muscle mass

• IV directly after reconstituting as for IM, inject into distal port of running IV line of D_5W, 0.9% NaCl, LR at 5 mg/min or less
• With food or milk to decrease GI symptoms PO

Evaluate:
• Therapeutic response: absence of breast engorgement, reversal of menopause, or decrease in tumor size in prostatic cancer

Teach patient/family:
• To avoid breast-feeding, since drug is excreted in breast milk
• To weigh weekly, report gain >5 lb
• To report breast lumps, vaginal bleeding, edema, jaundice, dark urine, clay-colored stools, dyspnea, headache, blurred vision, abdominal pain, numbness or stiffness in legs, chest pain; male to report impotence or gynecomastia
• To avoid sunlight or wear sunscreen; burns may occur

estrone (℞)

(ess'trone)

Aquest, Estrone Aqueous, Estrone-5, Estronol, Femogen Forte*, Kestrone-5, Theelin Aqueous

Func. class.: Estrogen

Chem. class.: Nonsteroidal synthetic estrogen

Action: Needed for adequate functioning of female reproductive system; affects release of pituitary gonadotropins, inhibits ovulation, promotes adequate calcium use in bone structures

Uses: Menopause, prostatic cancer, atrophic vaginitis, hypogonadism, primary ovarian failure

Dosage and routes:

Menopause/atrophic vaginitis
• *Adult:* IM 0.1-0.5 mg 2-3 ×/wk

Prostatic cancer
• *Adult:* IM 2-4 mg 2-3 ×/wk

Female hypogonadism/primary ovarian failure
• *Adult:* IM 0.1-1 mg qwk in one dose or divided doses

Available forms: Inj 2, 5 mg/ml

Side effects/adverse reactions:

CNS: Dizziness, headache, migraine, depression

CV: Hypotension, thrombophlebitis, edema, ***thromboembolism, stroke, pulmonary embolism, myocardial infarction***

GI: Nausea, vomiting, diarrhea, anorexia, pancreatitis, cramps, constipation, increased appetite, increased weight, ***cholestatic jaundice***

EENT: Contact lens intolerance, increased myopia, astigmatism

GU: Amenorrhea, cervical erosion, breakthrough bleeding, dysmenorrhea, vaginal candidiasis, breast changes, *gynecomastia, testicular atrophy, impotence*

INTEG: Rash, urticaria, acne, hirsutism, alopecia, oily skin, seborrhea, purpura, melasma

META: Folic acid deficiency, hypercalcemia, hyperglycemia

Contraindications: Breast cancer, thromboembolic disorders, reproductive cancer, genital bleeding (abnormal, undiagnosed), pregnancy (X)

Precautions: Hypertension, asthma, blood dyscrasias, gallbladder disease, CHF, diabetes mellitus, bone disease, depression, migraine headache, convulsive disorders, hepatic disease, renal disease, family history of cancer of the breast or reproductive tract

Pharmacokinetics:

IM: Degraded in liver; excreted in urine, breast milk; crosses placenta;

* Available in Canada only

Interactions:
• Decreased action of anticoagulants, oral hypoglycemics
• Toxicity: tricyclic antidepressants
• Decreased action of estrone: anticonvulsants, barbiturates, phenylbutazone, rifampin
• Increased action of corticosteroids

NURSING CONSIDERATIONS
Assess:
• Blood glucose in diabetic patient
• Weight daily, notify prescriber of weekly weight gain >5 lb; if increase, diuretic may be ordered
• B/P q4h, watch for increase caused by H_2O, Na retention
• I&O ratio; be alert for decreasing urinary output, increasing edema
• Liver function studies, including AST (SGOT), ALT (SGPT), bilirubin, alk phosphatase
• Hypertension, cardiac symptoms, jaundice, hypercalcemia
• Mental status: affect, mood, behavioral changes, aggression

Administer:
• Titrated dose; use lowest effective dose
• IM injection deep in large muscle mass

Evaluate:
• Therapeutic response: absence of breast engorgement, reversal of menopause, or decrease in tumor size in prostatic cancer

Teach patient/family:
• To weigh weekly, report gain >5 lb
• To report breast lumps, vaginal bleeding, edema, jaundice, dark urine, clay-colored stools, dyspnea, headache, blurred vision, abdominal pain, numbness or stiffness in legs, chest pain; male to report impotence or gynecomastia
• To avoid sunlight or wear sunscreen, burns may occur

ethacrynate/ethacrynic (℞)

(eth-a-kri′nate)
Edecrin, Edecrin Sodium
Func. class.: Loop diuretic
Chem. class.: Ketone derivative

Action: Acts on loop of Henle by increasing excretion of chloride, sodium

Uses: Pulmonary edema, edema in CHF, liver disease, nephrotic syndrome, ascites

Dosage and routes:
• *Adult:* PO 50-200 mg/day; may give up to 200 mg bid
• *Child:* PO 25 mg, increased by 25 mg/day until desired effect occurs

Pulmonary edema
• *Adult:* IV 50-100 mg given over several minutes or 0.5-1 mg/kg

Available forms: Tabs 25, 50 mg; powder for inj 50 mg

Side effects/adverse reactions:
GU: Polyuria, ***renal failure,*** glycosuria
ELECT: Hypokalemia, hypochloremic alkalosis, hypomagnesemia, hyperuricemia, hypocalcemia, hyponatremia, decreased glucose tolerance
CNS: Headache, fatigue, weakness, vertigo
GI: Nausea, ***severe diarrhea,*** dry mouth, vomiting, anorexia, cramps, upset stomach, abdominal pain, ***acute pancreatitis,*** jaundice, ***GI bleeding;*** abdominal distention
EENT: Loss of hearing, ear pain, tinnitus, blurred vision
INTEG: Rash, pruritus, purpura, ***Stevens-Johnson syndrome,*** sweating, photosensitivity
MS: Cramps, arthritis, stiffness
ENDO: Hyperglycemia
HEMA: ***Thrombocytopenia, agranulocytosis, leukopenia, neutropenia***

CV: ***Chest pain,*** hypotension, ***circulatory collapse,*** ECG changes

Contraindications: Hypersensitivity to sulfonamides, anuria, hypovolemia, lactation, electrolyte depletion, infants

Precautions: Dehydration, ascites, severe renal disease, pregnancy (D), hypoproteinemia

Pharmacokinetics:

PO: Onset ½ hr, peak 2 hr, duration 6-8 hr

IV: Onset 5 min, peak 15-30 min, duration 2 hr

Excreted by kidneys; crosses placenta; half-life 30-70 min

Interactions:

• Increased hypotension: antihypertensives

• Decreased diuretic effect: indomethacin, NSAIDs

• Increased ototoxicity: cisplatin, aminoglycosides, rancomycin

• Increased toxicity: lithium, nondepolarizing skeletal muscle relaxants, digitalis

• Increased anticoagulant activity: warfarin

• Incompatible with hydralazine, procainamide, reserpine, tolazine, triflupromazine, blood, blood products

NURSING CONSIDERATIONS

Assess:

• Weight, I&O daily to determine fluid loss; effect of drug may be decreased if used qd

• Rate, depth, rhythm of respiration, effect of exertion

• B/P lying, standing; postural hypotension may occur

• Electrolytes: K, Na, Cl; include BUN, blood sugar, CBC, serum creatinine, blood pH, ABGs, uric acid, Ca, Mg

• Glucose in urine if diabetic

• Hearing if high IV doses

• Improvement in CVP q8h

• Signs of metabolic alkalosis: drowsiness, restlessness

• Signs of hypokalemia: postural hypotension, malaise, fatigue, tachycardia, leg cramps, weakness

• Rashes, fever qd

• Confusion, especially in elderly; take safety precautions if needed

Administer:

• IV after diluting with 50 ml NaCl inj; give through Y-tube or 3-way stopcock or heplock; give 10 mg or less over 1 min or run infusion over ½ hr; do not add to IV sol

• In AM to avoid interference with sleep if using drug as a diuretic

• K replacement if K less than 3

• With food if nausea occurs; absorption may be decreased slightly

• PO, IV only; do not give IM/SC

Evaluate:

• Therapeutic response: improvement in edema of feet, legs, sacral area daily if being used in CHF

Teach patient/family:

• To increase fluid intake to 2-3 L/day unless contraindicated; to rise slowly from lying or sitting position

• About adverse reactions: muscle cramps, weakness, nausea, dizziness

• To take with food or milk for GI symptoms

• To take early in day to prevent nocturia

• To use sunscreen for photosensitivity

Treatment of overdose: Lavage if taken orally; monitor electrolytes; give dextrose in saline; monitor hydration, CV, renal status

ethambutol (℞)

(e-tham'byoo-tole)

Etibi*, Myambutol

Func. class.: Antitubercular

Chem. class.: Diisopropylethylene diamide derivative

Action: Inhibits RNA synthesis, decreases tubercle bacilli replication

Uses: Pulmonary tuberculosis, as an adjunct, other mycobacterial infections

Dosage and routes:

• *Adult and child >13 yr:* PO 15-25 mg/kg/day as a single dose

Retreatment

• *Adult and child >13 yr:* PO 25 mg/kg/day as single dose × 2 mo with at least 1 other drug, then decrease to 15 mg/kg/day as single dose

Available forms: Tabs 100, 400 mg

Side effects/adverse reactions:

GI: Abdominal distress, anorexia, nausea, vomiting

INTEG: Dermatitis, pruritis

CNS: Headache, confusion, fever, malaise, dizziness, disorientation, hallucinations

EENT: Blurred vision, optic neuritis, photophobia, decreased visual acuity

META: Elevated uric acid, acute gout, liver function impairment

MISC: ***Thrombocytopenia,*** joint pain, bloody sputum

Contraindications: Hypersensitivity, optic neuritis, child <13 yr

Precautions: Pregnancy (D), lactation, renal disease, diabetic retinopathy, cataracts, ocular defects, hepatic and hematopoictic disorders

Pharmacokinetics:

PO: Peak 2-4 hr, half-life 3 hr; metabolized in liver; excreted in urine (unchanged drug/inactive metabolites, unchanged drug in feces)

Interactions:

• Increased renal toxicity: aminoglycosides, cisplatin

• Delayed absorption of ethambutol: aluminum salts

NURSING CONSIDERATIONS

Assess:

• Liver studies qwk: ALT (SGOT), AST (SGPT), bilirubin

• Signs of anemia: Hct, Hgb, fatigue

• Mental status often: affect, mood, behavioral changes; psychosis may occur

• Hepatic status: decreased appetite, jaundice, dark urine, fatigue

• C&S including sputum before treatment

Administer:

• With meals or antacids to decrease GI symptoms

• Antiemetic if vomiting occurs

• After C&S is completed; qmo to detect resistance

Evaluate:

• Therapeutic response: decreased symptoms of TB

Teach patient/family:

• To avoid alcohol products

• That compliance with dosage schedule, duration is necessary

• That scheduled appointments must be kept or relapse may occur

ethchlorvynol (℞)

(eth-klor-vi'nole)

Placidyl

Func. class.: Sedative-hypnotic

Chem. class.: Tertiary acetylenic alcohol

Controlled Substance Schedule IV (USA), Schedule F (Canada)

Action: Produces cerebral depression; exact action is unknown

Uses: Sedation, insomnia

Dosage and routes:

Sedation

• *Adult:* PO 100-200 mg bid or tid

Insomnia

• *Adult:* PO 500 mg-1g ½ hr before hs; may repeat 100-200 mg prn

• *Geriatric:* PO 500 mg ½ hr before hs

Medication for EEG

• *Child:* PO 25 mg/kg in one dose not to exceed 1 g

Available forms: Caps 100, 200, 500, 750 mg

Side effects/adverse reactions:

HEMA: ***Thrombocytopenia***

CNS: Fatigue, drowsiness, dizziness, sedation, ataxia, nightmares, hangover, giddiness, weakness, hysteria

GI: Nausea, vomiting

INTEG: *Rash,* urticaria

EENT: Blurred vision, bitter aftertaste

CV: Hypotension

Contraindications: Hypersensitivity to this drug, severe pain, porphyria

Precautions: Depression, hepatic disease, renal disease, suicidal individual, pregnancy (3rd trimester) (C), lactation, elderly

Pharmacokinetics:

PO: Onset 15-30 min, peak 1-1½ hr, duration 5 hr; metabolized by liver; excreted by kidneys; half-life 10-20 hr, 21-100 hr terminal

Interactions:

• Decreased hypoprothrombinemic effect: dicumarol, warfarin

• Increased CNS effects of ETOH, barbiturates, other CNS depressants, MAOIs

Lab test interferences: Clinitest

NURSING CONSIDERATIONS

Assess:

• Blood studies: Hct, Hgb, RBCs before and after treatment if blood dyscrasias are suspected

• Hepatic studies: AST (SGOT), ALT (SGPT), bilirubin if hepatic disease is present

• Mental status: mood, sensorium, affect, memory (long, short)

• Physical tolerance: more frequent requests for medication, shakes, anxiety

• Toxicity: hypotension, hypothermia, weakness, poor muscle coordination, visual problems; drug should be discontinued

• Respiratory dysfunction: depression, character, rate, rhythm; hold drug if respirations <10/min or if pupils dilated (rare)

• Blood dyscrasias: fever, sore throat, bruising, rash, jaundice, epistaxis (rare)

• Allergy to tartrazine: this drug contains tartrazine and should not be used by patients allergic to this dye

Administer:

• After removal of cigarettes to prevent fires

• After trying conservative measures for insomnia

• ½-1 hr before hs for sleeplessness

• With food or meals to decrease dizziness, giddiness

• For only 1 wk; not intended for long-term treatment

Perform/provide:

• Assistance with ambulation after receiving dose, especially elderly

• Safety measures: side rails, night-light, call bell within easy reach

• Checking to see PO medication swallowed

• Storage in tight, light-resistant container in cool environment

Evaluate:

• Therapeutic response: ability to sleep at night, less early AM awakening if taking for insomnia

Teach patient/family:

• To avoid driving, other activities requiring alertness

---

* Available in Canada only

• To avoid alcohol ingestion, CNS depressants; serious CNS depression may result
• That effects may take 2 nights for benefits to be noticed
• Alternative measures to improve sleep: reading, exercise several hours before hs, warm bath, warm milk, TV, self-hypnosis, deep breathing
Treatment of overdose: Lavage, activated charcoal; monitor electrolytes, vital signs

ethinyl estradiol (℞)

(eth'in-il ess-tra-dye'ole)
Estinyl, Feminone
Func. class.: Estrogen
Chem. class.: Nonsteroidal synthetic estrogen

Action: Needed for adequate functioning of female reproductive system; affects release of pituitary gonadotropins, inhibits ovulation, promotes adequate calcium use in bone structures
Uses: Menopause, prostatic cancer, breast cancer (5 yrs or more after menopause), breast engorgement, hypogonadism
Dosage and routes:
Menopause
• *Adult:* PO 0.02-0.5 mg qd 3wk on, 1 wk off
Prostatic cancer
• *Adult:* PO 0.15-2 mg qd
Hypogonadism
• *Adult:* PO 0.05 mg qd-tid × 2 wk/mo, then 2 wk progesterone, then 3-6 mo cycles, then 2 mo off
Breast cancer
• *Adult:* PO 1 mg tid
Breast engorgement
• *Adult:* PO 0.5-1 mg qd × 3 days, then tapered off over 7 days
Available forms: Tabs 0.02, 0.05, 0.5 mg
Side effects/adverse reactions:
CNS: Dizziness, headache, migraine, depression
CV: Hypotension, thrombophlebitis, edema, ***thromboembolism, stroke, pulmonary embolism, myocardial infarction***
GI: Nausea, vomiting, diarrhea, anorexia, pancreatitis, cramps, constipation, increased appetite, increased weight, ***cholestatic jaundice***
EENT: Contact lens intolerance, increased myopia, astigmatism
GU: Amenorrhea, cervical erosion, breakthrough bleeding, dysmenorrhea, vaginal candidiasis, breast changes, *gynecomastia, testicular atrophy, impotence*
INTEG: Rash, urticaria, acne, hirsutism, alopecia, oily skin, seborrhea, purpura, melasma
META: Folic acid deficiency, hypercalcemia, hyperglycemia
Contraindications: Thromboembolic disorders, reproductive cancer, genital bleeding (abnormal, undiagnosed), pregnancy (X)
Precautions: Hypertension, asthma, blood dyscrasias, gallbladder disease, CHF, diabetes mellitus, bone disease, depression, migraine headache, convulsive disorders, hepatic disease, renal disease, family history of cancer of breast or reproductive tract
Pharmacokinetics:
PO: Degraded in liver; excreted in urine, breast milk; crosses placenta
Interactions:
• Decreased action of anticoagulants, oral hypoglycemics
• Toxicity: tricyclic antidepressants
• Decreased action of estradiol: anticonvulsants, barbiturates, phenylbutazone, rifampin
• Increased action of corticosteroids
NURSING CONSIDERATIONS
Assess:
• Blood glucose of diabetic patient

• Weight daily, notify physician of weekly weight gain >5 lb; if increase, diuretic may be ordered
• B/P q4h; watch for increase caused by H_2O, Na retention
• I&O ratio; be alert for decreasing urinary output, increasing edema
• Liver function studies: AST (SGOT), ALT (SGPT), bilirubin, alk phosphatase
• Hypertension, cardiac symptoms, jaundice, hypercalcemia
• Mental status: affect, mood, behavioral changes, aggression

Administer:
• Titrated dose; use lowest effective dose
• IM injection deep in large muscle mass
• With food or milk to decrease GI symptoms

Evaluate:
• Therapeutic response: absence of breast engorgement, reversal of menopause, or decrease in tumor size in prostatic cancer

Teach patient/family:
• To weigh weekly, report gain >5 lb
• To report breast lumps, vaginal bleeding, edema, jaundice, dark urine, clay-colored stools, dyspnea, headache, blurred vision, abdominal pain, numbness or stiffness in legs, chest pain; male to report impotence or gynecomastia

ethionamide (℞)

(e-thye-on-am′ide)
Trecator-SC
Func. class.: Antitubercular
Chem. class.: Thiomine derivative

Action: Bacteriostatic against *M. tuberculosis*
Uses: Pulmonary, extrapulmonary TB when other antitubercular drugs have failed

Dosage and routes:
• *Adult:* PO 500 mg-1 g qd in divided doses, with another antitubercular drug and pyridoxine
• *Child:* PO 15-20 mg/kg/day in 3-4 doses, not to exceed 1g

Available forms: Tabs 250 mg

Side effects/adverse reactions:
INTEG: Dermatitis, alopecia, acne
CV: Severe postural hypotension
CNS: Headache, drowsiness, tremors, ***convulsions,*** depression, psychosis, dizziness, peripheral neuritis
GI: ***Anorexia, nausea, vomiting,*** *diarrhea,* metallic taste
EENT: Blurred vision, optic neuritis
HEMA: ***Thrombocytopenia,*** purpura
MISC: Gynecomastia, impotence, menorrhagia, difficulty managing diabetes mellitus

Contraindications: Hypersensitivity, severe hepatic disease
Precautions: Pregnancy (D), lactation, renal disease, diabetic retinopathy, cataracts, ocular defects, child <13 yr

Pharmacokinetics:
PO: Peak 3 hr, duration 9 hr, half-life 3 hr; metabolized in liver; excreted in urine (unchanged drug/inactive); crosses placenta

Interactions:
• Increased neurotoxicity: cycloserine, ethyl alcohol
• Increased adverse reactions: TB test agents, anti-TB drugs

NURSING CONSIDERATIONS
Assess:
• Signs of anemia: Hgb, Hct, fatigue
• Liver studies qwk: ALT (SGOT), AST (SGPT), bilirubin
• Mental status often: affect, mood, behavioral changes; psychosis may occur

* Available in Canada only

• Hepatic status: decreased appetite, jaundice, dark urine, fatigue
Administer:
• With meals or antacids to decrease GI symptoms
• Antiemetic if vomiting occurs
• After C&S is completed, qmo to detect resistance
• Pyridoxine to prevent neuritis
Evaluate:
• Therapeutic response: decreased symptoms of TB
Teach patient/family:
• That compliance with dosage schedule, duration are necessary
• To avoid alcohol while taking this drug
• To notify prescriber of depression, mood changes, which are symptoms of toxicity

ethosuximide (℞)

(eth-oh-sux′i-mide)
Zarontin
Func. class.: Anticonvulsant
Chem. class.: Succinimide

Action: Inhibits spike, wave formation in absence seizures (petit mal), decreases amplitude, frequency, duration, spread of discharge in minor motor seizures
Uses: Absence seizures, partial seizures, tonic-clonic seizures
Dosage and routes:
• *Adult and child >6 yr:* PO 250 mg bid initially; may increase by 250 mg q4-7d, not to exceed 1.5 g/day
• *Child 3-6 yr:* PO 250 mg/day or 125 mg bid; may increase by 250 mg q4-7d, not to exceed 1.5 g/day
Available forms: Caps 250 mg, syr 250 mg/5 ml
Side effects/adverse reactions:
HEMA: ***Agranulocytosis, aplastic anemia, thrombocytopenia, leukocytosis, eosinophilia, pancytopenia***
CNS: Drowsiness, dizziness, fatigue, euphoria, lethargy, anxiety, aggressiveness, irritability, depression, insomnia, headache
GI: Nausea, vomiting, heartburn, anorexia, diarrhea, abdominal pain, cramps, dry mouth, constipation, hiccups, weight loss, gum hypertrophy, tongue swelling
GU: Vaginal bleeding, pink, brown urine
INTEG: Urticaria, pruritic erythema, hirsutism, ***Stevens-Johnson syndrome***
EENT: Myopia, blurred vision
Contraindications: Hypersensitivity to succinimide derivatives
Precautions: Lactation, pregnancy (C), hepatic disease, renal disease
Pharmacokinetics:
PO: Peak 1-7 hr, steady state 4-7 days; metabolized by liver; excreted in urine, bile, feces; half-life 24-60 hr
Interactions:
• Antagonist effect: tricyclic antidepressants (imipramine, doxepin)
• Decreased effects of estrogens, oral contraceptives
Lab test interferences:
False positive: Direct Coombs' test
NURSING CONSIDERATIONS
Assess:
• Renal studies: urinalysis, BUN, urine creatinine
• Blood studies: CBC, Hct, Hgb, reticulocyte counts qwk for 4 wk, then qmo
• Hepatic studies: AST (SGOT), ALT (SGPT), bilirubin
• Drug levels during initial treatment, therapeutic range (40-100 μg/ml)
• Mental status: mood, sensorium, affect, behavioral changes; if mental status changes, notify prescriber
• Eye problems: need for ophthalmic examinations before, during, after

treatment (slit lamp, fundoscopy, tonometry)
• Allergic reaction: red raised rash, exfoliative dermatitis; if these occur, drug should be discontinued
• Blood dyscrasias: fever, sore throat, bruising, rash, jaundice
• Toxicity: bone marrow depression, nausea, vomiting, ataxia, diplopia, cardiovascular collapse, Stevens-Johnson syndrome

Administer:
• With food, milk to decrease GI symptoms

Perform/provide:
• Hard candy, frequent rinsing, gum for dry mouth
• Assistance with ambulation early in treatment; dizziness occurs
• Seizure precautions: padded side rails, move objects that could harm patient

Evaluate:
• Therapeutic response: decreased seizure activity; document on patient's chart

Teach patient/family:
• To carry ID card or Medic Alert bracelet stating patient's name, drugs taken, condition, prescriber's name, phone number
• To avoid driving, other activities that require alertness
• To avoid alcohol ingestion, CNS depressants; increased sedation may occur
• Not to discontinue medication quickly after long-term use; absence seizures may occur
• To continue regular dental checkups to identify gingival hyperplasia

Treatment of overdose: Lavage, activated charcoal; monitor electrolytes, VS

ethotoin (℞)

(eth'oh-toyin)
Peganone
Func. class.: Anticonvulsant
Chem. class.: Hydantoin derivative

Action: Inhibits nerve impulses in the motor cortex by decreasing sodium ion influx, limiting tetanic stimulation

Uses: Generalized tonic-clonic or complex-partial seizures

Dosage and routes:
• *Adult:* PO 250 mg qid pc initially; may increase over several days to 3 g/day in divided doses
• *Child:* PO 250 mg bid; may increase by 250 mg qid

Available forms: Tabs 250, 500 mg

Side effects/adverse reactions:
HEMA: ***Agranulocytosis, thrombocytopenia, leukopenia, pancytopenia, megaloblastic anemia,*** lymphadenopathy
CNS: Fatigue, insomnia, numbness, fever, headache, dizziness
GI: Nausea, vomiting, diarrhea, gingival hypertrophy
INTEG: Rash
EENT: Nystagmus, diplopia
CV: Chest pain

Contraindications: Hypersensitivity to hydantoins, blood dyscrasias, hematologic disease, hepatic disease, pregnancy (D), lactation

Pharmacokinetics: Metabolized by liver; excreted in urine; half-life 3-9 hr

Interactions:
• Decreased effects of rifampin, chronic alcohol, barbiturates, antihistamines, antacids, other anticonvulsants, antineoplastics, calcium products, folic acid, oxacillin
• Increased effects of benzodiazepines, cimetidine, salicylates, sul-

fonamide, pyrazolones, phenothiazines, estrogens, disulfiram, chloramphenicol, anticoagulants
• Seizures: valproic acid
• Paranoia: Phenacemide
• Myocardial depressions: lidocaine, propranolol, sympathomimetics

Lab test interferences:
Increase: Serum glucose, urine glucose, BSP, alk phosphatase
Decrease: Urinary steroids, PBI, dexamethasone/metyrapone tests

NURSING CONSIDERATIONS

Assess:
• Renal studies: urinalysis, BUN, urine creatinine
• Blood studies: RBC, Hct, Hgb, reticulocyte counts qwk for 4 wk then qmo
• Hepatic studies: AST (SGOT), ALT (SGPT), bilirubin, creatinine periodically
• For signs, symptoms of infection: sore throat, fever, bruising, petechiae
• Drug levels during initial treatment, therapeutic level (15-50 μg/ml)
• Mental status: mood, sensorium, affect, behavioral changes; if mental status changes, notify prescriber
• Eye problems: need for ophthalmic examinations before, during, after treatment (slit lamp, fundoscopy, tonometry)
• Allergic reaction: red raised rash; drug should be discontinued
• Blood dyscrasias: fever, sore throat, bruising, rash, jaundice
• Toxicity: bone marrow depression, nausea, vomiting, ataxia, diplopia, cardiovascular collapse, Stevens-Johnson syndrome, lupus-like syndrome

Administer:
• With food, milk for GI symptoms
• After meals

Perform/provide:
• Hard candy, frequent rinsing, gum for dry mouth
• Assistance with ambulation early in treatment; dizziness occurs
• Seizure precautions: padded side rails, removing items that may harm patient

Evaluate:
• Therapeutic response: decreased seizure activity, document on patient's chart

Teach patient/family:
• To carry ID card or Medic Alert bracelet stating patient's name, drugs taken, condition, prescriber's name, phone number
• To avoid driving, other activities that require alertness
• To avoid alcohol ingestion, CNS depressants; increased sedation may occur
• Notify dentist; use good oral hygiene; monitor gums
• Not to discontinue medication quickly after long-term use; taper off over several wk

Treatment of overdose: Lavage, activated charcoal; monitor electrolytes, VS

E

ethylnorepinephrine (℞)

(eth-il nor-ep-i-nef'rin)
Bronkephrine
Func. class.: Adrenergic
Chem. class.: Catecholamine

Action: α-Stimulation with vasoconstriction, pressor response, nasal decongestion and β_2-stimulation with vasodilation and bronchial dilation

Uses: Bronchospasm

Dosage and routes:
• *Adult:* IM/SC 0.5-1 ml
• *Child:* IM/SC 0.1-0.5 ml

Available forms: Inj 2 mg/ml
Side effects/adverse reactions:
CNS: Tremors, anxiety, insomnia, headache, dizziness, confusion,
CV: Palpitations, tachycardia, hypertension, chest pain, ***dysrhythmias***
GI: Anorexia, nausea, vomiting
Contraindications: Hypersensitivity to sympathomimetics, narrow-angle glaucoma
Precautions: Pregnancy (C), lactation, cardiac disorders, hyperthyroidism, diabetes mellitus, prostatic hypertrophy
Pharmacokinetics:
IM/SC: Onset 6-12 min, duration 1-2 hr
Interactions:
• Do not use with MAOIs or tricyclic antidepressants; hypertensive crisis may occur
• Decreased effect of ethylnorepinephrine when used with methyldopa, urinary acidifiers, rauwolfia alkaloids
• Increased effect of ethylnorepinephrine when used with urinary alkalizers
NURSING CONSIDERATIONS
Assess:
• B/P and pulse q5min after parenteral route
Perform/provide:
• Storage of reconstituted sol refrigerated no longer than 24 hr
• Do not use discolored sol
Evaluate:
• Therapeutic response: ease of breathing after several min
Teach patient/family:
• Reason to take drug

etidocaine (℞)
(et-ee′doe-kane)
Duranest HCl
Func. class.: Local anesthetic
Chem. class.: Amide

Action: Competes with calcium for sites in nerve membrane that control sodium transport across cell membrane; decreases rise of depolarization phase of action potential
Uses: Peripheral nerve block, caudal anesthesia, central neural block, vaginal block
Dosage and routes:
Varies with route of anesthesia
Available forms: Inj 1%, 1.5%
Side effects/adverse reactions:
CNS: Anxiety, restlessness, ***convulsions, loss of consciousness,*** drowsiness, disorientation, tremors, shivering
CV: ***Myocardial depression, cardiac arrest, dysrhythmias,*** bradycardia, hypotension, hypertension, ***fetal bradycardia***
GI: Nausea, vomiting
EENT: Blurred vision, tinnitus, pupil constriction
INTEG: Rash, urticaria, allergic reactions, edema, burning, skin discoloration at injection site, tissue necrosis
RESP: ***Status asthmaticus, respiratory arrest, anaphylaxis***
Contraindications: Hypersensitivity, child <12 yr, elderly, severe liver disease
Precautions: Severe drug allergies, pregnancy (B)
Pharmacokinetics: Onset 2-8 min, duration 3-6 hr; metabolized by liver, excreted in urine (metabolites)
Interactions:
• Dysrhythmias: epinephrine, halothane, enflurane

• Hypertension: MAOIs, tricyclic antidepressants, phenothiazines
• Decreased action of etidocaine: chloroprocaine

NURSING CONSIDERATIONS
Assess:
• B/P, pulse, respiration during treatment
• Fetal heart tones during labor
• Allergic reactions: rash, urticaria, itching
• Cardiac status: ECG for dysrhythmias, pulse, B/P during anesthesia

Administer:
• Only with crash cart, resuscitative equipment nearby
• Only drugs without preservatives for epidural or caudal anesthesia

Perform/provide:
• Use of new sol; discard unused portions

Evaluate:
• Therapeutic response: anesthesia necessary for procedure

Treatment of overdose: Airway, O_2, vasopressor, IV fluids, anticonvulsants for seizures

---

etidronate (℞)
(eh-tih-droe′nate)
Didronel, Didronel IV
Func. class.: Parathyroid agent (calcium regulator)
Chem. class.: Diphosphate

Action: Decreases bone resorption and new bone development (accretion)

Uses: Paget's disease, heterotopic ossification, hypercalcemia of malignancy

Dosage and routes:
Paget's disease
• *Adult:* PO 5-10 mg/kg/day 2 hr ac with H_2O, not to exceed 20 mg/kg/day, max 6 mo or 11-20 mg/kg/day for max of 3 mo

Heterotropic ossification
• *Adult:* PO 20 mg/kg qd × 2 wk, then 10 mg/kg/day for 10 wk, total 12 wk

Hypercalcemia
• *Adult:* IV 7.5 mg/kg/day × 3 days, then 20 mg/kg/day (PO)

Heterotopic ossification/hip replacement
• *Adult:* PO 20 mg/kg/day × 4 wk before and 3 mo after surgery

Available forms: Tabs 200, 400 mg; inj 300 mg/6 ml

Side effects/adverse reactions:
GI: Nausea, diarrhea
MS: Bone pain, hypocalcemia, decreased mineralization of nonaffected bones
GU: Nephrotoxicity

Contraindications: Pathologic fractures, children, colitis, severe renal disease with creatinine >5 mg/dl

Precautions: Pregnancy (B), renal disease, lactation, restricted Vit D/calcium

Pharmacokinetics: Not metabolized; excreted in urine/feces; therapeutic response: 1-3 mo

NURSING CONSIDERATIONS
Assess:
• I&O ratio; check for decreased output in renal patients
• BUN, creatinine, uric acid, phosphate chloride, albumin, pH, urine Ca, Mg, alk phosphatase, urinalysis; Ca should be kept at 9-10 mg/dl, Vit D 50-135 IU/dl
• Muscle spasm, laryngospasm, paresthesias, facial twitching, colic; may indicate hypocalcemia
• Nutritional status, diet for sources of Vit D (milk, some seafood), Ca (dairy products, dark green vegetables), phosphates—adequate intake is necessary
• Persistent nausea or diarrhea

Administer:
• On empty stomach with H_2O 2 hr ac

• Drug therapy should not last longer than 6 mo
• IV after diluting in 250 ml or more NS; give over 2 hr or longer
• Food, especially high in Ca; vitamins with mineral supplements or antacids high in metals should not be given within 2 hr of dose

Evaluate:
• Therapeutic response: prevention of bone deficiencies

Teach patient/family:
• To avoid OTC products
• That therapeutic response may take 1-3 mo; effects persist for months after drug is discontinued
• That adequate intake of Ca^+, Vit D is necessary

etodolac (℞)

(e-toe-doe'lak)
Lodine
Func. class.: Nonsteroidal antiinflammatory

Action: Inhibits prostaglandin synthesis by decreasing an enzyme needed for biosynthesis; analgesic, antiinflammatory, antipyretic
Uses: Mild to moderate pain, osteoarthritis
Dosage and routes:
Osteoarthritis
• *Adult:* PO 800-1200 mg/day in divided doses initially, then adjust dose to 600-1200 mg/day in divided doses; do not exceed 1200 mg/day; patients <60 kg not to exceed 20 mg/kg
Analgesia
• *Adult:* PO 200-400 mg q6-8h prn for acute pain; do not exceed 1200 mg/day; patients <60 kg, not to exceed 20 mg/kg
• ***Available forms:*** Caps 200, 300 mg
Side effects/adverse reactions:
CV: Tachycardia, peripheral edema, fluid retention, palpitations, dysrhythmias, CHF
GU: ***Nephrotoxicity: dysuria, hematuria, oliguria, azotemia,*** cystitis, urinary tract infection
HEMA: ***Blood dyscrasias***
INTEG: Erythema, urticaria, purpura, rash, pruritus, sweating
GI: Nausea, anorexia, vomiting, diarrhea, jaundice, ***cholestatic hepatitis,*** constipation, flatulence, cramps, dry mouth, peptic ulcer, dyspepsia, ***GI bleeding***
CNS: Dizziness, headache, drowsiness, fatigue, tremors, confusion, insomnia, anxiety, depression, lightheadedness, vertigo
EENT: Tinnitus, hearing loss, blurred vision
Contraindications: Hypersensitivity; patients in whom aspirin, iodides, or other nonsteroidal antiinflammatories have produced asthma, rhinitis, urticaria, nasal polyps, angioedema, bronchospasm
Precautions: Pregnancy (C); lactation; children; bleeding; GI, cardiac disorders; elderly; renal, hepatic disorders
Pharmacokinetics:
PO: Peak 1-2 hr, serum protein binding >90%, half-life 7 hr; metabolized by liver (metabolites excreted in urine)
Interactions:
• Increased action of coumarin, phenytoin, cyclosporin, lithium
• Decreased antihypertensive effects: β-blockers
• Decreased plasma concentration of etodolac: salicylates
• Increased concentration and toxicity of etodolac: probenecid

NURSING CONSIDERATIONS
Assess:
• Blood, renal, liver studies: BUN, creatinine, AST (SGOT), ALT (SGPT), Hgb, before treatment, periodically thereafter

• Audiometric, ophthalmic examination before, during, after treatment
• For eye, ear problems: blurred vision, tinnitus; may indicate toxicity

Administer:
• With food to decrease GI symptoms, since extent of absorption is not affected by food

Perform/provide:
• Storage at room temp

Evaluate:
• Therapeutic response: decreased pain, stiffness, swelling in joints, ability to move more easily

Teach patient/family:
• To report blurred vision or ringing, roaring in ears; may indicate toxicity
• To avoid driving, other hazardous activities if dizziness or drowsiness occurs
• To report change in urine pattern, weight increase, edema, pain increase in joints, fever, blood in urine; indicates nephrotoxicity
• That therapeutic effects may take up to 1 mo
• To avoid aspirin, alcoholic beverages while taking this medication

etomidate (℞)

(e-tom'I-date)
Amidate
Func. class.: General anesthetic
Chem. class.: Nonbarbiturate hypnotic

Action: Acts at level of reticular-activating system to produce anesthesia

Uses: Induction of general anesthesia

Dosage and routes:
• *Adult and child >10 yr:* IV 0.2-0.6 mg/kg over ½-1 min

Available forms: Inj 2 mg/ml

Side effects/adverse reactions:
GI: Nausea, vomiting (postoperatively)
CNS: Tonic movements, myoclonic movements, averting movements
CV: Tachycardia, hypotension, hypertension, bradycardia
ENDO: Decreases steroid production
RESP: ***Laryngospasm***
INTEG: Pain on administration

Contraindications: Hypersensitivity, labor/delivery

Precautions: Pregnancy (C), child <10 yr, lactation, liver disease

Pharmacokinetics:
IV: Onset 20 sec, peak 1 min, duration 3-5 min; half-life 75 min; metabolized in liver; excreted in urine

NURSING CONSIDERATIONS

Assess:
• I&O ratio for increasing urine output
• VS q10min during IV administration
• Plasma cortisol levels if administered over several hours (5-20 μg/100 ml normal level of cortisol)
• Increasing or decreasing heart rate or dysrhythmias shown on ECG

Administer:
• Corticosteroids for severe hypotension
• Only with crash cart, resuscitative equipment nearby
• IV slowly only; muscular twitching is reduced with fentanyl before anesthesia induction

Evaluate:
• Therapeutic response: induction of anesthesia

etoposide (℞)

(e-toe-poe'side)
VePesid
Func. class.: Antineoplastic
Chem. class.: Semisynthetic podophyllotoxin

Action: Inhibits mitotic activity through metaphase to mitosis; also inhibits cells from entering mitosis, depresses DNA, RNA synthesis
Uses: Leukemias, lung, testicular cancer, lymphomas, neuroblastoma, melanoma, ovarian cancer
Dosage and routes:
• *Adult:* IV 45-75 mg/m^2/day × 3-5 days given q3-5wk or 200-250 mg/m^2/wk, or 125-140 mg/m^2/day 3 × wk, q5wk
Available forms: Inj 20 mg/ml; caps 50 mg
Side effects/adverse reactions:
HEMA: ***Thrombocytopenia, leukopenia, myelosuppression, anemia***
GI: Nausea, vomiting, anorexia, ***hepatotoxicity***
INTEG: Rash, alopecia, phlebitis at IV site
RESP: ***Bronchospasm***
CV: Hypotension
CNS: Headache, *fever*
GU: ***Nephrotoxicity***
Contraindications: Hypersensitivity, bone marrow depression, severe hepatic disease, severe renal disease, bacterial infection, pregnancy (D)
Precautions: Renal disease, hepatic disease, lactation, children, gout
Pharmacokinetics: Half-life 3 hr, terminal 15 hr; metabolized in liver; excreted in urine; crosses placental barrier
Interactions:
• Increased pro-time: warfarin
Y-site compatibilities: Ondansetron, fludarabine, sargramostim, melphalan, paclitaxel
Additive compatibilities: Cisplatin, floxuridine, fluorouracil, ifosfamide
NURSING CONSIDERATIONS
Assess:
• CBC, differential, platelet count weekly; withhold drug if WBC is <4000 or platelet count is <75,000; notify prescriber
• Renal function studies: BUN, serum uric acid, urine CrCl, electrolytes before, during therapy
• I&O ratio; report fall in urine output to <30 ml/hr; check blood pressure bid and report any significant decrease
• Monitor temp q4h; may indicate beginning infection
• Liver function tests before, during therapy (bilirubin, AST [SGOT], ALT [SGPT], LDH) as needed or monthly
• RBC, Hct, Hgb; may be decreased
• Bleeding: hematuria, guaiac stools, bruising or petechiae, mucosa or orifices q8h
• Food preferences; list likes, dislikes
• Effects of alopecia on body image; discuss feelings about body changes
• Yellowing of skin and sclera, dark urine, clay-colored stools, itchy skin, abdominal pain, fever, diarrhea
• Buccal cavity q8h for dryness, sores or ulceration, white patches, oral pain, bleeding, dysphagia
• Local irritation, pain, burning, discoloration at injection site
• Symptoms indicating severe allergic reaction: rash, pruritus, urticaria, purpuric skin lesions, itching, flushing
• Symptoms of anaphylaxis: flushing, restlessness, coughing, difficulty breathing
• Frequency of stools, characteristics: cramping, acidosis; signs of de-

hydration: rapid respirations, poor skin turgor, decreased urine output, dry skin, restlessness, weakness

Administer:

- After diluting 100 mg/250 ml or more D_5W or NaCl to 0.2-0.4 mg/ml, infuse over 30-60 min
- Antiemetic 30-60 min before giving drug and prn to prevent vomiting
- Allopurinol or sodium bicarbonate to maintain uric acid levels, alkalinization of urine
- Hyaluronidase 150 U/ml to 1 ml NaCl to infiltration area, ice compress for vesicant activity
- Transfusion for anemia
- Antispasmodic

Perform/provide:

- Liquid diet: carbonated beverages, Jell-O; dry toast or crackers may be added if patient is not nauseated or vomiting
- Increase fluid intake to 2-3 L/day to prevent urate deposits, calculi formation
- Diet low in purines: organ meats (kidney, liver), dried beans, peas to maintain alkaline urine
- Nutritious diet with iron, vitamin supplements
- HOB raised to facilitate breathing

Evaluate:

- Therapeutic response: decreased tumor size, spread of malignancy

Teach patient/family:

- To report any complaints or side effects to nurse or prescriber
- To report any changes in breathing or coughing
- That hair may be lost during treatment; a wig or hairpiece may make patient feel better; tell patient that new hair may be different in color, texture
- To make position changes slowly to prevent fainting

etretinate (℞)

(e-tret′i-nate)

Tegison

Func. class.: Systemic antipsoriatic

Chem. class.: Retinol derivative

Action: Unknown; drug is related to retinol

Uses: Severe recalcitrant psoriasis, including erythrodermic and generalized pustular types

Dosage and routes:

- *Adult:* PO 0.75-1 mg/kg/day in divided doses, not to exceed 1.5 mg/kg/day; maintenance dose 0.5-0.75 mg/kg/day generally beginning after 8-16 wk of therapy

Available forms: Caps 10, 25 mg

Side effects/adverse reactions:

INTEG: Alopecia; peeling of palms, soles, fingertips; itching; rash; dryness; red scaling face; bruising; sunburn; pyogenic granuloma; paronychia; onycholysis; perspiration change, nail changes

CNS: Fatigue, headache, dizziness, fever, pain, anxiety, amnesia, depression

EENT: Eye irritation, pain, double vision, change in lacrimation, earache, otitis externa, dry nose, eyes, mouth, nosebleed, cheilitis, sore tongue

GI: Anorexia, abdominal pain, nausea, ***hepatitis,*** constipation, diarrhea, flatulence, weight loss

CV: Edema, ***CV obstruction, atrial fibrillation,*** chest pain, coagulation disorders

RESP: Dyspnea, cough

GU: WBC in urine, ***proteinuria,*** glycosuria, *increased BUN, creatinine,* ***hematuria,*** *casts,* ***acetonuria, hemoglobinuria, dysuria***

META: Increase or decrease K, Ca, P, Na, Cl

MS: Hyperostosis, bone pain, cramps, myalgia, gout, hypertonia
Contraindications: Pregnancy (X)
Precautions: Lactation, children, hepatic disease, diabetes, obesity
Pharmacokinetics: 99% plasma protein binding; excreted in bile, urine; terminal half-life 120 days; stored in fatty tissue
Interactions:
• Increased absorption of etretinate: milk

NURSING CONSIDERATIONS
Assess:
• For pseudotumor cerebri: headache, nausea, vomiting, visual problems, papilledema
• Hepatic studies: AST, ALT, LDH, since hepatotoxicity may occur
• Visual problems: blurring, decreased night vision, poor visual acuity; drug should be discontinued and ophthalmologist consulted
• Lipids before, q1-2wk during treatment; after discontinuing treatment, lipids will return to normal
Evaluate:
• Therapeutic response: decrease in scaling, itching, amount of psoriasis
Teach patient/family:
• To take with food
• Not to use during pregnancy; contraception must be used for 1 mo before and after therapy
• Not to take Vit A supplements
• That contact lens intolerance is common

factor IX complex (human)/factor IV (human) (℞)

Konyne 80, Proplex T, Proplex SX-T, Profilnine Heat-Treated/ Alpha Nine, Alpha-Nine SD, Mononine

Func. class.: Hemostatic

Chem. class.: Factors II, VII, IX, X

Action: Causes an increase in blood levels of clotting factors II, VII, IX, X; factor IX (Human) has IX activity
Uses: Hemophilia B (Christmas disease), factor IX deficiency, anticoagulant reversal, control of bleeding in patients with factor VIII inhibitors, reversal of overdose of anticoagulants in emergencies
Dosage and routes:
Factor IX complex (human) bleeding in hemophilia B
• *Adult/child:* IV: establish 25% of normal factor IX or 60-75 U/kg, then 10-20 U/kg/day ×/wk
Prophylaxis for bleeding in hemophilia B
• *Adult/child:* IV 10-20 U/kg 1-2 ×/wk
Bleeding in hemophilia A/Inhibitors of factor VIII
• *Adult/child:* IV 75 U/kg, repeat in 12 hr
Oral anticoagulant reversal
• *Adult/child:* IV 15 U/kg
Factor VII Deficiency (use Proplex T only)
• *Adult/child:* IV 0.5 U/kg × weight (kg) × desired factor IX increase (% of normal); repeat q4-6 hr if needed
Factor IX (human) minor-moderate hemorrhage
(Use only Alpha Nine, Alpha Nine SD)

* Available in Canada only

• *Adult/child:* IV Dose to increase factor IX level to 20%-30% in one dose

Serious hemorrhage

• *Adult/child:* IV Dose to increase factor IX to 30% 50% as daily Inf

Minor hemorrhage Mononine only

• *Adult/child:* IV Dose to increase factor IX to 15%-25% (20-30 U/kg) repeat in 24 hr if needed

Major hemorrhage

• *Adult/child:* IV dose to increase factor IX to 25%-50% (75 U/kg) q 18-30 hr × 10 day or less

Available forms: Inj (number of units noted on label)

Side effects/adverse reactions:

GI: Nausea, vomiting, abdominal cramps, jaundice, ***viral hepatitis***

INTEG: Rash, flushing, *urticaria*

CNS: Headache, dizziness, malaise, paresthesia, *lethargy, chills, fever, flushing*

HEMA: ***Thrombosis, hemolysis, AIDS, DIC***

CV: Hypotension, tachycardia, *MI,* ***venous thrombosis, pulmonary embolism***

RESP: ***Bronchospasm***

Contraindications: Hypersensitivity, hepatic disease, DIC, elective surgery, mild factor IX deficiency

Precautions: Neonates/infants, pregnancy (C)

Pharmacokinetics:

IV: Half-life factor VII—3-6 hr, factor IX—24-36 hr; rapidly cleared from plasma

Interactions:

• Incompatible with protein products

• Increased risk of thrombosis: aminocaproic acid; do not administer

NURSING CONSIDERATIONS

Assess:

• Blood studies (coagulation factors assays by % normal: 5% prevents spontaneous hemorrhage, 30%-50% for surgery, 80%-100% for severe hemorrhage)

• Increased B/P, pulse

• For bleeding q15-30min, immobilize and apply ice to affected joints

• I&O; if urine becomes orange or red, notify prescriber

• Allergic or pyrogenic reaction: fever, chills, rash, itching, slow infusion rate if not severe

• DIC: bleeding, ecchymosis, hypersensitivity, changes in coagulation tests

Administer:

• IV after warming to room temp 3 ml/min or less, with plastic syringe only; do not admix

• After dilution with provided diluent, 50 U/ml or 25 U/ml; do not exceed 10 ml/min; decrease rate if fever, headache, flushing, tingling occur

• After crossmatch if patient has blood type A, B, AB, to determine incompatibility with factor

Perform/provide:

• Storage of reconstituted sol for 3 hr at room temp or up to 2 yr refrigeration (powder); check expiration date

Evaluate:

• Therapeutic response: prevention of hemorrhage

Teach patient/family:

• To report any signs of bleeding: gums, under skin, urine, stools, emesis

• Risk of viral hepatitis, AIDS; to be tested q2-3mo for HIV

• That immunization for hepatitis B may be given first

• To carry ID identifying disease; avoid salicylates, inform other health professionals of condition

F

famciclovir (℞)

(fam-cy'clo-veer)
Famvir
Func. class.: Antiviral
Chem. class.: Guanosine nucleoside

Action: Inhibits DNA polymerase and viral DNS synthesis by conversion of this guanosine nucleoside to penciclovir
Uses: Treatment of acute herpes zoster, genital herpes
Dosage and routes:
Adult: PO 500 mg q8h; in renal disease, if CrCl is ≥60 ml/min/1.73 m^2, 500 mg q8h; if 40-59 ml/min/1.73 m^2, 500 mg q12h; if 20-39 ml/min/1.73 m^2, 500 mg q24hr
Available forms: Tabs 500 mg
Side effects/adverse reactions:
MS: Back pain, arthralgia
GU: Decreased sperm count
CNS: Headache, fatigue, dizziness, paresthesia, somnolence
RESP: Pharyngitis, sinusitis
GI: Nausea, vomiting, diarrhea, constipation, abdominal pain
INTEG: Pruritis
Contraindications: Hypersensitivity to this drug, penciclovir
Precautions: Renal disease, pregnancy (B), hypersensitivity to acyclovir, ganciclovir, lactation
Pharmacokinetics: Unknown
Interactions:
- Decreased renal excretion: theophylline

NURSING CONSIDERATIONS
Assess:
- For number, distribution of lesions; burning, itching, pain, which are early symptoms of herpes infection
- Renal function studies: urine CrCl, BUN before and during treatment if decreased renal function; dose may have to be lowered
- Bowel pattern before, during treatment; diarrhea may occur

Administer:
- With or without meals; absorption does not appear to be lowered when taken with food

Evaluate:
- Therapeutic response: decreased size, spread of lesions

Teach patient/family:
- How to recognize beginning infection
- How to prevent spread of infection
- Reason for medication, expected results

famotodine (℞)

(fa-moe'ti-deen)
Pepcid AC acid controller, Pepcid, Pepcid IV
Func. class.: H_2 histamine receptor antagonist

Action: Competitively inhibits histamine at histamine H_2 receptor site, decreasing gastric secretion while pepsin remains at a stable level
Uses: Short-term treatment of active duodenal ulcer, maintenance therapy for duodenal ulcer, Zollinger-Ellison syndrome, multiple endocrine adenomas, gastric ulcers; gastroesophageal reflux disease, heartburn
Dosage and routes:
Duodenal ulcer
- *Adult:* PO 40 mg qd hs × 4-8 wk, then 20 mg qd hs if needed (maintenance); IV 20 mg q12h if unable to take PO

Hypersecretory conditions
- *Adult:* PO 20 mg q6h; may give 160 mg q6h if needed; IV 20 mg q12h if unable to take PO

Heartburn relief/prevention
Adult: PO 10 mg with water or 1 hr before eating
Available forms: Tabs 10, 20, 40 mg; powder for oral susp 40 mg/5 ml; inj 10 mg/ml, 20 mg/50 ml 0.9% NaCl
Side effects/adverse reactions:
HEMA: ***Thrombocytopenia***
CNS: Headache, dizziness, paresthesia, ***seizure,*** depression, anxiety, somnolence, insomnia, fever
EENT: Taste change, tinnitus, orbital edema
GI: Constipation, nausea, vomiting, anorexia, cramps, abnormal liver enzymes
INTEG: Rash
MS: Myalgia, arthralgia
RESP: ***Bronchospasm***
Contraindications: Hypersensitivity
Precautions: Pregnancy (B), lactation, children <12 yr, severe renal disease, severe hepatic function, elderly
Pharmacokinetics: Absorption 50% (PO)
PO: Onset 30-60 min, duration 6-12 hr, peak 1-3 hr
IV: Onset immediate, peak 30-60 min, duration 6-12 hr, plasma protein-binding 15%-20%; metabolized in liver 30% (active metabolites), 70% excreted by kidneys, half-life 2½-3½ hr
Interactions:
• Decreased absorption: ketoconazole
• Decreased absorption of famotidine: antacids
Y-site compatibilities: Aminophylline, ampicillin, ampicillin/sulbactam, amrinone, atropine, bretylium, calcium gluconate, cefazolin, cefoperazone, cefotaxime, cefotetan, cefoxitin, ceftazidime, ceftizoxime, cefuroxime, cephalotin, cephapirin, dexamethasone, dextran 40, digoxin, dobutamine, dopamine, enalaprilat, epinephrine, erythromycin lactobionate, esmolol, folic acid, furosemide, gentamicin, haloperidol, heparin, hydrocortisone sodium succinate, imipenem/cilastatin, insulin, isoproterenol, labetalol, lidocaine, magnesium sulfate, melphalan, methylprednisolone, metoclopramide, mezlocillin, nitroglycerin, norepinephrine, ondansetron, oxacillin, paclitaxel, perphenazine, phenylephrine, phenytoin, phytonadione, piperacillin, potassium chloride, potassium phosphate, procainamide, sodium bicarbonate, sodium nitroprusside, theophylline, thiamine, ticarcillin, verapamil

NURSING CONSIDERATIONS

Assess:
• Blood counts during therapy; watch for decreasing platelets; if low, therapy may have to be discontinued and restarted after hematologic recovery
• For bleeding, hematuria, hematuresis, occult blood in stools
• Blood dyscrasias (thrombocytopenia): bruising, fatigue, bleeding, poor healing
Administer:
• Antacids 1 hr before or 2 hr after famotidine; may be given with foods or liquids
• After shaking oral suspension
• IV direct after diluting 2 ml of drug (10 mg/ml) in 0.9% NaCl to total volume of 5-10 ml; inject over 2 min to prevent hypotension
• IV intermittent infusion after diluting 2 mg of drug in 100 ml of LR, 0.9% NaCl, D_5W, $D_{10}W$; run over 15-30 min
Perform/provide:
• Storage in cool environment (oral); IV sol is stable for 48 hr at room temp; do not use discolored sol; discard unused oral sol after 1 mo

F

Evaluate:
• Therapeutic response: decreased abdominal pain
Teach patient/family:
• That drug must be continued for prescribed time in prescribed method to be effective; do not double dose
• To report bleeding, bruising, fatigue, malaise, since blood dyscrasias occur
• About possibility of decreased libido, reversible after discontinuing therapy
• To avoid irritating foods, alcohol, aspirin and extreme temp of foods that may irritate GI system
• That smoking should be avoided; diminishes effectiveness of drug
• To avoid tasks requiring alertness; dizziness, drowsiness may occur
• To increase bulk and fluids in the diet to prevent constipation

fat emulsions (℞)

Intralipid 10%, Intralipid 20%, Liposyn II 10%, Liposyn II 20%, Liposyn III 10%, Liposyn III 20%, Soyacal 20%

Func. class.: Caloric
Chem. class.: Fatty acid, long chain

Action: Needed for energy, heat production; consist of neutral triglycerides, primarily unsaturated fatty acids
Uses: Increase calorie intake, fatty acid deficiency, prevention
Dosage and routes:
Deficiency
• *Adult and child:* IV 8%-10% of required calorie intake (intralipid)
Adjunct to TPN
• *Adult:* IV 1 ml/min over 15-30 min (10%) or 0.5 ml/min over 15-30 min (20%); may increase to 500 ml over 4-8 hr if no adverse reactions occur; not to exceed 2.5 g/kg
• *Child:* IV 0.1 ml/min over 10-15 min (10%) or 0.05 ml/min over 10-15 min (20%); may increase to 1 g/kg over 4 hr if no adverse reactions occur; not to exceed 4 g/kg
Prevention of deficiency
• *Adult:* IV 500 ml 2 ×/wk (10%), given 1 ml/min for 30 min, not to exceed 500 ml over 6 hr
• *Child:* IV 5-10 ml/kg/day (10%), given 0.1 ml/min for 30 min, not to exceed 100 ml/hr
Available forms: Inj 10% (50, 100, 200, 250, 500 ml), 20% (50, 100, 200, 250, 500 ml)
Side effects/adverse reactions:
CNS: Dizziness, headache, drowsiness, focal seizures
CV: ***Shock***
GI: Nausea, vomiting, ***hepatomegaly***
RESP: Dyspnea, ***fat in lung tissue***
HEMA: ***Hyperlipemia, hypercoagulation, thrombocytopenia, leukopenia, leukocytosis***
Contraindications: Hypersensitivity, hyperlipemia, lipid necrosis, acute pancreatitis accompanied by hyperlipemia, hyperbilirubinemia of the newborn
Precautions: Severe liver disease, diabetes mellitus, thrombocytopenia, gastric ulcers, premature, term newborns, pregnancy (C), sepsis
Y-site compatibilities: Aldesleukin, ampicillin, cefamandole, cefazolin, cefoxitin, cephapirin, clindamycin, digoxin, dopamine, erythromycin lactobionate, furosemide, gentamicin, isoproterenol, lidocaine, kanamycin, norepinephrine, oxacillin, penicillin G potassium, ticarcillin, tobramycin
Additive compatibilities: Intralipid with FreAmine I 8.5%, FreAmine III 8.5%, Travasol without electrolytes 8.5% and 10%, or

Dextrose Injection 10% and 70%, nizatidine

NURSING CONSIDERATIONS

Assess:

- Triglycerides, free fatty acid levels, platelet counts daily to prevent fat overload, thrombocytopenia
- Liver function studies: AST (SGOT), ALT (SGPT) Hct, Hgb; notify prescriber if abnormal
- Nutritional status: calorie count by dietitian; monitor weight daily

Administer:

- By intermittent inf at 10% (1 ml/min); 20% (0.5 ml/min) initially × 15-30 min, may increase 10% (120 ml/hr); 20% (62.5 ml/hr) if no adverse reaction; do not give more than 500 ml/1st day
- After changing IV tubing at each infusion: infection may occur with old tubing
- With infusion pump at prescribed rate; do not use in-line filter sized for lipid emulsion; clogging will occur

Perform/provide:

- Do not use mixed sol separated or oily looking

Evaluate:

- Therapeutic response: increased weight

Teach patient/family

- Reason for use of lipids

felbamate (℞)

(fell-ba′mate)

Felbatol

Func. class.: Anticonvulsant

Chem. class.: Carbamate derivative

Action: Mechanism of action unknown; may increase seizure threshold; has weak inhibitory effects on GABA-receptor and benzodiazepine-receptor binding

Uses: Partial seizures, with or without generalization in adults; partial and generalized seizures in children with Lennox-Gastaut syndrome

Dosage and routes:

Adjunctive therapy

- *Adult:* PO add 1.2 g/day in 3-4 divided doses; reduce other anticonvulsants (valproic acid, phenytoin, carbamazepine and derivatives) by 20% to control plasma concentrations; may increase felbamate 1.2 g/day increments qwk, up to 3.6 g/day

Monotherapy

Adult: PO 1.2 g/day in 3-4 divided doses; titrate with close supervision; increase dose by 600-mg increments q2wk to 3.6 g/day if needed

Lennox-Gastaut syndrome

Adjunctive therapy

Child (2-14 yr): PO add 15 mg/kg/day in 3-4 divided doses; reduce other anticonvulsants (valproic acid, phenytoin, carbamazepine and derivatives) by 20% to control plasma concentrations; may increase felbamate 15 mg/kg/day qwk up to 45 mg/day

Available forms: Tabs 400, 600 mg; susp 600 mg/5 ml

Side effects/adverse reactions:

CNS: Dizziness, fatigue, headache, insomnia, anxiety, tremor, unsteady gait, depression, paresthesia

CV: Chest pain

EENT: Dry mouth, blurred vision, diplopia

GI: Nausea, constipation, diarrhea, anorexia, vomiting, abdominal pain, increased liver enzymes, hiccups

GU: Urinary incontinence, intramenstrual bleeding, *UTI*

HEMA: Purpura, ***leukopenia***

INTEG: Rash, acne

RESP: Upper respiratory tract infection, rhinitis, sinusitis, pharyngitis, coughing

Contraindications: Hypersensitivity to this drug, other carbamates
Precautions: Hepatic, renal, cardiac disease, psychosis, pregnancy (C), lactation, child <6 yr, elderly
Pharmacokinetics:
PO: Well absorbed, metabolized by liver, excreted in urine (40%-50% unchanged); crosses placenta, excreted in breast milk, terminal half-life 20-23 hr; protein binding (22%-25% to albumin)
Interactions:
• Increased levels of phenytoin, valproic acid
• Decreased levels: carbamazepine

NURSING CONSIDERATIONS
Assess:
• Renal studies: urinalysis, BUN, urine creatinine q3mo
• Hepatic studies: ALT (SGPT), AST (SGOT), bilirubin
• Description of seizures
• Mental status: mood, sensorium, affect, behavioral changes; if mental status changes, notify prescriber
• Eye problems: need for ophthalmic examinations before, during, after treatment (slit lamp, fundoscopy, tonometry)
• Allergic reaction: purpura, red raised rash; drug should be discontinued
Administer:
• With food, milk to decrease GI symptoms
• Shake susp well
Perform/provide:
• Storage at room temp away from heat and light
• Hard candy, frequent rinsing of mouth, gum for dry mouth
• Assistance with ambulation during early part of treatment; dizziness occurs
• Seizure precautions: padded side rails, move objects that may harm patient
Evaluate:
• Therapeutic response: decreased seizure activity; document on patient's chart
Teach patient/family:
• To carry Medic Alert ID stating patient's name, drugs taken, condition, prescriber's name, phone number
• To avoid driving, other activities that require alertness
• Not to discontinue medication quickly after long-term use
Treatment of overdose:
Lavage, VS

felodipine (℞)
(fell-oh'di-peen)
Plendil
Func. class.: Calcium channel blocker
Chem. class.: Dihydropyridine

Action: Inhibits calcium ion influx across cell membrane, resulting in dilation of peripheral arteries
Uses: Essential hypertension, alone or with other antihypertensives
Dosage and routes:
• *Adult:* PO 5 mg qd initially, usual range 5-10 mg qd; do not exceed 20 mg qd; do not adjust dosage at intervals of <2 wk
Available forms: Ext rel tabs 5, 10 mg
Side effects/adverse reactions:
CV: Dysrhythmia, edema, CHF, hypotension, palpitations, ***MI, pulmonary edema,*** tachycardia, syncope, AV block, angina
GI: Nausea, vomiting, diarrhea, gastric upset, constipation, increased liver function studies, dry mouth
GU: Nocturia, polyuria
INTEG: Rash, pruritus
MISC: Flushing, sexual difficulties, cough, nasal congestion, shortness

* Available in Canada only

of breath, wheezing, epistaxis, respiratory infection, chest pain
CNS: Headache, fatigue, drowsiness, dizziness, anxiety, depression, nervousness, insomnia, light-headedness, paresthesia, tinnitus, psychosis, somnolence
HEMA: Anemia
Contraindications: Hypersensitivity, sick sinus syndrome, 2nd or 3rd degree heart block
Precautions: CHF, hypotension <90 mm Hg systolic, hepatic injury, pregnancy (C), lactation, children, renal disease, elderly
Pharmacokinetics: Peak plasma levels 2.5-5 hr; highly protein bound, >99% metabolized in liver, 0.5% excreted unchanged in urine; elimination half-life 11-16 hr
Interactions:
• Increased effects of β-blockers, antihypertensives, digitalis
• Increased felodipine level: cimetidine, ranitidine
NURSING CONSIDERATIONS
Assess:
• Cardiac status: B/P, pulse, respiration, ECG
Administer:
• Once daily as whole tablet
Evaluate:
• Therapeutic response: decreased B/P
Teach patient/family:
• To swallow whole; do not crush or chew
• To avoid hazardous activities until stabilized on drug, dizziness is no longer a problem
• To limit caffeine consumption
• To avoid OTC drugs unless directed by a prescriber
• Importance of complying with all areas of medical regimen: diet, exercise, stress reduction, drug therapy
Treatment of overdose: Defibrillation, atropine for AV block, vasopressor for hypotension

fenofibrate (℞)
(fen-oh-fee′brate)
Lipidil
Func. class.: Antilipemic
Chem. class.: Aryloxisobutyric acid derivative

Action: Inhibits biosynthesis of low-density and very low density lipoproteins, which are responsible for triglyceride development; mobilizes triglycerides from tissue; increases excretion of neutral sterols
Uses: Types IV, V hyperlipidemia
Dosage and routes:
• *Adult:* PO 100 mg/day
Available forms: Caps 100 mg
Side effects/adverse reactions:
CNS: Fatigue, weakness, drowsiness, dizziness
CV: Angina, dysrhythmias, thrombophlebitis, ***pulmonary emboli***
GI: Nausea, vomiting, dyspepsia, increased liver enzymes, stomatitis, flatulence, hepatomegaly, gastritis, increased cholethiasis, weight gain
GU: Decreased libido, impotence, dysuria, proteinuria, oliguria, ***hematuria***
HEMA: ***Leukopenia,*** anemia, ***eosinophilia,*** bleeding
INTEG: Rash, urticaria, pruritus, dry hair and skin, alopecia
MISC: Polyphagia, weight gain
MS: Myalgias, arthralgias
Contraindications: Severe hepatic disease, severe renal disease, primary biliary cirrhosis
Precautions: Peptic ulcer, pregnancy (C), lactation
Pharmacokinetics: Not known
Interactions:
• Increased effects of sulfonylureas, insulin
• Increased toxicity of fenofibrate: probenecid

• Increased anticoagulant effects of oral anticoagulants
• Decreased effects of fenofibrate: rifampin

Lab test interferences:
Increase: Liver function studies, CPK, BSP, thymol turbidity

NURSING CONSIDERATIONS

Assess:
• Renal and hepatic levels if patient is on long-term therapy

Administer:
• Drug with meals if GI symptoms occur

Evaluate:
• Therapeutic response: decreased triglycerides, diarrhea, pruritus (excess bile acids)
• Bowel pattern daily; increase bulk, water in diet if constipation develops

Teach patient/family:
• That compliance is needed, since toxicity may result if doses are missed
• That risk factors should be decreased: high-fat diet, smoking, alcohol consumption, absence of exercise
• That birth control should be practiced while on this drug
• To report GU symptoms: decreased libido, impotence, dysuria, proteinuria, oliguria, hematuria

---

fenoprofen (℞)

(fen-oh-proe′fen)
fenoprofen, Nalfon

Func. class.: Nonsteroidal anti-inflammatory

Chem. class.: Propionic acid derivative

Action: Inhibits prostaglandin synthesis by decreasing enzyme needed for biosynthesis; analgesic, antiinflammatory, antipyretic

Uses: Mild to moderate pain, osteoarthritis, rheumatoid arthritis, acute gout, arthritis, ankylosing spondylitis, inflammation, dysmenorrhea

Dosage and routes:

Pain
• *Adult:* PO 200 mg q4-6h prn

Arthritis
• *Adult:* PO 300-600 mg qid, not to exceed 3.2 g/day

Available forms: Caps 200, 300 mg; tabs 600 mg

Side effects/adverse reactions:
GI: Nausea, anorexia, vomiting, diarrhea, jaundice, ***cholestatic hepatitis,*** constipation, flatulence, cramps, dry mouth, peptic ulcer
CNS: Dizziness, headache, drowsiness, fatigue, tremors, confusion, insomnia, anxiety, depression
CV: Tachycardia, peripheral edema, palpitations, dysrhythmias
INTEG: Purpura, rash, pruritus, sweating
GU: ***Nephrotoxicity: dysuria, hematuria, oliguria, azotemia***
HEMA: ***Blood dyscrasias***
EENT: Tinnitus, hearing loss, blurred vision

Contraindications: Hypersensitivity, asthma, severe renal disease, severe hepatic disease

Precautions: Pregnancy (B) 1st and 2nd trimester, lactation, children, bleeding disorders, GI disorders, cardiac disorders, hypersensitivity to other antiinflammatory agents

Pharmacokinetics:
PO: Peak 2 hr, half-life 3-3½ hr; metabolized in liver; excreted in urine (metabolites), breast milk; 99% plasma protein binding

Interactions:
• May increase the action of coumarin, sulfonamides, salicylates
• May decrease effects of fenoprofen: phenobarbital, probenecid

---

* Available in Canada only

NURSING CONSIDERATIONS
Assess:
• Renal, liver, blood studies: BUN, creatinine, AST (SGOT), ALT (SGPT), Hgb, before treatment, periodically thereafter
• Audiometric, ophthalmic examination before, during, after treatment
• For eye, ear problems: blurred vision, tinnitus; may indicate toxicity
Administer:
• With food for GI symptoms; however, best to take on empty stomach to facilitate absorption
Perform/provide:
• Storage at room temp
Evaluate:
• Therapeutic response: decreased pain, stiffness in joints, decreased swelling in joints, ability to move more easily
Teach patient/family:
• To report blurred vision, ringing, roaring in ears; may indicate toxicity
• To avoid driving, other hazardous activities if dizziness, drowsiness occurs
• To report change in urine pattern, increased weight, edema, increased pain in joints, fever, blood in urine; indicates nephrotoxicity
• That therapeutic effects may take up to 1 mo
• To take with a full glass of water to enhance absorption
• To avoid concurrent use of alcohol, aspirin, acetaminophen, other OTC meds without consulting prescriber

fentanyl (℞)
(fen'ta-nill)
Fentanyl, Sublimaze
Func. class.: Narcotic analgesic
Chem. class.: Opiate, synthetic phenylpiperidine derivative

Controlled Substance Schedule II
Action: Inhibits ascending pain pathways in CNS, increases pain threshold, alters pain perception by binding to opiate receptors
Uses: Preoperatively, postoperatively; adjunct to general anesthetic, when combined with droperidol
Dosage and routes:
Anesthetic
• *Adult:* IV 0.05-0.1 mg q2-3min prn
Preoperatively
• *Adult:* IM 0.05-0.1 mg q30-60 min before surgery
Postoperatively
• *Adult:* IM 0.05-0.1 mg ql-2h prn
• *Child:* IM 0.02-0.03 mg/9 kg
Available forms: Inj 0.05 mg/ml
Side effects/adverse reactions:
CNS: Dizziness, delirium, euphoria
GI: Nausea, vomiting
MS: Muscle rigidity
EENT: Blurred vision, miosis
CV: ***Bradycardia, arrest,*** hypotension or hypertension
RESP: ***Respiratory depression, arrest, laryngospasm***
Contraindications: Hypersensitivity to opiates, myasthenia gravis
Precautions: Elderly, respiratory depression, increased intracranial pressure, seizure disorders, severe respiratory disorders, cardiac dysrhythmias, pregnancy (C), lactation
Pharmacokinetics:
IM: Onset 7-15 min, peak 30 min, duration 1-2 hr
IV: Onset immediate, peak 3-5 min, duration ½-1 hr; metabolized by

liver; excreted by kidneys; crosses placenta; excreted in breast milk; half-life 2½-4 hr; 80% bound to plasma proteins

Interactions:

• Effects may be increased with other CNS depressants: alcohol, narcotics, sedative/hypnotics, antipsychotics, skeletal muscle relaxants

Syringe compatibilities: Atropine, butorphanol, chlorpromazine, cimetidine, dimenhydrinate, diphenhydramine, droperidol, heparin, hydromorphone, hydroxyzine, meperidine, metoclopramide, midazolam, morphine, pentazocine, perphenazine, prochlorperazine edisylate, promazine, promethiazine, ranitidine, scopolamine

Y-site compatibilities: Atracurium, enalaprilat, esmolol, heparin, hydrocortisone sodium succinate, labetalol, nafcillin, pancuronium, potassium chloride, vecuronium

Additive compatibility: Bupivacaine

Solution compatibilities: D_5W, 0.9% NaCl

NURSING CONSIDERATIONS

Assess:

• VS after parenteral route; note muscle rigidity, drug history, liver, kidney function test

• CNS changes: dizziness, drowsiness, hallucinations, euphoria, LOC, pupil reaction

• Allergic reactions: rash, urticaria

• Respiratory dysfunction: respiratory depression, character, rate, rhythm; notify prescriber if respirations are <10/min

Administer:

• By injection (IM, IV); give slowly to prevent rigidity

• Only with resuscitative equipment available

• IV undiluted by anesthesiologist or diluted with 5 ml or more sterile H_2O or 0.9% NaCl given through Y-tube or 3-way-stopcock at 0.1 mg or less/1-2 min

Perform/provide:

• Storage in light-resistant area at room temp

• Coughing, turning, deep breathing for postoperative patients

• Safety measures: side rails, nightlight, call bell within reach

Evaluate:

• Therapeutic response: induction of anesthesia

---

fentanyl/droperidol combination (℞)

(fen'ta-nil) (droe-per'i-dole)

Innovar

Func. class.: General anesthetic/narcotic analgesic

Chem. class.: Phenylpiperone derivative

Controlled Substance Schedule II

Action: Action at subcortical levels to reduce motor activity, produces analgesia

Uses: Premedication, adjunct to general anesthesia, maintenance of anesthesia

Dosage and routes:

Induction

• *Adult:* IV 1 ml/20-25 lb

• *Child:* IV 0.5 ml/20 lb

Premedication

• *Adult:* IM 0.5-2 ml 45-60 min before surgery or procedure

• *Child:* IM 0.25 ml/20 lb 45-60 min before surgery or procedure

Available forms: Inj 0.05 mg fentanyl, 2.5 mg droperidol/ml

Side effects/adverse reactions:

RESP: ***Laryngospasm, bronchospasm, respiratory arrest***

CNS: Dystonia, akathisia, flexion of arms, fine tremors, dizziness, anxiety, drowsiness, restlessness, hallu-

---

* Available in Canada only

cination, depression, muscular rigidity, EPS
CV: Tachycardia, hypotension, circulatory depression
EENT: Upward rotation of eyes, oculogyric crisis, blurred vision
INTEG: Chills, facial sweating, shivering, diaphoresis
GI: Nausea, vomiting
Contraindications: Hypersensitivity, child < 2 yr, myasthenia gravis
Precautions: Elderly, increased intracranial pressure, cardiovascular disease (bradydysrhythmias), renal disease, liver disease, Parkinson's disease, COPD, pregnancy (C)
Pharmacokinetics:
IV: Onset 20 sec, peak 2-10 min, duration ½-2 hr; tranquilizing effect may last up to 12h
IM: Onset 7 min, duration 1-2 hr; metabolized in liver; excreted in urine metabolites (90%)
Interactions:
• Increased CNS depression: alcohol, narcotics, barbiturates, antipsychotics, other CNS depressants
• Decreased effects of amphetamines, anticonvulsants, anticoagulants
• Increased intraocular pressure: anticholinergics, antiparkinson drugs
• Increased side effects of lithium
• Incompatible with diazepam, methohexitol, nafcillin, phenobarbital, phenytoin, $NaCO_3$, thiopental in sol or syringe
NURSING CONSIDERATIONS
Assess:
• VS q10min during IV administration, q30min after IM dose
• Liver functions test and BUN, creatinine, $Paco_2$
• Rigidity of skeletal muscles
• EPS: dystonia, akathisia
• Increasing heart rate or decreasing B/P by >10% from baseline; notify prescriber at once; do not place patient in Trendelenburg position or sympathetic blockade may occur, causing respiratory arrest
Administer:
• Anticholinergics (benztropine, diphenhydramine) for EPS
• Only with crash cart, resuscitative equipment nearby; narcotic antagonist for severe respiratory depression, cardiac monitor
• IV direct undiluted through Y-tube or 3-way stopcock; give each 1 ml undiluted drug/1min or more; 0.1 ml/kg may be diluted in 250 ml D_5W and given as IV inf over 5-10 min; titrate to response
Perform/provide:
• Slow movement of patient to avoid orthostatic hypotension
Evaluate:
• Therapeutic response: decreased anxiety, absence of vomiting, maintenance of anesthesia
Teach patient/family:
• To use deep breathing, turning, coughing after surgery to prevent increased secretions in lungs

fentanyl transdermal (℞)

Duragesic-25, Duragesic-50, Duragesic-75, Duragesic-100
Func. class.: Narcotic analgesic
Chem. class.: Opiate, synthetic phenylpiperidine

Controlled Substance Schedule II
Action: Inhibits ascending pain pathways in CNS, increases pain threshold, alters pain perception by binding to opiate receptors
Uses: Management of chronic pain for those requiring opioid analgesia
Dosage and routes:
Adult: 25 μg/hr; may increase until pain relief occurs; apply patch to flat surface on upper torso and wear

for 72 hr; apply new patch on different site for continued relief

Available forms: Patch 2.5, 5, 7.5, 10 mg/hr

Side effects/adverse reactions:

CNS: Dizziness, delirium, euphoria, light-headedness, sedation, dysphoria, agitation, anxiety

GI: Nausea, vomiting, diarrhea, cramps

EENT: Blurred vision, miosis

CV: Bradycardia, ***cardiac arrest,*** hypotension or hypertension, facial flushing, chills

RESP: ***Respiratory depression, laryngospasm, bronchospasm***; depresses cough; hypoventilation

Contraindications: Hypersensitivity to opiates, myasthenia gravis, children <12 yr, patient <18 yr with weight <110 lbs

Precautions: Elderly, respiratory depression, increased intracranial pressure, seizure disorders, severe respiratory disorders, cardiac dysrhythmias, pregnancy (C), fever

Interactions:

• Effects may be increased with other CNS depressants: alcohol, narcotics, sedative/hypnotics, antipsychotics, skeletal muscle relaxants

NURSING CONSIDERATIONS

Assess:

• Pain contol; check for duration, site, character of pain, fever; use pain and sedation scoring

• CNS changes: dizziness, drowsiness, hallucinations, euphoria, LOC, pupil reaction

• Allergic reactions: rash, urticaria

• Respiratory dysfunction: respiratory depression, character, rate, rhythm; notify prescriber if respirations are <10/min

Administer:

• q72h for continuous pain relief; dosage is adjusted after at least 2 applications

• Give short-acting analgesics until patch takes effect (24 hrs)

Perform/provide:

• Safety measures: side rails, night-light, call bell within reach

Evaluate:

• Therapeutic response: decreased pain

Teach patient/family:

• Avoid activities that require alertness

ferrous fumarate/ ferrous gluconate/ ferrous sulfate (℞)

(fer'us)

Femiron, Feostat, Ferrets, Ferrous Fumarate, Fumasorb, Fumerin, Hemocyte, Ircon, Nephro-Fer, Span-FF, Fergon, Ferralet, Ferralet S.R., Ferrous Gluconate, Simron, Feosol, Feratab, Fer-In-Sol, Fer-Iron, Fero-Gradumet, Ferospace, Ferralyn, Ferra-TD, Ferrous Sulfate, Mol-Iron, Slow-Fe

Func. class.: Hematinic

Chem. class.: Iron preparation

Combination products: Fermalox: ferrous SO_4 200 mg, magnesium hydroxide, dried aluminum hydroxide gel 200 mg; Ferocyl: iron (fumarate) 50 mg, docusate sodium 100 mg; Ferro-Sequels: iron (fumarate) 50 mg, docusate sodium 100 mg; Simron: iron (gluconate) 10 mg, polysorbate 20, 400 mg

Action: Replaces iron stores needed for red blood cell development, energy and O_2 transport, utilization; fumarate contains 33% elemental iron; gluconate, 12%; sulfate, 20%; iron, 30%; ferrous sulfate exsiccated

* Available in Canada only

Uses:
Iron deficiency anemia, prophylaxis for iron deficiency in pregnancy

Dosage and routes:

Fumarate
• *Adult:* PO 200 mg tid-qid
• *Child:* 2-12 yr: PO 3 mg/kg/day (elemental iron) tid-qid
• *Child 6 mo-2 yr:* PO up to 6 mg/kg/day (elemental iron) tid-qid
• *Child: 6 mo-2 yr:* PO 6 mg/kg/day in 3-4 divided doses
• *Infants:* PO 10-25 mg/day (elemental iron) in 3-4 divided doses

Gluconate
• *Adult:* PO 200-600 mg tid
• *Child 6-12 yr:* PO 300-900 mg qd
• *Child <6 yr:* PO 100-300 mg qd

Sulfate
• *Adult:* PO 0.75-1.5 g/day in divided doses tid
• *Child 6-12 yr:* PO 600 mg/day in divided doses

Pregnancy
• *Adult:* PO 300-600 mg/day in divided doses

Available forms:

Fumarate
Tabs 63, 195, 200, 324, 325 mg; tabs chewable 100 mg; tabs controlled-release 300 mg; oral susp 100 mg/5 ml, 45 mg/0.6 ml

Gluconate
Tabs 300, 320, 325 mg; caps 86, 325, 435 mg; tabs film-coated 300 mg; elix 300 mg/5 ml

Sulfate
Tabs, 195, 300, 325 mg; tabs enteric-coated 325 mg; tabs extended-release, time-release caps, 525 mg

Side effects/adverse reactions:
GI: Nausea, constipation, epigastric pain, black and red tarry stools, vomiting, diarrhea
INTEG: Temporarily discolored tooth enamel and eyes

Contraindications: Hypersensitivity, ulcerative colitis/regional enteritis, hemosiderosis/hemochromatosis, peptic ulcer disease, hemolytic anemia, cirrhosis

Precautions: Anemia (long-term), pregnancy (A)

Pharmacokinetics:
PO: Excreted in feces, urine, skin, breast milk; enters bloodstream; bound to transferrin; crosses placenta

Interactions:
• Decreased absorption of: penicillamine, levodopa, methyldopa, quinolone, tetracycline
• Decreased absorption of iron preparations: antacids, tetracycline, vit E
• Increased absorption of iron preparation: ascorbic acid, chloramphenicol

Lab test interferences:
False-positive: Occult blood

NURSING CONSIDERATIONS

Assess:
• Blood studies: Hct, Hgb, reticulocytes, bilirubin before treatment, at least monthly
• Toxicity: nausea, vomiting, diarrhea (green, then tarry stools), hematemesis, pallor, cyanosis, shock, coma
• Elimination; if constipation occurs, increase water, bulk, activity
• Nutrition: amount of iron in diet (meat, dark green leafy vegetables, dried beans, dried fruits, eggs)
• Cause of iron loss or anemia, including salicylates, sulfonamides, antimalarials, quinidine

Administer:
• Only with vit E supplements to infants or hemolytic anemia may occur
• Between meals for best absorption; may give with juice; do not give with antacids or milk, delay at least 1 hr; if GI symptoms occur, give pc even if absorption is decreased; eggs, milk products, choco-

late, caffeine interfere with absorption
• Through plastic straw to avoid discoloration of tooth enamel; dilute thoroughly
• At least 1 hr before hs, since corrosion may occur in stomach
• For <6 months for anemia

Perform/provide:
• Storage in tight, light-resistant container

Evaluate:
• Therapeutic response: improvement in Hct, Hgb, reticulocytes, decreased fatigue, weakness

Teach patient/family:
• That iron will change stools black or dark green
• That iron poisoning may occur if increased beyond recommended level
• Not to crush; swallow tablet whole
• To keep out of reach of children
• Not to substitute one iron salt for another; elemental iron content differs (e.g., 300 mg ferrous fumarate contains about 100 mg elemental iron; 300 mg ferrous gluconate contains only about 30 mg elemental iron)
• To avoid reclining position for 15-30 min after taking drug to avoid esophageal corrosion
• To follow diet high in iron

Treatment of overdose: Induce vomiting; give eggs, milk until lavage can be done

fibrinolysin/desoxyribonuclease (℞)

(fye-brin-oh-lye′sin/dez-ox-ee-rye-boo-nuke′lee-ase)
Elase
Func. class.: Enzyme
Chem. class.: Proteolytic-bovine

Action: Dissolves fibrin in clots and fibrinous exudates; attacks DNA in areas of disintegrating cells

Uses: Debridement of wounds, vaginitis, cervicitis, ulcerative colitis, 2nd, 3rd degree burns; irrigating wounds, topically

Dosage and routes:

Debridement/intravaginally
• *Adult:* OINT 5 g × 5 applications

Irrigating
• *Adult:* IRIG dilution depends on type of wound

Available forms: Fibrinolysin with desoxyribonuclease 666.6 U/g; powder for reconstitution fibrinolysin 25 U/desoxyribonuclease 15,000 U

Side effects/adverse reactions:
INTEG: Hyperemia

Contraindications: Hypersensitivity to bovine or mercury products, hematoma

Precautions: Pregnancy (C)

NURSING CONSIDERATIONS

Assess:
• For signs of irritation and inflammation; drug should be discontinued
• Wound: drainage, color, odor, size, depth

Administer:
• After reconstituting with 10 ml sterile NaCl sol; use only fresh sol
• After removing necrotic debris, dry eschar
• Wet dressing by mixing 1 vial elase/10-50 ml NS; saturate gauze with sol; pack area; remove in 6-8 hr; repeat tid-qid

Perform/provide:
• Cleansing of wound using aseptic technique; cover with drug, then dressing; change at least qid

Evaluate:
• Therapeutic response: decrease in wound scarring, tissue necrosis

* Available in Canada only

filgrastim (℞)

(fill-grass'stim)

Neupogen, G-CSF, granulocyte colony stimulator

Func. class.: Biologic modifier

Chem. class.: Granulocyte colony-stimulating factor

Action: Stimulates proliferation and differentiation of neutrophils

Uses: To decrease infection in patients receiving antineoplastics that are myelosuppressive; to increase WBC in patients with drug-induced neutropenia; bone marrow transplantation

Dosage and routes:

• *Adult:* IV/SC 5 μg/kg/day in a single dose; may increase by 5 μg/kg in each chemotherapy cycle; give qd for up to 2 wk until the absolute neutrophil count (ANC) 10,000/mm^3; response to G-CSF is much greater with SC than IV therapy

Available forms: Inj 300 μg/ml

Side effects/adverse reactions:

RESP: Respiratory distress syndrome

CNS: Fever

HEMA: ***Thrombocytopenia***

INTEG: Alopecia, exacerbation of skin conditions

MS: Osteoporosis, skeletal pain

GI: Nausea, vomiting, diarrhea, mucositis, anorexia

Contraindications: Hypersensitivity to proteins of *E. coli*

Precautions: Pregnancy (C), lactation, cardiac conditions, children, myeloid malignancies

Pharmacokinetics: Metabolism, excretion, distribution not known

Interactions:

• Do not use this drug concomitantly with antineoplastics

Lab test interferences:

Increase: Uric acid, lactate dehydrogenase, alk phosphatase

NURSING CONSIDERATIONS

Assess:

• Blood studies: CBC, platelet count before treatment and twice weekly; neutrophil counts may be increased for 2 days after therapy

Administer:

• 300 μg/ml or 480 μg/1.6 ml; allow to warm to room temp; give single dose over 1 min or less through Y-tube or medport

• Using single-use vials; after dose is withdrawn, do not reenter vial

• For 2 wk or until ANC is 10,000/mm^3 after the expected chemotherapy neutrophil nadir

Perform/provide:

• Storage in refrigerator; do not freeze; may store at room temp; up to 6 hr

• Avoid shaking

Evaluate:

• Therapeutic response: absence of infection

Teach patient/family:

• Technique for self-administration: dose, side effects, disposal of containers and needles; provide instruction sheet

finasteride (℞)

(fin-ass'te-ride)

Proscar

Func. class.: Androgen hormone inhibitor

Chem. class.: 5-α-reductase inhibitor

Action: Inhibits 5-α-reductase and reduction in DHT; DHT induces androgenic effects by binding to androgen receptors in the cell nuclei of the prostate gland, liver, skin; produces lower levels of 5-α-reductase which prevents development of BHP

Uses: Symptomatic benign prostatic hyperplasia

F

Dosage and routes:
• *Adult:* PO 5 mg qd × 6-12 mo
Available forms: Tab 5 mg
Side effects/adverse reactions:
GU: Impotence, decreased libido, decreased volume of ejaculate
Contraindications: Hypersensitivity, children, women
Precautions: Large residual urinary volume, severely diminished urinary flow, liver function abnormalities
Pharmacokinetics: Bioavailability 63%, plasma protein binding 90%; metabolized in the liver; excreted in urine (metabolites) 39%, feces (57%); crosses blood-brain barrier
Interactions:
• Increases theophylline clearance
NURSING CONSIDERATIONS
Assess:
• Urinary patterns, residual urinary volume, severely diminished urinary flow
• PSA levels and digital rectal exam prior to initiating therapy and periodically thereafter
• Liver function studies prior to treatment; extensively metabolized in liver
Administer:
• Without regard to meals
Perform/provide:
• Storage <86° F (30° C); protect from light; keep container tightly closed
Evaluate:
• Therapeutic response: increased urinary flow, decreased postvoiding dribbling, frequency, nocturia
Teach patient/family:
• Pregnant women should not touch crushed tablets or come into contact with semen of a patient taking this drug; may adversely affect developing male fetus
• That volume of ejaculate may be decreased during treatment; impotence and decreased libido may also occur

---

flavoxate (℞)
(fla-vox'ate)
Urispas
Func. class.: Spasmolytic
Chem. class.: Flavone derivative

Action: Relaxes smooth muscles in urinary tract
Uses: Relief of nocturia, incontinence, suprapubic pain, dysuria, frequency associated with urologic conditions (symptomatic only)
Dosage and routes:
• *Adult and child >12 yr:* PO 100-200 mg tid-qid
Available forms: Tabs 100 mg
Side effects/adverse reactions:
HEMA: ***Leukopenia, eosinophilia***
CNS: Anxiety, restlessness, dizziness, ***convulsions,*** headache, drowsiness, confusion, decreased concentration
CV: Palpitations, sinus tachycardia, hypotension
GI: Nausea, vomiting, anorexia, abdominal pain, constipation
GU: Dysuria
INTEG: Urticaria, dermatitis
EENT: Blurred vision, increased intraocular tension, dry mouth, throat
Contraindications: Hypersensitivity, GI obstruction, GI hemorrhage, GU obstruction
Precautions: Pregnancy (B), lactation, suspected glaucoma, children <12 yr
Pharmacokinetics: Excreted in urine
NURSING CONSIDERATIONS
Assess:
• Urinary status: dysuria, frequency, nocturia, incontinence

---

* Available in Canada only

• Allergic reactions: rash, urticaria; drug should be discontinued

Evaluate:

• Therapeutic response: decreased dysuria

Teach patient/family

• To avoid hazardous activities; dizziness may occur

flecainide (℞)

(flek-ay′nide)

Tambocor

Func. class.: Antidysrhythmic (Class IC)

Action: Decreases conduction in all parts of the heart, with greatest effect on His-Purkinje system, which stabilizes cardiac membrane

Uses: Life-threatening ventricular dysrhythmias, sustained ventricular tachycardia, supraventicular tachydysrhythmias

Dosage and routes:

• *Adult:* PO 50-100 mg q12h; may increase q4d by 50 mg q12h to desired response, not to exceed 400 mg/day

Available forms: Tabs 50, 100, 150 mg

Side effects/adverse reactions:

CNS: Headache, dizziness, involuntary movement, confusion, psychosis, restlessness, irritability, paresthesias, ataxia, flushing, somnolence, depression, anxiety, malaise

EENT: Tinnitus, *blurred vision,* hearing loss

GI: Nausea, vomiting, anorexia, constipation, abdominal pain, flatulence, change in taste

CV: Hypotension, bradycardia, angina, PVCs, ***heart block, cardiovascular collapse, arrest,*** *dysrhythmias,* ***CHF, fatal ventricular tachycardia***

RESP: Dyspnea, ***respiratory depression***

INTEG: Rash, urticaria, edema, swelling

HEMA: Leukopenia, thrombocytopenia

GU: Impotence, decreased libido, polyuria, urinary retention

Contraindications: Hypersensitivity, severe heart block, cardiogenic shock, nonsustained ventricular dysrhythmias, frequent PVCs, non-life-threatening dysrhythmias

Precautions: Pregnancy (C), lactation, children, renal disease, liver disease, CHF, respiratory depression, myasthenia gravis

Pharmacokinetics:

PO: Peak 3 hr; half-life 12-27 hr; metabolized by liver; excreted unchanged by kidneys (10%); excreted in breast milk

Interactions:

• Increased levels of both drugs: propranolol

• Increased level of flecainide: amiodarone, cimetidine

• Increased negative inotropic effects: disopyramide, verapamil

• Increased digoxin level: digoxin

Lab test interferences:

Increase: CPK

NURSING CONSIDERATIONS

Assess:

• For hypokalemia, hyperkalemia before administration; correct electrolytes

• Blood levels: trough (0.2-1 μg/ml)

• B/P, ECG continuously for fluctuations

• Malignant hyperthermia: tachypnea, tachycardia, changes in B/P, increased temp

• Cardiac rate, respiration: rate, rhythm, character, continuously

• Respiratory status: rate, rhythm, lung fields for rales

• CNS effects: dizziness, confusion, psychosis, paresthesias, convulsions; drug should be discontinued

• Increased respiration, increased pulse; drug should be discontinued
Administer:
• Reduced dosage as soon as dysrhythmia is controlled
Evaluate:
• Therapeutic response: decreased dysrhythmias
Teach patient/family:
• To change position slowly from lying or sitting to standing to minimize orthostatic hypotension
• To take as prescribed, not to skip or double dose
• To avoid hazardous activities that require alertness until response is known
Treatment of overdose: O_2, artificial ventilation, ECG, dopamine for circulatory depression, diazepam or thiopental for convulsions, treat ventricular dysrhythmias

---

floxuridine (℞)

(flox-yoor'i-deen)
Floxuridine, FUDR
Func. class.: Antineoplastic, antimetabolite
Chem. class.: Pyrimidine antagonist

Action: Inhibits DNA synthesis; interferes with cell replication by competitively inhibiting thymidylate synthesis S phase of cell cycle
Uses: GI adenocarcinoma metastatic to liver; cancer of breast, head, neck, liver, brain, gallbladder, bile duct
Dosage and routes:
• *Adult:* INTRAARTERIAL by continuous inf 0.1-0.6 mg/kg/day × 1-6 wk; HEPATIC ARTERY INJ 0.4-0.6 mg/kg/day × 1-6 wk
Available forms: Powder for inj 500 mg/5 ml vial
Side effects/adverse reactions:
HEMA: ***Thrombocytopenia, leukopenia, myelosuppression, anemia***
GI: Anorexia, diarrhea, nausea, vomiting, ***hemorrhage, stomatitis***
GU: ***Renal failure***
EENT: Epistaxis
INTEG: Rash, fever, alopecia
CNS: Lethargy, malaise, weakness
Contraindications: Hypersensitivity, myelosuppression, pregnancy (D), poor nutritional status, serious infections
Precautions: Renal disease, hepatic disease, bone marrow depression
Pharmacokinetics: Half-life 10-20 min, 20 hr terminal; metabolized in liver; excreted in urine (active metabolite); crosses blood-brain barrier
Interactions:
• Increased toxicity: radiation, other antineoplastics
• Increased adverse reaction: live virus vaccines
Additive compatibilities: Carboplatin, cisplatin, cisplatin with etoposide, cisplatin with leucovorin, etoposide, fluorouracil, fluorouracil with leucovorin, leucovorin
Y-site compatibilities: Fludarabine, melphalan, ondansetron, sargramostim, paclitaxel, vinorelbine
Lab test interferences:
Increase: Liver function studies
NURSING CONSIDERATIONS
Assess:
• CBC, differential, platelet count qwk; withhold drug if WBC is $<3500/mm^3$ or platelet count is $<100,000/mm^3$; notify prescriber of these results; drug should be discontinued
• Renal function studies: BUN, serum uric acid, urine CrCl, electrolytes before, during therapy
• I&O ratio: report fall in urine output to <30 ml/hr
• Monitor temp q4h; fever may indicate beginning infection

• Liver function tests before, during therapy: bilirubin, alk phosphatase, AST (SGOT), ALT (SGPT), LDH; prn or qmo
• Bleeding: hematuria, guaiac, bruising or petechiae, mucosa or orifices q8h
• Food preferences; list likes, dislikes
• Inflammation of mucosa, breaks in skin
• Buccal cavity q8h for dryness, sores or ulceration, white patches, oral pain, bleeding, dysphagia
• Symptoms indicating severe allergic reaction: rash, urticaria, itching, flushing
• GI symptoms: frequency of stools, cramping; low-residue diet with elimination of milk products when used in conjunction with 5FUDR/ radiation therapy
• Acidosis, signs of dehydration: rapid respirations, poor skin turgor, decreased urine output, dry skin, restlessness, weakness

Administer:
• By intraarterial infusion pump after diluting 5 ml drug/5 ml sterile H_2O for inj, dilute further with D_5W or NS to required dilution
• Antiemetic 30-60 min before giving drug and prn
• Antibiotics for prophylaxis of infection
• Topical or systemic analgesics for pain
• Transfusion for anemia
• Antispasmodic for diarrhea

Perform/provide:
• Wrap sol; do not expose to light
• Strict asepsis and protective isolation if WBC levels are low
• Increased fluid intake to 2-3 L/day to prevent dehydration unless contraindicated
• Rinsing of mouth tid-qid with water, club soda, brushing of teeth bid-tid with soft brush or cotton-tipped applicators for stomatitis; use unwaxed dental floss
• Nutritious diet with iron, vitamin supplements, low fiber, and no dairy products as ordered

Evaluate:
• Therapeutic response: decreased tumor size, spread of malignancy

Teach patient/family:
• Why protective isolation is necessary
• To report signs of infection: fever, sore throat, flu symptoms
• To report signs of anemia: fatigue, headache, faintness, shortness of breath, irritability
• To report bleeding: avoid use of razors, commercial mouthwash
• To avoid use of aspirin products, ibuprofen
• To report stomatitis: any bleeding, white spots, ulcerations in mouth; tell patient to examine mouth qd, report symptoms

fluconazole (℞)

(floo-kon'a-zole)
Diflucan
Func. class.: Antifungal

Action: Inhibits ergosterol biosynthesis, causes direct damage to membrane phospholipids

Uses: Oropharyngeal candidiasis in AIDS patients, chronic mucocutaneous candidiasis, urinary candidiasis, cryptococcal meningitis

Dosage and routes:

Vaginal candidiasis
• *Adult:* PO 150 mg as a single dose

Serious fungal infections
• Adult: PO/IV 50-400 mg initially, then 200 mg qd for 4 wk

Oropharyngeal candidiasis in AIDS patients
• *Adult:* PO 200 mg initially, then 100 mg qd for at least 2 wk

Available forms: Tabs 50, 100, 200 mg; inj 200, 400 mg

Side effects/adverse reactions:

GI: Nausea, vomiting, diarrhea, cramping, flatus, increased AST, ALT, ***hepatotoxicity***

CNS: Headache

INTEG: ***Stevens-Johnson Syndrome***

Contraindications: Hypersensitivity

Precautions: Renal disease, pregnancy (B), lactation

Interactions:

- Potentiation of anticoagulation: warfarin
- Increased renal dysfunction: cyclosporines

Y-site compatibilities: Acyclovir, amikacin, aminophylline, ampicillin/sulbactam, aztreonam, benztropine, cefazolin, cefotetan, cefoxitin, chlorpromazine, cimetidine, dexamethasone sodium phosphate, diphenhydramine, droperidol, famotidine, fludarabine, foscarnet, ganciclovir, gentamicin, heparin, hydrocortisone, immune globulin, leucovorin, meperidine, metoclopramide, metronidazole, midazolam, morphine, nafcillin, ondansetron, oxacillin, penicillin G, potassium, phenytoin, prochlorperazine, promethazine, sargramostim, ticarcillin/clavulanate, tobramycin, vancomycin, zidovudine

NURSING CONSIDERATIONS

Assess:

- VS q15-30min during first infusion; note changes in pulse, B/P
- I&O ratio; watch for decreasing urinary output, change in specific gravity; discontinue drug to prevent renal damage
- Weight weekly; if weight gain >2 lb/wk and edema is present, renal damage should be considered
- Renal toxicity: increasing BUN, serum creatinine; if BUN is >40 mg/dl or if serum creatinine is >3 mg/dl, drug may be discontinued or dosage reduced
- For hepatotoxicity: increasing AST (SGOT), ALT (SGPT), alk phosphatase, bilirubin

Administer:

- After diluting according to package directions; run at 200 mg/hr or less; do not use plastic containers in connections
- IV using an in-line filter, using distal veins; check for extravasation and necrosis q2h
- Drug only after C&S confirms organism, drug needed to treat condition

Perform/provide:

- Storage protected from moisture and light, diluted sol is stable 24 hr

Evaluate:

- Therapeutic response: decreasing oral candidiasis, fever, malaise, rash; negative C&S for infection organism

Teach patient/family:

- That long-term therapy may be needed to clear infection

---

flucytosine (℞)

(floo-sye'toe-seen)

Ancobon, Ancotil*

Func. class.: Antifungal

Chem. class.: Pyrimidine (fluorinated)

Action: Converted to fluorouracil after entering fungi; inhibits RNA, DNA synthesis; synergisim action when used with amphotericin B in some fungal infections

Uses: *Candida* infections (septicemia, endocarditis, pulmonary, UTI), *Cryptococcus* (meningitis, pulmonary, urinary tract infections)

Dosage and routes:

- *Adult and child >50 kg:* PO 50-150 mg/kg/day q6h

* Available in Canada only

• *Adult and child <50 kg:* PO 1.5-4.5 g/m^2/day in 4 divided doses

Available forms: Caps 250, 500 mg

Side effects/adverse reactions:

INTEG: Rash

CNS: Headache, confusion, dizziness, sedation, vertigo

GI: Nausea, vomiting, anorexia, diarrhea, abdominal distention, cramps, enterocolitis, increased AST (SGOT), ALT (SGPT), alk phosphatase, ***bowel perforation*** (rare)

HEMA: ***Thrombocytopenia, agranulocytosis, anemia, leukopenia, pancytopenia***

GU: Increased BUN, creatinine

Contraindications: Hypersensitivity

Precautions: Renal disease, impaired hepatic function, bone marrow depression, blood dyscrasias, radiation/chemotherapy, pregnancy (C), lactation

Pharmacokinetics:

PO: Peak 2½-6 hr, half-life 3-6 hr, excreted in urine (unchanged), well distributed to CSF, aqueous humor, joints

Interactions:

• Synergisim: amphotericin B

Lab test interferences:

False increase: Creatinine

NURSING CONSIDERATIONS

Assess:

• VS q15-30min during first infusion; note changes in pulse, B/P

• Blood studies: CBC, including platelets

• Drug level during treatment (therapeutic level 25-100 μg/ml); if renal impairment is present, level usually kept <100 μg/ml

• For renal toxicity: increasing BUN, serum creatinine; if serum creatinine >1.7 mg/100 dl, dosage may be reduced

• For hepatotoxicity: increasing AST (SGOT), ALT (SGPT), alk phosphatase

• For allergic reaction: dermatitis, rash; drug should be discontinued, antihistamines (mild reaction) or epinephrine (severe reaction) administered

• For blood dyscrasias, fatigue, bruising, malaise, dark urine

Administer:

• Drug only after C&S confirms organism, drug needed to treat condition

• Few caps at a time to decrease nausea, vomiting over 15 min

Perform/provide:

• Symptomatic treatment as ordered for adverse reactions: aspirin, antihistamines, antiemetics, antispasmodics

• Storage in tight, light-resistant container at room temp

Evaluate:

• Therapeutic response: decreased fever, malaise, rash, negative C&S for infecting organism

Teach patient/family:

• That long-term therapy may be needed to clear infection (1-2 mo depending on type of infection)

• To report symptoms of blood dyscrasias: fatigue, bruising, malaise, dark urine

fludarabine (℞)

(floo-dar'a-been)

Fludara

Func. class.: Antineoplastic, antimetabolite

Chem. class.: Vidarabine derivative

Action: Competes with physiologic substrate that inhibits DNA synthesis

Uses: Chronic lymphocytic leukemia, non-Hodgkin's lymphoma

Dosage and routes:

• *Adult:* IV 25 mg/m^2 over 30 min qd × 5 days, may repeat q28 days;

reconstitute with 2 ml of sterile water for inj; dissolution should occur in <15 sec

Available forms: Lyophilized powder for reconstitution 50 mg/vial

Side effects/adverse reactions:

SYST: Fever, chills, malaise, fatigue

META: Hyperuricemia, hyperphosphatemia, hypocalcemia, metabolic acidosis, hyperkalemia

HEMA: Thrombophlebitis, bleeding, ***thrombocytopenia, leukopenia, myelosuppression, anemia***

GI: Nausea, vomiting, anorexia, diarrhea, stomatitis, ***hepatotoxicity,*** abdominal pain, hematemesis, ***hemorrhage***

EENT: Visual disturbances, sinusitis

GU: Dysuria, infection

INTEG: Rash

RESP: ***Pneumonia,*** dyspnea, cough, interstitial pulmonary infiltrate

CV: Edema

CNS: Weakness, confusion, headache, depression, sleep disorder, impaired mentation, ***coma,*** peripheral neuropathy

Contraindications: Hypersensitivity, pregnancy (D), lactation

Precautions: Renal disease, hepatic disease, infants

Pharmacokinetics: Rapidly converted to active metabolite; half-life of metabolite 10 hr; mean plasma clearance of metabolite 8.9 L/hr/m^2; 23% excreted in urine as unchanged metabolite

Interactions:

• Increased toxicity: radiation, other antineoplastics

• Increased adverse reactions: live virus vaccines

Y-site incompatibilities: Acyclovir, amphotericin B, chlorpromazine, daunorubicin, ganciclovir, hydroxyzine, melphalan, miconazole, prochloperazine, vinorelbine

NURSING CONSIDERATIONS

Assess:

• CBC (RBC, Hct, Hgb), differential, platelet count weekly; withhold drug if CBC <4000/mm^3, platelet count is <75,000/mm^3, or RBC, Hct, Hgb are low; notify prescriber of these results

• Renal function studies: BUN, uric acid, urine CrCl, electrolytes before and during therapy

• I&O ratio; report fall in urine output to <30 ml/hr

• Temp q4h; fever may indicate beginning infection; no rectal temp

• Liver function tests before, during therapy: bilirubin, ALT (SGOT), AST (SGPT), alk phosphatase, prn or qmo

• Blood uric acid levels during therapy

• Bleeding: hematuria, guaiac, bruising or petechiae, mucosa or orifices q8h

• Dyspnea, rales, nonproductive cough, chest pain, tachypnea, fatigue, increased pulse, pallor, lethargy, personality changes with high doses

• Food preferences: list likes, dislikes

• Edema in feet, joint pain, stomach pain, shaking

• Inflammation of mucosa, breaks in skin

• Yellowing of skin and sclera, dark urine, clay-colored stools, itchy skin, abdominal pain, fever, diarrhea

• Buccal cavity q8h for dryness, sores or ulceration, white patches, oral pain, bleeding, dysphagia

• Local irritation, pain, burning, discoloration at injection site

• GI symptoms: frequency of stools, cramping

• Acidosis, signs of dehydration: rapid respirations, poor skin turgor, decreased urine output, dry skin, restlessness, weakness

Administer:
• Antiemetic 30-60 min before giving drug and prn
• Allopurinol or sodium bicarbonate to maintain uric acid levels and alkalinization of the urine; prevent hyperuricemia
• Antibiotics for prophylaxis of infection
• Topical or systemic analgesics for pain
• Transfusion for anemia
• Antispasmodic for GI symptoms

Perform/provide:
• Strict asepsis and protective isolation if WBC levels are low
• Increase fluid intake to 2-3 L/day to prevent urate deposits and calculi formation, unless contraindicated
• Diet low in purines: absence of organ meats (kidney, liver), dried beans, peas to prevent increased urate deposits
• Rinsing of mouth tid-qid with water, club soda; brushing of teeth bid-tid with soft brush or cotton-tipped applicators for stomatitis; use unwaxed dental floss
• HOB raised to facilitate breathing if dyspnea or pneumonia occurs
• Storage in refrigerator

Evaluate:
• Therapeutic response: decrease in tumor size, spread of malignancy

Teach patient/family:
• Why protective isolation is necessary
• To report any coughing, chest pain, changes in breathing; may indicate beginning pneumonia
• To avoid foods with citric acid, hot or rough texture if stomatitis is present
• To report stomatitis: any bleeding, white spots, ulcerations in mouth; tell patient to examine mouth qd, report any symptoms
• To report signs of anemia: fatigue, headache, faintness, shortness of breath, irritability
• To report bleeding; avoid use of razors or commercial mouthwash
• To avoid use of aspirin products, ibuprofen

Overdose treatment: Discontinue drug, use supportive therapy

fludrocortisone (℞)

(floo-droe-kor′ti-sone)
Florinef Acetate
Func. class.: Corticosteroid
Chem. class.: Mineralocorticoid

Action: Promotes increased reabsorption of sodium and loss of potassium, water, hydrogen from distal renal tubules

Uses: Adrenal insufficiency, salt-losing adrenogenital syndrome

Dosage and routes:
• *Adult:* PO 0.1-0.2 mg qd

Available forms: Tabs 0.1 mg

Side effects/adverse reactions:
CNS: Flushing, sweating, headache
CV: Hypertension, ***circulatory collapse, thrombophlebitis, embolism,*** tachycardia
MS: Fractures, osteoporosis, weakness

Contraindications: Hypersensitivity, acute glomerulonephritis, amebiasis

Precautions: Pregnancy (C), osteoporosis, CHF

Pharmacokinetics:
PO: Half-life 3.5 hr, metabolized by liver, excreted in urine

Interactions:
• Decreased action of fludrocortisone: cholestyramine, colestipol, barbiturates, rifampin, ephedrine, phenytoin, theophylline
• Decreased effects of: diuretics, potassium-sparing diuretics, potassium supplements

• Increased side effects: sodium-containing food or medication, digitalis preparations

Lab test interferences:

Increase: Potassium, sodium

Decrease: Hematocrit

NURSING CONSIDERATIONS

Assess:

• K, while on long-term therapy; hypokalemia

• Weight daily; notify prescriber of weekly gain >5 lb

• B/P q4h, pulse; notify prescriber if chest pain occurs

• I&O ratio; be alert for decreasing urinary output, increasing edema

• K depletion: paresthesias, fatigue, nausea, vomiting, depression, polyuria, dysrhythmias, weakness

• Edema, hypertension, cardiac symptoms

Administer:

• Titrated dose; use lowest effective dose

• With food or milk to decrease GI symptoms

Perform/provide:

• Assistance with ambulation in patient with bone tissue disease to prevent fractures

Evaluate:

• Therapeutic response: correction of adrenal insufficiency

Teach patient/family:

• That ID as steroid user should be carried

• Not to discontinue this medication abruptly

flumazenil (℞)

(flu-maz′ee-nill)

Mazicon, Romazicon

Func. class.: Benzodiazepine receptor antagonist

Chem. class.: Imidazobenzodiazepine derivative

Action: Antagonizes actions of benzodiazepines on CNS, competitively inhibits activity at benzodiazepine recognition site on GABA/benzodiazepine receptor complex

Uses: Reversal of sedative effects of benzodiazepines

Dosage and routes:

Reversal of conscious sedation or in general anesthesia

• *Adult:* IV 0.2 mg (2 ml) given over 15 sec; wait 45 sec, then give 0.2 mg (2 ml) if consciousness does not occur; may be repeated at 60-sec intervals prn, up to 4 additional times (max total dose 1 mg); dose is to be individualized

Management of suspected benzodiazepine overdose

• *Adult:* IV 0.2 mg (2 ml) given over 30 sec; wait 30 sec, then give 0.3 mg (3 ml) over 30 sec if consciousness does not occur; further doses of 0.5 mg (5 ml) can be given over 30 sec at intervals of 1 min up to cumulative dose of 3 mg

Available forms: Inj 0.1 mg/ml

Side effects/adverse reactions:

EENT: Abnormal vision, blurred vision, tinnitus

CV: Hypertension, palpitations, cutaneous vasodilation, dysrhythmias, bradycardia, tachycardia, chest pain

GI: Nausea, vomiting, hiccups

CNS: Dizziness, agitation, emotional lability, confusion, ***convulsions,*** somnolence

SYST: Headache, injection site pain, increased sweating, fatigue, rigors

Contraindications: Hypersensitivity to this drug or benzodiazepines, serious cyclic antidepressant overdose, patients given benzodiazepine for control of life-threatening condition

Precautions: Pregnancy (C), lactation, children, elderly, renal disease, seizure disorders, head injury, labor and delivery, hepatic disease, hypo-

* Available in Canada only

ventilation, panic disorder, drug and alcohol dependency, ambulatory patients

Pharmacokinetics: Terminal half-life 41-79 min; metabolized in liver

Interactions:

- Toxicity: mixed drug overdosage
- Ingestion of food during IV INF: increased flumazenil clearance

NURSING CONSIDERATIONS

Assess:

- Cardiac status using continuous monitoring
- For seizures; protect patient from injury
- GI symptoms: nausea, vomiting; place in side-lying position to prevent aspiration
- Allergic reactions: flushing, rash, urticaria, pruritus

Administer:

- Give IV directly undiluted or diluted with 0.9% NaCl, D_5W, LR, give over 15 sec
- Check airway and IV access before administration

Evaluate:

- Therapeutic response: decreased sedation, respiratory depression, toxicity

Teach patient/family:

- That amnesia may continue
- Not to engage in hazardous activities for 18-24 hr after discharge
- Not to take any alcohol or nonprescription drugs for 18-24 hr

flunisolide (℞)

(floo-nis′oh-lide)

AeroBid, Nasalide

Func. class.: Corticosteroid

Chem. class.: Glucocorticoid

Action: Decreases inflammation by suppression of migration of polymorphonuclear leukocytes, fibroblasts, reversal of increased capillary permeability and lysosomal stabilization; does not depress hypothalamus

Uses: Rhinitis, allergies, nasal polyps

Dosage and routes:

- *Adult and child >6 yr:* SPRAY 2 puffs bid, not to exceed 4 puffs bid

Available forms: Nasal sol 25 μg/metered dose (Nasalide), 250 μg/metered dose (AeroBid)

Side effects/adverse reactions:

CNS: Headache, nervousness, restlessness

EENT: Hoarseness, *Candida* infection of oral cavity, sore throat

GI: Nausea, vomiting, dry mouth

Contraindications: Hypersensitivity, child <6 yr

Precautions: Nonasthmatic bronchial disease, bacterial, fungal, viral infections of mouth, throat, lungs, respiratory TB, untreated fungal, bacterial, or viral infections, pregnancy (C), glaucoma

Pharmacokinetics:

INH: Duration 1 hr

NURSING CONSIDERATIONS

Assess:

- Infection: increased temperature, WBC, even after withdrawal of medication; drug masks infection

Administer:

- Titrated dose; use lowest effective dose

Evaluate:

- Therapeutic response: ease of respirations, decreased inflammation

Teach patient/family:

- To use gum; rinse mouth after each dose
- That ID as steroid user should be carried
- To notify prescriber if therapeutic response decreases; dosage adjustment may be needed
- Proper administration technique; shake well before use
- Compliance to therapy

• Teach patient about cushingoid symptoms
• Symptoms of adrenal insufficiency: nausea, anorexia, fatigue, dizziness, dyspnea, weakness, joint pain

fluocinonide (℞)

(floo-oh-sin'oh-nide)
Flucinolone, Fluocinolone Acetonide, Fluonid, Flurosyn, Synalar, Synalar-HP, Synemol, Fluocinonide, Lidemol*, Lidex, Lidex-E, Vasoderm, Vasoderm E
Func. class.: Topical corticosteroid
Chem. class.: Synthetic fluorinated agent, group II potency

Action: Antipruritic, antiinflammatory
Uses: Psoriasis, eczema, contact dermatitis, pruritus
Dosage and routes:
• *Adult and child:* Apply to affected area tid-qid
Available forms: Oint, cream, sol, gel: 0.05%
Side effects/adverse reactions:
INTEG: Burning, dryness, itching, irritation, acne, folliculitis, hypertrichosis, perioral dermatitis, hypopigmentation, atrophy, striae, miliaria, allergic contact dermatitis, secondary infection
Contraindications: Hypersensitivity to corticosteroids; fungal infections
Precautions: Pregnancy (C), lactation, viral, bacterial infections
NURSING CONSIDERATIONS
Assess:
• Temperature: if fever develops, drug should be discontinued
Administer:
• Only to affected areas; do not get in eyes
• Medication, then cover with occlusive dressing (only if prescribed), seal to normal skin, change q12h; use occlusive dressings with extreme caution
• Only to dermatoses; do not use on weeping, denuded, infected area
Perform/provide:
• Cleansing before application
• Treatment for a few days after area has cleared
• Storage at room temp
Evaluate:
• Therapeutic response: absence of severe itching, patches on skin, flaking
Teach patient/family:
• To avoid sunlight on affected area; burns may occur

fluoride (OTC)

ACT, Checkmate, Fluor-A-Day*, Fluorigard, Fluorinse, Fluoritab, Fluotic*, Flura, Flura-Drops, Flura-Loz, Gel II, Gel-Kam, Gel-Tin, Karidium, Karigel, Karigel-N, Listermint with Fluoride, Loz-Tabs, Luride, Luride-SF, Luride Lozi-Tabs, Luride 0.25 Lozi-Tabs, Luride 0.5 Lozi-Tabs, Minute-Gel, Pediaflor, Pharmaflur, Pharmaflur 1.1, Pharmaflur df, Phos-Flur, Point-Two, Prevident, Sodium Fluoride, Stop, Thera-Flur, Thera-Flur-N
Func. class.: Trace elements
Chem. class.: Fluorideion

Action: Needed for hard tooth enamel and for resistance to periodontal disease; reduces acid production by dental bacteria
Uses: Prevention of dental caries
Dosage and routes:
• *Adult and child >12 yr:* TOP 10 ml 0.2% sol qd after brushing teeth,

* Available in Canada only

rinse mouth for >1 min with sol
• *Child 6-12 yr:* TOP 5 ml 0.2% sol
• *Child >3 yr:* PO 1 mg qd
• *Child <3 yr:* PO 0.5 mg
Available forms: Tabs chewable 0.25 mg; tabs 0.5, 1 mg, tabs effervescent 10 mg; drops 0.125, 0.25, 0.5 mg/ml; rinse supplements 0.2 mg/ml, rinse 0.01%, 0.02%, 0.09%; gel 0.1%, 0.5%, 1.23%
Side effects/adverse reactions:
ACUTE OVERDOSE: ***Black tarry stools, bloody vomit, diarrhea, decreased respiration, increased salivation, watery eyes***
CHRONIC OVERDOSE: ***Hypocalcemia and tetany, respiratory arrest, sores in mouth, constipation, loss of appetite, nausea, vomiting, weight loss, discoloration of teeth*** (white, black, brown)
Contraindications: Hypersensitivity, pregnancy (D)
Precautions: Child < 6 yr
Pharmacokinetics:
PO: Excreted in urine and feces; crosses placenta, breast milk
Interactions:
• Avoid use with dairy products
NURSING CONSIDERATIONS
Assess:
• Use in children
• Nutritional status: increase fluoride content of water, decrease carbohydrate snacks, increase fish, tea, mineral water
Administer:
• Drops after meals with fluids or undiluted tablets; may be chewed; do not swallow whole; may be given with water or juice; avoid milk
Evaluate:
• Therapeutic response: absence of dental caries
Teach patient/family:
• To monitor children using gel or rinse; not to be swallowed
• Not to drink, eat, or rinse mouth for at least ½ hr
• Not to use during pregnancy
• To apply after brushing and flossing hs
• To store out of children's reach

fluorometholone (℞)

(flure-oh-meth'oh-lone)
Flarex, Fluor-Op, FML, FML Forte, FML S.O.P.
Func. class.: Ophthalmic anti-inflammatory

Action: Decreases inflammation, resulting in decreased pain, photophobia, hyperemia, cellular infiltration
Uses: Inflammation of eye, lids, conjunctiva, cornea, uveitis, iridocyclitis, allergic condition, burns, foreign bodies, postoperatively in cataract, graft rejection
Dosage and routes:
• *Adult and child:* INSTILL 1-2 gtts into conjunctival sac qh × 2 days, if needed, then bid-qid
Available forms: Oint 0.1%; ophthalmic susp 0.1%, 0.25%
Side effects/adverse reactions:
EENT: ***Increased intraocular pressure,*** poor corneal wound healing, increased possibility of corneal infections, glaucoma exacerbation, ***optic nerve damage,*** decreased acuity, visual field, cataracts
Contraindications: Hypersensitivity, acute superficial herpes simplex, fungal/viral diseases of the eye or conjunctiva, active diabetes mellitus, ocular TB, infections of the eye
Precautions: Corneal abrasions, glaucoma, pregnancy (C), lactation, children
NURSING CONSIDERATIONS
Evaluate:
• Therapeutic response: absence of swelling, redness, exudate

F

Administer:
- After shaking suspension

Perform/provide:
- Storage in tight, light-resistant container

Teach patient/family:
- Instillation method: pressure on lacrimal duct for 1 min
- Not to share eye medications
- Not to touch applicator to eye
- Not to use if purulent drainage is present
- Not to discontinue steroids abruptly; taper over 1-2 wk

fluorouracil (℞)

(flure-oh-yoor'a-sil)

Efudex, Fluoroplex

Func. class.: Topical antineoplastic

Chem. class.: Antimetabolite

Action: Inhibits synthesis of DNA, RNA in susceptible cells

Uses: Keratosis (multiple/actinic), basal cell carcinoma

Dosage and routes:
- *Adult and child:* TOP apply to affected area bid

Available forms: Sol 1%, 2%, 5%; cream 1%, 5%

Side effects/adverse reactions:

INTEG: Rash, irritation, pain, burning, contact dermatitis, scaling, swelling, soreness, hyperpigmentation, pruritus

Contraindications: Hypersensitivity, pregnancy (D)

NURSING CONSIDERATIONS

Assess:
- WBC, platelets at least qmo
- Area of body involved for redness, swelling
- Check oral cavity qd for stomatitis; if present discontinue drug

Administer:
- Only 5% sol/cream for basal cell carcinoma
- Using gloves or applicator
- A low-residue diet with no dairy products where radiation is also used

Perform/provide:
- Covering of lesion with porous gauze dressing only
- Hand washing after application if gloves or applicator not used
- Storage at room temp

Evaluate:
- Therapeutic response: decreased size of lesion

Teach patient/family:
- To avoid application on normal skin or getting cream in eyes
- To discontinue use if rash or irritation occurs
- To avoid sunlight or use sunscreen; photosensitivity may occur
- To wash hands after application
- Not to change application; use exactly as prescribed
- That lesion will disappear in 1-2 mo

fluorouracil (5-fluorouracil) (℞)

(flure-oh-yoor'a-sil)

Adrucil, 5-FU

Func. class.: Antineoplastic, antimetabolite

Chem. class.: Pyrimidine antagonist

Action: Inhibits DNA synthesis; interferes with cell replication by competitively inhibiting thymidylate synthesis, S phase of cell cycle-specific vesicant

Uses: Cancer of breast, colon, rectum, stomach, pancreas

Dosage and routes:
- *Adult:* IV 12 mg/kg/day × 4 days, not to exceed 800 mg/day; may repeat with 6 mg/kg on day 6, 8, 10, 12; maintenance is 10-15 mg/kg/

wk as a single dose, not to exceed 1 g/wk

Available forms: Inj IV 50 mg/ml

Side effects/adverse reactions:

CV: Myocardial ischemia, angina

HEMA: ***Thrombocytopenia, leukopenia, myelosuppression, anemia, agranulocytosis***

GI: Anorexia, stomatitis, diarrhea, nausea, vomiting, ***hemorrhage,*** *enteritis glossitis*

GU: ***Renal failure***

EENT: Epistaxis

INTEG: Rash, fever

CNS: Lethargy, malaise, weakness

Contraindications: Hypersensitivity, myelosuppression, pregnancy (D), poor nutritional status, serious infections

Precautions: Renal disease, hepatic disease, bone marrow depression, angina, lactation, children

Pharmacokinetics: Half-life 10-20 min, 20 hr terminal; metabolized in the liver; excreted in the urine; crosses blood-brain barrier

Interactions:

- Increased toxicity: radiation or other antineoplastics

Syringe compatibilities: Bleomycin, cisplatin, cyclophosphamide, doxorubicin, furosemide, heparin, leucovorin, methotrexate, metoclopramide, mitomycin, vinblastine, vincristine

Y-site compatibilities: Bleomycin, cisplatin, cyclophosphamide, doxorubicin, furosemide, heparin, leucovorin, mannitol, melphalan, methotrexate, metoclopramide, mitomycin, paclitaxel, vinblastine, vincristine, sargramostim

Additive compatibilities: Bleomycin, cephalothin, etoposides, floxuridine, ifosfamide, leucovorin, methotrexate, prednisolone, vincristine, cyclophosphamide, cyclophosphamide mitoxantrone

Solution compatibilities: Amino acids 4.25%/D_{25}, D_5/LR, $D_{3.3}$/0.3 NaCl, D_5W, 0.9% NaCl, TPN #23

Lab test interferences:

Increase: Liver function studies, 6-HIAA

Decrease: Albumin

NURSING CONSIDERATIONS

Assess:

- CBC, differential, platelet count weekly; withhold drug if WBC is <3500/mm^3 or platelet count is <100,000/mm^3; notify prescriber of these results; drug should be discontinued
- Renal function studies: BUN, serum uric acid, urine CrCl, electrolytes before, during therapy
- I&O ratio; report fall in urine output to <30 ml/hr
- Temp q4h; fever may indicate beginning infection
- Liver function tests before, during therapy: bilirubin, alk phosphatase, AST (SGOT), ALT (SGPT), LDH; prn or qmo
- Bleeding: hematuria, guaiac, bruising or petechiae, mucosa or orifices q8h
- Food preferences: list likes, dislikes
- Inflammation of mucosa, breaks in skin
- Buccal cavity q8h for dryness, sores or ulceration, white patches, oral pain, bleeding, dysphagia
- Symptoms indicating severe allergic reaction: rash, urticaria, itching, flushing
- GI symptoms: frequency of stools, cramping
- Acidosis, signs of dehydration: rapid respirations, poor skin turgor, decreased urine output, dry skin, restlessness, weakness

Administer:

- IV undiluted; may inject through Y-tube or 3-way stopcock; give over

1-3 min; may be diluted in NS, D_5W, given over 2-8 hr as IV inf
• Antiemetic 30-60 min before giving drug to prevent vomiting
• Antibiotics for prophylaxis of infection
• Topical or systemic analgesics for pain
• Transfusion for anemia
• Antispasmodic for diarrhea

Perform/provide:
• Protection from light
• Strict asepsis, protective isolation if WBC levels are low
• Increase fluid intake to 2-3 L/day to prevent dehydration, unless contraindicated
• Changing of IV site q48h
• Rinsing of mouth tid-qid with water, club soda; brushing of teeth bid-tid with soft brush or cotton-tipped applicator for stomatitis; use unwaxed dental floss
• Nutritious diet with iron, vitamin supplements, low fiber, few dairy products, especially when combined with radiotherapy as ordered

Evaluate:
• Therapeutic response: decreased tumor size, spread of malignancy

Teach patient/family:
• Why protective isolation is necessary
• To avoid foods with citric acid, hot or rough texture if stomatitis is present; to drink adequate fluids
• To report stomatitis: any bleeding, white spots, ulcerations in mouth; tell patient to examine mouth qd, report symptoms
• To report signs of infection: fever, sore throat, flu symptoms
• To report signs of anemia: fatigue, headache, faintness, shortness of breath, irritability
• To report bleeding: avoid use of razors, commercial mouthwash
• To avoid use of aspirin products or ibuprofen
• To use contraception during therapy (men and women)

fluoxetine (℞)

(floo-ox'e-teen)
Prozac
Func. class.: Bicyclic antidepressant

Action: Inhibits CNS neuron uptake of serotonin but not of norepinephrine
Uses: Major depressive disorder
Investigational uses: Obsessive-compulsive disorder
Dosage and routes:
• *Adult:* PO 20 mg qd in AM; after 4 wk if no clinical improvement is noted, dose may be increased to 20 mg bid in AM, PM, not to exceed 80 mg/day
Available forms: Pulvules 20 mg; cap 10 mg; liquid 20 mg/5 ml
Side effects/adverse reactions:
CNS: Headache, nervousness, insomnia, drowsiness, anxiety, tremor, dizziness, fatigue, sedation, poor concentration, abnormal dreams, agitation, ***convulsions,*** apathy, euphoria, hallucinations, delusions, psychosis
GI: Nausea, diarrhea, dry mouth, anorexia, dyspepsia, constipation, cramps, vomiting, taste changes, flatulence, decreased appetite
INTEG: Sweating, rash, pruritus, acne, alopecia, urticaria
RESP: Infection, pharyngitis, nasal congestion, sinus headache, sinusitus, cough, dyspnea, bronchitis, asthma, hyperventilation, pneumonia
CV: Hot flashes, palpitations, angina pectoris, ***hemorrhage,*** hypertension, tachycardia, first-degree AV

* Available in Canada only

block, bradycardia, *MI,* thrombophlebitis
MS: Pain, arthritis, twitching
GU: Dysmenorrhea, decreased libido, urinary frequency, UTI, amenorrhea, cystitis, impotence, urine retention
EENT: Visual changes, ear/eye pain, photophobia, tinnitus
SYST: Asthenia, viral infection, fever, allergy, chills

Contraindications: Hypersensitivity

Precautions: Pregnancy (B), lactation, children, elderly, diabetes mellitus

Pharmacokinetics:
PO: Peak 6-8 hr; metabolized in liver; excreted in urine; half-life 2-7 days

Interactions:
- Do not use with MAOIs
- Increased side effects: highly protein-bound drugs (i.e., fluoxetine)
- Increased half-life of diazepam

Lab test interferences:
Increase: Serum bilirubin, blood glucose, alk phosphatase
Decrease: VMA, 5-HIAA
False increase: Urinary catecholamines

NURSING CONSIDERATIONS

Assess:
- Mental status: mood, sensorium, affect, suicidal tendencies, increase in psychiatric symptoms, depression, panic
- B/P (lying/standing), pulse q4h; if systolic B/P drops 20 mm Hg, hold drug, notify prescriber; take vital signs q4h in patients with cardiovascular disease
- Blood studies: CBC, leukocytes, differential, cardiac enzymes if patient is receiving long-term therapy
- Hepatic studies: AST (SGOT), ALT (SGPT), bilirubin, creatinine
- Weight qwk; appetite may decrease with drug
- ECG for flattening of T wave, bundle branch, AV block, dysrhythmias in cardiac patients
- EPS primarily in elderly: rigidity, dystonia, akathisia
- Urinary retention, constipation
- Withdrawal symptoms: headache, nausea, vomiting, muscle pain, weakness; not usual unless drug discontinued abruptly
- Alcohol consumption; if alcohol is consumed, hold dose until AM

Administer:
- Increased fluids, bulk in diet if constipation, urinary retention occur
- With food or milk for GI symptoms
- Crushed if patient is unable to swallow medication whole
- Dosage hs if oversedation occurs during the day; may take entire dose hs; elderly may not tolerate once/day dosing
- Gum, hard candy, frequent sips of water for dry mouth

Perform/provide:
- Storage at room temp; do not freeze
- Assistance with ambulation during therapy, since drowsiness, dizziness occur
- Safety measures including side rails, primarily in elderly
- Checking to see PO medication swallowed

Evaluate:
- Therapeutic response: decreased depression

Teach patient/family:
- That therapeutic effect may take 2-3 wk
- To use caution in driving, other activities requiring alertness because of drowsiness, dizziness, blurred vision
- Not to discontinue medication

F

quickly after long-term use; may cause nausea, headache, malaise

• To avoid alcohol ingestion, other CNS depressants

• To notify prescriber if pregnant or plan to become pregnant or breast-feed

fluoxymesterone (℞)

(floo-ox-ee-mess′te-rone)

Fluoxymesterone, Halotestin

Func. class.: Androgenic anabolic steroid

Chem. class.: Halogenated testosterone derivative

Action: Increases weight by building body tissue, increases potassium, phosphorus, chloride, nitrogen levels, bone development

Uses: Impotence from testicular deficiency, hypogonadism; breast engorgement; palliative treatment of female breast cancer

Dosage and routes:

Hypogonadism/impotence

• *Adult:* PO 2-10 mg qd

Breast engorgement

• *Adult:* PO 2.5 mg qd, then 5-10 mg qd × 5 days

Breast cancer

• *Adult:* PO 15-30 mg qd in divided doses until therapeutic effect occurs, then dosage should be reduced

Available forms: Tabs 2, 5, 10 mg

Side effects/adverse reactions:

INTEG: Rash, acneiform lesions, oily hair, skin, flushing, sweating, acne vulgaris, alopecia, hirsutism

CNS: Dizziness, headache, fatigue, tremors, paresthesias, flushing, sweating, anxiety, lability, insomnia, carpal tunnel syndrome

MS: Cramps, spasms

CV: Increased B/P

GU: ***Hematuria,*** amenorrhea, vaginitis, decreased libido, decreased breast size, clitoral hypertrophy, testicular atrophy

GI: Nausea, vomiting, constipation, weight gain, ***cholestatic jaundice***

EENT: Conjunctional edema, nasal congestion

ENDO: Abnormal GTT

Contraindications: Severe renal, severe cardiac, severe hepatic disease, hypersensitivity, pregnancy (X), lactation, genital bleeding (abnormal), children

Precautions: Diabetes mellitus, CV disease, MI

Pharmacokinetics:

PO: Metabolized in liver; excreted in urine; crosses placenta; excreted in breast milk

Interactions:

• Increased effects of oral antidiabetics, oxyphenbutazone

• Increased PT: anticoagulants

• Edema: ACTH, adrenal steroids

• Decreased effects of: insulin

Lab test interferences:

Increase: Serum cholesterol, blood glucose, urine glucose

Decrease: Serum Ca, serum K, T_4, T_3, thyroid ^{131}I uptake test, urine 17-OHCS, 17-KS, PBI, BSP

NURSING CONSIDERATIONS

Assess:

• Weight daily; notify prescriber if weekly weight gain is >5 lb

• B/P q4h

• I&O ratio; be alert for decreasing urinary output, increasing edema

• Growth rate in children; growth rate may be uneven (linear/bone growth) if used for extended periods

• Electrolytes: K, Na, Cl, cholesterol

• Liver function studies: ALT (SGPT), AST (SGOT), bilirubin

• Edema, hypertension, cardiac symptoms, jaundice

• Mental status: affect, mood, behavioral changes, aggression

• Signs of masculinization in female: increased libido, deepening of voice, breast tissue, enlarged clitoris, menstrual irregularities; male: gynecomastia, impotence, testicular atrophy
• Hypercalcemia: lethargy, polyuria, polydipsia, nausea, vomiting, constipation; drug may have to be decreased
• Hypoglycemia in diabetics, since oral antidiabetic action is increased

Administer:
• Titrated dose, use lowest effective dose
• With food or milk to decrease GI symptoms

Perform/provide:
• Diet with increased calories, protein; decrease Na if edema occurs

Evaluate:
• Therapeutic response: increased appetite, stamina

Teach patient/family:
• That drug must be combined with complete health plan: diet, rest, exercise
• To notify prescriber if therapeutic response decreases
• Not to discontinue abruptly
• About change in sex characteristics
• Females to report menstrual irregularities
• That 1-3 mo course is necessary for response in breast cancer
• That steroids should not be used for body building

fluphenazine (℞)

(floo-fen′a-zeen)
Permitil, Prolixin, fluphenazine decanoate, Prolixin Decanoate, Prolixin Enanthate, fluphenazine HCl
Func. class.: Antipsychotic/neuroleptic
Chem. class.: Phenothiazine, piperazine

Action: Depresses cerebral cortex, hypothalamus, limbic system, which control activity and aggression; blocks neurotransmission produced by dopamine at synapse; exhibits strong α-adrenergic and anticholinergic blocking action; mechanism for antipsychotic effects is unclear

Uses: Psychotic disorders, schizophrenia

Dosage and routes:

Enanthate, decanoate
• *Adult and child >12 yr:* SC 12.5-25 mg ql-3wk

HCl
• *Adult:* PO 2.5-10 mg, in divided doses q6-8h, not to exceed 20 mg qd; IM initially 1.25 mg then 2.5-10 mg in divided doses q6-8h
• *Child:* PO 0.25-3.5 mg qd in divided doses q 4-6h, max 10 mg/qd

Available forms: HCl tabs 1, 2.5, 5, 10 mg; elix 2.5 mg/5 ml; conc 5 mg/ml; inj IM 10 mg/ml, enanthate, decanoate, inj SC, IM 25 mg/ml

Side effects/adverse reactions:
RESP: ***Laryngospasm,*** dyspnea, ***respiratory depression***
CNS: EPS: pseudoparkinsonism, akathisia, dystonia, tardive dyskinesia, drowsiness, headache, ***seizures, neuroleptic malignant syndrome***
HEMA: Anemia, ***leukopenia, leukocytosis, agranulocytosis***

INTEG: Rash, photosensitivity, dermatitis
EENT: Blurred vision, glaucoma, dry eyes
GI: Dry mouth, nausea, vomiting, anorexia, constipation, diarrhea, jaundice, weight gain, ***paralytic ileus, hepatitis***
GU: Urinary retention, urinary frequency, enuresis, impotence, amenorrhea, gynecomastia
CV: Orthostatic hypotension, hypertension, ***cardiac arrest,*** ECG changes, ***tachycardia***

Contraindications: Hypersensitivity, circulatory collapse, liver damage, cerebral arteriosclerosis, coronary disease, severe hypertension/hypotension, blood dyscrasias, coma, child <12 yr, brain damage, bone marrow depression, alcohol and barbiturate withdrawal

Precautions: Pregnancy (C), lactation, seizure disorders, hypertension, hepatic disease, cardiac disease

Pharmacokinetics:
PO/IM (HCl): Onset 1 hr, peak 2-4 hr, duration 6-8 hr
SC (enanthate): Onset 1-2 days, peak 2-3 days, duration 1-3 wk, half-life 3.5-4 days; decanoate: onset 1-3 days, peak 1-2 days, duration over 4 wk, single-dose half-life 6.8-9.6 days; multiple dose, 14.3 days; metabolized by liver; excreted in urine (metabolites); crosses placenta; enters breast milk

Interactions:
- Oversedation: other CNS depressants, alcohol, barbiturate anesthetics
- Toxicity: epinephrine
- Decreased effects of levodopa, lithium
- Decreased effects of fluphenazine: smoking, phenobarbital
- Increased effects of both drugs: β-adrenergic blockers, alcohol
- Increased effects: anticholinergics

Lab test interferences:
Increase: Liver function tests, cardiac enzymes, cholesterol, blood glucose, prolactin, bilirubin, PBI, cholinesterase
Decrease: Hormones (blood and urine)
False positive: Pregnancy tests, PKU
False negative: Urinary steroids, 17-OHCS, pregnancy tests

NURSING CONSIDERATIONS

Assess:
- Swallowing of PO medication; check for hoarding, giving of medication to other patients
- I&O ratio; palpate bladder if low urinary output occurs
- Bilirubin, CBC, liver function studies monthly
- Urinalysis is recommended before and during prolonged therapy
- Affect, orientation, LOC, reflexes, gait, coordination, sleep pattern disturbances
- B/P standing and lying; take pulse and respirations q4h during initial treatment; establish baseline before starting treatment; report drops of 30 mm Hg
- Dizziness, faintness, palpitations, tachycardia on rising
- EPS including akathisia (inability to sit still, no pattern to movements), tardive dyskinesia (bizarre movements of jaw, mouth, tongue, extremities), pseudoparkinsonism (rigidity, tremors, pill rolling, shuffling gait)
- Skin turgor qd
- Constipation, urinary retention qd; if these occur, increase bulk, H_2O in diet

Administer:
- Concentrate with juice, milk, or uncaffeinated drinks

• Antiparkinsonian agent if EPS occur
• IM injection into large muscle mass; to minimize postural hypotension, give injection and have patient remain seated or recumbent for ½ hr
• Use dry needle, or solution will become cloudy; use 21/G or larger due to viscosity

Perform/provide:
• Decreased noise input by dimming lights, avoiding loud noises
• Supervised ambulation until stabilized on medication; do not involve in strenuous exercise; fainting is possible; patient should not stand still for long periods
• Increased fluids to prevent constipation
• Sips of water, candy, gum for dry mouth
• Storage in tight, light-resistant container in cool environment

Evaluate:
• Therapeutic response: decrease in emotional excitement, hallucinations, delusions, paranoia, reorganization of patterns of thought, speech

Teach patient/family:
• That orthostatic hypotension occurs often; to rise from sitting or lying position gradually; avoid hazardous activities until stabilized on medication
• To avoid hot tubs, hot showers, tub baths, since hypotension may occur
• To avoid abrupt withdrawal of this drug, or EPS may result; drug should be withdrawn slowly
• To avoid OTC preparations (cough, hay fever, cold) unless approved by prescriber; serious drug interactions may occur; avoid use with alcohol, CNS depressants; increased drowsiness may occur
• To use a sunscreen to prevent burns
• Regarding compliance with drug regimen
• About EPS and necessity for meticulous oral hygiene, since oral candidiasis may occur
• To report sore throat, malaise, fever, bleeding, mouth sores; if these occur, CBC should be drawn and drug discontinued
• That in hot weather, heat stroke may occur; take extra precautions to stay cool
• That urine may turn pink to reddish-brown

Treatment of overdose: Lavage; if orally ingested, provide an airway; *do not induce vomiting*

flurandrenolide (℞)

(flure-an-dren'oh-lide)

Cordran, Cordran SP, Cordran Tape, Drenison ¼*, Drenison Tape*

Func. class.: Topical corticosteroid

Chem. class.: Synthetic fluorinated agent

Action: Antipruritic, antiinflammatory

Uses: Corticosteroid-responsive dermatoses, pruritus

Dosage and routes:
• *Adult and child:* TOP apply to affected area tid-qid; apply tape q12-24h

Available forms: Oint 0.025%, 0.05%; cream 0.025%, 0.05%; lotion 0.05%; tape 4 μg/cm^2

Side effects/adverse reactions:

INTEG: Burning, dryness, itching, irritation, acne, folliculitis, hypertrichosis, perioral dermatitis, hypopigmentation, atrophy, striae, miliaria, allergic contact dermatitis, secondary infection

F

Contraindications: Hypersensitivity to corticosteroids, fungal infections, viral infections

Precautions: Pregnancy (C), lactation, viral infections, bacterial infections

NURSING CONSIDERATIONS

Assess:

- Temp; if fever develops, drug should be discontinued
- Systemic absorption: fever, infection, irritation

Administer:

- Only to affected areas; do not get in eyes
- Then cover with occlusive dressing if ordered; seal to normal skin; change q12h; systemic absorption may occur
- Only to dermatoses; do not use on weeping, denuded, or infected area
- Tape after cutting with scissors; apply only to clean, dry wounds

Perform/provide:

- Cleansing before application
- Treatment for a few days after area has cleared
- Storage at room temp

Evaluate:

- Therapeutic response: absence of severe itching, patches on skin, flaking

Teach patient/family:

- To avoid sunlight on affected area; burns may occur

flurazepam (℞)

(flure-az′e-pam)

Dalmane, flurazepam, Somnol*

Func. class.: Sedative-hypnotic

Chem. class.: Benzodiazepine derivative

Controlled Substance Schedule IV (USA), Schedule F (Canada)

Action: Produces CNS depression at the limbic, thalamic, hypothalamic levels of CNS; may be mediated by neurotransmitter γ-aminobutyric acid (GABA); results are sedation, hypnosis, skeletal muscle relaxation, anticonvulsant activity, anxiolytic action

Uses: Insomnia

Dosage and routes:

- *Adult:* PO 15-30 mg hs; may repeat dose once if needed
- *Geriatric:* PO 15 mg hs; may increase if needed

Available forms: Caps 15, 30 mg

Side effects/adverse reactions:

HEMA: ***Leukopenia, granulocytopenia*** (rare)

CNS: Lethargy, drowsiness, daytime sedation, dizziness, confusion, lightheadedness, headache, anxiety, irritability

GI: Nausea, vomiting, diarrhea, heartburn, abdominal pain, constipation

CV: Chest pain, pulse changes

Contraindications: Hypersensitivity to benzodiazepines, pregnancy, lactation, intermittent porphyria, uncontrolled pain

Precautions: Anemia, hepatic disease, renal disease, suicidal individuals, drug abuse, elderly, psychosis, child <15 yr

Pharmacokinetics:

PO: Onset 15-45 min, duration 7-8 hr; metabolized by liver; excreted by kidneys (inactive/active metabolites); crosses placenta; excreted in breast milk; half-life 47-100 hr, additional 100 hr for active metabolites

Interactions:

- Increased effects of flurazepam: cimetidine, disulfiram, probenicid, isoniazid
- Increased action of both drugs: alcohol, CNS depressants
- Decreased effect of flurazepam: antacids, theophylline, rifampin, smoking

* Available in Canada only

Lab test interferences:
Increase: AST (SGOT), ALT (SGPT), serum bilirubin
False increase: Urinary 17-OHCS
Decrease: RAI uptake

NURSING CONSIDERATIONS

Assess:
- Blood studies: Hct, Hgb, RBC (if on long-term therapy)
- Hepatic studies: AST (SGOT), ALT (SGPT), bilirubin
- Mental status: mood, sensorium, affect, memory (long, short)
- Blood dyscrasias: fever, sore throat, bruising, rash, jaundice, epistaxis (rare)
- Type of sleep problem: falling asleep, staying asleep

Administer:
- After removal of cigarettes to prevent fires
- After trying conservative measures for insomnia
- ½-1 hr before hs for sleeplessness
- On empty stomach for fast onset, but may be taken with food if GI symptoms occur

Perform/provide:
- Assistance with ambulation after receiving dose
- Safety measure: side rails, nightlight, call bell within easy reach
- Checking to see PO medication has been swallowed
- Storage in tight container in cool environment

Evaluate:
- Therapeutic response: ability to sleep at night, decreased amount of early morning awakening if taking drug for insomnia

Teach patient/family:
- To avoid driving or other activities requiring alertness until drug is stabilized
- To avoid alcohol ingestion or CNS depressants; serious CNS depression may result
- That effects may take 2 nights for benefits to be noticed
- Alternative measures to improve sleep: reading, exercise several hours before hs, warm bath, warm milk, TV, self-hypnosis, deep breathing
- That hangover is common in elderly but less common than with barbiturates

Treatment of overdose: Lavage, activated charcoal; monitor electrolytes, vital signs

flurbiprofen (℞)

(flure-bi′proe-fen)

Ansaid, Froben*, Ocufen

Func. class.: Nonsteroidal anti-inflammatory ophthalmic

Chem. class.: Phenylalkanoic acid

Action: Inhibits enzyme system necessary for biosynthesis of prostaglandins; inhibits miosis

Uses: Inhibition of intraoperative miosis, corneal edema

Dosage and routes:
- *Adult:* Opth 1 gtt q½h beginning 2 hr before surgery (4 gtt total); PO 200-300 mg qd in 2-4 divided doses; max 300 mg/day or 100 mg/dose

Available forms: Sol 0.03%; tabs 50, 100 mg

Side effects/adverse reactions:
EENT: Burning, stinging in the eye, irritation, bleeding or redness

Contraindications: Hypersensitivity, epithelial herpes simplex keratitis

Precautions: Pregnancy (C), lactation, child, aspirin or nonsteroidal antiinflammatory drug hypersensitivity, allergy, bleeding disorder

Interactions:
- Ineffective action of acetylcholine, carbachol

NURSING CONSIDERATIONS

Administer:

- Excess sol must be wiped away promptly to prevent flow into lacrimal system, producing systemic symptoms
- Give PO dose ½ hr before or 2 hr pc

Perform/provide:

- Protect sol from sun

Evaluate:

- Therapeutic response: absence of corneal edema, intraoperative miosis

Teach patient/family:

- To report change in vision, blurring, or loss of sight during miosis
- To avoid hazardous activities if dizziness or drowsiness occurs
- Not to use for any other condition than prescribed

---

flutamide (℞)

(floo′-ta-mide)

Eulexin

Func. class.: Antineoplastic, hormone

Chem. class.: Antiandrogen

Action: Interferes with testosterone uptake in the nucleus or testosterone activity in target tissues; arrests tumor growth in androgen-sensitive tissue, i.e., prostate gland; prostatic carcinoma is androgen-sensitive, so tumor growth is arrested

Uses: Metastatic prostatic carcinoma, stage D2 in combination with LHRH agonistic analogs (leuprolide)

Dosage and routes:

- *Adult:* PO 250 mg q8h tid, for a daily dosage of 750 mg

Available forms: Cap 125 mg

Side effects/adverse reactions:

CNS: Hot flashes, drowsiness, confusion, depression, anxiety

GU: Decreased libido, impotence, gynecomastia

GI: Diarrhea, nausea, vomiting, increased liver function studies, ***hepatitis,*** anorexia

INTEG: Irritation at site, rash, photosensitivity

MISC: Edema, hematopoietic symptoms, neuromuscular and pulmonary symptoms, hypertension

Contraindications: Hypersensitivity, pregnancy (D)

Pharmacokinetics: Rapidly and completely absorbed; excreted in urine and feces as metabolites; half-life 6 hr, geriatric half-life 8 hr; 94% bound to plasma proteins

NURSING CONSIDERATIONS

Assess:

- Liver function studies: AST (SGOT), ALT (SGPT), alk phosphatase, which may be elevated
- For CNS symptoms including: drowsiness, confusion, depression, anxiety

Evaluate:

- Therapeutic response: decrease in prostatic tumor size, decrease in spread of cancer

Teach patient/family:

- To report side effects: decreased libido, impotence, breast enlargement, hot flashes, diarrhea
- That this drug is taken with leuprolide

Treatment of overdose: Induce vomiting, provide supportive care

---

fluvoxamine (℞)

(flu-vox′a-meen)

Luvox

Func. class.: Antidepressant—Misc.

Action: Inhibits CNS neuron uptake of serotonin but not of norepinephrine

Uses: Major depressive disorder, obsessive-compulsive disorder

Dosage and routes:

• *Adult:* PO 50-300 mg qd or in 2 divided doses

Available forms: Tabs 50, 100 mg

Side effects/adverse reactions:

CNS: Headache, drowsiness, dizziness, convulsions, sleep disorders

GI: Nausea, anorexia, constipation, hepatotoxicity, vomiting, diarrhea

INTEG: Rash, sweating

GU: Decreased libido

Contraindications: Hypersensitivity

Precautions: Pregnancy (B), lactation, child, elderly

Pharmacokinetics: Crosses blood-brain barrier, 77% protein binding, metabolism by the liver, terminal half-life 16.9 hr, peak 2-8 hr

Interactions:

• Increased CNS depression: alcohol, barbiturates, benzodiazipines

• Increased toxicity: tricyclic antidepressants, theophylline, lithium

• Drug/smoking: Increased metabolism, decreased effects

NURSING CONSIDERATIONS

Assess:

• Hepatic studies: AST (SGOT), ALT (SGPT), bilirubin

• Mental status: mood, sensorium, affect, suicidal tendencies; increase in psychiatric symptoms: depression, panic

• Constipation; most likely in elderly

• For withdrawal symptoms: headache, nausea, vomiting, muscle pain, weakness; not usual unless discontinued abruptly

Administer:

• With food, milk for GI symptoms

Perform/provide:

• Storage at room temp; do not freeze

Evaluate:

• Therapeutic response: decrease in depression

Teach patient/family:

• That therapeutic effects may take 2-3 wk

• To use caution in driving, other activities requiring alertness because of drowsiness, dizziness that may occur

• Not to discontinue medication quickly after long-term use: may cause nausea, headache, malaise

• To increase bulk in diet if constipation occurs, especially elderly

• To take gum, hard sugarless candy, or frequent sips of water for dry mouth

folic acid (vit B_9) (OTC)

(foe'lik a'sid)

Apo-Folic, Folate, Folvite, Novofolacid*, Vitamin B_9

Func. class.: Vit B complex group

Action: Needed for erythropoiesis; increases RBC, WBC, platelet formation in megaloblastic anemias

Uses: Megaloblastic or macrocytic anemia caused by folic acid deficiency; liver disease, alcoholism, hemolysis, intestinal obstruction, pregnancy

Dosage and routes:

Supplement

• *Adult:* PO/IM/SC/IV 0.1 mg qd

• *Child:* PO/IM/SC/IV 0.05 mg qd

Megaloblastic/macrocytic anemia

• *Adult and child >4 yr:* PO/SC/IM/IV 1 mg qd × 4-5 days

• *Child <4 yr:* PO/SC/IM/IV 0.3 mg or less qd

• *Pregnancy/lactation:* PO/SC/IM/IV 0.8 mg qd

Prevention of megaloblastic/macrocytic anemia

• *Pregnancy:* PO/SC/IM/IV 1 mg qd

Available forms: Tabs 0.1, 0.4, 0.8, 1 mg; inj 5, 10 mg/ml

Side effects/adverse reactions:

RESP: ***Bronchospasm***

INTEG: Flushing

Contraindications: Hypersensitivity, anemias other than megaloblastic/macrocytic anemia, vit B_{12} deficiency anemia, uncorrected pernicious anemia

Precautions: Pregnancy (A)

Pharmacokinetics:

PO: Peak ½-1 hr; bound to plasma proteins; excreted in breast milk; methylated in liver; excreted in urine (small amounts)

Interactions:

- Decreased folate levels: chloramphenicol
- Increased metabolism of: phenobarbitol, hydantoins
- Do not use with methotrexate unless leucovorin rescue is available

Syringe incompatibility: Doxapram

Y-site compatibility: Famotidine

Solution compatibility: $D_{20}W$

NURSING CONSIDERATIONS

Assess:

- For fatigue, dyspnea, weakness, SOB that are signs of megaloblastic anemia
- Hgb, Hct and reticulocyte count
- Folate levels: 6-15 µg/ml
- Nutritional status: bran, yeast, dried beans, nuts, fruits, fresh vegetables, asparagus
- Drugs currently taken: alcohol, oral contraceptives, hydantoins, trimethoprim; these drugs may cause increased folic acid use by body and contribute to a deficiency

Administer:

- IV direct undiluted 5 mg or less/1 min or may be added to most IV sol or TPN

Perform/provide:

- Storage in light-resistant container

Evaluate:

- Therapeutic response: increased weight, oriented well-being; absence of fatigue

Teach patient/family:

- To take drug exactly as prescribed
- To notify prescriber of side effects

foscarnet (℞)

(foss-kar′net)

Foscavir

Func. class.: Antiviral

Chem. class.: Inorganic pyrophosphate organic analog

Action: Antiviral activity is produced by selective inhibition at the pyrophosphate binding site on virus-specific DNA polymerases and reverse transcriptases at concentrations that do not affect cellular DNA polymerases

Uses: Treatment of CMV retinitis

Dosage and routes:

- *Adult:* IV INF 60 mg/kg given over at least 1 hr, q8hr × 2-3 wk initially, then 90-120 mg/kg/day over 2 hr, usually give with at least 750-1000 ml NS qd

In renal abnormalities:

- *Adult:* IV

Male:

$$\frac{140 - \text{age}}{\text{serum creatinine} \times 72} = \text{Ccr}$$

Female: 0.85 × above value

Dose based on table provided in package insert

Available forms: Inj 24 mg/ml

Side effects/adverse reactions:

CNS: Fever, dizziness, headache, ***seizures,*** fatigue, neuropathy, tremor, ataxia, dementia, stupor, EEG abnormalities, vertigo, ***coma,*** abnormal gait, hypertonia, EPS, hemiparesis, ***paralysis,*** hyperreflexia,

* Available in Canada only

paraplegia, ***tetany,*** hyporeflexia, neuralgia, neuritis, cerebral edema, paresthesia, depression, confusion, anxiety, insomnia, somnolence, amnesia, hallucinations, agitation
GI: Nausea, vomiting, anorexia, abdominal pain, constipation, dysphagia, rectal hemorrhage, dry mouth, melena, flatulence, ulcerative stomatitis, pancreatitis, enteritis, enterocolitis, glossitis, proctitis, stomatitis, increased amylases, gastroenteritis, ***pseudomembranous colitis,*** duodenal ulcer, ***paralytic ileus, esophageal ulceration,*** abnormal A-G ratio, increased AST (SGOT), ALT (SGPT), cholecystitis, ***hepatitis,*** dyspepsia, tenesmus, hepatosplenomegaly, jaundice
INTEG: Rash, sweating, pruritus, skin ulceration, seborrhea, skin discoloration, alopecia, acne, dermatitis, pain/inflammation at injection site, facial edema, dry skin, urticaria
HEMA: Anemia, ***granulocytopenia, leukopenia, thrombocytopenia,*** platelet abnormalities, ***thrombosis, pulmonary embolism, coagulation disorders, decreased prothrombin, hypochromic anemia, pancytopenia, hemolysis, leukocytosis,*** lymphadenopathy, epistaxis, lymphopenia
SYST: Hypokalemia, hypocalcemia, hypomagnesemia, increased alk phosphatase, LDH, BUN, acidosis, hypophosphatemia, hyperphosphatemia, dehydration, glycosuria, increased creatine phosphokinase, hypervolemia, infection, ***sepsis, death, ascites,*** hyponatremia, hypochloremia, hypercalcemia
GU: ***Acute renal failure,*** decreased Ccr and increased serum creatinine, ***glomerulonephritis, toxic nephropathy, nephrosis, renal tubular disorders, pyelonephritis, uremia, hematuria, albuminuria,*** dysuria, polyuria

RESP: Coughing, dyspnea, pneumonia, sinusitis, pharyngitis, ***pulmonary infiltration,*** stridor, ***pneumothorax, hemoptysis, bronchospasm,*** bronchitis, ***respiratory depression, pleural effusion, pulmonary hemorrhage,*** rhinitis
EENT: Visual field defects, vocal cord paralysis, speech disorders, taste perversion, eye pain, conjunctivitis, tinnitus, otitis
CV: Hypertension, palpitations, ECG abnormalities, 1st degree AV block, nonspecific ST-T segment changes, hypotension, cerebrovascular disorder, cardiomyopathy, ***cardiac arrest,*** bradycardia, dysrhythmias
MS: Arthralgia, myalgia

Contraindications: Hypersensitivity

Precautions: Pregnancy (C), lactation, children, elderly, renal disease, seizure disorders, electrolyte/mineral imbalances, severe anemia

Pharmacokinetics: 14%-17% plasma protein bound, half-life 2-8 hr in normal renal function

Interactions:

- Nephrotoxicity: aminoglycosides, amphotericin B, IV pentamidine
- Hypocalcemia: pentamidine
- Increased anemia: zidovudine

Y-site compatibilities: Aminophylline, amikacin, ampicillin, aztreonam, benzquinamide, cephalosporins, dexamethasone, dopamine, erythromycin lactobionate, fluconazole, flucytosine, furosemide, gentamicin, heparin, hydromorphone, hydroxyzine, metronidazole, miconazole, morphine, nafcillin, oxacillin, penicillin G potassium, phenytoin, piperacillin, rantidine, tobramycin

NURSING CONSIDERATIO

Assess:

- Culture should be don treatment (blood, urine, t

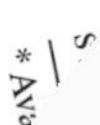

• Ophthalmic exam should confirm diagnosis
• Kidney, liver function studies: BUN, creatinine, AST (SGOT), ALT (SGPT)
• I&O ratio, urine pH
• Blood counts q2wk; watch for decreasing granulocytes, Hgb; if low, therapy may have to be discontinued and restarted after hematologic recovery; blood transfusions may be required
• GI symptoms: nausea, vomiting, diarrhea; severe symptoms may necessitate discontinuing drug
• Electrolytes and minerals: Ca, P, Mg, Na, K; watch closely for tetany during first administration
• Blood dyscrasias (anemia, granulocytopenia); bruising, fatigue, bleeding, poor healing
• Allergic reactions: flushing, rash, urticaria, pruritus

Administer:
• Increased fluids before and during drug administration to induce diuresis and minimize renal toxicity
• Using infusion device, at no more than 1 mg/kg/min; do not give by rapid or bolus IV; give by CVP or peripheral vein; standard 24 mg/ml solution may be used without dilution if using by CVP; dilute the 24 mg/ml sol to 12 mg/ml with D_5W or NS if using peripheral vein

Perform/provide:
• Regular ophthalmologic exams
• Close monitoring during therapy if tingling, numbness, paresthesias; if these occur, stop infusion, obtain lab sample for electrolytes

Evaluate:
• Therapeutic response: improvement in CMV retinitis

Teach patient/family:
• To call prescriber if sore throat, swollen lymph nodes, malaise, fever occur, since other infections may occur
• To report perioral tingling, numbness in extremities, and paresthesias
• That serious drug interactions may occur if OTC products are ingested; check first with prescriber
• That drug is not a cure but will control symptoms

fosinopril (℞)

(foss-in-o′pril)
Monopril
Func. class.: Antihypertensive
Chem. class.: Angiotensin-converting enzyme (ACE) inhibitor

Action: Selectively suppresses renin-angiotensin-aldosterone system; inhibits ACE; prevents conversion of angiotensin I to angiotensin II; results in dilation of arterial, venous vessels

Uses: Hypertension, alone or in combination with thiazide diuretics

Dosage and routes:
• *Adult:* PO 10 mg qd initially, then 20-40 mg/day divided bid or qd

Available forms: Tabs 10, 20 mg

Side effects/adverse reactions:
CV: Hypotension, chest pain, palpitations, angina, orthostatic hypotension
GU: ***Proteinuria,*** increased BUN, creatinine, decreased libido
HEMA: Decreased Hct, Hgb, ***eosinophilia, leukopenia, neutropenia***
INTEG: ***Angioedema,*** rash, flushing, sweating, photosensitivity, pruritus
RESP: Cough, sinusitis, dyspnea, ***bronchospasm***
META: Hyperkalemia
GI: Nausea, constipation, vomiting, diarrhea

CNS: Insomnia, paresthesia, headache, dizziness, fatigue, memory disturbance, tremor, mood change
MS: Arthralgia, myalgia
Contraindications: Hypersensitivity to ACE inhibitors, pregnancy (D), lactation, children
Precautions: Impaired liver function, hypovolemia, blood dyscrasias, CHF, COPD, asthma, elderly
Pharmacokinetics:
PO: Peak 3 hr; serum protein binding 97%; half-life 12 hr; metabolized by liver (metabolites excreted in urine, feces)
Interactions:
• Increased hypotension: diuretics, other antihypertensives, ganglionic blockers, adrenergic blockers
• Increased toxicity: vasodilators, hydralazine, prazosin, K-sparing diuretics, sympathomimetics
• Decreased absorption: antacids
• Decreased antihypertensive effect: indomethacin
• Increased serum levels of digoxin, lithium
• Increased hypersensitivity: allopurinol
Lab test interferences:
False positive: Urine acetone
NURSING CONSIDERATIONS
Assess:
• Blood studies: neutrophils, decreased platelets
• B/P, orthostatic hypotension, syncope
• Renal studies: protein, BUN, creatinine; increased levels may indicate nephrotic syndrome
• Baselines in renal, liver function tests before therapy begins
• K levels, although hyperkalemia rarely occurs
• Dipstick of urine for protein qd in first morning specimen; if protein is increased, a 24-hr urinary protein should be collected
• Edema in feet, legs daily
• Allergic reactions: rash, fever, pruritus, urticaria; drug should be discontinued if antihistamines fail to help
• Renal symptoms: polyuria, oliguria, frequency, dysuria
Administer:
• IV infusion of 0.9% NaCl (as ordered) to expand fluid volume if severe hypotension occurs
Perform/provide:
• Storage in tight container at 86° F (30° C) or less
• Supine or Trendelenburg position for severe hypotension
Evaluate:
• Therapeutic response: decrease in B/P
Teach patient/family:
• Not to discontinue drug abruptly
• Not to use OTC products (cough, cold, allergy) unless directed by prescriber; not to use salt substitutes containing potassium without consulting prescriber
• Importance of complying with dosage schedule, even if feeling better
• To rise slowly to sitting or standing position to minimize orthostatic hypotension
• To notify prescriber of mouth sores, sore throat, fever, swelling of hands or feet, irregular heart beat, chest pain
• To report excessive perspiration, dehydration, vomiting, diarrhea; may lead to fall in B/P
• That drug may cause dizziness, fainting, light-headedness during 1st few days of therapy
• That drug may cause skin rash or impaired perspiration
• How to take B/P; normal readings for age group
Treatment of overdose: 0.9% NaCl IV INF, hemodialysis

F

furosemide (℞)

(fur-oh'se-mide)

Fumide, Furomide M.D., furosemide, Lasix, Luramide, Novosemide*, Uritol*

Func. class.: Loop diuretic

Chem. class.: Sulfonamide derivative

Action: Inhibits reabsorption of sodium and chloride at proximal and distal tubule and in the loop of Henle

Uses: Pulmonary edema; edema in CHF, liver disease, nephrotic syndrome, ascites, hypertension

Investigational uses: Hypercalcemia in malignancy

Dosage and routes:

- *Adult:* PO 20-80 mg/day in AM; may give another dose in 6 hr up to 600 mg/day; IM/IV 20-40 mg, increased by 20 mg q2h until desired response
- *Child:* PO/IM/IV 2 mg/kg; may increase by 1-2 mg/kg/q6-8h up to 6 mg/kg

Pulmonary edema

- *Adult:* IV 40 mg given over several minutes, repeated in 1 hr; increase to 80 mg if needed

Hypertensive crisis/acute renal failure

- *Adult:* IV 100-200 mg over 1-2 min

Available forms: Tabs 20, 40, 80 mg; oral sol 8, 10, 500 mg/ml; inj IM, IV 10 mg/ml

Side effects/adverse reactions:

CNS: Headache, fatigue, weakness, vertigo, paresthesias

CV: Orthostatic hypotension, chest pain, ECG changes, ***circulatory collapse***

EENT: ***Loss of hearing,*** ear pain, tinnitus, blurred vision

ELECT: Hypokalemia, hypochloremic alkalosis, hypomagnesemia, hyperuricemia, hypocalcemia, hyponatremia, metabolic alkalosis

ENDO: Hyperglycemia

GI: Nausea, diarrhea, dry mouth, vomiting, anorexia, cramps, oral, gastric irritations, pancreatitis

GU: Polyuria, ***renal failure,*** glycosuria

HEMA: ***Thrombocytopenia, agranulocytosis, leukopenia, neutropenia, anemia***

INTEG: Rash, pruritus, purpura, ***Stevens-Johnson syndrome,*** sweating, photosensitivity, urticaria

MS: Cramps, stiffness

Contraindications: Hypersensitivity to sulfonamides, anuria, hypovolemia, infants, lactation, electrolyte depletion

Precautions: Diabetes mellitus, dehydration, severe renal disease, pregnancy (C)

Pharmacokinetics:

PO: Onset 1 hr, peak 1-2 hr, duration 6-8 hr; absorbed 70%

IV: Onset 5 min, peak ½ hr, duration 2 hr (metabolized by the liver 30%) Excreted in urine, some as unchanged drug, feces; crosses placenta; excreted in breast milk; half-life ½-1 hr

Interactions:

- Increased toxicity: lithium, nondepolarizing skeletal muscle relaxants, digitalis
- Increased K action of antihypertensives, oral anticoagulants, nitrates
- Increased ototoxicity: aminoglycosides, cisplatin, vancomycin
- Decreased antihypertensive effect of furosemide: indomethacin, metolazone

Y-site compatibilities: Amikacin sulfate, cisplatin, cyclophosphamide, dobuternine, fumotidine, fludarabine, fluorouracil, foscarnet, heparin, hydrocortisone dintrate, sodium

* Available in Canada only

succinate, kanamycin, leucovorin, methotrexate, mitomycin, potassium chloride, sargramostim, tobramycin, tolazoline, vitamin B complex with C

Additive compatibilities: Amikacin, aminophylline, amiodarone, ampicillin, atropine, flumetanide, calcium gluconate, cefumandole, cefuroxime, cimetidine, cloxacillin, digoxin, epinephrine, heparin, isosorbide, kanamycin, lidocaine, morphine, nitroglycerin, tobramycin, verapamil, ranitidine, sodium bicarbonate

Lab test interferences:

Interference: GTT

NURSING CONSIDERATIONS

Assess:

- Signs of metabolic alkalosis: drowsiness, restlessness
- Signs of hypokalemia: postural hypotension, malaise, fatigue, tachycardia, leg cramps, weakness
- Rashes, temperature elevation qd
- Confusion, especially in elderly; take safety precautions if needed
- Hearing, including tinnitus and hearing loss, when giving high doses for extended periods
- Weight, I&O qd to determine fluid loss; effect of drug may be decreased if used qd
- Rate, depth, rhythm of respiration, effect of exertion, lung sounds
- B/P lying, standing; postural hypotension may occur
- Electrolytes: K, Na, Cl; include BUN, blood sugar, CBC, serum creatinine, blood pH, ABGs, uric acid, Ca, Mg
- Skin turgor, edema, condition of mucous membranes in mouth and nose
- Glucose in urine if patient is diabetic
- Allergies to sulfonamides, thiazides

Administer:

- IV undiluted; may be given through Y-tube or 3-way stopcock; give 20 mg or less/min; may be added to NS or D_5W if large doses are required and given as IV INF, not to exceed 4 mg/min; use infusion pump
- In AM to avoid interference with sleep if using drug as a diuretic
- K replacement if K <3
- PO with food if nausea occurs; absorption may be decreased slightly; tablets may be crushed

Evaluate:

- Therapeutic response: improvement in edema of feet, legs, sacral area daily if medication is being used CHF

Teach patient/family:

- To discuss the need for a high-K diet or K replacement with prescriber
- To increase fluid intake 2-3 L/day unless contraindicated
- To rise slowly from lying or sitting position; orthostatic hypotension may occur
- Adverse reactions that may occur: muscle cramps, weakness, nausea, dizziness
- Regarding entire regimen, including exercise, diet, stress relief for hypertension
- To take with food or milk for GI symptoms
- To use sunscreen or protective clothing to prevent photosensitivity
- To take early in day to prevent sleeplessness
- To avoid OTC medication unless directed by prescriber

Treatment of overdose: Lavage if taken orally; monitor electrolytes; administer dextrose in saline; monitor hydration, CV, renal status

gabapentin (℞)

(gab'a-pen-tin)
Neurontin
Func. class.: Anticonvulsant

Action: Mechanism unknown; may increase seizure threshold; structurally similar to GABA; gabapentin binding sites in neocortex, hippocampus

Uses: Adjunct treatment of partial seizures, with or without generalization in adults

Dosage and routes:

• *Adult:* PO 900-1800 mg/day in 3 divided doses; may titrate by giving 300 mg on the first day, 300 mg bid on second day, 300 mg tid on third day; may increase to 1800 mg/day by adding 300 mg on subsequent days

Available forms: Caps 100, 300, 400 mg

Side effects/adverse reactions:

CNS: Dizziness, fatigue, anxiety, somnolence, ataxia, amnesia, abnormal thinking, unsteady gait, depression

CV: Vasodilation

EENT: Dry mouth, blurred vision, diplopia

GI: Constipation, increased appetite, dental abnormalities

GU: Impotence, bleeding, *UTI*

HEMA: ***Leukopenia,*** decreased WBC

INTEG: Pruritis, abrasion

MS: Myalgia

RESP: Rhinitis, pharyngitis, coughing

Contraindications: Hypersensitivity to this drug

Precautions: Hepatic disease, renal disease, pregnancy (C), lactation, child <6 yr, elderly

Pharmacokinetics:

Largely unbound to plasma proteins; not metabolized; excreted in urine (unchanged); elimination half-life 5-7 hr

Interactions:

• Decreased levels of gabapentin: antacids

NURSING CONSIDERATIONS

Assess:

• Renal studies: urinalysis, BUN, urine creatinine q3mo
• Hepatic studies: ALT (SGPT), AST (SGOT), bilirubin
• Description of seizures
• Mental status: mood, sensorium, affect, behavioral changes; if mental status changes, notify prescriber
• Eye problems, need for ophthalmic examinations before, during, after treatment (slit lamp, fundoscopy, tonometry)
• Allergic reaction: purpura, red raised rash; if these occur, drug should be discontinued

Administer:

• With food, milk to decrease GI symptoms

Perform/provide:

• Storage at room temp away from heat and light
• Hard candy, frequent rinsing of mouth, gum for dry mouth
• Assistance with ambulation during early part of treatment; dizziness occurs
• Seizure precautions: padded side rails; move objects that may harm patient
• Increased fluids, bulk in diet for constipation

Evaluate:

• Therapeutic response: decreased seizure activity; document on patient's chart

Teach patient/family:

• To carry Medic Alert ID stating patient's name, drugs taken, condition, prescriber's name and phone number
• To avoid driving, other activities that require alertness

• Not to discontinue medication quickly after long-term use

Treatment of overdose: Lavage, VS

gallamine (℞)

(gal'a-meen)

Flaxedil

Func. class.: Neuromuscular blocker (nondepolarizing)

Action: Inhibits transmission of nerve impulses by binding with cholinergic receptor sites, antagonizing action of acetylcholine

Uses: Facilitation of endotracheal intubation, skeletal muscle relaxation during mechanical ventilation, surgery, general anesthesia

Dosage and routes:

• *Adult and child >1 mo:* IV 1 mg/kg, not to exceed 100 mg, then 0.5-1 mg/kg q30-40 min

• *Child <1 mo, >5 kg:* IV 0.25-0.75 mg/kg, then 0.01-0.05 mg/kg q30-40 min

Available forms: Inj 20 mg/ml

Side effects/adverse reactions:

CV: Bradycardia, tachycardia, increased, decreased B/P

RESP: ***Prolonged apnea, bronchospasm, cyanosis, respiratory depression***

EENT: Increased secretions

INTEG: Rash, flushing, pruritus, urticaria

CNS: ***Malignant hyperthermia***

GI: Decreased motility

Contraindications: Hypersensitivity to iodides

Precautions: Pregnancy (C), thyroid disease, collagen disease, cardiac disease, lactation, children <2 yr, electrolyte imbalances, dehydration, neuromuscular disease (myasthenia gravis), respiratory disease, renal disease

Pharmacokinetics:

IV: Onset 2 min, duration 20-60 min; half-life 2 min, 29 min (terminal); excreted in urine, feces (metabolites); crosses placenta

Interactions:

• Increased neuromuscular blockade: aminoglycosides, clindamycin, lincomycin, quinidine, local anesthetics, polymyxin antibiotics, lithium, narcotic analgesics, thiazides, enflurane, isoflurane; used with cyclopropane, may provoke ventricular dysrhythmias

• Dysrhythmias: theophylline

• Incompatible with anesthetics, barbiturates in sol; incompatible with any other drug in syringe

NURSING CONSIDERATIONS

Assess:

• For electrolyte imbalances (K, Mg); may lead to increased action of this drug

• Vital signs (B/P, pulse, respirations, airway) q15min until fully recovered; rate, depth, pattern of respirations, strength of hand grip

• I&O ratio; check for urinary retention, frequency, hesitancy

• Recovery: decreased paralysis of face, diaphragm, leg, arm, rest of body

• Allergic reactions: rash, fever, respiratory distress, pruritus; drug should be discontinued

Administer:

• Using nerve stimulator by anesthesiologist to determine neuromuscular blockade

• Anticholinesterase to reverse neuromuscular blockade

• IV undiluted over 1-2 min (only by qualified person, usually an anesthesiologist)

• Only slightly discolored sol

Perform/provide:

• Storage in light-resistant, cool area

• Reassurance if communication is difficult during recovery from neuromuscular blockade

Evaluate:
• Therapeutic response: paralysis of jaw, eyelid, head, neck, rest of body
Treatment of overdose: Edrophonium or neostigmine, atropine; monitor VS; may require mechanical ventilation

---

gallium (℞)

(gal'ee-yum)
Ganite
Func. class.: Electrolyte modifier
Chem. class.: Hypocalcemic drug

Action: Lowers serum calcium levels by inhibiting calcium resorption from bone
Uses: Cancer-related hypercalcemia
Dosage and routes:
• *Adult:* IV 100-200 mg/m^2 qd × 5 days; infuse over 24 hr
Available forms: 25 mg/ml inj
Side effects/adverse reactions:
HEMA: ***Anemia, leukopenia***
CV: Tachycardia
EENT: Blurred vision, optic neuritis, hearing loss
GU: ***Nephrotoxicity,*** increased BUN, creatinine
META: *Hypophosphatemia,* hypocalcemia, decreased serum bicarbonate
Contraindications: Hypersensitivity, severe renal disease
Precautions: Pregnancy (C), lactation, children, mild renal disease
Pharmacokinetics:
IV: Onset 12-24 hr, peak 5 days, duration 8 days
Interactions:
• Increased nephrotoxicity: aminoglycosides, amphotericin B
NURSING CONSIDERATIONS
Assess:
• Renal status: BUN, creatinine, urine output; if creatinine level is 2.5 mg/dl or more, drug should be discontinued
• Monitor Ca, phosphate, bicarbonate, since all levels may be decreased and supplements of phosphate may be needed
• For hypercalcemia: nausea, vomiting, fatigue, weakness, thirst, dehydration, dysrhythmias, change in mental status
• For hypocalcemia: dysrhythmias; paresthesia; twitching; colic; laryngospasm; Trousseau's, Chvostek's sign; tremors
• For hypophosphatemia: confusion, decreased reflexes, joint stiffness and pain, portal hypotension
Administer:
• Adequate hydration with IV saline, 2 L/day during treatment
• After dilution of dose/1 L 0.9% NaCl or D_5W, run over 24 hr, use infusion pump
Perform/provide:
• Storage of solution 48 hr at room temp, 1 wk in refrigerator
Evaluate:
• Therapeutic response: decreased serum Ca levels
Teach patient/family:
• To follow dietary guidelines given by prescriber, including adequate Ca (dairy products, broccoli) and Vit D (fortified milk, grain products, fish oil)

---

ganciclovir (DHPG) (℞)

(gan-sye'kloe-vir)
Cytovene
Func. class.: Antiviral
Chem. class.: Synthetic nucleoside analog

Action: Inhibits replication of herpesviruses in vitro, in vivo by se-

*Available in Canada only

lective inhibition of the human CMV DNA polymerase and by direct incorporation into viral DNA
Uses: Cytomegalovirus (CMV) retinitis in immunocompromised persons, including those with AIDS, after indirect ophthalmoscopy con firms diagnosis
Dosage and routes:
Prevention of CMV
• *Adult:* IV 5 mg/kg q12hr × 1-2 wks, then 5 mg/kg/day or 6 mg/kg × 5 days each wk
Induction treatment
• *Adult:* IV 5 mg/kg given over 1 hr, q12h × 2-3 wk
Maintenance treatment
• *Adult:* IV INF 5 mg/kg given over 1 hr, qd × 7 days/wk; or 6 mg/kg qd × 5 days/wk; intraviteral IV 200 μg qwk
• Dosage must be reduced in renal impairment
Available forms: Powder 500 mg/vial ganciclovir
Side effects/adverse reactions:
HEMA: ***Granulocytopenia, thrombocytopenia, irreversible neutropenia, anemia, eosinophilia***
GI: Abnormal LFTs, nausea, vomiting, anorexia, diarrhea, abdominal pain, ***hemorrhage***
INTEG: Rash, alopecia, pruritis, urticaria, pain at site, phlebitis
CNS: Fever, chills, ***coma***, confusion, abnormal thoughts, dizziness, bizarre dreams, headache, psychosis, tremors, somnolence, paresthesia
CV: Dysrhythmia, hypertension/hypotension
RESP: Dyspnea
EENT: Retinal detachment in CMV retinitis
GU: ***Hematuria,*** increased creatinine, BUN
Contraindications: Hypersensitivity to acyclovir or ganciclovir
Precautions: Preexisting cytopenias, renal function impairment, pregnancy (C), lactation, children <6 mo, elderly, platelet count <25,000/mm
Pharmacokinetics: Half-life 3-4½ hr; excreted by the kidneys (unchanged drug); crosses blood-brain barrier, CSF
Interactions:
• Decreased renal clearance of ganciclovir: probenecid
• Increased toxicity: dapsone, pentamidine, flucytosine, vincristine, vinblastine, adriamycin, doxorubicin, amphotericin B, trimethoprim-sulfa combinations, or other nucleoside analogs
• Severe granulocytopenia: zidovudine; do not give together
• Increased seizures: imipenem/cilastatin
Y-site compatibilities: Enalaprilat, fluconazole, melphalan, paclitaxel

NURSING CONSIDERATIONS

Assess:
• For leukopenia/neutropenia/thrombocytopenia: WBCs, platelets q2d during 2 ×/d dosing and q1wk thereafter
• For leukopenia with qd WBC count in patients with prior leukopenia with other nucleoside analogs or for whom leukopenia counts are <1000 cells/mm^3 at start of treatment
• Serum creatinine or CrCl at least q2wk
Administer:
• Mixed in biologic cabinet, using gown, gloves, mask
• IV after diluting 500 mg/10 ml sterile H_2O for injection (50 mg/ml); shake; further dilute in 100 ml D_5W, 0.9% NaCl, LR and run over 1 hr; use infusion pump
• Slowly; do not give by bolus IV, IM, SC injection
• Using diluted sol within 12 hr; do not refrigerate or freeze

Evaluate:
• Therapeutic response: decreased symptoms of CMV

Teach patient/family:
• That drug does not cure condition, that regular ophthalmologic examinations are necessary
• That major toxicities may necessitate discontinuing drug
• To use contraception during treatment and that infertility may occur; men should use barrier contraception for 90 days after treatment

Treatment of overdose: Discontinue drug, use hemodialysis, and increase hydration

---

gemfibrozil (℞)

(gem-fi'broe-zil)
Lopid
Func. class.: Antilipemic
Chem. class.: Aryloxisobutyric acid derivative

Action: Inhibits biosynthesis of VLDL, LDL, which are responsible for cholesterol development

Uses: Type III/IV, V hyperlipidemia as adjunct with diet therapy

Dosage and routes:
• *Adult:* PO 1200 mg in divided doses bid 30 min before meals

Available forms: Caps 300, 600 mg

Side effects/adverse reactions:
GI: Nausea, vomiting, dyspepsia, diarrhea, abdominal pain
INTEG: Rash, urticaria, pruritus
HEMA: ***Leukopenia, anemia, eosinophilia***
CNS: Dizziness, blurred vision

Contraindications: Severe hepatic disease, preexisting gallbladder disease, severe renal disease, primary biliary cirrhosis, hypersensitivity

Precautions: Monitor hematologic and hepatic function, pregnancy (B), lactation

Pharmacokinetics:
PO: Peak 1-2 hr; plasma protein binding >90%; half-life 1.5 hr; excreted in urine; metabolized in liver

Interactions:
• May increase anticoagulant properties: oral anticoagulants
• Increased risk of myositis, myalgia: lovastatin

Lab test interferences:
Increase: Liver function studies, CPK, BSP, thymol turbidity, glucose
Decrease: Hgb, Hct, WBC

NURSING CONSIDERATIONS

Assess:
• Triglycerides, cholesterol; if cholesterol increases, drug should be discontinued
• Renal, hepatic levels if patient is on long-term therapy
• Bowel pattern daily; increase bulk, water in diet if constipation develops, especially elderly

Administer:
• 30 min before morning and evening meals

Evaluate:
• Therapeutic response: decreased cholesterol levels

Teach patient/family:
• That compliance is needed for positive results; do not double or skip dose
• That risk factors should be decreased: high-fat diet, smoking, alcohol consumption, absence of exercise
• To notify prescriber of diarrhea, nausea, vomiting, chills, fever, sore throat

---

* Available in Canada only

gentamicin (℞)

(jen-ta-mye'sin)

Alcomicin*, Apogen, Cidomycin*, Garamycin, Garamycin Intrathecal, Garamycin IV Piggyback, Garamycin Pediatric, gentamicin sulfate, Gentamicin Sulfate IV Piggyback, Jenamicin, Pediatric Gentamicin Sulfate

Func. class.: Antibiotic

Chem. class.: Aminoglycoside

Action: Interferes with protein synthesis in bacterial cell by binding to ribosomal subunit, causing misreading of genetic code; inaccurate peptide sequence forms in protein chain, causing bacterial death

Uses: Severe systemic infections of CNS, respiratory, GI, urinary tract, bone, skin, soft tissues caused by susceptible strains of *P. aeruginosa, Proteus, Klebsiella, Serratia, E. coli, Enterobacter, Citrobacter, Staphylococcus, Shigella, Salmonella*

Dosage and routes:

Severe systemic infections

- *Adult:* IV INF 3-5 mg/kg/day in 3 divided doses q8h; dilute in 50-200 ml NS or D_5W given over 30 min-2 hr; IM 3 mg/kg/day in divided doses q8h
- Adult: INTRATHECAL 4-8 mg qd
- *Child:* IV/IM 2-2.5 mg/kg q8h
- *Neonates and infants:* IV/IM 2.5 mg/kg q8h
- *Neonates <1 wk:* 2.5 mg/kg q12h
- *Infants and child >3 months:* INTRATHECAL 1-2 mg qd

Dental/respiratory procedures/ GI/GU surgery (prophylaxis endocarditis)

- *Adult:* IM 1.5 mg/kg ½-1 hr before procedure with ampicillin
- *Child:* IM 2.5 mg/kg ½-1 hr before procedure with ampicillin

Available forms: Inj IM, IV 10, 40, 60, 80, 100 mg; intrathecal 2 mg/ml

Side effects/adverse reactions:

GU: ***Oliguria, hematuria, renal damage, azotemia, renal failure, nephrotoxicity***

CNS: Confusion, depression, numbness, tremors, ***convulsions,*** muscle twitching, ***neurotoxicity,*** dizziness, vertigo

EENT: ***Ototoxicity,*** *deafness,* visual disturbances, tinnitus

HEMA: ***Agranulocytosis, thrombocytopenia, leukopenia, eosinophilia,*** anemia

GI: Nausea, vomiting, anorexia, increased ALT, AST, bilirubin, hepatomegaly, ***hepatic necrosis,*** splenomegaly

CV: Hypotension, hypertension, palpitations

INTEG: Rash, burning, urticaria, dermatitis, alopecia

Contraindications: Severe renal disease, hypersensitivity

Precautions: Neonates, mild renal disease, pregnancy (C), hearing deficits, myasthenia gravis, lactation, elderly, Parkinson's disease

Pharmacokinetics:

IM: Onset rapid, peak 1-2 hr

IV: Onset immediate, peak 1-2 hr

Plasma half-life 1-2 hr; duration 6-8 hr; not metabolized; excreted unchanged in urine; crosses placental barrier

Interactions:

- Increased ototoxicity, neurotoxicity, nephrotoxicity: other aminoglycosides, amphotericin B, polymyxin, vancomycin, ethacrynic acid, furosemide, mannitol, methoxyflurane, cisplatin, cephalosporins, bacitracin, enflurane
- Increased effects: nondepolarizing neuromuscular blockers

Y-site compatibilities: Acyclovir, aldesleukin, atracurium, cyclophosphamide, enalaprilat, esmolol, famotidine, fluconazole, fludarabine, foscarnet, hydromorphone, insulin, labetalol, hydromorphone, magnesium sulfate, meperidine, morphine, multivitamins, ondansetron, pancuronium, vecuronium, vitamin B with C, zidovudine

Additive compatibility: Ciprofloxacin

NURSING CONSIDERATIONS

Assess:

- Weight before treatment; calculation of dosage is usually based on ideal body weight, but may be calculated on actual body weight
- I&O ratio, urinalysis daily for proteinuria, cells, casts; report sudden change in urine output; toxicity is increased in patients with decreased renal function if high doses are given
- VS during infusion; watch for hypotension, change in pulse
- IV site for thrombophlebitis, including pain, redness, swelling, q30min, change site if needed; apply warm compresses to discontinued site
- Serum peak, drawn at 30-60 min after IV infusion or 60 min after IM injection, and trough level drawn just before next dose; blood level should be 2-4 times bacteriostatic level; peak = 4-10 μg/ml, trough = 1-2 μg/ml
- Urine pH if drug is used for UTI; urine should be kept alkaline
- Renal impairment by securing urine for CrCl testing, BUN, serum creatinine; lower dosage should be given in renal impairment (CrCl <80 ml/min)
- Deafness by audiometric testing, ringing, roaring in ears, vertigo; assess hearing before, during, after treatment
- Dehydration: high specific gravity, decrease in skin turgor, dry mucous membranes, dark urine
- Overgrowth of infection including fever, malaise, redness, pain, swelling, perineal itching, diarrhea, stomatitis, change in cough or sputum
- C&S before starting treatment to identify infecting organism
- Vestibular dysfunction: nausea, vomiting, dizziness, headache; drug should be discontinued if severe
- Injection sites for redness, swelling, abscesses; use warm compresses at site

Administer:

- IV after diluting in 50-200 ml NS or D_5W; sol concentration should be 1 mg/ml or less; decrease vol of diluent in child; maintain 0.1% sol run over ½-1 hr (adults) or up to 2 hr (children); flush IV line with NS or D_5W after administration
- IM injection in large muscle mass; rotate injection sites
- Drug in evenly spaced doses to maintain blood level
- Bicarbonate to alkalinize urine if ordered for UTI, as drug is most active in alkaline environment

Perform/provide:

- Adequate fluids of 2-3 L/day, unless contraindicated, to prevent irritation of tubules
- Supervised ambulation, other safety measures with vestibular dysfunction

Evaluate:

- Therapeutic response: absence of fever, draining wounds, negative C&S after treatment

Teach patient/family:

- To report headache, dizziness, symptoms of overgrowth of infection, renal impairment
- To report loss of hearing, ringing, roaring in ears or feeling of fullness in head

Treatment of overdose: Hemodialysis; monitor serum levels of drug

gentamicin (ophthalmic) (℞)

(jen-ta-mye'sin)

Garamycin Ophthalmic, Genoptic Ophthalmic, Genoptic S.O.P., Gentacidin, Gent-AK, gentamicin, Gentamicin Ophthalmic Liquifilm, Gentak

Func. class.: Antiinfective ophthalmic

Action: Inhibits bacterial protein synthesis

Uses: Infection of external eye

Dosage and routes:

• *Adult and child:* INSTILL 1 or 2 gtt q2-4h; TOP apply oint to conjunctival sac bid-qid

Available forms: Oint, sol 3%

Side effects/adverse reactions:

EENT: Poor corneal wound healing, temporary visual haze, overgrowth of nonsusceptible organisms

Contraindications: Hypersensitivity, vaccina, varicella, mycobacterial, fungal infections of eye, epithelial herpes simplex keratitis

Precautions: Antibiotic hypersensitivity, pregnancy (C)

NURSING CONSIDERATIONS

Assess:

• Allergy: itching, lacrimation, redness, swelling, photosensitivity

Administer:

• After washing hands; cleanse crusts or discharge from eye before application

Perform/provide:

• Storage at room temp

Evaluate:

• Therapeutic response: absence of redness, inflammation, tearing

Teach patient/family:

• To use drug exactly as prescribed
• Not to use eye makeup, towels, washcloths, eye medication of others; reinfection may occur
• That drug container tip should not be touched to eye
• To report itching, increased redness, burning, stinging, swelling; drug should be discontinued
• That drug may cause blurred vision when ointment is applied

gentamicin (topical) (℞)

(jen-ta-mye'sin)

G-Myticin, Garamycin, gentamicin

Func. class.: Local antiinfective

Chem. class.: Aminoglycoside

Action: Interferes with bacterial protein synthesis

Uses: Superficial skin infections; burns, skin ulcers

Dosage and routes:

• *Adult and child:* TOP rub into affected area tid-qid

Available forms: Cream, oint 0.1%

Side effects/adverse reactions:

INTEG: Rash, urticaria, stinging, burning, photosensitivity, pruritus

Contraindications: Hypersensitivity, impaired renal function

Precautions: Pregnancy (C), lactation

NURSING CONSIDERATIONS

Assess:

• Allergic reaction: burning, stinging, swelling, redness, photosensitivity

Administer:

• Enough medication to cover lesions completely; may cover with gauze dressing
• After cleansing with soap, water before each application; dry well

Perform/provide:

• Storage at room temp in dry place

Evaluate:

• Therapeutic response: decrease in size, number of lesions

G

Teach patient/family:

- To wash hands before, after each application
- To apply with glove to prevent further infection
- To avoid use of OTC creams, ointments, lotions unless directed by prescriber
- To avoid sunlight or wear sunscreen to prevent burns
- Not to use in eyes or external ear if eardrum is perforated
- To notify prescriber if condition worsens
- That overuse may lead to resistant organisms
- To avoid use on large skin lesions or over wide areas
- In impetigo, to remove crusts before applying

glipizide (℞)

(glip-i'zide)

Glucotrol

Func. class.: Antidiabetic

Chem. class.: Sulfonylurea (2nd generation)

Action: Causes functioning β-cells in pancreas to release insulin, leading to drop in blood glucose levels; may improve insulin binding to insulin receptors or increase the number of insulin receptors with prolonged administration; may also reduce basal hepatic glucose secretion; not effective if patient lacks functioning β-cells

Uses: Stable adult-onset diabetes mellitus (type II) NIDDM

Dosage and routes:

- *Adult:* PO 5 mg initially, then increase to desired response; max 40 mg/day in divided doses or 15 mg/dose
- *Elderly hepatic disease:* PO 2.5 mg initially, then increase to desired response; max 40 mg/day in divided doses or 15 mg/dose

Available forms: Tabs 5, 10 mg scored

Side effects/adverse reactions:

CNS: Headache, weakness, dizziness, drowsiness, tinnitus, fatigue, vertigo

GI: ***Hepatotoxicity, cholestatic jaundice,*** nausea, vomiting, diarrhea, heartburn

HEMA: ***Leukopenia, thrombocytopenia, agranulocytosis, aplastic anemia,*** increased AST, ALT, alk phosphatase, ***pancytopenia, hemolytic anemia***

INTEG: Rash, allergic reactions, pruritus, urticaria, eczema, photosensitivity, erythema

ENDO: ***Hypoglycemia***

Contraindications: Hypersensitivity to sulfonylureas, juvenile or brittle diabetes

Precautions: Pregnancy (C), elderly, cardiac disease, severe renal disease, severe hepatic disease, thyroid disease

Pharmacokinetics:

PO: Completely absorbed by GI route, onset 1-1½ hr, duration 10-24 hr, half-life 2-4 hr; metabolized in liver; excreted in urine; 90%-95% is plasma protein bound

Interactions:

- Increased hypoglycemic effects: insulin, MAOIs, cimetidine, chloramphenicol, guanethidine, methyldopa, nonsteroidal antiinflammatories, salicylates, probenecid
- Decreased action of glipizide: calcium channel blockers, corticosteroids, oral contraceptives, thiazide diuretics, thyroid preparations, estrogens, phenothiazines, phenytoin, rifampin, isoniazide, phenobarbital, sympathomimetics
- Disulfiram-like reaction: alcohol

• Decreased effects of both drugs: diazoxide

NURSING CONSIDERATIONS

Assess:

• Blood, urine glucose levels during treatment to determine diabetes control

• Hypo/hyperglycemic reaction that can occur soon after meals

Administer:

• Drug 30 min before meals

Perform/provide:

• Storage in tight light-resistant container at room temp

Evaluate:

• Therapeutic response: decrease in polyuria, polydipsia, polyphagia, clear sensorium, absence of dizziness, stable gait

Teach patient/family:

• Not to drink alcohol; explain disulfiram reaction

• To check for symptoms of cholestatic jaundice: dark urine, pruritus, yellow sclera; prescriber should be notified

• To use a capillary blood glucose test while on this drug

• To test blood glucose levels 3 ×/day

• The symptoms of hypo/hyperglycemia, what to do about each; to have glucagon emergency kit available

• That drug must be continued on daily basis; explain consequence of discontinuing drug abruptly

• To take drug in morning to prevent hypoglycemic reactions at night

• To avoid OTC medications unless ordered by prescriber

• That diabetes is a life-long illness; drug will not cure disease

• That all food in diet plan must be eaten to prevent hypoglycemia

• To carry Medic Alert ID for emergency purposes

• To test urine for glucose/ketones tid if this drug is replacing insulin

• To continue weight control, dietary restrictions, exercise, hygiene

Treatment of overdose: Glucose 25g IV via dextrose 50% solution 50 ml or 1 mg glucagon

glutethimide (℞)

(gloo-teth'i-mide)

Doriden, glutethimide

Func. class.: Sedative-hypnotic

Chem. class.: Piperidine derivative

Controlled Substance Schedule II (USA), Schedule F (Canada)

Action: Depresses activity in brain cells primarily in reticular activating system in brain stem, also selectively depresses neurons in posterior hypothalamus, limbic structures; pronounced anticholinergic activity; suppresses REM sleep

Uses: Insomnia

Dosage and routes:

• *Adult:* PO 250-500 mg hs; may repeat dose >4 hr before usual awakening, not to exceed 1 g

Available forms: Tabs 500 mg

Side effects/adverse reactions:

HEMA: ***Thrombocytopenia, aplastic anemia, leukopenia, megaloblastic anemia***

CNS: Residual sedation, dizziness, ataxia, stimulation, headache, hangover

GI: Nausea, vomiting, hiccups, diarrhea, jaundice

GU: Porphyria

INTEG: Rash, urticaria, purpura, ***exfoliative dermatitis*** (rare)

EENT: Dry mouth, blurred vision

Contraindications: Hypersensitivity to this drug or piperidine derivatives, severe pain, severe renal disease, porphyria

Precautions: Depression, suicidal individuals, drug abuse, cardiac dysrhythmias, narrow-angle glaucoma, prostatic hypertrophy, stenosed peptic ulcer, pyloroduodenal/bladder neck obstruction, pregnancy (C)

Pharmacokinetics:

PO: Onset 30 min, peak 1-2 hr, duration 4-8 hr; metabolized by liver; excreted by kidneys (metabolites); crosses placenta; excreted in breast milk; half-life 4 hr, 10-20 hr terminal

Interactions:

• Decreased hypoprothrombinemic effect: oral anticoagulants

• Increased CNS depression: alcohol and other CNS depressants

• Increased anticholinergic effect: tricyclic antidepressants

Lab test interferences:

Interferences: 17-OHCS

NURSING CONSIDERATIONS

Assess:

• Blood studies: Hct, Hgb, RBCs (if on long-term therapy)

• Hepatic studies: AST (SGOT), ALT (SGPT), bilirubin

• Mental status: mood, sensorium, affect, memory (long, short)

• Blood dyscrasias: fever, sore throat, bruising, rash, jaundice, epistaxis (rare)

• Type of sleep problem: falling asleep, staying asleep

Administer:

• After removal of cigarettes to prevent fires

• After trying conservative measures for insomnia

• ½-1 hr before hs for sleeplessness

• Several hours before patient is to arise (to avoid hangover)

Perform/provide:

• Assistance with ambulation after receiving dose

• Safety measures: side rails, nightlight, call bell within easy reach

• Checking to see PO medication has been swallowed

• Storage in tight container in cool environment

Evaluate:

• Therapeutic response: ability to sleep at night, decreased amount of early morning awakening

Teach patient/family:

• To avoid driving, other activities requiring alertness until stabilized

• To avoid alcohol ingestion or CNS depressants; serious CNS depression may result

• Not to discontinue medication quickly after long-term use; drug should be tapered over 1-2 wk

• That effects may take 2 nights for benefits to be noticed

• Alternate measures to improve sleep: reading, exercise several hours before hs, warm bath, warm milk, TV, self-hypnosis, deep breathing

• That hangover is common in elderly but less common than with barbiturates

• Symptoms of withdrawal: nausea, vomiting, anxiety, hallucinations, insomnia, tachycardia, fever, cramps, tremors, seizures

• Blood dyscrasias: fever, sore throat, bruising, rash, jaundice (rare)

• Allergic reaction: rash; discontinue drug if rash occurs

Treatment of overdose: Lavage, activated charcoal; monitor electrolytes, vital signs

glyburide (℞)

(glye'byoor-ide)

DiaBeta*, Glynase Prestab, Micronase

Func. class.: Antidiabetic

Chem. class.: Sulfonylurea (2nd generation)

Action: Causes functioning β-cells in pancreas to release insulin, leading to drop in blood glucose levels;

* Available in Canada only

may improve insulin binding to insulin receptors and increase number of insulin receptors with prolonged administration; may also reduce basal hepatic glucose secretion; not effective if patient lacks functioning β-cells

Uses: Stable adult-onset diabetes mellitus (type II) NIDDM

Dosage and routes:

• *Adult:* PO 2.5-5 mg initially, then increased to desired response

• *Elderly:* PO 1.25 mg initially, then increased to desired response; max 20 mg/day, maintenance 1.25-20 mg/qd

Available forms: Tabs 1.25, 2.5, 5 mg

Side effects/adverse reactions:

CNS: Headache, weakness, paresthesia, tinnitus, fatigue, vertigo

GI: Nausea, fullness, heartburn, ***hepatotoxicity, cholestatic jaundice,*** vomiting, diarrhea

HEMA: ***Leukopenia, thrombocytopenia, agranulocytosis, aplastic anemia,*** increased AST, ALT, alk phosphatase

INTEG: Rash, allergic reactions, pruritus, urticaria, eczema, photosensitivity, erythema

ENDO: ***Hypoglycemia***

MS: Joint pains

Contraindications: Hypersensitivity to sulfonylureas, juvenile or brittle diabetes

Precautions: Pregnancy (B), elderly, cardiac disease, severe renal disease, severe hepatic disease, thyroid disease, severe hypoglycemic reactions

Pharmacokinetics:

PO: Completely absorbed by GI route; onset 2-4 hr, peak 2-8 hr, duration 24 hr; half-life 10 hr; metabolized in liver; excreted in urine, feces (metabolites); crosses placenta; 90%-95% is plasma protein bound

Interactions:

• Both drugs' effects may be decreased: diazoxide

• Decreased digoxin level: digoxin

• Increased hypoglycemic effects: insulin, MAOIs, cimetidine, oral anticoagulants, chloramphenicol, guanethidine, methyldopa, nonsteroidal antiinflammatories, salicylates, probenecid

• Decreased action of glyburide: calcium channel blockers, corticosteroids, oral contraceptives, thiazide diuretics, thyroid preparations, estrogens, phenothiazines, phenytoin, rifampin, isoniazide, phenobarbital, sympathomimetics

• Disulfiram-like reaction: alcohol

NURSING CONSIDERATIONS

Assess:

• Hypo/hyperglycemic reaction that can occur soon after meals

Administer:

• With breakfast

Perform/provide:

• Storage in tight container in cool environment

Evaluate:

• Therapeutic response: decrease in polyuria, polydipsia, polyphagia, clear sensorium, absence of dizziness, stable gait

Teach patient/family:

• Not to drink alcohol; explain disulfiram reaction

• To check for symptoms of cholestatic jaundice: dark urine, pruritus, yellow sclera; if these occur, notify prescriber

• To use a capillary blood glucose test while on this drug

• The symptoms of hypo/hyperglycemia, what to do about each

• That drug must be continued on daily basis; explain consequence of discontinuing drug abruptly

• To take drug in morning to prevent hypoglycemic reactions at night

• To avoid OTC medications unless ordered by prescriber
• That diabetes is a lifelong illness; drug will not cure disease
• That all food included in diet plan must be eaten to prevent hypoglycemia; to have glucagon emergency kit available
• To carry a Medic Alert ID for emergency purposes

Treatment of overdose: Glucose 25 g IV via dextrose 50% solution, 50 ml or 1 mg glucagon

glycerin (OTC)

(gli'ser-in)

Fleet Babylax, Glycerin USP, Glycerol, Osmoglyn, Sani-Supp

Func. class.: Laxative, hyperosmotic

Chem. class.: Trihydric alcohol

Action: Increases osmotic pressure, draws fluid into colon, lumen from extravascular spaces to intravascular

Uses: Constipation

Dosage and routes:

Laxative

• *Adult and child >6 yr:* REC SUPP 3 g; ENEMA 5-15 ml
• *Child <6 yr:* REC SUPP 1-1.5 g; ENEMA 2-5 ml

Intraocular pressure reduction

• *Adult:* PO 1-1.5 g/kg once, then may be given 500 mg/kg q6h
• *Child:* PO 1-1.5 g/kg once, then 500 mg/kg 4-8 hr after 1st dose

Available forms: Rec sol 4 ml/applicator; supp; oral sol 0.6 g/ml

Side effects/adverse reactions:

CNS: Headache, confusion, ***convulsions***

GI: Nausea, vomiting, diarrhea

META: Dehydration

Contraindications: Hypersensitivity

Precautions: Pregnancy (C)

NURSING CONSIDERATIONS

Assess:

• Cause of constipation; identify whether fluids, bulk, or exercise is missing from lifestyle
• Cramping, rectal bleeding, nausea, vomiting; if these symptoms occur, drug should be discontinued

Administer:

• Insert supp; may cause evacuation in ½ hr
• Enema: use 4 ml applicator; patient should be in side-lying position
• Pour oral sol over cracked ice and sip through a straw
• To prevent cerebral dehydration, headache, patient should be recumbent during and after administration

Perform/provide:

• Storage in cool environment; do not freeze

Evaluate:

• Therapeutic response: decrease in constipation

Teach patient/family:

• Not to use laxatives for long-term therapy; bowel tone will be lost
• That normal bowel movements do not always occur daily
• Not to use in presence of abdominal pain, nausea, vomiting
• To notify prescriber if constipation unrelieved or if symptoms of electrolyte imbalance occur: muscle cramps, pain, weakness, dizziness, excessive thirst

glycerin, anhydrous (℞)

(gli'ser-in)

Ophthalgan Ophthalmic

Func. class.: Ophthalmic

Chem. class.: Trihydric alcohol

Action: Reduces corneal edema by osmosis of water through corneal

* Available in Canada only

epithelium, which is semipermeable

Uses: Reduce corneal edema

Dosage and routes:

• *Adult:* INSTILL 1-2 gtt after local anesthetic

Available forms: Sol

Side effects/adverse reactions:

EENT: Eye pain

CNS: Headache

Contraindications: Hypersensitivity

Precautions: Pregnancy (C), lactation, children

Pharmacokinetics: Onset 10 min, peak 20 min, duration 6-8 hr

NURSING CONSIDERATIONS

Administer:

• Anesthetic (tetracaine or proparacaine) before instillation to decrease pain

Perform/provide:

• Storage in tight container; discard 6 mo after opening

Evaluate:

• Therapeutic response: decreased corneal edema

Teach patient/family:

• Method of instillation, including pressure on lacrimal sac for 1 min, and not to touch dropper to eye

glycopyrrolate (℞)

(glye-koe-pye′roe-late)

glycopyrrolate, Robinul, Robinul Forte

Func. class.: Cholinergic blocker

Chem. class.: Quaternary ammonium compound

Action: Inhibits the action of acetylcholine at receptor sites in autonomic nervous system, which controls secretions, free acids in stomach

Uses: Decreased secretions before surgery, reversal of neuromuscular blockade, peptic ulcer disease, irritable bowel syndrome

Dosage and routes:

Preoperatively

• *Adult:* IM 0.002 mg/kg ½-1 hr before surgery

• *Child 2-12 yr:* IM 0.002-0.004 mg/kg

• *Child <2 yr:* IM 0.004 mg/kg

Reversal of neuromuscular blockade

• *Adult:* IV 0.2 mg for each 1 mg of neostigmine or 5 mg IV of pyridostigmine simultaneously

GI disorders

• *Adult:* PO 1-2 mg bid-tid; IM/IV 0.1-0.2 mg tid-qid, titrated to patient response

Available forms: Tabs 1, 2 mg; inj 0.2 mg/ml

Side effects/adverse reactions:

INTEG: Urticaria, allergic reactions

MISC: Suppression of lactation, nasal congestion, decreased sweating

CNS: Confusion, anxiety, restlessness, irritability, delusions, hallucinations, headache, sedation, depression, incoherence, dizziness, lethargy, flushing, weakness

EENT: Blurred vision, photophobia, dilated pupils, difficulty swallowing, increased intraocular pressure, mydriasis, cycloplegia

CV: Palpitations, tachycardia, postural hypotension, paradoxical bradycardia

GI: Dryness of mouth, constipation, nausea, vomiting, abdominal distress, paralytic ileus, altered taste perception

GU: Hesitancy, retention, impotence

Contraindications: Hypersensitivity, narrow-angle glaucoma, myasthenia gravis, GI/GU obstruction, child <3 yr, tachycardia, myocardial ischemia, hepatic disease, ulcerative colitis, toxic megacolon

Precautions: Pregnancy (C), elderly, lactation, prostatic hypertrophy, renal disease, CHF, pulmonary disease, hyperthyroidism
Pharmacokinetics:
PO: Peak 1 hr, duration 8-12 hr
IM: Peak 30-45 min, duration 2-7 hr
IV: Peak 10-15 min, duration 2-7 hr
Excreted in urine (50%), (unchanged); half-life 1-2 hr
Interactions:

• Increased anticholinergic effect: alcohol, antihistamines, phenothiazines, amantadine, tricyclics
• Decreased absorption of glycopyrrolate: antacids, antidiarrheals

Syringe compatibilities: Atropine, benzquinamide, butorphanol, chlorpromazine, cimetidine, codeine, dimenhydrinate, diphenhydramine, droperidol, fentanyl, glycopyrrolate, heparin, hydromorphone, hydroxyzine, levorphanol, lidocaine, meperidine, midazolam, morphine, nalbuphine, pentazocine, prochlorperazine, promazine, promethazine, proprionmazine, ranitidine, scopolamine

NURSING CONSIDERATIONS
Assess:

• I&O ratio; retention commonly causes decreased urinary output
• Urinary hesitancy, retention: palpate bladder if retention occurs
• Constipation; increase fluids, bulk, exercise if this occurs
• For tolerance over long-term therapy; dose may have to be increased or changed
• Mental status: affect, mood, CNS depression, worsening of mental symptoms during early therapy

Administer:

• IV undiluted, give through a Y-tube or 3-way stopcock; give 0.2 mg or less over 1-2 min
• Parenteral dose with patient recumbent to prevent postural hypotension
• Parenteral dose slowly; keep in bed for at least 1 hr after dose; monitor vital signs
• After checking dose carefully; even slight overdose may lead to toxicity
• With or after meals to prevent GI upset; may give with fluids other than water

Perform/provide:

• Storage at room temp
• Hard candy, frequent drinks, sugarless gum to relieve dry mouth

Evaluate:

• Therapeutic response: decreased secretions

Teach patient/family:

• Not to discontinue this drug abruptly; to taper off over 1 wk
• To avoid driving, other hazardous activities; drowsiness may occur
• To avoid OTC medication: cough, cold preparations with alcohol, antihistamines unless directed by prescriber

gonadorelin acetate (℞)

(goe-nad-oh-rell'in)
Lutrepulse
Func. class.: Gonadotropin hormone
Chem. class.: Synthetic endogenous gonadotropin-releasing hormone (GnRH)

Action: Induces ovulation in women by release of LH in the anterior pituitary gland
Uses: Primary hypothalamic amenorrhea to produce ovulation
Dosage and routes:

• IV Pump: 25-50 μg/q1½ hr, × 21 days; after three treatment intervals, it may be necessary to raise the dose in a stepwise program

* Available in Canada only

Available forms: Powder for inj, 0.8, 3.2 mg/vial to use with Lutrepulse pump
Side effects/adverse reactions:
INTEG: Inflammation at injection site, phlebitis, hematoma at catheter site
SYST: ***Anaphylaxis (bronchospasm, tachycardia, flushing, urticaria, induration of injection site)***
REPRO: Ovarian hyperstimulation, multiple pregnancy
Contraindications: Hypersensitivity; ovarian cysts, hormonally dependent tumors; causes of anovulation not of hypothalamic origin
Precautions: Pregnancy (B)
Pharmacokinetics: Metabolized by the liver to inactive compounds; excreted by kidneys, half-life (initial) 2-10 min, (terminal 10-40 min)
Interaction:
- Ovulation stimulators should not be used with this drug

NURSING CONSIDERATIONS
Assess:
- Effects by ovarian ultrasound: baseline, after 1 wk, after 2 wk, midluteal phase serum progesterone

Administer:
- Using Lutrepulse pump only; detailed instructions with pump
- After reconstituting 8 ml of diluent provided and transferring to plastic reservoir, withdraw 8 ml of diluent and inject into lyophile drug cake; shake, fill reservoir bag with reconstituted solution, and administer IV using pump provider; 8 ml = 1 wk supply; set pump to 25-50 μg/sol/min and pulse frequency of 1½ hr

Perform/provide:
- Storage at room temp; use prepared sol within 24 hr

Evaluate:
- Therapeutic response: absence of amenorrhea; return of ovulation with drug use

Teach patient/family:
- To report inflammation, redness at IV site
- On proper use of drug and pump; provide demonstration, return demonstration

gonadorelin HCl (℞)
(goe-nad-oh-rell'in)
Factrel
Func. class.: Gonadotropin hormone
Chem. class.: Synthetic luteinizing hormone–releasing hormone

Action: Combination luteinizing hormone (releasing hormone) that acts on anterior pituitary
Uses: Evaluation of response of gonadotropic hormone
Dosage and routes:
- *Women:* SC/IV 100 μg usually given between day 1-7 of menstrual cycle

Available forms: Powder for inj 100, 500 μg/vial
Side effects/adverse reactions:
CNS: Dizziness, headache, flushing
GI: Nausea
INTEG: Inflammation at injection site
SYST: ***Anaphylaxis*** antibody formation (large doses)
Contraindications: Hypersensitivity
Precautions: Pregnancy (B)
Pharmacokinetics: Metabolized to inactive compound; excreted by kidneys; half-life up to 40 min
Interactions:
- Increased level of gonadorelin: levodopa, spironolactone
- Decreased level of gonadorelin: digoxin, oral contraceptives, phenothiazines, dopamine antagonists

Lab test interferences:
False results when used with androgens, glucocorticoids, estrogens, progestins

NURSING CONSIDERATIONS

Assess:
- Test result: pituitary/hypothalamus dysfunction (decreased LH); postmenopausal (increased LH)

Administer:
- After reconstituting with sterile diluent (1 ml)/100 μg or 500 μg/2 ml enclosed in package; give over 30 sec
- Repeated doses may be necessary to elevate pituitary gonadotropin reserve

Perform/provide:
- Discard of unused portions

Teach patient/family:
- To report rash, hives, difficult breathing, flushing

---

goserelin (℞)

(goe'se-rel-lin)
Zoladex

Func. class.: Gonadotropin-releasing hormone
Chem. class.: Synthetic decapeptide analog of LHRH

Action: Inhibitor of pituitary gonadotropin secretion; initially increases LH and FSH, with increases in testosterone, reduction in sex steroid levels

Uses: Advanced prostate cancer

Dosage and routes:
- *Adult:* SC 3.6 mg q28d

Available forms: Depot inj 3.6 mg

Side effects/adverse reactions:

CNS: Headaches, ***spinal cord compression,*** anxiety, depression

CV: ***Dysrhythmia, cerebrovascular accident,*** hypertension, ***MI***, chest pain

ENDO: Gynecomastia, breast tenderness, hot flashes

GI: Nausea, vomiting, constipation, diarrhea, ulcer

GU: Spotting, breakthrough bleeding, decreased libido, renal insufficiency, urinary obstruction, urinary tract infection

INTEG: Rash, pain on injection

MS: Osteoneuralgia

Contraindications: Hypersensitivity, pregnancy (X)

Pharmacokinetics: Peak serum concentrations in 14-28 days; half-life 4½ hr

Lab test interferences:
Increased: Alk phosphatase, estradiol, FSH, LH, testosterone levels
Decreased: Testosterone levels, progesterone

NURSING CONSIDERATIONS

Assess:
- I&O ratios; palpate bladder for distention in urinary obstruction
- For relief of bone pain (back pain)

Administer:
- SC using implant, inserted by qualified person into upper subcutaneous tissue in abdominal wall q28d

Evaluate:
- Therapeutic response: more normal levels of prostate-specific antigen, acid phosphatase, alk phosphatase; testosterone level of <25 ng/dl

Teach patient/family:
- That gynecomastia and postmenopausal symptoms may occur but will decrease after treatment is discontinued

---

* Available in Canada only

granisetron (℞)

(grane-iss'e-tron)

Kytril

Func. class.: Antiemetic

Chem. class.: 5-HT_3 receptor antagonist

Action: Prevents nausea, vomiting by blocking serotonin peripherally, centrally, and in the small intestine

Uses: Prevention of nausea, vomiting associated with cancer chemotherapy including high-dose cisplatin

Dosage and routes:

• *Adult:* IV 10 μg/kg over 5 min, 30 min before the start of cancer chemotherapy; PO 1 mg bid, give 1st dose 1 hr before chemotherapy and next dose 12 hr after 1st

Available forms: Inj 1 mg/ml; tab 1 mg

Side effects/adverse reactions:

CNS: Headache

GI: Diarrhea, constipation, increased AST (SGOT), ALT (SGPT)

MISC: Rash, ***bronchospasm***

Contraindications: Hypersensitivity

Precautions: Pregnancy (B), lactation, children, elderly

Pharmacokinetics: Not known

Interactions: Unknown

NURSING CONSIDERATIONS

Assess:

• For absence of nausea, vomiting during chemotherapy

• Hypersensitive reaction: rash, bronchospasm

Administer:

• IV directly over 5 min

Perform/provide:

• Storage at room temp for 48 hr after dilution

Evaluate:

• Therapeutic response: absence of nausea, vomiting during cancer chemotherapy

Teach patient/family:

• To report diarrhea, constipation, rash, changes in respirations

griseofulvin microsize/ griseofulvin ultramicrosize (℞)

(gris-ee-oh-ful'vin)

Fulvicin-U/F, Grifulvin V, Grisactin, Grisactin 500, Fulvicin P/G, Grisactin-Ultra, Gris-PEG

Func. class.: Antifungal

Chem. class.: Penicillium griseofulvum derivative

Action: Arrests fungal cell division at metaphase; binds to human keratin, making it resistant to disease

Uses: Mycotic infections: tinea corporis, tinea pedis, tinea cruris, tinea barbae, tinea capitis, tinea unguium if caused by *Epidermophyton, Microsporum, Trichophyton*

Dosage and routes:

• *Adult:* PO 500-1000 mg qd in single or divided doses (microsize), 125-165 mg bid (ultramicrosize) or 250-330 mg qd; may need 500-660 mg in divided doses for severe infections

• *Child:* PO 10 mg/kg/day or 30 mg/m^2/day (microsize) or 5 mg/kg/day (ultramicrosize)

Available forms: Microcaps 125, 250 mg; tabs 250, 500 mg; oral susp 125 mg/ml; ultratabs 125, 165, 250, 330 mg

Side effects/adverse reactions:

INTEG: Rash, urticaria, photosensitivity, lichen planus

CNS: Headache, peripheral neuritis, paresthesias, confusion, dizziness, fatigue

EENT: Transient hearing loss

GU: Proteinuria, cylinduria, precipitate porphyria, increased thirst
GI: Nausea, vomiting, anorexia, diarrhea, cramps, dry mouth, flatulence
HEMA: ***Leukopenia, granulocytopenia, neutropenia, monocytosis***

Contraindications: Hypersensitivity, porphyria, hepatic disease, lupus erythematosus

Precautions: Penicillin sensitivity, pregnancy (C)

Pharmacokinetics:
PO: Peak 4 hr, half-life 9-24 hr, metabolized in liver; excreted in urine (inactive metabolites), feces, perspiration

Interactions:
- Tachycardia: alcohol
- Decreased action of griseofulvin: barbiturates
- Decreased action of warfarin, anticoagulants (oral)

NURSING CONSIDERATIONS

Assess:
- I&O ratio
- Liver studies qwk (ALT [SGPT], AST [SGOT], bilirubin, alk phosphatase)
- Renal studies: BUN, serum creatinine
- Blood studies: CBC, platelets, q2wk
- Drug level during treatment
- For history of penicillin allergy; may be cross-sensitive to this drug
- For renal toxicity: increasing BUN, serum creatinine, proteinuria, cylinduria
- For hepatotoxicity: increasing ALT (SGPT), AST (SGOT), bilirubin, alk phosphatase
- For blood dyscrasias: fatigue, malaise, dark urine, bruising

Administer:
- Drug carefully, making sure there is no confusion with dosage form (microsize vs ultramicrosize)
- With meals to decrease GI symptoms; fatty meals for better absorption
- Until 3 separate cultures are negative for infective organism

Perform/provide:
- Storage in tight, light-resistant containers at room temp

Evaluate:
- Therapeutic response: decreased fever, malaise, rash, negative C&S for infecting organism

Teach patient/family:
- That long-term therapy may be needed to clear infection (2 wk-6 mo depending on organism)
- Proper hygiene: hand-washing technique, nail care, use of concomitant topical agents if prescribed
- Importance of compliance even after feeling better
- To avoid alcohol, since nausea, vomiting, hypertension may occur
- To use sunscreen or avoid direct sunlight to prevent photosensitivity
- To notify prescriber of sore throat, fever, skin rash, which may indicate overgrowth of organisms
- To use nonhormonal contraception

guaifenesin (OTC, ℞)

(gwye-fen'e-sin)

Amonidrin, Anti-tuss, Balminil*, Breonesin, Fenesin, Gee-Gee, Genatuss, GG-Cen, Glyate, Glycotuss, Glytuss, Guaifenesin, Guiatuss, Halotussin, Humibid, Humibid L.A., Hytuss, Hytuss 2X, Malotuss, Mytussin, Naldecon Senior EX, Resyl*, Robitussin, Scot-Tussin Expectorant, Sinumist-SR, UniTussin

Func. class.: Expectorant

Combination products: Entex: guaifenesin 200 mg with phenylephrine HCl 5 mg with phenylpro-

* Available in Canada only

panolamine HCl 45 mg; Entex LA: guaifenesin 400 mg with phenylpropanolamine HCl 75 mg

Action: Acts as an expectorant by stimulating a gastric mucosal reflex to increase the production of lung mucus

Uses: Dry, nonproductive cough

Dosage and routes:

- *Adult:* PO 100-400 mg q4-6h, not to exceed 1.2 g/day; SUS REL 600-1200 mg q12h, not to exceed 2.4 g/day
- *Child 6-12 yr:* PO 100-200 mg q4h; 600 mg q12h (SUS REL) not to exceed 1.2 g/day
- *Child 2-6 yr:* PO 50-100 mg q4h; not to exceed 600 mg/day

Available forms: Tabs 100, 200 mg; caps 200 mg; syr 100 mg/5 ml

Side effects/adverse reactions:

CNS: Drowsiness

GI: Nausea, anorexia, vomiting

Contraindications: Hypersensitivity, persistent cough

Precautions: Pregnancy (C)

NURSING CONSIDERATIONS

Assess:

- Cough: type, frequency, character, including sputum; fluids should be increased to 2 L/day

Perform/provide:

- Storage at room temp
- Increased fluids, room humidification to liquefy secretions

Evaluate:

- Therapeutic response: absence of cough

Teach patient/family:

- To avoid driving, other hazardous activities if drowsiness occurs (rare)
- To avoid smoking, smoke-filled room, perfumes, dust, environmental pollutants, cleansers

guanabenz (℞)

(gwan'a-benz)

Wytensin

Func. class.: Antihypertensive

Chem. class.: Central α_2-adrenergic agonist

Action: Stimulates central α_2-adrenergic receptors in the CNS resulting in decreased sympathetic outflow from brain with decreased peripheral resistance

Uses: Hypertension

Dosage and routes:

- *Adult:* PO 4 mg bid, increasing in increments of 4-8 mg/day q1-2wk, not to exceed 32 mg bid

Available forms: Tabs 4, 8 mg

Side effects/adverse reactions:

RESP: Dyspnea

CV: ***Severe rebound hypertension,*** chest pain, dysrhythmias, palpitations, hypotension

CNS: Drowsiness, dizziness, sedation, headache, depression, weakness

EENT: Nasal congestion, blurred vision

GI: Nausea, diarrhea, constipation, dry mouth, anorexia, abnormal taste

GU: Impotence, frequency, gynecomastia

MS: Backache, extremities pain

Contraindications: Hypersensitivity to guanabenz

Precautions: Pregnancy (C), lactation, children <12 yr, severe coronary insufficiency, recent myocardial infarction, cerebrovascular disease, severe hepatic or renal failure

Pharmacokinetics:

PO: Onset 1 hr, Peak 2-4 hr; half-life 4-14 hr; excreted in urine

Interactions:

- Increased sedation: CNS depressants

NURSING CONSIDERATIONS

Assess:

• Renal studies: protein, BUN, creatinine; watch for increased levels
• Baselines in renal, liver function tests before therapy begins
• B/P during beginning treatment, periodically thereafter
• Edema in feet and legs daily
• Allergic reaction: rash, fever, pruritus, urticaria; drug should be discontinued if antihistamines fail to help
• Renal symptoms: polyuria, oliguria, frequency

Administer:

• In AM, at hs

Evaluate:

• Therapeutic response: decrease in B/P

Teach patient/family:

• To avoid hazardous activities; sedation may occur
• Not to discontinue drug abruptly, or withdrawal symptoms may occur: anxiety, increased B/P, headache, insomnia, increased pulse, tremors, nausea, sweating
• Not to use OTC (cough, cold, or allergy) products unless directed by prescriber
• Importance of complying with dosage schedule even if feeling better
• To notify prescriber of swelling of hands or feet, irregular heart beat, chest pain
• About excessive perspiration, dehydration, vomiting, diarrhea; may lead to fall in blood pressure; consult prescriber if these occur
• That drug may cause dizziness, fainting; light-headedness may occur during 1st few days of therapy
• That compliance is necessary; not to skip or stop drug unless directed by prescriber
• That drug may cause skin rash or impaired perspiration

Treatment of overdose: Administer vasopressor, discontinue drug; supine position

guanadrel (℞)

(gwahn′a-drel)

Hylorel

Func. class.: Antihypertensive

Chem. class.: Adrenergic blocker; peripheral guanethidine derivative

Action: Inhibits sympathetic vasoconstriction by inhibiting release of norepinephrine, depletes norepinephrine stores in adrenergic nerve endings, adrenal medulla

Uses: Hypertension (moderate to severe as an adjunct)

Dosage and routes:

• *Adult:* PO 5 mg bid, adjusted to desired response weekly or monthly; may need 20-75 mg/day in divided doses; higher doses are given tid or qid

Available forms: Tabs 10, 25 mg

Side effects/adverse reactions:

CV: Orthostatic hypotension, bradycardia, ***CHF,*** palpitations, chest pain, tachycardia, dysrhythmias

CNS: Drowsiness, fatigue, weakness, feeling of faintness, insomnia, dizziness, mental changes, memory loss, hallucinations, *depression,* anxiety, *confusion, paresthesias, headache*

GI: Nausea, cramps, diarrhea, constipation, dry mouth, anorexia, indigestion

INTEG: Rash, purpura, alopecia

EENT: Nasal stuffiness, tinnitus, visual changes, sore throat, double vision, dry burning eyes

GU: Ejaculation failure, impotence, dysuria, nocturia, frequency

RESP: ***Bronchospasm,*** dyspnea, cough, rales, SOB

* Available in Canada only

MS: Leg cramps, aching, pain, inflammation

Contraindications: Hypersensitivity, pregnancy (B), pheochromocytoma, lactation, CHF, child <18 yr

Precautions: Elderly, bronchial asthma, peptic ulcer, electrolyte imbalances, vascular disease

Pharmacokinetics:

PO: Onset 0.5-2 hr, peak 4-6 hr, duration 8 hr; half-life 10-12 hr; metabolized in liver 50%; excreted in urine (50% unchanged)

Interactions:

- Increased hypotension: diuretics, other antihypertensives
- Do not use with MAOIs
- Increased orthostatic hypotension: alcohol, opioids
- Decreased hypotensive effect: tricyclic antidepressants, phenothiazines, ephedrine, phenylpropanolamine

NURSING CONSIDERATIONS

Assess:

- Renal function studies in renal impairment (BUN, creatinine)
- Bleeding time; check for ecchymosis, thrombocytopenia, purpura
- I&O in renal disease patient
- Cardiac status: B/P lying and standing, pulse; watch for hypotension
- Edema in feet, legs daily; take weight daily
- Skin turgor, dryness of mucous membranes for hydration status
- Symptoms of CHF: edema, dyspnea, wet rales

Perform/provide

- Storage in air-tight container

Evaluate:

- Therapeutic response: decreased B/P

Teach patient/family:

- To avoid driving and performing hazardous activities if drowsiness occurs
- Not to discontinue drug abruptly
- Not to use OTC cough, cold preparations unless directed by prescriber
- To report bradycardia, dizziness, confusion, depression, fever or sore throat
- That impotence, gynecomastia may occur but are reversible
- To rise slowly to sitting or standing position to minimize orthostatic hypotension
- That therapeutic effect may take 2-4 wk

guanethidine (℞)

(gwahn-eth′i-deen)

Apo-Guanethidine*, guanethidine sulfate, Ismelin

Func. class.: Antihypertensive

Chem. class.: Antiadrenergic agent, peripheral

Combination products: Esimil: guanethidine monosulfate 10 mg (equivalent to guanethidine sulfate 8.4 mg) with hydrochlorothiazide 25 mg

Action: Inhibits norepinephrine release, depleting norepinephrine stores in adrenergic nerve endings

Uses: Moderate to severe hypertension

Dosage and routes:

- *Adult:* PO 10-12.5 mg qd, increase by 10 mg qwk; may require 25-50 mg qd
- *Adult:* (hospitalized) 25-50 mg; may increase by 25-50 mg/day or every other day
- *Child:* PO 0.2 mg/kg/day; (6 mg/m^2/day) increase q7-10d, 0.2 mg/kg or 6 mg/m^2/day not to exceed 3000 µg/kg/24 hr

Available forms: Tabs 10, 25 mg

Side effects/adverse reactions:

CV: Orthostatic hypotension, dizziness, weakness, bradycardia, ***CHF,***

fatigue, angina, heart block, chest paresthesia
CNS: Depression
GI: Nausea, vomiting, *diarrhea,* constipation, dry mouth, weight gain, anorexia, abdominal pain
INTEG: Dermatitis, loss of scalp hair
EENT: Nasal congestion, ptosis, blurred vision
GU: Ejaculation failure, impotence, nocturia, edema, *retention,* increased BUN, *frequency*
RESP: Dyspnea, cough, shortness of breath

Contraindications: Hypersensitivity, pheochromocytoma, recent MI, CHF, cardiac failure, sinus bradycardia

Precautions: Pregnancy (B), lactation, peptic ulcer, asthma

Pharmacokinetics:
PO: Therapeutic level: 1-3 wk; half-life 5 days; metabolized by liver; excreted in urine (metabolites), breast milk

Interactions:
- Increased hypotension: diuretics, other antihypertensives
- Do not use with MAOIs
- Increased orthostatic hypotension: alcohol
- Decreased hypotensive effect: tricyclic antidepressants, phenothiazines, ephedrine, phenylpropanolamine, oral contraceptives, thiothixine, doxepin, haloperidol, amphetamines

Lab test interferences:
Increase: BUN
Decrease: Blood glucose, VMA excretion, urinary norepinephrine

NURSING CONSIDERATIONS

Assess:
- Renal function studies in renal impairment (BUN, creatinine)
- Bleeding time; check for ecchymosis, thrombocytopenia, purpura
- I&O in renal disease patient
- Cardiac status: B/P, pulse; watch for hypotension
- Edema in feet, legs daily; take weight daily
- Skin turgor, dryness of mucous membranes for hydration status
- Symptoms of CHF: edema, dyspnea, wet rales

Evaluate:
- Therapeutic response: decreased B/P

Teach patient/family:
- To avoid driving, hazardous activities if drowsiness occurs
- Not to discontinue drug abruptly
- Not to use OTC cough, cold preparations unless directed by prescriber
- To report bradycardia, dizziness, confusion, depression, fever, sore throat
- That impotence, gynecomastia may occur but are reversible
- To rise slowly to sitting or standing position to minimize orthostatic hypotension; more common in AM, hot weather, during exercise, or when using alcohol
- That therapeutic effect may take 2-4 wk
- Notify prescriber of severe diarrhea

Treatment of overdose: Lavage, vasopressors given cautiously

guanfacine (℞)
(gwahn'fa-seen)
Tenex
Func. class.: Antihypertensive
Chem. class.: α_2-Adrenergic receptor agonist

Action: Stimulates central α-adrenergic receptors, resulting in decreased sympathetic outflow from brain

Uses: Hypertension in individual using a thiazide diuretic

* Available in Canada only

Dosage and routes:
• *Adult:* PO 1 mg/day hs; may increase dose in 2-3 wk to 2-3 mg/day
Available forms: Tabs 1 mg
Side effects/adverse reactions:
GI: Dry mouth, constipation, cramps, nausea, diarrhea
CNS: Somnolence, dizziness, headache, fatigue
GU: Impotence, urinary incontinence
EENT: Taste change, tinnitus, vision change, rhinitis, nasal congestion
MS: Leg cramps
RESP: Dyspnea
INTEG: Dermatitis, pruritus, purpura
CV: Bradycardia, chest pain
Contraindications: Hypersensitivity
Precautions: Pregnancy (B), lactation, children <12 yr, severe coronary insufficiency, recent MI, renal or hepatic disease, CVA
Pharmacokinetics:
Peak 1-4 hr; 70% bound to plasma proteins; half-life 17 hr; eliminated via kidneys unchanged and as metabolites
Interactions:
• Increased sedation: CNS depressants, other antihypertensives
• Decreased hypotensive effect: tricyclic antidepressants
NURSING CONSIDERATIONS
Assess:
• Blood studies: neutrophils, decrease in platelets
• Baselines in renal, liver function tests before therapy begins
• B/P before, during, after treatment; notify prescriber of significant changes
• Edema in feet, legs daily
• Allergic reaction: rash, fever, pruritus, urticaria; drug should be discontinued if antihistamines fail to help
• Symptoms of CHF: edema, dyspnea, wet rales, B/P
• Renal symptoms: polyuria, oliguria, frequency
Perform/provide:
• Storage of tablets in tight container
Evaluate:
• Therapeutic response: decreased B/P in hypertension
Teach patient/family:
• To avoid hazardous activities
• Not to discontinue drug abruptly or withdrawal symptoms may occur: anxiety, increased B/P, headache, insomnia, increased pulse, tremors, nausea, sweating
• Not to use OTC (cough, cold, or allergy) products unless directed by prescriber
• To avoid sunlight or to wear sunscreen; photosensitivity may occur
• Importance of complying with dosage schedule even if feeling better

haemophilus b vaccines (℞)

(hee-moef'ii lus)
Hib-Imune, HibVAX (polysaccharide), b-Capsa 1, ProHIBIT (conjugate)
Func. class.: Vaccine
Chem. class.: H. influenzae capsular polysaccharide

Action: Stimulates antibody production to *H. influenzae b*
Uses: Polysaccharide immunization of children 2-6 yr against *H. influenzae b,* conjugate immunization of child 1½-5 yr against invasive disease of *H. influenzae b*
Dosage and routes:
• *Child:* SC 0.5 ml (polysaccharide), IM 0.5 mg (conjugate)
Available forms: Polysaccharide powder for injection 25 μg/0.5 ml after reconstituting; conjugate powder for injection 25 μg polysaccha-

ride and 18 μg conjugated diphtheria toxoid/0.5 ml

Side effects/adverse reactions:

INTEG: Redness, soreness at injection site, rash

SYST: Low-grade fever, acute febrile reactions

Contraindications: Hypersensitivity, febrile illness, active infection

Precautions: Pregnancy (C)

Lab test interferences:

Interference: Latex agglutination, countercurrent immunoelectrophoresis

NURSING CONSIDERATIONS

Assess:

• For skin reactions: swelling, rash, urticaria

• For anaphylaxis: inability to breathe, bronchospasm

Administer:

• After diluting with 0.6 ml diluent, which will yield 10 doses of 0.5 ml

• Only with epinephrine 1:1000 on unit to treat laryngospasm

• Only by SC or IM route

Perform/provide:

• Storage in refrigerator

• Written record of immunization

Evaluate:

• For history of allergies, skin conditions (eczema, psoriasis, dermatitis), reactions to vaccinations

Teach patient/family:

• That usually one dose is required

halazepam (℞)

(hal-az′e-pam)

Paxipam

Func. class.: Sedative-hypnotic

Chem. class.: Benzodiazepine

Controlled Substance Schedule IV

Action: Depresses subcortical levels of CNS, including limbic system, reticular formation

Uses: Anxiety

Dosage and routes:

• *Adult:* PO 20-40 mg tid-qid

• *Geriatric:* PO 20 mg qd-bid

Available forms: Tabs 20, 40 mg

Side effects/adverse reactions:

CNS: Dizziness, drowsiness, confusion, headache, anxiety, tremors, stimulation, fatigue, depression, insomnia, hallucinations

GI: Constipation, dry mouth, nausea, vomiting, anorexia, diarrhea

INTEG: Rash, dermatitis, itching

CV: Orthostatic hypotension, ***ECG changes, tachycardia,*** hypotension

EENT: Blurred vision, tinnitus, mydriasis

Contraindications: Hypersensitivity to benzodiazepines, narrow-angle glaucoma, psychosis, pregnancy (D), lactation, child <18 yr

Precautions: Elderly, debilitated, hepatic disease, renal disease

Pharmacokinetics:

PO: Peak 1-3 hr, duration 3-6 hr; metabolized by liver; excreted by kidneys; crosses placenta, breast milk; half-life 14 hr

Interactions:

• Decreased effects of halazepam: oral contraceptives, valproic acid

• Increased effects of halazepam: CNS depressants, alcohol, disulfiram, oral contraceptives, cimetidine

• Increased risk of digoxin toxicity: digoxin

Lab test interferences:

Increase: AST (SGOT), ALT (SGPT), serum bilirubin

False increase: 17-OHCS

Decrease: RAIU

NURSING CONSIDERATIONS

Assess:

• B/P (lying, standing), pulse; if systolic B/P drops 20 mm Hg, hold drug, notify prescriber

• Blood studies: CBC during long-term therapy; blood dyscrasias have occurred rarely

* Available in Canada only

• Hepatic studies: AST (SGOT), ALT (SGPT), bilirubin, creatinine, LDH, alk phosphatase
• Mental status: mood, sensorium, affect, sleeping pattern, drowsiness, dizziness
• Physical dependency, withdrawal symptoms: headache, nausea, vomiting, muscle pain, weakness after long-term use
• Suicidal tendencies

Administer:

• With food or milk for GI symptoms
• Crushed if patient is unable to swallow medication whole
• Sugarless gum, hard candy, frequent sips of water for dry mouth

Perform/provide:

• Assistance with ambulation during beginning therapy, since drowsiness/dizziness occurs
• Safety measures, including side rails
• Check to see PO medication has been swallowed

Evaluate:

• Therapeutic response: decreased anxiety, restlessness, sleeplessness

Teach patient/family:

• That drug may be taken with food
• Not to be used for everyday stress or used longer than 4 mo unless directed by prescriber; not to take more than prescribed amount; may be habit forming
• To avoid OTC preparations (hay fever, cough, cold) unless approved by prescriber
• To avoid driving or other activities that require alertness; drowsiness may occur
• To avoid alcohol ingestion or other psychotropic medications unless prescribed by prescriber
• Not to discontinue medication abruptly after long-term use
• To rise slowly or fainting may occur
• That drowsiness may worsen at beginning of treatment

Treatment of overdose: Lavage, VS, supportive care, flumazenil

halcinonide (℞)

(hal-sin'oh-nide)
Halog, Halog-E

Func. class.: Corticosteroid, synthetic

Chem. class.: Fluorinated corticosteroid

Action: Antiinflammatory, antipruritic, vasoconstrictor actions

Uses: Inflammation of corticosteroid-responsive dermatoses

Dosage and routes:

• *Adult:* TOP apply to affected area bid-tid

Available forms: Cream 0.025%, 0.1%; oint 0.1%; sol 0.1%

Side effects/adverse reactions:

INTEG: Acne, atrophy, epidermal thinning, purpura, striae

Contraindications: Hypersensitivity, viral infections, fungal infections

Precautions: Pregnancy (C)

NURSING CONSIDERATIONS

Assess:

• Infection: increased temp, WBC, even after withdrawal of medication; may be systemically absorbed

Administer:

• Using an occlusive dressing; systemic absorption may occur
• For 3-5 days after lesions are gone

Perform/provide:

• Washing of skin before application
• Dressing change qd; check area for redness, rash, inflammation, discoloration; do not leave dressing in place over 16 hr

Evaluate:

• Therapeutic response: decreased inflammation

Teach patient/family:

• Not to get drug in eyes or mucous membranes

---

halofantrene (℞)

(hal-o-fan′-trine)

Halfan

Func. class.: Antimalarial

Chem. class.: Synthetic 4-aminoquinoline derivative

Action: Inhibits parasite replications, transcription of DNA to RNA by forming complexes with DNA of parasite

Uses: Malaria caused by *P. vivax, P. malariae, P. ovale, P. falciparum* (multidrug resistant)

Dosage and routes:

• *Adult:* 500 mg PO q6h × 3 doses

• *Children <40 kg:* 8 mg/kg q6h × 3 doses

Available forms: Tablets 500 mg

Side effects/adverse reactions:

CV: Hypotension, heart block, ***asystole with syncope,*** ECG changes

INTEG: Pruritus, pigmentary changes, skin eruptions, lichen planus-like eruptions, eczema, exfoliative dermatitis, alopecia

CNS: Headache, stimulation, fatigue, irritability, ***convulsion,*** bad dreams, dizziness, confusion, psychosis, decreased reflexes

EENT: Blurred vision, corneal changes, retinal changes, difficulty focusing, tinnitus, vertigo, deafness, photophobia, corneal edema

GI: Nausea, vomiting, anorexia, diarrhea, cramps, weight loss, stomatitis

HEMA: ***Thrombocytopenia, agranulocytosis, hemolytic anemia, leukopenia***

Contraindications: Hypersensitivity, retinal field changes, porphyria, children (long-term)

Precautions: Pregnancy (C), children, blood dyscrasias, severe GI disease, neurologic disease, alcoholism, hepatic disease, G6PD deficiency, psoriasis, eczema

Pharmacokinetics:

PO: Peak 1-2 hr, half-life 3-5 days; metabolized in the liver; excreted in urine, feces, breast milk; crosses placenta

Interactions:

• Decreased action of chloroquine: magnesium, aluminum compounds, kaolin

NURSING CONSIDERATIONS

Assess:

• Ophthalmic test if long-term treatment or drug dosage 150 mg/day

• Liver studies qwk: AST (SGOT), ALT (SGPT), bilirubin

• Blood studies: CBC, since blood dyscrasias occur

• For decreased reflexes: knee, ankle

• ECG during therapy

• Watch for depression of T waves, widening of QRS complex

• Allergic reactions: pruritus, rash, urticaria

• Blood dyscrasias: malaise, fever, bruising, bleeding (rare)

• For ototoxicity (tinnitus, vertigo, change in hearing); audiometric testing should be done before, after treatment

• For toxicity: blurring vision, difficulty focusing, headache, dizziness, knee, ankle reflexes; drug should be discontinued immediately

Administer:

• Before or after meals at same time each day to maintain drug level

• IM after aspirating to avoid injection into blood system, which may cause hypotension, asystole, heart block; rotate injection sites

---

Perform/provide:
- Storage in tight, light-resistant containers at room temperature; injection should be kept in cool environment

Evaluate:
- Therapeutic response: decreased symptoms of infection

Teach patient/family:
- To use sunglasses in bright sunlight to decrease photophobia
- That urine may turn rust or brown
- To report hearing, visual problems, fever, fatigue, bruising, bleeding, which may indicate blood dyscrasias

Treatment of overdose: Induce vomiting; gastric lavage; administer barbiturate (ultrashort-acting), vasopressin; tracheostomy may be necessary

haloperidol (℞)

(ha-loe-per'idole)

Apo-Haloperidol*, Haldol, Haldol L.A.*, haloperidol, Haloperidol Decanoate 50, Haloperidol 100, Novoperidol*, Peridol*

Func. class.: Antipsychotic/neuroleptic

Chem. class.: Butyrophenone

Action: Depresses cerebral cortex, hypothalamus, limbic system, which control activity and aggression; blocks neurotransmission produced by dopamine at synapse; exhibits strong α-adrenergic, anticholinergic blocking action; mechanism for antipsychotic effects unclear

Uses: Psychotic disorders, control of tics, vocal utterances in Gilles de la Tourette's syndrome, short-term treatment of hyperactive children showing excessive motor activity, prolonged parenteral therapy in chronic schizophrenia

Dosage and routes:

Psychosis
- *Adult:* PO 0.5-5 mg bid or tid initially depending on severity of condition; dose is increased to desired dose, max 100 mg/day; IM 2-5 mg q1-8h
- *Child 3-12 yr:* PO/IM 0.05-0.15 mg/kg/day
- *Decanoate:* Initial dose IM is 10-15 × daily oral dose at 4 wk interval; do not administer IV; not to exceed 100 mg

Chronic schizophrenia
- *Adult:* IM 10-15 times PO dose q4wk (decanoate)
- *Child 3-12 yr:* PO/IM 0.05-0.15 mg/kg/day

Tics/vocal utterances
- *Adult:* PO 0.5-5 mg bid or tid, increased until desired response occurs
- *Child 3-12 yr:* PO 0.05-0.075 mg/kg/day

Hyperactive children
- *Child 3-12 yr:* PO 0.05-0.075 mg/kg/day

Available forms: Tabs 0.5, 1, 2, 5, 10, 20 mg; conc 2 mg/ml; inj 5 mg/ml

Side effects/adverse reactions:

RESP: ***Laryngospasm,*** dyspnea, ***respiratory depression***

CNS: EPS: pseudoparkinsonism, akathisia, dystonia, tardive dyskinesia, drowsiness, headache, ***seizures, neuroleptic malignant syndrome,*** confusion

INTEG: Rash, photosensitivity, dermatitis

EENT: Blurred vision, glaucoma, dry eyes

GI: Dry mouth, nausea, vomiting, anorexia, constipation, diarrhea, jaundice, weight gain, ***ileus, hepatitis***

GU: Urinary retention, urinary frequency, enuresis, impotence, amenorrhea, gynecomastia

CV: Orthostatic hypotension, hypertension, ***cardiac arrest,*** ECG changes, ***tachycardia***

Contraindications: Hypersensitivity, blood dyscrasias, coma, child <3 yr, brain damage, bone marrow depression, alcohol and barbiturate withdrawal states, Parkinson's disease, angina, epilepsy, urinary retention, narrow-angle glaucoma

Precautions: Pregnancy (C), lactation, seizure disorders, hypertension, hepatic disease, cardiac disease

Pharmacokinetics:

PO: Onset erratic, peak 2-6 hr, half-life 24 hr

IM: Onset 15-30 min, peak 15-20 min, half-life 21 hr

IM (Decanoate): Peak 4-11 days, half-life 3 wk

Metabolized by liver; excreted in urine, bile; crosses placenta; enters breast milk

Interactions:

- Oversedation: other CNS depressants, alcohol, barbiturate anesthetics
- Toxicity: epinephrine
- Toxicity: lithium, neurotoxicity and brain damage possible
- Decreased effects of lithium, levodopa
- Increased effects of both drugs: β-adrenergic blockers, alcohol
- Increased anticholinergic effects: anticholinergics
- Decreased effects of haloperidol: phenobarbital

Syringe incompatibility: Heparin

Y-site compatibilities: Cimetidine, dobustamine, dopamine, famotidine, fludarabine, lidocaine, melphalan, nitroglycerin, norepinephrine, ondansetron, paclitaxel, phenylephrine, theophylline, vinorelbine

Lab test interferences:

Increase: Liver function tests, cardiac enzymes, cholesterol, blood glucose, prolactin, bilirubin, PBI, cholinesterase

Decrease: Hormones (blood, urine)

False positive: Pregnancy tests, PKU

False negative: Urinary steroids

NURSING CONSIDERATIONS

Assess:

- Swallowing of PO medication; check for hoarding or giving of medication to other patients
- I&O ratio; palpate bladder if low urinary output occurs
- Bilirubin, CBC, liver function studies monthly
- Urinalysis is recommended before and during prolonged therapy
- For depression in bipolar patients; rapid mood swings may occur with this drug
- Affect, orientation, LOC, reflexes, gait, coordination, sleep pattern disturbances
- B/P standing and lying; take pulse and respirations q4h during initial treatment; establish baseline before starting treatment; report drops of 30 mm Hg
- Dizziness, faintness, palpitations, tachycardia on rising
- EPS including akathisia (inability to sit still, no pattern to movements), tardive dyskinesia (bizarre movements of jaw, mouth, tongue, extremities), pseudoparkinsonism (rigidity, tremors, pill rolling, shuffling gait)
- Skin turgor daily
- For neuroleptic malignant syndrome: hyperthermia, muscle rigidity, altered mental status, increased CPK
- Constipation, urinary retention daily; if these occur, increase bulk, water in diet

Administer:

- Reduced dose to elderly
- Antiparkinsonian agent, to be used if EPS occur

---

* Available in Canada only

• IM injection into large muscle mass, use 21/G, 2″ needle; give no more than 3 ml/injection site; patient should remain recumbent for ½ hr
• Oral liquid: use calibrated dropper; do not mix in coffee or tea
• PO with food or milk

Perform/provide:
• Decreased noise input by dimming lights, avoiding loud noises
• Supervised ambulation until stabilized on medication; do not involve in strenuous exercise program because fainting is possible; patient should not stand still for long periods
• Increased fluids to prevent constipation
• Sips of water, candy, gum for dry mouth
• Storage in tight, light-resistant container

Evaluate:
• Therapeutic response: decrease in emotional excitement, hallucinations, delusions, paranoia, reorganization of patterns of thought, speech

Teach patient/family:
• That orthostatic hypotension occurs often and to rise from sitting or lying position gradually
• To avoid hazardous activities until stabilized on medication
• To remain lying down after IM injection for at least 30 min
• To avoid hot tubs, hot showers, tub baths, since hypotension may occur
• To avoid abrupt withdrawal of this drug, or EPS may result; drug should be withdrawn slowly
• To avoid OTC preparations (cough, hay fever, cold) unless approved by prescriber, since serious drug interactions may occur; avoid use with alcohol, CNS depressants; increased drowsiness may occur
• To use a sunscreen to prevent burns
• Regarding compliance with drug regimen
• About EPS and necessity for meticulous oral hygiene, since oral candidiasis may occur
• To report impaired vision, jaundice, tremors, muscle twitching
• That in hot weather, heat stroke may occur; take extra precautions to stay cool

Treatment of overdose: Activated charcoal lavage if orally ingested; provide an airway; *do not induce vomiting*

---

haloprogin (℞)

(ha-loe-proe′jin)
Halotex
Func. class.: Local antiinfective, antifungal
Chem. class.: Iodinated phenolic ester

Action: Interferes with fungal cell membrane permeability
Uses: Tinea pedis, tinea cruris, tinea corporis, tinea manus, tinea versicolor
Dosage and routes:
• *Adult and child:* TOP apply to affected area bid × 14-28 days
Available forms: Cream, sol 1%
Side effects/adverse reactions:
INTEG: Rash, urticaria, stinging, burning, vesiculation, pruritus, erythema, scaling, folliculitis sensitization
Contraindications: Hypersensitivity
Precautions: Pregnancy (B), lactation, children

NURSING CONSIDERATIONS
Assess:
• Allergic reaction: burning, sting-

ing, swelling, redness, vesiculation, scaling

Administer:

• After cleansing with soap, water before each application; dry well

• Enough medication to cover lesions completely

Perform/provide:

• Storage at room temp in dry place

Evaluate:

• Therapeutic response: decrease in size, number of lesions

Teach patient/family:

• To use asepsis (hand washing) before, after each application

• To apply with glove to prevent further infection

• To avoid use of OTC creams, ointments, lotions unless directed by prescriber

• To avoid contact with eyes

• To continue even though condition improves

• To use for full duration even if condition subsides or irritation increases; if condition does not improve after 4 wk, another treatment should be considered

heparin (℞)

(hep'a-rin)

Calcilean*, Calciparine, Hepalean*, Heparin Sodium and 0.45% Sodium Chloride, Heparin Sodium and 0.9% Sodium Chloride, Heparin Leo*, Heparin Lock Flush, heparin sodium, Hep-Lock, Hep-Lock U/P, Liquaemin Sodium

Func. class.: Anticoagulant

Action: Prevents conversion of fibrinogen to fibrin and prothrombin to thrombin by enhancing inhibitory effects of antithrombin III

Uses: Deep-vein thrombosis, pulmonary emboli, myocardial infarction, open heart surgery, disseminated intravascular clotting syndrome, atrial fibrillation with embolization, as an anticoagulant in transfusion and dialysis procedures, prevention of DVT/PE

Dosage and routes:

Deep-vein thrombosis/MI

• *Adult:* IV PUSH 5000-7000 U q4h then titrated to PTT or ACT level; IV BOL 5000-7500 U, then IV INF; IV INF; after bolus dose, then 1000 U/hr titrated to PTT or ACT level

• *Child:* IV INF 50 U/kg, maintenance 100 U/kg q4h or 20,000 U/m^2 qd

Pulmonary embolism

• *Adult:* IV PUSH 7500-10,000 U q4h then titrated to PTT or ACT level; IV BOL 7500-10,000, then IV INF; IV INF after bolus dose, then 1000 U/hr titrated to PTT or ACT level

• *Child:* IV INF 50 U/kg, maintenance 100 U/kg q4h or 20,000 U/m^2 qd

Open heart surgery

• *Adult:* IV INF 150-300 U/kg

Prophylaxis for DVT/PE

• *Adult SC:* 5,000 U q8-12h

Heparin flush

• *Adult, Child:* IV 10-100 U

Available forms: Heparin sodium inj 10, 1000, 5000, 10,000, 20,000, 40,000 U/ml; heparin calcium inj 5000 U/0.2 ml

Side effects/adverse reactions:

CNS: Fever, chills

GI: Diarrhea, nausea, vomiting, anorexia, stomatitis, abdominal cramps, ***hepatitis***

GU: ***Hematuria***

HEMA: ***Hemorrhage, thrombocytopenia***

INTEG: Rash, dermatitis, urticaria, alopecia, pruritus

Contraindications: Hypersensitivity, hemophilia, leukemia with bleeding, peptic ulcer disease, thrombo-

* Available in Canada only

cytopenic purpura, hepatic disease (severe), renal disease (severe), blood dyscrasias, severe hypertension, subacute bacterial endocarditis, acute nephritis
Precautions: Alcoholism, elderly, pregnancy (C)
Pharmacokinetics: Well absorbed (SC)
IV: Peak 5 min, duration 2-6 hr
SC: Onset 20-60 min, duration 8-12 hr
Half-life 1½ hr, excreted in urine, 95% bound to plasma proteins, does not cross placenta or alter breast milk; removed from the system via the lymph and spleen
Interactions:
• Decreased action of corticosteroids
• Increased action of diazepam
• Decreased action of heparin: digitalis, tetracyclines, antihistamines
• Increased action of heparin: oral anticoagulants, salicylates, dextran, steroids, nonsteroidal antiinflammatories
Y-site compatibilities: Acyclovir, aminophylline, ampicillin, atracurium, atropine, betamethasone, bleomycin, calcium gluconate, cephalothin, cephapirin, chlordiazepoxide, chlorpromazine, cimetidine, cisplatin, conjugated estrogens, cyancobalamin, cyclophosphamide, dexamethasone, digoxin, diphenhydramine, dopamine, edrophonium, enalaprilat, epinephrine, esmolol, ethacrynate, famotidine, fentanyl, fluconazole, fludarabine, fluorouracil, foscarnet, furosemide, hydralazine, insulin, isoproterenol, kanamycin, labetalol, leucovorin, lidocaine, magnesium sulfate, melphalan, menadiol sodium, meperidine, methicillin, methotrexate, methoxamine, methylergonovine, metoclopramide, minocycline, mitomycin, morphine, neostigmine, norepinephrine, ondansetron, oxacillin, oxytocin, paclitaxel, pancuronium, penicillin G potassium, pentazocine, phytonadione, prednisolone, procainamide, prochlorperazine, propranolol, pyridostigmine, ranitidine, sargramostim, scopolamine, sodium bicarbonate, streptokinase, succinylcholine, trimethophan camsylate, trimethobenzamide, vecuronium, vinblastine, vincristine, vinorelbine, zidovudine
Additive compatibilities: Amphotericin, calcium gluconate, cephalothin, cephapirin, chloramphenicol, clindamycin, colistimethate, dimenhydrinate, erythromycin gluceptate, furosemide, methyldopate methylprednisolone, nafcillin, octreotide, potassium chloride, prednisolone, promazine, ranitidine, sodium bicarbonate, verapamil, vitamin B complex, vitamin B complex with C
Lab test interferences:
False increase: T_3 uptake, serum thyroxine, BSP
Decrease: Uric acid
False negative: ^{125}I fibrinogen uptake

NURSING CONSIDERATIONS

Assess:
• Blood studies (Hct, occult blood in stools) q3mo
• Partial prothrombin time, which should be 1.5-2 × control, PTT often done qd, also APTT, ACT
• Platelet count q2-3d; thrombocytopenia may occur on 4th day of treatment
• Bleeding gums, petecchiae, ecchymosis, black tarry stools, hematuria, epistaxis, decrease in Hct, B/P; indicate bleeding and possible hemorrhage
• Fever, skin rash, urticaria
• Needed dosage change q1-2wk

Administer:
• IV diluted in 0.9% NaCl, dextrose, Ringer's sol and given by direct, intermittent, or continuous infusion; give 1000 U or less over 1 min; then 5000 U or less over 1 min; infusion may run from 4-24 hr; use infusion pump
• Blood after adding 7500 U/100 ml NaCl inj, add 6-8 ml of this sol/100 ml of whole blood
• At same time each day to maintain steady blood levels
• SC deep with 25G ⅜″ needle; do not massage area or aspirate when giving SC injection; give in abdomen between pelvic bone, rotate sites; do not pull back on plunger, leave in for 10 sec; apply gentle pressure for 1 min
• Changing needles is not recommended
• Avoiding all IM injections that may cause bleeding

Perform/provide:
• Storage in tight container

Evaluate:
• Therapeutic response: decrease of deep-vein thrombosis, PTT 1.5-2.5 × control, free flowing IV

Teach patient/family:
• To avoid OTC preparations that may cause serious drug interactions unless directed by prescriber
• That drug may be held during active bleeding (menstruation), depending on condition
• To use soft-bristle toothbrush to avoid bleeding gums, avoid contact sports, use electric razor, avoid IM injection
• To carry a Medic Alert ID identifying drug taken
• To report any signs of bleeding: gums, under skin, urine, stools

Treatment of overdose: Withdraw drug, protamine SO_4 1:1 solution

hepatitis B vaccine (℞)

Gammagee, H-BIG, Hep-B, HyperHep

Func. class.: Vaccine

Action: Provides active immunity to hepatitis B

Uses: Prevention of hepatitis B virus in exposed patients, including passive immunity in neonates born to HB_sAg+ mother

Dosage and routes:
• *Adult and child >10 yr:* IM 1 ml, then 1 ml after 1 mo, then 1 ml 6 mo after initial dose
• *Child 3 mo-10 yr:* IM 0.5 ml, then 0.5 ml after 1 mo, then 0.5 ml 6 mo after initial dose
• *Patients with decreased immunity:* IM 2 ml, then 2 ml after 1 mo, then 2 ml 6 mo after initial dose

Available forms: Inj 10 mg/0.5 ml, 20 μg/ml

Side effects/adverse reactions:
INTEG: Soreness at injection site, urticaria, erythema, swelling
SYST: Induration
CNS: Headache, dizziness, fever
GI: Nausea, vomiting
SYST: ***Anaphylaxis, angioedema***

Contraindications: Hypersensitivity to immune globulins, thimerosal, glycine

Precautions: Pregnancy, elderly, lactation, children; active infection, IgA deficiency

NURSING CONSIDERATIONS

Assess:
• For history of allergies, skin conditions (eczema, psoriasis, dermatitis), reactions to vaccinations
• For skin reactions: rash, induration, urticaria
• For anaphylaxis: inability to breathe, bronchospasm, hypoten-

sion, wheezing, diaphoresis, fever, flushing

Administer:

- After rotating vial; do not shake
- Only with epinephrine 1:1000 on unit to treat laryngospasm
- In deltoid for better absorption; give 2 ml dose in two different sites

Perform/provide:

- Written record of immunization
- Comfort measures

Evaluate:

- Prevention of hepatitis B

hetastarch (℞)

(het'a-starch)

Hespan

Func. class.: Plasma expander

Chem. class.: Synthetic polymer

Action: Similar to human albumin, which expands plasma volume by colloidal osmotic pressure

Uses: Plasma volume expander, leukapheresis

Dosage and routes:

- *Adult:* IV INF 500-1000 ml (30-60g), total dose not to exceed 1500 ml/day, not to exceed 20 ml/kg/hr (hemorrhagic shock)

Leukapheresis

- *Adult:* IV INF 250-700 ml infused at 1:8 ratio with whole blood, may be repeated 2/wk up to 10 treatments

Available forms: 6% hetastarch/0.9% NaCl inj

Side effects/adverse reactions:

HEMA: Decreased hematocrit, platelet function, increased bleeding/coagulation times, increased sed rate

INTEG: Rash, urticaria, pruritus, angioedema, chills, fever, flushing, peripheral edema

RESP: Wheezing, dyspnea, ***bronchospasm, pulmonary edema***

GI: Nausea, vomiting

EENT: Periorbital edema

SYST: ***Anaphylaxis***

CNS: Headache

Contraindications: Hypersensitivity, severe bleeding disorders, renal failure, CHF (severe)

Precautions: Pregnancy (C), liver disease, pulmonary edema

Pharmacokinetics:

IV: Expands blood volume 1-2 × amount infused, excreted in urine

Y-site compatibilities: Cimetidine, doxycycline, enalaprilat

Additive compatibility: Cloxacillin

Lab test interferences:

False increase: Bilirubin

NURSING CONSIDERATIONS

Assess:

- VS q5min × 30 min; CVP during infusion (5-10 cm H_2O normal range), PCWP
- Monitor CBC with differential, Hgb, Hct, Pro-time, PTT, platelet count, clotting time during treatment; Hct may drop; do not allow to drop >30% by vol
- Urine output q1h, watch for increase in urinary output, which is common; if output does not increase, infusion should be decreased or discontinued
- I&O ratio and specific gravity, urine osmolarity; if specific gravity is very low, renal clearance is low; drug should be discontinued
- Allergy: rash, urticaria, pruritus, wheezing, dyspnea, bronchospasm; drug should be discontinued immediately
- For circulatory overload: increased pulse, respirations, SOB, wheezing, chest tightness, chest pain
- For dehydration after infusion: decreased output, fever, poor skin turgor, increased specific gravity, dry skin

Administer:

• IV inf undiluted, run at 20 ml/kg/hr (1.2 g/kg); reduced rate in septic shock, burns

Perform/provide:

• Storage at room temp; discard unused portion, do not freeze, do not use if turbid or deep brown or if precipitate forms

Evaluate:

• Therapeutic response: increased plasma volume

hexamethylmelamine

(℞)

Hexalen

Func. class.: Antineoplastic, alkylating agent

Action: Responsible for inhibition of cell DNA and RNA synthesis, cell death; rapidly degraded; cell cycle nonspecific

Uses: Resistant or recurrent ovarian cancer; may be used alone or in combination

Dosage and routes:

• *Adult:* PO 260 mg/m^2; average dose 400 mg qd × 14 days, then rest for 14 days; cycle should continue until patient no longer responds

Available forms: Caps 50 mg

Side effects/adverse reactions:

EENT: Tinnitus, hearing loss

HEMA: ***Thrombocytopenia, leukopenia***

GI: Nausea, vomiting, diarrhea, stomatitis, weight loss, colitis, hepatotoxicity, anorexia

CNS: Headache, dizziness, drowsiness, paresthesia, peripheral neuropathy, coma, hyporeflexia, muscle weakness

INTEG: Alopecia, pruritus, herpes zoster

Contraindications: Lactation, pregnancy (1st trimester) (D), myelosuppression, acute herpes zoster, hypersensitivity

Precautions: Radiation therapy, leukopenia, thrombocytopenia

Pharmacokinetics: Metabolized in liver, excreted in urine

Interactions:

• Increased toxicity: antineoplastics, radiation

• Reduced efficiency: influenza vaccine, pneumococcal vaccine

NURSING CONSIDERATIONS

Assess:

• CBC, differential, platelet count weekly; withhold drug if WBC is <4000 or platelet count is <75,000; notify prescriber

• Renal function studies: BUN, serum uric acid, urine CrCl before, during therapy

• I&O ratio; report fall in urine output to <30 ml/hr

• Monitor temp q4h; fever may indicate beginning infection; no rectal temps

• Liver function tests before, during therapy: (bilirubin, AST [SGOT], ALT [SGPT], LDH) prn or qmo

• Bleeding: hematuria, guaiac, bruising, or petechiae, mucosa or orifices q8h

• Food preferences: list likes, dislikes

• Yellowing of skin and sclera, dark urine, clay-colored stools, itchy skin, abdominal pain, fever, diarrhea

• Effects of alopecia on body image; discuss feelings about body changes

• Inflammation of mucosa, breaks in skin

• Buccal cavity q8h for dryness, sores, or ulceration, white patches, oral pain, bleeding, dysphagia

• Symptoms indicating severe allergic reaction: rash, pruritus, urti-

* Available in Canada only

caria, purpuric skin lesions, itching, flushing

Administer:

- As divided daily doses 1-2 hr pc and hs
- Antiemetic 30-60 min before giving drug and prn
- Topical or systemic analgesics for pain
- Local or systemic drugs for infection

Perform/provide:

- Storage at room temp in dry form
- Strict medical asepsis, protective isolation if WBC levels are low
- Special skin care
- Increase fluid intake to 2-3 L/day to prevent urate deposits, calculi formation
- Diet low in purines: organ meats (kidney, liver), dried beans, peas to maintain alkaline urine
- Rinsing of mouth tid-qid with water, club soda; brushing of teeth bid-tid with soft brush or cotton-tipped applicators for stomatitis; use unwaxed dental floss

Evaluate:

- Therapeutic response: decreased tumor size, decreased spread of malignancy

Teach patient/family:

- About protective isolation
- That sterility, amenorrhea can occur; reversible after discontinuing treatment
- That hair may be lost during treatment; a wig or hairpiece may make patient feel better; new hair may be different in color, texture
- To avoid foods with citric acid, hot or rough texture
- To report any bleeding, white spots, or ulcerations in mouth to prescriber; tell patient to examine mouth qd
- To report signs of infection: fever, sore throat, flu symptoms
- To report signs of anemia: fatigue, headache, faintness, shortness of breath, irritability

---

homatropine (℞)

(hoe'ma-troe-peen)

Homatropine HBr Ophthalmic, Isopto

Func. class.: Mydriatic

Chem. class.: Synthetic alkaloid

Action: Blocks response of iris sphincter muscle, ciliary muscle of the lens to cholinergic stimulation, resulting in dilation, paralysis of accommodation

Uses: Uveitis, iritis, mydriatic, cycloplegic for refraction

Dosage and routes:

- *Adult and child:* INSTILL 1-2 gtt; repeat in 5-10 min for refraction or q3-4h for uveitis; use only 2% strength in children

Available forms: Sol 2%, 5%

Side effects/adverse reactions:

CV: Tachycardia

CNS: Confusion, somnolence, flushing, fever, restlessness, seizures, ataxic gait, psychiatric disturbances in children

EENT: Blurred vision, photophobia, increased intraocular pressure, irritation, edema

Contraindications: Hypersensitivity, children <6 yr, narrow-angle glaucoma, increased intraocular pressure, infants

Precautions: Children, elderly, hypertension, hyperthyroidism, diabetes, pregnancy (C), Down syndrome

Pharmacokinetics:

INSTILL: Peak ½-1 hr, duration 1-3 days

NURSING CONSIDERATIONS

Assess:

- Eye pain; discontinue use

Evaluate:
• Therapeutic response: decrease in inflammation or cycloplegic refraction

Teach patient/family:
• To report change in vision, blurring or loss of sight, trouble breathing, sweating, flushing
• Method of instillation: pressure on lacrimal sac for 1 min; not to touch dropper to eye
• That blurred vision will decrease with repeated use of drug
• Not to engage in hazardous activities until able to see
• To wait 5 min to use other drops
• Not to blink more than usual

hyaluronidase (℞)

(hye-al-yoor-on'i-dase)
Wydase
Func. class.: Enzyme

Action: Hydrolyzes hyaluronic acid within areas filled with exudates
Uses: Hypodermoclysis, subcutaneous urography; adjunct to dispersion of other drugs
Dosage and routes:
Adjunct
• *Adult and child:* INJ 150 U with other drug
Urography
• *Adult and child:* SC 75 U over scapula, then contrast medium injected at same site
Hypodermoclysis
• *Adult and child >3 yr:* SC 150 U/L of clysis sol
Available forms: Inj powder 150, 1500 U; inj sol 150 U/ml
Side effects/adverse reactions:
INTEG: Rash, urticaria, itching
OTHER: Overhydration (hyperdermoclysis)
Contraindications: Hypersensitivity to bovine products, CHF, hypoproteinemia, around infected/inflamed or cancerous area
Precautions: Pregnancy (C)
Interactions:
• Systemic reactions: local anesthetics

NURSING CONSIDERATIONS
Assess:
• Site before administration (hypodermoclysis)
• For overhydration in child <3 yr
Administer:
• After test dose: 0.02 ml of 150 U/ml sol is injected; if wheal develops or itching occurs, test is positive
• Right after mixing; sol is unstable
• To child <3 yr, not exceeding 200 ml; in neonates not exceeding 2 ml/min
Evaluate:
• Therapeutic response: absence of swelling, pain after hypodermoclysis

hydralazine (℞)

(hye'dral'a-zeen)
Alazine, Apresoline, Pralzine, Hydralazine HCl, novo-Hylazin*, Rolzine
Func. class.: Antihypertensive, direct-acting peripheral vasodilator
Chem. class.: Phthalazine

Combination products: Cherapas, Ser-A-Gen, Ser-Ap-Es, Serathide, Serpazide, Tri-Hydroserpine, Unipres: reserpine 0.1 mg with hydralazine HCl 25 mg, hydrochlorothiazide 15 mg; Ser-a-Gen: hydrochlorothiazide 15 mg, hydralazine hydrochloride 25 mg, reserpine 0.1 mg; Serpasil-Apresoline HCl No. 1: hydralazine HCl 25 mg, reserpine 0.1 mg; Serpasil-Apresoline HCl No. 2: hydralazine HCl 25 mg, reserpine 0.2 mg

Action: Vasodilates arteriolar smooth muscle by direct relaxation; reduction in blood pressure with reflex increases in cardiac function

Uses: Essential hypertension; *parenteral:* severe essential hypertension, CHF

Dosage and routes:

• *Adult:* PO 10 mg qid 2-4 days, then 25 mg for rest of 1st wk, then 50 mg qid individualized to desired response, not to exceed 300 mg qd; IV/IM BOL 20-40 mg q4-6h, administer PO as soon as possible; IM 20-40 mg q4-6h

• *Child:* PO 0.75-3 mg/kg/day in 4 divided doses; max 7.5 mg/kg/24 hr; IV BOL 0.1-0.2 mg/kg q4-6h; IM 0.1-0.2 mg/kg q4-6h

Available forms: Inj IV, IM 20 mg/ml; tabs 10, 25, 50, 100 mg

Side effects/adverse reactions:

MISC: Nasal congestion, muscle cramps, *lupuslike symptoms*

CV: Palpitations, reflex tachycardia, angina, ***shock,*** edema, rebound hypertension

CNS: Headache, tremors, dizziness, anxiety, peripheral neuritis, depression

GI: Nausea, vomiting, anorexia, diarrhea, constipation

INTEG: Rash, pruritus

HEMA: ***Leukopenia, agranulocytosis,*** anemia

GU: Impotence, urinary retention, Na, H_2O retention

Contraindications: Hypersensitivity to hydralazines, coronary artery disease, mitral valvular rheumatic heart disease, rheumatic heart disease

Precautions: Pregnancy (C), CVA, advanced renal disease

Pharmacokinetics:

PO: Onset 20-30 min, peak 1 hr, duration 2-4 hr

IM: Onset 5-10 min, peak 1 hr, duration 2-4 hr

IV: Onset 5-20 min, peak 10-80 min, duration 2-6 hr; half-life 2-8 hr; metabolized by liver; less than 10% present in urine

Interactions:

• Increased tachycardia, angina: sympathomimetics (epinephrine, norepinephrine)

• Increased effects of β-blockers

• Use MAOIs with caution in patients receiving hydralazine

Y-site compatibilities: Heparin, hydrocortisone, potassium chloride, verapamil, vitamin B with C

Additive compatibility: Dobutamine

NURSING CONSIDERATIONS

Assess:

• B/P q5min × 2 hr, then q1h × 2 hr, then q4h

• Pulse, jugular venous distention q4h

• Electrolytes, blood studies: K, Na, Cl, CO_2, CBC, serum glucose

• Weight daily, I&O

• LE prep, ANA titer before starting therapy

• Edema in feet, legs daily

• Skin turgor, dryness of mucous membranes for hydration status

• Rales, dyspnea, orthopnea

• IV site for extravasation, rate

• Fever, joint pain, tachycardia, palpitations, headache, nausea

• Mental status: affect, mood, behavior, anxiety; check for personality changes

Administer:

• Give with meals (PO) to enhance absorption

• IV undiluted; give through Y-tube or 3-way stopcock each 10 mg or less/min

• To recumbent patient, keep for 1 hr after administration

Evaluate:

• Therapeutic response: decreased B/P

Teach patient/family:

• To take with food to increase bioavailability

• To avoid OTC preparations unless directed by prescriber

• To notify prescriber if chest pain, severe fatigue, fever, muscle or joint pain occurs

Treatment of overdose: Administer vasopressors, volume expanders for shock; if PO, lavage or give activated charcoal, digitalization

hydrochlorothiazide (℞)

(hye-droe-klor-oh-thye'a-zide)

Diaqua, Diuchlor H*, Esidrix, Ezide, Hydro-Chlor, hydrochlorothiazide, HydroDiuril, Hydromal, Hydro-Par, Hydro-T, Hydrozide*, Neo-Codema*, Novohydrazide*, Oretic, Thiuretic, Urozide*

Func. class.: Thiazide diuretic

Chem. class.: Sulfonamide derivative

Combination products: CAM-AP-ES: hydrochlorothiazide 15 mg, hydralazine 25 mg, reserpine 0.1 mg; Dyazide: hydrochlorothiazide 25 mg with triamterene 50 mg; Maxzide: hydrochlorothiazide 50 mg with triamterene 75 mg; Oreticyl 25: deserpidine 0.125 mg with hydrochlorothiazide 25 mg; Oreticyl 50: deserpidine 0.125 mg with hydrochlorothiazide 50 mg; Oreticyl Forte: deserpidine 0.25 mg with hydrochlorothiazide 50 mg; Spironazide: spironolactone 25 mg, hydrochlorothiazide 25 mg; Spirozide: spironolactone 25 mg, hydrochlorothiazide 25 mg; Timolide 10/25: timolol maleate 10 mg with hydrochlorothiazide 25 mg; Unipres: hydrochlorothiazide 15 mg, reserpine 0.1 mg, hydralazine hydrochloride 25 mg; Urisedamine: methenamine mandelate 500 mg, hyoscyamine 0.15 mg

Action: Acts on distal tubule and cortical thick ascending limb of loop of Henle by increasing excretion of water, sodium, chloride, potassium

Uses: Edema, hypertension, diuresis, CHF; edema in corticosteroid, estrogen therapy

Dosage and routes:

• *Adult:* PO 25-100 mg/day

• *Child >6 mo:* PO 2.2 mg/kg/day in divided doses

• *Child <6 mo:* PO up to 3.3 mg/kg/day in divided doses

Available forms: Tabs 25, 50, 100 mg; sol 50 mg/5 ml, 100 mg/ml

Side effects/adverse reactions:

GU: Frequency, polyuria, ***uremia, glucosuria,*** hyperurecemia

CNS: Drowsiness, paresthesia, depression, headache, *dizziness, fatigue, weakness,* fever

GI: Nausea, vomiting, anorexia, constipation, diarrhea, cramps, pancreatitis, GI irritation, ***hepatitis***

EENT: Blurred vision

INTEG: Rash, urticaria, purpura, photosensitivity

META: Hyperglycemia, hyperuricemia, increased creatinine, BUN

HEMA: ***Aplastic anemia, hemolytic anemia, leukopenia, agranulocytosis, thrombocytopenia, neutropenia***

CV: Irregular pulse, orthostatic hypotension, palpitations, volume depletion

ELECT: Hypokalemia, hypercalcemia, hyponatremia, hypochloremia, hypomagnesemia

Contraindications: Hypersensitivity to thiazides or sulfonamides,

* Available in Canada only

anuria, renal decompensation, hypomagnesemia
Precautions: Hypokalemia, renal disease, pregnancy (B), lactation, hepatic disease, gout, COPD, lupus erythematosus, diabetes mellitus, hyperlipidemia
Pharmacokinetics:
PO: Onset 2 hr, peak 4 hr, duration 6-12 hr; excreted unchanged by kidneys; crosses placenta; enters breast milk
Interactions:
- Increased toxicity of lithium, nondepolarizing skeletal muscle relaxants, digitalis
- Decreased effects of antidiabetics
- Decreased absorption of thiazides: cholestyramine, colestipol
- Decreased hypotensive response: indomethacin, NSAIDs
- Hyperglycemia, hyperuricemia, hypotension: diazoxide

Lab test interferences:
Increase: BSP retention, amylase, parathyroid test
Decrease: PBI, PSP
NURSING CONSIDERATIONS
Assess:
- Weight, I&O daily to determine fluid loss; effect of drug may be decreased if used qd
- Rate, depth, rhythm of respiration, effect of exertion
- B/P lying, standing; postural hypotension may occur
- Electrolytes: K, Mg, Na, Cl; include BUN, blood sugar, CBC, serum creatinine, blood pH, ABGs, uric acid, Ca
- Glucose in urine if patient is diabetic
- Signs of metabolic alkalosis: drowsiness, restlessness
- Signs of hypokalemia: postural hypotension, malaise, fatigue, tachycardia, leg cramps, weakness, dehydration
- Rashes, temp qd
- Confusion, especially in elderly; take safety precautions if needed

Administer:
- In AM to avoid interference with sleep if using drug as a diuretic
- K replacement if K <3 mg/dl
- With food; if nausea occurs, absorption may be decreased slightly

Evaluate:
- Therapeutic response: improvement in edema of feet, legs, sacral area qd if medication is being used in CHF

Teach patient/family:
- To increase fluid intake to 2-3 L/day unless contraindicated; to rise slowly from lying or sitting position
- To notify prescriber of muscle weakness, cramps, nausea, dizziness
- That drug may be taken with food or milk
- To use sunscreen for photosensitivity
- That blood sugar may be increased in diabetics
- To take early in day to avoid nocturia

Treatment of overdose: Lavage if taken orally; monitor electrolytes; administer dextrose in saline; monitor hydration, CV, renal status

hydrocodone (℞)

(hye-droe-koe′done)
Hycodan, Robidone*
Func. class.: Narcotic analgesic
Chem. class.: Opiate

Combination products: Bancap HC, Dolacet, Hydrocet, Zydone: hydrocodone bitartrate 5 mg with acetaminophen 500 mg; Co-Gesic, Damacet-P, Duradyne, Hy-Phen, Norcet, Vicodin: hydrocodone bitartrate 5 mg with acetaminophen 500 mg; Damason-P: hydrocodone

H

bitartrate 5 mg with aspirin 224 mg, caffeine 32 mg; Hydrogesic: hydrocodone bitartrate 7.5 mg with acetaminophen 650 mg; T-Gesic: hydrocodone bitartrate 5 mg with acetaminophen 325 mg, butalbital 30 mg, caffeine 40 mg

---

Controlled Substance Schedule III

Action: Acts directly on cough center in medulla to suppress cough

Uses: Hyperactive and nonproductive cough, mild pain

Dosages and routes:

• *Adults:* PO 5 mg q4h prn or 10 mg q12h (long-acting)

• *Child:* PO 2-12 mg 1.25-5 mg q4h prn

Available forms: Caps 5 mg, susp 5 mg/ml, tabs 5 mg, 10 mg (long-acting)

Side effects/adverse reactions:

CNS: Drowsiness, dizziness, lightheadedness, confusion, headache, sedation, euphoria, dysphoria, weakness, hallucinations, disorientation, mood changes, dependence, ***convulsions***

GI: Nausea, vomiting, anorexia, constipation, cramps, dry mouth

GU: Increased urinary output, dysuria, urinary retention

INTEG: Rash, urticaria, flushing, pruritus

EENT: Tinnitus, blurred vision, miosis, diplopia

CV: Palpitations, tachycardia, bradycardia, change in B/P, ***circulatory depression,*** syncope

RESP: ***Respiratory depression***

Contraindications: Hypersensitivity, addiction (narcotic)

Precautions: Addictive personality, pregnancy (C), lactation, increased intracranial pressure, MI (acute), severe heart disease, respiratory depression, hepatic disease, renal disease, child <18 yr

Pharmacokinetics: Onset 10-20 min, duration 3-6 hr, half-life 3-4 hr; metabolized in liver; excreted in urine; crosses placenta

Interactions:

• Increased CNS depression: alcohol, narcotics, sedative/hypnotics, phenothiazines, skeletal muscle relaxants, general anesthetics, tricyclic antidepressants

Lab test interferences:

Increase: Amylase, lipase

NURSING CONSIDERATIONS

Assess:

• I&O ratio; check for decreasing output; may indicate urinary retention

• CNS changes: dizziness, drowsiness, hallucinations, euphoria, LOC, pupil reaction

• Allergic reactions: rash, urticaria

• Respiratory dysfunction: respiratory depression, character, rate, rhythm; notify prescriber if respirations are <10/min

• Need for pain medication, physical dependence

Administer:

• With antiemetic after meals if nausea or vomiting occurs

Perform/provide:

• Storage in light-resistant area at room temp

• Assistance with ambulation

• Safety measures: side rails, nightlight, call bell within easy reach

Evaluate:

• Therapeutic response: decrease in pain or cough

Teach patient/family:

• To report any symptoms of CNS changes, allergic reactions

• That physical dependency may result when used for extended periods

• Withdrawal symptoms may occur: nausea, vomiting, cramps, fever, faintness, anorexia

---

* Available in Canada only

Treatment of overdose: Naloxone HCl (Narcan) 0.2-0.8 mg IV, O_2, IV fluids, vasopressors

hydrocortisone/hydrocortisone acetate

(hye-droe kor'ti-sone)

Cortamed*, Otall

Func. class.: Otic

Chem. class.: Synthetic steroid

Action: Antiinflammatory, antipruritic

Uses: Ear canal inflammation

Dosage and routes:

• *Adult and child:* INSTILL 3-4 gtt bid-qid

Available forms: Otic sol 0.25%, 0.5%, 1%

Side effects/adverse reactions:

EENT: Itching, irritation in ear

INTEG: Rash, urticaria

Contraindications: Hypersensitivity, perforated eardrum

Precautions: Pregnancy (C)

NURSING CONSIDERATIONS

Assess:

• For redness, swelling, fever, pain in ear, which indicates infection

Administer:

• After removing impacted cerumen by irrigation

• After cleaning stopper with alcohol

• After restraining child if necessary

• Warming sol to body temp

Evaluate:

• Therapeutic response: decreased ear pain, inflammation

Teach patient/family:

• Method of instillation using aseptic technique, including not touching dropper to ear

• That dizziness may occur after instillation

hydrocortisone/hydrocortisone acetate/hydrocortisone valerate (Topical) (OTC)

(hye-droe-kor'ti-sone)

Acticort 100, Aeroseb-HC, Ala-Cort, Ala-Scalp, Alphaderm, Bactine Hydrocortisone, Caldecort Anti-Itch, Cetacort, Cortaid, Cortaid Maximum Strength, Cort-Dome, Cortef Feminine Itch, Cortizone-5, Cortizone-10, Cortril, Delacort, Delcort, Dermacort, Dermicort, Dermolate Anti-Itch, Dermtex HC, Hi-Cor 1.0, Hi-Cor 2.5, Hycort, HydroTex, Hytone, Lacticare-HC, Nutracort, Penecort, 1% HC, S-T Cort, Synacort, Tega-Cort, Tega-Cort Forte, Texacort, Westcort

Func. class.: Topical corticosteroid

Chem. class.: Natural nonfluorinated, group IV potency (valerate), group VI potency (acetate and plain)

Action: Antipruritic, antiinflammatory

Uses: Psoriasis, eczema, contact dermatitis, pruritus

Dosage and routes:

• *Adult and child >2 yr:* Apply to affected area qd-qid

Available forms: *Hydrocortisone* oint 0.5%, 1%, 2.5%; cream 0.25%, 0.5%, 1%, 2.5%; lotion 0.25%, 0.5%, 1%, 2%, 2.5%; gel 1%; sol 1%; aerosol/pump spray 0.5%; *acetate* oint 0.5%, 1%, 2.5%; cream 0.5%; lotion 0.05%; aerosol 1%; *valerate* oint 0.2%; cream 0.2% (many others)

Side effects/adverse reactions:

INTEG: Burning, dryness, itching, irritation, acne, folliculitis, hypertrichosis, perioral dermatitis, hypopigmentation, atrophy, striae, miliaria, allergic contact dermatitis, secondary infection

Contraindications: Hypersensitivity to corticosteroids; fungal infections

Precautions: Pregnancy (C), lactation, viral, bacterial infections

NURSING CONSIDERATIONS

Assess:

• Temp; if fever develops, drug should be discontinued

• For systemic absorption: fever, inflammation, irritation

Administer:

• Only to affected areas; do not get in eyes

• Medication, then cover with occlusive dressing if prescribed; seal to intact skin; change q12h; systemic absorption may occur; use gloves

• Only to dermatoses; do not use on weeping, denuded, infected area

• Apply aerosol from 6 in (15 cm) for 1-2 sec

Perform/provide:

• Cleansing before application

• Treatment for a few days after area has cleared

• Storage at room temp

Evaluate:

• Therapeutic response: absence of severe itching, patches on skin, flaking

Teach patient/family:

• To avoid sunlight on affected area; burns may occur

• Not to use other OTC products unless approved by prescriber

hydrocortisone/hydrocortisone acetate/hydrocortisone sodium phosphate/hydrocortisone sodium succinate (℞)

(hye-dro-kor'ti-sone)

Cortef, Hydrocortone/Cortef Acetate, Hydrocortone Acetate/Hydrocortone Phosphate/A-Hydrocort, Solu-Cortef, Cortenema

Func. class.: Corticosteroid

Chem. class.: Short-acting glucocorticoid

Action: Decreases inflammation by suppression of migration of polymorphonuclear leukocytes, fibroblasts, reversal of increased capillary permeability and lysosomal stabilization

Uses: Severe inflammation, septic shock, adrenal insufficiency, ulcerative colitis, collagen disorders

Dosage and routes:

Adrenal insufficiency/inflammation

• *Adult:* PO 5-30 mg bid-qid; IM/IV 100-250 mg (succinate), then 50-100 mg IM as needed; IM/IV 15-240 mg q12h (phosphate)

Shock

• *Adult:* 500 mg-2 g q2-6h (succinate)

• *Child:* IM/IV 0.16-1 mg/kg bid-tid (succinate)

Colitis

• *Adult:* ENEMA 100 mg nightly for 21 days

Available forms: Tabs 5, 10, 20 mg; inj 25, 50 mg/ml; enema 100 mg/60 ml; acetate-inj 25*, 50 mg/ml*, enema 10% aerosol foam; supp 25 mg; cypionate-oral susp 10 mg/5 ml; phosphate-inj 50 mg/ml; succinate-

* Available in Canada only

inj 100 mg*, 250 mg*, 500 mg*, 1000 mg/vial*

Side effects/adverse reactions:
CNS: Depression, flushing, sweating, headache, mood changes
CV: Hypertension, ***circulatory collapse, thrombophlebitis, embolism***, tachycardia, edema
EENT: Fungal infections, increased intraocular pressure, blurred vision
GI: Diarrhea, nausea, abdominal distention, ***GI hemorrhage***, increased appetite, ***pancreatitis***
HEMA: ***Thrombocytopenia***
INTEG: Acne, poor wound healing, ecchymosis, petechiae
MS: Fractures, osteoporosis, weakness

Contraindications: Psychosis, hypersensitivity, idiopathic thrombocytopenia, acute glomerulonephritis, amebiasis, fungal infections, nonasthmatic bronchial disease, child <2 yr, AIDS, TB

Precautions: Pregnancy (C), lactation, diabetes mellitus, glaucoma, osteoporosis, seizure disorders, ulcerative colitis, CHF, myasthenia gravis, renal disease, esophagitis, peptic ulcer

Pharmacokinetics:
PO: Onset 1-2 hr, peak 1 hr, duration 1-1½ days
IM/IV: Onset 20 min, peak 4-8 hr, duration 1-1½ days
REC: Onset 3-5 days
Metabolized by liver, excreted in urine (17-OHCS, 17-KS), crosses placenta

Interactions:
• Decreased action of hydrocortisone: cholestyramine, colestipol, barbiturates, rifampin, ephedrine, phenytoin, theophylline
• Decreased effects of anticoagulants, anticonvulsants, antidiabetics, ambenonium, neostigmine, isoniazid, toxoids, vaccines, anticholinesterases, salicylates, somatrem
• Increased side effects: alcohol, salicylates, indomethacin, amphotericin B, digitalis, cyclosporine, diuretics
• Increased action of hydrocortisone: salicylates, estrogens, indomethacin, oral contraceptives, ketoconazole, macrolide antibiotics

Sodium phosphate preparations
Syringe compatibilities: Fluconazole, fludarabine, metoclopramide
Additive compatibilities: Amphotericin B, bleomycin, dacarbazine

Sodium succinate preparations
Syringe compatibilities: Metoclopramide, thiopental
Y-site compatibilities: Acyclovir, aminophylline, ampicillin, amrinone, atracurium, atropine, betamethasone, calcium gluconate, cephalothin, cephapirin, chlordiazepoxide, chlorpromazine, cyanocobalamin, dexamethasone, digoxin, diphenhydramine, dopamine, droperidol, edrophonium, enalaprilat, epinephrine, esmolol, conjugated estrogens, ethacrynate, famotidine, fentanyl, fentanyl/droperidol, fludarabine, fluorouracil, foscarnet, furosemide, hydralazine, insulin, isoproterenol, kanamycin, lidocaine, magnesium sulfate, melphalan, menadiol, methicillin, methoxamine, methylergonovine, minocycline, morphine, neostigmine, norepinephrine, ondansetron, oxacillin, oxytocin, paclitaxel, pancuronium, penicillin G potassium, pentazocine, phytonadione, prednisolone, procainamide, prochlorperazine, propranolol, pyridostigmine, scopolamine, sodium bicarbonate, succinylcholine, trimethobenzamide, trimethaphan camsylate, vecuronium, vinrelobine
Additive compatibilities: Aminophylline, amphotericin, daunorubi-

cin, mitoxantrone, potassium chloride

Lab test interferences:

Increase: Cholesterol, Na, blood glucose, uric acid, Ca, urine glucose

Decrease: Ca, K, T_4, T_3, thyroid ^{131}I uptake test, urine 17-OHCS, 17-KS, PBI

False negative: Skin allergy tests

NURSING CONSIDERATIONS

Assess:

- K, blood sugar, urine glucose while on long-term therapy; hypokalemia and hyperglycemia
- Weight daily, notify prescriber of weekly gain >5 lb
- B/P q4h, pulse; notify prescriber of chest pain
- I&O ratio; be alert for decreasing urinary output, increasing edema
- Plasma cortisol levels during long-term therapy (normal level: 138-635 nmol/L SI units when drawn at 8 AM)
- Infection: increased temp, WBC, even after withdrawal of medication; drug masks infection
- K depletion: paresthesias, fatigue, nausea, vomiting, depression, polyuria, dysrhythmias, weakness
- Edema, hypertension, cardiac symptoms
- Mental status: affect, mood, behavioral changes, aggression

Administer:

- Daily dose in AM for better results
- **Phosphate:** IV undiluted or added to dextrose or saline inj and given by infusion; give 25 mg or less/min
- **Succinate:** IV in mix-o-vial, or reconstitute 250 mg or less/2 ml bacteriostatic H_2O for inj; mix gently; give direct IV over 1 min or more; may be further diluted in 100, 250, 500, or 1000 ml of D_5W, D_5 0.9%, NaCl 0.9% given over ordered rate
- IM inj deep in large mass; rotate sites; avoid deltoid; use 21G needle
- In one dose in AM to prevent adrenal suppression; avoid SC administration; may damage tissue
- With food or milk for GI symptoms
- Rectal: telling patient to retain for 20 min if possible

Perform/provide:

- Assistance with ambulation in patient with bone tissue disease to prevent fractures

Evaluate:

- Therapeutic response: ease of respirations, decreased inflammation

Teach patient/family:

- That ID as steroid user should be carried
- To notify prescriber if therapeutic response decreases; dosage adjustment may be needed
- Not to discontinue abruptly, or adrenal crisis can result; drug should be tapered off
- To avoid OTC products: salicylates, alcohol in cough products, cold preparations unless directed by prescriber
- About cushingoid symptoms of adrenal insufficiency: nausea, anorexia, fatigue, dizziness, dyspnea, weakness, joint pain

hydromorphone (℞)

(hye-droe-mor'fone)

Dilaudid, Dilaudid HP, hydromorphone HCl

Func. class.: Narcotic analgesics

Chem. class.: Opiate, semisynthetic phenanthrene

Controlled Substance Schedule II

Action: Inhibits ascending pain pathways in CNS, increases pain threshold, alters pain perception

Uses: Moderate to severe pain

* Available in Canada only

Dosage and routes:
• *Adult:* PO 1-6 mg q4-6h prn; IM/SC/IV 2-4 mg q4-6h; REC 3 mg hs prn
Available forms: Inj IM, IV 1, 2, 3, 4 mg/ml; tabs 1, 2, 3, 4 mg; rec supp 3 mg
Side effects/adverse reactions:
CNS: Drowsiness, dizziness, confusion, headache, sedation, euphoria
GI: Nausea, vomiting, anorexia, constipation, cramps
GU: Increased urinary output, dysuria, urinary retention
INTEG: Rash, urticaria, bruising, flushing, diaphoresis, pruritus
EENT: Tinnitus, blurred vision, miosis, diplopia
CV: Palpitations, bradycardia, change in B/P
RESP: ***Respiratory depression***
Contraindications: Hypersensitivity, addiction (narcotic)
Precautions: Addictive personality, pregnancy (C), lactation, increased intracranial pressure, MI (acute), severe heart disease, respiratory depression, hepatic disease, renal disease, child <18 yr
Pharmacokinetics:
Onset 15-30 min, peak ½-1½ hr, duration 4-5 hr; metabolized by liver; excreted by kidneys; crosses placenta; excreted in breast milk
Interactions:
• Effects may be increased with other CNS depressants: alcohol, narcotics, sedative/hypnotics, antipsychotics, skeletal muscle relaxants
Syringe compatibilities: Atropine, chlorpromazine, cimetidine, diphenhydramine, fentanyl, glycopyrrolate, hydroxyzine, midazolam, pentazocine, pentobarbital, promethazine, ranitidine, scopolamine, tetracaine, tiethylperazine, trimethobenzamide
Y-site compatibilities: Acyclovir, amikacin, ampicillin, cefamandole, cefazolin, cefoperazone, ceforanide, cefotaxime, ceftazidine, cefoxitin, ceftizoxime, cefuroxime, cephalothin, cephapirin, chloramphenicol, clindamycin, doxycycline, erythromycin lactobionate, fludarabine, foscarnet, gentamicin, kanamycin, magnesium sulfate, melphalan, metronidazole, mezlocillin, moxalactam, nafcillin, ondansetron, oxacillin, paclitaxel, penicillin G potassium, piperacillin, ticarcillin, tobramycin, trimethoprim/sulfamethoxazole, vancomycin, vinorelbine
Solution compatibilities: D_5W, D_5/0.45% NaCl, D_5/0.9% NaCl, D_5/LR, D_5/Ringer's sol, 0.45% NaCl, 0.9% NaCl, Ringer's and lactated Ringer's sol
Lab test interferences:
Increase: Amylase

NURSING CONSIDERATIONS
Assess:
• I&O ratio; check for decreasing output; may indicate urinary retention
• CNS changes: dizziness, drowsiness, hallucinations, euphoria, LOC, pupil reaction
• Allergic reactions: rash, urticaria
• Respiratory dysfunction: respiratory depression, character, rate, rhythm; notify prescriber if respirations are <10/min
• Need for pain medication, physical dependence
• Pain control, sedation by scoring
Administer:
• IV direct diluted with 5 ml sterile H_2O or NS; give through Y-tube or 3-way stopcock; give 2 mg or less/5 min
• IV INF: Dilute each 0.1-1 mg/ml NS (0.1-1 mg/m) deliver by narcotic syringe infusor; may be diluted in D_5W, D_5NaCl, 0.45% NaCl

H

or NS for larger amounts and delivery through an infusion pump
• With antiemetic if nausea, vomiting occur
• When pain is beginning to return; determine interval by response

Perform/provide:
• Storage in light-resistant area at room temp
• Assistance with ambulation
• Safety measures: side rails, nightlight, call bell within easy reach

Evaluate:
• Therapeutic response: decrease in pain

Teach patient/family:
• To report any symptoms of CNS changes, allergic reactions
• That physical dependency may result when used for extended periods
• Withdrawal symptoms may occur: nausea, vomiting, cramps, fever, faintness, anorexia

Treatment of overdose: Naloxone HCl (Narcan) 0.2-0.8 mg IV, O_2, IV fluids, vasopressors

hydromorphone/guaifenesin/alcohol (℞)

(hye-droe-mor′fone)
Dilaudid Cough Syrup
Func. class.: Antitussive, narcotic
Chem. class.: Phenanthrene derivative, guaifenesin

Controlled Substance Schedule II
Action: Increases respiratory tract fluid by decreasing surface tension, adhesiveness, which increases removal of mucus; analgesic, antitussive
Uses: Cough
Dosage and routes:
• *Adult:* PO 1 mg q3-4h prn
• *Child 6-12 yr:* PO 0.5 mg q3-4h prn

Available forms: Syr 1 mg/5 ml
Side effects/adverse reactions:
CNS: Dizziness, drowsiness
GI: Nausea, constipation, vomiting, anorexia
CV: Hypotension
INTEG: Urticaria, rash
RESP: ***Respiratory depression***
Contraindications: Hypersensitivity, increased intracranial pressure, status asthmaticus
Precautions: Hypothyroidism, Addison's disease, CNS depression, brain tumor, asthma, hepatic disease, renal disease, COPD, psychosis, alcoholism, convulsive disorders, pregnancy (C), lactation
Pharmacokinetics: Metabolized by liver; half-life 2-4 hr
Interactions:
• Enhanced CNS depression: barbiturates, narcotics, antipsychotics, antidepressants

NURSING CONSIDERATIONS

Assess:
• VS, cardiac status, including hypotension
• Respiratory rate, depth
• Cough: type, frequency, character, including sputum

Administer:
• Decreased dose to elderly patients; metabolism may be slowed

Perform/provide:
• Storage at room temp
• Increased fluids, bulk, exercise to decrease constipation

Evaluate:
• Therapeutic response: absence of cough

Teach patient/family:
• To avoid driving, other hazardous activities until patient stabilized on medication if drowsiness occurs
• To avoid alcohol, other CNS depressants; will enhance sedating properties of this drug

hydroquinone (℞)

(hye'droe-kwin-one)

Cocrema Mercolized, Eldopaque, Eldopaque-Forte, Eldoquin, Eldoquin-Forte, Esoterica Facial, Esoterica Fortified, Esoterica Regular, Melanex, Porcelana, Porcelana With Sunscreen, Solaquin, Solaquin Forte

Func. class.: Depigmentating agent

Chem. class.: Enzyme inhibitor

Action: Inhibits production of tyrosine, which is needed in formation of melanin

Uses: Bleaching skin, including age spots, freckles, lentigo, chloasma

Dosage and routes:

• *Adult and child:* TOP apply to affected area qd-bid

Available forms: Top cream 2%, 4%; top lotion 2%; gel 4%; sol 3%

Side effects/adverse reactions:

INTEG: Rash, dryness, fissures, stinging, contact dermatitis, erythema, irritation

Contraindications: Hypersensitivity, inflamed skin, prickly heat, sunburn

Precautions: Pregnancy (C), lactation, child <1 yr

NURSING CONSIDERATIONS

Assess:

• Area of body involved, including time involved; what helps or aggravates condition

Administer:

• Topical corticosteroid for irritation

• Test dose to be applied to area 25 mm in diameter; check site after 24 hr; if itching or excessive inflammation occurs, drug should not be used

Perform/provide:

• Storage at room temp in tight container

Evaluate:

• Therapeutic response: fading of spots over time

Teach patient/family:

• To avoid application on normal skin, getting cream in eyes

• To use opaque sunscreen during day on exposed areas, or bleaching effect may be reversed

• That minor redness is not a contraindication

• To continue to use sunscreen after bleaching is complete

hydroxocobalamin (vit B_{12}) (℞)

Acti-B_{12}*, Alphamin, Hydrobexan, Hydro-Crysti 12, Hydroxo-12, hydroxycobalamin, LA-12

Func. class.: Vitamin

Chem. class.: B_{12}—water-soluble vitamin

Action: Needed for adequate nerve functioning, protein and carbohydrate metabolism, normal growth, RBC development

Uses: Vit B_{12} deficiency, pernicious anemia, vit B_{12} malabsorption syndrome, Schilling test

Dosage and routes:

• *Adult:* IM 30-100 μg qd × 5-10 days, maintenance 100-200 mg IM qmo

• *Child:* IM 1-30 μg qd × 5-10 days, maintenance 60 μg IM qmo or more often

Pernicious anemia/malabsorption syndrome

• *Adult:* IM 100-1000 μg qd × 2 wk, then 100-1000 μg IM qmo

H

• *Child:* IM 1000-5000 μg × 2 wk or more given in 100-500 μg doses, then 60 μg IM/SC qmo

Schilling test

• *Adult and child:* IM 1000 μg in one dose

Available forms: Inj IM 100, 120, 1000 μg/ml

Side effects/adverse reactions:

CNS: Flushing, optic nerve atrophy

GI: Diarrhea

CV: ***CHF,*** peripheral vascular thrombosis, ***pulmonary edema***

INTEG: Itching, rash

Contraindications: Hypersensitivity, optic nerve atrophy, cardiac disease

Precautions: Pregnancy (A), lactation, children

Pharmacokinetics: Stored in liver, kidneys, stomach; 50%-90% excreted in urine; crosses placenta, breast milk

Interactions:

• Decreased absorption of hydroxocobalamin: aminoglycosides, anticonvulsants, colchicine, chloramphenicol, antineoplastics, cimetidine, alcohol, vit C, K preparations

• Increased absorption of this drug: prednisone

Lab test interferences:

False positive: Intrinsic factor

NURSING CONSIDERATIONS

Assess:

• K levels during beginning treatment

• CBC for increased reticulocyte count during 1st week of therapy, followed by increase in RBC and hemoglobin

• Nutritional status: egg yolks, fish, organ meats, dairy products, clams, oysters, which are good sources of vit B_{12}

• For pulmonary edema or worsening of CHF in cardiac patients

Administer:

• By IM inj for pernicious anemia unless contraindicated

Evaluate:

• Therapeutic response: decreased anorexia, dyspnea on excretion, palpitations, paresthesias, psychosis, visual disturbances

Teach patient/family

• That treatment must continue for life for pernicious anemia

• Importance of well-balanced diet

• To avoid persons with infections

---

hydroxychloroquine (℞)

(hye-drox-ee-klor′oh-kwin)

Plaquenil Sulfate

Func. class.: Antimalarial

Chem. class.: 4-aminoquinoline derivative

Action: Inhibits parasite replications, transcription of DNA to RNA by forming complexes with DNA in parasite

Uses: Malaria caused by *P. vivax, P. malariae, P. ovale, P. falciparum* (some strains): lupus erythematosus, rheumatoid arthritis

Dosage and routes:

Malaria

• *Adult and child:* PO 5 mg/kg/wk on same day of week, not to exceed 400 mg; treatment should begin 2 wk before entering endemic area, continue 8 wk after leaving; if treatment begins after exposure, 800 mg for adult, 10 mg/kg for children in 2 divided doses 6 hr apart

Lupus erythematosus

• *Adult:* PO 400 mg qd-bid; length depends on patient response; maintenance 200-400 mg qd

Rheumatoid arthritis

• *Adult:* PO 400-600 mg qd, then 200-300 mg qd after good response

* Available in Canada only

Available forms: Tabs 200 mg (base 155 mg)

Side effects/adverse reactions:

CV: Hypotension, heart block, ***asystole with syncope***

INTEG: Pruritus, pigmentation changes, skin eruptions, lichen planus-like eruptions, eczema, ***exfoliative dermatitis,*** alopecia

CNS: Headache, stimulation, fatigue, irritability, ***convulsion,*** bad dreams, dizziness, confusion, psychosis, decreased reflexes

EENT: Blurred vision, corneal changes, retinal changes, difficulty focusing, tinnitus, vertigo, deafness, photophobia, corneal edema

GI: Nausea, vomiting, anorexia, diarrhea, cramps

HEMA: ***Thrombocytopenia, agranulocytosis, hemolytic anemia, leukopenia***

Contraindications: Hypersensitivity, retinal field changes, porphyria, children (long-term)

Precautions: Blood dyscrasias, severe GI disease, neurologic disease, alcoholism, hepatic disease, G6PD deficiency, psoriasis, eczema, pregnancy (C), lactation

Pharmacokinetics:

PO: Peak 1-2 hr, half-life 3-5 days; metabolized in liver; excreted in urine, feces, breast milk; crosses placenta

Interactions:

- Decreased action of hydroxychloroquine: Mg or Al compounds
- Increased levels of digoxin
- Increased antibody titer: rabies vaccine

NURSING CONSIDERATIONS

Assess:

- Ophthalmic test if long-term treatment or drug dosage >150 mg/day
- Liver studies qwk: AST (SGOT), ALT (SGPT), bilirubin
- Blood studies: CBC, platelets; WBC, RBC, platelets may be decreased
- For decreased reflexes: knee, ankle
- ECG during therapy
- Watch for depression of T waves, widening of QRS complex
- Allergic reactions: pruritus, rash, urticaria
- Blood dyscrasias: malaise, fever, bruising, bleeding (rare)
- For ototoxicity (tinnitus, vertigo, change in hearing); audiometric testing should be done before, after treatment
- For toxicity: blurring vision, difficulty focusing, headache, dizziness, knee, ankle reflexes; drug should be discontinued immediately

Administer:

- Before or after meals or with milk; at same time each day to maintain drug level
- IM after aspirating to avoid injection into blood system, which may cause hypotension, asystole, heart block; rotate injection sites

Perform/provide:

- Storage in tight, light-resistant container at room temp; keep injection in cool environment

Evaluate:

- Therapeutic response: decreased symptoms of malaria

Teach patient/family:

- To use sunglasses in bright sunlight to decrease photophobia
- That urine may turn rust or brown
- To report hearing, visual problems, fever, fatigue, bruising, bleeding, which may indicate blood dyscrasias

Treatment of overdose: Induce vomiting; gastric lavage; administer barbiturate (ultrashort-acting), vasopressin, ammonium chloride; tracheostomy may be necessary

H

hydroxyprogesterone (℞)

(hye-drox-ee-pro-jess'te-rone)

Delalutin, Duralutin, Gesterol L.A. 250, Hylutin, Hyprogest 250, Hyproval PA, Prodrox, Pro-Depo

Func. class.: Progestin, hormone

Action: Inhibits secretion of pituitary gonadotropins, which prevents follicular maturation, ovulation, stimulates growth of mammary tissue, antineoplastic action against endometrial cancer

Uses: Uterine carcinoma, menstrual disorders (abnormal uterine bleeding, amenorrhea)

Dosage and routes:

Menstrual disorders

• *Adult:* IM 125-375 mg q4wk; discontinue after 4 cycles

Uterine cancer

• *Adult:* IM 1-5 g/wk

Available forms: Inj IM 125, 250 mg/ml

Side effects/adverse reactions:

CNS: Dizziness, headache, migraines, depression, fatigue

CV: Hypotension, thrombophlebitis, edema, ***thromboembolism, stroke, pulmonary embolism, myocardial infarction***

GI: Nausea, vomiting, anorexia, cramps, increased weight, ***cholestatic jaundice***

EENT: Diplopia

GU: Amenorrhea, cervical erosion, breakthrough bleeding, dysmenorrhea, vaginal candidiasis, breast changes, *gynecomastia, testicular atrophy, impotence,* endometriosis, ***spontaneous abortion***

INTEG: Rash, urticaria, acne, hirsutism, alopecia, oily skin, seborrhea, purpura, melasma, photosensitivity

META: Hyperglycemia

Contraindications: Breast cancer, hypersensitivity, thromboembolic disorders, genital bleeding (abnormal, undiagnosed), pregnancy (X)

Precautions: Lactation, hypertension, asthma, blood dyscrasias, gallbladder disease, HF, diabetes mellitus, bone disease, depression, migraine headache, convulsive disorders, hepatic disease, renal disease, family history of breast cancer

Pharmacokinetics:

IM: Half-life 5 min, duration 24 hr; excreted in urine, feces; metabolized in liver

Lab test interferences:

Increase: Alk phosphatase, nitrogen (urine), pregnanediol, amino acids

Decrease: GTT, HDL

Interference: Thyroid hormone assays

NURSING CONSIDERATIONS

Assess:

• Weight daily; notify prescriber of weekly weight gain >5 lb

• B/P at beginning of treatment and periodically

• I&O ratio; be alert for decreasing urinary output, increasing edema

• Liver function studies: ALT (SGPT), AST (SGOT), bilirubin, periodically during long-term therapy

• Edema, hypertension, cardiac symptoms, jaundice

• Mental status: affect, mood, behavioral changes, depression

Administer:

• Titrated dose; use lowest effective dose

• Oil solution deeply in large muscle mass (IM), rotate sites

• In one dose in AM

• With food or milk to decrease GI symptoms

• After warming to dissolve crystals

Perform/provide:

• Storage in dark area

Evaluate:

• Therapeutic response: decreased abnormal uterine bleeding, absence of amenorrhea

Teach patient/family:

• To avoid sunlight or use sunscreen; photosensitivity can occur

• To report breast lumps, vaginal bleeding, edema, jaundice, dark urine, clay-colored stools, dyspnea, headache, blurred vision, abdominal pain, numbness or stiffness in legs, chest pain; male to report impotence or gynecomastia

• To report suspected pregnancy

---

hydroxyurea (℞)

(hye-drox'ee-yoo-ree-ah)

Hydrea

Func. class.: Antineoplastic, antimetabolite

Chem. class.: Synthetic urea analog

Action: Acts by inhibiting DNA synthesis without interfering with RNA or protein synthesis; incorporates thymidine into DNA, causing direct damage to DNA strands; S phase specific of cell cycle

Uses: Melanoma, chronic myelocytic leukemia, recurrent or metastatic ovarian cancer, squamous cell carcinoma of the head and neck

Dosage and routes:

Solid tumors

• *Adult:* PO 80 mg/kg as a single dose q3d or 20-30 mg/kg as a single dose qd

In combination with radiation

• *Adult:* PO 80 mg/kg as a single dose q3d; should be started 7 days before irradiation

Resistant chronic myelocytic leukemia

• *Adult:* PO 20-30 mg/kg/day as a single daily dose

Available forms: Caps 500 mg

Side effects/adverse reactions:

HEMA: ***Leukopenia, anemia, thrombocytopenia***

GI: Nausea, vomiting, anorexia, diarrhea, stomatitis, constipation

GU: Increased BUN, uric acid, creatinine, temporary renal function impairment

INTEG: *Rash,* urticaria, pruritus, dry skin

CV: Angina, ischemia

CNS: Headache, confusion, hallucinations, dizziness, ***convulsions***

Contraindications: Hypersensitivity, leukopenia (<2500/mm^3), thrombocytopenia (<100,000/mm^3), anemia (severe), pregnancy (D), lactation

Precautions: Renal disease (severe)

Pharmacokinetics: Readily absorbed when taken orally, peak level in 2 hr; degraded in liver; excreted in urine, almost totally eliminated in 24 hr; readily crosses blood-brain barrier

Interactions:

• Increased toxicity: radiation or other antineoplastics

Lab test interferences:

Increase: Renal function studies

NURSING CONSIDERATIONS

Assess:

• CBC, differential, platelet count qwk; withhold drug if WBC is <3500/mm^3 or platelet count is <100,000/mm^3; notify prescriber; drug should be discontinued

• Renal function studies: BUN, serum uric acid, urine CrCl, electrolytes before, during therapy

• I&O ratio; report fall in urine output to <30 ml/hr

• Monitor temp q4h; fever may indicate beginning infection

• Liver function tests before, during therapy: bilirubin, alk phosphatase, AST (SGOT), ALT (SGPT), LDH; prn or qmo

• B/P q3-4h; check for chest pain; angina, ischemia may occur
• Bleeding: hematuria, guaiac, bruising or petechiae, mucosa or orifices q8h
• Food preferences; list likes, dislikes
• Inflammation of mucosa, breaks in skin
• Buccal cavity q8h for dryness, sores or ulceration, white patches, oral pain, bleeding, dysphagia
• Symptoms indicating severe allergic reaction: rash, urticaria, itching, flushing
• Neurotoxicity: headaches, hallucinations, convulsions, dizziness

Administer:
• Allopurinol or $NaHCO_3$ concurrently to prevent high uric acid levels; extra fluids
• Antiemetic 30-60 min before giving drug and prn
• Antibiotics for prophylaxis of infection
• Transfusion for anemia

Perform/provide:
• Rinsing of mouth tid-qid with water, club soda; brushing of teeth bid-tid with soft brush or cotton-tipped applicators for stomatitis; use unwaxed dental floss
• Nutritious diet with iron, vitamin supplements as ordered

Evaluate:
• Therapeutic response: decreased tumor size, spread of malignancy

Teach patient/family:
• To report signs of infection: elevated temperature, sore throat, flulike symptoms
• To report signs of anemia: fatigue, headache, faintness, shortness of breath, irritability
• To report bleeding: avoid use of razors, commercial mouthwash
• To avoid use of aspirin products, ibuprofen
• To avoid foods with citric acid, hot or rough texture if stomatitis is present
• To report stomatitis: any bleeding, white spots, ulcerations in the mouth; tell patient to examine mouth qd, report symptoms
• That contraceptive measures are recommended during therapy
• To drink 10-12 (8 oz) glasses of fluid/day
• To notify prescriber of fever, chills, sore throat, nausea, vomiting, anorexia, diarrhea, bleeding, bruising; may indicate blood dyscrasias

hydroxyzine (℞)

(hye-drox′i-zeen)

Anxanil, Apo-Hydroxyzine*, Atarax, Atarax 100, Atozine, Durel, Durrex, E-Vista, Hydroxacen, hydroxyzine HCl, hydroxyzine pamoate, Hyzine-50, Multipax*, Novohydroxyzine*, Quiess, Vamate, Vistacon, Vistaject-25, Vistaject-50, Vistaquel 50, Vistaril, Vistazine 50

Func. class.: Sedative-hypnotic

Chem. class.: Piperazine derivative

Action: Depresses subcortical levels of CNS, including limbic system, reticular formation

Uses: Anxiety preoperatively, postoperatively to prevent nausea, vomiting, to potentiate narcotic analgesics; sedation; pruritus

Dosage and routes:
• *Adult:* PO 25-100 mg tid-qid
• *Child >6 yr:* 50-100 mg/day in divided doses
• *Child <6 yr:* 50 mg/day in divided doses

Preoperatively/postoperatively
• *Adult:* IM 25-100 mg q4-6h

* Available in Canada only

• *Child:* IM 1.1 mg/kg q4-6h

Available forms: Tabs 10, 25, 50, 100 mg; caps 25, 50, 100 mg; syrup 100 mg/5 ml; oral susp 25 mg/5 ml; IM inj 25, 50 mg/ml

Side effects/adverse reactions:

CNS: Dizziness, drowsiness, confusion, headache, tremors, fatigue, depression, ***convulsions***

GI: Dry mouth

Contraindications: Hypersensitivity, acute asthma

Precautions: Elderly, debilitated, hepatic disease, renal disease, narrow-angle glaucoma, COPD, prostatic hypertrophy, pregnancy (C)

Pharmacokinetics:

PO: Onset 15-30 min, duration 4-6 hr, half-life 3 hr

Interactions:

• Increased CNS depressant effect: barbiturates, narcotics, analgesics, alcohol

Syringe compatibilities: Atropine, benzquinamide, butorphanol, chlorpromazine, cimetidine, codeine, diphenhydramine, doxapram, droperidol, fentanyl, glycopyrrolate, hydromorphone, lidocaine, meperidine, metoclopromide, morphine, nalbuphine, oxymorphone, pentazocine, procaine, prochlorperazine, promazine, ranitidine, scopolamine

Y-site compatibilities: Melphan, vinorelbine

Lab test interferences:

False increase: 17-OHCS

NURSING CONSIDERATIONS

Assess:

• B/P (lying, standing), pulse; if systolic B/P drops 20 mm Hg, hold drug, notify prescriber

• Blood studies: CBC

• Hepatic studies: AST, ALT, bilirubin, creatinine

• Mental status: mood, sensorium, affect

• Increased sedation

Administer:

• By Z-track injection in large muscle for IM to decrease pain, chance of necrosis

• With food or milk for GI symptoms

• Crushed if patient is unable to swallow medication whole

• Gum, hard candy, frequent sips of water for dry mouth

Perform/provide:

• Assistance with ambulation during beginning therapy, since drowsiness/dizziness occurs

• Safety measures, including side rails

• Checking to see PO medication has been swallowed

Evaluate:

• Therapeutic response: decreased anxiety

Teach patient/family:

• Not to be used for everyday stress or used longer than 4 mo

• Avoid OTC preparations (cold, cough, hay fever) unless approved by prescriber

• To avoid driving, activities that require alertness

• To avoid alcohol ingestion, other psychotropic medications

• Not to discontinue medication quickly after long-term use

• To rise slowly or fainting may occur

Treatment of overdose: Lavage if orally ingested; VS, supportive care; IV norepinephrine for hypotension

H

hyoscyamine (℞)

(hye-oh-sye'a-meen)

Anaspaz, Cystospaz, Cystospaz-M, Gastrosed, Levsin, Levsin Drops, Levsinex Timecaps, Neoquess

Func. class.: GI anticholinergic

Chem. class.: Belladonna alkaloid

Combination products: Levsin with Phenobarbital Tablets, Anaspaz: hyoscyamine sulfate 0.125 mg with phenobarbital; Levsinex with Phenobarbital Elixir: hyoscyamine sulfate 0.125 mg/5 ml with phenobarbital 1.5 mg/5 ml; Levsinex with Phenobarbital Time-caps: hyoscyamine sulfate 0.375 mg with phenobarbital 45 mg; Levsin-PB: hyoscyamine sulfate 0.125 mg/ml with phenobarbital 15 mg/ml

Action: Inhibits muscarinic actions of acetylcholine at postganglionic parasympathetic neuroeffector sites

Uses: Treatment of peptic ulcer disease in combination with other drugs; other GI disorders, other spastic disorders

Dosage and routes:

- *Adult:* PO/SL 0.125-0.25 mg tid-qid ac, hs; TIME REL 0.375 q12h; IM/SC/IV 0.25-0.5 mg q6h
- *Child 2-10 yr:* ½ adult dose
- *Child <2 yr:* ¼ adult dose

Available forms: Tabs 0.125, 0.13, 0.15 mg; caps time rel 0.375 mg; sol 0.125 mg/ml; elix 0.125 mg/5 ml; inj 0.5 mg/ml

Side effects/adverse reactions:

CNS: Confusion, stimulation in elderly, headache, insomnia, dizziness, drowsiness, anxiety, weakness, hallucination

GI: Dry mouth, constipation, paralytic ileus, heartburn, nausea, vomiting, dysphagia, absence of taste

GU: Hesitancy, retention, impotence

CV: Palpitations, tachycardia

EENT: Blurred vision, photophobia, mydriasis, cycloplegia, increased ocular tension

INTEG: Urticaria, rash, pruritus, anhidrosis, fever, allergic reactions

Contraindications: Hypersensitivity to anticholinergics, narrow-angle glaucoma, GI obstruction, myasthenia gravis, paralytic ileus, GI atony, toxic megacolon, prostatic hypertrophy

Precautions: Hyperthyroidism, coronary artery disease, dysrhythmias, CHF, ulcerative colitis, hypertension, hiatal hernia, hepatic disease, renal disease, pregnancy (C), urinary retention

Pharmacokinetics:

PO: Duration 4-6 hr; metabolized by liver; excreted in urine; half-life 3.5 hr

Interactions:

- Decreased effect of hyoscyamine: antacids
- Increased anticholinergic effect: amantadine, tricyclic antidepressants, MAOIs, H_1 antihistamines
- Decreased effect of phenothiazines, levodopa, ketoconazole

NURSING CONSIDERATIONS

Assess:

- VS, cardiac status: checking for dysrhythmias, increased rate, palpitations
- I&O ratio; check for urinary retention or hesitancy
- GI complaints: pain, bleeding (frank or occult), nausea, vomiting, anorexia

Administer:

- ½ hr ac for better absorption
- Decreased dose to elderly patients; metabolism may be slowed
- Gum, hard candy, frequent rinsing of mouth for dryness of oral cavity

Perform/provide:
- Storage in tight container protected from light
- Increased fluids, bulk, exercise to decrease constipation

Evaluate:
- Therapeutic response: absence of epigastric pain, bleeding, nausea, vomiting

Teach patient/family:
- To avoid driving, other hazardous activities until stabilized on medication
- To avoid alcohol or other CNS depressants; will enhance sedating properties of this drug
- To avoid hot environments; heat stroke may occur; drug suppresses perspiration
- To use sunglasses when outside to prevent photophobia; may cause blurred vision

ibuprofen (OTC, ℞)

(eye-byoo'proe-fen)

Aches N Pain, Actiprofen*, Advil, Amersol*, Apo-Ibuprofen*, Children's Advil, Excedrin IS, Genpril, Haltran, Ibuprin, ibuprofen, Ibuprohm, IBU-Tab, Medipren, Menadol, Midol-200, Motrin, Motrin IB, Novo-profen*, Nuprin, Pamprin-IB, Rufen, Saleto-200, Saleto-400, Saleto-600, Saleto-800, Trendar

Func. class.: Nonsteroidal antiinflammatory

Chem. class.: Propionic acid derivative

Action: Inhibits prostaglandin synthesis by decreasing enzyme needed for biosynthesis; analgesic, antiinflammatory, antipyretic

Uses: Rheumatoid arthritis, osteoarthritis, primary dysmenorrhea, gout, dental pain, musculoskeletal disorders, fever

Dosage and routes:

Analgesic
- *Adult:* PO 200-400 mg q4-6h, not to exceed 3.2 g/day

Antipyretic
- *Child 6 mo-12 yr:* PO 5 mg/kg (temp <102.5°F or 39.2°C) 10 mg/kg (temp >102.5°F) may repeat q4-6h, max 40 mg/kg/day

Antiinflammatory
- *Adult:* PO 300-800 mg tid-qid, max 3.2 gm/day
- *Child:* PO 30-40 mg/kg/day in 3-4 divided doses, max 50 mg/kg/day

Available forms: Tabs 200, 300, 400, 600, 800 mg; oral susp 100 mg/5 ml

Side effects/adverse reactions:

CV: Tachycardia, peripheral edema, palpitations, dysrhythmias, hypertension

CNS: Dizziness, drowsiness, fatigue, tremors, confusion, insomnia, anxiety, depression

EENT: Tinnitus, hearing loss, blurred vision

GI: Nausea, anorexia, vomiting, diarrhea, jaundice, ***cholestatic hepatitis***, constipation, flatulence, cramps, dry mouth, peptic ulcer

GU: ***Nephrotoxicity;*** dysuria, hematuria, oliguria, azotemia

HEMA: ***Blood dyscrasias***

INTEG: Purpura, rash, pruritus, sweating

Contraindications: Hypersensitivity, asthma, severe renal disease, severe hepatic disease

Precautions: Pregnancy (B) 1st and 2nd trimester, lactation, children, bleeding disorders, GI disorders, cardiac disorders, hypersensitivity to other antiinflammatory agents

Pharmacokinetics: Well absorbed (PO)

PO: Onset ½ hour; peak 1-2 hr, half-life 2-4 hr, metabolized in liver (inactive metabolites), excreted in urine (inactive metabolites), 90%-99% plasma protein binding, does not enter breast milk

Interactions:

• May increase action of coumarin, phenytoin, sulfonamides

• Decreased action of ibuprofen: salicylates

NURSING CONSIDERATIONS

Assess:

• Renal, liver, blood studies: BUN, creatinine, AST (SGOT), ALT (SGPT), Hgb, before treatment, periodically thereafter

• Pain: note type, duration, location and intensity with ROM

• Audiometric, ophthalmic examination before, during, after treatment; for eye, ear problems: blurred vision, tinnitus; may indicate toxicity

• Cardiac status: edema (peripheral), tachycardia, palpitations; monitor B/P, pulse for character, quality, rhythm

• For history of peptic ulcer disorder; asthma, aspirin, hypersensitivity, check closely for allergic reactions and lupus

Administer:

• With food, milk or antacid to decrease GI symptoms; however, best to take on empty stomach to facilitate absorption; if nausea and vomiting occur/persist, notify prescriber

Perform/provide:

• Storage at room temp

Evaluate:

• Therapeutic response: decreased pain, stiffness in joints; decreased swelling in joints; ability to move more easily; reduction in fever or menstrual cramping

Teach patient/family:

• To report blurred vision, ringing, roaring in ears; may indicate toxicity; eye and hearing tests should be done during long-term therapy

• To avoid driving, other hazardous activities if dizziness or drowsiness occurs

• To report change in urine pattern, increased weight, edema, increased pain in joints, fever, blood in urine; indicate nephrotoxicity

• That therapeutic inflammatory effects may take up to 1 mo

• To avoid alcohol, salicylates; bleeding may occur

• To avoid sun, sunlamp

idarubicin (℞)

(eye-dah-roob′ih-sin)

Idamycin

Func. class.: Antineoplastic, antibiotic

Chem. class.: Anthracycline glycoside

Action: Inhibits DNS synthesis by binding to DNA, avesicant derived from daunorubicin by binding to DNA, which causes strand splitting; cell cycle specific (S phase); a vesicant

Uses: Used in combination with other antineoplastics for acute myelocytic leukemia in adults

Dosage and routes:

Adult: IV 12 mg/m^2/day × 3 days in combination with cytosine arabinoside, or 25 mg/m^2 IV bolus followed by 200 mg/m^2/day × 5 days by continuous INF

Available forms: Inj 5, 10 mg vials

Side effects/adverse reactions:

HEMA: ***Thrombocytopenia, leukopenia, anemia***

GI: Nausea, vomiting, abdominal pain, mucositis, diarrhea, ***hepatotoxicity***

INTEG: Rash, extravasation, dermatitis, reversible alopecia, urticaria, thrombophlebitis at injection site

CV: ***Dysrhythmias, CHF, pericarditis, myocarditis,*** peripheral edema

CNS: Fever, chills, headache

Contraindications: Hypersensitivity, pregnancy (D), lactation

Precautions: Renal and hepatic disease, gout, bone marrow depression, children

Pharmacokinetics: Half-life 22 hr; metabolized by liver; crosses placenta; excreted in bile, urine (primarily as metabolites)

Interactions:

- Increased toxicity: other antineoplastics or radiation

Y-site compatibilities: Amikacin, cimetidine, cyclophosphamide, cytarabine, diphenhydramine, droperidol, erythromycin lactobionate, heparin, magnesium sulfate, mannitol, melphalan, metoclopromide, potassium chloride, ranitidine, vinorelbine

Solution compatibilities: $D_{3.3}$/0.3% NaCl, D_5/0.9% NaCl, D_5W, Ringer's, 0.9% NaCl

Lab test interferences:

Increase: Uric acid

NURSING CONSIDERATIONS

Assess:

- CBC, differential, platelet count weekly; withhold drug if WBC is <4000/mm^3 or platelet count is <75,000/mm^3; notify physician of these results
- Blood, urine, uric acid levels
- Renal function studies: BUN, serum uric acid, urine CrCl, electrolytes before, during therapy
- I&O ratio; report fall in urine output to <30 ml/hr
- Monitor temp q4h; fever may indicate beginning infection
- Liver function tests before, during therapy: bilirubin, AST (SGOT), ALT (SGPT), alk phosphatase prn or qmo
- ECG: watch for ST-T wave changes, low QRS and T, possible dysrhythmias (sinus tachycardia, heart block, PVCs)
- Bleeding: hematuria, guaiac stools, bruising or petechiae, mucosa or orifices q8h
- Food preferences: list likes, dislikes
- Effects of alopecia on body image; discuss feelings about body changes
- Inflammation of mucosa, breaks in skin
- Yellowing of skin, sclera, dark urine, clay-colored stools, itchy skin, abdominal pain, fever, diarrhea
- Buccal cavity q8h for dryness, sores, ulceration, white patches, oral pain, bleeding, dysphagia
- Local irritation, pain, burning at injection site
- GI symptoms: frequency of stools, cramping
- Acidosis, signs of dehydration: rapid respirations, poor skin turgor, decreased urine output, dry skin, restlessness, weakness
- Cardiac status: B/P, pulse, character, rhythm, rate

Administer:

- After preparing in biologic cabinet wearing gown, gloves, mask
- Antiemetic 30-60 min before giving drug and 6-10 hr after treatment to prevent vomiting
- After reconstituting 5 mg vial with 5 ml 0.9% NaCl (1 mg/1 ml); give over 10-15 min through Y-tube or 3-way stopcock of inf of D_5 or NS; discard unused portion
- Allopurinol or sodium bicarbonate to reduce uric acid levels, alkalinization of urine
- Transfusion for anemia
- Hydrocortisone for extravasation; apply ice compress after stopping infusion

Perform/provide:
- Strict hand-washing technique, gloves, protective clothing
- Liquid diet: carbonated beverages, gelatin may be added if patient is not nauseated or vomiting
- Increase fluid intake to 2-3 L/day to prevent urate and calculi formation
- Diet low in purines: absence of organ meats (kidney, liver), dried beans, peas to reduce uric acid level
- Rinsing of mouth tid-qid with water, club soda; brushing of teeth tid-qid with soft brush or cotton-tipped applicators for stomatitis; use unwaxed dental floss
- Storage at room temp for 3 days after reconstituting or 7 days refrigerated

Evaluate:
- Therapeutic response: decreased tumor size, spread of malignancy

Teach patient/family:
- To report any complaints, side effects to nurse or prescriber
- That hair may be lost during treatment and wig or hairpiece may make patient feel better; tell patient that new hair may be different in color, texture
- To avoid foods with citric acid, hot or rough texture
- To report any bleeding, white spots, ulcerations in mouth; tell patient to examine mouth qd
- That urine may be red-orange for 48 hr

idoxuridine-IDU (℞)

(eye-dox-yoor′i-deen)
Herplex, Stoxil
Func. class.: Antiviral
Chem. class.: Pyrimidine nucleoside

Action: Inhibits viral replication by interfering with viral DNA synthesis

Uses: Herpes simplex keratitis, CMV, varicella zoster alone or with corticosteroids

Dosage and routes:
- *Adult and child:* INSTILL 1 gtt q1h during day and 2 hr during night

Available forms: Sol 0.1%, oint 0.5%

Side effects/adverse reactions:
EENT: Poor corneal wound healing, temporary visual haze, overgrowth of nonsusceptible organisms

Contraindications: Hypersensitivity

Precautions: Antibiotic hypersensitivity, pregnancy (C)

Interactions:
- Do not use boric acid with this drug

NURSING CONSIDERATIONS

Assess:
- For infection: redness, crusts, drainage, inflammation
- Allergy: itching, lacrimation, redness, swelling

Administer:
- After washing hands; cleanse crusts or discharge from eye before application

Perform/provide:
- Storage in refrigerator in light-resistant container until used

Evaluate:
- Therapeutic response: absence of redness, inflammation, tearing, photophobia

Teach patient/family:
- To use drug exactly as prescribed
- Not to use eye makeup, towels, washcloths, eye medication of others; reinfection may occur
- That drug container tip should not be touched to eye
- To report itching, increased redness, burning, stinging, swelling; drug should be discontinued

• That drug may cause blurred vision when ointment is applied

ifosfamide (℞)

(i-foss'fa-mid)

Ifex

Func. class.: Antineoplastic alkylating agent

Chem. class.: Nitrogen mustard

Action: Alkylates DNA, RNA, inhibits enzymes that allow synthesis of amino acids in proteins; also responsible for cross-linking DNA strands; activity is not cell cycle stage specific

Uses: Testicular cancer

Dosage and routes:

• *Adult:* IV 1.2 g/m^2/day × 5 days, repeat course q3wk, given with mesna

Available forms: Inj 1, 3 g

Side effects/adverse reactions:

CNS: Facial paresthesia, fever, malaise, somnolence, confusion, depression, hallucinations, dizziness, disorientation, ***seizures, coma***

GI: Nausea, vomiting, anorexia, ***hepatotoxicity,*** stomatitis, constipation

INTEG: Dermatitis, alopecia, pain at injection site

GU: ***Hematuria, nephrotoxicity, hemorrhagic cystitis,*** dysuria, urinary frequency

HEMA: ***Thrombocytopenia, leukopenia, anemia***

Contraindications: Hypersensitivity, bone marrow suppression

Precautions: Renal disease, pregnancy (D), lactation, children

Pharmacokinetics: Metabolized by liver; saturation occurs at high doses; excreted in urine; half-life 7-15 hr

Syringe compatibility: Mesna

Y-site compatibilities: Fludarabine, melphalan, paclitaxel, ondansetron, sargramostim, vinorelbine

Additive compatibilities: Carboplatin, cisplatin, epirubicin, etoposide, fluorouracil, mesna

NURSING CONSIDERATIONS

Assess:

• Liver function studies before, during therapy (bilirubin, AST, ALT, LDH) as needed or monthly

• CBC, differential, platelet count weekly; withhold drug if WBC <4000 or platelet count <75,000; notify prescriber

• Monitor temp q4h (may indicate beginning infection)

• Blood dyscrasias (anemia, granulocytopenia); bruising, fatigue, bleeding, poor healing

• Allergic reactions: dermatitis, exfoliative dermatitis, pruritus, urticaria

• Bleeding: hematuria, guaiac, bruising or petechiae, mucosa or orifices q8h

• Food preferences; list likes, dislikes

• Effects of alopecia on body image, discuss feelings about body changes

• Yellowing of skin, sclera, dark urine, clay-colored stools, itchy skin, abdominal pain, fever, diarrhea

• Inflammation of mucosa, breaks in skin

Administer:

• IV after diluting 1 g/20 ml sterile or bacteriostatic H_2O for inj with parabens or benzyl only; shake; may be diluted further with D_5W, LR, NS, sterile H_2O for inj; 1 g/20 ml = 50 mg/ml; 1 g/50ml = 20 mg/ml; 1 g/200 ml = 5 mg/ml; give over 30 min

• Antiemetic 30-60 min before giving drug to prevent vomiting

• Antibiotics for prophylaxis of infection
• Always give with mesna to prevent ifosfamide-induced hemorrhagic cystitis

Perform/provide:
• Storage of powder at room temp
• Strict medical asepsis, protective isolation if WBC levels are low
• Increase fluid intake to 2-3 L/day to prevent urate deposits, calculi formation
• Warm compresses at injection site for inflammation

Evaluate:
• Therapeutic response: decrease in size and spread of tumor

Teach patient/family:
• To notify prescriber of sore throat, swollen lymph nodes, malaise, fever; other infections may occur
• About protective isolation
• That hair may be lost during treatment; a wig or hairpiece may make the patient feel better; new hair may be different in color, texture
• To report signs of anemia: fatigue, headache, faintness, shortness of breath, irritability
• To report bleeding; avoid use of razors, commercial mouthwash
• To avoid use of aspirin products or ibuprofen
• To use contraceptive measures during therapy

imipenem/ cilastatin (℞)

(i-me-pen'em sye-la-stat'in)
Primaxin IM, Primaxin IV
Func. class.: Antiinfective-misc. penicillin

Action: Interferes with cell wall replication of susceptible organisms; osmotically unstable cell wall swells, bursts from osmotic pressure; addition of cilastatin prevents renal inactivation that occurs with high urinary concentrations of imipenem

Uses: Serious infections caused by gram-positive: *S. pneumoniae,* group A β-hemolytic streptococci, *S. aureus,* enterococcus; gram-negative: *Klebsiella, Proteus, E. coli, Acinetobacter, Serratia, P. aeruginosa; Salmonella, Shigella*

Dosage and routes:
• *Adult:* IV 250-500 mg q6h; severe infections may require 1 g q6h; may give IM q12h (total daily IM dosage >1500 mg not recommended)

Available forms: Inj 250, 500 mg (IV); inj 500, 750 mg (IM)

Side effects/adverse reactions:
CNS: Fever, somnolence, ***seizures,*** dizziness, weakness, myoclonia
GI: Diarrhea, nausea, vomiting, ***pseudomembranous colitis, hepatitis,*** glossitis
CV: Hypotension, palpitations
HEMA: ***Eosinophilia, neutropenia,*** decreased Hgb, Hct
INTEG: Rash, urticaria, pruritus, pain at injection site, phlebitis, erythema at injection site
SYST: ***Anaphylaxis***
RESP: Chest discomfort, dyspnea, hyperventilation

Contraindications: Hypersensitivity, IM hypersensitivity to local anesthetics of the amide type

Precautions: Pregnancy (C), lactation, elderly, hypersensitivity to penicillins, seizure disorders, renal disease, children

Pharmacokinetics:
IV: Onset immediate, peak ½-1 hr, half-life 1 hr

Interactions:
• Increased imipenem plasma levels: probenecid

Y-site compatibilities: Acyclovir, famotidine, fludarabine, foscarnet, idarubicin, regular insulin, melphalan, ondansetron, vinorelbine, zidovudine

Lab test interferences:
Increase: AST (SGOT), ALT (SGPT), LDH, BUN, alk phosphatase, bilirubin, creatinine
False positive: Direct Coombs' test

NURSING CONSIDERATIONS

Assess:
- Sensitivity to penicillin, other cephalosporins
- Renal disease: lower dose may be required
- Bowel pattern qd; if severe diarrhea occurs, drug should be discontinued; may indicate pseudomembranous colitis
- Allergic reactions: rash, urticaria, pruritus; may occur few days after therapy begins
- Overgrowth of infection: perineal itching, fever, malaise, redness, pain, swelling, drainage, rash, diarrhea, change in cough, sputum

Administer:
- After reconstitution of 250 or 500 mg with 10 ml of diluent and shake; add to at least 100 ml of same inf sol
- 250-500 mg over 20-30 min; 1 g over 40-60 min; give through Y-tube or 3-way stopcock; do not give by IV bolus or if cloudy
- After C&S is taken

Evaluate:
- Therapeutic response: negative C&S

Teach patient/family:
- To report severe diarrhea; may indicate pseudomembranous colitis
- To report sore throat, bruising, bleeding, joint pain; may indicate blood dyscrasias (rare)

Treatment of overdose: Epinephrine, antihistamines; resuscitate if needed (anaphylaxis)

imipramine (℞)

(im-ip'ra-meen)

Apo-Imipramine*, imipramine HCl, Impril*, Janimine, Novo-Pramine*, SK-Pramine, Tofranil, Tofranil PM, Tripramine

Func. class.: Antidepressant—tricyclic

Chem. class.: Dibenzazepine—tertiary amine

Action: Blocks reuptake of norepinephrine, serotonin into nerve endings, increasing action of norepinephrine, serotonin in nerve cells

Uses: Depression, enuresis in children

Investigational uses: Chronic pain, migraine headaches, cluster headaches as adjunct

Dosage and routes:
- *Adult:* PO/IM 75-100 mg/day in divided doses, may increase by 25-50 mg to 200 mg, not to exceed 300 mg/day; may give daily dose hs
- *Child:* PO 25-75 mg/day

Available forms: Tabs 10, 25, 50 mg; inj 25 mg/2 ml; caps 75, 100, 125, 150 mg

Side effects/adverse reactions:

HEMA: ***Agranulocytosis, thrombocytopenia, eosinophilia, leukopenia***

CNS: Dizziness, drowsiness, confusion, headache, anxiety, tremors, stimulation, weakness, insomnia, nightmares, EPS (elderly), increased psychiatric symptoms, paresthesia

GI: Diarrhea, dry mouth, nausea, vomiting, ***paralytic ileus,*** increased appetite, cramps, epigastric distress, jaundice, ***hepatitis,*** stomatitis

GU: Retention, ***acute renal failure***

INTEG: Rash, urticaria, sweating, pruritus, photosensitivity

CV: Orthostatic hypotension, ECG changes, tachycardia, ***hypertension,*** palpitations
EENT: Blurred vision, tinnitus, mydriasis
Contraindications: Hypersensitivity to tricyclic antidepressants, recovery phase of MI, convulsive disorders, prostatic hypertrophy
Precautions: Suicidal patients, severe depression, increased intraocular pressure, narrow-angle glaucoma, urinary retention, cardiac disease, hepatic disease, hyperthyroidism, electroshock therapy, elective surgery, elderly, pregnancy (C), lactation
Pharmacokinetics:
PO: Steady state 2-5 days; metabolized by liver; excreted in urine, breast milk, feces; crosses placenta; half-life 6-20 hr
Interactions:
- Decreased effects of guanethidine, clonidine, indirect-acting sympathomimetics (ephedrine)
- Increased effects of direct-acting sympathomimetics (epinephrine), alcohol, barbiturates, benzodiazepines, CNS depressants
- Hyperpyretic crisis, convulsions, hypertensive episode: MAOI (pargyline [Eutonyl])

Lab test interferences:
Increase: Serum bilirubin, alk phosphatase, blood glucose
Decrease: 5-HIAA, VMA, urinary catecholamines

NURSING CONSIDERATIONS
Assess:
- B/P (lying, standing), pulse q4h; if systolic B/P drops 20 mm Hg, hold drug, notify prescriber; take vital signs q4h in patients with cardiovascular disease
- Blood studies: CBC, leukocytes, differential, cardiac enzymes if patient is receiving long-term therapy
- Hepatic studies: AST (SGOT), ALT (SGPT), bilirubin
- Weight qwk; appetite may increase with drug
- ECG for flattening of T wave, bundle branch block, AV block, dysrhythmias in cardiac patients
- EPS primarily in elderly: rigidity, dystonia, akathisia
- Mental status: mood, sensorium, affect, suicidal tendencies, increase in psychiatric symptoms: depression, panic
- Urinary retention, constipation; constipation is more likely to occur in children, elderly
- Withdrawal symptoms: headache, nausea, vomiting, muscle pain, weakness; not usual unless drug discontinued abruptly
- Alcohol consumption; if alcohol is consumed, hold dose until morning

Administer:
- Increased fluids, bulk in diet for constipation, urinary retention
- With food or milk for GI symptoms
- Dosage hs if oversedation occurs during day; may take entire dose hs; elderly may not tolerate once/day dosing
- Gum, hard candy, or frequent sips of water for dry mouth
- In route after running warm water over ampule to dissolve crystals

Perform/provide:
- Storage in tight container at room temp; do not freeze
- Assistance with ambulation during beginning therapy, since drowsiness/dizziness occurs
- Safety measures, including side rails, primarily in elderly
- Checking to see PO medication swallowed

Evaluate:
- Therapeutic response: decreased depression, enuresis

Teach patient/family:
• That therapeutic effects may take 2-3 wk
• Dispensed in small amounts because of suicide potential, especially in beginning of therapy
• To use caution in driving, other activities requiring alertness because of drowsiness, dizziness, blurred vision
• To avoid alcohol ingestion, other CNS depressants
• Not to discontinue medication quickly after long-term use; may cause nausea, headache, malaise
• To wear sunscreen or large hat, since photosensitivity occurs
Treatment of overdose: ECG monitoring; induce emesis; lavage, activated charcoal; administer anticonvulsant

immune globulin (℞)

gamma globulin, IG, IGIV, ISG, Gamimune N, Gammagard, Gammar-IV, Gammar, Gamastan, Iveegam, Sandoglobulin, Venoglobulin-S, immune serum globulin
Func. class.: Immune serum
Chem. class.: IgG

Action: Provides passive immunity to hepatitis A, measles, varicella, rubella, immune globulin deficiency; contains gamma globulin antibodies (IgG)
Uses: Agammaglobulinemia, hepatitis A exposure, measles exposure, measles vaccine complications, purpura, rubella exposure, chickenpox exposure
Dosage and routes:
• *Adult:* IM 30-50 ml qmo; IV 100 mg/kg qmo, 0.01-0.02 ml/ kg/min × ½ hr (Gamimune); IV 200 mg/kg qmo, 0.05-1 ml/min × 15-30 min, then increase to 1.5-2.5 ml/min (Sandoglobulin)
• *Child:* IM 20-40 ml qmo
Hepatitis A exposure
• *Adult and child:* IM 0.02-0.04 ml/kg or 0.1 mg/kg if treatment is delayed
Hepatitis B exposure
• *Adult and child:* IM 0.06 ml/kg within 1 wk, qmo
Measles (post exposure)
• *Child:* IM 0.25 ml/kg within 6 days
Immunoglobulin deficiency
• *Adult and child:* IM 1.3 ml/kg, then 0.66 ml/kg after 2-4 wk and q2-4wk thereafter
Idiopathic thrombocytopenia purpura
• *Adult and child:* IV 0.4 g/kg × 5 days or 1 g/kg/day × 1-2 days
Available forms: Inj 2, 10 ml/vial; 5% sol, 0.5, 1, 2.5, 3, 6, 10 g vials
Side effects/adverse reactions:
INTEG: Pain at injection site, rash, pruritus, chills, chest pain
MS: Arthralgia
SYST: Lymphadenopathy, ***anaphylaxis***
CNS: Headache, fatigue, malaise
GI: Abdominal pain
Contraindications: Hypersensitivity
Precautions: Pregnancy (C)
Interactions:
• Do not administer live virus vaccines within 3 mo of this drug
• Incompatible with any other drug in sol or syringe
NURSING CONSIDERATIONS
Assess:
• For exposure date: this drug should be given within 6 days of measles, 7 days of hepatitis B, 14 days of hepatitis A

• For anaphylaxis: diaphoresis, wheezing, chest tightness, hypotension

Administer:

• **Gamimune:** IV undiluted or dilute with D_5; give 0.01 ml/kg/ min; may increase to 0.02-0.04 ml/kg/ min

• **Sandoglobulin:** IV diluted with provided diluent; give 0.5-1 ml/min × 15-30 min; may increase to 1.5-2.5 ml/min

• **Venoglobulin-I:** (50 mg/ml sol) give 0.01-0.02 ml/kg/min if no adverse reaction in ½ hr, increase to 0.04 ml/kg/min, store at room temp

• **Gammagald:** reconstitute with sterile H_2O for inj (50 mg protein/ ml); give 0.5 ml/kg/hr, may increase to 4 ml/kg/hr, use infusion set provided

• **Gamma-IV:** give 0.01 ml/kg/min (50 mg/ml sol) × 15-30 min, may increase to 0.02 ml/kg/min, may increase to 0.03-0.06 ml/kg/min

• IM ≤3ml in one site, use large muscle mass

• Only with epinephrine 1:1000, resuscitative equipment available

• Only within 2 wk of exposure to hepatitis A

Perform/provide:

• Storage at 36°-46° F (2°-8° C)

Evaluate:

Prevention of infection, increased platelets

Teach patient/family:

• That passive immunity is temporary

• Treatment of anaphylaxis: epinephrine, diphenhydramine, O_2, vasopressors, corticosteroids

indapamide (℞)

(in-dap'a-mide)

Lozol, Lozide*

Func. class.: Diuretic—thiazide-like

Chem. class.: Indoline

Action: Acts on proximal section of distal renal tubule by inhibiting reabsorption of sodium; may act by direct vasodilation caused by blocking of calcium channel

Uses: Edema, hypertension, diuresis

Investigational uses: May be used alone or in combination with other antihypertensives for edema in CHF

Dosage and routes:

Edema

• *Adult:* PO 2.5 mg qd in AM; may be increased to 5 mg qd if needed

Antihypertensive

1.25-5 mg qd

Available forms: Tabs 1.25, 2.5 mg

Side effects/adverse reactions:

GU: Polyuria, dysuria, frequency, impotence

ELECT: Hypochloremic alkalosis, hypomagnesemia, hyperuricemia, hypercalcemia, hyponatremia, hypokalemia, hyperglycemia

CNS: Headache, dizziness, fatigue, weakness, paresthesias, depression

GI: Nausea, diarrhea, dry mouth, vomiting, anorexia, cramps, constipation, pancreatitis, abdominal pain, jaundice, hepatitis

EENT: Loss of hearing, tinnitus, blurred vision, nasal congestion, increased intraocular pressure

INTEG: Rash, pruritus, photosensitivity, alopecia, urticaria

MS: Cramps

CV: Orthostatic hypotension, volume depletion, palpitations, dysrhythmias

* Available in Canada only

Contraindications: Hypersensitivity, anuria
Precautions: Hypokalemia, dehydration, ascites, hepatic disease, severe renal disease, pregnancy (B), lactation
Pharmacokinetics:
PO: Onset 1-2 hr, peak 2 hr, duration up to 36 hr; excreted in urine, feces; half-life 14-18 hr
Interactions:
- Hyperglycemia, hyperuricemia, hypotension: diazoxide
- Muscle relaxants, steroids, lithium, digitalis
- Decreased K: steroids
- Decreased effects: antidiabetics
- Decreased absorption: cholestyramine, colestipol
- Decreased hypotensive effect: indomethacin, NSAIDs

Lab test interferences:
Increase: Ca, parathyroid test glucose, uric acid

NURSING CONSIDERATIONS
Assess:
- Weight daily, I&O daily to determine fluid loss; effect of drug may be decreased if used qd
- Rate, depth, rhythm of respiration, effect of exertion
- B/P lying, standing; postural hypotension may occur
- Electrolytes: K, Mg, Na, Cl: include BUN, CBC, serum creatinine, blood pH, ABGs, uric acid, Ca, glucose
- Signs of metabolic alkalosis
- Signs of hypokalemia
- Rashes, fever qd
- Confusion, especially in elderly; take safety precautions if needed
- Hydration: skin turgor, thirst, dry mucous membranes

Administer:
- In AM to avoid interference with sleep
- With food; if nausea occurs, absorption may be decreased slightly

Evaluate:
- Therapeutic response: improvement in edema of feet, legs, sacral area daily if medication is being used in CHF

Teach patient/family:
- To increase fluid intake to 2-3 L/day unless contraindicated; diet high in K; to rise slowly from lying or sitting position
- Adverse reactions: muscle cramps, weakness, nausea, dizziness
- To take with food or milk for GI symptoms
- To use sunscreen for photosensitivity
- To take early in day to prevent nocturia

Treatment of overdose: Lavage if taken orally; monitor electrolytes, administer IV fluids; monitor hydration, CV, renal status

indecainide (℞)

(in-de-kane′ide)
Decabid
Func. class.: Antidysrhythmic, (Class Ic)

Action: Unknown; able to slow conduction, reduce membrane responsiveness; inhibits automaticity, increases ratio of effective refractory period to action potential duration
Uses: Life-threatening dysrhythmias, sustained ventricular tachycardia
Dosage and routes:
- *Adult:* PO 100-200 mg/day in divided dose q12h; 50 mg q12h initially, then increase dose by 25 mg increments q4d, max 400 mg/day

Available forms: Ext rel tabs 50, 75, 100 mg
Side effects/adverse reactions:
CV: ***Dysrhythmias, CHF***
CNS: *Headache, dizziness,* lightheadedness

GI: Constipation, nausea
GU: Impotence
EENT: Blurred vision, diplopia
Contraindications: 2nd or 3rd degree AV block, right bundle branch block, cardiogenic shock, hypersensitivity
Precautions: Severe CHF, hypokalemia, hyperkalemia, sick-sinus syndrome, pregnancy (B), lactation, children, hepatic or renal disease
Pharmacokinetics:
Half-life 9-10 hr; metabolized by liver; 63% of drug recovered in urine
Interactions:
• Increased effect of indecainide: cimetidine
• Increased serum concentrations of: digoxin
Lab test interferences:
Increase: CPK
NURSING CONSIDERATIONS
Assess:
• GI status: bowel pattern, number of stools
• Cardiac rate: respiration, rate, rhythm, character continuously
• Chest x-ray film, pulmonary function test during treatment
• I&O ratio; check for decreasing output
• B/P for fluctuations
• Lung fields; bilateral rales may occur in CHF patient
• Increased respiration, increased pulse; drug should be discontinued
Evaluate:
• Therapeutic response: absence of dysrhythmias
Treatment of overdose: O_2, artificial ventilation, ECG, administer dopamine for circulatory depression, diazepam or thiopental for convulsions

indomethacin (℞)
(in-doe-meth'a-sin)
Apo-Indomethacin*, Indameth, Indocid*, Indomethacin, Indocin, Indocin IV, Indocin PDA*, Indocin SR, Novomethacin*
Func. class.: Nonsteroidal antiinflammatory (NSAID)
Chem. class.: Propionic acid derivative

Action: Inhibits prostaglandin synthesis by decreasing enzyme needed for biosynthesis; analgesic, antiinflammatory, antipyretic
Uses: Rheumatoid arthritis, ankylosing rheumatoid spondylitis, acute gouty arthritis, closure of patent ductus arteriosus in premature infants
Dosage and routes:
Arthritis/antiinflammatory
• *Adult:* PO/REC 25 mg bid-tid; may increase by 25 mg/day qwk, not to exceed 200 mg/day; SUS REL 75 mg qd, may increase to 75 mg bid
Acute arthritis
• *Adult:* PO/REC 50 mg tid; use only for acute attack, then reduce dose
Patent ductus arteriosus
• *Infant <2 days:* IV 0.2 mg/kg, then 0.1 mg/kg q12-24h
• *Infant 2-7 days:* IV 0.2 mg/kg, then 0.2 mg × 2 doses after 12, 24h
• *Infant >7 days:* IV 0.2 mg/kg, then 0.25 mg/kg × 2 doses after 12, 24 hr
Available forms: Caps 25, 50 mg; caps sus rel 75 mg; susp 25 mg/5 ml; rec supp 50 mg; inj 1 mg vial
Side effects/adverse reactions:
GI: Nausea, anorexia, vomiting, diarrhea, jaundice, ***cholestatic hepatitis,*** constipation, flatulence, cramps, dry mouth, peptic ulcer, ***ulceration, perforation***

* Available in Canada only

CNS: Dizziness, drowsiness, fatigue, tremors, confusion, insomnia, anxiety, depression
CV: Tachycardia, peripheral edema, palpitations, dysrhythmias, hypertension
INTEG: Purpura, rash, pruritus, sweating
GU: ***Nephrotoxicity: dysuria, hematuria, oliguria, azotemia***
HEMA: ***Blood dyscrasias***
EENT: Tinnitus, hearing loss, blurred vision

Contraindications: Hypersensitivity, asthma, severe renal disease, severe hepatic disease, ulcer disease

Precautions: Pregnancy, lactation, children, bleeding disorders, GI disorders, cardiac disorders, hypersensitivity to other antiinflammatory agents, pregnancy (B) 1st and 2nd trimesters, lactation, depression

Pharmacokinetics:
PO: Onset 1-2 hr, peak 3 hr, duration 4-6 hr; metabolized in liver, kidneys; excreted in urine, bile, feces; crosses placenta; excreted in breast milk; 99% plasma protein binding

Interactions:
- Increased action of coumarin, phenytoin, sulfonamides
- Toxicity: lithium, methotrexate
- Decreased action of triamterene
- Do not give with antacids

NURSING CONSIDERATIONS

Assess:
- Renal, liver, blood studies: BUN, creatinine, AST (SGOT), ALT (SGPT), Hgb, before treatment, periodically thereafter
- Audiometric, ophthalmic exam before, during, after treatment
- For eye, ear problems: blurred vision, tinnitus; may indicate toxicity
- For confusion, mood changes, hallucinations

Administer:
- IV after diluting 1 mg/ml or more NS or sterile H_2O for inj without preservative; give over 5-10 sec
- With food to decrease GI symptoms and prevent ulcerations; do not crush, chew, or break sus rel cap

Perform/provide:
- Storage at room temp

Evaluate:
- Therapeutic response: decreased pain, stiffness in joints, decreased swelling in joints, ability to move more easily

Teach patient/family:
- To report blurred vision, ringing, roaring in ears; may indicate toxicity
- To avoid driving, other hazardous activities if dizziness, drowsiness occurs
- To report change in urine pattern, increased weight, edema, increased pain in joints, fever, blood in urine; indicate nephrotoxicity; to report mood changes: anxiety, depression
- That therapeutic antiinflammatory effects may take up to 1 mo
- To avoid alcohol, salicylates; bleeding may occur

---

influenza virus vaccine, trivalent A & B (whole virus/split virus) (℞)

Fluzone, Fluogen, Fluviral*, Influenza Virus vaccine, Trivalent, FluShield, Fluvirin

Func. class.: Vaccine

Action: Produces antibodies to influenza virus; split virus vaccine causes less adverse reactions

Uses: Prevention of Russian, Chile, Philippine influenza

Dosage and routes:
- *Adult and child >12 yr:* IM 0.5 ml in 1 dose

• *Child 3-12 yr:* IM 0.5 ml, repeat in 1 mo (split) unless 1978-1985 vaccine was given
• *Child 6 mo to 3 yr:* IM 0.25 ml, repeat in 1 mo (split) unless 1978-1985 vaccine was given
Available forms: Inj IM (varies)
Side effects/adverse reactions:
CNS: Fever, Guillain-Barré syndrome
INTEG: Urticaria, induration, erythema
SYST: ***Anaphylaxis,*** malaise
MS: Myalgia
Contraindications: Hypersensitivity, active infection, chicken, egg allergy, Guillain-Barré syndrome
Precautions: Elderly, immunosuppression, pregnancy (B)
NURSING CONSIDERATIONS
Assess:
• For skin reactions: rash, induration, erythema
• For anaphylaxis: inability to breathe, bronchospasm
Administer:
• Only with epinephrine 1:1000 on unit to treat laryngospasm
• Only IM
Perform/provide:
• Written record of immunization
• At least 2 mo after measles virus vaccine; do not administer at same time as DPT
Evaluate:
• For history of allergies, skin conditions (eczema, psoriasis, dermatitis), reactions to vaccinations

insulin, isophane suspension (NPH) (℞)

NPH Iletin II, Humulin N, Iletin NPH*, Insulatard NPH, Lentard, Novolin N*, NPH Insulin, NPH Purified

Func. class.: Pancreatic hormone
Chem. class.: Exogenous unmodified insulin

Action: Decreases blood sugar; indirectly increases blood pyruvate, lactate; decreases phosphate, potassium
Uses: Ketoacidosis, type I (IDDM), type II (NIDDM) diabetes mellitus
Dosage and routes:
• *Adult:* SC dosage individualized by blood, urine glucose, usual dose 7-26 U; may increase by 2-10 U/day if needed
Available forms: 100 U/ml
Side effects/adverse reactions:
EENT: Blurred vision, dry mouth
META: ***Hypoglycemia***, rebound hyperglycemia (Somogyi effect)
INTEG: Flushing, rash, urticaria, warmth, *lipodystrophy,* lipohypertrophy, swelling, redness
SYST: ***Anaphylaxis***
Contraindications: Hypersensitivity to protamine
Precautions: Pregnancy (B)
Interactions:
• Increased hypoglycemia: salicylate, alcohol, β-blockers, anabolic steroids, fenfluramine, phenylbutazone, sulfinpyrazone, guanethidine, oral hypoglycemics, MAOIs, tetracycline
• Decreased hypoglycemia: thiazides, thyroid hormones, oral contraceptives, corticosteroids, estrogens, dobutamine, epinephrine
Pharmacokinetics:
SC: Onset 1-2 hr, peak 4-12 hr, duration 18-24 hr

* Available in Canada only

Metabolized by liver, muscle, kidneys; excreted in urine

Lab test interferences:
Increase: VMA
Decrease: K, Ca
Interference: Liver function studies, thyroid function studies

NURSING CONSIDERATIONS

Assess:

- Fasting blood glucose, 2 hr PP (80-150 mg/dl normal fasting level) (70-130 mg/dl-normal 2 hr level)
- Urine ketones during illness; insulin requirements may increase during stress, illness
- Hypoglycemic reaction that can occur during peak time

Administer:

- After warming to room temp by rotating in palms to prevent injecting cold insulin
- Increased doses if tolerance occurs
- Human insulin to those allergic to beef or pork

Perform/provide:

- Storage at room temp for <1 mo, keep away from heat and sunlight, refrigerate all other supply, do not use if discolored; do not freeze
- Rotation of injection sites within one area: abdomen, upper back, thighs, upper arm, buttocks; keep record of sites

Evaluate:

- Therapeutic response: decrease in polyuria, polydipsia, polyphagia, clear sensorium, absence of dizziness, stable gait

Teach patient/family:

- That blurred vision occurs; not to change corrective lenses until vision is stabilized 1-2 mo
- To keep insulin, equipment available at all times
- That drug does not cure diabetes but controls symptoms
- To carry Medic Alert ID as diabetic
- Hypoglycemia reaction: headache, tremors, fatigue, weakness
- Dosage, route, mixing instructions, if any diet restrictions, disease process
- To carry candy or lump sugar to treat hypoglycemia; have glucagon emergency kit available
- Symptoms of ketoacidosis: nausea, thirst, polyuria, dry mouth, decreased B/P, dry, flushed skin, acetone breath, drowsiness, Kussmaul respirations
- That a plan is necessary for diet, exercise; all food on diet should be eaten; exercise routine should not vary
- To avoid OTC drugs unless directed by prescriber

Treatment of overdose: Glucose 25g IV, via dextrose 50% sol, 50 ml or 1 mg glucagon

insulin, isophane suspension and regular insulin (℞)

Humulin 70/30, Mixtard, Novolin 70/30

Func. class.: Pancreatic hormone
Chem. class.: Exogenous unmodified insulin

Action: Decreases blood sugar, indirectly increases blood pyruvate, lactate, decreases phosphate, potassium

Uses: Ketoacidosis, type I (IDDM), type II (NIDDM) diabetes mellitus

Dosage and routes:

- *Adult:* SC individualized dose

Available forms: 70 U/ml isophane insulin with 30 U/ml regular insulin = 100 U/ml

Side effects/adverse reactions:
EENT: Blurred vision, dry mouth
META: ***Hypoglycemia,*** rebound hyperglycemia (Somogyi effect)

INTEG: Flushing, rash, urticaria, warmth, *lipodystrophy,* lipohypertrophy, swelling, redness
SYST: ***Anaphylaxis***
Contraindications: Hypersensitivity to protamine
Precautions: Pregnancy (B)
Interactions:
• Increased hypoglycemia: salicylate, alcohol, β-blockers, anabolic steroids, fenfluramine, guanethidine, sulfinpyrazone, oral hypoglycemics, MAOIs, tetracycline
• Decreased hypoglycemia: thiazides, thyroid hormones, oral contraceptives, corticosteroids, estrogens, dobutamine, epinephrine, smoking, levothyroxine
Pharmacokinetics:
SC: Onset 30 min, peak 4-8 hr, duration 12-24 hr
Metabolized by liver, muscle, kidneys; excreted in urine
Lab test interferences:
Increase: VMA
Decrease: K, Ca
Interference: Liver function studies, thyroid function studies

NURSING CONSIDERATIONS
Assess:
• Fasting blood glucose, 2 hr PP (80-150 mg/dl normal fasting level) (70-130 mg/dl normal 2 hr level)
• Urine ketones during illness; insulin requirement increases during stress, illness
• Hypoglycemic reaction that can occur during peak time
Administer:
• After warming to room temp by rotating in palms to prevent injecting cold insulin
• Increased doses if tolerance occurs
• Human insulin to those allergic to beef or pork
Perform/provide:
• Storage at room temp for <1 mo, keep cool and away from heat, refrigerate all other supply, do not use if discolored
• Rotation of injection sites within one area: abdomen, upper back, thighs, upper arm, buttocks; keep record of sites
Evaluate:
• Therapeutic response: decrease in polyuria, polydipsia, polyphagia, clear sensorium, absence of dizziness, stable gait
Teach patient/family:
• That blurred vision occurs; not to change corrective lens until vision is stabilized 1-2 mo
• To keep insulin, equipment available at all times
• That drug does not cure diabetes but controls symptoms
• To carry Medic Alert ID as diabetic
• Hypoglycemia reaction: headache, tremors, fatigue, weakness
• Dosage, route, mixing instructions, if any diet restrictions, disease process
• To carry candy or lump sugar to treat hypoglycemia
• Symptoms of ketoacidosis: nausea, thirst, polyuria, dry mouth, decreased B/P, dry, flushed skin, acetone breath, drowsiness, Kussmaul respirations
• That a plan is necessary for diet, exercise; all food on diet should be eaten; exercise routine should not vary
• About blood glucose testing; make sure patient is able to determine glucose level
• To avoid OTC drugs unless directed by prescriber
Treatment of overdose: Glucose 25 g IV, via dextrose 50% sol, 50 ml or glucagon 1 mg

---
* Available in Canada only

insulin, regular (℞)

Actrapid, Iletin II, Humulin R, Iletin I, Novolin R, Velosulin

Func. class.: Pancreatic hormone

Chem. class.: Exogenous unmodified insulin

Action: Decreases blood sugar, indirectly increases blood pyruvate, lactate, decreases phosphate, potassium

Uses: Adult-onset diabetes, juvenile diabetes, ketoacidosis type I, II, NIDDM, IDDM

Dosage and routes:

Ketoacidosis

• *Adult:* IV 5-10 U, then 5-10 U/hr until desired response, then switch to SC dose; IV/INF 2-12 U (50 U/500 ml of normal saline)

• *Child:* IV 0.1 U/kg

Replacement

• *Adult:* SC dosage individualized by blood, urine glucose levels, up to qid given ½ hr before meals

Available forms: Inj U 100/ml

Side effects/adverse reactions:

EENT: Blurred vision, dry mouth

INTEG: Flushing, rash, urticaria, warmth, *lipodystrophy,* lipohypertrophy, swelling, redness

META: ***Hypoglycemia,*** rebound hyperglycemia (Somogyi effect)

SYST: ***Anaphylaxis***

Contraindications: Hypersensitivity

Precautions: Pregnancy (B)

Interactions:

• Increased hypoglycemia: salicylate, alcohol, β-blockers, anabolic steroids, fenfluramine, guanethidine, oral hypoglycemics, MAOIs, tetracycline, sulfinpyrazone

• Decreased hypoglycemia: thiazides, thyroid hormones, oral contraceptives, corticosteroids, estrogens, dobutamine, epinephrine, dextrothyroxine, smoking

• Mask signs/symptoms of hypoglycemia: β-blocker

Syringe compatibility: Metoclopramide

Y-site compatibilities: Dobutamine, famotidine, heparin, ampicillin, ampicillin/sulbactam, aztreonam, cefazolin, cefotetan, gentamicin, imipenen/cilastatin, magnesium sulfate, oxytocin, ritodrine, terbutalin, ticarcillin, ticarcillin/clavulanate, tobramycin, vancomycin, vitamin B with C, indomethacin sodium trihydrate, meperidine, morphine, pentobarbital, potassium chloride, regular insulin, sodium bicarbonate

Additive compatibilities: Bretylium, cimetidine, lidocaine, verapamil

Pharmacokinetics:

SC: Onset 30-60 min, peak 2-3 hr, duration 5-7 hr

IV: Onset 10-30 min, peak 30-60 min, duration 1-2 hr, half-life 3-5 min; metabolized by liver, muscle, kidneys, excreted in urine

Lab test interferences:

Increase: VMA

Decrease: K, Ca

Interference: Liver function studies, thyroid function studies

NURSING CONSIDERATIONS

Assess:

• Hypoglycemic / hyperglycemic reaction that can occur soon after meals

• Fasting blood glucose, 2 hr PP (60-100 mg/dl normal fasting level); (70-130 mg/dl normal 2 hr level)

• Urine ketones during illness; insulin requirements increase during times of stress, illness

Administer:

• After warming to room temp by rotating in palms to prevent lipodystrophy from injecting cold insulin

• SC at 90-degree angle (½″ needle), 45-degree angle (⅝″ needle); apply pressure; do not massage
• ½ hr ac, so peak action coincides with peak sugar level
• Increased doses if tolerance occurs
• Human insulin to those allergic to beef or pork
• IV undiluted through Y-tube or 3-way stopcock; give 50 U or less/min; may be diluted in 0.9% NS or 0.45% saline for INF; run at rate ordered; use infusion pump; drug rate should be decreased if serum glucose level is 250 mg/100 ml; large single IV doses should not be given

Perform/provide:
• Storage at room temp for 1 mo; keep in cool area; refrigerate all other supply; do not freeze; do not use discolored or cloudy sol; discard open vials not used in 1 mo
• Rotation of injection sites: abdomen, upper back, thighs, upper arm, buttocks; keep record of sites

Evaluate:
• Therapeutic response: decrease in polyuria, polydipsia, polyphagia; clear sensorium, absence of dizziness, stable gait

Teach patient/family:
• That blurred vision occurs; not to change corrective lenses until vision is stabilized 1-2 mo
• To keep insulin, equipment available at all times; provide instructions for using automatic injector if needed
• That drug does not cure diabetes, but controls symptoms
• To carry Medic Alert ID as diabetic
• Hypoglycemic reaction: headache, tremors, fatigue, weakness, sweating
• Dosage, route; mixing instructions if any diet restrictions; disease process
• To carry candy or lump sugar to treat hypoglycemia
• Symptoms of ketoacidosis: nausea, thirst, polyuria, dry mouth, decrease in B/P, dry flushed skin, acetone breath, drowsiness, Kussmaul respirations
• That a plan is necessary for diet, exercise; all food on diet should be eaten; exercise routine should not vary
• About blood glucose testing; make sure patient is able to determine glucose level
• That pregnant patients should use glucose oxidase reagents
• To avoid OTC drugs unless directed by prescriber
• To identify lipotrophy; make chart of rotation sites

Treatment of overdose: Glucose 25 g IV, via dextrose 50% sol, 50 ml or 1 mg glucagon

insulin, regular concentrated (℞)

Regular (concentrated) Iletin II U-500

Func. class.: Pancreatic hormone

Chem. class.: Exogenous unmodified insulin

Action: Decreases blood sugar, indirectly increases blood pyruvate, lactate, decreases phosphate, potassium

Uses: Treatment of diabetic patients with marked insulin resistance (>200 U/day)

Dosage and routes:
• *Adult:* SC dosage individualized by blood, urine glucose qd-tid

Available forms: Inj 500 U/ml

Side effects/adverse reactions:
EENT: Blurred vision

META: ***Hypoglycemia,*** rebound hyperglycemia (Somogyi effect)
INTEG: Flushing, rash, urticaria, warmth, *lipodystrophy,* lipohypertrophy, swelling, redness
SYST: ***Anaphylaxis***
Contraindications: Hypersensitivity
Precautions: Pregnancy (B)
Pharmacokinetics:
SC: Onset 30-60 min, peak 2-5 hr, duration 5-7 hr
Metabolized by liver, muscle, kidneys; excreted in urine
Interactions:
• Increased hypoglycemia: salicylate, alcohol, β-blockers, anabolic steroids, fenfluramine, guanethidine, oral hypoglycemics, MAOIs, tetracycline, sulfinpyrazone
• Decreased hypoglycemia: thiazides, thyroid hormones, oral contraceptives, corticosteroids, estrogens, smoking, dextrothyroxine, dobutamine, epinephrine
Lab test interferences:
Increase: VMA
Decrease: K, Ca
Interference: Liver function studies, thyroid function studies
NURSING CONSIDERATIONS
Assess:
• Fasting blood glucose, 2 hr PP (60-100 mg/dl normal fasting level); (70-130 mg/dl normal 2 hr level)
• Urine ketones during times of illness; insulin requirements increase during stress, illness
• Hypoglycemic/hyperglycemic reaction that can occur soon after meals or suddenly while on therapy
Administer:
• After warming to room temp by rotating in palms, to prevent lipodystrophy from injecting cold insulin
• ½ hr ac, so peak action coincides with peak sugar level
• Increased doses if tolerance occurs
Perform/provide:
• Storage in refrigerator; do not freeze; do not use discolored or cloudy sol
• Rotation of injection sites: abdomen, upper back, thighs, upper arms, buttocks; keep record of sites
Evaluate:
• Therapeutic response: decrease in polyuria, polydipsia, polyphagia; clear sensorium; absence of dizziness; stable gait
Teach patient/family:
• That blurred vision occurs; not to change corrective lenses until vision is stabilized 1-2 mo
• To keep insulin, equipment available at all times
• That drug does not cure diabetes but controls symptoms
• To carry Medic Alert ID as diabetic
• Hypoglycemia reaction: headache, tremors, fatigue, weakness
• Dosage, route, mixing instructions if any diet restrictions, disease process
• To carry candy or lump sugar to treat hypoglycemia
• Symptoms of ketoacidosis: nausea, thirst, polyuria, dry mouth, decreased B/P, dry, flushed skin, acetone breath, drowsiness, Kussmaul respirations
• That a plan is necessary for diet, exercise; all food on diet should be eaten; exercise routine should not vary
• About blood glucose testing; make sure patient is able to determine glucose level
• To avoid OTC drugs unless directed by prescriber
Treatment of overdose: Glucose 25 g IV, via dextrose 50% sol, 50 ml or 1 mg glucagon

I

insulin, zinc suspension (Lente) (℞)

Humulin L, Lentard Monotard*, Lente Iletin II, Lente Insulin, Lente Iletin I, Lente Purified Pork Insulin, Novolin L

Func. class.: Pancreatic hormone

Chem. class.: Exogenous unmodified insulin

Action: Decreases blood sugar, indirectly increases blood pyruvate, lactate, decreases phosphate, potassium

Uses: Ketoacidosis, type I (IDDM), type II (NIDDM) diabetes mellitus

Dosage and routes:

- *Adult:* SC individualized

Available forms: 100 U/ml

Side effects/adverse reactions:

EENT: Blurred vision, dry mouth

META: ***Hypoglycemia,*** rebound hyperglycemia (Somogyi effect)

INTEG: Flushing, rash, urticaria, warmth, *lipodystrophy,* lipohypertrophy, swelling, redness

SYST: ***Anaphylaxis***

Contraindications: Hypersensitivity to protamine

Precautions: Pregnancy (B)

Pharmacokinetics:

SC: Onset 1-2½ hr, peak 7-15 hr, duration 12-24 hr

Metabolized by liver, muscle, kidneys; excreted in urine

Interactions:

- Increased hypoglycemia: salicylate, alcohol, β-blockers, anabolic steroids, fenfluramine, guanethidine, oral hypoglycemics, MAOIs, tetracycline, sulfinpyrazone
- Hyperglycemia: thiazides, thyroid hormones, oral contraceptives, corticosteroids, estrogens, dobutamine, epinephrine, smoking, levothyroxine

Lab test interferences:

Increase: VMA

Decrease: K, Ca

Interference: Liver function studies, thyroid function studies

NURSING CONSIDERATIONS

Assess:

- Fasting blood glucose, 2 hr PP (80-150 mg/dl normal fasting level); (70-130 mg/dl normal 2 hr level)
- Urine ketones during illness; insulin requirements increase during illness, stress
- Hypoglycemic reaction that can occur during peak time

Administer:

- After warming to room temp by rotating in palms to prevent injecting cold insulin
- Increased doses if tolerance occurs
- Human insulin to those allergic to beef or pork

Perform/provide:

- Storage at room temp for <1 mo; keep in cool area; refrigerate all other supply; do not use if discolored
- Rotation of injection sites within one area: abdomen, upper back, thighs, upper arm, buttocks; keep record of sites

Evaluate:

- Therapeutic response: decrease in polyuria, polydipsia, polyphagia; clear sensorium, absence of dizziness, stable gait

Teach patient/family:

- That blurred vision occurs; not to change corrective lenses until vision is stabilized 1-2 mo
- To keep insulin, equipment available at all times
- That drug does not cure diabetes but controls symptoms
- To carry Medic Alert ID as diabetic
- About hypoglycemia reaction: headache, tremors, fatigue, weakness

* Available in Canada only

• Dosage, route, mixing instructions; if any diet restrictions; disease process
• To carry candy or lump sugar to treat hypoglycemia
• Symptoms of ketoacidosis: nausea, thirst, polyuria, dry mouth, decreased B/P, dry, flushed skin, acetone breath, drowsiness, Kussmaul respirations
• That a plan is necessary for diet, exercise; all food on diet should be eaten; exercise routine should not vary
• About blood glucose testing, make sure patient is able to determine glucose level
• To avoid OTC drugs unless directed by prescriber

Treatment of overdose: Glucose 25 g IV, via dextrose 50% sol, 50 ml or 1 mg glucagon

insulin, zinc suspension extended (Ultralente) (℞)

Ultralente*, Untralente Iletin I, Ultralente Insulin

Func. class.: Pancreatic hormone

Chem. class.: Exogenous unmodified insulin

Action: Decreases blood sugar, indirectly increases blood pyruvate, lactate, decreases phosphate, potassium

Uses: Ketoacidosis, type I (IDDM), type II (NIDDM) diabetes mellitus

Dosage and routes:
• *Adult:* SC individualized

Available forms: 100 U/ml

Side effects/adverse reactions:
EENT: Blurred vision, dry mouth
META: ***Hypoglycemia,*** rebound hyperglycemia (Somogyi effect)
INTEG: Flushing, rash, urticaria, warmth, *lipodystrophy,* lipohypertrophy, redness, swelling
SYST: ***Anaphylaxis***

Contraindications: Hypersensitivity to protamine

Precautions: Pregnancy (C)

Pharmacokinetics:
SC: Onset 4-8 hr, peak 10-30 hr, duration 7-36 hr
Metabolized by liver, muscle, kidneys, excreted in urine

Interactions:
• Increased hypoglycemia: salicylate, alcohol, β-blockers, anabolic steroids, fenfluramine, guanethidine, oral hypoglycemics, MAOIs, tetracycline, sulfinpyrazone
• Decreased hypoglycemia: thiazides, thyroid hormones, oral contraceptives, corticosteroids, estrogens, dobutamine, epinephrine, smoking, levothyroxine

Lab test interferences:
Increase: VMA
Decrease: K, Ca
Interference: Liver function studies, thyroid function studies

NURSING CONSIDERATIONS

Assess:
• Fasting blood glucose, 2 hr PP (80-150 mg/dl normal fasting level); (70-130 mg/dl normal 2 hr level)
• Urine ketones during illness; insulin requirements increase during stress, illness
• Hypoglycemic reaction that can occur during peak time

Administer:
• After warming to room temp by rotating in palms to prevent injecting cold insulin
• Increased doses if tolerance occurs

Perform/provide:
• Storage at room temp for <1 mo; refrigerate all other supply; do not use if discolored

• Rotation of injection sites within one area: abdomen, upper back, thighs, upper arm, buttocks; keep record of sites

Evaluate:

• Therapeutic response: decrease in polyuria, polydipsia, polyphagia; clear sensorium, absence of dizziness, stable gait

Teach patient/family:

• That blurred vision occurs; not to change corrective lenses until vision is stabilized 1-2 mo

• To keep insulin, equipment available at all times

• That drug does not cure diabetes but controls symptoms

• To carry Medic Alert ID as diabetic

• Hypoglycemia reaction: headache, tremors, fatigue, weakness

• Dosage, route, mixing instructions; if any diet restrictions; disease process

• To carry candy or lump sugar to treat hypoglycemia

• Symptoms of ketoacidosis: nausea, thirst, polyuria, dry mouth, decreased B/P, dry, flushed skin, acetone breath, drowsiness, Kussmaul respirations

• That a plan is necessary for diet, exercise; all food on diet should be eaten; exercise routine should not vary

• About blood glucose testing; make sure patient is able to determine glucose level

• That pregnant patients should use glucose oxidase reagents

• To avoid OTC drugs unless directed by prescriber

Treatment of overdose: Glucose 25 g IV, via dextrose 50% sol, 50 ml or 1 mg glucagon

insulin, zinc suspension, prompt (semilente) (℞)

Semilente Iletin I, Semilente Insulin

Func. class.: Pancreatic hormone

Chem. class.: Exogenous unmodified insulin

Action: Decreases blood sugar; indirectly increases blood pyruvate, lactate, decreases phosphate, potassium

Uses: Ketoacidosis, type I (IDDM), type II (NIDDM) diabetes mellitus

Dosage and routes:

• *Adult:* SC dosage individualized by blood, urine glucose qd-tid

Available forms: 100 U/ml

Side effects/adverse reactions:

EENT: Blurred vision, dry mouth

META: ***Hypoglycemia,*** rebound hyperglycemia (Somogyi effect)

INTEG: Flushing, rash, urticaria, warmth, *lipodystrophy,* lipohypertrophy, swelling, redness

SYST: ***Anaphylaxis***

Contraindications: Hypersensitivity to protamine

Precautions: Pregnancy (B)

Pharmacokinetics:

SC: Onset 1-1½ hr, peak 5-10 hr, duration 12-16 hr

Metabolized by liver, muscle, kidneys; excreted in urine

Interactions:

• Increased hypoglycemia: salicylate, alcohol, β-blockers, anabolic steroids, fenfluramine, guanethidine, oral hypoglycemics, MAOIs, tetracycline, sulfinpyrazone

• Hyperglycemia: thiazides, thyroid hormones, oral contraceptives, corticosteroids, estrogens, dobutamine, epinephrine, smoking, levothyroxine

* Available in Canada only

Lab test interferences:
Increase: VMA
Decrease: K, Ca
Interference: Liver function studies, thyroid function studies

NURSING CONSIDERATIONS

Assess:

- Fasting blood glucose, 2 hr PP (80-150 mg/dl normal fasting level); (70-130 mg/dl normal 2 hr level)
- Urine ketones during illness; insulin requirements increase during stress, illness
- Hypoglycemic reaction that can occur during peak time

Administer:

- After warming to room temp by rotating in palms, to prevent injecting cold insulin
- Increased doses if tolerance occurs

Perform/provide:

- Storage at room temp for <1 mo in cool area; refrigerate all other supply; do not use if discolored
- Rotation of injection sites within one area: abdomen, upper back, thighs, upper arm, buttocks; keep record of sites

Evaluate:

- Therapeutic response: decrease in polyuria, polydipsia, polyphagia; clear sensorium, absence of dizziness, stable gait

Teach patient/family:

- That blurred vision occurs; not to change corrective lenses until vision is stabilized 1-2 mo
- To keep insulin, equipment available at all times
- That drug does not cure diabetes but controls symptoms
- To carry Medic Alert ID as diabetic
- Hypoglycemic reaction: headache, tremors, fatigue, weakness
- Dosage, route, mixing instructions; if any diet restrictions; disease process
- To carry candy or lump sugar to treat hypoglycemia
- Symptoms of ketoacidosis: nausea, thirst, polyuria, dry mouth, decreased B/P, dry, flushed skin, acetone breath, drowsiness, Kussmaul respirations
- That a plan is necessary for diet, exercise; all food on diet should be eaten; exercise routine should not vary
- Blood glucose testing; make sure patient is able to determine glucose level
- That pregnant patients should use glucose oxidase reagents
- To avoid OTC drugs unless directed by prescriber

Treatment of overdose: Glucose 25 g IV, via dextrose 50% sol, 50 ml or 1 mg glucagon

---

interferon alfa-2a/interferon alfa-2b (℞)

(in-ter-fer'on)
Roferon-a/Intron-a, a-2-interferon

Func. class.: Miscellaneous antineoplastic
Chem. class.: Protein product

Action: Antiviral action inhibits viral replication by reprogramming virus; antitumor action suppresses cell proliferation; immunomodulating action phagocytizes target cells

Uses: Hairy cell leukemia in persons >18 yr, condylomata acuminata, metastatic melanoma, AIDS

Dosage and routes:

- *Adult:* SC/IM (interferon alfa-2a) 3 million IU × 16-24 wk, then 3 million IU 3 × wk maintenance

Hairy cell leukemia

2 million IU/m^2 3 × wk; if severe adverse reactions occur, dose should be skipped or reduced by ½

Condylomata acuminata
Interferon 2b 1 million IU/lesion 3 × /wk × 3 wk
Kaposi's sarcoma
30 million IU/m^2 3 × /wk
Available forms: alfa-2a inj 3, 6, 36 million IU/ml; alfa-2b inj 3, 5, 10, 18, 25, 50 million U/vial
Side effects/adverse reactions:
CNS: Dizziness, confusion, numbness, paresthesias, hallucinations, ***convulsions, coma,*** amnesia, anxiety, mood changes
CV: Edema, hypotension, hypertension, chest pain, palpitations, dysrhythmias, ***CHF, MI, CVA***
INTEG: Rash, dry skin, itching, alopecia, flushing
GI: Weight loss, taste changes
GU: Impotence
MISC: Flulike syndrome; fever, fatigue, myalgias, headache, chills
Contraindications: Hypersensitivity
Precautions: Severe hypotension, dysrhythmia, tachycardia, pregnancy (C), lactation, children, severe renal or hepatic disease, convulsion disorder
Pharmacokinetics:
Half-life (interferon alfa-2a) 3.7-8.5 hr, peak 3-4 hr; half-life (interferon alfa-2b) 2-7 hr, peak 6-8 hr
Lab test interferences:
Interference: AST (SGOT), ALT (SGPT), LDH, alk phosphatase, WBC, platelets, granulocytes, creatinine

NURSING CONSIDERATIONS
Assess:
- For symptoms of infection; may be masked by drug fever
- CNS reaction: LOC, mental status, dizziness, confusion

Administer:
- IM/SC after reconstituting 3-5 million IU/1 ml, 10 million IU/2 ml, 25 million IU/5 ml, of diluent provided, mix gently
- Intralesional after reconstituting 10 million IU/1 ml bacteriostatic water for inj; no more than 5 lesions can safely be treated at a time
- At hs to minimize side effects
- Acetaminophen as ordered to alleviate fever and headache

Perform/provide:
- Storage of reconstituted sol for 1 mo in refrigerator
- Increased fluid intake to 2-3 L/day

Evaluate:
- Therapeutic response: decrease in size, number of lesions

Teach patient/family:
- To avoid hazardous tasks, since confusion, dizziness may occur
- That brands of this drug should not be changed; each form is different, with different doses
- That fatigue is common; activity may have to be altered
- Not to become pregnant while taking drug; possible mutagenic effects
- To report signs of infection: sore throat, fever, diarrhea, vomiting
- That impotence may occur during treatment but is temporary
- Emotional lability is common; notify prescriber if severe or incapacitating

interferon alfa-n 3 (℞)
(in-ter-feer′on)
Alferon N
Func. class.: Antineoplastic
Chem. class.: Human interferon α-protein

Action: Binds interferon to membrane receptors on cell surface with high specificity; this produces protein synthesis, inhibition of virus replication, suppression of cell proliferide, increased phagocytosis

Uses: Condylomata acuminata (veneral/genital warts)
Dosages and routes:
• *Adult:* 0.05 ml (250,000 IU) per wart, given 2 × /wk × 8 wk; not to exceed 0.5 ml (2.5 million IU); inject into base of wart
Available forms: Inj 5 m IU/1 ml vial with 3.3 mg/ml phenol and 1 mg/ml human albumin
Side effects/adverse reactions:
CNS: Fever, headache, sweating, vasovagal reaction, chills, fatigue, dizziness, insomnia, sleepiness, depression
GI: Nausea, vomiting, heartburn, diarrhea, constipation, anorexia, stomatitis, dry mouth
MS: Myalgias, arthralgia, back pain
INTEG: Pain at injection site, pruritis
CV: Chest pain, hypotension
Contraindications: Hypersensitivity to this product, egg protein, IgG, neomycin
Precautions: Pregnancy (C), lactation, children, CHF, angina (unstable), COPD, diabetes mellitus with ketoacidosis, hemophilia, pulmonary embolism, thrombophlebitis, bone marrow depression, convulsive disorder
Pharmacokinetics: Unable to detect
Lab test interferences:
Interferences: AST (SGOT), ALT (SGPT), LDH, alk phosphatase, WBC, platelets, granulocytes, creatinine
NURSING CONSIDERATIONS
Assess:
• For symptoms of infection; may be masked by drug fever
• CNS reaction: LOC, mental status, dizziness, confusion
• For body image disturbance
Administer:
• Acetaminophen to alleviate fever and headache
Perform/provide:
• Storage of reconstituted sol for 1 mo in refrigerator
• Increased fluid intake to 2-3 L/day
Evaluate:
• Therapeutic response: decrease in wart size
Teach patient/family:
• To avoid hazardous tasks, since confusion, dizziness may occur
• That brands of this drug should not be changed; each form is different, with different doses
• That fatigue is common; activity may have to be altered
• Not to become pregnant while taking drug; possible mutagenic effects
• To report signs of infection: sore throat, fever, diarrhea, vomiting
• Signs of hypersensitivity: liver, urticaria, wheezing, dyspnea; notify prescriber immediately

---

interferon β-1b (℞)
(in-ter-feer′on)
Betaseron
Func. class.: Multiple sclerosis agent
Chem. class.: E. coli derivative

Action: Antiviral, immunoregulatory; action not clearly understood; biologic response modifying properties mediated through specific receptors on cells, inducing expression of interferon-induced gene products
Uses: Ambulatory patients with relapsing or remitting multiple sclerosis
Investigational uses: May be useful in treatment of AIDS, AIDS-related Kaposi's sarcoma, malignant melanoma, metastatic renal cell carcinoma, cutaneous T cell lym-

phoma, acute non-A, non-B hepatitis

Dosage and routes:

Relapsing/remitting multiple sclerosis

• *Adult:* SC 0.25 mg (8 IU) qod

Available forms: Powder for inj lyophilized 0.3 mg (9.6 mIU)

Side effects/adverse reactions:

CNS: Headache, fever, pain, chills, mental changes, hypertonia, ***suicide attempts***

CV: Migraine, palpitations, hypertension, tachycardia, peripheral vascular disorders

EENT: Conjunctivitis, blurred vision

GI: Diarrhea, constipation, vomiting, abdominal pain

GU: Dysmenorrhea, irregular menses, metrorrhagia, cystitis, breast pain

HEMA: ***Decreased lymphocytes, ANC, WBC;*** *lymphadenopathy*

INTEG: Sweating, inj site reaction

MS: Myalgia, ***myasthenia***

RESP: Sinusitis, dyspnea

Contraindications: Hypersensitivity to natural or recombinant interferon-β or human albumin

Precautions: Pregnancy (C), lactation, child <18 yr, chronic progressive MS, depression, mental disorders

NURSING CONSIDERATIONS

Assess:

• Blood, renal, hepatic studies: CBC, differential, platelet counts, BUN, creatinine ALT, urinalysis

• CNS symptoms: headache, fatigue, depression

• GI status: diarrhea or constipation, vomiting, abdominal pain

• Cardiac status: Increased B/P, tachycardia

Administer:

• Acetaminophen for fever, headache

• SC only; do not give IM or IV

Perform/provide:

• Storage in refrigerator; do not freeze

Evaluate:

• Therapeutic response: decreased symptoms of multiple sclerosis

Teach patient/family:

• To provide patient or family member with written, detailed information about the drug

• That blurred vision, sweating may occur

• Women patients that irregular menses, dysmenorrhea, or metrorrhagia as well as breast pain may occur

---

interferon gamma-1b (℞)

(in-ter-fer′on)

Actimmune

Func. class.: Biologic response modifier

Chem. class.: Lymphokine, interleukin type

Action: Species-specific protein synthesized in response to viruses, potent phagocyte-activating effects; can mediate killing of *S. aureus, T. gondii, L. donovani, L. monocytogenes, M. avium-intracellulare;* enhances oxidative metabolism of macrophages, enhances antibody-dependent cellular cytotoxicity

Uses: Serious infections associated with chronic granulomatous disease

Dosage and routes:

• *Adult:* SC 50 $\mu g/m^2$ (1.5 million U/m^2) for patients with surface area >0.5 m^2; 1.5 µg/kg/dose for patient with surface area <0.5 m^2; give Monday, Wednesday, Friday for 3 × /wk dosing

Available forms: Inj 100 µg (3 million U)/single-dose vial

Side effects/adverse reactions:
GI: Nausea, anorexia, abdominal pain, weight loss, diarrhea, vomiting
CNS: Headache, fatigue, depression, fever, chills
INTEG: Rash, pain at injection site
MS: Myalgia, arthralgia
Contraindications: Hypersensitivity to interferon gamma, *E. coli*-derived products
Precautions: Pregnancy (C), cardiac disease, seizure disorders, CNS disorders, myelosuppression, lactation, children
Pharmacokinetics:
SC: Dose absorbed 89%, elimination half-life 5.9 hr, peak 7 hr
Interactions:
• Increased myelosuppression: other myelosuppressive agents
NURSING CONSIDERATIONS
Assess:
• Blood, renal, hepatic studies: CBC, differential, platelet counts, BUN, creatinine, ALT (SGPT), urinalysis
• CNS symptoms: headache, fatigue, depression
Administer:
• At hs to minimize adverse reactions; administer acetaminophen for fever, headache
• 50% of dose if severe reactions occur or discontinue treatment until reactions subside
• Using sterilized glass or plastic disposable syringes
• In right and left deltoid and anterior thigh
• Warm to room temp before use; do not leave at room temp over 12 hr (unopened vial)
Perform/provide:
• Storage in refrigerator upon receipt; do not freeze; do not shake
Evaluate:
• Therapeutic response: decreased serious infections, improvement in existing infections and inflammatory conditions
Teach patient/family:
• Method of administration if family members will be giving medication
• Provide patient or family member with written, detailed information about drug

iodoquinol (℞)
(eye-oh-do-kwin′ole)
Diodoquin*, Yodoxin
Func. class.: Amebicide
Chem. class.: Dihalogenated derivative of 8-hydroxyquinoline

Action: Direct-acting amebicide; action occurs in intestinal lumen
Uses: Intestinal amebiasis
Dosage and routes:
• *Adult:* PO 630-650 mg tid × 20 days, not to exceed 2 g/day
• *Child:* PO 30-40 mg/kg/day in 2-3 divided doses × 20 days, not to exceed 1.95 g/24 hr × 20 days; do not repeat treatment before 2-3 wk
Available forms: Tabs 210, 650 mg; powder
Side effects/adverse reactions:
HEMA: ***Agranulocytosis*** (rare)
INTEG: Rash; pruritus; discolored skin, hair, nails; alopecia
CNS: Malaise, headache, agitation, peripheral neuropathy
MISC: Fever, chills, vertigo, thyroid enlargement
EENT: Blurred vision, sore throat, retinal edema, subacute myelo-optic neuropathy
GI: Anorexia, nausea, vomiting, diarrhea, epigastric distress, gastritis, constipation, abdominal cramps, rectal irritation, anal itch
Contraindications: Hypersensitivity to this drug or iodine, renal disease, hepatic disease, severe thyroid

disease, preexisting optic neuropathy
Precautions: Pregnancy (C), lactation
Lab test interferences:
Interfere: Thyroid function test
False positive: PKU
Increase: PBI
Decrease: ^{131}I uptake test
NURSING CONSIDERATIONS
Assess:
- Stools during entire treatment; should be clear at end of therapy; stools should be free of parasites for 1 yr before patient is considered cured
- I&O, stools for number, frequency, character
- Iodism: skin eruption, urticaria, discoloring of hair, nails
- Allergic reaction: fever, rash, itching, chills; drug should be discontinued
- Blurred vision; patient should have periodic eye exams during treatment
- Superinfection, fever, monilial growth, fatigue, malaise
- Diarrhea for 2-3 days

Administer:
- PO after meals to avoid GI symptoms

Perform/provide:
- Storage in tight container

Evaluate:
- Therapeutic response: decreased diarrhea, symptoms in amebiasis

Teach patient/family:
- Proper hygiene after BM: handwashing technique
- To avoid contact of drug with eyes, mouth, nose, other mucous membranes
- About need for compliance with dosage schedule, duration of treatment

ipecac (℞, OTC)
(ip′e-kak)
Func. class.: Emetic
Chem. class.: Cephaelis ipecacuanha derivative

Action: Acts on chemoreceptor trigger zone to induce vomiting; irritates gastric mucosa
Uses: In poisoning to induce vomiting
Dosage and routes:
- *Adult:* PO 15-30 ml, then 200-300 ml water
- *Child >1 yr:* PO 15 ml, then 200-300 ml water
- *Child <1 yr:* PO 5-10 ml, then 100-200 ml water; may repeat dose if needed

Available forms: Liq
Side effects/adverse reactions:
CNS: ***Depression, convulsions, coma***
GI: Nausea, vomiting, bloody diarrhea
CV: ***Circulatory failure, atrial fibrillation, fatal myocarditis, dysrhythmias***
Contraindications: Hypersensitivity, unconscious/semiconscious, depressed gag reflex, poisoning with petroleum products or caustic substances, convulsions
Precautions: Lactation, pregnancy (C)
Pharmacokinetics:
PO: Onset 15-30 min
Interactions:
- Do not administer with activated charcoal; effect will be decreased

NURSING CONSIDERATIONS
Assess:
- VS, B/P; check patients with cardiac disease more often
- Type of poisoning; do not administer if petroleum products or caus-

tic substances have been ingested: kerosene, gasoline, lye, Drano
• Respiratory status before, during, after administration; check rate, rhythm, character; respiratory depression can occur rapidly with elderly or debilitated patients

Administer:
• **Ipecac *syrup*, not ipecac,** which is 14 times stronger; death may occur
• Activated charcoal after vomiting completed; may begin lavage after 10-15 min after 2 doses of ipecac syrup with no result

Evaluate:
• Therapeutic response: vomiting

ipratropium (℞)

(i-pra-troe'pee-um)
Atrovent
Func. class.: Anticholinergic, bronchodilator
Chem. class.: Synthetic quaternary ammonium compound

Action: Inhibits interaction of acetylcholine at receptor sites on the bronchial smooth muscle, resulting in decreased cGMP and bronchodilation
Uses: Bronchodilation during bronchospasm in those with COPD
Dosage and routes:
• *Adult:* 2 INH 4 × day, not to exceed 12 INH/24 hr
Available forms: Aerosol 18 μg/actuation
Side effects/adverse reactions:
GI: Nausea, vomiting, cramps
EENT: Dry mouth, blurred vision
CNS: Anxiety, dizziness, headache, nervousness
RESP: Cough, worsening of symptoms, ***bronchospasms***
INTEG: Rash
CV: Palpitation
Contraindications: Hypersensitivity to this drug, atropine, soya lecithin
Precautions: Pregnancy (B), lactation, children <12 yr, narrow-angle glaucoma, prostatic hypertrophy, bladder neck obstruction
Pharmacokinetics:
Half-life 2 hr; does not cross blood-brain barrier

NURSING CONSIDERATIONS

Assess:
• For palpitations; if severe, drug may have to be changed
• For tolerance over long-term therapy; dose may have to be increased or changed

Perform/provide:
• Storage at room temp
• Hard candy, frequent drinks, sugarless gum to relieve dry mouth

Evaluate:
• Therapeutic response: ability to breathe adequately

Teach patient/family:
• That compliance is necessary with number of inhalations/24 hr, or overdose may occur
• To shake before using
• Correct method of inhalation and cleaning of equipment daily

iron dextran* (℞)

Imferon, In Fed
Func. class.: Hematinic
Chem. class.: Ferric hydroxide complex with dextran

Action: Iron is carried by transferrin to the bone marrow, where it is incorporated into hemoglobin
Uses: Iron deficiency anemia
Dosage and routes:
• *Adult and child:* IM 0.5 ml as a test dose by Z-track, then no more than the following per day
• *Adult <50 kg:* IM 100 mg

• *Adult >50 kg:* IM 250 mg
• *Infant <5 kg:* IM 25 mg
• *Child <9 kg:* IM 50 mg
• *Adult:* IV 0.5 ml test dose, then 100 mg qd after 2-3 days; IV 250/1000 ml of NaCl; give 25 mg test dose, wait 5 min, then infuse over 6-12 hr or follow equation

$$\frac{0.3 \times \text{wt (lb)} \times 100\text{-Hgb (g/dl)} \times 100}{14.8} = \text{mg iron}$$

<30 lb (66 kg) should be given 80% of above formula dose

Available forms: Inj IM/IV 50 mg/ml, inj IM only 50 mg/ml

Side effects/adverse reactions:

CNS: Headache, paresthesia, dizziness, shivering, weakness, ***seizures***

GI: Nausea, vomiting, metallic taste, abdominal pain

INTEG: Rash, pruritus, urticaria, fever, sweating, chills, brown skin discoloration, pain at injection site, necrosis, sterile abscesses, phlebitis

CV: Chest pain, ***shock,*** hypotension, tachycardia

RESP: Dyspnea

HEMA: ***Leukocytosis***

OTHER: ***Anaphylaxis***

Contraindications: Hypersensitivity, all anemias excluding iron deficiency anemia, hepatic disease

Precautions: Acute renal disease, children, asthma, lactation, rheumatoid arthritis (IV), infants <4 mo, pregnancy (C)

Pharmacokinetics:

IM: Excreted in feces, urine, bile, breast milk; crosses placenta; most absorbed through lymphatics; can be gradually absorbed over weeks/months from fixed locations

Interactions:

• Not to mix with other drugs in syringe or sol
• Decreased reticulocyte response: chloramphenicol
• Increased toxicity: oral iron—do not use

Lab test interferences:

False increase: Serum bilirubin
False decrease: Serum Ca
False positive: ^{99m}Tc diphosphate bone scan, iron test (large doses > 2 ml)

NURSING CONSIDERATIONS

Assess:

• Blood studies: Hct, Hgb, reticulocytes, bilirubin before treatment, at least monthly
• Allergy: ***anaphylaxis***, rash, pruritus, fever, chills, wheezing; notify prescriber immediately
• Cardiac status: anginal pain, hypotension, tachycardia
• Nutrition: amount of iron in diet (meat, dark green leafy vegetables, dried beans, dried fruits, eggs)
• Cause of iron loss or anemia, including use of salicylates, sulfonamides

Administer:

• D/C oral iron before parenteral; give only after test dose of 25 mg by preferred route; wait at least 1 hr before giving remaining portion
• IM deeply in large muscle mass; use Z-track method and a 19-20G 2-3″ needle; ensure needle is long enough to place drug deep in muscle, change needles after withdrawing and before injecting to prevent skin, tissue staining
• IV after flushing with 10 ml 0.9% NaCl; give undiluted; may be diluted in 50-250 NS for infusion; give 1 ml (50 mg) or less over 1 min or more; flush line after use with 10 ml 0.9% NaCl; patient should remain recumbent for ½-1 hr
• IV injection requires single-dose vial without preservative; verify on label IV use is approved

* Available in Canada only

• Only with epinephrine available in case of anaphylactic reaction during dose

Perform/provide:

• Storage at room temp in cool environment

• Recumbent position 30 min after IV injection to prevent orthostatic hypotension

Evaluate:

• Therapeutic response: increased serum iron levels, Hct, Hgb

Teach patient/family:

• That iron poisoning may occur if increased beyond recommended level; not to take oral iron preparation

• That delayed reaction may occur 1-2 days after administration and last 3-4 days (IV) 3-7 days (IM); report fever, chills, malaise, muscle, joint aches, nausea, vomiting, backache

Treatment of overdose:
Discontinue drug, treat allergic reaction, give diphenhydramine or epinephrine as needed, give iron-chelating drug in acute poisoning

isocarboxazid (℞)

(eye-soe-kar-box'a-zid)

Marplan

Func. class.: Antidepressant—MAOI

Chem. class.: Hydrazine

Action: Increases concentrations of endogenous epinephrine, norepinephrine, serotonin, dopamine in storage sites in CNS by inhibition of MAO; increased concentration reduces depression

Uses: Depression when uncontrolled by other means

Dosage and routes:

• *Adult:* PO 30 mg/day in divided doses; reduce dose to lowest effective dose when condition improves

Available forms: Tabs 10 mg

Side effects/adverse reactions:

HEMA: Anemia

CNS: Dizziness, drowsiness, confusion, headache, anxiety, tremors, stimulation, weakness, hyperreflexia, mania, insomnia, fatigue, weight gain

GI: Constipation, dry mouth, nausea, vomiting, *anorexia,* diarrhea, weight gain

GU: Change in libido, frequency

INTEG: Rash, flushing, increased perspiration, jaundice

CV: Orthostatic hypotension, hypertension, dysrhythmias, hypertensive crisis

EENT: Blurred vision

ENDO: ***SIADH-like syndrome***

Contraindications: Hypersensitivity to MAOIs, elderly, hypertension, CHF, severe hepatic disease, pheochromocytoma, severe renal disease, severe cardiac disease

Precautions: Suicidal patients, convulsive disorders, severe depression, schizophrenia, hyperactivity, diabetes mellitus, pregnancy (C)

Pharmacokinetics:

PO: Duration up to 2 wk; metabolized by liver; excreted by kidneys

Interactions:

• Increased pressor effects: guanethidine, clonidine, indirect-acting sympathomimetics (ephedrine)

• Increased effects of direct-acting sympathomimetics (epinephrine), alcohol, barbiturates, benzodiazepines, CNS depressants, levodopa

• Hyperpyretic crisis, convulsions, hypertensive episode: tricyclic antidepressants, meperidine

• Hypoglycemic effect: increased insulin

NURSING CONSIDERATIONS

Assess:

• B/P (lying, standing), pulse; if systolic B/P drops 20 mm Hg, hold drug, notify prescriber

• Blood studies: CBC, leukocytes, cardiac enzymes if patient is receiving long-term therapy
• Hepatic studies: ALT (SGPT), AST (SGOT), bilirubin, creatinine; hepatotoxicity may occur
• Toxicity: increased headache, palpitation; discontinue drug immediately; prodromal signs of hypertensive crisis
• Mental status: mood, sensorium, affect, memory (long, short), increase in psychiatric symptoms
• Urinary retention, constipation, edema; take weight qwk
• Withdrawal symptoms: headache, nausea, vomiting, muscle pain, weakness

Administer:
• Increased fluids, bulk in diet for constipation, urinary retention
• With food or milk for GI symptoms
• Crushed if patient is unable to swallow medication whole
• Dosage hs if oversedation occurs during day
• Gum, hard candy, or frequent sips of water for dry mouth
• Phentolamine for severe hypertension

Perform/provide:
• Storage in tight container in cool environment, away from children
• Assistance with ambulation during beginning therapy, since drowsiness/dizziness occurs
• Safety measures, including side rails
• Checking to see PO medication swallowed

Evaluate:
• Therapeutic response: decreased depression

Teach patient/family:
• That therapeutic effects may take 1-4 wk
• To avoid driving, other activities requiring alertness; hypotension may be increased in the elderly
• To avoid alcohol ingestion, CNS depressants, OTC medications (cold, weight-control, hay fever, cough syrup)
• Not to discontinue medication quickly after long-term use
• To avoid high-tyramine foods: cheese (aged), sour cream, beer, wine, pickled products, liver, raisins, bananas, figs, avocados, meat tenderizers, chocolate, yogurt; not to increase caffeine
• Report headache, palpitation, neck stiffness

Treatment of overdose: Lavage, activated charcoal; monitor electrolytes, vital signs; diazepam IV, $NaHCO_3$

isoetharine (℞)

(eye-soe-eth'a-reen)
Arm-a-Med, isoetharine HCl, Beta-2, Bronkometer, Bronkosol
Func. class.: Adrenergic β_2-agonist

Action: Causes bronchodilation by β_2 stimulation, resulting in increased levels of cAMP, causing relaxation of bronchial smooth muscle with very little effect on heart rate

Uses: Bronchospasm, asthma

Dosage and routes:
• *Adult:* INH 3-7 puffs undiluted, IPPB 0.5 ml diluted 1:3 with NS

Available forms: Sol for nebulization 0.06%, 0.08%, 0.1%, 0.125%, 0.17%, 0.2%, 0.25%, 0.5%, 1.0%

Side effects/adverse reactions:
CNS: Tremors, anxiety, insomnia, headache, dizziness, stimulation
CV: Palpitations, tachycardia, hypertension, ***cardiac arrest,*** dysrhythmias

* Available in Canada only

GI: Nausea
META: Hyperglycemia
Contraindications: Hypersensitivity to sympathomimetics, narrow-angle glaucoma
Precautions: Pregnancy (C), cardiac disorders, hyperthyroidism, diabetes mellitus, prostatic hypertrophy
Pharmacokinetics:
INH: Onset immediate, peak 5-15 min, duration 1-4 hr, metabolized in liver, GI tract, lungs, excreted in urine
Interactions:
• Increased effects of both drugs: other sympathomimetics
• Decreased action when used with other β-blockers
• Hypertensive crisis: MAOIs
NURSING CONSIDERATIONS
Assess:
• Respiratory function: vital capacity, forced expiratory volume, ABGs, pulse, B/P
• Paresthesias and coldness of extremities; peripheral blood flow may decrease
Administer:
• 2 hr before hs to avoid sleeplessness
Perform/provide:
• Storage at room temp; do not use sol if brown or contains a precipitate
Evaluate:
• Therapeutic response: ease of breathing
Teach patient/family:
• Not to use OTC medications; extra stimulation may occur
• Use of inhaler; review package insert with patient
• To avoid getting aerosol in eyes
• To wash inhaler in warm water and dry qd
• About all aspects of drug; avoid smoking, smoke-filled rooms, persons with respiratory infections

isoflurophate (℞)

(eye-soe-flure'oh-fate)
Floropryl
Func. class.: Miotic
Chem. class.: Cholinesterase inhibitor, irreversible

Action: Prevents breakdown of neurotransmitter acetylcholine, which accumulates, causing enhancement, prolongation of physiologic effects
Uses: Open-angle glaucoma, accommodative esotropia, conditions obstructing aqueous outflow
Dosage and routes:
• *Adult and child:* INSTILL ¼ in strip of 0.025% oint in conjunctival sac q8-72 hr for glaucoma or qhs × 2 wk for esotropia
Available forms: Only as ophthalmic ointment 0.025%
Side effects/adverse reactions:
CNS: Headache
CV: Hypotension, bradycardia, paradoxic tachycardia
RESP: ***Bronchospasm,*** dyspnea, bronchoconstriction, wheezing
EENT: Blurred vision, lacrimation, conjunctival congestion, lid muscle twitching, stinging, burning
GU: Urinary incontinence
GI: Abdominal cramps, diarrhea, increased salivation, nausea, vomiting
Contraindications: Hypersensitivity, uveal inflammation
Precautions: History of retinal detachment, asthma, bradycardia, parkinsonism, peptic ulcer, recent MI, epilepsy, myasthenia gravis
Pharmacokinetics:
Miosis: Onset 5-10 min, duration 1-4 wk
Intraocular pressure: Peak 24 hr, duration 1 wk
Interactions:
• Increased effects of both drugs:

I

succinylcholine, systemic anticholinesterase

NURSING CONSIDERATIONS

Administer:

• Ointment to conjunctival sac with patient supine

Evaluate:

• Therapeutic response: decreased aqueous outflow

Teach patient/family:

• That top of tube must not come in contact with moisture; keep tube closed, dry, away from tears or cornea; to wash hands after application
• To report change in vision, blurring or loss of sight, trouble breathing, sweating, flushing
• That long-term therapy may be required
• That blurred vision will decrease with repeated use of drug
• To minimize effects of blurred vision, apply at bedtime
• To observe for signs/symptoms of systemic absorption (i.e., diarrhea, weakness)
• To observe eyes for irritation
• To monitor for cardiac, respiratory, or GI problems

isoniazid (℞)

(eye-soe-nye'a-zid)

INH, isoniazid, Isotamine*, Laniazid, Laniazid C.T., Nydrazid, PMS-Isoniazid*, Tubizid

Func. class.: Antitubercular

Chem. class.: Isonicotinic acid hydrazide

Combination products: Rifamate: isoniazid 150 mg with rifampin 300mg; Rimactane: isoniazid 2 capsules, rifampin 300 mg

Action: Bactericidal interference with lipid, nucleic acid biosynthesis

Uses: Treatment, prevention of tuberculosis

Dosage and routes:

Treatment

• *Adult:* PO/IM 5 mg/kg qd as single dose for 9 mo to 2 yr, not to exceed 300 mg/day
• *Child and infants:* PO/IM 10-20 mg/kg qd as single dose for 18-24 mo, not to exceed 300 mg/day

Prevention

• *Adult* PO 300 mg qd as single dose × 12 mo
• *Child and infants:* PO/IM 10 mg/kg qd as single dose for 12 mo, not to exceed 300 mg/day

Available forms: Tabs 50, 100, 300 mg; inj 100 mg/ml; powder, syrup 50 mg/5 ml

Side effects/adverse reactions:

Hypersensitivity: fever, skin eruptions, lymphadenopathy, vasculitis
CNS: Peripheral neuropathy, memory impairment, ***toxic encephalopathy, convulsions,*** psychosis
EENT: Blurred vision, optic neuritis
HEMA: ***Agranulocytosis, hemolytic, aplastic anemia, thrombocytopenia, eosinophilia, methemoglobinemia***
MISC: Dyspnea, B_6 deficiency, pellagra, hyperglycemia, metabolic acidosis, gynecomastia, rheumatic syndrome, SLE-like syndrome
GI: Nausea, vomiting, epigastric distress, ***jaundice, fatal hepatitis***

Contraindications: Hypersensitivity, optic neuritis

Precautions: Pregnancy (C), renal disease, diabetic retinopathy, cataracts, ocular defects, hepatic disease, child <13 yr

Pharmacokinetics:

PO: Peak 1-2 hr, duration 6-8 hr
IM: Peak 45-60 min
Metabolized in liver; excreted in urine (metabolites); crosses placenta; excreted in breast milk

* Available in Canada only

Interactions:

• Increased toxicity: tyramine foods, alcohol, cycloserine, ethionamide, rifampin, carbamazepine

• Decreased absorption: aluminum antacids

• Decreased effectiveness of BCG vaccine

NURSING CONSIDERATIONS

Assess:

• Liver studies qwk: ALT (SGPT), AST (SGOT), bilirubin

• Renal status: before, qmo: BUN, creatinine, output, sp gr, urinalysis

• Mental status often: affect, mood, behavioral changes; psychosis may occur

• Hepatic status: decreased appetite, jaundice, dark urine, fatigue

Administer:

• With meals to decrease GI symptoms; better to take on empty stomach 1 hr ac or 2 hr pc

• Antiemetic if vomiting occurs

• After C&S is completed; qmo to detect resistance

• IM deep in large muscle mass, massage, rotate inj site

Evaluate:

• Therapeutic response: decreased symptoms of TB

Teach patient/family:

• That compliance with dosage schedule, duration is necessary, not to skip or double dose

• That scheduled appointments must be kept or relapse may occur

• To avoid alcohol while taking drug

• That if diabetic, use blood glucose monitor to obtain correct result

• To report weakness, fatigue, loss of appetite, nausea, vomiting, yellowing of skin or eyes, tingling/numbness of hands/feet

isoproterenol (℞)

(eye-soe-proe-ter′e-nole)

Aerolone, Dispos-a-Med isoproterenol HCl, Isuprel, Isoproterenol HCl, Isuprel Glossets, Isuprel Mistometer, Medihaler-Iso, Vapo-Iso

Func. class.: β-Adrenergic agonist

Chem. class.: Catecholamine

Combination products: DUO-Medihaler: isoproterenol HCl 160 μg/metered spray with phenylephrine bitartrate 240 μg/metered spray

I

Action: Has β_1 and β_2 action; relaxes bronchial smooth muscle and dilates the trachea and main bronchi by increasing levels of cAMP, which relaxes smooth muscles; causes increased contractility and heart rate by acting on β-receptors in heart

Uses: Bronchospasm, asthma, heart block, ventricular dysrhythmias, shock

Dosage and routes:

Asthma, bronchospasm

• *Adult:* SL 10-20 mg q6-8h; INH 1 puff, may repeat in 2-5 min, maintenance 1-2 puffs 4-6 × /day; IV 10-20 μg during anesthesia

• *Child:* SL 5-10 mg q6-8h; INH 1 puff, may repeat in 2-5 min, maintenance 1-2 puffs 4-6 × /d

Heart block/ventricular dysrhythmias

• *Adult:* IV 0.02-0.06, then 0.01-0.2 mg or 5 μg/min HCl; 0.2 mg, then 0.02-1 mg as needed HCl

• *Child:* IV ½ beginning adult dose

Shock

• *Adult:* IV INF 0.5-5 μg/min 1 mg/500 ml D_5W, titrate to B/P, CVP, hourly urine output

Available forms: Sol for nebulization 1:400 (0.25%), 1:200 (0.5%),

1:100 (1%); aerosol 0.25%, 0.2%; powd for INH 0.1 mg/cart; inj 1:5000 (0.2 mg/ml) glossets (SL) 10, 15 mg

Side effects/adverse reactions:
CNS: Tremors, anxiety, insomnia, headache, dizziness, stimulation
CV: Palpitations, tachycardia, hypertension, ***cardiac arrest***
GI: Nausea, vomiting
RESP: Bronchial irritation, edema, dryness of oropharynx, ***bronchospasms*** (overuse)
META: Hyperglycemia

Contraindications: Hypersensitivity to sympathomimetics, narrow-angle glaucoma

Precautions: Pregnancy (C), cardiac disorders, hyperthyroidism, diabetes mellitus, prostatic hypertrophy

Pharmacokinetics:
IV: Onset rapid, duration 10 min
INH/SL: Onset 1-2 hr
REC: Onset 2-4 hr
Metabolized in liver, lungs, GI tract

Interactions:
- Increased effects of both drugs: other sympathomimetics
- Decreased action when used with β-blockers

Y-site compatibilities: Amiodarone, amrinone, atracurium, bretyllium, famotidine, heparin, hydrocortisone sodium succinate, pancuronium, potassium chloride, vecuronium, vitamin B with C

Syringe compatibility: Ranitidine

Additive compatibilities: Calcium chloride, calcium gluceptate, cephalothin, cimetidine, dobutamine, floxacillin, heparin, magnesium sulfate, multivitamins, netilmicin, potassium chloride, succinylchloride, tetracycline, verapamil, vitamin B with C

NURSING CONSIDERATIONS

Assess:
- Resp function: B/P, pulse, lung sounds
- Blood studies (CBC, WBC, differential), since blood dyscrasias may occur (rare)
- I&O ratio; check for urinary retention, frequency, hesitancy
- For paresthesias and coldness of extremities; peripheral blood flow may decrease
- Injection site: tissue sloughing; administer phentolamine mixed with 0.9% NaCl

Administer:
- IV direct dilute 0.2 mg/10 ml 0.9% NaCl (1:50,000 sol); give over 1 min; IV INF 2 mg (1:5000 sol)/ 500 ml of D_5W; run each 1 ml (1: 250,000) sol/min; may be increased; use infusion pump, intracardiac, 1:5000 sol undiluted
- With meals for GI symptoms
- SL tab by rectal route if needed

Perform/provide:
- Storage at room temp; do not use discolored sol

Evaluate:
- Therapeutic response: increased B/P with stabilization, ease of breathing

Teach patient/family:
- To rinse mouth after use
- Use of inhaler; review package insert with patient
- To avoid getting aerosol in eyes
- To wash inhaler in warm water and dry qd
- About all aspects of drug; avoid smoking, smoke-filled rooms, persons with respiratory infections

Treatment of overdose: Administer a β-blocker

isosorbide (℞)

(eye-soe-sor′bide)
Ismotic
Func. class.: Miscellaneous ophthalmic agent

Action: Increases osmotic gradient

* Available in Canada only

between plasma and ocular fluids, decreasing intraocular pressure
Uses: Reduces intraocular pressure from glaucoma and cataract surgery
Dosage and routes:
- *Adult:* PO 1.5 g/kg, then increase to 1-3 g/kg bid-qid

Available forms: Sol 45%
Side effects/adverse reactions:
CNS: Headache, light-headedness, irritability, lethargy, syncope, confusion, dizziness, vertigo, disorientation
GI: Nausea, vomiting, anorexia, diarrhea, cramps, thirst
INTEG: Rash
META: Hypernatremia, hyperosmolarity
Contraindications: Hypersensitivity, anuria, severe renal disease, pulmonary edema, hemorrhagic glaucoma, dehydration
Precautions: Pregnancy (C), patients on Na-restricted diet

NURSING CONSIDERATIONS
Assess:
- I&O; report decrease in urinary output
- Electrolytes during treatment

Administer:
- After pouring over ice (oral)

Evaluate:
- Therapeutic response: decreased intraocular pressure

isosorbide dinitrate (℞)

(eye-soe-sor'bide)
Apo-ISDN*, Cedocard-SR*, Coronex*, Dilatrate-SR, ISDN, Iso-Bid, Isonate, Isorbid, Isordil Tembids, Isordil Titradose, isosorbide dinitrate, Isotrate Timecelles, Novasorbide, Sorbitrate, Sorbitrate SA, Isordil, Isosorbide Dinitrate, Sorbitrate
Func. class.: Antianginal
Chem. class.: Nitrate

Action: Decreases preload, afterload, which is responsible for decreasing left ventricular end-diastolic pressure, systemic vascular resistance and reducing cardiac O_2 demand
Uses: Chronic stable angina pectoris, prophylaxis of angina pain
Dosage and routes:
- *Adult:* PO 5-40 mg qid; SL 2.5-10 mg, may repeat q2-3h; CHEW TAB 5-10 mg prn or q2-3h as prophylaxis; SUS REL 40-80 mg q8-12h

Available forms: Caps sus rel 40 mg; tabs 5, 10, 20, 30, 40 mg; chew tabs 5, 10 mg; SL tabs 2.5, 5, 10 mg
Side effects/adverse reactions:
MISC: Twitching, hemolytic anemia, ***methemoglobinemia***
CV: *Postural hypotension,* tachycardia, ***collapse,*** syncope
GI: Nausea, vomiting
INTEG: Pallor, sweating, rash
CNS: *Vascular headache, flushing, dizziness*, weakness, faintness
Contraindications: Hypersensitivity to this drug or nitrates, severe anemia, increased intracranial pressure, cerebral hemorrhage, acute MI
Precautions: Postural hypotension, pregnancy (C), lactation, children
Pharmacokinetics:
Sus action: Duration 6-8 hr

PO: Onset 15-30 min, duration 4-6 hr
SL: Onset 2-5 min, duration 1-4 hr
Chew tab: Onset 3 min, duration ½-3 hr
Metabolized by liver, excreted in urine as metabolites (80%-100%)
Interactions:
• Increased effects: β-blockers, diuretics, antihypertensives, alcohol products
NURSING CONSIDERATIONS
Assess:
• B/P, pulse, respirations during beginning therapy
• Pain: duration, time started, activity being performed, character
• Tolerance if taken over long period
• Headache, light-headedness, decreased B/P; may indicate a need for decreased dosage
Administer:
• After checking expiration date
• With 8 oz H_2O on empty stomach (oral tablet); do not crush SR or SL drug
Evaluate:
• Therapeutic response: decrease or prevention of anginal pain
Teach patient/family:
• To leave tabs in original container
• To avoid alcohol products
• That drug may cause headache, but tolerance usually develops; taking with meals may reduce or eliminate headache
• That drug may be taken before stressful activity (exercise, sexual activity)
• That SL may sting when drug comes in contact with mucous membranes
• To avoid hazardous activities if dizziness occurs
• Importance of complying with complete medical regimen
• To make position changes slowly to prevent orthostatic hypotension
• Not to crush, chew SL or sus rel tabs

isosorbide mononitrate

(eye-soe-sor'bide)
ISMO
Func. class.: Antianginal
Chem. class.: Nitrate

Action: Decreases preload, afterload, resulting in decreased left ventricular end-diastolic pressure, systemic vascular resistance
Uses: Prevention of angina pectoris due to coronary artery disease
Dosage and routes:
• *Adult:* PO 20 mg bid, 7 hr apart
Available forms: Tabs 20 mg
Side effects/adverse reactions:
MISC: Twitching, hemolytic anemia, methemoglobinemia
CV: Postural hypotension, tachycardia, ***collapse,*** syncope
GI: Nausea, vomiting
INTEG: Pallor, sweating, rash
CNS: Vascular headache, flushing, dizziness, weakness, faintness
Contraindications: Hypersensitivity to nitrates, severe anemia, increased intracranial pressure, cerebral hemorrhage, acute MI, closed-angle glaucoma
Precautions: Postural hypotension, pregnancy (C), lactation, children, glaucoma
Pharmacokinetics: Metabolized by liver; excreted in urine as metabolites (80%-100%); half-life 4 hr
Interactions:
• Increased effects: β-blockers, diuretics, antihypertensives, alcohol, calcium channel blockers
NURSING CONSIDERATIONS
Assess:
• B/P, pulse, respirations during beginning therapy

* Available in Canada only

• Headache, light-headedness, decreased B/P; may indicate a need for decreased dosage
Administer:
• With 8 oz H_2O on empty stomach (oral tablet)
Evaluate:
• Therapeutic response: absence of anginal pain
Teach patient/family:
• That drug may cause headache, but tolerance usually develops; taking with meals may reduce or eliminate headache
• To avoid hazardous activities if dizziness occurs
• To make position changes slowly to prevent fainting
• Not to use alcohol products

isotretinoin (℞)

(eye-soe-tret′i-noyn)
Accutane, Accutane Roche*
Func. class.: Dermatologic—antiacne agent
Chem. class.: Retinoic acid isomer, vitamin A derivative

Action: Decreases sebum secretion; improves cystic acne
Uses: Severe recalcitrant cystic acne
Dosage and routes:
• *Adult:* PO 0.5-2 mg/kg/day in 2 divided doses × 15-20 wk; if relapse occurs, repeat after 2 mo off drug
Available forms: Caps 10, 20, 40 mg
Side effects/adverse reactions:
INTEG: Dry skin, pruritus, cheilosis, joint pain, hair loss, photosensitivity, urticaria, bruising, hirsutism, petechiae, hypo/hyperpigmentation, nail brittleness
MS: Hyperostosis, arthralgia, bone, joint, muscle pain
CV: Chest pain, palpitation, tachycardia
GI: Nausea, vomiting, anorexia, increased liver enzymes, regional ileus, abdominal pain, weight loss
EENT: Eye irritation, conjunctivitis, epistaxis, dry nose, mouth, contact lens intolerance, optic neuritis, photophobia
GU: ***Hematuria, proteinuria,*** hypouricemia, white cells in urine
HEMA: ***Thrombocytopenia,*** decreased Hgb, Hct, WBC, reticulocyte count
CNS: Lethargy, fatigue, headache, depression, ***pseudotumor cerebri***
Contraindications: Hypersensitivity, inflamed skin, pregnancy (X)
Precautions: Lactation, diabetes, photosensitivity, hepatic disease, inflammatory bowel disease, obesity
Pharmacokinetics:
PO: Peak 2.9-3.2 hr, half-life 10-20 hr; metabolized in liver, excreted in urine, feces
Interactions:
• Additive toxic effects: Vit A; do not use together
• Pseudotumor cerebri: minocycline or tetracycline
• Increased triglyceride levels: alcohol
Lab test interferences:
Increase: Sedimentation rate, triglyceride, liver function studies
Decrease: RBC/WBC count
NURSING CONSIDERATIONS
Assess:
• Triglyceride levels, cholesterol, high-density lipoproteins AST (SGOT), ALT (SGPT), alk phosphatase before, during treatment
• Urinalysis qwk for protein, blood; CBC, SMA CPK; blood glucose in diabetics periodically
• Area of body involved, including time involved, what helps or aggravates condition
• Pseudotumor cerebri: headache, vomiting, nausea, visual disturbance; discontinue drug

Administer:
• Whole; do not crush; give with meals
• Second course of treatment if needed after waiting 2 mo

Perform/provide:
• Storage in tight, light-resistant container

Evaluate:
• Therapeutic response: decrease in size and number of lesions

Teach patient/family:
• To avoid sunlight or wear sunscreen; photosensitivity may occur
• That an increase in acne may occur during initial treatment, decrease in 4-6 wk
• Not to become pregnant while taking drug
• Not to take Vit A supplements; to take drug with meals
• Not to crush
• To minimize or eliminate alcohol consumption, triglycerides may increase

isoxsuprine (℞)

(eye-sox'syoo-preen)
isoxsuprine HCl, Vasodilan, Voxsuprine

Func. class.: Peripheral vasodilator

Chem. class.: Nylidrin-related agent

Action: α-Adrenoreceptor antagonist with β-adrenoreceptor stimulating properties; may also act directly on vascular smooth muscle; causes cardiac stimulation, uterine relaxation

Uses: Symptoms of cerebrovascular insufficiency, peripheral vascular disease including arteriosclerosis obliterans, thromboangiitis obliterans, Raynaud's disease

Dosage and routes:
• *Adult:* PO 10-20 mg tid or qid

Available forms: Tabs 10, 20 mg

Side effects/adverse reactions:
CV: Hypotension, ***tachycardia,*** palpitations, chest pain
CNS: Dizziness, weakness, tremors, anxiety
GI: Nausea, vomiting, abdominal pain, distention
INTEG: Severe rash, flushing

Contraindications: Hypersensitivity, postpartum, arterial bleeding

Precautions: Pregnancy (C), tachycardia

Pharmacokinetics:
PO: Peak 1 hr, duration 3 hr, half-life 1¼ hr; excreted in urine; crosses placenta

NURSING CONSIDERATIONS

Assess:
• B/P, pulse during treatment until stable; take B/P lying, standing; orthostatic hypotension is common

Administer:
• With meals to reduce GI upset

Perform/provide:
• Storage at room temp

Evaluate:
• Therapeutic response: ability to walk without pain, increased pulse volume, increased temp in extremities, improved orientation, long- and short-term memory

Teach patient/family:
• That medication is not cure; may have to be taken continuously depending on condition; therapeutic response may not be evident for 2-3 mo
• That it is necessary to quit smoking to prevent excessive vasoconstriction
• To avoid hazardous activities until stabilized on medication; dizziness may occur
• To make position changes slowly, or fainting will occur

- To discontinue drug, notify prescriber if rash develops
- To report palpitations, flushing if severe
- To avoid changes in temp; extremities should be kept warm to promote better circulation

isradipine (℞)

(is-ra′di-peen)

DynaCirc

Func. class.: Calcium channel blocker

Chem. class.: Dihydropyridine

Action: Inhibits calcium ion influx across cell membrane during cardiac depolarization; produces relaxation of coronary vascular smooth muscle, peripheral vascular smooth muscle; dilates coronary vascular arteries; increases myocardial oxygen delivery in patients with vasospastic angina

Uses: Essential hypertension, angina

Dosage and routes:

Adult: PO 2.5 mg bid; increase at 3-4 wk intervals up to 10 mg bid

Available forms: Caps 2.5, 5 mg

Side effects/adverse reactions:

HEMA: ***Thrombocytopenia, leukopenia, anemia***

CV: Peripheral edema, tachycardia, hypotension, chest pain

GI: Nausea, vomiting, diarrhea, gastric upset, constipation, hepatitis

GU: Nocturia, polyuria, ***acute renal failure***

INTEG: Rash, pruritus, urticaria, photosensitivity, hair loss

CNS: Headache, fatigue, dizziness, fainting, sleep disturbances

MISC: Flushing

Contraindications: Sick sinus syndrome, 2nd or 3rd degree heart block, hypotension less than 90 mm Hg systolic, hypersensitivity

Precautions: CHF, hypotension, hepatic disease, pregnancy (C), lactation, children, renal disease, elderly

Pharmacokinetics: Metabolized in liver; metabolites excreted in urine, feces; secreted in breast milk, peak plasma levels at 2-3 hr

Interactions:

- Increased effects of: digitalis, neuromuscular blocking agents, cyclosporine
- Increased effects of isradipine: cimetidine, carbamazepine

NURSING CONSIDERATIONS

Assess:

- B/P, pulse rate, chest pain; monitor ECG periodically during therapy
- Cardiac status: B/P, pulse, respiration, ECG

Evaluate:

- Therapeutic response: decreased anginal pain, decreased B/P

Teach patient/family:

- To avoid hazardous activities until stabilized on drug, dizziness is no longer a problem
- To limit caffeine consumption
- To avoid OTC drugs unless directed by prescriber
- Importance of compliance in all areas of medical regimen: diet, exercise, stress reduction, drug therapy
- To notify prescriber of irregular heartbeat, shortness of breath, swelling of feet and hands, pronounced dizziness, constipation, nausea, hypotension

Treatment of overdose: Defibrillation, β-agonists, IV Ca inotropic agents, diuretics, atropine for AV block, vasopressor for hypotension

itraconazole (℞)

(it-ra-con'a-zol)

Sporanox

Func. class.: Antifungal, systemic

Chem. class.: Triazole derivative

Action: Alters cell membranes and inhibits several fungal enzymes

Uses: Systemic candidiasis, chronic mucocandidiasis, oral thrush, candiduria, coccidioidomycosis, histoplasmosis, chromomycosis, paracoccidioidomycosis, blastomycosis (pulmonary and extrapulmonary)

Dosage and routes:

• *Adult:* PO 200 mg tid × 3 days with food; may increase to 400 mg qd if needed

Available forms: Caps 100 mg

Side effects/adverse reactions:

GU: Gynecomastia, impotence, decreased libido

INTEG: Pruritus, fever, rash,

CNS: Headache, dizziness, insomnia, somnolence, depression

GI: Nausea, vomiting, anorexia, diarrhea, cramps, abdominal pain, flatulence, ***GI bleeding, hepatotoxicity***

MISC: Edema, fatigue, malaise, hypertension, hypokalemia, tinnitus

Contraindications: Hypersensitivity, lactation, fungal meningitis, coadministration with terfenadine

Precautions: Hepatic disease, achlorhydria or hypochlorhydine (drug-induced), children, pregnancy (C)

Pharmacokinetics:

PO: Peak 3-5 hr, half-life 60 hr; metabolized in liver; excreted in bile, feces; requires acid pH for absorption; distributed poorly to CSF; highly protein bound

Interactions:

• Do not use with terfenadine: may result in rare instance of life-threatening dysrhythmias and death

• Hepatotoxicity: other hepatotoxic drugs

• Itraconazole increases levels of cyclosporine

• Decreased action of itraconazole: antacids, H_2-receptor antagonists, isoniazid, rifampin

• Increased anticoagulant effect: coumarin anticoagulants

• Severe hypoglycemia: oral hypoglycemics

• Concomitant administration with phenytoin may result in decreased levels of itraconazole; effects of phenytoin may be increased

NURSING CONSIDERATIONS

Assess:

• I&O ratio

• Liver studies (ALT [SGPT], AST [SGOT], bilirubin) if on long-term therapy

• For allergic reaction: rash, photosensitivity, urticaria, dermatitis

• For hepatotoxicity: nausea, vomiting, jaundice, clay-colored stools, fatigue

Administer:

• In the presence of acid products only; do not use alkaline products or antacids within 2 hr of drug; may give coffee, tea, acidic fruit juices

• With food for GI symptoms

• With hydrochloric acid if achlorhydria is present

Perform/provide:

• Storage in tight container at room temp

Evaluate:

• Therapeutic response: decreased fever, malaise, rash, negative C&S for infecting organism

Teach patient/family:

• That long-term therapy may be needed to clear infection (1 wk-6 mo depending on infection)

• To avoid hazardous activities if dizziness occurs
• To take 2 hr ac administration of other drugs that increase gastric pH (antacids, H_2-blockers, anticholinergics)
• Importance of compliance with drug regimen
• To notify prescriber of GI symptoms, signs of liver dysfunction (fatigue, nausea, anorexia, vomiting, dark urine, pale stools)

kanamycin (℞)

(kan-a-mye'sin)
kanamycin sulfate, Kantrex
Func. class.: Antiinfective
Chem. class.: Aminoglycoside

Action: Interferes with protein synthesis in bacterial cell by binding to the 30s ribosomal subunit, causing inaccurate peptide sequence to form in protein chain, causing bacterial death

Uses: Severe systemic infections of CNS, respiratory, GI, urinary tract, bone, skin, soft tissues caused by *E. coli, Acinetobacter, Proteus, K. pneumoniae,* also used as adjunct in hepatic coma, peritonitis, preoperatively to sterilize bowel; decreases ammonia-producing bacteria in bowel and intraperitoneally after fecal spill during surgery

Dosage and routes:

Severe systemic infections
• *Adult and child:* IV INF 15 mg/kg/d in divided doses q8-12h; diluted 500 mg/200 ml of NS or D_5W given over 30-60 min, not to exceed 1.5 g/d; IM 15 mg/kg/d in divided doses q8-12h, not to exceed 1.5 g/d, irrigation not to exceed 1.5 g/d

Hepatic coma
• *Adult:* PO 8-12 g/d in divided doses

Preoperative bowel sterilization
• *Adult:* PO 1 g qh × 4 doses, then q6h × 36-72 hr

Available forms: Inj 75, 500 mg/2ml, 1 g/3 ml; cap 500 mg

Side effects/adverse reactions:
GU: ***Oliguria, hematuria, renal damage, azotemia, renal failure, nephrotoxicity***
CNS: Confusion, depression, numbness, tremors, ***convulsions,*** muscle twitching, ***neurotoxicity***
RESP: Respiratory depression
EENT: ***Ototoxicity,*** deafness, visual disturbances, dizziness, vertigo, tinnitus
HEMA: ***Agranulocytosis, thrombocytopenia, leukopenia, eosinophilia, anemia***
GI: Nausea, vomiting, anorexia, increased ALT, AST, bilirubin, hepatomegaly, ***hepatic necrosis,*** splenomegaly
CV: Hypotension
INTEG: Rash, burning, urticaria, dermatitis, alopecia

Contraindications: Bowel obstruction, severe renal disease, hypersensitivity

Precautions: Neonates, myasthenia gravis, hearing deficits, mild renal disease, pregnancy (D), lactation, Parkinson's disease

Pharmacokinetics:
IM: Onset rapid, peak 1-2 hr
IV: Onset immediate, peak 1-2 hr
Plasma half-life 2-3 hr; not metabolized; excreted unchanged in urine; crosses placenta

Interactions:
• Increased ototoxicity, neurotoxicity, nephrotoxicity: other aminoglycosides, amphotericin B, polymyxin, vancomycin, ethacrynic acid, furosemide, mannitol, methoxyflurane, cisplatin, cephalosporins, bacitracin

K

• Do not mix in sol or syringe: carbenicillin, ticarcillin, amphotericin B, cephalothin, erythromycin, heparin
• Increased effects: nondepolarizing muscle relaxants, succinylcholine
• Decreased effects of oral anticoagulants

Additive compatibilities: Ascorbic acid, cefoxitin, chloramphenicol, clindamycin, dopamine, furosemide, polymyxin B, sodium bicarbonate, tetracycline; admixing is not recommended

Y-site compatibilities: Cyclophosphamide, furosemide, heparin with hydrocortisone, sodium succinate, hydromorphone, magnesium sulfate, meperidine, morphine, perphenazine, potassium chloride

NURSING CONSIDERATIONS

Assess:

• Weight before treatment; dosage is usually calculated on ideal body weight, but may be calculated on actual body weight
• I&O ratio, urinalysis daily for proteinuria, cells, casts; report sudden change in urine output
• VS during infusion; watch for hypotension, change in pulse
• IV site for thrombophlebitis, including pain, redness, swelling q30min; change site if needed; apply warm compresses to discontinued site
• Serum peak, drawn at 30-60 min after IV infusion or 60 min after IM injection; trough level drawn just before next dose; blood level should be 2-4 × bacteriostatic level; trough = 5-10 mEq/ml, peak = <30 mEq/ml
• Urine pH if drug is used for UTI; urine should be kept alkaline
• Renal impairment by CrCl, BUN, serum creatinine testing of urine; lower dosage should be given in renal impairment (CrCl <80 ml/min)
• Deafness by audiometric testing, ringing, roaring in ears, vertigo; assess hearing before, during, after treatment
• Dehydration: high specific gravity, decrease in skin turgor, dry mucous membranes, dark urine
• Superinfection: fever, malaise, redness, pain, swelling, perineal itching, diarrhea, stomatitis, change in cough, sputum
• C&S before starting treatment to identify infecting organism
• Vestibular dysfunction: nausea, vomiting, dizziness, headache; drug should be discontinued if severe
• Injection sites for redness, swelling, abscesses; use warm compresses at site

Administer:

• IV after diluting 500 mg or less/100 ml of D_5W, D_5/NaCl, 0.9% NaCl, LR or more; give 3-4 ml/min or less; flush line after use
• IM inj in large muscle mass; rotate injection sites
• Penicillins at least 1 hr before or after this drug
• Drug in evenly spaced doses to maintain blood level
• Bicarbonate to alkalinize urine if ordered in treating UTI, as drug is most active in alkaline environment

Perform/provide:

• Adequate fluids of 2-3 L/day unless contraindicated to prevent irritation of tubules
• Flush of IV line with NS or D_5W after infusion
• Supervised ambulation, other safety measures with vestibular dysfunction

Evaluate:

• Therapeutic effect: absence of fever, draining wounds, negative C&S after treatment

* Available in Canada only

Teach patient/family:
- To report headache, dizziness, symptoms of overgrowth of infection, renal impairment
- To report loss of hearing, ringing, roaring in ears or feeling of fullness in head

Treatment of overdose: Hemodialysis; monitor serum levels of drug

kaolin, pectin (OTC)
(kay'oh-lin pek'tin)

Func. class.: Antidiarrheal
Chem. class.: Hydrous magnesium aluminum silicate

Combination products: Donnagel Suspension: kaolin 6 g, pectin 142.8 mg, hyoscyamine SO_4 0.1037 mg, atropine SO_4 0.0194 mg, scopolamine hydrobromide 0.0065 mg, alcohol 3.8%/30 ml susp

Action: Decreases gastric motility, H_2O content of stool; adsorbent, demulcent

Uses: Diarrhea (cause undetermined)

Dosage and routes:
- *Adult:* PO 60-120 ml (30 ml conc) after each loose BM
- *Child >12 yr:* PO 60 ml after each loose BM
- *Child 6-12 yr:* PO 30-60 ml (15 ml conc) after each loose BM
- *Child 3-6 yr:* PO 15-30 ml (75 ml conc) after each loose BM

Available forms: Susp kaolin 0.87 g/5 ml, pectin 43 mg/5 ml; kaolin 0.98 g/5 ml, pectin 21.7 mg/5 ml

Side effects/adverse reactions:
GI: Constipation (chronic use)

Precautions: Pregnancy (C)

Interactions:
- Decreased action of all other drugs

NURSING CONSIDERATIONS

Assess:
- Bowel pattern before; for rebound constipation
- Dehydration in children

Administer:
- After shaking suspension
- For 48 hr only

Evaluate:
- Therapeutic response: decreased diarrhea

Teach patient/family:
- Not to exceed recommended dose
- To shake well before administration

ketamine (℞)
(keet'a-meen)
Ketalar

Func. class.: General anesthetic
Chem. class.: Phencyclidine derivative

Action: Acts on limbic system, cortex to provide anesthesia

Uses: Short anesthesia for diagnostic/surgical procedures

Dosage and routes:
- *Adult and child:* IV 1-4.5 mg/kg over 1 min
- *Adult and child:* IM 6.5-13 mg/kg

Available forms: Inj 10, 50, 100 mg/ml vial

Side effects/adverse reactions:
CNS: Hallucinations, confusion, delirium, tremors, polyneuropathy, fasciculations, pseudoconvulsions
CV: Increased BP, hypotension, bradycardia
EENT: Diplopia, salivation, small increase in intraocular pressure
INTEG: Rash, pain at injection site

Contraindications: Hypersensitivity, CVA, increased intracranial pressure, severe hypertension, cardiac decompensation, child <2 yr

Precautions: Pregnancy (C), seizure disorders, elderly, psychiatric disorders

Pharmacokinetics:

IV: Peak 40 sec, duration 10 min

IM: Peak 3-8 min, duration 25 min

Interactions:

• Increased action of ketamine: narcotics or atropine

• Respiratory depression: antihypertensives with CNS depressant effects

• Hypertension, tachycardia: thyroid hormones

• Increased action of tubocurarine

Syringe compatibility: Benzequinamide

NURSING CONSIDERATIONS

Assess:

• VS q10min during IV administration, q30min after IM dose

• For hallucinations, delusions, separation from environment

• For EPS: dystonia, akathisia

• For increasing heart rate or decreasing B/P; notify prescriber at once

Administer:

• IV after diluting 100 mg/ml with equal parts of D_5W, 0.9% NaCl, sterile H_2O for inj, give over 1 min; may be diluted 10 ml (50 mg/ml)/500 ml of 0.9% NaCl or D_5W = 1 mg/ml; run at 1-2 mg/min; titrate to response

• Anticholinergic preoperatively to decrease secretions

• Only with crash cart, resuscitative equipment available

• Narcotic or diazepam to control recovery symptoms

Perform/provide:

• Quiet environment for recovery to decrease psychotic symptoms

Evaluate:

• Therapeutic response: maintenance of anesthesia

ketoconazole (℞)

(kee-toe-koe'na-zole)

Nizoral

Func. class.: Antifungal

Chem. class.: Imidazole derivative

Action: Alters cell membranes and inhibits several fungal enzymes

Uses: Systemic candidiasis, chronic mucocandidiasis, oral thrush, candiduria, coccidioidomycosis, histoplasmosis, chromomycosis, paracoccidioidomycosis, blastomycosis; tinea cruris, tinea corporis, tinea versicolor, *Pityrosporum ovale*

Investigational uses: Cushing's syndrome, advanced prostatic cancer

Dosage and routes:

• *Adult:* PO 200-400 mg qd

• *Children:* PO: >2 years: 3.3-6.6 mg/kg/day as single daily dose; <2 years, daily dose not established

• *Adult and child:* TOP 2% cream applied qd or bid

• *Adult:* Shampoo massage into scalp 1 min, reapply × 3 min, rinse, continue treatment 2 × /wk × 1 mo, no more than q3d

Available forms: Tabs 200 mg; cream 2%; shampoo 2%

Side effects/adverse reactions:

GU: Gynecomastia, impotence

INTEG: Pruritus, fever, chills, photophobia, rash, dermatitis, purpura, urticaria

CNS: Headache, dizziness, somnolence

SYST: Anaphylaxis

GI: Nausea, vomiting, anorexia, diarrhea, abdominal pain, hepatotoxicity

HEMA: Thrombocytopenia, leukopenia, hemolytic anemia

Contraindications: Hypersensitiv-

* Available in Canada only

ity, lactation, fungal meningitis; coadministration with terfenadine

Precautions: Renal disease, hepatic disease, achlorhydria (drug-induced), pregnancy, children <2 years, other hepatotoxic agents including terfenadine

Pharmacokinetics:

PO: Peak 1-2 hr, half-life 2 hr, terminal 8 hr; metabolized in liver; excreted in bile, feces; requires acid pH for absorption; distributed poorly to CSF; highly protein bound

Interactions:

• Do not use with terfenadine; may result in rare instances of life-threatening dysrhythmias and death
• Hepatotoxicity: other hepatotoxic drugs (including terfenadine)
• Ketoconazole increases concentration of cyclosporine and corticosteroids
• Decreased action of ketoconazole: antacids, H_2-receptor antagonists, isoniazid, rifampin
• Increased anticoagulant effect, coumarin anticoagulants
• Ketoconazole may decrease theophylline effect

NURSING CONSIDERATIONS

Assess:

• I&O ratio
• Liver studies (ALT, AST, bilirubin) if on long-term therapy
• For allergic reaction: rash, photosensitivity, urticaria, dermatitis
• For hepatotoxicity: nausea, vomiting, jaundice, clay-colored stools, fatigue

Administer:

• In the presence of acid products only; do not use alkaline products or antacids within 2 hr of drug; may give coffee, tea, acidic fruit juices
• With food to decrease GI symptoms
• With HCl if achlorhydria is present

Perform/provide:

• Storage in tight container at room temp

Evaluate:

• Therapeutic response: decreased fever, malaise, rash, negative C&S for infecting organism, absence of scaling

Teach patient/family:

• That long-term therapy may be needed to clear infection (1 wk-6 mo depending on infection)
• To avoid hazardous activities if dizziness occurs
• To take 2 hr ac administration of other drugs that increase gastric pH (antacids, H_2-blockers, anticholinergics)
• Importance of compliance with drug regimen
• To notify prescriber of GI symptoms, signs of liver dysfunction (fatigue, nausea, anorexia, vomiting, dark urine, pale stools)

---

ketoprofen (℞)

(ke-to-proe′fen)
ketoprofen, Orudis, Orudis-E*, Oruvail

Func. class.: Nonsteroidal antiinflammatory (NSAID)
Chem. class.: Propionic acid derivative

Action: Inhibits prostaglandin synthesis by decreasing enzyme needed for biosynthesis; analgesic, antiinflammatory, antipyretic

Uses: Mild to moderate pain, osteoarthritis, rheumatoid arthritis, dysmenorrhea

Dosage and routes:

Antiinflammatory

• *Adult:* PO 150-300 mg in divided doses tid-qid, not to exceed 300 mg/day

Analgesic
• *Adult:* PO 25-50 mg q6-8hr
Available forms: Caps 25, 50, 75 mg
Side effects/adverse reactions:
GI: Nausea, anorexia, vomiting, diarrhea, jaundice, ***cholestatic hepatitis,*** constipation, flatulence, cramps, dry mouth, peptic ulcer
CNS: Dizziness, drowsiness, fatigue, tremors, confusion, insomnia, anxiety, depression
CV: Tachycardia, peripheral edema, palpitations, dysrhythmias, hypertension
INTEG: Purpura, rash, pruritus, sweating
GU: ***Nephrotoxicity: dysuria, hematuria, oliguria, azotemia***
HEMA: ***Blood dyscrasias***
EENT: Tinnitus, hearing loss, blurred vision
Contraindications: Hypersensitivity, asthma, severe renal disease, severe hepatic disease, ulcer disease
Precautions: Pregnancy (B), lactation, children, bleeding disorders, GI disorders, cardiac disorders, hypersensitivity to other antiinflammatory agents, elderly
Pharmacokinetics:
PO: Peak 2 hr, half-life 3-3½ hr; metabolized in liver; excreted in urine (metabolites); excreted in breast milk; 99% plasma protein binding
Interactions:
• Increased action of coumarin, streptokinase, probenecid
NURSING CONSIDERATIONS
Assess:
• Renal, liver, blood studies: BUN, creatinine, AST (SGOT), ALT (SGPT), Hgb, before treatment, periodically thereafter
• Audiometric, ophthalmic examination before, during, after treatment
• For eye, ear problems: blurred vision, tinnitus; may indicate toxicity
Administer:
• Whole; do not crush, break or open capsules
• With food to decrease GI symptoms; however, best to take on empty stomach to facilitate absorption
Perform/provide:
• Storage at room temp
Evaluate:
• Therapeutic response: decreased pain, stiffness in joints, decreased swelling in joints, ability to move more easily
Teach patient/family:
• To report blurred vision, ringing, roaring in ears; may indicate toxicity
• To avoid driving, other hazardous activities if dizziness, drowsiness occurs, especially elderly
• To report change in urine pattern, increased weight, edema, increased pain in joints, fever, blood in urine; indicate nephrotoxicity
• That therapeutic effects may take up to 1 mo
• To avoid aspirin, alcohol, steroids

ketorolac (℞)
(kee-toe'role-ak)
Acular, Toradol
Func. class.: Nonsteroidal antiinflammatory
Chem. class.: Pyrrolo-pyrrole

Action: Inhibits prostaglandin synthesis by decreasing an enzyme needed for biosynthesis; analgesic, antiinflammatory, antipyretic effects
Uses: Mild to moderate pain; seasonal allergic conjunctivitis (ophth)
Dosage and routes:
• *Adult (multiple dosing):* IV BOL/IM 30 mg q6h max 120 mg/day, with transition of 20 mg PO (1st

* Available in Canada only

dose), then 10 mg q4-6h; ≥65 yr, renal impairment, or weight <50 kg 15 mg q6hr, max 60 mg

• *Adult (single dosing):* IV BOL/IM 30 mg IV or 60 mg IM, then 20 mg transition dose, not to exceed 40 mg/day then 10 mg q4-6h; ≥65 yr, renal impairment or weight <50 kg 30 mg IM or 15 mg IV

• *Adult:* OPHTH 1 gtt qid

Available forms: Inj 15, 30 mg/ml (prefilled syringes); ophth 0.5% sol; tab 10 mg

Side effects/adverse reactions:

CV: Hypertension, flushing, syncope, pallor

CNS: Dizziness, drowsiness, tremors

EENT: Tinnitus, hearing loss, blurred vision

GI: Nausea, anorexia, vomiting, diarrhea, constipation, flatulence, cramps, dry mouth, peptic ulcer, ***GI bleeding, perforation***

GU: ***Nephrotoxicity: dysuria, hematuria, oliguria, azotemia***

HEMA: ***Blood dyscrasias***

INTEG: Purpura, rash, pruritus, sweating

Contraindications: Hypersensitivity, asthma, severe renal disease, severe hepatic disease, peptic ulcer disease, L&D, lactation, CV bleeding

Precautions: Pregnancy (C), children, bleeding disorders, GI disorders, cardiac disorders, hypersensitivity to other antiinflammatory agents, elderly

Pharmacokinetics:

IM: Peak 50 min, half-life 6 hr

Interactions:

• Increased action of ketorolac: phenytoin, sulfonamides

• Compatible in 0.9% NaCl, D_5, Ringer's, LR, Plasmalate, aminophylline, lidocaine, morphine, meperidine, dopamine, insulin, heparin, promethazine, hydroxyzine. These meds should not be mixed in syringe

NURSING CONSIDERATIONS

Assess:

• Eyes: redness, swelling, tearing, itching (ophth)

• Renal, liver, blood studies: BUN, creatinine, AST (SGOT), ALT (SGPT), Hgb before treatment, periodically thereafter

• Bleeding times; check for bruising, bleeding; test for occult blood in urine

• For eye, ear problems: blurred vision, tinnitus (may indicate toxicity)

• Hepatic dysfunction: jaundice, yellow sclera and skin, clay-colored stools

• Audiometric, ophthalmic exam before, during, after treatment

• GI condition, hypertension, cardiac conditions

Administer:

• IM/IV for 5 days or less

Perform/provide:

• Storage at room temp

Evaluate:

• Therapeutic response: decreased pain, stiffness, swelling in joints, ability to move more easily; decreased ocular itching (ophth)

Teach patient/family:

• To report blurred vision or ringing, roaring in ears (may indicate toxicity)

• To avoid driving, other hazardous activities if dizziness or drowsiness occurs

• To report change in urine pattern, weight increase, edema, pain increase in joints, fever, blood in urine (indicates nephrotoxicity)

• To avoid alcohol, ASA

• This drug may cause redness, burning if soft contact lens are worn (ophth)

K

labetalol (℞)

(la-bet′a-lole)

Normodyne, Trandate

Func. class.: Antihypertensive

Chem. class.: Nonselective β-blocker

Combination products: Normozide 100/25: labetalol hydrochloride 100 mg, hydrochlorothiazide 25 mg; Normozide 200/25: labetalol hydrochloride 200 mg, hydrochlorothiazide 25 mg; Normozide 300/25: labetalol hydrochloride 300 mg, hydrochlorothiazide 25 mg

Action: Produces falls in B/P without reflex tachycardia or significant reduction in heart rate through mixture of α-blocking, β-blocking effects; elevated plasma renins are reduced

Uses: Mild to moderate hypertension; treatment of severe hypertension (IV)

Investigational uses: Angina pectoris (PO), hypotension during surgery (IV)

Dosage and routes:

Hypertension

• *Adult:* PO 100 mg bid; may be given with a diuretic; may increase to 200 mg bid after 2 days; may continue to increase q1-3 days; max 400 mg bid

Hypertensive crisis

• *Adult:* IV INF 200 mg/160 ml D_5W, run at 2 ml/min; stop infusion at desired response, repeat q6-8h as needed; IV BOL 20 mg over 2 min, may repeat 40-80 mg q10min, not to exceed 300 mg

Available forms: Tabs 100, 200, 300 mg; inj 5 mg/ml in 20 ml amps

Side effects/adverse reactions:

CV: Orthostatic hypotension, bradycardia, ***CHF,*** chest pain, ***ventricular dysrhythmias***, AV block

CNS: Dizziness, mental changes, drowsiness, fatigue, headache, catatonia, depression, anxiety, nightmares, paresthesias, lethargy

GI: Nausea, vomiting, diarrhea

INTEG: Rash, alopecia, urticaria, pruritus, fever

HEMA: ***Agranulocytosis, thrombocytopenia, purpura*** (rare)

EENT: Tinnitus, visual changes, sore throat, double vision, dry burning eyes

GU: Impotence, dysuria, ejaculatory failure

RESP: ***Bronchospasm,*** dyspnea, wheezing

Contraindications: Hypersensitivity to β-blockers, cardiogenic shock, heart block (2nd or 3rd degree), sinus bradycardia, CHF, bronchial asthma

Precautions: Major surgery, pregnancy (C), lactation, diabetes mellitus, renal disease, thyroid disease, COPD, well-compensated heart failure, CAD, nonallergic bronchospasm

Pharmacokinetics:

PO: Onset ½-2 hr, peak 2-4 hr, duration 8-12 hr

IV: Onset 5 min, peak 15 min, duration 2-4 hr

Half-life 6-8 hr; metabolized by liver (metabolites inactive); excreted in urine; crosses placenta; excreted in breast milk

Interactions:

• Increased bronchodilation: β-adrenergic agonists

• Increased hypotension: diuretics, other antihypertensives, halothane, cimetidine, nitroglycerin

• Decreased effects: sympathomimetics, lidocaine, indomethacin, theophylline, cimetidine

• Increased hypoglycemia: insulin

Y-site compatibilities: Amikacin, aminophylline, ampicillin, butorphanol, calcium gluconate, cefazolin, ceftazidine, ceftizoxine, chloramphenicol, cimetidine, clindamycin, co-trimoxazole, dopamine, enalaprilat, erythromycin lactobionate, famotidine, fentanyl, gentamicin, heparin, lidocaine, magnesium sulfate, meperidine, metronidazole, morphine, oxacillin, penicillin G potassium, piperacillin, potassium chloride, potassium phosphate, ranitidine, sodium acetate, tobramycin, vancomycin

Solution compatibilities: D_5R, D_5LR, $D_2½/0.45\%$ NaCl, $D_5/0.2\%$ NaCl, $D_5/0.33\%$ NaCl, $D_50.9\%$ NaCl, D_5W, Ringer's, LR

Lab test interferences:

False increase: Urinary catecholamines

NURSING CONSIDERATIONS

Assess:

- I&O, weight daily
- B/P during beginning treatment, periodically thereafter, pulse q4h; note rate, rhythm, quality
- Apical/radial pulse before administration; notify prescriber of any significant changes
- Baselines in renal, liver function tests before therapy begins
- Edema in feet, legs daily
- Skin turgor, dryness of mucous membranes for hydration status

Administer:

- IV undiluted or diluted in LR, D_5W, D_5 in 0.2%, 0.9%, 0.33% NaCl or Ringer's inj, give undiluted 20 mg or less/2 min; infusion is titrated to patient response; 200 mg of drug/160 ml sol = 1 mg/ml; 300 mg of drug/240 ml sol = 1 mg/ml; 200 mg of drug/250 ml sol = 2 mg/3 ml; use infusion pump
- PO ac, hs; tablet may be crushed or swallowed whole
- Reduced dosage in renal dysfunction
- IV, keep patient recumbent for 3 hr

Perform/provide:

- Storage in dry area at room temp; do not freeze

Evaluate:

- Therapeutic response: decreased B/P after 1-2 wk

Teach patient/family:

- Not to discontinue drug abruptly; taper over 2 wk; may cause precipitate angina
- Not to use OTC products containing α-adrenergic stimulants (nasal decongestants, OTC cold preparations) unless directed by prescriber
- To report bradycardia, dizziness, confusion, depression, fever
- To take pulse at home, advise when to notify prescriber
- To avoid alcohol, smoking, Na intake
- To comply with weight control, dietary adjustments, modified exercise program
- To carry Medic Alert ID to identify drug, allergies
- To avoid hazardous activities if dizziness is present
- To report symptoms of CHF: difficult breathing, especially on exertion or when lying down, night cough, swelling of extremities
- To take medication at bedtime to prevent effect of orthostatic hypotension
- To wear support hose to minimize effects of orthostatic hypotension

Treatment of overdose: Lavage, IV atropine for bradycardia, IV theophylline for bronchospasm, digitalis, O_2, diuretic for cardiac failure; hemodialysis is useful for removal, hypotension; administer vasopressor (norepinephrine)

lactulose (℞)

(lak'tyoo-lose)

Cephulac, Cholac, Chronulac, Constilac, Constulose, Duphalac, Emulose, Enulose Lactulax*

Func. class.: Laxative (hyperosmotic); ammonia detoxicant

Chem. class.: Lactose synthetic derivative

Action: Prevents absorption of ammonia in colon; increases water in stool

Uses: Chronic constipation, portal-systemic encephalopathy in patients with hepatic disease

Dosage and routes:

Constipation

• *Adult:* PO 15-60 ml qd

Encephalopathy

• *Adult:* PO 20-30 g tid or qid until stools are soft; RET ENEMA 30-45 ml in 100 ml of fluid

Available forms: Oral sol, rec sol 3.33 g/5 ml

Side effects/adverse reactions:

GI: Nausea, vomiting, anorexia, abdominal cramps, diarrhea, flatulence, distention, belching

Contraindications: Hypersensitivity, low-galactose diet

Precautions: Pregnancy (C), lactation, diabetes mellitus, elderly, debilitated patients

Pharmacokinetics: Metabolized in intestine, excreted by kidneys onset 1-2 days, peak unknown, duration unknown

Interactions:

• Decreased effects of lactulose: neomycin, other oral antiinfectives

NURSING CONSIDERATIONS

Assess:

• Stool: amount, color, consistency

• Blood ammonia level (30-70 mg/100 ml); may decrease ammonia level by 25%-50%

• Blood, urine electrolytes if drug is used often; may cause diarrhea, hypokalemia, hyponatremia

• I&O ratio to identify fluid loss

• Cause of constipation; determine whether fluids, bulk, or exercise is missing from lifestyle

• Cramping, rectal bleeding, nausea, vomiting; if these symptoms occur, drug should be discontinued

• Clearing of confusion, lethargy, restlessness, irritability

Administer:

• With 8 oz fruit juice, water, milk to increase palatability of oral form

• Retention enema by diluting 300 ml lactose/700 ml of water; administer by rectal balloon catheter

• Increase fluids to 2 L/day; do not give with other laxatives; if diarrhea occurs, reduce dosage

Evaluate:

• Therapeutic response: decreased constipation, decreased blood ammonia level, clearing of mental state

Teach patient/family:

• Not to use laxatives long-term

• To dilute with water or fruit juice to counteract sweet taste

• To store in cool environment; do not freeze

• To take on an empty stomach for rapid action

• To report diarrhea; may indicate overdose

lamotrigine (℞)

(la-mot'ri-geen)

Lamictal

Func. class.: Anticonvulsant

Chem. class.: Phenyltriazine

Action: Unknown, may inhibit voltage-sensitive sodium channels

* Available in Canada only

Uses: Adjunct in the treatment of partial seizures
Dosage and routes:
No valproic acid
• *Adult:* 50 mg/day for wks 1-2, then increase to 100 mg divided bid for wks 3-4; maintenance, 300-500 mg/day
With valproic acid
• *Adult:* 25 mg qod wks 1-4, then 150 mg/day in divided doses
Available forms: Tabs 25, 100, 150, 200 mg
Side effects/adverse reactions:
CNS: ***Dizziness,*** ataxia, ***headache,*** fever, insomnia, tremor, depression, anxiety
EENT: Nystagmus, ***diplopia, blurred vision***
GI: ***Nausea, vomiting, anorexia, abdominal pain,*** hepatotoxicity
GU: ***Dysmenorrhea***
INTEG: ***Rash,*** alopecia, photosensitivity
Contraindications: Hypersensitivity
Precautions: Pregnancy (C), lactation, child <16, renal, hepatic disease
Pharmacokinetics: Half-life varies depending on dose
Interactions:
• Increased metabolic clearance: carbenazine, phenobarbital, phenytoin
• Decreased metabolic clearance: valproic acid
NURSING CONSIDERATIONS
Assess:
• For seizure activity: duration, type, intensity, halo before seizure
Evaluate:
• Therapeutic response: decrease in severity of seizures
Teach patient/family:
• To take PO doses divided with or after meals to decrease adverse effects, not to discontinue drug abruptly; seizures may occur
• To avoid hazardous activities until stabilized on drug
• To carry Medic Alert ID, to notify prescriber of skin rash or increased seizure activity, to use sunscreen and protective clothing if photosensitivity occurs
• To notify prescriber if pregnant or intend to become pregnant

leucovorin (℞)
(loo-koe-vor'in)
leucovorin calcium, Wellcovorin
Func. class.: Vitamin/folic acid antagonist antidote
Chem. class.: Tetrahydrofolic acid derivative

Action: Needed for normal growth patterns; prevents toxicity during antineoplastic therapy by protecting normal cells
Uses: Megaloblastic or macrocytic anemia caused by folic acid deficiency, overdose of folic acid antagonist, methotrexate toxicity, toxicity caused by pyrimethamine or trimethoprim, pneumocystosis, toxoplasmosis
Dosage and routes:
Megaloblastic anemia caused by enzyme deficiency
• *Adult and child:* PO/IV/IM up to 1 mg/day
Megaloblastic anemia caused by deficiency of folate
• *Adult and child:* IM 1 mg or less qd until adequate response
Methotrexate toxicity
• *Adult and child:* PO/IM/IV given 6-36 hr after dose of methotrexate 10 mg/m^2, then 10 mg/m^2 q6hr × 72 hr
Pyrimethamine toxicity
• *Adult and child:* PO/IM 5 mg qd

L

Trimethoprim toxicity
• *Adult and child:* PO/IM 400 mg qd
Available forms: Tabs 5, 10, 15, 25 mg; inj 3, 5 mg/ml; powder for inj 10 mg/ml
Side effects/adverse reactions:
RESP: Wheezing
INTEG: Rash, pruritus, erythema, thrombocytosis, urticaria
Contraindications: Hypersensitivity, anemias other than megaloblastic not associated with Vit B_{12} deficiency
Precautions: Pregnancy (C)
Interactions:
• Decreased folate levels: chloramphenicol
• Increased metabolism of phenobarbitol, hydantoins
Syringe/Y-site compatibilities: Bleomycin, cisplatin, cyclophosphamide, doxorubicin, fluorouracil, furosemide, heparin, methotrexate, metoclopramide, mitomycin, vinblastine, vincristine
Additive compatiblilities: Cisplatin, floxuridine, fluorouracil
NURSING CONSIDERATIONS
Assess:
• CrCl before leucovorin rescue and qd to detect nephrotoxicity
• I&O; watch for nausea and vomiting
• Nutritional status: bran, yeast, dried beans, nuts, fruits, fresh vegetables, asparagus, which have high folic acid levels
• Other drugs taken: alcohol, hydantoins, trimethoprim may cause increased folic acid use by body
Administer:
• Within 1 hr of folic acid antagonist
• For IV reconstitute 50 mg/5 ml bacteriostatic or sterile H_2O for inj (10 mg/ml) or (100 mg/10 ml) use immediately if sterile H_2O is used
• Give by direct IV over 60 mg/min or less
• Give by intermittent inf after diluting in 100-500 ml of 0.9% NaCl, D_5W, $D_{10}W$, LR, Ringer's sol
Perform/provide:
• Increase fluid intake if used to treat folic acid inhibitor overdose
• Protection from light and heat
Evaluate:
• Therapeutic response: increased weight; improved orientation, well-being; absence of fatigue
Teach patient/family:
• For leucovorin rescue have patient drink 3L fluid qd of rescue
• For folic acid deficiency to eat folic acid rich foods: bran, yeast, dried beans, nuts, fresh green leafy vegetables
• To take drug exactly as prescribed
• To notify prescriber of side effects
• To report signs of hyposensitivity reaction immediately

leuprolide (℞)

(loo-proe'lide)
Leupron Depo Ped, Lupron, Lupron Depot
Func. class.: Antineoplastic hormone
Chem. class.: Gonadotropin-releasing hormone

Action: Causes initial increase in circulating levels of LH, FSH; continuous administration results in decreased LH, FSH; in men, testosterone is reduced to castrate levels; in premenopausal women, estrogen is reduced to menopausal levels
Uses: Metastatic prostate cancer, management of endometriosis
Dosage and routes:
• *Adult:* SC 1 mg/day
Available forms: Inj IM (depot) 3.75 mg, 7.5 mg single dose, multiple

dose vials (5 mg/ml), pediatric depot 7.5, 11.25, 15 mg

Side effects/adverse reactions:
GU: Edema, hot flashes, impotence, decreased libido, amenorrhea, vaginal dryness, gynecomastia

Contraindications: Hypersensitivity to GnRH or analogs, thromboembolic disorders, pregnancy (X), lactation, undiagnosed vaginal bleeding

Precautions: Edema, hepatic disease, CVA, MI, seizures, hypertension, diabetes mellitus

Pharmacokinetics: SC: onset 1-2 wk, peak 2-4 wk; absorbed rapidly (SC), slowly (IM depot); half-life 3 hr

NURSING CONSIDERATIONS

Assess:
• For symptoms of endometriosis (lower abdominal pain)
• Liver function tests before, during therapy (bilirubin, AST [SGOT], ALT [SGPT], LDH) as needed or monthly
• Pituitary gonadotropic and gonadal function during therapy and 4-8 wk after therapy is decreased
• Worsening of signs and symptoms; normal during beginning therapy
• Fatigue, increased pulse, pallor, lethargy
• Food preferences; list likes, dislikes
• Edema in feet, joints; stomach pain; shaking
• Symptoms indicating severe allergic reaction: rash, pruritus, urticaria, purpuric skin lesions, itching, flushing
• For central precocious puberty (CPP) if treatment is for this condition; secondary S4 characteristics to child <9 yr, estradiol/testosterone levels, GnRH test, tomography of head, adrenal steroids, chorionic gonadotropin, wrist x-ray, height, weight

Administer:
• IM/SC using syringe and drug packaged together, give deep in large muscle mass, rotate sites
• Use depot IM only
• Reconstitute vial (single dose)/1 ml of diluent, shake, use immediately

Perform/provide:
• Nutritious diet with iron, vitamin supplements as ordered
• Storage in tight container at room temp

Evaluate:
• Therapeutic response: decreased tumor size and spread of malignancy

Teach patient/family:
• To notify prescriber if menstruation continues; menstruation should stop
• To use a nonhormonal method of contraception during therapy
• That bone pain will disappear after 1 wk
• To report any complaints, side effects to nurse or prescriber
• How to prepare, give; to rotate sites for SC injections
• To keep accurate records of dose
• That tumor flare may occur: increase in size of tumor, increased bone pain, will subside rapidly; may take analgesics for pain; premenopausal women must use mechanical birth control; ovulation may be induced

---

levamisole (℞)

(lee-vam′i-sol)

Ergamisol

Func. class.: Antineoplastic-Immunomodulator

Action: May increase the action of macrophages, monocytes, T cells, which will restore immune function; complete action unknown

Uses: Treatment of Dukes' stage C colon cancer given with fluorouracil after surgical resection

Investigational uses: Malignant melanoma (advanced)

Dosage and routes:

• *Adult:* PO 50 mg q8h × 3d; begin treatment at least 1 wk but no more than 4 wk after resection; given with fluorouracil 450 mg/m^2/d; IV given daily × 5d beginning 21-34d after resection; maintenance is 50 mg q8h × 3d q2wk × 1 yr; given with fluorouracil 45 mg/m^2/d by IV push qwk starting 28d after the initial 5-d course × 1 yr

Available forms: Tab 50 mg (base), IV

Side effects/adverse reactions:

CNS: Dizziness, headache, paresthesia, somnolence, depression, anxiety, fatigue, fever, mental changes, ataxia, insomnia

GI: Nausea, vomiting, anorexia, diarrhea, stomatitis, constipation, flatulence, dyspepsia, abdominal pain

INTEG: Rash, pruritus, alopecia, dermatitis, urticaria

HEMA: ***Granulocytopenia, leukopenia, thrombocytopenia***

CV: Chest pain, edema

META: Hyperbilirubinemia

EENT: Blurred vision, conjunctivitis

OTHER: Rigors, infection, altered sense of smell, arthralgia, myalgia

Contraindications: Hypersensitivity

Precautions: Pregnancy (C), lactation, children, blood dyscrasias

Pharmacokinetics: Peak 1.5-2 hr, elimination half-life 3-4 hr; metabolized by the liver

Interactions:

• Increased plasma levels: phenytoin

• Disulfiram-like reaction: alcohol

NURSING CONSIDERATIONS

Assess:

• Kidney, liver function studies: BUN, creatinine, AST (SGOT), ALT (SGPT), alk phosphatase, bilirubin

• Baseline blood counts with differential, platelets, electrolyte, repeat q3mo for 1 yr; if platelets are <100,000/mm^3, therapy should be discontinued and restarted after recovery; fluorouracil should not be given if WBC is 2500-3500/mm^3; after WBC is >3500/mm^3, dose should be reduced by 20%; if WBC <2500/mm^3 for 10 days, discontinue levamisole

• Stomatitis or GI symptoms: drug may have to be discontinued; then start fluorouracil 28 days after the start of 1st course

• Blood dyscrasias (anemia, granulocytopenia); bruising, fatigue, bleeding, poor healing

• Allergic reactions: dermatitis, exfoliative dermatitis, pruritus, urticaria

Administer:

• 7-20 days after surgery; start fluorouracil with 2nd course of levamisole; begin no sooner than 21d and no later than 35d after surgery; if levamisole therapy begins 21-30d after resection, fluorouracil should be given with 1st course; apply pressure to venipuncture sites for 10 min, especially if platelets are low

Evaluate:

• Therapeutic response: decrease in size and spread of tumor

Teach patient/family:

• To call prescriber if sore throat, swollen lymph nodes, malaise, fever occur, since other infections may occur

• To use contraception during therapy and 4 mo after

• To avoid alcohol; disulfiram re-

---

* Available in Canada only

action can occur; also to avoid tyramine-containing products
• To avoid use of products containing aspirin, ibuprofen; to report bleeding
• To report signs of anemia or CNS reactions
• That hair may be lost during treatment; a wig or hairpiece may be worn

levodopa (℞)

(lee'voe-doe-pa)

Dopar, Larodopa, L-Dopa

Func. class.: Antiparkinson agent

Chem. class.: Catecholamine

Action: Decarboxylation to dopamine, which increases dopamine levels in brain

Uses: Parkinsonism

Dosage and routes:

• *Adult:* PO 0.5-1 g qd divided bid-qid with meals; may increase by up to 0.75 g q3-7d not to exceed 8 g/d unless closely supervised

Available forms: Caps 100, 250, 500 mg; tabs 100, 250, 500 mg

Side effects/adverse reactions:

HEMA: ***Hemolytic anemia, leukopenia, agranulocytosis***

CNS: Involuntary choreiform movements, hand tremors, fatigue, headache, anxiety, twitching, numbness, weakness, confusion, agitation, insomnia, nightmares, psychosis, hallucination, hypomania, severe depression, dizziness

GI: Nausea, vomiting, anorexia, abdominal distress, dry mouth, flatulence, dysphagia, bitter taste, diarrhea, constipation

INTEG: Rash, sweating, alopecia

CV: Orthostatic hypotension, tachycardia, hypertension, palpitation

EENT: Blurred vision, diplopia, dilated pupils

MISC: Urinary retention, incontinence, weight change, dark urine

Contraindications: Hypersensitivity, narrow-angle glaucoma, undiagnosed skin lesions

Precautions: Renal disease, cardiac disease, hepatic disease, respiratory disease, MI with dysrhythmias, convulsions, peptic ulcer, pregnancy (C), asthma, endocrine disease, affective disorders, psychosis, lactation, children <12 yr, peptic ulcer

Pharmacokinetics:

PO: Peak 1-3 hr, excreted in urine (metabolites)

Interactions:

• Hypertensive crisis: MAOIs, furazolidone
• Decreased effects of levodopa: anticholinergics, hydantoins, methionine, papaverine, pyridoxine, tricyclics, benzodiazepines
• Increased effects of levodopa: antacids, metoclopramide

Lab test interferences:

False positive: Urine ketones, urine glucose, Coombs' test

False negative: Urine glucose (glucose oxidase)

False increase: Uric acid, urine protein

Decrease: VMA

NURSING CONSIDERATIONS

Assess:

• Liver function enzymes: AST (SGOT), ALT (SGPT), alk phosphatase, LDH, bilirubin, CBC
• Involuntary movements in parkinsonism: akinesia, tremors, staggering gait, muscle rigidity, drooling
• Levodopa toxicity: mental, personality changes, increased twitching, grimacing, tongue protrusion
• B/P, respiration during initial treatment, hypo/hypertension should be reported

• Mental status: affect, mood, behavioral changes, depression; complete suicide assessment

Administer:

• Drug until NPO before surgery
• Adjust dosage to patient response
• With meals; limit protein taken with drug
• Only after MAOIs have been discontinued for 2 wk

Perform/provide:

• Assistance with ambulation during beginning therapy
• Testing for diabetes mellitus, acromegaly if on long-term therapy

Evaluate:

• Therapeutic response: decrease in akathisia, increased mood

Teach patient/family:

• That therapeutic effects may take several weeks to a few months
• To change positions slowly to prevent orthostatic hypotension
• To report side effects: twitching, eye spasms; indicate overdose
• To use drug exactly as prescribed; if drug is discontinued abruptly, parkinsonian crisis may occur
• That urine, sweat may darken
• To avoid Vit B_6 preparations, vitamin-fortified foods containing B_6; these foods can reverse effects of levodopa

levomethydyle (℞)

(le'vo-meth'y-dyle)

ORLAMM

Func. class.: Narcotic agonist analgesic

Action: Depresses pain impulse transmission at the spinal cord level by interacting with opioid receptors

Uses: Management of opiate dependency

Dosage and routes:

Opiate withdrawal

Usually given 3×/wk (Monday, Wednesday, Friday or Tuesday, Thursday, Saturday)

• *Initial dose:* 20-40 mg each dose at 48 or 72 hr; may be adjusted in increments of 5-10 mg until steady state occurs (1-2 wk); patients dependent on methadone may require larger doses
• *Maintenance:* 60-90 mg 3×/wk
• *Transfer to methadone:* Initial treatment given after 48 hr; may give increased or decreased (5-10 mg) in the daily methadone dose (symptoms of withdrawal)

Available forms: Oral sol 10 mg/ml

Side effects/adverse reactions:

CNS: Drowsiness, dizziness, confusion, headache, sedation, euphoria

CV: Palpitations, bradycardia, change in B/P

EENT: Tinnitus, blurred vision, miosis, diplopia

GI: Nausea, vomiting, anorexia, constipation, cramps, biliary tract spasm

GU: Increased urinary output, dysuria, urinary retention

INTEG: Rash, urticaria, bruising, flushing, diaphoresis, pruritus

RESP: ***Respiratory depression***

Contraindications: Hypersensitivity

Precautions: Addictive personality, pregnancy (B), lactation, increased intracranial pressure, MI (acute), severe heart disease, respiratory depression, hepatic disease, renal disease, child <18 yr

Pharmacokinetics:

PO: Onset 30-60 min, duration 6-8 hr, cumulative 22-48 hr

Metabolized by liver, excreted by kidneys, crosses placenta, excreted in breast milk

Interactions:

• Increased effects with other CNS depressants: alcohol, narcotics, sedative/hypnotics, antipsychotics, skeletal muscle relaxants, rifampin, phenytoin

NURSING CONSIDERATIONS

Assess:

• I&O ratio; check for decreasing output; may indicate urinary retention

Administer:

• With antiemetic for nausea, vomiting

Perform/provide:

• Storage in light-resistant container at room temp

Evaluate:

• Therapeutic response: decreased dependence on opiate
• CNS changes: dizziness, drowsiness, hallucinations, euphoria, LOC, pupil reaction
• Allergic reactions: rash, urticaria
• Respiratory dysfunction: depression, character, rate, rhythm

Teach patient/family:

• To report any symptoms of CNS changes, allergic reactions
• That physical dependency may result after extended period of use
• That withdrawal symptoms may occur: nausea, vomiting, cramps, fever, faintness, anorexia

levonorgestrel implant (℞)

(lee-voe-nor-jess'trel)
Norplant System
Func. class.: Contraceptive system
Chem. class.: Synthetic progestin

Action: As a progestin, transforms proliferative endometrium into secretory endometrium; inhibits secretion of pituitary gonadotropins, which prevents follicular maturation and ovulation

Uses: Prevention of pregnancy for 5 yr

Dosage and routes:

• *Adult:* 6 caps subdermally implanted in the upper arm during 1st 7 days after onset of menses

Available forms: Kit of 6 cap, 36 mg/cap

Side effects/adverse reactions:

CNS: Dizziness, headache, nervousness

GU: Amenorrhea, cervical erosion, breakthrough bleeding, dysmenorrhea, vaginal candidiasis, breast changes, vaginitis

GI: Nausea, abdominal discomfort

INTEG: Alopecia, dermatitis, hirsutism, acne, hypertrichosis, infection at site, pain/itching at site

OTHER: Change in appetite, weight gain

Contraindications: Hypersensitivity, pregnancy (X), thrombophlebitis, undiagnosed genital bleeding, liver tumors, breast carcinoma, liver disease

Precautions: Depression, psychosis, lactation, fluid retention, contact lens wearers

Pharmacokinetics: Max concentration at 24 hr

Interactions:

• Decreased contraception: phenytoin, carbamazepine

NURSING CONSIDERATIONS

Assess:

• Blood studies: cholesterol, triglycerides; may be increased or decreased; sex hormone–binding globulin, thyroxine, T_3 uptake
• Menstrual irregularities: spotting, prolonged bleeding, amenorrhea; usually diminish
• For jaundice, thrombophlebitis; implants should be removed
• For acne, dermatitis, hirsutism, alopecia

Administer:

• 8 cm (3 in) above the crease of the elbow; implantation should be during first 7 days after onset of menses; implantation should be fanlike, 15 degrees apart

Evaluate:

• Therapeutic response: absence of pregnancy

Teach patient/family:

• That if vision problems occur, an ophthalmologist should be seen

• That physical examinations are necessary

---

levorphanol (℞)

(lee-vor'fa-nole)

Levo-Dromoran

Func. class.: Narcotic analgesic (opioid analgesic agonist)

Chem. class.: Opiate, synthetic morphine derivative

Controlled Substance Schedule II

Action: Depresses pain impulse transmission at the spinal cord level by interacting with opioid receptors

Uses: Moderate to severe pain

Dosage and routes:

• *Adult:* PO/SC/IV 2-3 mg q4-5h prn

Available forms: Inj 2 mg/ml; tabs 2 mg

Side effects/adverse reactions:

CNS: Drowsiness, dizziness, confusion, headache, sedation, euphoria

GI: Nausea, vomiting, anorexia, constipation, cramps

GU: Urinary retention, dysuria

INTEG: Rash, urticaria, diaphoresis, pruritus

EENT: Tinnitus, blurred vision, miosis, diplopia

CV: Palpitations, bradycardia, change in B/P

RESP: ***Respiratory depression***

Contraindications: Hypersensitivity, addiction (narcotic)

Precautions: Addictive personality, pregnancy (B), lactation, increased intracranial pressure, MI (acute), severe heart disease, respiratory depression, hepatic disease, renal disease, child <18 yr

Pharmacokinetics:

PO: Onset up to 60 min, peak 1½-2 hr, duration 4-5 hr

SC: Peak 1½ hr, duration 4-5 hr

IV: Peak 20 min, duration 4-5 hr; metabolized by liver; excreted by kidneys; crosses placenta; excreted in breast milk; half-life 11 hr

Interactions:

• Effects may be increased with other CNS depressants: alcohol, narcotics, sedative/hypnotics, antipsychotics, skeletal muscle relaxants

Syringe compatibility: Glycopyrrolate

Lab test interferences:

Increase: Amylase

NURSING CONSIDERATIONS

Assess:

• I&O ratio; check for decreasing output; may indicate urinary retention

• CNS changes: dizziness, drowsiness, hallucinations, euphoria, LOC, pupil reaction

• Allergic reactions: rash, urticaria

• Respiratory dysfunction: respiratory depression, character, rate, rhythm; notify prescriber if respirations are <10/min

• Need for pain medication, physical dependence

Administer:

• With antiemetic if nausea, vomiting occur

• When pain is beginning to return; determine dosage interval by patient response

• IV directly through Y-tube or 3-way stopcock over 5 min; do not give rapidly; circulatory collapse may occur

Perform/provide:

• Storage in light-resistant area at room temp

- Assistance with ambulation
- Safety measures: side rails, night-light, call bell within easy reach

Evaluate:

- Therapeutic response: decrease in pain

Teach patient/family:

- To report any symptoms of CNS changes, allergic reactions
- That physical dependency may result from extended period of use
- Withdrawal symptoms may occur: nausea, vomiting, cramps, fever, faintness, anorexia

Treatment of overdose: Naloxone (Narcan) 0.2-0.8 mg IV, O_2, IV fluids, vasopressors

levothyroxine (℞)

(lee-voe-thye-rox'een)

Levothroid, levothyroxine sodium, Levoxine, Synthroid, T_4

Func. class.: Thyroid hormone

Chem. class.: Levoisomer of thyroxine

Combination products: Euthroid-½: levothyroxine sodium 30 µg, liothyronine sodium 7.5 µg; Euthroid-1: levothyroxine sodium 60 µg, liothyronine sodium 15 µg; Euthroid-2: levothyroxine sodium 120 µg, liothyronine sodium 30 µg; Euthroid-3: levothyroxine sodium 180 µg, liothyronine sodium 45 µg; Thyrolar-¼: levothyroxine sodium 12.5 mg, liothyronine sodium 3.1 µg; Thyrolar-½: levothyroxine sodium 25 µg, liothyronine sodium 6.25 µg; Thyrolar-1: levothyroxine sodium 50 µg, liothyronine sodium 12.5 µg; Thyrolar-2: levothyroxine sodium 100 µg, liothyronine sodium 25 µg; Thyrolar-3: levothyroxine sodium 150 µg, liothyronine sodium 37.5 µg

Action: Increases metabolic rate, controls protein synthesis, increases cardiac output, renal blood flow, O_2 consumption, body temp, blood volume, growth, development at cellular level

Uses: Hypothyroidism, myxedema coma, thyroid hormone replacement, cretinism, thyrotoxicosis

Dosage and routes:

Severe hypothyroidism

- *Adult:* PO 12.5-50 µg qd, increased by 50-100 µg q1-4 wk until desired response, maintenance dose 75-125 µg qd; IM/IV 50-100 µg/day as a single dose
- *Child >12 yr:* PO 2-3 µg/kg/day as a single dose AM
- *Child 6-12 yr:* PO 4-5 µg/kg/day as a single dose AM
- *Child 1-5 yr:* PO 5-6 µg/kg/day as a single dose AM
- *Child 6-12 mo:* PO 6-8 µg/kg/day as a single dose AM
- *Child to 6 mo:* PO 8-10 µg/kg/day as a single dose AM

Myxedema coma

- *Adult:* IV 200-500 µg, may increase by 100-300 µg after 24 hr; place on oral medication as soon as possible

Available forms: Inj 50, 200, 500 µg/vial; tabs 0.025, 0.05, 0.075, 0.088, 0.1, 0.112, 0.125, 0.15, 0.175, 0.2, 0.3 mg

Side effects/adverse reactions:

CNS: Anxiety, insomnia, tremors, headache, ***thyroid storm***

CV: Tachycardia, palpitations, angina, dysrhythmias, hypertension, ***cardiac arrest***

GI: Nausea, diarrhea, increased or decreased appetite, cramps

MISC: Menstrual irregularities, weight loss, sweating, heat intolerance, fever

Contraindications: Adrenal insufficiency, myocardial infarction, thyrotoxicosis

L

Precautions: Elderly, angina pectoris, hypertension, ischemia, cardiac disease, pregnancy (A), lactation

Pharmacokinetics:

PO: Onset unknown, peak 1-3 wk, duration 1-3 wk

IV: Onset 6-8 hr, peak 24 hr, duration unknown

Half-life 6-7 days; distributed throughout body tissues

Interactions:

- Decreased absorption of levothyroxine: cholestyramine
- Increased effects of anticoagulants, sympathomimetics, tricyclic antidepressants
- Decreased effects of digitalis drugs, insulin, hypoglycemics
- Decreased effects of levothyroxine: estrogens
- Considered to be incompatible in syringe with all other drugs

Lab test interferences:

Increase: CPK, LDH, AST (SGOT), PBI, blood glucose

Decrease: TSH, ^{131}I uptake test, uric acid, triglycerides

NURSING CONSIDERATIONS

Assess:

- B/P, pulse before each dose
- I&O ratio
- Weight qd in same clothing, using same scale, at same time of day
- Height, growth rate of a child
- T_3, T_4, FTIs, which are decreased; radioimmunoassay of TSH, which is increased; radio uptake, which is increased if patient is on too low a dose of medication
- Pro-time may require decreased anticoagulant, check for bleeding, bruising
- Increased nervousness, excitability, irritability, which may indicate too high dose of medication, usually after 1-3 wk of treatment
- Cardiac status: angina, palpitation, chest pain, change in VS

Administer:

- IV after diluting with provided diluent 0.5 mg/5 ml; shake; give through Y-tube or 3-way stopcock; give 0.1 mg or less over 1 min; do not add to IV inf; 0.1 mg = 1 ml
- In AM if possible as a single dose to decrease sleeplessness
- At same time each day to maintain drug level
- Only for hormone imbalances; not to be used for obesity, male infertility, menstrual conditions, lethargy
- Lowest dose that relieves symptoms; lower dose to the elderly and in cardiac diseases

Perform/provide:

- Storage in tight, light-resistant container; sol should be discarded if not used immediately
- Withdrawal of medication 4 wk before RAIU test

Evaluate:

- Therapeutic response: absence of depression; increased weight loss, diuresis, pulse, appetite; absence of constipation, peripheral edema, cold intolerance, pale, cool dry skin, brittle nails, alopecia, coarse hair, menorrhagia, night blindness, paresthesias, syncope, stupor, coma, rosy cheeks

Teach patient/family:

- That hair loss will occur in child, is temporary
- To report excitability, irritability, anxiety, which indicate overdose
- Not to switch brands unless approved by prescriber
- That drug may be discontinued after giving birth, thyroid panel evaluated after 1-2 mo
- That hypothyroid child will show almost immediate behavior/personality change
- That drug is not to be taken to reduce weight

• To avoid OTC preparations with iodine; read labels
• To avoid iodine food, iodized salt, soybeans, tofu, turnips, some seafood, some bread
• That drug is not a cure but controls symptoms and treatment is lifelong

lidocaine (topical) (OTC, ℞)

(lye'doe-kane)

Aloe Extra, Anestacon, Burn Relief, Derma Flex, lidocaine HCl topical, lidocaine viscous, Solarcaine, Xylocaine, Xylocaine Viscous, Zilactin-L

Func. class.: Topical anesthetic

Chem. class.: Aminoacylamide

Action: Inhibits nerve impulses from sensory nerves, which produces anesthesia

Uses: Pruritus, sunburn, toothache, sore throat, cold sores, oral pain

Dosage and routes:

• *Adult and child:* TOP apply q3-4h to affected area; INSTILL 15 ml (male) or 5 ml (female) into urethra

Available forms: Liquid 2.5%, 5%; ointment 2.5, 5%; cream 0.5%; gel 0.5, 2.5%; spray 0.5%; spray-oral 10%; sol 2%, 4%; jelly 2%

Side effects/adverse reactions:

INTEG: Rash, irritation, sensitization

Contraindications: Hypersensitivity, application to large areas

Precautions: Sepsis, pregnancy (B), denuded skin

NURSING CONSIDERATIONS

Assess:

• Allergy: rash, irritation, reddening, swelling
• Infection: if affected area is infected, do not apply

Administer:

• After cleansing and drying of affected area

Evaluate:

• Therapeutic response: absence of pain, itching, burning of affected area

Teach patient/family:

• To report rash, irritation, redness, swelling
• How to apply ointment

lidocaine (℞)

(lye-doe-kane)

Anestacon, Baylocaine, L-Caine, Lidopen Auto-Injector, Xylocaine HCl IM for Cardiac Arrythmias, lidocaine HCl IV for Cardiac Arrhythmias, Xylocaine HCl IV for Cardiac Arrhythmias

Func. class.: Antidysrhythmic (Class IB)

Chem. class.: Aminoacyl amide

Action: Increases electrical stimulation threshold of ventricle, His-Purkinje system, which stabilizes cardiac membrane, decreases automaticity

Uses: Ventricular tachycardia, ventricular dysrhythmias during cardiac surgery, myocardial infarction, digitalis toxicity, cardiac catheterization

Dosage and routes:

• *Adult:* IV BOL 50-100 mg (1 mg/kg) over 2-3 min, repeat q3-5min, not to exceed 300 mg in 1 hr; begin IV INF; IV INF 20-50 μg/kg/min; IM 200-300 mg (4.3 mg/kg) in deltoid muscle, may repeat in 1-1½ hr if needed
• *Elderly, CHF reduced liver function:* IV BOL give ½ adult dose
• *Child:* IV BOL 1 mg/kg, then IV INF 30 μg/kg/min

Available forms: IV INF 0.2% (2 mg/ml), 0.4% (4 mg/ml), 0.8% (8 mg/ml); IV Ad 4% (40 mg/ml), 10% (100 mg/ml), 20% (200 mg/ml); IV dir 1% (10 mg/ml), 2% (20 mg/ml); IM 300 mg/ml, 10%

Side effects/adverse reactions:

CNS: Headache, dizziness, involuntary movement, confusion, tremor, drowsiness, euphoria, ***convulsions***

EENT: Tinnitus, blurred vision

GI: Nausea, vomiting, anorexia

CV: Hypotension, bradycardia, ***heart block, cardiovascular collapse, arrest***

RESP: Dyspnea, ***respiratory depression***

INTEG: Rash, urticaria, edema, swelling

MISC: Febrile response, phlebitis at injection site

Contraindications: Hypersensitivity to amides, severe heart block, supraventricular dysrhythmias, Adams-Stokes syndrome, Wolff-Parkinson-White syndrome

Precautions: Pregnancy (B), lactation, children, renal disease, liver disease, CHF, respiratory depression, malignant hyperthermia

Pharmacokinetics:

IV: Onset 2 min, duration 20 min

IM: Onset 5-15 min, duration 1½ hr; half-life 8 min, 1-2 hr (terminal); metabolized in liver; excreted in urine; crosses placenta

Interactions:

• Increased neuromuscular blockade of neuromuscular blockers, tubocurarine

• Increased effects of lidocaine: cimetidine, phenytoin, propranolol, metoprolol

• Decreased effects of lidocaine: barbiturates

Solution compatibilities: D_5W, D_5/0.9% NaCl, D_5/0.45% NaCl, D_5/LR, LR, 0.9% NaCl, 0.45% NaCl

Syringe compatibilities: Carbenicillin, glycopyrrolate, heparin, hydroxyzine, methicillin, metoclopramide, milrinone, moxalactam, nalbuphine

Y-site compatibilities: Altaplase, amiodarone, amrinone, cefazolin, diltiazem, dobutamine, enalaprilat, famotidine, haloperidol, heparin with hydrocortisone sodium succinate, labetalol, meperidine, morphine, nitroglycerin, nitroprusside, potassium chloride, streptokinase, vitamin B with C

Additive compatibilities: Aminophylline, amiodarone, bretylium, calcium chloride, calcium gluceptate, calcium gluconate, chloramphenicol, chlorothiazide, cimetidine, dexamethasone, digoxin, diphenhydramine, dobutamine, dopamine, ephedrine, erythromycin lactobionate, floxacillin, furosemide, heparin, hydrocortisone sodium succinate, hydroxyzine, regular insulin, mephentermine, metaraminol, nitroglycerin, penicillin G potassium, oxytetracycline, pentobarbital, phenylephrine, potassium chloride, procainamide, prochlorperazine, promazine, ranitidine, sodium bicarbonate, tetracycline, verapamil, vitamin B with C

Lab test interferences:

Increase: CPK

NURSING CONSIDERATIONS

Assess:

• ECG continuously to determine increased PR or QRS segments; if these develop, discontinue or reduce rate; watch for increased ventricular ectopic beats; may have to rebolus

• IV infusion rate using infusion pump; run at less than 4 mg/min

• Blood levels (therapeutic level: 1.5-6 μg/ml)

• B/P continuously for fluctuations in cardiac rate

• I&O ratio, electrolytes (K, Na, Cl)
• Malignant hyperthermia: tachypnea, tachycardia, changes in B/P, increased temp
• Respiratory status: rate, rhythm, lung fields for rales, watch for respiratory depression
• CNS effects: dizziness, confusion, psychosis, paresthesias, convulsions; drug should be discontinued
• Lung fields, bilateral rales may occur in CHF patient
• Increased respiration, increased pulse; drug should be discontinued

Administer:

• IV bolus undiluted (1%, 2% only) give 50 mg or less over 1 min or dilute 1 g/250-500 ml of D_5W; titrate to patient response; use infusion pump; pediatric inf is 120 mg of lidocaine/100 ml D_5W; 1-2.5 ml/kg/hr = 20-50 μg/kg/min; use only 1%, 2% sol for IV bol
• IM injection in deltoid; aspirate to avoid intravascular administration; check site daily for infiltration or extravasation

Evaluate:

• Therapeutic response: decreased dysrhythmias

Teach patient/family:

• Use of automatic lidocaine injection device if ordered

Treatment of overdose: O_2, artificial ventilation, ECG; administer dopamine for circulatory depression, diazepam or thiopental for convulsions; decrease drug if needed

lidocaine (local) (℞)

(lye'doe-kane)

Dalcaine, Dilocaine, Duo-Trach Kit, L-Caine, lidocaine HCl, Lidoject-1, Lidoject-2, Nervocaine 1%, Nervocaine 2%, Octocaine HCl, Xylocaine HCl

Func. class.: Local anesthetic

Chem. class.: Amide

Action: Competes with calcium for sites in nerve membrane that control sodium transport across cell membrane; decreases rise of depolarization phase of action potential

Uses: Peripheral nerve block; caudal anesthesia; epidural, spinal, surgical anesthesia

Dosage and routes:

Varies by route of anesthesia

Available forms: Inj 0.5%, 1%, 1.5%, 2%, 4%, 5%; inj with epinephrine 0.5%, 1%, 1.5%, 2%

Side effects/adverse reactions:

CNS: Anxiety, restlessness, ***convulsions, loss of consciousness,*** drowsiness, disorientation, tremors, shivering

CV: ***Myocardial depression, cardiac arrest, dysrhythmias,*** bradycardia, hypotension, hypertension, fetal bradycardia

GI: Nausea, vomiting

EENT: Blurred vision, tinnitus, pupil constriction

INTEG: Rash, urticaria, allergic reactions, edema, burning, skin discoloration at injection site, tissue necrosis

RESP: ***Status asthmaticus, respiratory arrest, anaphylaxis***

Contraindications: Hypersensitivity, child <12 yr, elderly, severe liver disease

Precautions: Elderly, severe drug allergies, pregnancy (C)

L

Pharmacokinetics:
Onset 4-17 min, duration 3-6 hr; metabolized by liver, excreted in urine (metabolites)
Interactions:
• Dysrhythmias: epinephrine, halothane, enflurane
• Hypertension: MAOIs, tricyclic antidepressants, phenothiazines
• Decreased action of lidocaine: chloroprocaine
NURSING CONSIDERATIONS
Assess:
• B/P, pulse, respiration during treatment
• Fetal heart tones if drug is used during labor
• For allergic reactions: rash, urticaria, itching
• Cardiac status: ECG for dysrhythmias, pulse, B/P during anesthesia
Administer:
• Only with crash cart, resuscitative equipment nearby
• Only drugs without preservatives for epidural or caudal anesthesia
Perform/provide:
• Use of new sol; discard unused portions
Evaluate:
• Therapeutic response: anesthesia necessary for procedure
Treatment of overdose: Airway, O_2, vasopressor, IV fluids, anticonvulsants for seizures

lincomycin (℞)
(lin-koe-mye'sin)
Lincocin, Lincorex
Func. class.: Antibacterial
Chem. class.: Lincomycin derivative

Action: Binds to 50S subunit of bacterial ribsomes, suppresses protein synthesis
Uses: Infections caused by group A β-hemolytic streptococci, pneumococci, staphylococci (respiratory tract, skin, soft tissue, urinary tract infections, osteomyelitis, septicemia)
Dosage and routes:
• *Adult:* PO 500 mg q6-8h, not to exceed 8 g/d; IM 600 mg/d or q12h; IV 600 mg-1 g q8-12h; dilute in 100 ml IV sol; infuse over 1 hr, not to exceed 8 g/day
• *Child >1 mo:* PO 30-60 mg/kg/d in divided doses q6-8h; IM 10 mg/kg/d q12h; IV 10-20 mg/kg/d in divided doses q8-12h; dilute to 100 ml IV sol; infuse over 1 hr
Available forms: Caps 500 mg; caps pediatric 250 mg; inj IM, IV 300 mg/ml
Side effects/adverse reactions:
HEMA: ***Leukopenia, eosinophilia, agranulocytosis, thrombocytopenia***
GI: Nausea, vomiting, abdominal pain, tenesmus, diarrhea, ***pseudomembranous colitis***
GU: Increased AST (SGOT), ALT (SGPT), bilirubin, alk phosphatase, jaundice, *vaginitis,* urinary frequency
EENT: Rash, urticaria, pruritus, erythema, pain, abscess at injection site
Contraindications: Hypersensitivity, ulcerative colitis/enteritis, infants <1 mo
Precautions: Renal disease, liver disease, GI disease, elderly, pregnancy (C), lactation
Pharmacokinetics:
PO: Peak 2-4 hr, duration 6 hr
IM: Peak 30 min, duration 8-12 hr, half-life 4-6 hr; metabolized in liver; excreted in urine, bile, feces as active, inactive metabolites; crosses placenta; excreted in breast milk

* Available in Canada only

Interactions:
• Increased neuromuscular blockade: nondepolarizing muscle relaxants
• Decreased absorption of lincomycin: kaolin
• Decreased action of chloramphenicol, erythromycin
• Incompatible with ampicillin, carbenicillin, kanamycin, novobiocin, phenytoin, in sol or syringe; incompatible after 4 hr with penicillin

Lab test interferences:
Increase: Alk phosphatase, bilirubin, CPK, AST (SGOT), ALT (SGPT)

NURSING CONSIDERATIONS

Assess:
• Signs of infection
• Any patient with compromised renal system; drug is excreted slowly in poor renal system function; toxicity may occur rapidly
• Liver studies: AST (SGOT), ALT (SGPT)
• Blood studies: WBC, RBC, Hct, Hgb, platelets, serum iron, reticulocytes; drug should be discontinued if bone marrow depression occurs
• Renal studies: urinalysis, protein, blood, BUN, creatinine
• C&S before drug therapy; drug may be given as soon as culture is taken
• Drug level in impaired hepatic, renal systems
• B/P, pulse in patient receiving drug parenterally
• Bowel pattern before, during treatment
• Skin eruptions, itching, dermatitis
• Respiratory status: rate, character, wheezing, tightness in chest
• Allergies before treatment, reaction of each medication; place allergies on chart in bright red letters; notify all people giving drugs

Administer:
• IV by infusion only; do not administer bolus dose; dilute 1g or less/100 ml or more D_5W, $D_{10}W$, 0.9% NaCl, LR, not to exceed 100 ml/hr; if more than 4 g of drug is to be given, add to 500 ml of sol
• IM deep injection; rotate sites
• Orally with at least 8 oz H_2O on empty stomach

Perform/provide:
• Storage at room temp (caps), up to 2 wk (reconstituted sol)
• Adrenalin, suction, tracheostomy set, endotracheal intubation equipment on unit
• Adequate intake of fluids (2 L) during diarrhea episodes

Evaluate:
• Therapeutic response: decreased temp, negative C&S

Teach patient/family:
• To take oral drug with full glass of water; may give with food if GI symptoms occur
• Aspects of drug therapy: complete entire course of medication to ensure organism death (10-14 days); culture may be taken after completed course of medication
• To report sore throat, fever, fatigue; may indicate superinfection
• That drug must be taken in equal intervals around clock to maintain blood levels
• To notify nurse of diarrhea

Treatment of hypersensitivity:
Withdraw drug; maintain airway; administer epinephrine, aminophylline, O_2, IV corticosteroids

L

lindane (℞)

(lin-dane)

GBH*, G-Well, Kwell, Kwellada*, Kwildane, lindane, Scabene, Thionex

Func. class.: Scabicide/Pediculicide

Chem. class.: Chlorinated hydrocarbon (synthetic)

Action: Stimulates nervous system of arthropods, resulting in seizures, death of organism

Uses: Scabies, lice (head/pubic/body), nits

Dosage and routes:

Lice

- *Adult and child:* CREAM/LOTION wash area with soap, water; remove visible crusts; apply to skin surfaces; remove with soap, water in 8-12 hr; may reapply in 1 wk if needed; shampoo using 30 ml: work into lather, rub for 5 min, rinse, dry with towel; comb with fine-toothed comb to remove nits

Scabies

- *Adult and child:* TOP apply 1% cream/lotion to skin, neck to bottom of feet, toes, repeat in 1 wk prn

Available forms: Lotion, shampoo, cream (1%)

Side effects/adverse reactions:

INTEG: Pruritus, rash, irritation, contact dermatitis

GI: Nausea, vomiting, diarrhea, liver damage (inhalation of vapors)

HEMA: ***Aplastic anemia*** (chronic inhalation of vapors)

CV: ***Ventricular fibrillation*** (chronic inhalation of vapors)

GU: ***Kidney damage*** (chronic inhalation of vapors)

CNS: Tremors, ***convulsions,*** stimulation, dizziness (chronic inhalation of vapors)

Contraindications: Hypersensitivity; premature neonate; patients with known seizure disorders, inflammation of skin, abrasions, or breaks in skin

Precautions: Pregnancy (B); avoid contact with eyes; children <10 yr, infants, lactation

Interactions:

- Oils may enhance absorption; if an oil-based hair dressing is used, shampoo, rinse, dry hair before applying lindane shampoo

NURSING CONSIDERATIONS

Assess:

- Head, hair for lice and nits before and after treatment; if scabies are present check all skin surfaces
- Identify source of infection: school, family, sexual contacts

Administer:

- To body areas, scalp only; do not apply to face, lips, mouth, eyes, any mucous membrane, anus, or meatus
- Topical corticosteroids as ordered to decrease contact dermatitis
- Antihistamines
- Lotions of menthol or phenol to control itching
- Topical antibiotics for infection

Perform/provide:

- Isolation until areas on skin, scalp have cleared and treatment is completed
- Removal of nits by using a fine-toothed comb rinsed in vinegar after treatment; use gloves

Evaluate:

- Therapeutic response: decreased crusts, nits, brownish trails on skin, itching papules in skin folds, decreased itching after several weeks

Teach patient/family:

- To wash all inhabitants' clothing, using insecticide; preventive treatment may be required of all persons living in same house, using lotion or shampoo to decrease spread of in-

* Available in Canada only

fection; use rubber gloves when applying drug
• That itching may continue for 4-6 wk
• That drug must be reapplied if accidently washed off, or treatment will be ineffective
• Not to apply to face; if accidental contact with eyes occurs, flush with water
• To treat sexual contacts simultaneously

Treatment of ingestion: Gastric lavage, saline laxatives, IV diazepam (Valium) for convulsions

liothyronine (T_3) (℞)

(lye-oh-thye'roe-neen)

Cytomel, liothyronine sodium, Triostat

Func. class.: Thyroid hormone

Chem. class.: Synthetic T_3

Action: Increases metabolic rates, cardiac output, O_2 consumption, body temp, blood volume, growth, development at cellular level

Uses: Hypothyroidism, myxedema coma, thyroid hormone replacement, cretinism, nontoxic goiter, T_3 suppression test

Dosage and routes:
• *Adult:* PO 25 μg qd, increased by 12.5-25 μg q1-2wk until desired response, maintenance dose 25-75 μg qd

Cretinism
• *Child >3 yr:* PO 50-100 μg qd
• *Child <3 yr:* PO 5 μg qd, increased by 5 μg q3-4d titrated to response

Myxedema, severe hypothyroidism
• *Adult:* PO 5 μg qd; may increase by 5-10 μg q1-2 wk; maintenance dose 50-100 μg qd

Nontoxic goiter
• *Adult:* PO 5 μg qd, increased by 12.5-25 μg q1-2 wk; maintenance dose 75 μg qd

Suppression test
• *Adult:* PO 75-100 μg qd × 1 wk; radioactive ^{131}I is given before and after 1 wk dose

Available forms: Tabs 5, 25, 50 μg; inj 10 μg/ml

Side effects/adverse reactions:
CNS: Insomnia, tremors, headache, ***thyroid storm***
CV: Tachycardia, palpitations, angina, dysrhythmias, hypertension, ***cardiac arrest***
GI: Nausea, diarrhea, increased or decreased appetite, cramps
MISC: Menstrual irregularities, weight loss, sweating, heat intolerance, fever

Contraindications: Adrenal insufficiency, myocardial infarction, thyrotoxicosis

Precautions: Elderly, angina pectoris, hypertension, ischemia, cardiac disease, pregnancy (A), lactation

Pharmacokinetics:
PO/IV: Peak 12-48 hr, duration 72 hr, half life 6-7 days

Interactions:
• Decreased absorption of liothyronine: cholestyramine
• Increased effects of anticoagulants, sympathomimetics, tricyclic antidepressants
• Decreased effects of digitalis drugs, insulin, hypoglycemics
• Decreased effects of liothyronine: estrogens

Lab test interferences:
Increase: CPK, LDH, AST (SGOT), PBI, blood glucose
Decrease: TSH, ^{131}I uptake test, uric acid, triglycerides

NURSING CONSIDERATIONS

Assess:
• B/P, pulse before each dose

• I&O ratio
• Weight qd in same clothing, using same scale, at same time of day
• Height, growth rate of child
• T_3, T_4, which are decreased; radioimmunoassay of TSH, which is increased; radio uptake, which is increased if patient is on too low a dose of medication
• Pro-time may require decreased anticoagulant; check for bleeding, bruising
• Increased nervousness, excitability, irritability, which may indicate too high dose of medication, usually after 1-3 wk of treatment
• Cardiac status: angina, palpitation, chest pain, change in VS

Administer:
• In AM if possible as a single dose to decrease sleeplessness
• At same time each day to maintain drug level
• Only for hormone imbalances; not to be used for obesity, male infertility, menstrual conditions, lethargy
• Lowest dose that relieves symptoms
• Liothyronine after discontinuing other thyroid preparation

Perform/provide:
• Removal of medication 4 wk before RAIU test

Evaluate:
• Therapeutic response: absence of depression; increased weight loss, diuresis, pulse, appetite; absence of constipation, peripheral edema, cold intolerance, pale, cool dry skin, brittle nails, alopecia, coarse hair, menorrhagia, night blindness, paresthesia, snycope, stupor, coma, rosy cheeks

Teach patient/family:
• That hair loss will occur in child but is temporary
• To report excitability, irritability, anxiety, which indicates overdose
• Not to switch brands unless approved by prescriber
• That hypothyroid child will show almost immediate behavior/personality change
• That drug is not to be taken to reduce weight
• To avoid OTC preparations with iodine; read labels
• To avoid iodine food, iodized salt, soybeans, tofu, turnips, some seafood, some bread
• That drug controls symptoms but does not cure; treatment is lifelong

liotrix (℞)

(lye'oh-trix)
Euthroid, Thyrolar, T_3/T_4
Func. class.: Thyroid hormone
Chem. class.: Levothyroxine/ liothyronine (synthetic T_4, T_3)

Action: Increases metabolic rates, cardiac output, O_2 consumption, body temp, blood volume, growth, development at cellular level

Uses: Hypothyroidism, thyroid hormone replacement

Dosage and routes:
• *Adult and child:* PO 15-30 mg qd, increased by 15-30 mg q1-2wk until desired response; may increase by 15-30 mg q2wk in child
• *Geriatric:* PO 15-30 mg, double dose q6-8wk until desired response

Available forms: Euthroid- ½, 1, 2, 3 gr; Thyrolar- ¼, ½, 1, 2, 3 gr; ½ gr = 30 mg

Side effects/adverse reactions:
CNS: Insomnia, tremors, headache, thyroid storm
CV: Tachycardia, palpitations, angina, dysrhythmias, hypertension, cardiac arrest
GI: Nausea, diarrhea, increased or decreased appetite, cramps

* Available in Canada only

MISC: Menstrual irregularities, weight loss, sweating, heat intolerance, fever

Contraindications: Adrenal insufficiency, myocardial infarction, thyrotoxicosis

Precautions: Elderly, angina pectoris, hypertension, ischemia, cardiac disease, pregnancy (A), lactation

Pharmacokinetics:

PO (T_4): Onset unknown, peak 1-3 wk, duration 1-3 wk

PO (T_3): Onset unknown, peak 24-72 hr, duration 72 hr, half-life 1 wk (T_4) 2 days (T_3)

Interactions:

- Decreased absorption of liotrix: cholestyramine, colestipol
- Increased effects of anticoagulants, sympathomimetics, tricyclic antidepressants, catecholamines
- Decreased effects of digitalis, insulin, hypoglycemics
- Decreased effects of liotrix: estrogens

Lab test interferences:

Increase: CPK, LDH, AST (SGOT), PBI, blood glucose

Decrease: TSH, ^{131}I uptake test, uric acid, triglycerides

NURSING CONSIDERATIONS

Assess:

- B/P, pulse before each dose
- I&O ratio
- Weight qd in same clothing, using same scale, at same time of day
- Height, growth rate of child
- T_3, T_4 FTIs, which are decreased; radioimmunoassay of TSH, which is increased; radio uptake, which is increased if patient is on too low a dose of medication
- Pro-time may require decreased anticoagulant; check for bleeding, bruising
- Increased nervousness, excitability, irritability, which may indicate too high dose of medication, usually after 1-3 wk of treatment
- Cardiac status: angina, palpitation, chest pain, change in VS

Administer:

- In AM if possible as a single dose to decrease sleeplessness
- At same time each day to maintain drug level
- Only for hormone imbalances; not to be used for obesity, male infertility, menstrual conditions, lethargy
- Lowest dose that relieves symptoms

Perform/provide:

- Withdrawal of medication 4 wk before RAIU test
- Storage in air-tight, light-resistant container

Evaluate:

- Therapeutic response: absence of depression; increased weight loss, diuresis, pulse, appetite; absence of constipation, peripheral edema, cold intolerance, pale, cool dry skin, brittle nails, coarse hair, menorrhagia, night blindness, paresthesias, syncope, stupor, coma, rosy cheeks

Teach patient/family:

- That hair loss will occur in child, is temporary
- To report excitability, irritability, anxiety, which indicate overdose
- Not to switch brands unless approved by prescriber
- That hypothyroid child will show almost immediate behavior/personality change
- That drug is not to be taken to reduce weight
- To avoid OTC preparations with iodine; read labels
- To avoid iodine food, iodized salt, soybeans, tofu, turnips, some seafood, some bread

• That drug does not cure, but controls symptoms, treatment is lifelong

lisinopril (℞)

(lyse-in'oh-pril)

Prinivil, Zestril

Func. class.: Angiotensin converting enzyme (ACE) inhibitor

Chem. class.: Enalaprilat lysine analog

Action: Selectively suppresses renin-angiotensin-aldosterone system; inhibits ACE, preventing conversion of angiotensin I to angiotensin II

Uses: Mild to moderate hypertension, adjunctive therapy of CHF

Dosage and routes:

Hypertension

• *Adult:* PO 10-40 mg qd; may increase to 80 mg qd if required

CHF

• Adult PO 5 mg initially with diuretics/digitalis

Available forms: Tabs 2.5, 5, 10, 20, 40 mg

Side effects/adverse reactions:

GI: Nausea, vomiting, anorexia, constipation, flatulence, GI irritation

GU: ***Proteinuria, renal insufficiency,*** sexual dysfunction, impotence

INTEG: Rash, pruritus

CNS: Vertigo, depression, stroke, insomnia, paresthesias, headache, *fatigue,* asthenia

EENT: Blurred vision, nasal congestion

RESP: Cough, dyspnea

Contraindications: Hypersensitivity

Precautions: Pregnancy (C), lactation, renal disease, hyperkalemia

Pharmacokinetics:
Onset 1 hr, peak 6-8 hr, duration 24 hr, excreted unchanged in urine

Interactions:

• Increased hypotensive effect: diuretics, other hypertensives, probenecid

• Decreased effects of lisinopril: aspirin, indomethacin

• Increased K levels: K salt substitutes, K-sparing diuretics, K supplements

• Increased effects of antihypertensives, reserpine, diuretics

• Increased hypersensitivity reactions: allopurinol

• Drug/food: high-potassium diet (bananas, orange juice, avocados, nuts, spinach) should be avoided; hyperkalemia may occur

Lab test interferences:

Interfere: Glucose/insulin tolerance tests

NURSING CONSIDERATIONS

Assess:

• B/P, pulse q4h; note rate, rhythm, quality

• Electrolytes: K, Na, Cl

• Apical/pedal pulse before administration; notify prescriber of any significant changes

• Baselines in renal, liver function tests before therapy begins

• Edema in feet, legs qd

• Skin turgor, dryness of mucous membranes for hydration status

• Symptoms of CHF: edema, dyspnea, wet rales

Evaluate:

• Therapeutic response: decreased B/P, CHF symptoms

Teach patient/family:

• Not to discontinue drug abruptly

• To rise slowly to sitting or standing position to minimize orthostatic hypotension

Treatment of overdose: Lavage, IV atropine for bradycardia, IV theophylline for bronchospasm, digitalis, O_2, diuretic for cardiac failure, hemodialysis

lithium (℞)

(li'thee-um)

Carbolith*, Cibalith-S, Duralith, Eskalith, Eskalith CR, Lithane, lithium carbonate, Lithizine*, Lithonate, Lithotabs

Func. class.: Antimanic

Chem. class.: Alkali metal ion salt

Action: May alter sodium, potassium ion transport across cell membrane in nerve, muscle cells; may balance biogenic amines of norepinephrine, serotonin in CNS areas involved in emotional responses

Uses: Manic-depressive illness (manic phase), prevention of bipolar manic-depressive psychosis

Dosage and routes:

• *Adult:* PO 300-600 mg tid, maintenance 300 mg tid or qid; slow rel tabs 300 mg bid; dose should be individualized to maintain blood levels at 0.5-1.5 mEq/L

• *Child:* PO 15-20 mg (0.4-0.5 mEq)/kg/day in 2-3 divided doses

Available forms: Caps 300, 600 mg; tabs 300 mg; tabs cont rel 450 mg; syrup 300 mg/5ml (8 mEq/5 ml); cap slow rel 150, 300 mg*

Side effects/adverse reactions:

CNS: Headache, drowsiness, dizziness, tremors, twitching, ataxia, ***seizure,*** slurred speech, restlessness, confusion, stupor, memory loss, clonic movements, fatigue

GI: Dry mouth, anorexia, nausea, vomiting, diarrhea, incontinence, abdominal pain, metallic taste

GU: ***Polyuria, glycosuria, proteinuria, albuminuria,*** urinary incontinence, polydipsia, edema

CV: Hypotension, ECG changes, dysrhythmias, ***circulatory collapse,*** edema

INTEG: Drying of hair, alopecia, rash, pruritus, hyperkeratosis, acneiform lesions, folliculitis

HEMA: ***Leukocytosis***

EENT: Tinnitus, blurred vision

ENDO: Hyponatremia, hypothyroidism, goiter, hyperglycemia, hyperthyroidism

MS: Muscle weakness

Contraindications: Hepatic disease, renal disease, brain trauma, OBS, pregnancy (D), lactation, children <12 yr, schizophrenia, severe cardiac disease, severe renal disease, severe dehydration

Precautions: Elderly, thyroid disease, seizure disorders, diabetes mellitus, systemic infection, urinary retention

Pharmacokinetics:

PO: Onset rapid, peak ½-4 hr, half-life 18-36 hr depending on age; crosses blood-brain barrier; 80% of filtered lithium is reabsorbed by the renal tubules, excreted in urine; crosses placenta; enters breast milk; well absorbed by oral method

Interactions:

• Increased hypothyroid effects: antithyroid agents, calcium iodide, potassium iodide, iodinated glycerol

• Brain damage: haloperidol, thioridazine

• Increased effects of neuromuscular blocking agents, phenothiazines

• Increased renal clearance: sodium bicarbonate, acetazolamide, mannitol, aminophylline

• Increased toxicity: indomethacin, diuretics, nonsteroidal antiinflammatories

• Decreased effects of lithium: theophyllines, urea, urinary alkalinizers

L

Lab test interferences:
Increase: K excretion, urine glucose, blood glucose, protein, BUN
Decrease: VMA, T_3, T_4, PBI, ^{131}I

NURSING CONSIDERATIONS

Assess:
- Weight qd; check for and report edema in legs, ankles, wrists
- Na intake; decreased Na intake with decreased fluid intake may lead to lithium retention; increased Na and fluids may decrease lithium retention
- Skin turgor at least qd
- Urine for albuminuria, glycosuria, uric acid during beginning treatment, q2mo thereafter
- Neuro status: LOC, gait, motor reflexes, hand tremors
- Serum lithium levels qwk initially, then q2mo (therapeutic level: 0.5-1.5 mEq/L)

Administer:
- Reduced dose to elderly
- With meals to avoid GI upset
- Adequate fluids (2-3 L/day) to prevent dehydration during initial treatment, 1-2 L/day during maintenance

Evaluate:
- Therapeutic response: decrease in excitement, manic phase

Teach patient/family:
- Symptoms of minor toxicity: vomiting, diarrhea, poor coordination, fine motor tremors, weakness, lassitude; major toxicity: coarse tremors, severe thirst, tinnitus, dilute urine
- To monitor urine specific gravity, emphasize need for follow-up care to determine lithium levels
- That contraception is necessary, since lithium may harm fetus
- Not to operate machinery until lithium levels are stable
- That beneficial effects may take 1-3 wks
- Provide a list of drugs that interact with lithium and discuss need for adequate salt and fluid intake

Treatment of overdose: Induce emesis or lavage, maintain airway, respiratory function; dialysis for severe intoxication

lomefloxacin (℞)

(lome-flox'a-sin)
Maxaquin
Func. class.: Antiinfective
Chem. class.: Fluoroquinolone

Action: Interferes with conversion of intermediate DNA fragments into high-molecular-weight DNA in bacteria; DNA gyrase inhibitor

Uses: Treatment of lower respiratory tract infections (pneumonia, bronchitis), genitourinary infections (prostatitis, UTIs), preoperatively to reduce UTIs in transurethral surgical procedures; gram negative bacteria: *Aeromonas, Citrobater, Enterobacter, Escherichia coli, Haemophilus influenzae, Klebsiella, Legionella, Moraxella catarrhalis, Morganella morganii, Proteus vulgaris, P. mirabilis, Providencia alcalifaciens, P. rettgeri, Pseudomonas aeruginosa, Serratia;* gram positive bacteria: *Staphylococcus aureus, S. epidermidis, S. saprophyticus*

Dosage and routes:
- *Adult:* PO 400 mg/day 7-14 day depending on type of infection

In renal impairment
- *Adult:* PO 200 mg/dose

Prophylaxis of UTI
- *Adult:* PO 400 mg 2-6 hr before surgery

Available forms: Tabs 400

Side effects/adverse reactions:
CNS: Dizziness, headache, somnolence, depression, insomnia, nervousness, confusion, agitation

* Available in Canada only

GI: Diarrhea, nausea, vomiting, anorexia, flatulence, heartburn, dry mouth, increased AST (SGOT), ALT (SGPT), constipation, abdominal pain, oral thrush, glossitis, stomatitis
INTEG: Rash, pruritus, urticaria, photosensitivity
EENT: Visual disturbances
Contraindications: Hypersensitivity to quinolones
Precautions: Pregnancy (C), lactation, children, elderly, renal disease, seizure disorders, excessive exposure to sunlight
Pharmacokinetics:
PO: Peak 1-2 hr, half-life 6-8 hr; excreted in urine as active drug, metabolites
Interactions:
• Decreased effects of lomefloxacin: antacids, nitrofurantoin, sucralfate, iron salts, zinc salts
• Increased lomefloxacin levels: probenecid, cimetidine
• Increased levels of cyclosporine, warfarin

NURSING CONSIDERATIONS
Assess:
• Kidney, liver function studies: BUN, creatinine, AST (SGOT), ALT (SGPT)
• I&O ratio, urine pH; <5.5 is ideal
• CNS symptoms: insomnia, vertigo, headache, agitation, confusion
• Allergic reactions: rash, flushing, urticaria, pruritus
Administer:
• After clean-catch urine for C&S
Perform/provide:
• Limited intake of alkaline foods, drugs; milk, dairy products, peanuts, vegetables, alkaline actacids, sodium bicarbonate
Evaluate:
• Therapeutic response: negative C&S
Teach patient/family:
• That fluids must be increased to 3L/day to avoid crystallization in kidneys
• That if dizziness or light-headedness occurs, to ambulate, perform activities with assistance
• To complete full course of drug therapy
• To contact prescriber if adverse reactions occur
• To avoid iron- or mineral-containing supplements within 2 hr before and after dosing
• That photosensitivity may occur and sunscreen should be used

lomustine (℞)

(loe-mus'teen)
CCNU, CeeNU
Func. class.: Antineoplastic alkylating agent
Chem. class.: Nitrosourea

Action: Responsible for cross-linking DNA strands, which leads to cell death; activity is not cell cycle phase specific
Uses: Hodgkin's disease, lymphomas, melanomas, multiple myeloma; brain, lung, bladder, kidney, colon cancer
Investigational uses: Brain, breast, renal, GI tract, bronchogenic carcinoma; melanomas
Dosage and routes:
• *Adult:* PO 130 mg/m^2 as a single dose q6wk; titrate dose to WBC; do not give repeat dose unless WBC >4000/mm^3, platelet count >100,000/mm^3
Available forms: Cap 10, 40, 100 mg
Side effects/adverse reactions:
HEMA: ***Thrombocytopenia, leukopenia, myelosuppression, anemia***

GI: Nausea, vomiting, anorexia, stomatitis, ***hepatotoxicity***
GU: ***Azotemia, renal failure***
INTEG: Burning at injection site
RESP: ***Fibrosis, pulmonary infiltrate***

Contraindications: Hypersensitivity, leukopenia, thrombocytopenia, pregnancy (D)

Precautions: Radiation therapy

Pharmacokinetics:
Metabolized in liver, excreted in urine; half-life 16-48 hr; 50% protein bound; crosses blood-brain barrier; appears in breast milk

Interactions:
- Increased toxicity: barbiturates, phenytoin, chloral hydrate
- Increased metabolism of lomustine: phenobarbital
- Potentiation of lomustine: succinylcholine
- Increased bone marrow depression: allopurinol

NURSING CONSIDERATIONS

Assess:
- CBC, differential, platelet count qwk; withhold drug if WBC <4000 or platelet count <75,000; notify prescriber
- Pulmonary function tests, chest x-ray films before, during therapy; chest film should be obtained q2wk during treatment
- Renal function studies: BUN, serum uric acid, urine CrCl before, during therapy
- I&O ratio; report fall in urine output of 30 ml/hr
- Monitor temp q4h (may indicate beginning infection); no rectal temps
- Liver function tests before, during therapy (bilirubin, AST [SGOT], ALT [SGPT], LDH) as needed or monthly
- Bleeding: hematuria, guaiac, bruising or petechiae, mucosa or orifices q8h
- Dyspnea, rales, unproductive cough, chest pain, tachypnea
- Food preferences; list likes, dislikes
- Yellowing of skin and sclera, dark urine, clay-colored stools, itchy skin, abdominal pain, fever, diarrhea
- Inflammation of mucosa, breaks in skin
- Buccal cavity q8h for dryness, sores or ulceration, white patches, oral pain, bleeding, dysphagia
- Local irritation, pain, burning, discoloration at injection site
- Symptoms indicating severe allergic reaction: rash, pruritus, urticaria, purpuric skin lesions, itching, flushing

Administer:
- Antiemetic 30-60 min before giving drug to prevent vomiting
- Antibiotics for prophylaxis of infection
- Topical or systemic analgesics for pain
- Local or systemic drugs for infection

Perform/provide:
- Storage in tight container at room temp
- Strict medical asepsis, protective isolation if WBC levels are low
- Special skin care
- Deep-breathing exercises with patient tid-qid; place in semi-Fowler's position
- Increase fluid intake to 2-3 L/day to prevent urate deposits, calculi formation
- Rinsing of mouth tid-qid with water, club soda; brushing of teeth bid-tid with soft brush or cotton-tipped applicators for stomatitis; use unwaxed dental floss

Evaluate:
- Therapeutic response: decreased tumor size, spread of malignancy

* Available in Canada only

Teach patient/family:
- About protective isolation
- To report any changes in breathing or coughing
- To avoid foods with citric acid, hot or rough texture if buccal inflammation is present
- To report any bleeding, white spots or ulcerations in mouth to prescriber; tell patient to examine mouth qd
- To report signs of infection: fever, sore throat, flu symptoms
- To report signs of anemia: fatigue, headache, faintness, shortness of breath, irritability
- To avoid use of razors, commercial mouthwash
- To avoid use of aspirin products or ibuprofen

loperamide (OTC, ℞)

(loe-per'a-mide)

A-D Kaopectate II Caplets, loperamide solution, Imodium, Imodium A-D, Imodium A-D Caplet, loperamide, Maalox Antidiarrheal Caplets, Pepto Diarrhea Control

Func. class.: Antidiarrheal

Chem. class.: Piperidine derivative

Action: Direct action on intestinal muscles to decrease GI peristalsis; reduces volume, increases bulk, electrolytes not lost

Uses: Diarrhea (cause undetermined), chronic diarrhea, ileostomy discharge

Dosage and routes:
- *Adult:* PO 4 mg, then 2 mg after each loose stool, not to exceed 16 mg/d
- *Child 2-5 yr:* PO 1 mg then 0.1 mg/kg after each loose stool
- *Child 5-8 yr:* PO 2 mg bid on day 1, then 0.1 mg/kg after each loose stool
- *Child 8-12 yr:* PO 2 mg tid on day 1, then 0.1 mg/kg after each loose stool

Available forms: Caps 2 mg; liq 1 mg/5 ml; tabs 2 mg

Side effects/adverse reactions:

CNS: Dizziness, drowsiness, fatigue, fever

GI: Nausea, dry mouth, vomiting, constipation, abdominal pain, anorexia, ***toxic megacolon***

INTEG: Rash

RESP: ***Respiratory depression***

Contraindications: Hypersensitivity, severe ulcerative colitis, pseudomembranous colitis, acute diarrhea associated with *E. coli*

Precautions: Pregnancy (B), lactation, children <2 yr, liver disease, dehydration, bacterial disease

Pharmacokinetics:

PO: Onset ½-1 hr, duration 4-5 hr, half-life 7-14 hr; metabolized in liver; excreted in feces as unchanged drug; small amount in urine

Interactions:
- Do not mix oral sol with other sols

NURSING CONSIDERATIONS

Assess:
- Stools: volume, color, characteristics
- Electrolytes (K, Na, Cl) if on long-term therapy
- Skin turgor q8h if dehydration is suspected
- Bowel pattern before; for rebound constipation
- Response after 48 hr; if no response, drug should be discontinued
- Dehydration in children
- Abdominal distention, toxic megacolon; may occur in ulcerative colitis

Administer:
- For 48 hr only, cont inf

Perform/provide:
• Storage in tight container
Evaluate:
• Therapeutic response: decreased diarrhea
Teach patient/family:
• To avoid OTC products unless directed by prescriber
• That ostomy patient may take this drug for extended time
• That if drowsiness occurs, not to operate machinery
• To use hard candy, sips of water for dry mouth

loracarbef (℞)

(lor-a-kar'beff)
Lorabid
Func. class.: Antiinfective
Chem. class.: Carbacephem

Action: Inhibits bacterial cell wall synthesis, which renders cell wall osmotically unstable
Uses: Gram-negative: *H. influenzae, E. coli, P. mirabilis, Klebsiella;* gram-positive: *S. pneumoniae, S. pyogenes, S. aureus;* upper and lower respiratory tract, urinary tract, skin infections; otitis media; pharyngitis, tonsillitis
Dosage and routes:
• *Adult and child >13:* PO 200-400 mg q12h
• *Child to 12 yr:* PO 15-30 mg/kg/day in 2 divided doses q12h
Available forms: Caps 200 mg; 100, 200 mg/5 ml oral susp
Side effects/adverse reactions:
CNS: Dizziness, headache, fatigue, paresthesia, fever, chills, confusion
GI: Diarrhea, nausea, vomiting, anorexia, dysgeusia, glossitis, bleeding, increased AST (SGOT), ALT (SGPT), bilirubin, LDH, alk phosphatase, abdominal pain, loose stools, flatulence, heartburn, stomach cramps, colitis, jaundice
INTEG: Rash, urticaria, dermatitis, ***anaphylaxis***
GU: Vaginitis, pruritus, candidiasis, increased BUN, ***nephrotoxicity, renal failure,*** pyuria, dysuria, reversible interstitial nephritis
HEMA: ***Leukopenia, thrombocytopenia, agranulocytosis,*** anemia, ***neutropenia, lymphocytosis, eosinophilia, pancytopenia, hemolytic anemia, leukocytosis, granulocytopenia***
RESP: Dyspnea
Contraindications: Hypersensitivity to cephalosporins or related antibiotics, seizures
Precautions: Pregnancy (B), lactation, children, renal disease
Pharmacokinetics:
PO: Peak 1 hr, half-life 1 hr; excreted in urine as unchanged drug
Interactions:
• Decreased effects: tetracyclines, erythromycins
• Increased effect/toxicity: aminoglycosides, furosemide, probenecid, ethacrynic acid, vancomycin
Lab test interferences:
Increase (false): Creatinine (serum urine), urinary 17-KS
False positive: Urinary protein, direct Coombs' test, urine glucose testing (clinitest)
Interference: Cross-matching
NURSING CONSIDERATIONS
Assess:
• Nephrotoxicity: increased BUN, creatinine
• I&O ratio
• Blood studies: AST (SGOT), ALT (SGPT), CBC, Hct, bilirubin, LDH, alk phosphatase, Coombs' test qmo if patient is on long-term therapy
• Electrolytes: K, Na, Cl qmo if patient is on long-term therapy
• Bowel pattern qd; if severe diarrhea occurs, drug should be discon-

tinued; may indicate pseudomembranous colitis
• Urine output; if decreasing, notify prescriber (may indicate nephrotoxicity)
• Allergic reactions: rash, flushing, urticaria, pruritus
• Bleeding: ecchymosis, bleeding gums, hematuria, stool guaiac daily
• Overgrowth of infection: perineal itching, fever, malaise, redness, pain, swelling, drainage, rash, diarrhea, change in cough, sputum

Administer:
• 1 hr before or 2 hr after a meal
• After C&S is completed
• For 7 days to ensure organism death, prevent superinfection

Evaluate:
• Therapeutic response: negative C&S

Teach patient/family:
• If diabetic use blood glucose testing
• Not to drink alcohol or take meds with alcohol or reaction may occur
• Complete full course of drug therapy
• Take on an empty stomach 1 hr before or 2 hr after a meal
• Notify prescriber if breast-feeding or of any side effects

Treatment of overdose: Epinephrine, antihistamines; resuscitate if needed (anaphylaxis)

loratadine (℞)

(lor-a'ti-deen)
Claritin

Func. class.: Antihistamine
Chem. class.: Selective histamine (H_1) receptor antagonist

Action: Binds to peripheral histamine receptors, providing antihistamine action without sedation
Uses: Seasonal rhinitis
Dosage and routes:
• *Adult:* PO 10 mg qd
Available forms: Tabs 10 mg
Side effects/adverse reactions:
CNS: Sedation (more common with increased doses)
Contraindications: Hypersensitivity, acute asthma attacks, lower respiratory tract disease
Precautions: Pregnancy (B), increased intraocular pressure, bronchial asthma
Pharmacokinetics:
Peak 1½ hr, elimination half-life 14½ hr; metabolized in liver to active metabolites, excreted in urine
Interactions:
• Additive CNS depressant effects: alcohol, other CNS depressants

NURSING CONSIDERATIONS
Perform/provide:
• Storage in tight container at room temp

Evaluate:
• Therapeutic response: absence of running or congested nose

Teach patient/family:
• To avoid driving, other hazardous activities if drowsiness occurs

lorazepam (℞)

(lor-a'ze-pam)
Alzapam, Apo-Lorazepam*, Ativan, Loraz, lorazepam, Novolorazem*

Func. class.: Sedative/hypnotic; antianxiety
Chem. class.: Benzodiazepine

Controlled Substance Schedule IV
Action: Potentiates the actions of GABA, especially in system and reticular formation
Uses: Anxiety, irritability in psychiatric or organic disorders, preoperatively, insomnia, adjunct in endoscopic procedures

Dosage and routes:
Anxiety
• Adult: PO 2-6 mg/day in divided doses, not to exceed 10 mg/day
Insomnia
• Adult: PO 2-4 mg hs; only minimally effective after 2 wk continuous therapy
Preoperatively
• *Adult:* IM 50 μg/kg 2 hr prior to surgery; IV 44 μg/kg 15-20 min prior to surgery
Available forms: Tabs 0.5, 1, 2 mg; inj 2, 4 mg/ml; conc sol 0.2 mg/ml
Side effects/adverse reactions:
CNS: Dizziness, drowsiness, confusion, headache, anxiety, tremors, stimulation, fatigue, depression, insomnia, hallucinations, weakness, unsteadiness
GI: Constipation, dry mouth, nausea, vomiting, anorexia, diarrhea
INTEG: Rash, dermatitis, itching
CV: Orthostatic hypotension, ***ECG changes, tachycardia,*** hypotension
EENT: Blurred vision, tinnitus, mydriasis
Contraindications: Hypersensitivity to benzodiazepines, narrow-angle glaucoma, psychosis, pregnancy (D), lactation, child <12 yr, history of drug abuse, COPD
Precautions: Elderly, debilitated, hepatic disease, renal disease
Pharmacokinetics:
PO: Onset ½ hr, peak 1-6 hr, duration 24-48 hr
IM: Onset 15-30 min, peak 1-1½ hr, duration 24-48 hr
IV: Onset 5-15 min, peak unknown, duration 24-48 hr
Metabolized by liver; excreted by kidneys; crosses placenta, breast milk; half-life 14 hr
Interactions:
• Decreased effects of lorazepam: oral contraceptives, valproic acid
• Increased effects of lorazepam: CNS depressants, alcohol, disulfiram, oral contraceptives
Syringe compatibility: Cimetidine
Y-site compatibilities: Acyclovir, atracurium, fludarabine, melphalan, paclitaxel, pancuronium, vecuronium, vinorelbine, zidovudine
Lab test interferences:
Increase: AST (SGOT), ALT (SGPT), serum bilirubin
Decrease: RAIU
False increase: 17-OHCS

NURSING CONSIDERATIONS
Assess:
• B/P (lying, standing), pulse; if systolic B/P drops 20 mm Hg, hold drug, notify prescriber; respirations q5-15 min if given IV
• Blood studies: CBC during long-term therapy; blood dyscrasias have occurred rarely
• Hepatic studies: AST (SGOT), ALT (SGPT), bilirubin, creatinine, LDH, alk phosphatase
• Mental status: mood, sensorium, affect, sleeping pattern, drowsiness, dizziness
• Physical dependency, withdrawal symptoms: headache, nausea, vomiting, muscle pain, weakness, tremors, convulsions, after long-term, excessive use
• Suicidal tendencies
Administer:
• With food or milk for GI symptoms
• Crushed if patient is unable to swallow medication whole
• Sugarless gum, hard candy, frequent sips of water for dry mouth
• IV after diluting in equal vol sterile H_2O, 5% dextrose or 0.9% NaCl for inj; give through Y-tube or 3-way stopcock; give at 2 mg or less over 1 min
• Deep into large muscle mass (IM inj)

* Available in Canada only

Perform/provide:

- Assistance with ambulation during beginning therapy, since drowsiness/dizziness occurs
- Safety measures, including side rails
- Check to see whether PO medication has been swallowed
- Refrigerate parenteral form

Evaluate:

- Therapeutic response: decreased anxiety, restlessness, insomnia

Teach patient/family:

- That drug may be taken with food
- Not to be used for everyday stress or used longer than 4 mo unless directed by prescriber
- Not to take more than prescribed amount; may be habit forming
- To avoid OTC preparations (cough, cold, hay fever) unless approved by prescriber
- To avoid driving, activities that require alertness, since drowsiness may occur
- To avoid alcohol ingestion, other psychotropic medications, unless directed by prescriber
- Not to discontinue medication abruptly after long-term use
- To rise slowly or fainting may occur, especially elderly
- That drowsiness may worsen at beginning of treatment
- To use birth control if child-bearing age

Treatment of overdose: Lavage, VS, supportive care, flumazenil

losartan

(lo-zar′tan)

Cozaar

Func. class.: Antihypertensive

Chem. class.: Angiotensin II receptor (Type AT_1)

Action: Blocks the vasoconstrictor and aldosterone-secreting effects of angiotensin II; selectively blocks the binding of angiotensin II to the AT_1 receptor found in tissues

Uses: Hypertension, alone or in combination

Dosage and routes:

- *Adult:* PO 50 mg qd alone or 25 mg qd when used in combination

Available forms: Tabs 25, 50 mg

Side effects/adverse reactions:

CNS: Dizziness, insomnia, anxiety, confusion, abnormal dreams, migraine, tremor, vertigo

CV: Angina pectoris, 2nd degree AV block, ***cerebrovascular accident,*** hypotension, *myocardial infarction, dysrhythmias*

EENT: Blurred vision, burning eyes, conjunctivitis, task perversion

GI: Diarrhea, dyspepsia, anorexia, constipation, dry mouth, flatulence, gastritis, vomiting

GU: Impotence, nocturia, urinary frequency, UTI

HEMA: Anemia

INTEG: Alopecia, dermatitis, dry skin, flushing, photosensitivity, rash, pruritus, sweating

META: Gout

MS: Cramps, myalgia, pain, stiffness

RESP: Cough, upper respiratory infection, congestion, dyspnea, bronchitis

Contraindications: Hypersensitivity

Precautions: Hypersensitivity to ACE inhibitors; Pregnancy (C) 1st trimester, (D) 2nd and 3rd trimesters; lactation, children, elderly

Pharmacokinetics: Extensively metabolized, half-life 2 hr, metabolite 6-9 hr, highly bound to plasma proteins, excreted in urine and feces

Interactions: None significant

NURSING CONSIDERATIONS

Assess:

- B/P, pulse q4h; note rate, rhythm, quality

• Electrolytes: K, Na, Cl
• Baselines in renal, liver function tests before therapy begins
• Edema in feet, legs qd
• Skin turgor, dryness of mucous membranes for hydration status

Administer:
• Without regard to meals

Evaluate:
• Therapeutic response: decreased B/P

Teach patient/family:
• To avoid sunlight or wear sunscreen if in sunlight; photosensitivity may occur
• To comply with dosage schedule, even if feeling better
• To notify prescriber of mouth sores, fever, swelling of hands or feet, irregular heartbeat, chest pain
• Excessive perspiration, dehydration, vomiting, diarrhea; may lead to fall in blood pressure; consult prescriber if these occur
• That drug may cause dizziness, fainting; light-headedness may occur
• To rise slowly to sitting or standing position to minimize orthostatic hypotension

lovastatin (℞)

(lo'va-sta-tin)
Mevacor
Func. class.: Cholesterol-lowering agent
Chem. class.: Aspergillus terreus strain derivative

Action: Inhibits HMG-COA reductase enzyme, which reduces cholesterol synthesis
Uses: As an adjunct in primary hypercholesterolemia (types IIa, IIb), mixed hyperlipidemia
Dosage and routes:
(Patient should first be placed on a cholesterol-lowering diet)
• *Adult:* PO 20 mg qd with evening meal; may increase to 20-80 mg/d in single or divided doses, not to exceed 80 mg/d; dosage adjustments should be made qmo
Available forms: Tabs 20, 40 mg
Side effects/adverse reactions:
GI: Nausea, constipation, diarrhea, dyspepsia, flatus, abdominal pain, heartburn, ***liver dysfunction***
MS: Muscle cramps, myalgia, ***myositis, rhabdomyolysis***
CNS: Dizziness, headache
INTEG: Rash, pruritus
EENT: Blurred vision, dysgeusia, lens opacities
Contraindications: Hypersensitivity, pregnancy (X), lactation, active liver disease
Precautions: Past liver disease, alcoholism, severe acute infections, trauma, hypotension, uncontrolled seizure disorders, severe metabolic disorders, electrolyte imbalances, visual disorder, children
Pharmacokinetics:
PO: Peak 2-4 hr, metabolized in liver (metabolites), highly protein bound, excreted in urine, feces, crosses placenta, excreted in breast milk
Interactions:
• Increased effects: bile acid sequestrants, coumadin
• Increased myalgia, myositis: cyclosporine, gemfibrozil, niacin
• Drug/food: increased levels of lovastatin with food
Lab test interferences:
Increase: CPK, liver function tests

NURSING CONSIDERATIONS
Assess:
• Cholesterol levels periodically during treatment
• Liver function studies q1-2mo during the first 1½ yr of treatment; AST (SGOT), ALT (SGPT), liver function tests may increase
• Renal function in patients with

compromised renal system: BUN, creatinine, I&O ratio
• Eyes with slit lamp before, 1 mo after treatment begins, annually; lens opacities may occur

Administer:
• In evening with meal; if dose is increased, take with breakfast and evening meal

Perform/provide:
• Storage in cool environment in airtight light-resistant container

Evaluate:
• Therapeutic response: cholesterol at desired level after 8 wk

Teach patient/family:
• That treatment will take several years
• That blood work and eye exam will be necessary during treatment
• To report blurred vision, severe GI symptoms, dizziness, headache
• That previously prescribed regimen will continue: low-cholesterol diet, exercise program

---

loxapine (℞)

(lox'a-peen)
Loxapac*, loxapine succinate, Loxitane IM, Loxitane, Loxitane-C
Func. class.: Antipsychotic/neuroleptic
Chem. class.: Dibenzoxazepine

Action: Depresses cerebral cortex, hypothalamus, limbic system, which control activity and aggression; blocks neurotransmission produced by dopamine at synapse; exhibits strong α-adrenergic, anticholinergic blocking action; mechanism for antipsychotic effects is unclear

Uses: Psychotic disorders

Investigational uses: Depression, anxiety

Dosage and routes:
• *Adult:* PO 10 mg bid-qid initially, may be rapidly increased depending on severity of condition, maintenance 60-100 mg/day; IM 12.5-50 mg q4-6hr or more until desired response, then start PO form

Available forms: Caps 5, 10, 25, 50 mg; conc 25 mg/ml; inj 50 mg/ml

Side effects/adverse reactions:
RESP: ***Laryngospasm,*** dyspnea, ***respiratory depression***
CNS: EPS: pseudoparkinsonism, akathisia, dystonia, tardive dyskinesia, drowsiness, headache, ***seizures,*** confusion
HEMA: ***Anemia, leukopenia, leukocytosis, agranulocytosis***
INTEG: Rash, photosensitivity, dermatitis
EENT: Blurred vision, glaucoma
GI: Dry mouth, nausea, vomiting, anorexia, constipation, diarrhea, jaundice, weight gain
GU: Urinary retention, urinary frequency, enuresis, impotence, amenorrhea, gynecomastia
CV: Orthostatic hypotension, ***cardiac arrest,*** ECG changes, tachycardia

Contraindications: Hypersensitivity, blood dyscrasias, coma, child <16 yr, brain damage, bone marrow depression, alcohol and barbiturate withdrawal states

Precautions: Pregnancy (C), lactation, seizure disorders, hepatic disease, cardiac disease, prostatic hypertrophy, cardiac conditions, child <16 yr

Pharmacokinetics:
PO: Onset 20-30 min, peak 2-4 hr, duration 12 hr
IM: Onset 15-30 min, peak 15-20 min, duration 12 hr
Metabolized by liver; excreted in urine; crosses placenta; enters breast milk; initial half-life 5 hr; terminal half-life 19 hr

L

Interactions:

- Toxicity: epinephrine
- Increased EPS: other antipsychotics
- Decreased effects: guanadrel, guanethidine
- Increased CNS depression: MAOIs, antidepressants

NURSING CONSIDERATIONS

Assess:

- Mental status before initial administration
- Swallowing of PO medication; check for hoarding or giving of medication to other patients
- I&O ratio; palpate bladder if low urinary output occurs
- Bilirubin, CBC, liver function studies qmo
- Urinalysis is recommended before and during prolonged therapy
- Affect, orientation, LOC, reflexes, gait, coordination, sleep pattern disturbances
- B/P standing and lying; take pulse and respirations q4h during initial treatment; establish baseline before starting treatment; report drops of 30 mm Hg
- Dizziness, faintness, palpitations, tachycardia on rising
- EPS including akathisia (inability to sit still, no pattern to movements), tardive dyskinesia (bizarre movements of the jaw, mouth, tongue, extremities), pseudoparkinsonism (rigidity, tremors, pill rolling, shuffling gait)
- Skin turgor qd
- For neuroleptic malignant syndrome: muscle rigidity, increased CPK, altered mental status, hyperthermia
- Constipation, urinary retention qd; if these occur, increase bulk, water in diet

Administer:

- Reduced dose to elderly
- Antiparkinsonian agent if EPS symptoms occur
- IM injection into large muscle mass
- Concentrate mixed in orange or grapefruit juice

Perform/provide:

- Decreased noise input by dimming lights, avoiding loud noises
- Supervised ambulation until stabilized on medication; do not involve in strenuous exercise program because fainting is possible; patient should not stand still for long periods
- Increased fluids to prevent constipation
- Sips of water, candy, gum for dry mouth
- Storage in air-tight, light-resistant container

Evaluate:

- Therapeutic response: decrease in emotional excitement, hallucinations, delusions, paranoia; reorganization of patterns of thought, speech

Teach patient/family:

- That orthostatic hypotension may occur and to rise from sitting or lying position gradually
- To remain lying down after IM injection for at least 30 min
- To avoid hot tubs, hot showers, tub baths; hypotension may occur
- To avoid abrupt withdrawal of this drug, or EPS may result; drug should be withdrawn slowly
- To avoid OTC preparations (cough, hay fever, cold) unless approved by prescriber; serious drug interactions may occur; avoid use with alcohol, CNS depressants; increased drowsiness may occur
- To avoid hazardous activities until stabilized on medication
- To use a sunscreen during sun exposure to prevent burns

• Regarding compliance with drug regimen; warn patient about avoiding OTC preparations
• About necessity for meticulous oral hygiene, since oral candidiasis may occur
• To report impaired vision, jaundice, tremors, muscle twitching
• That in hot weather heat stroke may occur; take extra precautions to stay cool

Treatment of overdose: Lavage if orally ingested; provide an airway

lypressin (℞)

(lye-press′in)

Diapid

Func. class.: Pituitary hormone

Chem. class.: Lysine vasopressin

Action: Promotes reabsorption of water by action on renal tubular epithelium

Uses: Nonnephrogenic diabetes insipidus

Dosage and routes:

• *Adult:* INTRANASAL 1-2 sprays in one or both nostrils qid, an extra dose hs if needed

Available forms: Intranasal 0.185 mg/ml

Side effects/adverse reactions:

EENT: Nasal irritation, congestion, rhinitis, conjunctivitis, rhinorrhea

CNS: Headache

GI: Nausea, heartburn, cramps

MISC: Chest tightness, cough, dyspnea

Precautions: CAD, pregnancy (B)

Pharmacokinetics:

Nasal: Onset 1 hr, duration 3-8 hr, half-life 15 min

Metabolized in liver, kidneys, excreted in urine

NURSING CONSIDERATIONS

Assess:

• Nares for irritation
• I&O ratio; weight qd; check for edema in extremities; if water retention is severe, diuretic may be prescribed
• Water intoxication: lethargy, behavioral changes, disorientation, neuromuscular excitability

Perform/provide:

• Storage at room temp

Evaluate:

• Therapeutic response: absence of severe thirst, decreased urine output, osmolality

Teach patient/family:

• To clear nasal passages before using drug, not to inhale spray
• To carry drug at all times

mafenide (topical) (℞)

(ma′fe-nide)

Sulfamylon

Func. class.: Local antiinfective

Chem. class.: Sulfonamide

Action: Interferes with bacterial cell wall synthesis

Uses: Adjunctive treatment in burns (2nd, 3rd degree)

Dosage and routes:

• *Adult and child:* TOP apply 1/16″ to affected area qd bid, reapply as needed

Available forms: Cream 85 mg/g as acetate

Side effects/adverse reactions:

INTEG: Rash, urticaria, stinging, burning, bleeding, excoriation of new skin, superinfections, pruritus, blisters, facial edema, hives, erythema

OTHER: Metabolic acidosis, tachypnea, ***bone marrow suppression, fatal hemolytic anemia, eosinophilia***

Contraindications: Hypersensitivity, inhalation injury

Precautions: Pregnancy (C), impaired pulmonary function, lactation, impaired renal function

M

• Allergic reaction: burning, stinging, swelling, redness
• Fluid loss: decreased urinary output

NURSING CONSIDERATIONS
Administer:
• Analgesic before application if needed
• Enough medication to cover burns completely; they must be covered at all times
• After cleansing debris from burn before each application
• Using aseptic technique to debrided areas

Perform/provide:
• Dry storage at room temp

Evaluate:
• Therapeutic response: appearance of granulation tissue

Teach patient/family:
• That therapy will continue until area is ready for grafting
• About signs of superinfection
• About changes in respiratory activity

magaldrate (hydroxymagnesium aluminate) (OTC)

(mag'al-drate)
Antiflux, Lowsium, Riopan, Riopan Extra Strength
Func. class.: Antacid
Chem. class.: Aluminum/magnesium hydroxide

Action: Neutralizes gastric acidity; drug is dissolved in gastric contents; combination of aluminum, magnesium
Uses: Antacid, peptic ulcer disease (adjunct), duodenal, gastric ulcers, reflux esophagitis, hyperacidity, indigestion, heartburn
Dosage and routes:
• *Adult:* PO 1-2 (480-1080 mg) between meals, hs, not to exceed 20 tabs/d; CHEW TAB 1-2 (480-960 mg) between meals, hs, not to exceed 20 tabs/d; SUSP 5-10 ml (400-800 mg) with H_2O between meals, hs, not to exceed 100 ml/d
Available forms: Tabs 480 mg; chew tabs 480 mg; susp 540 mg/5 ml, 480 mg/5 ml, 1080 mg/5 ml
Side effects/adverse reactions:
GI: Constipation, diarrhea
META: Hypermagnesemia, hypophosphatemia
Contraindications: Hypersensitivity to this drug or aluminum
Precautions: Elderly, fluid restriction, decreased GI motility, GI obstruction, dehydration, renal disease, Na-restricted diets, pregnancy (C)
Pharmacokinetics:
PO: Duration 60 min
Interactions:
• Decreased effectiveness of tetracyclines, ketoconazole
• Decreased absorption of anticholinergics, chlordiazepoxide, cimetidine, corticosteroids, iron salts, phenothiazines, phenytoin, salicylates

NURSING CONSIDERATIONS
Assess:
• GI status: location of pain, intensity, characteristics, heartburn, hemataenesis
• Serum Mg^{++} levels with impaired renal function
• Constipation: increase bulk in diet if needed

Administer:
• Laxatives or stool softeners if constipation occurs
• After shaking; give between meals and hs

Evaluate:
• Therapeutic response: absence of pain, decreased acidity

Teach patient/family:
• To separate enteric-coated drugs and antacid by 1 hr

• To notify prescriber immediately of coffee-ground emesis, emesis with flank blood, black tarry stools

magnesium (℞)

Func. class.: Anticonvulsant

Chem. class.: Magnesium product

Action: Decreases acetylcholine in motor nerve terminals, which is responsible for anticonvulsant properties; osmotically retains fluid, which increases amount of water in feces when used as laxative; reduces SA node impulse formation, prolongs conduction time in myocardium

Uses: Hypomagnesemic seizures, control of seizures in pregnancy-induced hypertension, seizures in acute nephritis

Dosage and routes:

Hypomagnesemic seizures

• *Adult:* IV 1-2 g over 15 min, then 1 g IM q4-6h, depending on response

Nephritis

• *Child:* IM 20-40 mg/kg in 20% sol, repeat as needed

Preeclampsia/eclampsia

• *Adult:* IV 4 g/250 ml D_5W and 4 g IM, then 4 g IM q4h prn; or 4 g IV loading dose, then 1-4 g IV inf qh, not to exceed 3 ml/min

Available forms: Inj IV, IM 10%, 12.5%, 25%, 50%; granules

Side effects/adverse reactions:

CNS: Sweating, depressed deep tendon reflexes, flushing, drowsiness, flaccid paralysis, hypothermia, weakness, sedation

RESP: ***Paralysis***

CV: Hypotension, ***circulatory collapse, heart block,*** decreased cardiac function

Contraindications: Hypersensitivity, myocardial infarction, renal disease

Precaution: Pregnancy (C)

Pharmacokinetics:

IV: Onset 1-5 min, duration 30 min

IM: Onset 1 hr, duration 3-4 hr

Excreted by kidneys

Interactions:

• Increased CNS depression: barbiturates, general anesthetics, narcotics, antipsychotics

• Increased effects of neuromuscular blockers

Y-site compatibilities: Acyclovir, amikacin, ampicillin, cefamandole, cefazolin, cefoperazone, ceforanide, cefotaxime, cefoxitin, cephalothin, cephapirin, chloramphenicol, clindamycin, dobutamine, doxycycline, enalaprilat, erythromycin, lactobionate, esmolol, famotidine, fludarabine, gentamicin, heparin, hydrocortisone, hydromorphone, idarubicin, insulin, kanamycin, labetalol, meperidine, metronidazole, minocycline, morphine, nafcillin, ondansetron, oxacillin, paclitaxel, penicillin G potassium, piperacillin, potassium chloride, sargramostim, ticarcillin, tobramycin, trimethoprim/sulfamethoxazole, vancomycin, vitamin B complex with C

Additive compatibilities: Calcium gluconate, cephalothin, chloramphenicol, cisplatin, hydrocortisone sodium succinate, methyldopate, penicillin G potassium, potassium phosphate, verapamil

NURSING CONSIDERATIONS

Assess:

• VS q15min after IV dose; do not exceed 150 mg/min

• Cardiac function: monitoring, Mg levels

• Timing of contractions; determine intensity; monitor fetal heart rate, reactivity; may decrease with this drug during labor

M

• I&O: should remain at 30 ml/hr or more; if less than this, notify prescriber
• Urine output before each dose; should be >100 ml/4 hr
• Mental status: mood, sensorium, affect, memory (long, short)
• Respiratory dysfunction: respiratory depression, character, rate, rhythm; hold drug if respirations are <16/min
• Hypermagnesemia: depressed patellar reflex, flushing, polydipsia, confusion, weakness, flaccid paralysis, hypothermia, dyspnea begin to appear at blood levels of 4 mEq/L
• Respiratory rate, rhythm of newborn if drug was given 24 hr before delivery or less; check reflexes of newborn whose mother received this drug before delivery
• Reflexes: knee jerk, patellar; decrease signals Mg^{++} toxicity; mild depression will occur in therapeutic range

Administer:
• Only when calcium gluconate available for magnesium toxicity
• IV undiluted 1.5 ml of 10% sol over 1 min; may dilute to 20% sol, infuse over 3 hr
• IV at less than 150 mg/min; circulatory collapse may occur
• IV as a single dose infused/3 hr in hypomagnesemia

Perform/provide:
• Seizure precautions: dark room with decreased stimuli, padded side rails

Evaluate:
• Therapeutic response; absence of seizures

Teach patient/family:
• Symptoms of hypermagnesemia

Treatment of overdose: Stop drug; administer calcium gluconate; monitor reflexes, Mg levels; ECG monitoring if Ca is administered

magnesium oxide (OTC)

Mag-Ox, Maox, Uro-Mag

Func. class.: Antacid

Chem. class.: Magnesium product

Action: Neutralizes gastric acidity

Uses: Constipation, hypomagnesemia, antacid

Dosage and routes:
• *Adult:* PO 250 mg-1 g pc, hs with 4-8 oz water

Laxative
• *Adult:* PO 2-4 g with water hs

Hypomagnesemia
• *Adult:* PO 650-1.3 g qd

Available forms: Caps 140 mg; tabs 400, 420 mg

Side effects/adverse reactions:

GU: Renal stones

GI: Diarrhea, flatulence, cramps, belching, nausea, vomiting

META: Hypermagnesemia: *weakness, lethargy, depression, decreased B/P, increased pulse,* ***respiratory depression, coma***

Contraindications: Hypersensitivity

Precautions: Severe renal disease, GI bleeding, diarrhea, intestinal obstruction, pregnancy (C)

Pharmacokinetics:

PO: Excreted in urine

Interactions:
• Decreased effectiveness of: tetracyclines, ketoconazole
• Decreased absorption of anticholinergics, chlordiazepoxide, cimetidine, corticosteroids, iron salts, phenothiazines, phenytoin

Lab test interferences:

Increase: Urinary pH, gastrin

Decrease: K^+

NURSING CONSIDERATIONS

Assess:
• Decreased constipation, characteristics of stools

Perform/provide:

• Storage in airtight container

Evaluate:

• Therapeutic response: absence of pain, decreased acidity

Teach patient/family:

• Not to change antacids unless directed by prescriber

magnesium salicylate (OTC, ℞)

Doan's pills, Magan, Mobidin

Func. class.: Nonnarcotic analgesic

Chem. class.: Salicylate

Action: Blocks pain impulses in CNS that occur in response to inhibition of prostaglandin synthesis; antipyretic action results from inhibition of hypothalamic heat-regulating center to produce vasodilation to allow heat dissipation

Uses: Mild to moderate pain or fever including arthritis, juvenile rheumatoid arthritis

Dosage and routes:

Arthritis

• *Adult:* PO not to exceed 4.8 g/d in divided doses

Pain/fever

• *Adult:* PO 600 mg tid or qid

Available forms: Tabs 325, 545, 600 mg

Side effects/adverse reactions:

HEMA: ***Thrombocytopenia, agranulocytosis, leukopenia, neutropenia, hemolytic anemia,*** increased pro-time

CNS: Stimulation, drowsiness, dizziness, confusion, ***convulsion,*** headache, flushing, hallucinations, coma

GI: Nausea, vomiting, GI bleeding, diarrhea, heartburn, anorexia, ***hepatitis***

INTEG: Rash, urticaria, bruising

EENT: Tinnitus, hearing loss

CV: Rapid pulse, ***pulmonary edema***

RESP: Wheezing, hyperpnea

ENDO: Hypoglycemia, hyponatremia, hypokalemia

Contraindications: Hypersensitivity to salicylates, GI bleeding, bleeding disorders, children <12 yr, vit K deficiency

Precautions: Anemia, hepatic disease, renal disease, Hodgkin's disease, pregnancy (C), lactation

Pharmacokinetics:

PO: Onset 15-30 min, peak 1-2 hr, duration 4-6 hr; metabolized by liver; excreted by kidneys; crosses placenta; excreted in breast milk; half-life 1-3½ hr

Interactions:

• Decreased effects of magnesium salicylate: antacids, steroids, urinary alkalizers

• Increased blood loss: alcohol, heparin

• Increased effects of anticoagulants, insulin, methotrexate

• Decreased effects of probenecid, spironolactone, sulfinpyrazone, sulfonylmides

• Toxic effects: PABA

• Decreased blood sugar levels: salicylates

Lab test interferences:

Increase: Coagulation studies, liver function studies, serum uric acid, amylase, CO_2, urinary protein

Decrease: Serum K, PBI, cholesterol, blood glucose

Interfere: Urine catecholamines, pregnancy test

NURSING CONSIDERATIONS

Assess:

• Liver function studies: AST, ALT, bilirubin, creatinine (long-term therapy)

• Renal function studies: BUN, urine creatinine (long-term therapy)

• Blood studies: CBC, Hct, Hgb, pro-time (long-term therapy)

M

• I&O ratio; decreasing output may indicate renal failure (long-term therapy)
• Hepatotoxicity: dark urine, clay-colored stools, yellow skin and sclera, itching, abdominal pain, fever, diarrhea (long-term therapy)
• Allergic reactions: rash, urticaria; if these occur, drug may have to be discontinued
• Renal dysfunction: decreased urine output
• Ototoxicity: tinnitus, ringing, roaring in ears; audiometric testing is needed before, after long-term therapy
• Visual changes: blurring, halos, corneal and retinal damage
• Edema in feet, ankles, legs
• Prior drug history; there are many drug interactions

Administer:
• To patient crushed or whole; chewable tablets may be chewed
• With food or milk to decrease gastric symptoms; give 30 min before or 2 hr after antacids
• With full glass of water

Evaluate:
• Therapeutic response: decreased pain, fever

Teach patient/family:
• To report any symptoms of hepatotoxicity, renal toxicity, visual changes, ototoxicity, allergic reactions, bleeding (long-term therapy)
• Not to exceed recommended dosage; acute poisoning may result
• To read label on other OTC drugs; many contain aspirin
• That therapeutic response takes 2 wk (arthritis)
• To avoid alcohol ingestion; GI bleeding may occur
• That if anticoagulants are given with this drug, both should be discontinued 2 wk before surgery

Treatment of overdose: Lavage, activated charcoal, monitor electrolytes, VS

magnesium salts (OTC)

Concentrated Phillip's Milk of Magnesia, Milk of Magnesia, Phillip's Milk of Magnesia

Func. class.: Laxative, saline; antacid

Action: Increases osmotic pressure, draws fluid into colon, neutralizes HCl

Uses: Constipation, bowel preparation before surgery or exam

Dosage and routes:

Laxative
• *Adult:* PO 30-60 ml hs (Milk of Magnesia), 300 mg
• *Adult and child >6 yr:* PO 15 g in 8 oz H_2O (magnesium sulfate); PO 10-20 ml (Concentrated Milk of Magnesia); PO 5-10 oz hs (magnesium citrate)
• *Child 2-6 yr:* 5-15 ml (Milk of Magnesia)

Available forms: Liquid 395 mg/5 ml; tabs chew 300, 600 mg; conc. liquid 1.2 gm/5 ml

Side effects/adverse reactions:
CNS: Muscle weakness, flushing, sweating, confusion, sedation, depressed reflexes, ***flaccidity, paralysis,*** hypothermia
GI: Nausea, vomiting, anorexia, cramps
CV: Hypotension, heart block, ***circulatory collapse***
META: Electrolyte, fluid imbalances

Contraindications: Hypersensitivity, renal diseases, abdominal pain, nausea/vomiting, obstruction, acute surgical abdomen, rectal bleeding

Precautions: Pregnancy (B)

Pharmacokinetics:
PO: Peak 1-2 hr; excreted in feces

* Available in Canada only

Interactions:
- Increased CNS depression: CNS depressants, barbiturates, narcotics, anesthetics

NURSING CONSIDERATIONS

Assess:
- I&O ratio; check for decrease in urinary output
- Causc of constipation; lack of fluids, bulk, exercise
- Cramping, rectal bleeding, nausea, vomiting; drug should be discontinued
- Mg toxicity: thirst, confusion, decrease in reflexes

Administer:
- With 8 oz H_2O

Evaluate:
- Therapeutic response: decreased constipation

Teach patient/family:
- Not to use laxatives for long-term therapy; bowel tone will be lost
- Chilling helps the taste of magnesium citrate
- Shake suspension well
- Do not give at hs as a laxative; may interfere with sleep
- Give citrus fruit after administering to counteract unpleasant taste

---

mannitol (℞)

(man'i-tole)
mannitol, Osmitrol, Resectial
Func. class.: Osmotic diuretic
Chem. class.: Hexahydric alcohol

Action: Acts by increasing osmolarity of glomerular filtrate, which raises osmotic pressure of fluid in renal tubules; decrease in reabsorption of water electrolytes, increase in urinary output, sodium, chloride excretion

Uses: Edema, promote systemic diuresis in cerebral edema, decrease intraocular pressure, improve renal function in acute renal failure, chemical poisoning

Dosage and routes:

Oliguria, prevention
- *Adult:* IV 50-100 g 5%-25% sol

Oliguria, treatment
- *Adult:* IV 300-400 mg/kg 20%-25% sol up to 100 g 15%-20% sol
- *Child:* IV 0.25-2 g/kg as 15%-20% sol run over 2-6 hr

Intraocular pressure/intracranial pressure
- *Adult:* IV 1.5-2 g/kg 15%-25% sol over ½-1 hr
- *Child:* IV 1-2 g/kg/30-60 g/m^2 as 15%-20% sol run over ½-1 hr

Renal failure
- *Adult:* IV 50-200 g/24 hr, adjusted to maintain output of 30-50 mg/hr

Diuresis in drug intoxication
- *Adult and child >12 yr:* 5%-10% sol continuously up to 200 g IV, while maintaining 100-500 ml urine output/hr

Available forms: Inj IV 5%, 10%, 15%, 20%, 25%

Side effects/adverse reactions:

GU: Marked diuresis, urinary retention, thirst

CNS: Dizziness, headache, ***convulsions, rebound increased ICP,*** confusion

GI: Nausea, vomiting, dry mouth, diarrhea

CV: Edema, thrombophlebitis, hypotension, hypertension, tachycardia, angina-like chest pains, fever, chills

RESP: Pulmonary congestion

ELECT: Fluid, electrolyte imbalances, ***acidosis,*** electrolyte loss, dehydration

EENT: Loss of hearing, blurred vision, nasal congestion, decreased intraocular pressure

M

Contraindications: Active intracranial bleeding, hypersensitivity, anuria, severe pulmonary congestion, edema, severe dehydration, progressive heart, renal failure

Precautions: Dehydration, pregnancy (C), severe renal disease, CHF, lactation

Pharmacokinetics:

IV: Onset 30-60 min for diuresis, ½-1 hr for intraocular pressure, 25 min for cerebrospinal fluid; duration 4-6 hr for intraocular pressure, 3-8 hr for cerebrospinal fluid; excreted in urine, half-life 100 min

Interactions:

- Decreased effect: lithium
- Increased effects of EDTA
- Drug/food: potassium foods: increased hyperkalemia

Y-site compatibilities: Ondansetron, fluorouracil, idarubicin, melphalan, paclitaxel, vinorelbine sulfate

Additive compatibilities: Amikacin, bretylium, cefamandole, cefoxitin, cimetidine, cisplatin, dopamine, gentamicin, metoclopramide, netilmicin, nizatidine, tobramycin, verapamil

Lab test interferences:

Interference: Inorganic phosphorus, ethylene glycol

NURSING CONSIDERATIONS

Assess:

- Weight, I&O qd to determine fluid loss; effect of drug may be decreased if used qd; output qh prn
- Rate, depth, rhythm of respiration, effect of exertion
- B/P lying, standing; postural hypotension may occur
- Electrolytes: K, Na, Cl; include BUN, CBC, serum creatinine, blood pH, ABGs
- Signs of metabolic acidosis: drowsiness, restlessness
- Signs of hypokalemia: postural hypotension, malaise, fatigue, tachycardia, leg cramps, weakness
- Rashes, temp qd
- Confusion, especially in elderly; take safety precautions if needed
- Hydration including skin turgor, thirst, dry mucous membranes

Administer:

- IV in 15%-25% sol with filter; give over ½-1½ hr; rapid infusion may worsen CHF; warm in hot water and shake to dissolve crystals
- Test dose in severe oliguria, 0.2 g/kg over 3-5 min; if no urine increase, give 2nd test dose; if no response, reassess patient

Evaluate:

- Therapeutic response: improvement in edema of feet, legs, sacral area daily if medication is being used in CHF; decreased intraocular pressure, prevention of hypokalemia, increased excretion of toxic substances

Teach patient/family:

- To rise slowly from lying or sitting position
- Reason for and method of treatment

Treatment of overdose: Discontinue infusion; correct fluid, electrolyte imbalances; hemodialysis; monitor hydration, CV, renal function

maprotiline (℞)

(ma-proe′ti-leen)

Ludiomil, maprotiline

Func. class.: Antidepressant

Chem. class.: Tetracyclic

Action: Blocks reuptake of norepinephrine, serotonin into nerve endings, increasing action of norepinephrine, serotonin in nerve cells

Uses: Depression, dysthymic disorder, bipolar disorder—depressed, agitated depression

* Available in Canada only

Dosage and routes:

• *Adult:* PO 75 mg/day in moderate depression, may increase to 150 mg/day; not to exceed 225 mg in hospitalized patients; severely depressed hospitalized patients may be given 300 mg/day

• *Elderly:* 50-75 mg/day

Available forms: Tabs 25, 50, 75 mg

Side effects/adverse reactions:

HEMA: ***Agranulocytosis, thrombocytopenia, eosinophilia, leukopenia***

CNS: Dizziness, drowsiness, confusion, headache, anxiety, tremors, stimulation, weakness, insomnia, nightmares, EPS (elderly), increased psychiatric symptoms, ***seizures***

GI: Diarrhea, dry mouth, nausea, vomiting, ***paralytic ileus,*** increased appetite, cramps, epigastric distress, jaundice, ***hepatitis,*** stomatitis

GU: Retention, ***acute renal failure***

INTEG: Rash, urticaria, sweating, pruritus, photosensitivity

CV: Orthostatic hypotension, ECG changes, tachycardia, ***hypertension,*** palpitations

EENT: Blurred vision, tinnitus, mydriasis

Contraindications: Hypersensitivity to tricyclic antidepressants, recovery phase of MI, convulsive disorders, prostatic hypertrophy

Precautions: Suicidal patients, severe depression, increased intraocular pressure, narrow-angle glaucoma, urinary retention, cardiac disease, hepatic disease, hypothyroidism, hyperthyroidism, electroshock therapy, elective surgery, elderly, pregnancy (B)

Pharmacokinetics:

PO: Onset 15-30 min, peak 12 hr, duration up to 3 wk, steady state 6-10 days; metabolized by liver; excreted in urine, feces; crosses placenta; half-life 21-25 hr

Interactions:

• Decreased effects of guanethidine, clonidine, indirect-acting sympathomimetics (ephedrine)

• Increased effects of direct-acting sympathomimetics (epinephrine), alcohol, barbiturates, benzodiazepines, CNS depressants

• Hyperpyretic crisis, convulsions, hypertensive episode: MAOI (pargyline [Eutonyl])

Lab test interferences:

Increase: Serum bilirubin, blood glucose, alk phosphatase

False increase: Urinary catecholamines

Decrease: VMA, 5-HIAA

NURSING CONSIDERATIONS

Assess:

• B/P (lying, standing), pulse q4h; if systolic B/P drops 20 mm Hg, hold drug, notify prescriber; take vital signs q4h in patients with cardiovascular disease

• Blood studies: CBC, leukocytes, differential, cardiac enzymes if patient is receiving long-term therapy

• Hepatic studies: AST (SGOT), ALT (SGPT), bilirubin, creatinine

• Weight qwk; appetite may increase with drug

• ECG for flattening of T wave, bundle branch block, AV block, dysrhythmias in cardiac patients

• EPS primarily in elderly: rigidity, dystonia, akathisia

• Mental status: mood, sensorium, affect, suicidal tendencies, increase in psychiatric symptoms: depression, panic

• Urinary retention, constipation; constipation is more likely to occur in children

• Withdrawal symptoms: headache, nausea, vomiting, muscle pain, weakness; do not usually occur unless drug was discontinued abruptly

• Alcohol consumption; if alcohol

M

is consumed, hold dose until morning

Administer:

• Increased fluids, bulk in diet for constipation, especially elderly
• With food, milk for GI symptoms
• Dosage hs if oversedation occurs during day; may take entire dose hs; elderly may not tolerate once/day dosing
• Gum, hard candy, or frequent sips of water for dry mouth
• Concentrate with fruit juice, water, or milk to disguise taste

Perform/provide:

• Storage in tight container at room temp; do not freeze
• Assistance with ambulation during beginning therapy, since drowsiness/dizziness occurs
• Safety measures, including side rails, primarily in elderly
• Checking to see PO medication swallowed

Evaluate:

• Therapeutic response: decreased depression

Teach patient/family:

• That therapeutic effects may take 2-3 wk
• Use of caution in driving, other activities requiring alertness, because of drowsiness, dizziness, blurred vision
• To avoid alcohol ingestion, other CNS depressants
• Not to discontinue medication quickly after long-term use; may cause nausea, headache, malaise
• To wear sunscreen or large hat, since photosensitivity occurs

Treatment of overdose: ECG monitoring, induce emesis; lavage, activated charcoal; administer anticonvulsant

masoprocol (℞)

(mas-o-proe'cole)
Actinex
Func. class.: Miscellaneous topical product

Action: Unknown
Uses: Actinic keratoses
Dosage and routes:
• *Adult:* TOP apply to lesion bid × 2-4 wk
Available forms: Cream 10%
Side effects/adverse reactions:
INTEG: Irritation, redness, flaking, itching, burning, tightness of the skin, edema, dryness, soreness
Contraindications: Hypersensitivity, children
Precautions: Avoid occlusive dressings, pregnancy (B), lactation
Pharmacokinetics: <2% absorption over 96-hr period

NURSING CONSIDERATIONS

Assess:

• Number and severity of lesions; inflammation, erythema, flaking, itching, burning, tightness, bleeding, edema

Administer:

• By covering lesion with cream; do not bandage

Perform/provide:

• Storage out of reach of children

Evaluate:

• Therapeutic response: decrease in size and number of lesions

Teach patient/family:

• To avoid all other medications unless directed by prescriber

mazindol (℞)

(may'zin-dole)
Mazanor, Sanorex
Func. class.: Anorexiant
Chem. class.: Imidazoisoindole derivative

Controlled Substance Schedule IV
Action: Acts on central adrenergic and dopaminergic pathways to stimulate satiety center in hypothalamic, limbic regions
Uses: Exogenous obesity
Dosage and routes:
• *Adult:* PO 1 mg ac, or 2 mg 1 hr ac lunch
Available forms: Tabs 1, 2 mg
Side effects/adverse reactions:
HEMA: ***Bone marrow depression, leukopenia, agranulocytosis***
EENT: Mydriasis, blurred vision, eye irritation
MISC: Hair loss, muscle pain, flushing, fever
CNS: Hyperactivity, insomnia, restlessness, dizziness, headache, stimulation, irritability, drowsiness, weakness, tremor, fatigue, malaise, euphoria, depression, confusion
GI: Nausea, anorexia, dry mouth, diarrhea, constipation, vomiting
GU: Impotence, change in libido, dysuria, menstrual irregularities, testicular pain, urinary frequency
CV: Palpitations, tachycardia, hypertension, dysrhythmias, pulmonary hypertension
INTEG: Urticaria, rash, pallor, shivering, sweating
Contraindications: Hypersensitivity to sympathomimetic amine, glaucoma, drug abuse, cardiovascular disease, children <12 yr, hypertension, severe arteriosclerosis, agitated states, hyperthyroidism
Precautions: Diabetes mellitus, convulsive disorders, pregnancy (C), lactation
Pharmacokinetics:
PO: Onset ½-1 hr, duration 8-15 hr; metabolized by liver, excreted by kidneys
Interactions:
• Hypertensive crisis: MAOIs or within 14 days of MAOIs, furazolidone
• Decreased effects of mazindol: tricyclics
• Decreased effects of guanethidine
• Increased effects of insulin

NURSING CONSIDERATIONS
Assess:
• VS, B/P; may reverse antihypertensives; check patients with cardiac disease more often
• CBC, urinalysis, in diabetes: blood sugar, urine sugar; insulin changes may have to be made, since eating will decrease
• Height, growth rate in children; growth rate may be decreased
• Mental status: mood, sensorium, affect, stimulation, insomnia, aggressiveness
• Physical dependency: not to be used for extended time; should be discontinued gradually; tolerance will occur after long-term use
• Withdrawal symptoms: headache, nausea, vomiting, muscle pain, weakness
Administer:
• At least 6 hr before hs to avoid sleeplessness, 1 hr ac meals
• For obesity only if patient is on weight reduction program including dietary changes, exercise; patient will develop tolerance, and weight loss won't occur without additional methods
• Gum, hard candy, frequent sips of water for dry mouth
Evaluate:
• Therapeutic response: decreased weight

M

Teach patient/family:

• To take with meals to avoid GI symptoms
• To decrease caffeine consumption (coffee, tea, cola, chocolate), which may increase irritability, stimulation
• Not to take more frequently than prescribed
• To avoid OTC preparations unless approved by prescriber
• To taper off drug over several weeks, or depression, increased sleeping, lethargy may ensue
• To avoid alcohol ingestion
• To avoid hazardous activities until patient is stabilized on medication
• To get needed rest; patient will feel more tired at end of day

Treatment of overdose: Administer fluids, chlorpromazine 1 mg/kg; antihypertensive for increased B/P; ammonium Cl for increased excretion

measles, mumps, and rubella vaccine (℞)

M-M-R-II

Func. class.: Vaccine

Action: Produces antibodies to measles, mumps, rubella

Uses: Prevention of measles, mumps, rubella

Dosage and routes:

• *Children >15 mos and adults:* SC 0.5 ml

Available forms: Inj SC measles 1000 $TCID_{50}$, mumps 20,000 $TCID_{50}$, rubella 1000 $TCID_{50}$ (0.5 ml)

Side effects/adverse reactions:

CNS: Fever, ***subacute sclerosing panencephalitis and blindness associated with optic neuritis,*** paresthesias

INTEG: Urticaria, erythema, burning, stinging at injection site

SYST: Lymphadenitis, ***anaphylaxis,*** malaise, sore throat, headache

MS: Osteomyelitis, arthralgia, arthritis

Contraindications: Hypersensitivity, blood dyscrasias, anemia, active infection, immunosuppression, egg, chicken allergy, pregnancy, febrile illness, neomycin allergy, neoplasms

Precautions: Elderly, lactation, children with TB

Interactions:

• Decreased response to TB skin test
• Other live virus vaccines

NURSING CONSIDERATIONS

Assess:

• For skin reactions: rash, induration, erythema
• For anaphylaxis: inability to breathe, bronchospasm

Administer:

• Only with epinephrine 1:1000 on unit to treat laryngospasm
• Only SC

Perform/provide:

• Storage at 39° F (4° C); protect from heat, light; do not give within 1 mo of other live virus vaccines
• Written record of immunization

Evaluate:

• For history of allergies, skin disorders (eczema, psoriasis, dermatitis), reactions to vaccinations

Teach patient/family:

• That fever may occur 5-12 days after vaccine given
• That joint pains, tingling in extremities may occur 5-12 days after vaccine given
• That pain and inflammation may occur
• To take acetaminophen for fever

mebendazole (℞)

(me-ben'da-zole)
Nemasole*, Vermox
Func. class.: Anthelmintic
Chem. class.: Carbamate

Action: Inhibits glucose uptake, degeneration of cytoplasmic microtubules in the cell; interferes with absorption, secretory function
Uses: Pinworms, roundworms, hookworms, whipworms, threadworms, pork tapeworms, dwarf tapeworms, beef tapeworms, hydatid cyst
Dosage and routes:
• *Adult and child >2 yr:* PO 100 mg as a single dose or bid × 3 days, depending on type of infection; course may be repeated in 3 wk if needed
Available forms: Tabs, chewable 100 mg
Side effects/adverse reactions:
CNS: Dizziness, fever
GI: Transient diarrhea, abdominal pain
Contraindications: Hypersensitivity
Precautions: Child <2 yr, lactation, pregnancy (1st trimester) (C)
Pharmacokinetics:
PO: Peak ½-7 hr; excreted in feces primarily (metabolites), small amount in urine (unchanged); highly bound to plasma proteins
Interactions:
• Decreased effect of mebendazole: carbamazine, hydantoins
NURSING CONSIDERATIONS
Assess:
• Stools during entire treatment; specimens must be sent to lab while still warm, also 1-3 wk after treatment is completed
• For allergic reaction: rash (rare)
• For diarrhea during expulsion of worms; avoid self-contamination with patient's feces
• For infection in other family members, since infection from person to person is common
• Blood studies: AST (SGOT), ALT (SGPT), alk phosphatase, BUN, CBC during treatment
Administer:
• May be crushed, chewed
• PO after meals to avoid GI symptoms, since absorption is not altered by food
• Second course after 3 wk if needed; usually recommended
Perform/provide:
• Storage in tight container
Evaluate:
• Therapeutic response: expulsion of worms and 3 negative stool cultures after completion of treatment
Teach patient/family:
• Proper hygiene after BM, including hand-washing technique; tell patient to avoid putting fingers in mouth; clean fingernails
• That infected person should sleep alone; do not shake bed linen, change bed linen qd, wash in hot water, change and wash undergarments daily
• To clean toilet qd with disinfectant (green soap solution)
• Need for compliance with dosage schedule, duration of treatment
• To wear shoes, wash all fruits and vegetables well before eating; use commercial fruit/vegetable cleaner

mecamylamine (℞)

(mek-a-mill'a-meen)
Inversine
Func. class.: Antihypertensive
Chem. class.: Ganglionic blocker

Action: Occupies receptor site, prevents acetylcholine from attaching

to postsynaptic nerve ending in sympathetic and parasympathetic ganglia
Uses: Moderate to severe hypertension, malignant hypertension
Dosage and routes:
- *Adult:* PO 2.5 mg bid, may increase in increments of 2.5 mg × 2 days until desired response; maintenance 25 mg/day in 3 divided doses

Available forms: Tabs 2.5 mg
Side effects/adverse reactions:
CV: Postural hypotension, irregular heart rate, ***CHF***
CNS: Drowsiness, sedation, headache, tremors, weakness, syncope, paresthesia, dizziness, ***convulsions***
EENT: Blurred vision, nasal congestion, dry mouth, dilated pupils
GU: Impotence, urinary retention, decreased libido
GI: Anorexia, glossitis, nausea, vomiting, constipation, ***paralytic ileus***
Contraindications: Hypersensitivity, MI, coronary insufficiency, renal disease, glaucoma, organic pyloric stenosis, uremia, uncooperative patients, mild/labile hypertension
Precautions: CVA, prostatic hypertrophy, bladder neck obstruction, urethral stricture, renal dysfunction (elevated BUN), cerebral dysfunction, pregnancy (C), lactation
Pharmacokinetics:
PO: Onset ½-2 hr, duration 6-12 hr; excreted in urine, feces, breast milk; crosses placenta
Interactions:
- Increased effects: thiazide diuretics, antihypertensives, CNS depressants (alcohol, anesthetics, MAOIs), bethanechol

NURSING CONSIDERATIONS
Assess:
- B/P lying and standing, other VS throughout treatment
- Weight qd, I&O
- Edema in feet, legs qd
- Skin turgor, dryness of mucous membranes for hydration status
- Tolerance to drug with prolonged use
- Constipation: number of stools, consistency; give stool softener as ordered or increase bulk in diet

Administer:
- Whole; do not chew or crush
- After meals for better absorption; give larger dose at noon and evening, smaller dose in AM
- Gum, frequent rinsing of mouth, hard candy for dry mouth

Evaluate:
- Therapeutic response: decreased B/P

Teach patient/family:
- To notify prescriber of tremor, seizure, signs of paralytic ileus
- To avoid OTC preparations unless directed by prescriber
- To rise slowly from sitting or lying position; orthostatic hypotension may occur
- That impotence may occur but is reversible after discontinuing drug

Treatment of overdose: Administer gastric lavage, discontinue drug, administer small doses of pressor amines for hypotension

---

mechlorethamine (℞)

(me-klor-eth'a-meen)
Mustargen, Nitrogen mustard
Func. class.: Antineoplastic alkylating agent
Chem. class.: Nitrogen mustard

Action: Responsible for cross-linking DNA strands leading to cell death; rapidly degraded, a vesicant; activity is not cell cycle specific
Uses: Hodgkin's disease, leukemias, lymphomas, lymphosarcoma; ovarian, breast, lung carcinoma; neoplastic effusions

Dosage and routes:

• *Adult:* IV 0.4 mg/kg or 10 mg/m^2 as 1 dose or 2-4 divided doses over 2-4 days; second course after 3 wk depending on blood cell count

Neoplastic effusions

• *Adult:* Intracavity 10-20 mg, may be 200-400 μg/kg

Available forms: Inj 10 mg; powder for inj

Side effects/adverse reactions:

EENT: Tinnitus, hearing loss

HEMA: ***Thrombocytopenia, leukopenia, agranulocytosis,*** anemia

GI: Nausea, vomiting, diarrhea, stomatitis, weight loss, colitis, ***hepatotoxicity***

CNS: Headache, dizziness, drowsiness, paresthesia, peripheral neuropathy, ***coma***

INTEG: Alopecia, pruritus, herpes zoster, extravasation

Contraindications: Lactation, pregnancy (1st trimester) (D), myelosuppression, acute herpes zoster

Precautions: Radiation therapy, chronic lymphocytic leukopenia

Pharmacokinetics:

Metabolized in liver, excreted in urine

Interactions:

• Increased toxicity: antineoplastics, radiation

• Blood dyscrasias: amphotericin B

Y-site compatibilities: Fludarubine, melphalan, ondansetron, sargramostim, vinorelbine

NURSING CONSIDERATIONS

Assess:

• CBC, differential, platelet count qwk; withhold drug if WBC is <4000 or platelet count is <75,000; notify prescriber

• Renal function studies: BUN, serum uric acid, urine CrCl before, during therapy

• I&O ratio; report fall in urine output of 30 ml/hr

• Monitor temp q4h (may indicate beginning infection); no rectal temps

• Liver function tests before, during therapy (bilirubin, AST [SGOT], ALT [SGPT], LDH) as needed or monthly

• Bleeding: hematuria, guaiac, bruising or petechiae, mucosa or orifices q8h

• Food preferences; list likes, dislikes

• Yellow skin and sclera, dark urine, clay-colored stools, itchy skin, abdominal pain, fever, diarrhea

• Effects of alopecia on body image; discuss feelings about body changes

• Inflammation of mucosa, breaks in skin

• Buccal cavity q8h for dryness, sores, ulceration, white patches, oral pain, bleeding, dysphagia

• Local irritation, pain, burning, discoloration at injection site

• Symptoms indicating severe allergic reaction: rash, pruritus, urticaria, purpuric skin lesions, itching, flushing

Administer:

• After using guidelines for preparation of cytotoxic drugs

• Antiemetic 30-60 min before giving drug and prn

• Antibiotics for prophylaxis of infection

• IV after diluting 10 mg/10 ml sterile H_2O or NaCl; leave needle in vial, shake, withdraw dose, give through Y-tube or 3-way stopcock or directly over 3-5 min

• Watch for infiltration; infiltrate area with isotonic sodium thiosulfate or 1% lidocaine; apply ice for 6-12 hr

• Topical or systemic analgesics for pain

• Local or systemic drugs for infection

M

Perform/provide:

• Storage at room temp in dry form
• Strict medical asepsis, protective isolation if WBC levels are low
• Special skin care
• Increase fluid intake to 2-3 L/day to prevent urate deposits, calculi formation
• Diet low in purines: organ meats (kidney, liver), dried beans, peas to maintain alkaline urine
• Preparation under hood using gloves and mask
• Rinsing of mouth tid-qid with water, club soda; brushing of teeth bid-tid with soft brush or cotton-tipped applicators for stomatitis; use unwaxed dental floss
• Warm compresses at injection site for inflammation

Evaluate:

• Therapeutic response: decreased tumor size, spread of malignancy

Teach patient/family:

• About protective isolation
• That sterility, amenorrhea can occur; reversible after discontinuing treatment
• That hair may be lost during treatment; a wig or hairpiece may make patient feel better; new hair may be different in color, texture
• To avoid foods with citric acid, hot or rough texture
• To report any bleeding, white spots, or ulcerations in mouth to prescriber; tell patient to examine mouth qd
• To report signs of infection: fever, sore throat, flu symptoms
• To report signs of anemia: fatigue, headache, faintness, shortness of breath, irritability
• To avoid use of razors, commercial mouthwash
• To avoid use of aspirin products, ibuprofen

meclizine (OTC, ℞)

(mek'li-zeen)

Antivert, Antivert/25, Antivert/25 Chewable, Antivert-50, Antrizine, Bonamine*, Bonine, Dizmiss, meclizine HCl, Meni-D, Ru-Vert-M

Func. class.: Antiemetic, antihistamine, anticholinergic

Chem. class.: H_1-receptor antagonist, piperazine derivative

Action: Acts centrally by blocking chemoreceptor trigger zone, which in turn acts on vomiting center

Uses: Dizziness, motion sickness

Dosage and routes:

• *Adult:* PO 25-100 mg qd in divided doses or 1 hr before traveling

Available forms: Tabs 12.5, 25, 50 mg; chew tabs 25 mg; tabs film coated 25 mg

Side effects/adverse reactions:

CNS: Drowsiness, fatigue, restlessness, headache, insomnia

GI: Nausea, anorexia

EENT: Dry mouth, blurred vision

Contraindications: Hypersensitivity to cyclizines, shock, lactation

Precautions: Children, narrow-angle glaucoma, glaucoma, urinary retention, lactation, prostatic hypertrophy, elderly, pregnancy (B)

Pharmacokinetics:

PO: Duration 8-24 hr, half-life 6 hr

Interactions:

• Increased effect of alcohol, tranquilizers, narcotics

Lab test interferences:

False negative: Allergy skin testing

NURSING CONSIDERATIONS

Assess:

• VS, B/P
• Signs of toxicity of other drugs or masking of symptoms of disease: brain tumor, intestinal obstruction

* Available in Canada only

• Observe for drowsiness, dizziness, LOC

Administer:

• Tablets may be swallowed whole, chewed, or allowed to dissolve

Evaluate:

• Therapeutic response: absence of dizziness, vomiting

Teach patient/family:

• That a false-negative result may occur with skin testing; these procedures should not be scheduled for 4 days after discontinuing use
• To avoid hazardous activities, activities requiring alertness; dizziness may occur; instruct patient to request assistance with ambulation
• To avoid alcohol, other depressants

meclofenamate (℞)

(me-kloe-fen-am'ate)

meclofenamate, meclofen, Meclomen

Func. class.: Nonsteroidal antiinflammatory

Chem. class.: Anthranilic acid derivative

Action: Inhibits prostaglandin synthesis by decreasing an enzyme needed for biosynthesis; analgesic, antiinflammatory, antipyretic

Uses: Mild to moderate pain, osteoarthritis, rheumatoid arthritis

Dosage and routes:

• *Adult:* PO 200-400 mg/day in divided doses tid-qid

Available forms: Caps 50, 100 mg

Side effects/adverse reactions:

GI: Nausea, anorexia, vomiting, diarrhea, jaundice, ***cholestatic hepatitis,*** constipation, flatulence, cramps, dry mouth, peptic ulcer, ***ulceration, perforation***

CNS: Dizziness, drowsiness, fatigue, tremors, confusion, insomnia, anxiety, depression

CV: Tachycardia, hypertension, peripheral edema, palpitations, dysrhythmias

INTEG: Purpura, rash, pruritus, sweating

GU: ***Nephrotoxicity: dysuria, hematuria, oliguria, azotemia***

HEMA: ***Blood dyscrasias***

EENT: Tinnitus, hearing loss, blurred vision

Contraindications: Hypersensitivity, asthma, severe renal, severe hepatic disease, ulcer disease

Precautions: Pregnancy (B), lactation, children, bleeding disorders, GI disorders, cardiac disorders, hypersensitivity to other antiinflammatory agents

Pharmacokinetics:

PO: Peak 2 hr, half-life 3-3½ hr; metabolized in liver, excreted in urine (metabolites), excreted in breast milk

Interactions:

• Increased action of coumarin, phenytoin, sulfonamides

NURSING CONSIDERATIONS

Assess:

• Renal, liver, blood studies: BUN, creatinine, AST (SGOT), ALT (SGPT), Hgb, Hct before treatment, periodically thereafter
• Audiometric and ophthalmic exam before, during, after treatment
• For history of peptic ulcer disease
• For eye, ear problems: blurred vision, tinnitus (may indicate toxicity)

Administer:

• With food to decrease GI symptoms; best to take on empty stomach to facilitate absorption

Perform/provide:

• Storage at room temp

Evaluate:

• Therapeutic response: decreased pain, stiffness, swelling in joints, ability to move more easily

Teach patient/family:
- To report increased GI symptoms; dose may have to be reduced
- To report blurred vision, ringing, roaring in ears (may indicate toxicity)
- To avoid driving, other hazardous activities for dizziness, drowsiness
- To report change in urine pattern, weight increase, edema, pain increase in joints, fever, blood in urine (indicates nephrotoxicity)
- That therapeutic effects may take up to 1 mo
- To take with full glass water
- To avoid other NSAIDs, alcohol, steroids

medium-chain triglycerides (℞)

MCT Oil

Func. class.: Caloric

Action: Needed for energy in body; more rapidly hydrolyzed than fat

Uses: Inadequate dietary fat intake or absorption

Dosage and routes:
- *Adult:* PO 15 ml tid-qid, not to exceed 100 ml/day

Available forms: Oil (115 calories/15 ml)

Side effects/adverse reactions:

CNS: Loss of consciousness (reversible)

GI: Nausea, vomiting, anorexia, cramps, diarrhea, distention

Contraindications: Hypersensitivity, severe hepatic disease, lipoproteinemia

Precautions: Portacaval shunts, pregnancy (C), pancreatitis, hyperlipemia

NURSING CONSIDERATIONS

Assess:
- Triglycerides, free-fatty-acid levels, platelet counts qd to prevent fat overload, thrombocytopenia
- Liver function: AST (SGOT), ALT (SGPT)
- Nutritional status: calorie count by dietitian

Evaluate:
- Therapeutic response: increased weight

Teach patient/family:
- Reason for use of lipids
- Methods of incorporating drug in food or beverages (salad dressings, chilled fruit juices)

medroxyprogesterone (℞)

(me-drox'ee-proe-jess'te-rone)

Amen, Curretab, Cycrin, Depo-Provera, medroxyprogesterone acetate, Provera

Func. class.: Progestogen

Chem. class.: Progesterone derivative

Action: Inhibits secretion of pituitary gonadotropins, which prevents follicular maturation and ovulation; stimulates growth of mammary tissue; antineoplastic action against endometrial cancer

Uses: Uterine bleeding (abnormal), secondary amenorrhea, endometrial cancer, renal cancer, contraceptive

Investigational uses: Pickwickian syndrome, sleep apnea

Dosage and routes:

Secondary amenorrhea
- *Adult:* PO 5-10 mg qd × 5-10 days

Endometrial/renal cancer
- *Adult:* 1M 400-1000 mg/wk

Uterine bleeding
- *Adult:* PO 5-10 mg qd × 5-10 days starting on 16th day of menstrual cycle

Contraceptive
- *Adult:* INJ q3mo

Available forms: Tabs 2.5, 10 mg; inj susp 100, 400 mg/ml, contraceptive injectable

Side effects/adverse reactions:

CNS: Dizziness, headache, migraines, depression, fatigue

CV: Hypotension, thrombophlebitis, edema, ***thromboembolism, stroke, pulmonary embolism, MI***

GI: Nausea, vomiting, anorexia, cramps, increased weight, ***cholestatic jaundice***

EENT: Diplopia

GU: Amenorrhea, cervical erosion, breakthrough bleeding, dysmenorrhea, vaginal candidiasis, breast changes, *gynecomastia, testicular atrophy, impotence,* endometriosis, ***spontaneous abortion***

INTEG: Rash, urticaria, acne, hirsutism, alopecia, oily skin, seborrhea, purpura, melasma, photosensitivity

META: Hyperglycemia

Contraindications: Breast cancer, hypersensitivity, thromboembolic disorders, reproductive cancer, genital bleeding (abnormal, undiagnosed), pregnancy (X)

Precautions: Lactation, hypertension, asthma, blood dyscrasias, gallbladder disease, CHF, diabetes mellitus, bone disease, depression, migraine headache, convulsive disorders, hepatic disease, renal disease, family history of cancer of breast or reproductive tract

Pharmacokinetics:

PO: Duration 24 hr, excreted in urine and feces, metabolized in liver

Lab test interferences:

Increase: Alk phosphatase, N (urine), pregnanediol, amino acids

Decrease: GTT, HDL

NURSING CONSIDERATIONS

Assess:

- Weight qd; notify prescriber of weekly weight gain >5 lb
- B/P at beginning of treatment and periodically
- I&O ratio; be alert for decreasing urinary output, increasing edema
- Liver function studies: ALT (SGPT), AST (SGOT), bilirubin, periodically during long-term therapy
- Edema, hypertension, cardiac symptoms, jaundice
- Mental status: affect, mood, behavioral changes, depression
- Hypercalcemia

Administer:

- Titrated dose; use lowest effective dose
- Oil solution deep in large muscle mass (IM), rotate sites
- After warming to dissolve crystals
- In one dose in AM
- With food or milk to decrease GI symptoms (PO)

Perform/provide:

- Storage in dark area

Evaluate:

- Therapeutic response: decreased abnormal uterine bleeding, absence of amenorrhea

Teach patient/family:

- To avoid sunlight or use sunscreen; photosensitivity can occur
- About cushingoid symptoms
- To report breast lumps, vaginal bleeding, edema, jaundice, dark urine, clay-colored stools, dyspnea, headache, blurred vision, abdominal pain, numbness or stiffness in legs, chest pain; male to report impotence or gynecomastia
- To report suspected pregnancy

M

mefenamic acid (℞)

(me-fe-nam′ik)

Ponstel

Func. class.: Nonsteroidal antiinflammatory

Chem. class.: Anthranilic acid derivative

Action: Inhibits prostaglandin synthesis by decreasing an enzyme needed for biosynthesis and interferes with prostaglandins at receptor sites; analgesic, antiinflammatory, antipyretic

Uses: Mild to moderate pain, dysmenorrhea, inflammatory disease

Dosage and routes:

• *Adult and child >14 yr:* PO 500 mg, then 250 mg q6h, use not to exceed 1 wk

Available forms: Caps 250 mg

Side effects/adverse reactions:

GI: Nausea, anorexia, vomiting, diarrhea, jaundice, ***cholestatic hepatitis,*** constipation, flatulence, cramps, dry mouth, peptic ulcer, ***ulceration, perforation***

CNS: Dizziness, drowsiness, fatigue, tremors, confusion, insomnia, anxiety, depression

CV: Tachycardia, peripheral edema, palpitations, dysrhythmias

INTEG: Purpura, rash, pruritus, sweating

GU: ***Nephrotoxicity: dysuria, hematuria, oliguria, azotemia***

HEMA: ***Blood dyscrasias***

EENT: Tinnitus, hearing loss, blurred vision

Contraindications: Hypersensitivity, asthma, severe renal disease, severe hepatic disease, ulcer disease

Precautions: Pregnancy (C), lactation, children, bleeding disorders, GI disorders, cardiac disorders, hypersensitivity to other antiinflammatory agents

Pharmacokinetics:

PO: Peak 2 hr, half-life 3-3½ hr; metabolized in liver, excreted in urine (metabolites), excreted in breast milk, extensive protein binding

Interactions:

• Increased action of coumarin, phenytoin, sulfonamides

NURSING CONSIDERATIONS

Assess:

• Renal, liver, blood studies: BUN, creatinine, AST (SGOT), ALT (SGPT), Hgb before treatment, periodically thereafter

• Audiometric, ophthalmic exam before, during, after treatment

• For eye, ear problems: blurred vision, tinnitus (may indicate toxicity)

Administer:

• With food to decrease GI symptoms; take on empty stomach to facilitate absorption

Perform/provide:

• Storage at room temp

Evaluate:

• Therapeutic response: decreased pain, stiffness, swelling in joints, ability to move more easily

Teach patient/family:

• To report blurred vision or ringing, roaring in ears (may indicate toxicity)

• To avoid driving, other hazardous activities if dizziness or drowsiness occurs

• To report change in urine pattern, weight increase, edema, pain increase in joints, fever, blood in urine (indicates nephrotoxicity)

• That therapeutic effects may take up to 1 mo

• To report diarrhea or skin rash: drug may be discontinued

• To take with full glass of water

• To avoid ASA, alcohol, steroids

mefloquine (℞)

(me-flow′quine)

Lariam

Func. class: Antimalarial

Chem. class.: Analog of quinine

Action: Exact mechanism not known; blood schizonticide

Uses: Treatment and prevention of *P. falciparum* malaria, *P. vivax*

Dosage and routes:

• *Adult:* PO 1250 mg as a single dose (treatment); 250 mg qwk × 4 wk, then 250 mg q2wk (prevention)

Available forms: Tabs 250 mg

Side effects/adverse reactions:

CV: Bradycardia, extrasystole

CNS: Dizziness, headache, syncope, *neuropsychiatric disturbances: disorientation, hallucinations,* ***coma, convulsions***

GI: Nausea, vomiting, loss of appetite, diarrhea, abdominal pain

INTEG: Itching, rash

MISC: Myalgia

Contraindications: Hypersensitivity

Precautions: Cardiac dysrhythmias, neurologic disease, lactation, children, pregnancy (C)

Pharmacokinetics:

Protein binding 98%, excreted in breast milk and urine, half-life 21 days (adults)

Interactions:

• Increased ECG abnormalities, possible cardiac arrest: β-blockers, quinine, quinidine

• Increased potential for convulsions: chloroquine, valproic acids

NURSING CONSIDERATIONS

Assess:

• B/P, pulse; watch for bradycardia

• Neuropsychiatric symptoms: disorientation, hallucinations; drug should be discontinued

• Liver studies qwk: ALT (SGPT), AST (SGOT), bilirubin

Administer:

• Do not take on an empty stomach; take medication with at least 8 oz water

Perform/provide:

• Storage in tight, light-resistant container

Evaluate:

• Therapeutic response: decreased symptoms of malaria

Teach patient/family:

• Do not take on empty stomach

megestrol (℞)

(me-jess′trole)

Megace, megestrol acetate

Func. class.: Antineoplastic

Chem. class.: Hormone, progestin

Action: Affects endometrium by antiluteinizing effect; this is thought to bring about cell death

Uses: Breast, endometrial cancer, renal cell cancer

Dosage and routes:

Endometrial/ovarian carcinoma

• *Adult:* PO 40-320 mg/day in divided doses

Breast carcinoma

• *Adult:* PO 40 mg qid

Anorexia (AIDS)

• *Adult:* PO 40 mg qid

Available forms: Tabs 20, 40 mg; oral susp 40 mg/ml

Side effects/adverse reactions:

GI: Nausea, vomiting, anorexia, diarrhea, abdominal cramps

GU: Gynecomastia, fluid retention, ***hypercalcemia***

CV: ***Thrombophlebitis***

INTEG: Alopecia, rash, pruritus, purpura, itching

CNS: Mood swings

Contraindications: Hypersensitivity, pregnancy (X)

Pharmacokinetics:

PO: Duration 1-3 days, half-life 60 min; metabolized in liver; excreted in feces, breast milk

Lab test interferences:

Increase: Alk phosphatase, urinary N, urinary pregnanediol, plasma amino acids

False positive: Urine glucose

Decrease: HDL, glucose tolerance test

NURSING CONSIDERATIONS

Assess:

- I&O ratio; weights
- Serum Ca levels
- Homan's sign
- Food preferences; list likes, dislikes
- Effects of alopecia on body image; discuss feelings about body changes
- Symptoms indicating severe allergic reaction: rash, pruritus, urticaria, purpuric skin lesions, itching, flushing
- Frequency of stools, characteristics: cramping, acidosis, signs of dehydration (rapid respirations, poor skin turgor, decreased urine output, dry skin, restlessness, weakness)
- Mood swings
- Anorexia, nausea, vomiting, constipation, weakness, loss of muscle tone

Administer:

- Antispasmodic
- Diuretics for increased fluids
- Oral susp for AIDS patients

Perform/provide:

- Increase fluid intake to 2-3 L/day to prevent dehydration and maintain normal Ca
- Nutritious diet with iron, vitamin supplements as ordered
- Limitation of Ca (dairy products)
- Storage in tight container at room temp

Evaluate:

- Therapeutic response: decreased tumor size, spread of malignancy; weight gain in AIDS patients

Teach patient/family:

- To report vaginal bleeding
- That nonhormonal contraception should be used during and 4 mo after treatment
- That gynecomastia can occur; reversible after discontinuing treatment
- To recognize and report signs of fluid retention, thromboemboli, hepatotoxicity

---

melphalan (℞)

(mel′fa-lan)

Alkeran, Alkeran IV, L-PAM, L-Sarcolysin

Func. class.: Antineoplastic alkylating agent

Chem. class.: Nitrogen mustard

Action: Responsible for cross-linking DNA strands leading to cell death; activity is not cell cycle specific

Uses: Multiple myeloma, breast cancer, reticulum cell sarcoma, testicular seminoma, malignant melanoma, advanced ovarian cancer

Investigational uses: Breast, testicular, prostate carcinoma; osteogenic sarcoma, chronic myelogenous leukemia

Dosage and routes:

Multiple myeloma

- *Adult:* PO 6 mg qd × 2-3 wk; stop drug for 4 wk or until WBC level begins to rise; do not administer if WBC <3000/mm^3 or platelets <100,000/mm^3; may be given 0.15 mg/kg/day × 7 days; wait until platelets and WBCs rise, then 0.05 mg/kg/day

---

* Available in Canada only

Ovarian carcinoma
• *Adult:* IV INF 16 mg/m^2, reduce in renal insufficiency, give over 15-20 min, give at 2 wk intervals × 4 doses, then at 4 wk intervals

Available forms: Tabs 2 mg, powder for inj 50 mg

Side effects/adverse reactions:
HEMA: ***Thrombocytopenia, neutropenia,*** leukopenia, anemia
GI: Nausea, vomiting, stomatitis, diarrhea
GU: Amenorrhea, hyperuricemia, gonadal suppression
INTEG: Rash, urticaria, alopecia, pruritus
RESP: ***Fibrosis, dysplasia***
SYST: ***Anaphylaxis,*** allergic reactions

Contraindications: Lactation, pregnancy (D), hypersensitivity to this drug or other nitrogen mustards

Precautions: Radiation therapy, bone marrow depression, infections, renal disease, children

Pharmacokinetics:
Metabolized in liver, excreted in urine, half-life 1½ hr

Interactions:
• Increased toxicity: antineoplastics, radiation

NURSING CONSIDERATIONS

Assess:
• CBC, differential, platelet count qwk; withhold drug if WBC is <4000 or platelet count is <75,000; notify prescriber
• Renal function studies: BUN, serum uric acid, urine CrCl before, during therapy
• I&O ratio; report fall in urine output of 30 ml/hr
• Monitor temp q4h (may indicate beginning infection); no rectal temps
• Liver function tests before, during therapy (bilirubin, AST [SGOT], ALT [SGPT], LDH) as needed or monthly
• Bleeding: hematuria, guaiac, bruising or petechiae, mucosa or orifices q8h
• Food preferences; list likes, dislikes
• Yellow skin and sclera, dark urine, clay-colored stools, itchy skin, abdominal pain, fever, diarrhea
• Inflammation of mucosa, breaks in skin
• Buccal cavity q8h for dryness, sores, ulceration, white patches, oral pain, bleeding, dysphagia
• Local irritation, pain, burning, discoloration at injection site
• Symptoms indicating severe allergic reaction: rash, pruritus, urticaria, purpuric skin lesions, itching, flushing

Administer:
• Antiemetic 30-60 min before giving drug to prevent vomiting
• Antibiotics for prophylaxis of infection
• Topical or systemic analgesics for pain
• Local or systemic drugs for infection

Perform/provide:
• Storage in air-tight, light-resistant container
• Strict medical asepsis, protective isolation if WBC levels are low
• Special skin care
• Increase fluid intake to 2-3 L/day to prevent urate deposits, calculi formation
• Diet low in purines: organ meats (kidney, liver), dried beans, peas to maintain alkaline urine
• Rinsing of mouth tid-qid with water, club soda; brushing of teeth bid-tid with soft brush or cotton-tipped applicators for stomatitis; use unwaxed dental floss
• Warm compresses at injection site for inflammation

Evaluate:

• Therapeutic response: decreased tumor size, spread of malignancy

Teach patient/family:

• About protective isolation

• That sterility, amenorrhea can occur; reversible after discontinuing treatment

• To avoid foods with citric acid, hot or rough texture

• To report any bleeding, white spots, or ulcerations in mouth to prescriber; tell patient to examine mouth qd

• To report signs of infection: fever, sore throat, flu symptoms

• To report signs of anemia: fatigue, headache, faintness, shortness of breath, irritability

• To avoid use of razors, commercial mouthwash

• To avoid use of aspirin products, ibuprofen

menadione/menadiol sodium diphosphate (Vit K_3) (℞)

(men-a-dye'one)

Synkavite*, Synkayvite

Func. class.: Vitamin, fat soluble

Action: Needed for adequate blood clotting (factors II, VII, IX, X)

Uses: Vit K malabsorption, hypoprothrombinemia

Dosage and routes:

• *Adult:* PO 2-10 mg (menadione)

• *Adult:* PO/IM/IV 5-15 mg (menadiol sodium diphosphate)

Available forms: Tabs 5 mg; inj 5, 10, 37.5 mg/ml

Side effects/adverse reactions:

CNS: Headache, ***brain damage*** (large doses)

GI: Nausea, decreased liver function tests

HEMA: ***Hemolytic anemia, hemoglobinuria, hyperbilirubinemia***

INTEG: Rash, urticaria

Contraindications: Hypersensitivity, severe hepatic disease, last few weeks of pregnancy (X)

Precautions: Neonates

Pharmacokinetics: Metabolized, crosses placenta

Interactions:

• Decreased action of menadione: oral antibiotics, cholestyramine, mineral oil

• Decreased action of oral anticoagulants

• Incompatible with alkaloids, codeine, levarterenol, levorphanol, meperidine, methadone, procaine

NURSING CONSIDERATIONS

Assess:

• Pro-time during treatment (2 sec deviation from control time, bleeding time, and clotting time), monitor for bleeding, pulse, and BP

• Nutritional status: liver (beef), spinach, tomatoes, coffee, asparagus, broccoli, cabbage, lettuce, greens

Administer:

• Deep IM, IV slowly over 7 min; may be given IV undiluted or added to infusions

Evaluate:

• Therapeutic response: decreased bleeding tendencies, decreased pro-time, decreased clotting time

Teach patient/family:

• Not to take other supplements unless directed by prescriber

• Necessary foods in diet

• To avoid use of mineral oil

• To avoid IM injections, activities leading to injury, use soft tooth brush, don't floss; use electric razor until coagulation defect corrected

• Not to take OTC drugs, especially containing aspirin or alcohol

• Importance of frequent lab tests to monitor coagulation factors

* Available in Canada only

menotropins (℞)

(men-oh-troe′pin)

Humegon, Pergonal

Func. class.: Gonadotropin

Chem. class.: Exogenous gonadotropin

Action: In women, increases follicular growth, maturation; in men, when given with HCG, stimulates spermatogenesis

Uses: Infertility, anovulation in women, stimulates spermatogenesis in men

Dosage and routes:

Infertility

- *Men:* IM 1 amp 3 × wk with HCG 2000 U 2 × wk × 4 mo
- *Women:* IM 75 IU FSH, LH qd × 9-12 days, then 10,000 U HCG 1 day after these drugs; repeat × 2 menstrual cycles, then increase to 150 IU FSH, LH qd × 9-12 days, then 10,000 U HCG 1 day after these drugs × 2 menstrual cycles

Anovulation

- *Women:* IM 75 IU FSH, LH qd × 9-12d, then 10,000 U HCG 1 day after last dose of these drugs; repeat × 1-3 menstrual cycles

Available forms: Powder for inj lyophilized 75 IU FSH, LH activity 150 IU FSH, LH activity

Side effects/adverse reactions:

CNS: Fever

CV: ***Hypovolemia***

GI: Nausea, vomiting, diarrhea, anorexia

GU: Ovarian enlargement, abdominal distention/pain, multiple births, ovarian hyperstimulation: sudden ovarian enlargement, ascites with or without pain, pleural effusion, gynecomastia in men

HEMA: ***Hemoperitoneum, arterial thromboembolism***

Contraindications: Primary ovarian failure, abnormal bleeding, thyroid/adrenal dysfunction, organic intracranial lesion, ovarian cysts, primary testicular failure

Precautions: Pregnancy (C)

NURSING CONSIDERATIONS

Assess:

- Weight qd; notify prescriber if weight increases rapidly
- Estrogen excretion level; if >100 μg/24 hr, drug is withheld; hyperstimulation syndrome may occur
- I&O ratio; be alert for decreasing urinary output
- Ovarian enlargement, abdominal distention/pain; report symptoms immediately

Administer:

- After reconstituting with 1-2 ml sterile saline inj; use immediately

Evaluate:

- Therapeutic response: ovulation, pregnancy

Teach patient/family:

- That multiple births are possible; if pregnancy occurs, usually 4-6 wk after start of treatment
- To keep appointment during treatment qd × 2 wk
- That daily intercourse is necessary from day preceding administration of gonadotropin until ovulation occurs

mepenzolate (℞)

(me-pen′zoe-late)

Cantil

Func. class.: GI anticholinergic

Chem. class.: Synthetic quaternary ammonium antimuscarinic

Action: Inhibits muscarinic actions of acetylcholine at postganglionic parasympathetic neuroeffector sites

Uses: Treatment of peptic ulcer disease, irritable bowel syndrome in combination with other drugs; for other GI disorders

Dosage and routes:

• *Adult:* PO 25-50 mg qid with meals, hs; titrate to patient response

Available forms: Tabs 25 mg

Side effects/adverse reactions:

CNS: Confusion, stimulation in elderly, headache, insomnia, dizziness, drowsiness, anxiety, weakness, hallucination

GI: Dry mouth, constipation, ***paralytic ileus,*** heartburn, nausea, vomiting, dysphagia, absence of taste

GU: Hesitancy, retention, impotence

CV: Palpitations, tachycardia

EENT: Blurred vision, photophobia, mydriasis, cycloplegia, increased ocular tension

INTEG: Urticaria, rash, pruritus, anhidrosis, fever, allergic reactions

Contraindications: Hypersensitivity to anticholinergics, narrow-angle glaucoma, GI obstruction, myasthenia gravis, paralytic ileus, GI atony, toxic megacolon

Precautions: Hyperthyroidism, coronary artery disease, dysrhythmias, CHF, ulcerative colitis, hypertension, hiatal hernia, hepatic disease, renal disease, pregnancy (C), elderly, urinary retention, prostatic hypertrophy

Pharmacokinetics:

PO: Onset 1 hr, duration 3-4 hr; metabolized by liver, excreted in urine

Interactions:

• Increased anticholinergic effect: amantadine, tricyclic antidepressants, MAOIs

• Decreased effect of phenothiazines, levodopa, ketoconazole

NURSING CONSIDERATIONS

Assess:

• VS, cardiac status: check for dysrhythmias, increased rate, palpitations

• I&O ratio; check for urinary retention or hesitancy

• GI complaints: pain, bleeding (frank or occult), nausea, vomiting, anorexia

Administer:

• ½-1 hr ac for better absorption

• Decreased dose to elderly patients; metabolism may be slowed

• Gum, hard candy, frequent rinsing of mouth for dry oral cavity

Perform/provide:

• Storage in tight container protected from light

• Increased fluids, bulk, exercise to decrease constipation

Evaluate:

• Therapeutic response: absence of epigastric pain, bleeding, nausea, vomiting

Teach patient/family:

• Avoid driving, other hazardous activities until stabilized on medication

• Avoid alcohol, other CNS depressants; will enhance sedating properties of this drug

• To avoid hot environments; heat stroke may occur; drug suppresses perspiration

• Use sunglasses when outside to prevent photophobia; may cause blurred vision

• To drink plenty of fluids

• To report dysphagia

meperidine (℞)

(me-per′i-deen)

Demerol, meperidine, Pethadol, Pethidine

Func. class.: Narcotic analgesic

Chem. class.: Opiate, phenylpiperidine derivative

Combination products: Mepergan: meperidine HCl 25 mg/ml with promethazine HCl 25 mg/ml; Me-

* Available in Canada only

pergan Fortis: meperidine HCl 50 mg with promethazine HCl 25 mg

Controlled Substance Schedule II
Action: Depresses pain impulse transmission at the spinal cord level by interacting with opioid receptors
Uses: Moderate to severe pain, preoperatively, postoperatively
Dosage and routes:
Pain
• *Adult:* PO/SC/IM 50-150 mg q3-4h prn; dose should be decreased if given IV
• *Child:* PO/SC/IM 1 mg/kg q4-6h prn, not to exceed 100 mg q4hr
Labor analgesia
• Adult: SC/IM 50-100 mg given when contractions are regularly spaced, repeat q1-3hr prn
Preoperatively
• *Adult:* IM/SC 50-100 mg q30-90 min before surgery; dose should be reduced if given IV
• *Child:* IM/SC 1-2.2 mg/kg 30-90 min before surgery
Available forms include: Inj 10, 50, 75, 100 mg/ml; tabs 50, 100 mg; syr 50 mg/5 ml
Side effects/adverse reactions:
CNS: Drowsiness, dizziness, confusion, headache, sedation, euphoria, ***increased intracranial pressure***
CV: Palpitations, bradycardia, change in B/P, tachycardia (IV)
EENT: Tinnitus, blurred vision, miosis, diplopia, depressed corneal reflex
GI: Nausea, vomiting, anorexia, constipation, cramps
GU: Urinary retention, dysuria
INTEG: Rash, urticaria, bruising, flushing, diaphoresis, pruritus
RESP: ***Respiratory depression***
Contraindications: Hypersensitivity, addiction (narcotic)
Precautions: Addictive personality, pregnancy (B), lactation, increased intracranial pressure, MI (acute), severe heart disease, respiratory depression, hepatic disease, renal disease, child <18 yr
Pharmacokinetics:
Absorption 50% (PO), well absorbed IM, SC
PO: Onset 15 min, peak 1 hr, duration 4-5 hr
SC/IM: Onset 10 min, peak 1 hr, duration 4-5 hr
IV: Onset 5 min, duration 2 hr
Metabolized by liver (to active/inactive metabolites), excreted by kidneys; crosses placenta, excreted in breast milk; half-life 3-6 hr; toxic by-product can result from regular use
Interactions:
• Increased effects with other CNS depressants: alcohol, narcotics, sedative/hypnotics, antipsychotics, skeletal muscle relaxants, MAOIs, chlorpromazine
Syringe compatibilities: Atropine, benzquinamide, butorphanol, chlorpromazine, cimetidine, dimenhydrinate, diphenhydramine, droperidol, fentanyl, glycopyrrolate, hydroxyzine, metochlopramide, midazolam, pentazocine, perphenazine, prochlorperazine, promazine, promethazine, ranitidine, scopolamine
Additive compatibilities: Scopolamine, triflupromazine
Y-site compatibilities: Amikacin, ampicillin, bumetanide, cefamandole, cefazolin, ceforanide, cefotaxime, cefotetan, cefoxitin, ceftizoxime, ceftriaxone, cefuroxime, cephalothin, cephapirin, chloramphenicol, clindamycin, dexamethasone, diphenhydramine, dobutamine, dopamine, doxycycline, droperidol, erythromycin lactobionate, famotidine, fluconazole, fludarabine, gentamicin, heparin, hydrocortisone, sodium succinate, insulin, kanamycin, labetalol, lidocaine, methyldo-

M

pate, magnesium sulfate, melphalan, methylprednisolone, metoclopramide, metoprolol, metronidazole, mezlocillin, minocycline, ondansetron, oxacillin, oxytocin, paclitaxel, penicillin G potassium, piperacillin, potassium chloride, propranolol, ranitidine, sargramostim, ticarcillin, ticarcillin/clavulanate, tobramycin, trimethoprim/sulfamethoxazole, vancomycin, verapamil, vinorelbine

Lab test interferences:
Increase: Amylase, lipase

NURSING CONSIDERATIONS

Assess:

• Pain: location, type, character; give before pain becomes extreme
• I&O ratio; check for decreasing output; may indicate urinary retention
• Need for drug
• For constipation; increase fluids, bulk in diet
• CNS changes: dizziness, drowsiness, hallucinations, euphoria, LOC, pupil reactions
• Allergic reactions: rash, urticaria
• Respiratory dysfunction: depression, character, rate, rhythm; notify prescriber if respirations are <12/min

Administer:

• IV after diluting with 5 ml or more sterile H_2O or NS; give directly over 4-5 min; may be further diluted in sol to 1 mg/ml during anesthesia in D_5W or NS; if diluted in NS, may be given through patient-controlled inf device
• Patient should remain recumbent for 1 hr after IM/SC route
• With antiemetic for nausea, vomiting
• When pain is beginning to return; determine dosage interval by patient response
• In gradually decreasing dose after long-term use; withdrawal symptoms may occur

Perform/provide:

• Storage in light-resistant container at room temp
• Assistance with ambulation
• Safety measures: side rails, nightlight, call bell within easy reach

Evaluate:

• Therapeutic response: decrease in pain

Teach patient/family:

• To report any symptoms of CNS changes, allergic reactions
• That physical dependency may result from extended use
• That drowsiness, dizziness may occur; to call for assistance
• Withdrawal symptoms may occur: nausea, vomiting, cramps, fever, faintness, anorexia
• To make position changes slowly; orthostatic hypotension can occur
• To avoid OTC medications, alcohol unless directed by prescriber

Treatment of overdose: Naloxone (Narcan) 0.2-0.8 mg IV, O_2, IV fluids, vasopressors

mephentermine (℞)

(me-fen′ter-meen)
Wyamine
Func. class.: Adrenergic, direct and indirect acting
Chem. class.: Substituted phenylethylamine

Action: Causes increased contractility and heart rate by acting on β-receptors in heart; also acts on α-receptors, causing vasoconstriction in blood vessels, cardiac output is elevated and systolic and diastolic pressures are increased

Uses: Shock and hypotension following variety of procedures

* Available in Canada only

Dosage and routes:
Hypotension
• *Adult:* IV 15-45 mg depending on procedure
Hypotension/shock
• *Adult:* IV 0.5 mg/kg
• *Child:* IV 0.4 mg/kg
Available forms: Inj IV 15, 30 mg/ml
Side effects/adverse reactions:
CV: Palpitations, tachycardia, hypertension
CNS: Tremors, drowsiness, confusion, incoherence
Contraindications: Hypersensitivity to sympathomimetics
Precautions: Pregnancy (B), cardiac disorders, hyperthyroidism, diabetes mellitus, prostatic hypertrophy
Pharmacokinetics:
IV: Onset immediate, duration ½-1 hr; metabolized in liver, excreted in urine
Interactions:
• Do not use with MAOIs or tricyclic antidepressants; hypertensive crisis may occur
• Decreased effect of mephentermine: methyldopa, urinary acidifiers, rauwolfia alkaloids
• Increased effect of mephentermine: urinary alkalizers
• Dysrhythmias: halothane, cyclopropaine, digitalis
• Incompatible with epinephrine, hydralazine

NURSING CONSIDERATIONS
Assess:
• I&O ratio; notify prescriber if output is <30 ml/hr
• ECG during administration continuously; if B/P increases, drug is decreased
• B/P, pulse q5min after parenteral route
• CVP or PWP during infusion if possible
Administer:
• Plasma expanders for hypovolemia
• IV undiluted 30 mg or less/1 min, or diluted 600 mg/500 ml D_5W, titrate to patient response, check site for extravasation; use an infusion pump
Perform/provide:
• Refrigerated storage of reconstituted sol no longer than 24 hr
• Do not use discolored sol
Evaluate:
• Therapeutic response: increased B/P with stabilization
Teach patient/family:
• Reason for drug administration

---

mephenytoin (℞)
(me-fen′i-toyn)
Mesantoin
Func. class.: Anticonvulsant
Chem. class.: Hydantoin derivative

Action: Reduces electrical discharges in motor cortex, reducing seizures; increases AV conduction velocity, prolongs refractory period
Uses: Generalized tonic-clonic, complex-partial seizures
Dosage and routes:
• *Adult:* PO 50-100 mg/day, may increase by 50-100 mg q7d, up to 200 mg tid
• *Child:* PO 50-100 mg/day or 100-450 mg/m^2/day in 3 divided doses, initially; then increase 50-100 mg q7d, up to 200 mg tid in divided doses q8h
Available forms: Tabs 100 mg
Side effects/adverse reactions:
HEMA: ***Agranulocytosis, neutropenia, leukopenia, pancytopenia, eosinophilia, lymphadenopathy***
CNS: Drowsiness, dizziness, fatigue, irritability, tremors, insomnia, depression

GI: Nausea, vomiting
INTEG: *Rash, **exfoliative dermatitis***
EENT: Photophobia, conjunctivitis, nystagmus, diplopia
RESP: ***Pulmonary fibrosis***
Contraindications: Hypersensitivity to hydantoins, sinus bradycardia, heart block, Adams-Stokes syndrome
Precautions: Alcoholism, hepatic disease, renal disease, blood dyscrasias, CHF, elderly, pregnancy (C), respiratory depression, diabetes mellitus
Pharmacokinetics:
PO: Onset 30 min, duration 24-48 hr, metabolized by liver, excreted by kidneys, half-life 144 hr
Interactions:
• Decreased effects: rifampin, chronic alcohol use, barbiturates, antihistamines, antacids, other anticonvulsants, antineoplastics, Ca products, folic acid, oxacillin
• Increased effects: benzodiazepines, cimetidine, salicylates, sulfonamide, pyrazolones, phenothiazines, estrogens, disulfiram, chloramphenicol, anticoagulants
• Seizures: valproic acid
• Myocardial depression: lidocaine, propanolol, sympathomimetics

NURSING CONSIDERATIONS
Assess:
• Blood studies: CBC, platelets q2 wk until stabilized, then qmo × 12, then q3mo; discontinue drug if neutrophils are <1600/mm^3, liver function tests with long-term use
• Drug level: therapeutic level 25-40 µg/ml
• Blood glucose may be increased
• Mental status: mood, sensorium, affect, behavioral changes; if mental status changes, notify prescriber
• Eye problems: need for ophthalmic examinations before, during, after treatment (slit lamp, fundoscopy, tonometry)
• Allergic reaction: red raised rash; drug should be discontinued
• Blood dyscrasias: fever, sore throat, bruising, rash, jaundice
• Toxicity: bone marrow depression, nausea, vomiting, ataxia, diplopia, cardiovascular collapse, Stevens-Johnson syndrome
Evaluate:
• Therapeutic response: decreased seizure activity
Teach patient/family:
• Not to discontinue drug quickly; should be tapered
• To avoid activities that require alertness if drowsiness, dizziness occurs
• That use of alcohol may decrease effects of drug
• To inform dentist; use good oral hygiene

---

mephobarbital (℞)
(me-foe-bar′bi-tal)
Mebaral
Func. class.: Anticonvulsant
Chem. class.: Barbiturate

Controlled Substance Schedule IV
Action: Depresses sensory cortex, motor activity; inhibits ascending conduction in reticular formation of thalamus
Uses: Generalized tonic-clonic (grand mal), absence (petit mal) seizures
Dosage and routes:
• *Adult:* PO 400-600 mg/day or in divided doses
• *Child:* PO 6-12 mg/kg/day in divided doses q6-8h
Available forms: Tabs 32, 50, 100, 200 mg
Side effects/adverse reactions:
HEMA: ***Thrombocytopenia, agranulocytosis, megaloblastic anemia***

---

* Available in Canada only

CNS: Dizziness, headache, hangover, paradoxic stimulation, drowsiness, increased pain
GI: Nausea, vomiting, epigastric pain
INTEG: Rash, urticaria, purpura, erythema multiforme, facial edema
EENT: Tinnitus, hearing loss
CV: Hypotension, bradycardia
RESP: Wheezing, hyperpnea
ENDO: Hypoglycemia, hyponatremia, hypokalemia
Contraindications: Hypersensitivity to barbiturates, pregnancy (D)
Precautions: Hepatic disease, renal disease, lactation, alcoholism, drug abuse, hyperthyroidism
Pharmacokinetics:
PO: Onset 20-60 min, duration 6-8 hr
Interactions:
• Increased effects: CNS depressants, chloramphenicol, valproic acid, disulfiram, nondepolarizing skeletal muscle relaxants, sulfonamides
• Increased orthostatic hypotension: furosemide

NURSING CONSIDERATIONS
Assess:
• Drug level, CBC, BUN, creatinine
• Mental status: mood, sensorium, affect, memory (long, short)
• Respiratory depression: respiration <10/min, shallow
• Blood dyscrasias: fever, sore throat, bruising, rash, jaundice
Perform/provide:
• Storage in light-resistant container
Evaluate:
• Therapeutic response: decreased seizure activity
Teach patient/family:
• Never to withdraw drug abruptly; notify prescriber of side effects
• To avoid hazardous activities until stabilized on drug
• That dreaming may increase when drug is discontinued

Treatment of overdose: Administer calcium gluconate IV

mepivacaine (℞)
(meep-ee'va-kane)
Carbocaine, Carbocaine with Neo-Cobefrin, Isocaine HCl, mepivicane HCl, Polocaine
Func. class.: Local anesthetic
Chem. class.: Amide

Action: Competes with calcium for sites in nerve membrane that control sodium transport across cell membrane; decreases rise of depolarization phase of action potential
Uses: Nerve block, caudal anesthesia, epidural, pain relief, paracervical block, transvaginal block or infiltration
Dosage and routes:
Varies with route of anesthesia
Available forms: Inj 1%, 1.5%, 2%, 3%
Side effects/adverse reactions:
CNS: Anxiety, restlessness, ***convulsions, loss of consciousness,*** drowsiness, disorientation, tremors, shivering
CV: ***Myocardial depression, cardiac arrest, dysrhythmias,*** bradycardia, hypotension, hypertension, ***fetal bradycardia***
GI: Nausea, vomiting
EENT: Blurred vision, tinnitus, pupil constriction
INTEG: Rash, urticaria, allergic reactions, edema, burning, skin discoloration at injection site, tissue necrosis
RESP: ***Status asthmaticus, respiratory arrest, anaphylaxis***
Contraindications: Hypersensitivity, child <12 yr, elderly, severe liver disease
Precautions: Elderly, severe drug allergies, pregnancy (C)

Pharmacokinetics:
Onset 15 min, duration 3 hr; metabolized by liver, excreted in urine (metabolites)

Interactions:
- Dysrhythmias: epinephrine, halothane, enflurane
- Hypertension: MAOIs, tricyclic antidepressants, phenothiazines
- Decreased action of mepivacaine: chloroprocaine

NURSING CONSIDERATIONS

Assess:
- B/P, pulse, respiration during treatment
- Fetal heart tones during labor
- Allergic reactions: rash, urticaria, itching
- Cardiac status: ECG for dysrhythmias, pulse, B/P during anesthesia

Administer:
- Only with crash cart, resuscitative equipment nearby
- Only drugs without preservatives for epidural or caudal anesthesia

Perform/provide:
- Use of new sol; discard unused portion

Evaluate:
- Therapeutic response: anesthesia necessary for procedure

Treatment of overdose: Airway, O_2, vasopressor, IV fluids, anticonvulsants for seizures

meprobamate (℞)

(me-proe-ba′mate)

Equanil, Meditran*, meprobamate, Meprospan, Miltown, Miltown 600, Neo-Tran*, Novomepro*, Saronil, Sedabamate, Tranhep

Func. class.: Sedative/hypnotic

Chem. class.: Propanediol carbamate derivative

Combination products: Deprol: meprobanate 400 mg with benactyzine HCl 1 mg; Epromate, Equagesic, Equazine-M, Hepto-M, Mepro Compound, Meprogesic, Micranin: meprobamate 200 mg with aspirin 325 mg; Milprem-200, PMB 200: meprobamate 200 mg with conjugated estrogens 0.45 mg; Milprem-400, PMB 400: meprobamate 400 mg with conjugated estrogens 0.45 mg; Robaxisal, Robomol/ASA: methocarbamol 400 mg, aspirin 325 mg

Controlled Substance Schedule IV

Action: Produces widespread depression of the CNS

Uses: Anxiety

Dosage and routes:
- *Adult:* PO 1.2-1.6 g/day in 2-3 divided doses, not to exceed 2.4 g/day or 800-1600 mg/day in 2 divided doses (SUS REL); max 2.4 g/day
- *Child 6-12 yr:* PO 100-200 mg bid-tid or 200 mg (SUS REL) bid

Available forms: Tabs 200, 400, 600 mg; caps 400 mg; sust rel caps 200, 400 mg

Side effects/adverse reactions:

HEMA: ***Thrombocytopenia, leukopenia, eosinophilia***

CNS: Dizziness, drowsiness, headache, ***convulsions,*** ataxia

GI: Nausea, vomiting, anorexia, diarrhea, stomatitis

INTEG: Urticaria, pruritus, maculopapular rash

CV: Hypotension, tachycardia, palpitations, ***hyperthermia***

EENT: Blurred vision, tinnitus, mydriasis, slurred speech

Contraindications: Hypersensitivity, renal failure, porphyria, pregnancy (D), history of drug abuse or dependence

Precautions: Suicidal patients, severe depression, renal disease, hepatic disease, elderly

Pharmacokinetics:
PO: Onset 1 hr; metabolized by liver;

* Available in Canada only

excreted in urine, in feces, breast milk; crosses placenta; half-life 6-16 hr

Interactions:

• Increased effects of meprobamate: CNS depressants, alcohol, tricyclic antidepressants

Lab test interferences:

False increase: 17-OHCS

False positive: Phentolamine test

NURSING CONSIDERATIONS

Assess:

• Sleep pattern; note sleep apnea, obstructed airway, pain/discomfort, urinary frequency other circumstances that interrupt sleep

• B/P (lying, standing), pulse; if systolic B/P drops 20 mm Hg, hold drug, notify prescriber

• Blood studies: CBC during long-term therapy; blood dyscrasias have occurred rarely

• Therapeutic blood levels 0.5-2 mg/100 ml

• Hepatic studies: AST (SGOT), ALT (SGPT), bilirubin, creatinine, LDH, alk phosphatase

• Mental status: mood, sensorium, affect, drowsiness, dizziness

• Tolerance, withdrawal symptoms: headache, nausea, vomiting, muscle pain, weakness, hyperthermia, death, convulsions after long-term use

• Suicidal tendencies

Administer:

• With food, milk for GI symptoms

• Crushed tabs if patient is unable to swallow medication whole; do not break, crush or chew sus rel cap

• Sugarless gum, hard candy, frequent sips of water for dry mouth

Perform/provide:

• Assistance with ambulation during beginning therapy, since drowsiness/dizziness occurs

• Safety measures, side rails

• Check to see PO medication has been swallowed

Evaluate:

• Therapeutic response: decreased anxiety, restlessness, insomnia

Teach patient/family:

• That drug may be taken with food

• Not to be used for everyday stress or used longer than 4 months unless directed by prescriber; not to take more than prescribed amount; may be habit forming

• To avoid OTC preparations (alcohol, cold, hay fever) unless approved by prescriber

• To avoid driving, activities that require alertness, since drowsiness may occur

• To avoid alcohol ingestion, other psychotropic medications unless directed by prescriber

• Not to discontinue medication abruptly after long-term use

• To rise slowly or fainting may occur, especially elderly

• That drowsiness may worsen at beginning of treatment

Treatment of overdose: Lavage, VS, supportive care

mercaptopurine (℞)

(mer-kap-toe-pyoor′een)

Purinethol, 6-MP

Func. class.: Antineoplastic-antimetabolite

Chem. class.: Purine analog

Action: Inhibits purine metabolism at multiple sites, which inhibits DNA and RNA synthesis, S phase of cell cycle specific

Uses: Chronic myelocytic leukemia, acute lymphoblastic leukemia in children, acute myelogenous leukemia

Investigational uses: Polycythemia vera, psoriatic arthritis, colitis, lymphoma

Dosage and routes:
• *Adult and child:* PO 2.5 mg/kg/day, not to exceed 5 mg/kg/day; maintenance 1.5-2.5 mg/kg/day
• *Child:* 70 mg/m^2/day
Available forms: Tabs 50 mg
Side effects/adverse reactions:
CNS: Fever, headache, weakness
HEMA: ***Thrombocytopenia, leukopenia, myelosuppression, anemia***
GI: Nausea, vomiting, anorexia, diarrhea, stomatitis, ***hepatotoxicity*** (high doses), jaundice, gastritis
GU: ***Renal failure,*** hyperuricemia, ***oliguria,*** crystalluria, ***hematuria***
INTEG: Rash, dry skin, urticaria
Contraindications: Patients with prior drug resistance, leukopenia (<2500/mm^3), thrombocytopenia (<100,000 / mm^3), anemia, pregnancy (D)
Precautions: Renal disease
Pharmacokinetics: Incompletely absorbed when taken orally; metabolized in liver, excreted in urine
Interactions:
• Increased toxicity: radiation or other antineoplastics
• Increased bone marrow depression: allopurinol
• Reversal of neuromuscular blockade: nondepolarizing muscle relaxants

NURSING CONSIDERATIONS
Assess:
• CBC, differential, platelet count qwk; withhold drug if WBC is <3500 or platelet count is <100,000; notify prescriber; drug should be discontinued
• Renal function studies: BUN, serum uric acid, urine CrCl, electrolytes before, during therapy
• I&O ratio; report fall in urine output to <30 ml/hr
• Monitor temp q4h; fever may indicate beginning infection; no rectal temps
• Liver function tests before, during therapy: bilirubin, alk phosphatase, AST (SGOT), ALT (SGPT), qwk during beginning therapy
• Bleeding: hematuria, guaiac, bruising, petechiae, mucosa or orifices q8h
• Food preferences; list likes, dislikes
• Inflammation of mucosa, breaks in skin
• Buccal cavity q8h for dryness, sores, ulceration, white patches, oral pain, bleeding, dysphagia
• Symptoms indicating severe allergic reaction: rash, urticaria, itching, flushing

Administer:
• Antacid before oral agent; give drug after evening meal before bedtime
• Allopurinol or sodium bicarbonate to maintain uric acid levels, alkalinization of urine
• Antibiotics for prophylaxis of infection
• Topical or systemic analgesics for pain
• Transfusion for anemia

Perform/provide:
• Strict medical asepsis, protective isolation if WBC levels are low
• Increase fluid intake to 2-3 L/day to prevent urate deposits, calculi formation, unless contraindicated
• Diet low in purines: absence of organ meats (kidney, liver), dried beans, peas to maintain alkaline urine
• Rinsing of mouth tid-qid with water, club soda; brushing of teeth bid-tid with soft brush or cotton-tipped applicators for stomatitis; use unwaxed dental floss
• Nutritious diet with iron, vitamin supplements as ordered
• Storage in tightly closed container in cool environment

---
* Available in Canada only

Evaluate:

- Therapeutic response: decreased size of tumor, spread of malignancy

Teach patient/family:

- To avoid foods with citric acid, hot or rough texture for stomatitis
- To report stomatitis: any bleeding, white spots, ulcerations in mouth; tell patient to examine mouth qd, report symptoms
- Contraceptive measures are recommended during therapy
- To drink 10-12 (8 oz) glasses of fluid/day
- To notify prescriber of fever, chills, sore throat, nausea, vomiting, anorexia, diarrhea, bleeding, bruising, which may indicate blood dyscrasias
- To report signs of infection: fever, sore throat, flu symptoms
- To report signs of anemia: fatigue, headache, faintness, shortness of breath, irritability
- To report bleeding: avoid use of razors, commercial mouthwash
- To avoid use of aspirin products, ibuprofen

mesalamine (℞)

(mez-al'a-meen)

Asacol, Pentusa, Rowasa Salofalk*

Func. class.: GI antiinflammatory

Chem. class.: 5-aminosalicylic acid

Action: May diminish inflammation by blocking cyclooxygenase, inhibiting prostaglandin production in colon; local action only

Uses: Mild to moderate active distal ulcerative colitis, proctosigmoiditis, proctitis

Dosage and routes:

- *Adult:* REC 60 ml (4 g) hs, retained for 8 hr × 3-6 wk; PO 800 mg tid for 6 wk; SUPP 500 mg bid for 3-6 wk

Available forms: Rec susp 4 g/60 ml; supp 500 mg, tab del rel 400 mg

Side effects/adverse reactions:

CV: Pericarditis, myocarditis

GI: Cramps, gas, nausea, diarrhea, rectal pain, constipation

CNS: Headache, fever, dizziness, insomnia, asthenia, weakness, fatigue

INTEG: Rash, itching, acne

SYST: Flu, malaise, back pain, peripheral edema, leg and joint pain, arthralgia, dysmenorrhea

EENT: Sore throat, cough, pharyngitis, rhinitis

Contraindications: Hypersensitivity to this drug or salicylates

Precautions: Renal disease, pregnancy (B), lactation, children, sulfite sensitivity

Pharmacokinetics:

REC: Primarily excreted in feces but some in urine as metabolite; half-life 1 hr, metabolite half-life 5-10 hr

NURSING CONSIDERATIONS

Assess:

- GI symptoms: cramps, gas, nausea, diarrhea, rectal pain; if severe, drug should be discontinued

Administer:

- May give orally, tabs should be swallowed whole
- Rectally; drug should be given hs, retained until morning

Perform/provide:

- Storage at room temp

Evaluate:

- Therapeutic response: absence of pain, bleeding from GI tract, decrease in number of diarrhea stools

Teach patient/family:

- That usual course of therapy is 3-6 wk
- To shake bottle well
- Method of rectal administration
- To inform prescriber of GI symptoms
- Not to crush tabs

M

• To report abdominal cramping, pain, diarrhea with blood, headache, fever, rash; drug should be discontinued

mesoridazine (℞)

(mez-oh-rid'a-zeen)

Serentil

Func. class.: Antipsychotic/ neuroleptic

Chem. class.: Phenothiazine, piperidine

Action: Depresses cerebral cortex, hypothalamus, limbic system, which control activity, aggression; blocks neurotransmission produced by dopamine at synapse; exhibits strong α-adrenergic, anticholinergic blocking action; mechanism for antipsychotic effects is unclear

Uses: Psychotic disorders, schizophrenia, anxiety, alcoholism, behavioral problems in mental deficiency, chronic brain syndrome

Dosage and routes:

Schizophrenia

• *Adult:* PO 50 mg tid, optimum dose 100-400 mg/day; IM 25 mg may repeat ½-1 hr; dosage range 25-200 mg/day

Behavior problems

• *Adult:* PO 25 mg tid; optimum dose 75-300 mg/day;

Alcoholism

• *Adult:* PO 25 mg bid; optimum dose 50-200 mg/day

Schizoaffective disorders

• *Adult:* PO 10 mg tid; optimum dose 30-150 mg/day

Available forms: Tabs 10, 25, 50, 100 mg; conc 25 mg/ml; inj 25 mg/ml

Side effects/adverse reactions:

RESP: ***Laryngospasm,*** dyspnea, ***respiratory depression***

CNS: EPS: pseudoparkinsonism, akathisia, dystonia, tardive dyskinesia, drowsiness, headache

HEMA: ***Anemia, leukopenia, leukocytosis, agranulocytosis***

INTEG: Rash, photosensitivity, dermatitis

EENT: Blurred vision, glaucoma

GI: Dry mouth, nausea, vomiting, anorexia, constipation, diarrhea, jaundice, weight gain

GU: Urinary retention, urinary frequency, enuresis, impotence, amenorrhea, gynecomastia

CV: Orthostatic hypotension, hypertension, ***cardiac arrest,*** ECG changes, tachycardia

Contraindications: Hypersensitivity, circulatory collapse, liver damage, cerebral arteriosclerosis, coronary disease, severe hypertension/ hypotension, blood dyscrasias, coma, brain damage, bone marrow depression, narrow-angle glaucoma

Precautions: Pregnancy (C), lactation, seizure disorders, hypertension, hepatic disease, cardiac disease, prostatic hypertrophy, intestinal obstruction, respiratory conditions

Pharmacokinetics:

PO: Onset erratic, peak 2 hr, duration 4-6 hr

IM: Onset 15-30 min, peak 30 min, duration 6-8 hr

Metabolized by liver, excreted in urine, crosses placenta, enters breast milk

Interactions:

• Oversedation: other CNS depressants, alcohol, barbiturate anesthetics

• Toxicity: epinephrine

• Decreased absorption: aluminum hydroxide, magnesium hydroxide antacids

• Decreased effects of lithium, levodopa

• Increased effects of both drugs: β-adrenergic blockers, alcohol

• Increased anticholinergic effects: anticholinergics

Lab test interferences:
Increase: Liver function tests, cardiac enzymes, cholesterol, blood glucose, prolactin, bilirubin, PBI, cholinesterase, ^{131}I
Decrease: Hormones (blood, urine)
False positive: Pregnancy tests, PKU
False negative: Urinary steroids, 17-OHCS

NURSING CONSIDERATIONS

Assess:
• Mental status before initial administration
• Swallowing of PO medication; check for hoarding or giving to other patients
• I&O ratio; palpate bladder if low urinary output occurs
• Bilirubin, CBC, liver function studies monthly
• Urinalysis is recommended before, during prolonged therapy
• Affect, orientation, LOC, reflexes, gait, coordination, sleep pattern disturbances
• B/P standing and lying, pulse, respirations q4h during initial treatment; establish baseline before starting treatment; report drops of 30 mm Hg
• Dizziness, faintness, palpitations, tachycardia on rising
• EPS including akathisia (inability to sit still, no pattern to movements), tardive dyskinesia (bizarre movements of jaw, mouth, tongue, extremities), pseudoparkinsonism (rigidity, tremors, pill rolling, shuffling gait)
• For neuroleptic malignant syndrome: hyperthermia, altered mental status, muscle rigidity, increased CPK
• Skin turgor daily
• Constipation, urinary retention daily; if these occur increase bulk, water in diet

Administer:
• Antiparkinsonian agent after securing order from prescriber for EPS
• Concentrate mixed in distilled water, orange, grape juice; do not prepare, store bulk dilutions
• IM inj into large muscle mass; do not use if precipitate present

Perform/provide:
• Decreased noise input by dimming lights, avoiding loud noises
• Supervised ambulation until stabilized on medication; do not involve in strenuous exercise program because fainting is possible; patient should not stand still for long periods
• Increased fluids to prevent constipation
• Sips of water, candy, gum for dry mouth
• Storage in air-tight, light-resistant container

Evaluate:
• Therapeutic response: decrease in emotional excitement, hallucinations, delusions, paranoia, and reorganization of patterns of thought, speech

Teach patient/family:
• That orthostatic hypotension is common and to rise from sitting or lying position gradually; to avoid hazardous activities until stabilized on medication
• To remain lying down for at least 30 min after IM injection
• To avoid hot tubs, hot showers, tub baths; hypotension may occur
• To avoid abrupt withdrawal of mesoridazine, or EPS may result; drug should be withdrawn slowly
• To avoid OTC preparations (cough, hay fever, cold) unless approved by prescriber; serious drug interactions may occur; to avoid use with alcohol, CNS depressants; increased drowsiness may occur

M

• To use sunscreen during sun exposure to prevent burns
• Regarding compliance with drug regimen
• About necessity for meticulous oral hygiene, since oral candidiasis may occur
• To report sore throat, malaise, fever, bleeding, mouth sores; if these occur, a CBC should be drawn and drug discontinued
• That in hot weather heat stroke may occur; take extra precautions to stay cool

Treatment of overdose: Lavage if orally ingested; provide an airway; *do not induce vomiting*

---

metaproterenol (℞)

(met-a-proe-ter′e-nole)
Alupent, Arm-A-Med Metaproterenol Sulfate, Metaprel
Func. class.: Selective β_2-agonist

Action: Relaxes bronchial smooth muscle by direct action on β_2-adrenergic receptors with increased levels of cAMP with increased bronchodilation, diuresis, cardiac CNS stimulation

Uses: Bronchial asthma, bronchospasm

Dosage and routes:
• *Adult and child>12 yr:* INH 2-3 puffs; may repeat q3-4h, not to exceed 12 puffs/day
• *Adult:* PO 20 mg q6-8h
• *Child >9 yr or >27 kg:* PO 20 mg q6-8h or 0.4-0.9 mg/kg tid
• *Child 6-9 yr or <27 kg:* PO 10 mg q6-8h or 0.4-0.9 mg/kg tid

Available forms: Tabs 10, 20 mg; aerosol 0.65 mg/dose; syrup 10 mg/5 ml; sol nebulizer 0.4, 0.6%, 5%

Side effects/adverse reactions:
CNS: Tremors, anxiety, insomnia, headache, dizziness, stimulation
CV: Palpitations, tachycardia, hypertension, dysrhythmias, ***cardiac arrest***
GI: Nausea, vomiting

Contraindications: Hypersensitivity to sympathomimetics, narrow-angle glaucoma

Precautions: Pregnancy (C), cardiac disorders, hyperthyroidism, diabetes mellitus, prostatic hypertrophy

Pharmacokinetics:
Well absorbed (PO)
PO: Onset 15-30 min, peak 1 hr, duration 4 hr, excreted in urine as metabolites
INH: Onset 5 min, peak 1 hr, duration 4 hr

Interactions:
• Increased effects of both drugs: other sympathomimetics
• Decreased action of β-blockers, oral hypoglycemics

Lab test interferences:
Decrease: K

NURSING CONSIDERATIONS

Assess:
• Respiratory function: vital capacity, forced expiratory volume, ABGs; also B/P; lung sounds, secretion before and after treatment
• Tolerance over long-term therapy; dose may have to be changed; check for rebound bronchospasm

Administer:
• 2 hr before hs to avoid sleeplessness
• PO with food for GI upset

Perform/provide:
• Storage at room temp; do not use discolored sol

Evaluate:
• Therapeutic response: absence of dyspnea, wheezing; improved ABGs

Teach patient/family:
• To increase fluid intake to liquefy secretions

---

* Available in Canada only

• Not to use OTC medications; extra stimulation may occur
• To notify prescriber of headaches, chest pain, weakness, dizziness, anxiety
• Use of inhaler; review package insert with patient
• To avoid getting aerosol in eyes
• To wash inhaler in warm water and dry qd
• On all aspects of drug; avoid smoking, smoke-filled rooms, persons with respiratory infections

metformin (℞)

(met-for'min)
Glucophage
Func. class.: Antidiabetic, oral
Chem. class.: Biguanide

Action: Inhibits hepatic glucose production and increases sensitivity of peripheral tissue to insulin
Uses: Stable adult-onset diabetes mellitus (type II) NIDDM
Dosage and routes:
• *Adult:* PO 500 mg bid initially, then increase to desired response 1-3 g; dosage adjustment q2-3 wk or 850 mg qd with morning meal with dosage increased every other week, max 2550 mg/day
Available forms: Tabs 500, 850 mg
Side effects/adverse reactions:
CNS: Headache, weakness, dizziness, drowsiness, tinnitus, fatigue, vertigo, *agitation*
GI: Nausea, vomiting, diarrhea, heartburn, anorexia, metallic taste
HEMA: ***Thrombocytopenia***
INTEG: Rash
ENDO: Lactic acidosis
Contraindications: Hypersensitivity, hepatic, renal disease, alcoholism, cardiopulmonary disease
Precautions: Pregnancy (UK), elderly, thyroid disease, previous hypersensitivity to phenformin or buformin
Pharmacokinetics: Excreted by the kidneys unchanged 35%-50%, half-life 1½-5 hr, terminal 9-17 hr, peak 1-3 hr
Interactions:
• Increased risk of lactic acidosis, ethanol, glucocorticoids
• Increased blood glucose levels: acetazolamide
• Increased hypoglycemia: cimetidine

NURSING CONSIDERATIONS
Assess:
• For hypoglycemic reactions (sweating, weakness, dizziness, anxiety, tremors, hunger), hyperglycemic reactions soon after meals
• CBC (baseline, q3mo) during treatment; check liver function tests periodically AST (SGOT), LDH, renal studies: BUN, creatinine during treatment
• For lactic acidosis
Administer:
• Conversion from other oral hypoglycemic agents; change may be made without gradual dosage change; monitor serum or urine glucose and ketones tid during conversion
• Twice a day give with meals to decrease GI upset and provide best absorption
• Tabs crushed and mixed with meal or fluids for patients with difficulty swallowing
Perform/provide:
• Storage in tight container in cool environment
Teach patient/family:
• To use capillary blood glucose test or Chemstrip tid
• Symptoms of hypo/hyperglycemia, what to do about each
• That drug must be continued on daily basis; explain consequence of discontinuing drug abruptly

M

• To take drug in morning to prevent hypoglycemic reactions at night
• To avoid OTC medications unless approved by the prescriber
• That diabetes is lifelong illness; that this drug is not a cure; only controls symptoms
• That all food included in diet plan must be eaten to prevent hypoglycemia
• To carry Medic Alert ID and glucagon emergency kit for emergencies

Evaluate:
• Therapeutic response: Decrease in polyuria, polydipsia, polyphagia; clear sensorium; absence of dizziness; stable gait, blood glucose at normal level

Treatment of overdose: Glucose 25 g IV via dextrose 50% sol, 50 ml or 1 mg glucagon

methadone (℞)

(meth'a-done)
Dolophine HCl, methadone, methadone HCl Diskets, methadone HCl Intensol
Func. class.: Narcotic analgesic
Chem. class.: Opiate, synthetic diphenylheptane derivative

Controlled Substance Schedule II
Action: Depresses pain impulse transmission at the spinal cord level by interacting with opioid receptors, produce CNS depression
Uses: Severe pain, narcotic withdrawal
Dosage and routes:
Pain
• *Adult:* PO/SC/IM 2.5-10 mg q4-12h prn
Narcotic withdrawal
• *Adult:* PO 15-40 mg/day individualized initially, then 20-120 mg/day titrated to patient response
Available forms: Inj 10 mg/ml; tabs 5, 10 mg; oral sol 5, 10 mg/5 ml; dispersible tabs 40 mg; oral conc 10 mg/ml
Side effects/adverse reactions:
CNS: Drowsiness, dizziness, confusion, headache, sedation, euphoria
GI: Nausea, vomiting, anorexia, constipation, cramps, biliary tract spasm
GU: Increased urinary output, dysuria, urinary retention
INTEG: Rash, urticaria, bruising, flushing, diaphoresis, pruritus
EENT: Tinnitus, blurred vision, miosis, diplopia
CV: Palpitations, bradycardia, change in B/P
RESP: ***Respiratory depression***
Contraindications: Hypersensitivity to this drug or chlorobutanol (inj), addiction (narcotic)
Precautions: Addictive personality, pregnancy (B), lactation, increased intracranial pressure, MI (acute), severe heart disease, respiratory depression, hepatic disease, renal disease, child <18 yr
Pharmacokinetics:
PO: Onset 30-60 min, duration 6-8 hr, cumulative 22-48 hr
SC/IM: Onset 10-20 min, peak 1 hr, duration 6-8 hr, cumulative 22-48 hr
Metabolized by liver; excreted by kidneys; crosses placenta; excreted in breast milk; half-life 1-1½ days; 90% bound to plasma proteins
Interactions:
• Increased effects with other CNS depressants: alcohol, narcotics, sedative/hypnotics, antipsychotics, skeletal muscle relaxants, rifampin, phenytoin
Lab test interferences:
Increase: Amylase

NURSING CONSIDERATIONS
Assess:
• I&O ratio; check for decreasing output; may indicate urinary retention
• CNS changes: dizziness, drowsiness, hallucinations, euphoria, LOC, pupil reaction
• Allergic reactions: rash, urticaria
• Respiratory dysfunction: respiratory depression, character, rate, rhythm; notify prescriber if respirations are <10/min
• Need for pain medication; possible physical dependence
Administer:
• With antiemetic if nausea/vomiting occurs
• When pain is beginning to return; determine dosage interval by patient response
• Rotating inj sites, give deep in large muscle mass (IM)
Perform/provide:
• Storage in light-resistant area at room temp
• Assistance with ambulation
• Safety measures: side rails, nightlight, call bell within easy reach
Evaluate:
• Therapeutic response: decrease in pain, successful narcotic withdrawal
Teach patient/family:
• To report any symptoms of CNS changes, allergic reactions
• That physical dependency may result from extended use
• Withdrawal symptoms may occur: nausea, vomiting, cramps, fever, faintness, anorexia
Treatment of overdose: Naloxone (Narcan) 0.2-0.8 mg IV, O_2, IV fluids, vasopressors

methamphetamine (℞)
(meth-am-fet'a-meen)
Desoxyn, Desoxyn Gradumet
Func. class.: Cerebral stimulant
Chem. class.: Amphetamine

Controlled Substance Schedule II
Action: Increases release of norepinephrine and dopamine in cerebral cortex to reticular activating system
Uses: Exogenous obesity, minimal brain dysfunction, attention deficit disorder with hyperactivity
Dosage and routes:
Attention deficit disorder
• *Child >6 yr:* 2.5-5 mg qd or bid increasing by 5 mg/wk
Obesity
• *Adult:* PO 2.5-5 mg, 30 min ac or 10-15 mg long-acting tab qd in AM
Available forms: Tabs 5 mg; tabs long-acting 5, 10, 15 mg
Side effects/adverse reactions:
CNS: Hyperactivity, insomnia, restlessness, talkativeness, dizziness, headache, chills, stimulation, dysphoria, irritability, aggressiveness, tremor
GI: Anorexia, dry mouth, diarrhea, constipation, weight loss, metallic taste, cramps
GU: Impotence, change in libido
CV: Palpitations, tachycardia, hypertension, decreased heart rate, dysrhythmia
INTEG: Urticaria
Contraindications: Hypersensitivity to sympathomimetic amines, hyperthyroidism, hypertension, glaucoma hypertrophy, severe arteriosclerosis, drug abuse, cardiovascular disease, anxiety
Precautions: Gilles de la Tourette's disorder, pregnancy (C), lactation, child <3 years
Pharmacokinetics:
PO: Duration 3-6 hr, metabolized

M

by liver, excreted by kidneys, crosses blood-brain barrier

Interactions:

• Hypertensive crisis: MAOIs or within 14 days of MAOIs

• Increased effect of methamphetamine: acetazolamide, antacids, sodium bicarbonate

• Decreased effects of methamphetamine: barbiturates, tricyclics, ascorbic acid, ammonium chloride

• Decreased effect of guanethidine

NURSING CONSIDERATIONS

Assess:

• VS, B/P; may reverse antihypertensives; check patients with cardiac disease more often

• CBC, urinalysis, in diabetes: blood sugar, urine sugar; insulin changes may have to be made, since eating will decrease

• Height, growth rate in children; growth rate may be decreased

• Mental status: mood, sensorium, affect, stimulation, insomnia, aggressiveness

• Physical dependency: should not be used for extended time; dose should be discontinued gradually; tolerance will occur (long-term use)

• Withdrawal symptoms: headache, nausea, vomiting, muscle pain, weakness

Administer:

• At least 6 hr before hs to avoid sleeplessness

• For obesity only if patient is on program including dietary changes, exercise; patient will develop tolerance; loss of weight won't occur without additional methods; give 2 hr before meals

• Gum, hard candy or frequent sips of water for dry mouth

Evaluate:

• Therapeutic response: decreased weight, decreased hyperactivity

Teach patient/family:

• To decrease caffeine consumption (coffee, tea, cola, chocolate), which may increase irritability, stimulation

• To avoid OTC preparations unless approved by presciber

• To taper off drug over several weeks, or depression, increased sleeping, lethargy may ensue

• To avoid alcohol ingestion

• To avoid hazardous activities until patient is stabilized on medication

• To get needed rest; patients will feel more tired at end of day

• Not to chew or crush sus rel forms

Treatment of overdose: Administer fluids, hemodialysis or peritoneal dialysis; antihypertensive for increased B/P; ammonium Cl for increased excretion

methantheline (℞)

(meth-an'tha-leen)

Banthine

Func. class.: GI anticholinergic

Chem. class.: Synthetic quaternary ammonium antimuscarinic

Combination products: Cystex: methenamine 165 mg, salicylamide 65 mg, sodium salicylate 97 mg, benzoic acid 32 mg; Hexalol: methenamine 40.8 mg, phenyl salicylate 18.1 mg, atropine SO_4 0.03, hyoscyamine 0.03 mg, benzoic acid 4.5 mg, methylene blue 5.4 mg; Thiacide: methenamine mandelate 500 mg, potassium acid phosphate 250 mg; TracTabs 2X: methenamine 120 mg, methylene blue 6 mg, phenyl salicylate 30 mg, atropine 0.06, hyoscyamine SO_4 0.03 mg, benzoic acid 7.5 mg; Uroquid-Acid No. 2: methenamine mandelate 500 mg, sodium acid phosphate 500 mg

* Available in Canada only

Action: Inhibits muscarinic actions of acetylcholine at postganglionic parasympathetic neuroeffector sites

Uses: Treatment of peptic ulcer disease, irritable bowel syndrome, pancreatitis, gastritis, biliary dyskinesia, pylorospasm, reflex neurogenic bladder in children

Dosage and routes:

- *Adult:* PO 50-100 mg q6h
- *Child >1 yr:* PO 12.5-50 mg qid
- *Child <1 yr:* PO 12.5-25 mg qid
- *Neonate:* PO 12.5 mg bid-tid

Available forms: Tabs 50 mg

Side effects/adverse reactions:

CNS: Confusion, stimulation in elderly, headache, insomnia, dizziness, drowsiness, anxiety, weakness, hallucination

GI: Dry mouth, constipation, paralytic ileus, heartburn, nausea, vomiting, dysphagia, absence of taste

GU: Hesitancy, retention, impotence

CV: Palpitations, tachycardia

EENT: Blurred vision, photophobia, mydriasis, cycloplegia, increased ocular tension

INTEG: Urticaria, rash, pruritus, anhidrosis, fever, allergic reactions

Contraindications: Hypersensitivity to anticholinergics, narrow-angle glaucoma, GI obstruction, myasthenia gravis, paralytic ileus, GI atony, toxic megacolon

Precautions: Hyperthyroidism, coronary artery disease, dysrhythmias, CHF, ulcerative colitis, hypertension, hiatal hernia, hepatic disease, renal disease, pregnancy (C), urinary retention, prostatic hypertrophy

Pharmacokinetics:

PO: Onset 30-45 min, duration 4-6 hr; metabolized by liver, excreted in urine, bile

Interactions:

- Increased anticholinergic effect: amantadine, tricyclic antidepressants, MAOIs, H_1 antihistamines
- Increased effect of nitrofurantoin
- Decreased effect of phenothiazines, levodopa

NURSING CONSIDERATIONS

Assess:

- VS, cardiac status: check for dysrhythmias, increased rate, palpitations
- I&O ratio; check for urinary retention, hesitancy
- GI complaints: pain, bleeding (frank or occult), nausea, vomiting, anorexia

Administer:

- ½-1 hr ac for better absorption
- Decreased dose to elderly patients; metabolism may be slowed
- Gum, hard candy, frequent rinsing of mouth for dryness of oral cavity

Perform/provide:

- Storage in tight container protected from light
- Increased fluids, bulk, exercise to decrease constipation

Evaluate:

- Therapeutic response: absence of epigastric pain, bleeding, nausea, vomiting

Teach patient/family:

- To avoid driving, other hazardous activities until stabilized on medication
- To avoid alcohol, other CNS depressants; will enhance sedating properties of this drug
- That drug may cause blurred vision

methazolamide (℞)

(meth-a-zoe′la-mide)

Neptazane

Func. class.: Carbonic anhydrase inhibitor diuretic

Chem. class.: Sulfonamide derivative

Action: Decreases production of

aqueous humor in eye, which lowers intraocular pressure

Uses: Open-angle glaucoma or preoperatively in narrow-angle glaucoma; can be used with miotic, osmotic agents

Dosage and routes:

• *Adult:* PO 50-100 mg bid or tid

Available forms: Tabs 25, 50 mg

Side effects/adverse reactions:

GU: Frequency, hypokalemia, polyuria, uremia, ***glucosuria, hematuria,*** dysuria, renal calculi

CNS: Drowsiness, paresthesia, anxiety, depression, headache, dizziness, confusion, stimulation, fatigue, ***convulsions***, sedation, nervousness

GI: Nausea, vomiting, anorexia, constipation, diarrhea, melena, weight loss, ***hepatic insufficiency,*** metallic taste in mouth

EENT: Myopia, tinnitus

INTEG: Rash, pruritus, urticaria, fever, photosensitivity, ***Stevens-Johnson syndrome***

ENDO: Hyperglycemia

HEMA: ***Aplastic anemia, hemolytic anemia, leukopenia, agranulocytosis, thrombocytopenia, purpura, pancytopenia***

Contraindications: Hypersensitivity to sulfonamides, severe renal disease, severe hepatic disease, electrolyte imbalances (hyponatremia, hypokalemia), hyperchloremic acidosis, Addison's disease, COPD

Precautions: Hypercalciuria, pregnancy (C), diabetes mellitus

Pharmacokinetics:

PO: Onset 2-4 hr, peak 6-8 hr, duration 10-18 hr; excreted in urine, crosses placenta

Interactions:

• Decreased effectiveness of lithium, barbiturates

• Increased action of amphetamines, procainamide, quinidine, flecainide, ephedrine, pseudoephedrine

• Hypokalemia: with other diuretics, corticosteroids, amphotericin B

• Toxicity: salicylates

Lab test interferences:

False positive: Urinary protein

NURSING CONSIDERATIONS

Assess:

• Weight, I&O daily to determine fluid loss; effect of drug may be decreased if used qd

• Rate, depth, rhythm of respiration, effect of exertion

• B/P lying, standing; postural hypotension may occur

• Electrolytes: K, Na, Cl; include BUN, blood sugar, CBC, serum creatinine, blood pH, ABGs, liver function tests

• Signs of metabolic acidosis: drowsiness, restlessness

• Signs of hypokalemia: postural hypotension, malaise, fatigue, tachycardia, leg cramps, weakness

• Rashes, temp qd

• Confusion, especially in elderly; take safety precautions if needed

Administer:

• In AM to avoid sleeplessness

• K replacement if K less than 3

• With food if nausea occurs; absorption may be decreased slightly

Evaluate:

• Therapeutic response: decrease in aqueous humor

Teach patient/family:

• To increase fluid intake to 2-3 L/day unless contraindicated; to rise slowly from lying or sitting position

• To use sunscreen for photosensitivity

• To notify prescriber of sore throat, unusual bleeding, bruising, paresthesias, tremors, flank pain, or skin rash

• To avoid hazardous activities if drowsiness occurs

Treatment of overdose: Lavage if taken orally; monitor electrolytes;

* Available in Canada only

administer dextrose in saline; monitor hydration, CV, renal status

methenamine (℞)

(meth-en'a-meen)

Hiprex, Hip-Rex*, Urex, Mandameth, Mandelamine, methenamine mandelate

Func. class.: Urinary antiinfective

Chem. class.: Methenamine, mandelic acid

Action: In acid urine, hydrolyzed to ammonia, formaldehyde, which are bactericidal

Uses: UTIs caused by *E. coli, Klebsiella, Enterobacter, P. mirabilis, P. morganii, Serratia, Citrobacter*

Dosage and routes:

• *Adult and child >12 yr:* PO 1 g q12h, maximum: 4 g/24 hr

• *Child 6-12 yr:* PO 500 mg-1 g q12h

Neurogenic bladder

• *Adult:* PO 1 g qid pc

• *Child 6-12 yr:* PO 500 mg qid pc

• *Child <6 yr:* PO 50 mg/kg in 4 divided doses pc

Available forms: Tabs 500 mg, 1 g; oral sol 500 mg, 1 g; susp 250, 500 mg/5 ml; tabs, enteric-coated 250, 500 mg, g; tabs, film-coated 500 mg, 1g

Side effects/adverse reactions:

CNS: Headache

INTEG: Pruritus, rash, urticaria

GI: Nausea, vomiting, anorexia, abdominal pain, increase AST (SGOT), ALT (SGPT)

GU: Dysuria, bladder irritation, ***albuminuria, hematuria,*** crystalluria

EENT: Tinnitus, stomatitis

Contraindications: Hypersensitivity, severe dehydration, renal insufficiency

Precautions: Renal disease, pregnancy (C), lactation

Pharmacokinetics:

PO: Excreted in urine, half-life 4 hr

Interactions:

• Insoluble precipitate in urine: sulfonamides

• Do not use with silver, iron, mercury salts

Lab test interferences:

Interfere: VMA, urinary catecholamines

False decrease: Urine estriol, 5HIAA

False increase: 17-OHCS

NURSING CONSIDERATIONS

Assess:

• I&O ratio; urine pH <5.5 is ideal; monitor for hematuria indicating crystalluria

• Periodic liver function test: AST (SGOT), ALT (SGPT), alk phosphatase

• C&S before treatment, after completion

• Allergy: fever, flushing, rash, urticaria, pruritus

Administer:

• After clean-catch urine for C&S

• Two daily doses if urine output is high or if patient has diabetes

• Up to 12 g of vit C if needed to acidify urine; cranberry, prune juice may be used

Perform/provide:

• Storage protected from heat

• Limited intake of alkaline foods or drugs: milk, dairy products, peanuts, vegetables, alkaline antacids, sodium bicarbonate

Evaluate:

• Therapeutic response: decreased pain, frequency, urgency, negative C&S, absence of infection

Teach patient/family:

• To keep urine acidic by eating meats, eggs, fish, gelatin products, prunes, plums, cranberries

• That fluids must be increased to 3 L/day to avoid crystallization in kidneys

M

• To complete full course of drug therapy; to take drug at evenly spaced intervals around clock for best results

methicillin (℞)

(meth-i-sill'in)

Staphcillin

Func. class.: Broad-spectrum antiinfective

Chem. class.: Penicillinase-resistant penicillin

Action: Interferes with cell wall replication of susceptible organisms; osmotically unstable cell wall swells, bursts from osmotic pressure

Uses: Effective for gram-positive cocci *(S. aureus, S. pyogenes, S. viridans, S. faecalis, S. bovis, S. pneumoniae)*, infections caused by penicillinase-producing *Staphylococcus*

Dosage and routes:

• *Adult:* IM/IV 4-12 g/day in divided doses q4-6h

• *Child:* IM/IV 50-300 mg/kg/day in divided doses q4-12h

Available forms: Powder for inj 1, 4, 6, 10 g; inf only 1 g

Side effects/adverse reactions:

HEMA: Anemia, increased bleeding time, ***bone marrow depression, granulocytopenia***

GI: Nausea, vomiting, diarrhea, increased AST (SGOT), ALT (SGPT), abdominal pain, glossitis, colitis, interstitial nephritis

GU: Oliguria, ***proteinuria, hematuria,*** *vaginitis, moniliasis,* ***glomerulonephritis***

CNS: Lethargy, hallucinations, anxiety, depression, twitching, ***coma, convulsions***

Contraindications: Hypersensitivity to penicillins

Precautions: Pregnancy (B), hypersensitivity to cephalosporins, neonates

Pharmacokinetics:

IM: Peak ½-1 hr, duration 4 hr

IV: Peak 15 min, duration 2 hr

Metabolized in liver; excreted in urine, bile, breast milk; crosses placenta

Interactions:

• Decreased antimicrobial effectiveness of methicillin: tetracyclines, erythromycins

• Increased methicillin concentrations: aspirin, probenecid

• Drug/food: decreased absorption: food, carbonated drinks, citrus fruit juices

Syringe compatibilities: Chloramphenicol, colistimethate, erythromycin, gentamicin, lidocaine, polymyxin B, procaine

Y-site compatibilities: Heparin, hydrocortisone sodium succinate, potassium chloride, verapamil, vitamin B with C

Additive compatibilities: Aminophylline, ascorbic acid, calcium chloride, gluconate, cephalothin, chloramphenicol, colistimethate, corticotropin, dimenhydrinate, diphenhydramine, erythromycin, gentamicin, pencillin G, polymyxin B, potassium chloride, prednisolone, procaine, verapamil

Lab test interferences:

False positive: Urine glucose, urine protein

NURSING CONSIDERATIONS

Assess:

• I&O ratio; report hematuria, oliguria, since penicillin in high doses is nephrotoxic

• Any patient with compromised renal system; drug is excreted slowly in poor renal system function; toxicity may occur rapidly

• Liver studies: AST (SGOT), ALT (SGPT)

• Blood studies: WBC, RBC, H&H, bleeding time
• Renal studies: urinalysis, protein, blood
• C&S before therapy; drug may be given as soon as culture is taken
• Bowel pattern before, during treatment
• Skin eruptions after administration of penicillin to 1 wk after discontinuing drug
• For thrombophlebitis at IV site, change IV site q48hr
• Respiratory status: rate, character, wheezing, tightness in chest
• Allergies before initiation of treatment, reaction of each medication; highlight allergies on chart

Administer:
• IV after diluting 1 g/1.8 ml sterile H_2O; further dilute each 500 mg/25 ml or more NaCl; give directly at 10 ml/min, added to D_5W, NS, LR, or by inf over ½-8 hr
• Drug after C&S completed

Perform/provide:
• Adrenalin, suction, tracheostomy set, endotracheal intubation equipment
• Adequate fluid intake (2 L) during diarrhea episodes
• Scratch test to assess allergy after securing order from prescriber; usually done when penicillin is only drug of choice
• Storage at room temp; reconstituted sol stable for 8 hr

Evaluate:
• Therapeutic response: absence of fever, draining wounds

Teach patient/family:
• That culture may be taken after completed course of medication
• To report sore throat, fever, fatigue (may indicate superinfection)
• To wear or carry Medic Alert ID if allergic to penicillins
• To notify nurse of diarrhea

Treatment of anaphylaxis: Withdraw drug; maintain airway; administer epinephrine, aminophylline, O_2, IV corticosteroids

methimazole (℞)

(meth-im'a-zole)
Tapazole
Func. class.: Thyroid hormone antagonist (antithyroid)
Chem. class.: Thioamide

Action: Inhibits synthesis of thyroid hormones by decreasing iodine use in manufacture of thyroglobin and iodothyronine; does not affect already formed hormones

Uses: Hyperthyroidism, preparation for thyroidectomy, thyrotoxic crisis, thyroid storm

Dosage and routes:

Hyperthyroidism
• *Adult:* PO 5-20 mg tid depending on severity of condition; continue until euthyroid; maintenance dose 5-10 mg qd-tid, maximal dose 150 mg qd
• *Child:* PO 0.4 mg/kg/day in divided doses q8h; continue until euthyroid; maintenance dose 0.2 mg/kg/day in divided doses q8h

Preparation for thyroidectomy
• *Adult and child:* PO same as above; iodine may be added × 10 days before surgery

Thyrotoxic crisis
• *Adult and child:* PO same as hyperthyroidism with iodine and propranolol

Available forms: Tabs 5, 10 mg

Side effects/adverse reactions:
ENDO: Enlarged thyroid
INTEG: Rash, urticaria, pruritus, alopecia, hyperpigmentation, lupus-like syndrome
GU: ***Nephritis***
CNS: Drowsiness, headache, vertigo, fever, paresthesias, neuritis

M

HEMA: ***Agranulocytosis, leukopenia, thrombocytopenia, hypothrombinemia, lymphadenopathy,*** bleeding, vasculitis
GI: Nausea, diarrhea, vomiting, ***jaundice, hepatitis,*** loss of taste
MS: Myalgia, arthralgia, nocturnal muscle cramps

Contraindications: Hypersensitivity, pregnancy (3rd trimester) (D), lactation

Precautions: Infection, bone marrow depression, hepatic disease, pregnancy (1st, 2nd trimester), >40 yr

Pharmacokinetics:

PO: Onset 1 wk, duration up to 10 wk, duration up to several mo, half-life 1-2 hr, excreted in urine, breast milk, crosses placenta

Lab test interferences:

Increase: Pro-time, AST (SGOT)/ ALT (SGPT), alk phosphatase

NURSING CONSIDERATIONS

Assess:

- Pulse, B/P, temp
- I&O ratio; check for edema: puffy hands, feet, periorbits; indicate hypothyroidism
- Weight qd; same clothing, scale, time of day
- T_3, T_4, which are increased; serum TSH, which is decreased; free thyroxine index, which is increased if dosage is too low; discontinue drug 3-4 wk before RAIU
- Blood work: CBC for blood dyscrasias: leukopenia, thrombocytopenia, agranulocytosis; LFTs
- Overdose: peripheral edema, heat intolerance, diaphoresis, palpitations, dysrhythmias, severe tachycardia, fever, delirium, CNS irritability
- Hypersensitivity: rash, enlarged cervical lymph nodes; drug may have to be discontinued
- Hypoprothrombinemia: bleeding, petechiae, ecchymosis
- Clinical response: after 3 wk should include increased weight, pulse; decreased T_4
- Bone marrow depression: sore throat, fever, fatigue

Administer:

- With meals to decrease GI upset
- At same time each day to maintain drug level
- Lowest dose that relieves symptoms; discontinue before RAI

Perform/provide:

- Storage in light-resistant container
- Fluids to 3-4 L/day, unless contraindicated

Evaluate:

- Therapeutic response: weight gain, decreased pulse, decreased T_4, B/P

Teach patient/family:

- Not to breast-feed
- To take pulse daily
- To report redness, swelling, sore throat, mouth lesions, which indicate blood dyscrasias
- To keep graph of weight, pulse, mood
- To avoid OTC products that contain iodine
- That seafood, other iodine products may be restricted
- Not to discontinue this medication abruptly; thyroid crisis may occur; stress patient response
- That response may take several months if thyroid is large
- Symptoms/signs of overdose: periorbital edema, cold intolerance, mental depression
- Symptoms of inadequate dose: tachycardia, diarrhea, fever, irritability

* Available in Canada only

methocarbamol (℞)

(meth-oh-kar′ba-mole)

Delaxin, Marbaxin 750, methocarbamol, Robaxin, Robaxin-750, Robomol-500, Robomol-750, Tresortil*

Func. class.: Skeletal muscle relaxant, Central acting

Chem. class.: Carbamate derivative

Action: Depresses multisynaptic pathways in the spinal cord, causing skeletal muscle relaxation

Uses: Adjunct for relief of spasm and pain in musculoskeletal conditions, tetanus management

Dosage and routes:

Pain

• *Adult:* PO 1.5 g × 2-3 days, then 1 g qid; IM 500 mg in each gluteal region, may repeat q8h; IV BOL 1-3 g/day at 3 ml/min; IV INF 1 gm/250 ml D_5W or NS, not to exceed 3 g/day

Tetanus

• *Adult:* IV INF 1-3 g/L of solution q6h; IV BOL 1-2 g injected into running IV

• *Child:* IV 15 mg/kg q6h

Available forms: Tabs 500, 750 mg; inj 100 mg/ml

Side effects/adverse reactions:

CNS: Dizziness, weakness, drowsiness, headache, tremor, depression, insomnia, ***seizures***

HEMA: Hemolysis, increased hemoglobin (IV only)

EENT: Diplopia, temporary loss of vision, blurred vision, nystagmus

CV: Postural hypotension, bradycardia

GI: Nausea, vomiting, hiccups, anorexia, metallic taste

GU: Brown, black, green urine

INTEG: Rash, pruritus, fever, facial flushing, urticaria

Contraindications: Hypersensitivity, child <12 yr, intermittent porphyria

Precautions: Renal disease, hepatic disease, addictive personalities, pregnancy (C), myasthenia gravis, epilepsy

Pharmacokinetics:

IM/IV: Onset rapid

PO: Onset ½ hr, peak 1-2 hr, half-life 1-2 hr

Metabolized in liver, excreted in urine unchanged, crosses placenta

Interactions:

• Increased CNS depression: alcohol, tricyclic antidepressants, narcotics, barbiturates, sedatives, hypnotics

• Considered incompatible with any drug in sol or syringe

Lab test interferences:

False increase: VMA, urinary 5-HIAA

NURSING CONSIDERATIONS

Assess:

• Blood studies: CBC, WBC, differential; blood dyscrasias may occur

• During and after injection: CNS effects, rash, conjunctivitis, nasal congestion may occur

• Liver function studies: AST (SGOT), ALT (SGPT), alk phosphatase; hepatitis may occur

• ECG in epileptic patients; poor seizure control has occurred

• Allergic reactions: rash, fever, respiratory distress

• Severe weakness, numbness in extremities

• Tolerance: increased need for medication, more frequent requests for medication, increased pain

• CNS depression: dizziness, drowsiness, psychiatric symptoms

Administer:

• With meals for GI symptoms

• IV undiluted over 1 min or more, give 300 mg or less/1 min or longer;

may be diluted in 250 ml or less D_5 or isotonic NaCl sol
• By slow IV to prevent phlebitis; keep recumbent for 15 min to prevent orthostatic hypotension; check for extravasation
• IM deep in large muscle mass; rotate sites

Perform/provide:
• Storage in tight container at room temp
• Assistance with ambulation if dizziness/drowsiness occurs

Evaluate:
• Therapeutic response: decreased pain, spasticity

Teach patient/family:
• Not to discontinue medication quickly; insomnia, nausea, headache, spasticity, tachycardia will occur; drug should be tapered off over 1-2 wk
• That urine may turn green, black, or brown
• Not to take with alcohol, other CNS depressants
• To avoid altering activities while taking this drug
• To avoid hazardous activities if drowsiness, dizziness occurs
• To avoid using OTC medication: cough preparations, antihistamines, unless directed by prescriber

Treatment of overdose: Induce emesis of conscious patient, lavage, dialysis; have epinephrine, antihistamines, and corticosteroids available

---

methohexital (℞)
(meth-oh-hex′i-tal)
Brevital Sodium, Brietal Sodium*
Func. class.: General anesthetic
Chem. class.: Barbiturate

Controlled Substance Schedule IV

Action: Acts in reticular-activating system to produce anesthesia; may be potentiated by GABA

Uses: General anesthesia for electroshock therapy, reduction of fractures, adjunct with other anesthetics, balanced anesthesia

Dosage and routes:
• *Adult and child:* IV 50-100 mg given 1 ml/5 sec

Maintenance
• *Adult and child:* IV 20-40 mg q4-7 min 0.1% sol; CONT IV 1 gtt/sec 0.2% sol

Available forms: Inj 500 mg, 2.5, 5g

Side effects/adverse reactions:
RESP: ***Respiratory depression, bronchospasm***
CNS: Retrograde amnesia, prolonged somnolence
CV: Tachycardia, hypotension, ***myocardial depression, dysrhythmias***
EENT: Sneezing, coughing
INTEG: Chills, *shivering,* necrosis, pain at injection site
MS: Muscle irritability

Contraindications: Hypersensitivity, status asthmaticus, hepatic/intermittent porphyrias, pregnancy (D)

Precautions: Severe cardiovascular disease, renal disease, hypotension, liver disease, myxedema, myasthenia gravis, asthma, increased intracranial pressure

Pharmacokinetics:
IV: Onset 30-40 sec; half-life 11.5 hr; crosses placenta

Interactions:
• Increased action: CNS depressants
• Do not mix with atropine or silicone in sol or syringe

NURSING CONSIDERATIONS

Assess:
• VS q3-5min during IV administration, after dose, q4hr postoperatively

---

* Available in Canada only

• Extravasation; use chloroprocaine to decrease pain, increase circulation
• Dysrhythmias, myocardial depression

Administer:
• After preparation with sterile water 0.9%, NaCl or 5% dextrose
• Only with crash cart, resuscitative equipment nearby
• IV slowly only by qualified persons

Evaluate:
• Therapeutic response: induction of anesthesia

---

methotrexate (amethopterin, MTX) (℞)

(meth-oh-trex'ate)

Folex PFS, methotrexate, Methotrexate LPF, Rheumatrex Dose Pack

Func. class.: Antineoplastic-antimetabolite

Chem. class.: Folic acid antagonist

Action: Inhibits an enzyme that reduces folic acid, which is needed for nucleic acid synthesis in all cells; S phase of cell cycle specific; immunosuppressive

Uses: Acute lymphocytic leukemia, in combination for breast, lung, head, neck carcinoma, lymphosarcoma, gestational choriocarcinoma, hydatidiform mole psoriasis, rheumatoid arthritis, mycosis fungoides

Investigational uses: Used investigationally to produce abortion

Dosage and routes:

Leukemia
• *Adult and child:* PO 3.3 mg/m²/day with prednisone IT 12 mg/m², maintenance 30 mg/m²/day 2× /wk; IV 2.5 mg/kg q2wk

Choriocarcinoma
• *Adult and child:* PO 15-30 mg/ m² qd × 5 days, then off 1 wk; may repeat

Osteosarcoma
• *Adult and child:* IV 12 g/m² given over 4 hr, then leucovorin rescue

Mycosis Fungoides
• *Adult:* PO 2.5-10 mg/day until cleared (may be many months); IM 50 mg qwk or 25 mg 2 × /wk

Psoriasis
• *Adult:* PO/IM/IV 10 mg qwk, may increase to 25 mg qwk

Available forms: Tabs, 2.5 mg; inj 25 mg/ml; powder for inj 20, 25, 50, 100, 250 mg, 1 g; sodium inj 2.5, 25 mg/ml

Side effects/adverse reactions:

HEMA: ***Leukopenia, thrombocytopenia, myelosuppression, anemia***

GI: Nausea, vomiting, anorexia, diarrhea, stomatitis, ***hepatotoxicity,*** cramps, ulcer, gastritis, ***GI hemorrhage,*** abdominal pain, hematemesis

GU: Urinary retention, ***renal failure,*** menstrual irregularities, defective spermatogenesis, ***hematuria, azotemia, uric acid nephropathy***

INTEG: Rash, alopecia, dry skin, urticaria, photosensitivity, folliculitis, vasculitis, petechiae, ecchymosis, acne, alopecia

CNS: Dizziness, ***convulsions,*** head ache, confusion, hemiparesis, malaise, fatigue, chills, fever

Contraindications: Hypersensitivity, leukopenia (<2500/mm³), thrombocytopenia (<100,000/mm³), anemia, psoriatic patients with severe renal/hepatic disease, pregnancy (D)

Precautions: Renal disease, lactation

Pharmacokinetics:
PO: Readily absorbed
PO/IM/IV: Onset 4-7 days; peak 1-2 wk; duration 3 wk

IT: Onset peak, duration unknown
Not metabolized; excreted in urine (unchanged); crosses placenta, blood-brain barrier; 50% plasma protein bound

Interactions:

- Increased toxicity: aspirin, sulfa drugs, other antineoplastics, radiation, alcohol, probenecid, phenytoin, phenylbutazone, pyrimethamine
- Decreased effect of oral digoxin
- Increased hypoprothrombinemia: oral anticoagulants
- Decreased effect of methotrexate: folic acid supplements
- Possible fatal interactions: nonsteroidal antiinflammatory drugs

Syringe compatibilities: Bleomycin, cisplatin, cyclophosphamide, doxapram, doxorubicin, fluorouracil, furosemide, leucovorin, mitomycin, vinblastine, vincristine

Y-site compatibilities: Bleomycin, cisplatin, cyclophosphamide, doxorubicin, fludarabine, fluorouracil, furosemide, heparin, leucovorin, metoclopramide, melphalan, mitomycin, ondansetron, paclitaxel, sargramostim, vancomycin, vinblastine, vincristine, vinorelbine

Additive compatibilities: Cephalothin, cyclophosphamide, cytarabine, fluorouracil, hydroxyzine, mercaptopurine, sodium bicarbonate, vincristine

Solution compatibilities: Amino acids, 4.25%/D_{25}, D_5W, sodium bicarbonate 0.05 mol/L

NURSING CONSIDERATIONS

Assess:

- CBC, differential, platelet count weekly; withhold drug if WBC is <3500/mm^3 or platelet count is <100,000/mm^3; notify prescriber; drug should be discontinued
- Renal function studies: BUN, serum uric acid, urine CrCl, electrolytes before, during therapy
- I&O ratio; report fall in urine output to <30 ml/hr
- Monitor temp q4h; fever may indicate beginning infection; no rectal temps
- Liver function tests before and during therapy: bilirubin, alk phosphatase, AST (SGOT), ALT (SGPT); liver biopsy should be done before start of therapy (psoriasis patients)
- Bleeding time, coagulation time during treatment
- Bleeding: hematuria, guaiac, bruising or petechiae, mucosa or orifices q8h
- Food preferences; list likes, dislikes
- Effects of alopecia on body image; discuss feelings about body changes
- Hepatotoxicity: yellow skin and sclera, dark urine, clay-colored stools, pruritus, abdominal pain, fever, diarrhea
- Buccal cavity q8h for dryness, sores, ulceration, white patches, oral pain, bleeding, dysphagia
- Symptoms indicating severe allergic reaction: rash, urticaria, itching, flushing

Administer:

- IV after diluting 5 mg/2 ml of sterile H_2O for inj; give through Y-tube or 3-way stopcock at 10 mg or less/min
- Antacid before oral agent; give drug after evening meal before bedtime
- Antiemetic 30-60 min before giving drug
- Allopurinol or sodium bicarbonate to maintain uric acid levels, alkalinization of urine, adequate fluids
- Leucovorin Ca within 12 hr of this drug to prevent tissue damage; check agency policy

• Antibiotics for prophylaxis of infection
• Topical or systemic analgesics for pain
• Transfusion for anemia

Perform/provide:
• Strict medical asepsis and protective isolation if WBC levels are low
• Liquid diet: carbonated beverage, Jell-O; dry toast, crackers may be added when patient is not nauseated or vomiting
• Increased fluid intake to 2-3 L/day to prevent urate deposits, calculi formation, unless contraindicated
• Diet low in purines: absence of organ meats (kidney, liver), dried beans, peas to maintain alkaline urine
• Rinsing of mouth tid-qid with water, club soda; brushing of teeth bid-tid with soft brush or cotton-tipped applicators for stomatitis; use unwaxed dental floss
• Nutritious diet with iron, vitamin supplements
• Storage in tightly closed container in cool environment; store injection, powder for injection in dark, dry area

Evaluate:
• Therapeutic response: decreased tumor size, spread of malignancy

Teach patient/family:
• About protective isolation
• To report any complaints, side effects to nurse or prescriber: black tarry stools, chills, fever, sore throat, bleeding, bruising, cough, shortness of breath, dark or bloody urine
• That hair may be lost during treatment; wig or hairpiece may make patient feel better; tell patient that new hair may be different in color, texture (alopecia is rare)
• To avoid foods with citric acid, hot or rough texture if stomatitis is present
• To report stomatitis: any bleeding, white spots, ulcerations in mouth to prescriber; tell patient to examine mouth qd, report symptoms to nurse
• That contraceptive measures are recommended during therapy for at least 8 wk following cessation of therapy
• To drink 10-12 glasses of fluid/day
• To avoid alcohol, salicylates
• To avoid use of razors, commercial mouthwash

---

methotrimeprazine (℞)

(meth-oh-trye-mep′ra-zeen)
Levoprome, Nozinan*
Func. class.: Nonnarcotic analgesic
Chem. class.: Aliphatic (propylamine-phenothiazine derivative)

Action: Depresses cerebral cortex, hypothalamus, limbic system; blocks neurotransmission produced by dopamine at synapse; exhibits strong α-adrenergic, anticholinergic blocking action, antihistamine

Uses: Sedation, analgesia, preoperative and postoperative analgesia, obstetric analgesia in nonambulatory patients

Dosage and routes:

Analgesia/sedation
• *Adult and child >12 yr:* IM 10-20 mg q4-6h prn
• *Elderly:* IM 5-10 mg q4-6h

Preoperative medication
• *Adult and child >12 yr:* IM 2-20 mg 45 min to 3 hr before surgery

Postoperative medication
• *Adult and child >12 yr:* IM 2.5-7.5 mg q4-6h titrated to patient's needs

Obstetric analgesia
• *Adult:* 15-20 mg, may be repeated

Available forms: Inj 20 mg/ml

M

Side effects/adverse reactions:
HEMA: ***Thrombocytopenia, agranulocytosis, leukopenia, neutropenia, hemolytic anemia*** (long-term, high dose)
CNS: *Weakness, dizziness,* drowsiness, confusion, delirium, euphoria, headache, sedation, EPS
GI: *Nausea, vomiting, abdominal pain, dry mouth,* jaundice (long-term use)
GU: ***Hematuria,*** dysuria, hesitancy, retention, uterine inertia (rare)
INTEG: Pain, edema at injection site, fever, chills
EENT: Nasal congestion, blurred vision, slurred speech
CV: *Orthostatic hypotension,* palpitations, tachycardia, bradycardia

Contraindications: Hypersensitivity to this drug, phenothiazines, bisulfite; seizures; severe hepatic disease; severe renal disease; severe cardiac disease; coma

Precautions: Elderly, pregnancy (C)

Pharmacokinetics:
IM: Onset 20-30 min, peak 1-2 hr, duration 4 hr; metabolized by liver, excreted by kidneys and in feces, crosses placenta, excreted in breast milk

Interactions:
- Increased sedation: CNS depressants, alcohol, barbiturates, reserpine, narcotics, general anesthetics, meprobamate

Syringe compatibilities: Atropine, hydroxyzine, metoclopramide, scopolamine

NURSING CONSIDERATIONS

Assess:
- Blood studies: CBC, ALT (SGPT), AST (SGOT), bilirubin
- VS q10min for 30 min; watch for decreasing B/P with increased pulse that may occur 10-30 min after injection; continue to monitor closely for 6-12 hr after several injections
- Effect on uterine contractions, fetal heart tones if using for labor

Administer:
- After removal of cigarettes to prevent fires
- IM inj in deep large muscle mass to prevent tissue sloughing; rotate sites
- Lowest dose, then gradually increase; lower doses are required after general anesthesia

Perform/provide:
- Bed rest for several hours after injection if orthostatic hypotension occurs
- Safety measure: side rails, nightlight, call bell within easy reach
- Storage in darkness; expires after 5 yr
- Assistance with ambulation for 6 hr after injection

Evaluate:
- Therapeutic response: decrease in pain, grimacing, absence of change in VS, ability to cough and breathe deep after surgery

Teach patient/family:
- To avoid ambulation without assistance for 6 hr after drug is given

Treatment of overdose: Monitor electrolytes, vital signs

methoxsalen (℞)

(meth-ox'a-len)
8-Mop, Oxsoralen, Oxsoralen Ultra
Func. class.: Pigmenting agent
Chem. class.: Psoralen derivative

Action: Decreases cell turnover by combining with epidermal cell DNA, causing photo damage when used with ultraviolet rays

Uses: Vitiligo, psoriasis

* Available in Canada only

Dosage and routes:
Vitiligo
• *Adult and child >12 yr:* PO 20 mg qd 2-4 hr before exposure to therapeutic ultraviolet rays; administer on alternate days; TOP apply 1-2 hr before exposure to UVA light; treatment intervals regulated by erythema response
Psoriasis
Adult PO: Dosage individualized to weight; taken 2 hr before exposure to therapeutic ultraviolet rays
Available forms: Lotion 1%; hard caps 10 mg; soft caps 10 mg; contains tartrazine
Side effects/adverse reactions:
CNS: Headache, depression, restlessness, anxiety, nervousness, vertigo, insomnia, malaise
GI: Nausea
INTEG: Rash, pruritus, burning, peeling, erythema, edema, urticaria, hypopigmentation
MISC: Leg cramps, hypotension, herpes simplex
Contraindications: Hypersensitivity, melanoma, LE, albinism, sunburn, cataracts, squamous cell cancer, child ≤12 yr, diseases associated with photosensitivity
Precautions: Hepatic disease, cardiac disease, children, lactation, pregnancy (C); contains tartrazine (FD&C #5), photosensitizing agents
Pharmacokinetics:
PO: Duration 8 hr, half-life 2 hr, metabolized in liver, excreted in urine
Interactions:
• Increased effects of methoxsalen: other photosensitizing agents, phenothiazines, thiazides, tetracyclines, griseofulvin, halogenated salicylanides, sulfonamides, coal tar derivatives, nalidixic acid
NURSING CONSIDERATIONS
Assess:
• Hepatic tests (AST [SGOT], ALT [SGPT], bilirubin), renal tests (BUN, protein), antinuclear antibodies during treatment
Administer:
• With food or milk to prevent GI upset
• To prevent extensive phototoxicity, qod
• Lotion to small areas; use systemic treatment for large areas
Perform/provide:
• Protection to eyes, lips during treatment
• Use of finger cot or gloves to apply lotion
Evaluate:
• Therapeutic response: increased pigmentation in vitiligo, decreased psoriatic areas
Teach patient/family:
• To avoid ultraviolet exposure for at least 24 hr after topical application and 8 hr after PO dose
• That sunscreen may be used for exposure to sunlight after treatment
• That repigmentation may require 6-9 mo
• Avoid furocoumarin-containing foods: limes, figs, parsley, parsnips, mustard, carrots, celery

methscopolamine (℞)

(meth-skoe-pol′a-meen)
Pamine
Func. class.: GI anticholinergic
Chem. class.: Synthetic quarternary ammonium antimuscarinic

Action: Inhibits muscarinic actions of acetylcholine at postganglionic parasympathetic neuroeffector sites
Uses: Peptic ulcer disease
Dosage and routes:
• *Adult:* PO 2.5-5 mg ½ hr ac, hs
Available forms: Tabs 2.5 mg
Side effects/adverse reactions:
CNS: Confusion, stimulation in elderly, headache, insomnia, dizzi-

ness, drowsiness, anxiety, weakness, hallucination
GI: Dry mouth, constipation, ***paralytic ileus,*** heartburn, nausea, vomiting, dysphagia, absence of taste
GU: Hesitancy, retention, impotence
CV: Palpitations, tachycardia
EENT: Blurred vision, photophobia, mydriasis, cycloplegia, increased ocular tension
INTEG: Urticaria, rash, pruritus, anhidrosis, fever, allergic reactions
Contraindications: Hypersensitivity to anticholinergics, narrow-angle glaucoma, GI obstruction, myasthenia gravis, paralytic ileus, GI atony, toxic megacolon
Precautions: Hyperthyroidism, coronary artery disease, dysrhythmias, CHF, ulcerative colitis, hypertension, hiatal hernia, hepatic disease, renal disease, pregnancy (C), urinary retention, prostatic hypertrophy
Pharmacokinetics:
PO: Onset 1 hr, duration 6-8 hr; metabolized by liver, excreted in urine
Interactions:
• Increased anticholinergic effect: amantadine, tricyclic antidepressants, MAOIs, H_1 antihistamines
• Decreased effect of phenothiazines, levodopa, ketoconazole
NURSING CONSIDERATIONS
Assess:
• VS, cardiac status: checking for dysrhythmias, increased rate, palpitations
• I&O ratio; check for urinary retention or hesitancy
• GI complaints: pain, bleeding (frank or occult), nausea, vomiting, anorexia
Administer:
• ½-1 hr ac for better absorption
• Decreased dose to elderly patients; metabolism may be slowed
• Gum, hard candy, frequent rinsing of mouth for dryness
Perform/provide:
• Storage in tight container protected from light
• Increased fluids, bulk, exercise to decrease constipation
Evaluate:
• Therapeutic response: absence of epigastric pain, bleeding, nausea, vomiting
Teach patient/family:
• To avoid driving or other hazardous activities until stabilized on medication
• To avoid alcohol or other CNS depressants; will enhance sedating properties of this drug
• To drink plenty of fluids
• To report dysphagia
• That drug may cause blurred vision

methsuximide (℞)

(meth-sux′i-mide)
Celontin, Kapseals
Func. class.: Anticonvulsant
Chem. class.: Succinimide

Action: Inhibits spike, wave formation in absence seizures (petit mal), decreases amplitude, frequency, duration, spread of discharge in minor motor seizures
Uses: Refractory absence seizures (petit mal)
Dosage and routes:
• *Adult and child:* PO 300 mg/day; may increase by 300 mg/wk, not to exceed 1.2 g/day in divided doses
Available forms: Caps, half-strength 150 mg; caps 300 mg
Side effects/adverse reactions:
HEMA: ***Agranulocytosis, aplastic anemia, thrombocytopenia, leukocytosis, eosinophilia, pancytopenia***
CNS: Drowsiness, dizziness, fatigue, euphoria, lethargy, irritability, de-

* Available in Canada only

pression, insomnia, anxiety, aggressiveness, ataxia, headache, confusion

GI: Nausea, vomiting, heartburn, anorexia, diarrhea, abdominal pain, cramps, constipation, gum hypertrophy, tongue swelling

GU: Vaginal bleeding, ***hematuria, renal damage***

INTEG: Urticaria, pruritic erythema, hirsutism, ***Stevens-Johnson syndrome***, systemic lupus erythematosus

EENT: Myopia, blurred vision

Contraindications: Hypersensitivity to succinimide derivatives

Precautions: Hepatic disease, renal disease, pregnancy (C), lactation

Pharmacokinetics:

PO: Onset 15-30 min, peak 1-2 hr, duration 4-6 hr

REC: Onset slow, duration 4-6 hr

Metabolized by liver, excreted by kidneys, half-life 2⅗-4 hr

Interactions:

• Antagonist effect: tricyclic antidepressants

• Decreased effects of estrogens, oral contraceptives

Lab test interferences:

Increase: Coombs' test

NURSING CONSIDERATIONS

Assess:

• Renal studies: urinalysis, BUN, urine creatinine

• Blood studies: CBC, Hct, Hgb, reticulocyte counts qwk for 4 wk then qmo

• Hepatic studies: ALT (SGPT), AST (SGOT), bilirubin, creatinine

• Drug levels during initial treatment, therapeutic range (10-40 μg/ml)

• Mental status: mood, sensorium, affect, behavioral changes; notify prescriber of changes

• Eye problems; need for ophthalmic exams before, during, after treatment (slit lamp, fundoscopy, tonometry)

• Allergic reaction: red raised rash; drug should be discontinued

• Blood dyscrasias: fever, sore throat, bruising, rash, jaundice

• Toxicity: bone marrow depression, nausea, vomiting, ataxia, diplopia

Administer:

• With food, milk to decrease GI symptoms

Perform/provide:

• Hard candy, frequent rinsing of mouth, gum for dry mouth

• Assistance with ambulation during early part of treatment; dizziness occurs

Evaluate:

• Therapeutic response: decreased seizure activity, document on chart

Teach patient/family:

• To avoid driving, other activities that require alertness

• To avoid alcohol ingestion, CNS depressants; increased sedation may occur

• Not to discontinue medication quickly after long-term use

• To call prescriber promptly if lupuslike syndrome occurs (enlarged lymph nodes, fever, bruising, sore throat)

• That drug may change urine to pink or brown

Treatment of overdose: Lavage, activated charcoal; monitor electrolytes, VS

M

methylcellulose (OTC)

(meth-ill-sell′yoo-lose)

Citrucel

Func. class.: Laxative, bulk

Chem. class.: Hydrophilic semisynthetic cellulose derivative

Action: Attracts water, expands in intestine to increase peristalsis; also

absorbs excess water in stool; decreases diarrhea
Uses: Constipation
Dosage and routes:
• *Adult:* PO 5-20 ml tid with 8 oz H_2O
• *Child:* PO 5-10 ml qd or bid with H_2O or 500 mg tid with 8 oz H_2O
Available forms: Powder 105 mg/g; sol 450 mg/5 ml; tab 500 mg
Side effects/adverse reactions:
GI: ***Obstruction,*** abdominal distention
Contraindications: Hypersensitivity, GI obstruction, hepatitis
Pharmacokinetics:
PO: Onset 12-24 hr, peak 1-3 days
Interactions:
• Decreased absorption: antibiotics, digitalis, nitrofurantoin, salicylates, tetracyclines, oral anticoagulants
NURSING CONSIDERATIONS
Assess:
• Blood, urine electrolytes if used often
• I&O ratio to identify fluid loss
• Cause of constipation; lack of fluids, bulk, exercise
• Cramping, rectal bleeding, nausea, vomiting; drug should be discontinued
Administer:
• Alone for better absorption; do not take within 1 hr of other drugs
• In morning or evening (oral dose)
Evaluate:
• Therapeutic response: decrease in constipation
Teach patient/family:
• To swallow tabs whole; do not chew, increase fluid intake
• That normal bowel movements do not always occur daily
• Not to use in presence of abdominal pain, nausea, vomiting
• To notify prescriber if constipation unrelieved or if symptoms of electrolyte imbalance occur: muscle cramps, pain, weakness, dizziness, excessive thirst

methyldopa/methyldopate (℞)

(meth-ill-doe'pa)
Aldomet, Amodopar, Apo-Methyldopa*, Dopamet*, methyldopa/methyldopate HCl, Novamedopa*
Func. class.: Antihypertensive
Chem. class.: Centrally acting α-adrenergic inhibitor

Action: Stimulates central inhibitory α-adrenergic receptors or acts as false transmitter, resulting in reduction of arterial pressure
Uses: Hypertension
Dosage and routes:
• *Adult:* PO 250-500 mg bid or tid, then adjusted q2d as needed, 0.5-3 g qd in 2-4 divided doses (maintenance), not to exceed 3 g/day; IV 250-500 mg in 100 ml D_5W q6h, run over 30-60 min, not to exceed 1 g q6h
• *Child:* PO 10 mg/kg/day in 2-4 divided doses, not to exceed 65 mg/kg or 3 g/day, whichever is less; IV 20-40 mg/kg/day in 4 divided doses, not to exceed 65 mg/kg
Available forms: Tabs 125, 250, 500 mg; oral susp 250 mg/5ml; inj 50 mg/ml (250 mg/5 ml)
Side effects/adverse reactions:
GI: Nausea, vomiting, diarrhea, constipation, hepatic dysfunction
CV: Bradycardia, myocarditis, orthostatic hypotension, angina, edema, weight gain
CNS: Drowsiness, weakness, dizziness, sedation, headache, depression, psychosis
EENT: Nasal congestion, eczema

* Available in Canada only

HEMA: ***Leukopenia, thrombocytopenia, hemolytic anemia,*** positive Coombs' test
INTEG: Lupuslike syndrome
GU: Impotence, failure to ejaculate
Contraindications: Active hepatic disease, hypersensitivity, blood dyscrasias
Precautions: Pregnancy (C), liver disease, eclampsia, severe cardiac disease
Pharmacokinetics:
PO: Peak 2-4 hr, duration 12-24 hr
IV: Peak 2 hr, duration 10-16 hr
Metabolized by liver, excreted in urine
Interactions:
- Increased pressor effect: sympathomimetic amines (norepinephrine, phenylpropanolamine)
- Increased hypotension: levodopa
- Increased sedation: haloperidol
- Increased action of anesthetics

Y-site compatibilities: Esmolol, meperidine, morphine
Additive compatibilities: Aminophylline, ascorbic acid, chloramphenicol, diphenhydramine, heparin, magnesium sulfate, multivitamins, netilmicin, potassium chloride, promazine, sodium bicarbonate, succinylcholine, verapamil, vitamin B with C
Solution compatibilities: D_5W, D_5/0.9% NaCl, Ringer's, sodium bicarbonate 5%, 0.9% NaCl, amino acids 4.25%/D_{25}, $Dextran_6$/0.9% NaCl, Normosol R, Normosol M/D_5W

NURSING CONSIDERATIONS
Assess:
- Blood studies: neutrophils, decreased platelets
- Baselines in renal, liver function tests before therapy begins
- B/P during beginning treatment, periodically thereafter
- Allergic reaction: rash, fever, pruritus, urticaria; drug should be discontinued if antihistamines fail to help
- Symptoms of CHF: edema, dyspnea, wet rales, B/P
- Renal symptoms: polyuria, oliguria, frequency

Administer:
- IV after diluting with 100-200 ml D_5W; run over ½-1 hr

Perform/provide:
- Storage of tabs in tight container

Evaluate:
- Therapeutic response: decrease in B/P in hypertension

Teach patient/family:
- To avoid hazardous activities
- To administer 1 hr before meals
- Not to discontinue drug abruptly, or withdrawal symptoms may occur: anxiety, increased B/P, headache, insomnia, increased pulse, tremors, nausea, sweating
- Not to use OTC (cough, cold, allergy) products unless directed by prescriber
- To avoid sunlight or wear sunscreen; photosensitivity may occur
- To comply with dosage schedule even if feeling better
- To rise slowly to sitting or standing position to minimize orthostatic hypotension
- To notify prescriber of mouth sores, sore throat, fever, swelling of hands or feet, irregular heartbeat, chest pain, signs of angioedema
- That excessive perspiration, dehydration, vomiting, diarrhea may lead to fall in blood pressure; consult prescriber
- That dizziness, fainting, lightheadedness may occur during 1st few days of therapy
- That compliance is necessary; not to skip or stop drug unless directed by prescriber
- That drug may cause skin rash or impaired perspiration

M

methylene blue (℞)

(meth'i-leen)

methylene blue, Urolene Blue

Func. class.: Urinary tract antiseptic

Chem. class.: Antiseptic dye

Action: Oxidation-reduction; has opposite action on hemoglobin depending on concentration; with increased concentration, converts ferrous ion of reduced hemoglobin to ferric form; methemoglobin is thus produced; prolonged administration accelerates destruction of erythrocytes

Uses: Oxalate urinary tract calculi; UTIs caused by *E. coli, Klebsiella, Enterobacter, P. mirabilis, P. vulgaris, P. morganii, Serratia, Citrobacter,* cyanide poisoning, methemoglobinemia

Dosage and routes:

• *Adult:* PO 65-130 mg pc with full glass of water

Cyanide poisoning/methemoglobinemia

• *Adult and child:* IV 1-2 mg/kg of 1% sol; inject slowly over 5 min or more

Available forms: Tabs 65 mg; inj 10 mg/ml

Side effects/adverse reactions:

CV: Cyanosis, CV abnormalities

INTEG: Pruritus, rash, urticaria, photosensitivity, profuse sweating

CNS: Dizziness, headache, drowsiness, mental confusion, fever with large doses

GI: Nausea, vomiting, abdominal pain, diarrhea

GU: Bladder irritation

Contraindications: Hypersensitivity to this drug, renal insufficiency

Precautions: Anemia, renal disease, hepatic disease, G6PD deficiency, pregnancy (C)

Pharmacokinetics:

PO/IV: Excreted in urine, bile, feces

NURSING CONSIDERATIONS

Assess:

• For cyanosis

• I&O ratio; urine pH <5.5 is ideal

• Hct, Hgb

• CNS symptoms: insomnia, headache, drowsiness, confusion

• Allergic reactions: fever, flushing, rash, urticaria, pruritus

Administer:

• After clean-catch urine is obtained for C&S

• Two daily doses if urine output is high or if patient has diabetes

Perform/provide:

• Limited intake of alkaline foods, drugs: milk, dairy products, peanuts, vegetables, alkaline antacids, sodium bicarbonate

Evaluate:

• Therapeutic response: decreased pain, frequency, urgency, C&S absence of infection

Teach patient/family:

• That anemia may result with continued administration

• That drug turns urine, sometimes stool, blue-green

• To notify prescriber if symptoms do not improve

• To notify prescriber of any sign/symptoms of side effects or adverse reactions

methylergonovine (℞)

(meth-ill-er-goe-noe'veen)

Methergine, Methylergobasine*, methylergonovine

Func. class.: Oxytocic

Chem. class.: Ergot alkaloid

Action: Stimulates uterine, vascular, smooth muscle, causing contractions; decreases bleeding

* Available in Canada only

Uses: Treatment of hemorrhage postpartum or postabortion, uterine contractions

Dosage and routes:

• *Adult:* IM 0.2 mg q2-5h, not to exceed 5 doses; IV 0.2 mg given over 1 min; PO 0.2-0.4 mg q6-12h × 2-7 days after initial IM or IV dose

Available forms: Inj 0.2 mg/ml; tabs 0.2 mg

Side effects/adverse reactions:

RESP: Dyspnea
GU: Cramping
CNS: Headache, dizziness
GI: Nausea, vomiting
CV: Chest pain, palpitation, *hypertension,* dysrhythmias
EENT: Tinnitus
INTEG: Sweating, rash, allergic reactions

Contraindications: Hypersensitivity to ergot preparations, indication of labor, before delivery of placenta, hypertension, pelvic inflammatory disease, respiratory disease, cardiac disease, peripheral vascular disease

Precautions: Pregnancy (C), severe hepatic disease, severe renal disease, jaundice, diabetes mellitus, convulsive disorders, sepsis

Pharmacokinetics:

PO: Onset 5-25 min, duration 3 hr
IM: Onset 2-5 min, duration 3 hr
IV: Onset immediate, duration 45 min
Metabolized in liver, excreted in urine

Interactions:

• Exercise caution: vasoconstrictors

Y-site compatibilities: Heparin, hydrocortisone sodium succinate, potassium chloride, vitamin B with C

NURSING CONSIDERATIONS

Assess:

• B/P, pulse, character and amount of vaginal bleeding; watch for indications of hemorrhage
• Respiratory rate, rhythm, depth; notify prescriber of abnormalities
• For uterine relaxation; observe for severe cramping
• Ergot toxicity: tinnitus, hypertension, palpitations, chest pain

Administer:

• IV undiluted through Y-tube or 3-way stopcock; give 0.2 mg or less/min
• Only during fourth stage of labor; not to be used to augment labor
• IM in deep muscle mass; rotate injection sites of additional doses
• With crash cart available on unit; IV route used only in emergencies

Evaluate:

• Therapeutic response: absence of hemorrhage

Teach patient/family:

• To report increased blood loss, severe abdominal cramps, fever or foul-smelling lochia

M

methylphenidate (℞)

(meth-ill-fen′i-date)
Methidate, Ritalin, Ritalin SR
Func. class.: Cerebral stimulant
Chem. class.: Piperidine derivative

Controlled Substance Schedule II

Action: Increases release of norepinephrine, dopamine in cerebral cortex to reticular activating system; exact action not known

Uses: Attention deficit hyperactivity disorder, narcolepsy

Dosage and routes:

Attention deficit hyperactivity disorder

• *Child >6 yr:* 5 mg before breakfast and lunch, increasing by 5-10 mg/wk, not to exceed 60 mg/day

Narcolepsy

• *Adult:* PO 10 mg bid-tid, 30-45 min before meals, may increase up to 40-60 mg/day

Available forms: Tabs 5, 10, 20 mg; tabs sus rel 20 mg

Side effects/adverse reactions:

MISC: Fever, arthralgia, scalp hair loss

CNS: Hyperactivity, insomnia, restlessness, talkativeness, dizziness, headache, akathisia, dyskinesia, Gilles de la Tourette's syndrome

GI: Nausea, anorexia, dry mouth, weight loss, abdominal pain

CV: Palpitations, tachycardia, B/P changes, angina, dysrhythmias, ***thrombocytopenic purpura***

INTEG: ***Exfoliative dermatitis,*** urticaria, rash, erythema multiforme

ENDO: Growth retardation

GU: ***Uremia***

HEMA: ***Leukopenia, anemia***

Contraindications: Hypersensitivity, anxiety, history of Gilles de la Tourette's syndrome; children <6 yrs, glaucoma

Precautions: Hypertension, depression, pregnancy (C), seizures, lactation, drug abuse

Pharmacokinetics:

PO: Onset ½-1 hr, duration 4-6 hr, metabolized by liver, excreted by kidneys

Interactions:

• Hypertensive crisis: MAOIs or within 14 days of MAOIs, vasopressors

• Decreased effect of guanethidine

NURSING CONSIDERATIONS

Assess:

• VS, B/P; may reverse antihypertensives; check patients with cardiac disease more often for increased B/P

• CBC, urinalysis, in diabetes: blood sugar, urine sugar; insulin changes may have to be made, since eating will decrease

• Height, growth rate q3mo in children; growth rate may be decreased

• Mental status: mood, sensorium, affect, stimulation, insomnia, aggressiveness

• Withdrawal symptoms: headache, nausea, vomiting, muscle pain, weakness

Administer:

• At least 6 hr before hs to avoid sleeplessness

• Gum, hard candy, frequent sips of water for dry mouth

Evaluate:

• Therapeutic response: decreased hyperactivity or ability to stay awake

Teach patient/family:

• To decrease caffeine consumption (coffee, tea, cola, chocolate); may increase irritability, stimulation

• Not to chew or crush timed-released medication

• To avoid OTC preparations unless approved by prescriber

• To taper off drug over several weeks, or depression, increased sleeping, lethargy will occur

• To avoid alcohol ingestion

• To avoid hazardous activities until stabilized on medication

• To get needed rest; patients will feel more tired at end of day

Treatment of overdose: Administer fluids; hemodialysis or peritoneal dialysis; antihypertensive for increased B/P; administer short-acting barbiturate before lavage

methylprednisolone/ methylprednisolone acetate/methylprednisolone sodium succinate (℞)

(meth-il-pred-niss'oh-lone)

Medrol/Depo-Medrol, Duralone, Medralone, Rep-Pred/A-Methapred, Solu-Medrol

Func. class.: Corticosteroid

Chem. class.: Glucocorticoid, immediate acting

Action: Decreases inflammation by suppression of migration of polymorphonuclear leukocytes, fibroblasts, reversal of increased capillary permeability and lysosomal stabilization

Uses: Severe inflammation, shock, adrenal insufficiency, collagen disorders

Dosage and routes:

Adrenal insufficiency/inflammation

• *Adult:* PO 2-60 mg in 4 divided doses; IM 40-80 mg (acetate); IM/IV 10-250 mg (succinate); intraarticular: 4-30 mg (acetate)

• *Child:* IV 117 μg-1.66 mg/kg in 3-4 divided doses (succinate)

Shock

• *Adult:* IV 100-250 mg q2-6h (succinate)

Available forms: Tabs 2, 4, 6, 8, 16, 24, 32 mg; inj 20, 40, 80 mg/ml acetate; inj 40, 125, 500, 1000 mg/vial succinate

Side effects/adverse reactions:

CNS: Depression, flushing, sweating, headache, mood changes

CV: Hypertension, ***circulatory collapse, thrombophlebitis, embolism***, tachycardia

EENT: Fungal infections, increased intraocular pressure, blurred vision

GI: Diarrhea, nausea, abdominal distention, GI hemorrhage, increased appetite, pancreatitis

HEMA: ***Thrombocytopenia***

INTEG: Acne, poor wound healing, ecchymosis, petechiae

MS: Fractures, osteoporosis, weakness

Contraindications: Psychosis, hypersensitivity, idiopathic thrombocytopenia, acute glomerulonephritis, amebiasis, fungal infections, nonasthmatic bronchial disease, child <2 yr, AIDS, TB

Precautions: Pregnancy (C), lactation, diabetes mellitus, glaucoma, osteoporosis, seizure disorders, ulcerative colitis, CHF, myasthenia gravis, renal disease, esophagitis, peptic ulcer

Pharmacokinetics: Well absorbed PO, IM

PO: Peak 1-2 hr, duration 1½ day

IM: Peak 4-8 days, duration 1-4 wk

Intraarticular: Peak 1 wk

Half-life >3½ hr; crosses placenta, enters breast milk in small amounts; metabolized in liver, excreted by kidneys (unchanged)

Interactions:

• Decreased action of methylprednisolone: cholestyramine, colestipol, barbiturates, rifampin, ephedrine, phenytoin, theophylline

• Decreased effects of anticoagulants, anticonvulsants, antidiabetics, ambenonium, neostigmine, isoniazid, toxoid, vaccines, anticholinesterases, salicylates, somatrem

• Increased side effects: alcohol, salicylates, indomethacin, amphotericin B, digitalis, cyclosporine, diuretics

• Increased action of methylprednisolone: salicylates, estrogens, indomethacin, oral contraceptives, ketoconazole, macrolide antibiotics

Y-site compatibilities: Acyclovir, amrinone, enalaprilat, famotidine,

M

fludarabine, melphalan, meperidine, morphine, vitamin B with C

Syringe compatibility: Metoclopramide

Lab test interferences:

Increase: Cholesterol, Na, blood glucose, uric acid, Ca, urine glucose

Decrease: Ca, K, T_4, T_3, thyroid ^{131}I uptake test, urine 17-OHCS, 17-KS, PBI

False negative: Skin allergy tests

NURSING CONSIDERATIONS

Assess:

• K depletion: parethesias, fatigue, nausea, vomiting, depression, polyuria, dysrhythmias, weakness

• Edema, hypertension, cardiac symptoms

• Mental status: affect, mood, behavioral changes, aggression

• K, blood sugar, urine glucose while on long-term therapy; hypokalemia and hyperglycemia

• Joint mobility, pain, edema if given intraarticularly

• Weight daily; notify prescriber of weekly gain >5 lb

• B/P q4hr, pulse; notify prescriber of chest pain, rales

• I&O ratio; be alert for decreasing urinary output, increasing edema

• Adrenal insufficiency: weight loss, nausea, vomiting, confusion, anxiety, hypotension, weakness

• Plasma cortisol levels during long-term therapy (normal level: 138-635 nmol/L SI units when drawn at 8 AM)

• Growth in children on long-term treatment

Administer:

• IV after diluting with diluent provided; agitate slowly; give 500 mg or less/1 min or longer; may be given as IV infusion in its own diluent over 10-20 min

• Titrated dose; use lowest effective dose

• IM inj deep in large muscle mass; rotate sites; avoid deltoid; use 21G needle; after shaking suspension (parenteral)

• In one dose in AM to prevent adrenal suppression; avoid SC administration; may damage tissue

• With food or milk to decrease GI symptoms (PO)

Perform/provide:

• Assistance with ambulation in patient with bone tissue disease to prevent fractures

Evaluate:

• Therapeutic response: ease of respirations, decreased inflammation; decreased symptoms of adrenal insufficiency

• Infection: increased temp, WBC, even after withdrawal of medication; drug masks infection

Teach patient/family:

• To increase intake of K, Ca, protein

• That ID as steroid user should be carried

• To notify prescriber if therapeutic response decreases; dosage adjustment may be needed

• Not to discontinue abruptly, or adrenal crisis can result

• To avoid OTC products: salicylates, alcohol in cough products, cold preparations unless directed by prescriber; to avoid vaccinations, since immunosuppression occurs

• About cushingoid symptoms

• Symptoms of adrenal insufficiency: nausea, anorexia, fatigue, dizziness, dyspnea, weakness, joint pain

* Available in Canada only

methylprednisolone (℞)

(meth-ill-pred-niss'oh-lone)

Depo-Medrol

Func. class.: Topical corticosteroid

Chem. class.: Synthetic nonfluorinated agent, group VI potency

Action: Antipruritic, antiinflammatory

Uses: Psoriasis, eczema, contact dermatitis, pruritus

Dosage and routes:

• *Adult and child:* Apply to affected area qd-qid

Available forms: Oint 0.25%, 1%

Side effects/adverse reactions:

INTEG: Burning, dryness, itching, irritation, acne, folliculitis, hypertrichosis, perioral dermatitis, hypopigmentation, atrophy, striae, miliaria, allergic contact dermatitis, secondary infection

Contraindications: Hypersensitivity to corticosteroids, fungal infections

Precautions: Pregnancy (C), lactation, viral or bacterial infections

NURSING CONSIDERATIONS

Assess:

• Temp: if fever develops, drug should be discontinued

• For systemic absorption: fever, inflammation, irritation

Administer:

• Only to affected areas; do not get in eyes

• Medication, then cover with occlusive dressing (only if prescribed), seal to normal skin, change q12h; systemic absorption may occur; use gloves

• Only to dermatoses; do not use on weeping, denuded, or infected area

Perform/provide:

• Cleansing before application

• Treatment for a few days after area has cleared

• Storage at room temp

Evaluate:

• Therapeutic response: absence of severe itching, patches on skin, flaking

Teach patient/family:

• To avoid sunlight on affected area; burns may occur

methyprylon (℞)

(meth-i-prye'lon)

Noludar

Func. class.: Sedative-hypnotic

Chem. class.: Piperidine derivative

Controlled Substance Schedule III (USA), Schedule F (Canada)

Action: Acts at level of thalamus to produce CNS mood alterations by interfering with nerve impulse transmission in sensory cortex by increasing threshold of arousal centers; suppresses REM sleep

Uses: Insomnia

Dosage and routes:

• *Adult:* PO 200-400 mg 15-30 min before hs

• *Child >12 yr:* PO 50 mg hs; may increase to 200 mg

Available forms: Caps 300 mg, tabs 50, 200 mg

Side effects/adverse reactions:

CNS: Residual sedation, dizziness, ataxia, stimulation, headache, pyrexia, nightmares, depression; REM rebound after discharge

GI: Nausea, vomiting, diarrhea, esophagitis, constipation

INTEG: Rash, pruritus

Contraindications: Hypersensitivity to piperidine derivatives, severe pain, severe renal or hepatic disease, porphyria

Precautions: Depression, suicidal individuals, drug abuse, cardiac dysrhythmias, narrow-angle glaucoma, prostatic hypertrophy, stenosed peptic ulcer, pyloroduodenal/bladder neck obstruction, pregnancy (B)

Pharmacokinetics:

PO: Onset 45 min, peak 1-2 hr, duration 5-8 hr; metabolized by liver, excreted by kidneys, crosses placenta, excreted in breast milk; half-life 3-6 hr

Interactions:

- Increased CNS depression: alcohol, barbiturates, narcotics, other CNS depressants

NURSING CONSIDERATIONS

Assess:

- Blood studies: Hct, Hgb, RBC (long-term therapy)
- Hepatic studies: AST (SGOT), ALT (SGPT), bilirubin (long-term therapy)
- Mental status: mood, sensorium, affect, memory (long, short)
- Type of sleep problem: falling asleep, staying asleep
- Physical dependency, including more frequent requests for medication, shakes, anxiety
- Withdrawal: nausea, vomiting, anxiety, hallucinations, insomnia, tachycardia, fever, cramps, tremors, seizures
- Allergic reaction: rash; discontinue drug if rash occurs

Administer:

- After removal of cigarettes to prevent fires
- After trying conservative measures for insomnia
- ½-1 hr before hs for sleeplessness
- On empty stomach for fast onset, but may be taken with food if GI symptoms occur
- Overdosing symptoms: respiratory depression, hypotension, confusion, coma, constricted pupils

Perform/provide:

- Assistance with ambulation after receiving dose
- Safety measures: side rails, nightlight, call bell within easy reach
- Checking to see PO medication has been swallowed; watch depressed, drug-dependent patients for hoarding, self-overdosing
- Storage in tight, light-resistant container in cool environment

Evaluate:

- Therapeutic response: ability to sleep at night, decreased amount of early morning awakening if taking drug for insomnia

Teach patient/family:

- To avoid driving, other activities requiring alertness until drug stabilizes
- To avoid alcohol ingestion or CNS depressants; serious CNS depression may result
- Not to discontinue medication quickly after long-term use; drug should be tapered over 1-2 wk
- That effects may take 2 nights for benefits to be noticed
- Alternative measures to improve sleep: reading, exercise several hours before hs, warm bath, warm milk, TV, self-hypnosis, deep breathing
- That hangover is common in elderly, but less common than with barbiturates

Treatment of overdose: Lavage, activated charcoal; monitor electrolytes, vital signs

* Available in Canada only

methysergide (℞)

(meth-i-ser'jide)

Sansert

Func. class.: Serotonin antagonist

Chem. class.: Ergot derivative

Action: Competitively blocks serotonin HT receptors in CNS and periphery; potent vasoconstrictor

Uses: Prophylaxsis for migraine and other vascular headaches

Dosage and routes:

• *Adult:* PO 2 mg bid with meals

Available forms: Tabs 2 mg

Side effects/adverse reactions:

CNS: Tremors, anxiety, insomnia, headache, dizziness, euphoria, confusion, depersonalization, hallucination, paresthesias, drowsiness

CV: ***Retroperitoneal fibrosis,*** valvular thickening, palpitations, tachycardia, postural hypertension, angina, ***thrombophlebitis,*** ECG changes, ***cardiac fibrosis***

GI: Nausea, vomiting, weight gain

MS: Arthralgia, myalgia

INTEG: Flushing, rash, alopecia

HEMA: ***Blood dyscrasias***

Contraindications: Hypersensitivity to ergot, tartrazine, occlusion (peripheral, vascular), CAD, hepatic disease, renal disease, peptic ulcer, hypertension, connective tissue disease, fibrotic pulmonary disease

Precautions: Pregnancy (C), lactation, children

Pharmacokinetics:

PO: Half-life 10 hr, metabolized by liver, excreted in urine (metabolites/unchanged drug)

Interactions:

• Increased vasoconstriction: β-blockers

• Decreased effect of: narcotic analgesics

NURSING CONSIDERATIONS

Assess:

• Weight daily, check for peripheral edema in feet, legs, B/P

• For stress, activity, recreation, coping mechanisms

• Neurologic status: LOC, blurring vision, nausea, vomiting, tingling in extremities that precede headache

• Ingestion of tyramine foods (pickled products, beer, wine, aged cheese), food additives, preservatives, colorings, artificial sweeteners, chocolate, caffeine may precipitate these types of headaches

Administer:

• At beginning of headache; dose must be titrated to patient response

• Give with or after meals to avoid GI symptoms

• Only to women who are not pregnant; harm to fetus may occur

Perform/provide:

• Storage in dark area

• Quiet, calm environment with decreased stimulation for noise, bright light, or excessive talking

Evaluate:

• Therapeutic response: decrease in frequency, severity of headache

Teach patient/family:

• Not to use OTC medications; serious drug interactions may occur

• To maintain dose at approved level, not to increase even if drug does not relieve headache

• To report side effects: increased vasoconstriction starting with cold extremities, then paresthesia, weakness

• That headaches may increase when drug discontinued after long-term use

• To keep drug out of reach of children; death may occur

• To report at once: dyspnea, paresthesias, urinary problems, pain in abdomen, chest, back, legs

M

• To use drug for less than 6 mo unless a 3-4 wk rest period has been taken
• That drug may cause drowsiness

metipranolol (℞)

(met-ee-pran′oh-lole)
Optipranolol
Func. class.: β-Adrenergic blocker
Chem. class.: l-isomer

Action: Reduces production of aqueous humor by unknown mechanism
Uses: Ocular hypertension, chronic open-angle glaucoma
Dosage and routes:
• *Adult:* INSTILL 1 gtt bid
Available forms: Sol 0.3%
Side effects/adverse reactions:
CNS: Weakness, fatigue, depression, anxiety, headache, confusion
GI: Nausea, anorexia, dyspepsia
EENT: Eye irritation, conjunctivitis, keratitis
INTEG: Rash, urticaria
CV: ***Bradycardia,*** hypertension
RESP: ***Bronchospasm,*** dyspnea, bronchitis, coughing, rhinitis
Contraindications: Hypersensitivity, asthma, 2nd or 3rd degree heart block, right ventricular failure, congenital glaucoma (infants)
Precautions: Pregnancy (C)
Pharmacokinetics:
INSTILL: Onset 15-30 min, peak 1-2 hr, duration 24 hr
Interactions:
• Increased effect: propranolol, metoprolol

NURSING CONSIDERATIONS
Assess:
• B/P, heart rate throughout treatment
• For increased intraocular pressure
• For eye irritation, conjunctivitis
Evaluate:
• Therapeutic response: decreased intraocular pressure
Teach patient/family:
• To report change in vision (blurring or loss of sight), trouble breathing, sweating, flushing
• Method of instillation, including pressure on lacrimal sac for 1 min, and not to touch dropper to eye
• That long-term therapy may be required
• That blurred vision will decrease with continued use of drug

metoclopramide (℞)

(met-oh-kloe-pra′mide)
Clopra, Emex*, Maxeran*, Maxolon, metoclopramide HCl, Octamide PFS, Reclomide, Reglan
Func. class.: Cholinergic
Chem. class.: Central dopamine receptor antagonist

Action: Enhances response to acetylcholine of tissue in upper GI tract, which causes contraction of gastric muscle, relaxes pyloric, duodenal segments, increases peristalsis without stimulating secretions
Uses: Prevention of nausea, vomiting induced by chemotherapy, radiation, delayed gastric emptying, gastroesophageal reflux
Dosage and routes:
Nausea/vomiting
• *Adult:* IV 2 mg/kg q2h × 5 doses 30 min before administration of chemotherapy
Delayed gastric emptying
• *Adult:* PO 10 mg 30 min ac, hs × 2-8 wk
Gastroesophageal reflux
• *Adult:* PO 10-15 mg qid 30 min ac
Available forms: Tabs 5, 10 mg; syr 5 mg/5 ml; inj 5 mg/ml

* Available in Canada only

Side effects/adverse reactions:
CNS: Sedation, fatigue, restlessness, headache, sleeplessness, dystonia, dizziness, drowsiness
GI: Dry mouth, constipation, nausea, anorexia, vomiting
GU: Decreased libido, prolactin secretion, amenorrhea, galactorrhea
CV: Hypotension, supraventricular tachycardia
INTEG: Urticaria, rash
Contraindications: Hypersensitivity to this drug or procaine or procainamide, seizure disorder, pheochromocytoma, breast cancer (prolactin dependent), GI obstruction
Precautions: Pregnancy (B), lactation, GI hemorrhage, CHF
Pharmacokinetics:
IV: Onset 1-3 min, duration 1-2 hr
PO: Onset ½-1 hr, duration 1-2 hr
IM: Onset 10-15 min, duration 1-2 hr
Metabolized by liver, excreted in urine, half-life 4 hr
Interactions:
- Decreased action of metoclopramide: anticholinergics, opiates
- Increased sedation: alcohol, other CNS depressants

Syringe compatibilities: Aminophylline, ascorbic acid, atropine, benztropine, bleomycin, chlorpromazine, cisplatin, cyclophosphamide, cytarabine, dexamethasone, dimenhydrinate, diphenhydramine, doxorubicin, droperidol, fentanyl, fluorouracil, heparin, hydrocortisone, hydroxyzine, regular insulin, leucovorin, lidocaine, magnesium sulfate, meperidine, methylprednisolone sodium succinate, midazolam, mitomycin, morphine, pentazocine, perphenazine, prochlorperazine, promazine, promethazine, ranitidine, scopolamine, vinblastine, vincristine
Additive compatibilities: Clindamycin, multivitamins, potassium, acetate, potassium chloride, potassium phosphate, verapamil
Lab test interferences:
Increase: Prolactin, aldosterone, thyrotropin

NURSING CONSIDERATIONS
Assess:
- For EPS and tardive dyskinesia
- Mental status: depression, anxiety, irritability
- GI complaints: nausea, vomiting, anorexia, constipation

Administer:
- IV undiluted if dose is $<$10 mg; give over 2 min; 10 mg or more may be diluted in 50 ml or more D_5W, NaCl, Ringer's, LR and given over 15 min or more
- ½-1 hr before meals for better absorption
- Gum, hard candy, frequent rinsing of mouth for dry oral cavity

Perform/provide:
- Protect from light with aluminum foil during infusion
- Discard open ampules

Evaluate:
- Therapeutic response: absence of nausea, vomiting, anorexia, fullness

Teach patient/family:
- To avoid driving, other hazardous activities until patient is stabilized on this medication
- To avoid alcohol, other CNS depressants that will enhance sedating properties of this drug

M

metocurine (℞)

(met-oh-kyoo'reen)

Metubine

Func. class.: Neuromuscular blocker (nondepolarizing)

Chem. class.: Methyl analog of tubocurarine

Action: Inhibits transmission of nerve impulses by binding with cholinergic receptor sites, antagonizing action of acetylcholine

Uses: Facilitation of endotracheal intubation, skeletal muscle relaxation during mechanical ventilation, surgery, or general anesthesia, reduction of fractures/dislocations

Dosage and routes:

Surgery

• *Adult:* IV 2-4 mg if given cyclopropane as an anesthetic; 1.5-3 mg if given ether as an anesthetic; 4-7 mg if given nitrous oxide

ECT (electroconvulsive therapy) adjunct

• *Adult:* IV 2-3 mg

Available forms: Inj 2 mg/ml

Side effects/adverse reactions:

CV: Bradycardia, tachycardia, increased, decreased B/P

RESP: ***Prolonged apnea, bronchospasm, cyanosis, respiratory depression***

EENT: Increased secretions

INTEG: Rash, flushing, pruritus, urticaria

Contraindications: Hypersensitivity to iodides

Precautions: Pregnancy (C), cardiac disease, hepatic disease, renal disease, lactation, children <2 yr, electrolyte imbalances, dehydration, neuromuscular disease (myasthenia gravis), respiratory disease, or when histamine release is a definite hazard (e.g., asthma)

Pharmacokinetics:

IV: Peak 3-5 min, duration 35-90 min, half-life 3½ hr; excreted in urine, bile (½ unchanged); crosses placenta

Interactions:

• Increased neuromuscular blockade: aminoglycosides, clindamycin, lincomycin, quinidine, local anesthetics, polymyxin antibiotics, lithium, narcotic analgesics, thiazides, enflurane, isoflurane, magnesium sulfate

• Dysrhythmias: theophylline

• Do not mix with barbiturates in sol or syringe; unstable in alkaline sol

NURSING CONSIDERATIONS

Assess:

• For electrolyte imbalances (K, Mg); may lead to increased action of this drug

• Vital signs (B/P, pulse, respirations, airway) until fully recovered; rate, depth, pattern of respirations (keep airway clear), strength of hand grip

• I&O ratio; check for urinary retention, frequency, hesitancy

• Recovery: decreased paralysis of face, diaphragm, leg, arm, rest of body

• Allergic reactions: rash, fever, respiratory distress, pruritus; drug should be discontinued

Administer:

• Using nerve stimulator by anesthesiologist to determine neuromuscular blockade

• Anticholinesterase to reverse neuromuscular blockade

• By slow IV over 1-2 min (only by qualified person, usually an anesthesiologist)

• Only slightly discolored sol

Perform/provide:

• Storage in light-resistant, cool area

• Reassurance if communication is

difficult during recovery from neuromuscular blockade
Evaluate:
• Therapeutic response: paralysis of jaw, eyelid, head, neck, rest of body
Teach patient/family: That postoperative stiffness is normal and will subside
Treatment of overdose: Edrophonium or neostigmine, atropine; monitor VS; may require mechanical ventilation

metolazone (℞)

(me-tole'a-zone)
Diulo, Mykrox, Zaroxolyn
Func. class.: Diuretic
Chem. class.: Thiazide like quinazoline derivative

Action: Acts on distal tubule and cortical thick ascending limb of the loop of Henle by increasing excretion of water, sodium, chloride, potassium, magnesium, bicarbonate
Uses: Edema, hypertension, CHF
Dosage and routes:
Edema
• *Adult:* PO 5-20 mg/day
Hypertension
• *Adult:* PO 2.5-5 mg/day (Diulo, Zaroxolyn)
• *Adult:* PO 0.5 mg (Mykrox) qd in AM, may increase to 1 mg
Available forms: Tabs 0.5, 2.5, 5, 10 mg
Side effects/adverse reactions:
GU: Frequency, polyuria, ***uremia, glucosuria***
CNS: Drowsiness, paresthesia, anxiety, depression, headache, *dizziness, fatigue, weakness*
GI: Nausea, vomiting, anorexia, constipation, diarrhea, cramps, pancreatitis, GI irritation, ***hepatitis***
EENT: Blurred vision
INTEG: Rash, urticaria, purpura, photosensitivity, fever
META: Hyperglycemia, increased creatinine, BUN
HEMA: ***Aplastic anemia, hemolytic anemia, leukopenia, agranulocytosis, neutropenia***
CV: Irregular pulse, orthostatic hypotension, palpitations, volume depletion
ELECT: Hypokalemia, hypomagnesemia, hypercalcemia, hyponatremia, hypochloremia, hypophosphatemia
Contraindications: Hypersensitivity to thiazides or sulfonamides, anuria, lactation
Precautions: Hypokalemia, renal disease, hepatic disease, gout, COPD, lupus erythematosus, diabetes mellitus, pregnancy (B)
Pharmacokinetics:
PO: Onset 1 hr, peak 2 hr, duration 12-24 hr; excreted unchanged by kidneys; crosses placenta; enters breast milk; half-life 8 hr
Interactions:
• Synergism: furosemide
• Increased toxicity of lithium, nondepolarizing skeletal muscle relaxants
• Decreased effects of antidiabetics, methenamine
• Decreased absorption of thiazides, cholestyramine, colestipol
• Decreased hypotensive response: indomethacin
• Hyperglycemia, hyperuricemia, hypotension: diazoxide
Lab test interferences:
Increase: BSP retention, Ca, amylase, parathyroid test
Decrease: PBI, PSP
NURSING CONSIDERATIONS
Assess:
• Weight, I&O daily to determine fluid loss; effect of drug may be decreased if used qd
• Rate, depth, rhythm of respiration, effect of exertion

M

• B/P lying, standing; postural hypotension may occur
• Electrolytes: K, Mg, Na, Cl; include BUN, blood sugar, CBC, serum creatinine, blood pH, ABGs, uric acid, Ca
• Glucose in urine of diabetic
• Improvement in edema of feet, legs, sacral area daily if medication is being used in CHF
• Improvement in CVP q8h
• Signs of metabolic alkalosis: drowsiness, restlessness
• Signs of hypokalemia: postural hypotension, malaise, fatigue, tachycardia, leg cramps, weakness
• Rashes, fever qd
• Confusion, especially in elderly; take safety precautions if needed

Administer:
• In AM to avoid interference with sleep if using drug as a diuretic
• K replacement if K <3
• With food; if nausea occurs, absorption may be decreased slightly
• Extended products are Diulo, Zaroxalyn; prompt product is Mykrox

Evaluate:
• Therapeutic response: decreased edema, B/P

Teach patient/family:
• To increase fluid intake to 2-3 L/day unless contraindicated, to rise slowly from lying or sitting position
• To notify prescriber of muscle weakness, cramps, nausea, dizziness
• That drug may be taken with food or milk
• To use sunscreen for photosensitivity
• That blood sugar may be increased in diabetics
• To take early in day to avoid nocturia

Treatment of overdose: Lavage if taken orally; monitor electrolytes; administer dextrose in saline; monitor hydration, CV, renal status

metoprolol (℞)

(met-oh'proe-lole)
Apo-Metoprolol*, Betaloc*, Betaloc Durules*, Lopresor*, Lopressor, Lopressor SR*, Novometoprol*, Toprol XL

Func. class.: Antihypertensive
Chem. class.: β_1-Blocker

Combination products: Lopressor HCT 50/25: metoprolol tartrate 50 mg with hydrochlorothiazide 25 mg; Lopressor HCT 100/25: metoprolol tartrate 100 mg with hydrochlorothiazide 25 mg

Action: Lowers B/P by β-blocking effects; elevated plasma renins are reduced; blocks β_2-adrenergic receptors in bronchial, vascular smooth muscle only at high doses

Uses: Mild to moderate hypertension, acute MI to reduce cardiovascular mortality, angina pectoris

Investigational uses: Dysrhythmias, hypertrophic cardiomyopathy, mitral valve prolapse, pheochromocytoma, tremors, prevention of vascular headaches, aggression

Dosage and routes:

Hypertension
• *Adult:* PO 50 mg bid, or 100 mg qd; may give up to 200-450 mg in divided doses; SUS REL give qd

Myocardial infarction
• *Adult:* (early treatment) IV BOL 5 mg q2min × 3, then 50 mg PO 15 min after last dose and q6h × 48 hr; (late treatment) PO maintenance 100 mg bid for 3 mo

Available forms: Tabs 50, 100 mg; inj 1 mg/ml; sus rel tab 50, 100, 200 mg

Side effects/adverse reactions:
CV: Hypotension, *bradycardia*
CHF: Palpitations, dysrhythmias, ***cardiac arrest, AV block***

* Available in Canada only

CNS: Insomnia, dizziness, mental changes, hallucinations, ***depression,*** anxiety, headaches, nightmares, confusion, fatigue
GI: Nausea, vomiting, colitis, cramps, ***diarrhea,*** constipation, flatulence, dry mouth, ***hiccups***
INTEG: Rash, purpura, alopecia, dry skin, urticaria, pruritus
HEMA: ***Agranulocytosis, eosinophilia, thrombocytopenia, purpura***
EENT: Sore throat, dry burning eyes
GU: Impotence
RESP: ***Bronchospasm,*** dyspnea, wheezing
Contraindications: Hypersensitivity to β-blockers, cardiogenic shock, heart block (2nd, 3rd degree), sinus bradycardia, CHF, bronchial asthma
Precautions: Major surgery, pregnancy (C), lactation, diabetes mellitus, renal disease, thyroid disease, COPD, heart failure, CAD, nonallergic bronchospasm, hepatic disease
Pharmacokinetics:
PO: Peak 2-4 hr, duration 13-19 hr; half-life 3-4 hr; metabolized in liver (metabolites); excreted in urine; crosses placenta; enters breast milk
Interactions:
- Increased hypotension, bradycardia: reserpine, hydralazine, methyldopa, prazosin
- Decreased antihypertensive effects: indomethacin, sympathomimetics
- Increased hypoglycemic effects: insulin
- Decreased bronchodilation: theophyllines, β-agonists

Y-site compatibilities: Alteplase, meperidine, morphine
Lab test interferences:
Increase: Liver function tests, renal function tests

NURSING CONSIDERATIONS
Assess:
- ECG directly when giving IV during initial treatment
- I&O, weight daily
- B/P during initial treatment, periodically thereafter; pulse q4h; note rate, rhythm, quality
- Apical/radial pulse before administration; notify prescriber of any significant changes
- Baselines in renal, liver function tests before therapy begins
- Edema in feet, legs daily
- Skin turgor, dryness of mucous membranes for hydration status

Administer:
- PO ac, hs, tablet may be crushed or swallowed whole
- IV, undiluted, give over 1 min, keep patient recumbent for 3 hr

Perform/provide:
- Storage in dry area at room temp, do not freeze

Evaluate:
- Therapeutic response: decreased B/P after 1-2 wk

Teach patient/family:
- To take with or immediately after meals
- Not to discontinue drug abruptly; taper over 2 wk; may cause precipitate angina
- Not to use OTC products containing α-adrenergic stimulants (nasal decongestants, OTC cold preparations) unless directed by prescriber
- To report bradycardia, dizziness, confusion, depression, fever, sore throat, shortness of breath to prescriber
- To take pulse at home; advise when to notify prescriber
- To avoid alcohol, smoking, Na intake
- To comply with weight control, dietary adjustments, modified exercise program

• To carry Medic Alert ID to identify drug, allergies
• To avoid hazardous activities if dizziness is present
• To report symptoms of CHF: difficult breathing, especially on exertion or when lying down, night cough, swelling of extremities
• To take medication hs to prevent effect of orthostatic hypotension
• To wear support hose to minimize effects of orthostatic hypotension

Treatment of overdose: Lavage, IV atropine for bradycardia, IV theophylline for bronchospasm, digitalis, O_2, diuretic for cardiac failure, hemodialysis, hypotension administer vasopressor (norepinephrine)

metronidazole (℞)

(me-troe-ni'da-zole)

Apo-Metronidazole*, Femazole, Flagyl, Flagyl IV, Flagyl IV RTU, Metro IV, metronidazole, metronidazole Redi-Infusion, Metryl, Neo-Metric*, Novonidazole*, PMS-Metronidazole*, Protostat, Satric, Trikacide*

Func. class.: Trichomonacide, amebicide; antiinfective

Chem. class.: Nitroimidazole derivative

Action: Direct-acting amebicide/trichomonacide binds, degrades DNA in organism

Uses: Intestinal amebiasis, amebic abscess, trichomoniasis, refractory trichomoniasis, bacterial anaerobic infections, giardiasis, septicemia, endocarditis, bone, joint infections, lower respiratory tract infections

Dosage and routes:

Trichomoniasis

• *Adult:* PO 250 mg tid × 7 days or 2 g in single dose; do not repeat treatment for 4-6 wk

Refractory trichomoniasis

• *Adult:* PO 250 mg bid × 10 days

Amebic abscess

• *Adult:* PO 500-750 mg tid × 5-10 days
• *Child:* PO 35-50 mg/kg/day in 3 divided doses × 10 days

Intestinal amebiasis

• *Adult:* PO 750 mg tid × 5-10 days
• *Child:* PO 35-50 mg/kg/day in 3 divided doses × 10 days; then oral iodoquinol

Anaerobic bacterial infections

• *Adult:* IV INF 15 mg/kg over 1 hr, then 7.5 mg/kg IV or PO q6h, not to exceed 4 g/day; first maintenance dose should be administered 6 hr following loading dose

Giardiasis

• *Adult:* PO 250 mg tid × 5 days
• *Child:* PO 5 mg/kg tid × 5 days

Available forms: Tabs 250, 500 mg; film-coated tabs 250, 1500 mg; inj 5 mg/vial; HCl inj 500 mg

Side effects/adverse reactions:

CV: Flat T waves

CNS: Headache, dizziness, confusion, irritability, restlessness, ataxia, depression, fatigue, drowsiness, insomnia, paresthesia, peripheral neuropathy, ***convulsions,*** incoordination, depression

EENT: Blurred vision, sore throat, retinal edema, dry mouth, metallic taste, furry tongue, glossitis, stomatitis

GI: Nausea, vomiting, diarrhea, epigastric distress, *anorexia,* constipation, *abdominal cramps,* metallic taste, ***pseudomembranous colitis***

GU: Darkened urine, vaginal dryness, polyuria, ***albuminuria,*** dysuria, cystitis, decreased libido, ***neurotoxicity,*** incontinence, dyspareunia

HEMA: ***Leukopenia, bone marrow, depression, aplasia***

* Available in Canada only

INTEG: Rash, pruritus, urticaria, flushing

Contraindications: Hypersensitivity to this drug, renal disease, hepatic disease, contracted visual or color fields, blood dyscrasias, pregnancy (1st trimester), lactation, CNS disorders

Precautions: Candida infections, pregnancy (2nd, 3rd trimesters) (B)

Pharmacokinetics:

IV: Onset immediate, peak end of inf

PO: Peak 1-2 hr, half-life 6-11 hr

Crosses placenta, enters breast milk, excreted in feces; absorbed PO (80%-85%)

Interactions:

- Disulfiram reaction: alcohol
- May increase action of warfarin
- Decreased action of metronidazole: phenobarbital
- Incompatible with any drug in syringe or sol

Lab test interferences:

Decrease: AST (SGOT), ALT (SGPT)

NURSING CONSIDERATIONS

Assess:

- For infection: WBC, wound symptoms, fever, skin or vaginal secretions; start treatment after C&S
- Stools during entire treatment; should be clear at end of therapy; stools should be free of parasites for 1 yr before patient is considered cured (amebiasis)
- Vision by ophthalmic exam during, after therapy; vision problems frequent
- I&O; weight daily; stools for number, frequency, character
- Neurotoxicity: peripheral neuropathy, seizures, dizziness, incoordination, pruritus, joint pains; may be discontinued
- Allergic reaction: fever, rash, itching, chills; drug should be discontinued if these symptoms occur
- Superinfection: fever, monilial growth, fatigue, malaise
- Renal and reproductive dysfunction: dysuria, polyuria, impotence, dyspareunia, decreased libido

Administer:

- IV prediluted; Flagyl IV, dilute with 4.4 ml sterile H_2O or 0.9% NaCl; must be diluted further with 8 mg/ml or more 0.9% NaCl, D_5W, or LR; must neutralize with 5 mEq Na_2CO_3/500 mg; CO_2 gas will be generated and may require venting; run over 1 hr; primary IV must be discontinued; may be given as continuous infusion; do not use aluminum products; IV may require venting
- PO with or after meals to avoid GI symptoms, metallic taste; crush tabs if needed

Perform/provide:

- Storage in light-resistant container; do not refrigerate

Evaluate:

- Therapeutic response: decreased symptoms of infection

Teach patient family:

- That urine may turn dark-reddish brown
- Proper hygiene after BM; handwashing technique
- To avoid hazardous activities, since dizziness can occur
- Need for compliance with dosage schedule, duration of treatment
- To use condoms if treatment for trichomoniasis, or cross-contamination may occur
- To use frequent sips of water, sugarless gum for dry mouth
- That treatment of both partners is necessary in trichomoniasis
- Not to drink alcohol or use preparations containing alcohol; disulfiram reaction can occur

M

metyrosine (℞)

(me-tye'roe-seen)
Demser
Func. class.: Antihypertensive
Chem. class.: Adrenergic blocker

Action: Inhibits enzyme tyrosine hydroxylase, resulting in decreased levels of catecholamines

Uses: Pheochromocytoma

Dosage and routes:

• *Adult and child >12 yr:* PO 250 mg qid, may increase by 250-500 mg qd to a max of 4 g/day in divided doses

Available forms: Caps 250 mg

Side effects/adverse reactions:

CNS: Sedation, drowsiness, dizziness, headache, depression, EPS, hallucinations, psychosis, agitation

INTEG: Rash, urticaria

EENT: Dry mouth, nasal stuffiness

GU: Dysuria, ***oliguria, hematuria,*** enuresis, impotence

GI: Nausea, vomiting, anorexia, diarrhea, abdominal pain

MISC: Breast swelling

Contraindications: Hypersensitivity, essential hypertension, children <12 yr

Precautions: Pregnancy (C), lactation, hepatic disease, renal disease

Pharmacokinetics:

PO: Onset 2 days, duration 3-4 days; half-life 3.4-3.7 hr, excreted in urine

Interactions:

• Increased sedation: CNS depressants: alcohol, barbiturates, antipsychotics

• Decreased effects of levodopa

• EPS: phenothiazines, haloperidol

Lab test interferences:

False increase: Urinary catecholamines

NURSING CONSIDERATIONS

Assess:

• Electrolytes: K, Na, Cl, CO_2

• Renal function studies: catecholamines, BUN, creatinine

• Hepatic function studies: AST (SGOT), ALT (SGPT), alk phosphatase

• B/P, ECG other VS throughout treatment

• Weight daily, I&O

• Change in behavior or personality: psychosis, anxiety, hallucinations, EPS

• Nausea, vomiting, diarrhea

• Edema in feet, legs daily

• Skin turgor, dryness of mucous membranes for hydration status

Administer:

• Antiemetic or antidiarrheals for vomiting, diarrhea

Perform/provide:

• Fluids to 2 L/day to prevent crystallization by kidneys

Evaluate:

• Therapeutic response: decreased B/P, decreased levels of catecholamines

Teach patient/family:

• To take each dose with a full glass of water; maintain sufficient daily intake

• Not to drive or perform hazardous tasks if behavioral changes, dizziness, or drowsiness occurs

• To avoid alcohol, other CNS depressants

• To notify prescriber of any of following: jaw stiffness, drooling, speech difficulty, tremors, disorientation, diarrhea, painful urination

Treatment of overdose: Administer vasopressors, discontinue drug

mexiletine (℞)

(mex-il′e-teen)

Mexitil

Func. class.: Antidysrhythmic (Class IB)

Chem. class.: Lidocaine analog

Action: Increases electrical stimulation threshold of ventricle, His-Purkinje system, which stabilizes cardiac membrane

Uses: Ventricular tachycardia, ventricular dysrhythmias during cardiac surgery, MI

Dosage and routes:

• *Adult:* PO 400 mg (loading dose), then 200 mg q8h, then 200-400 mg q8h

Available forms: Caps 150, 200, 250 mg

Side effects/adverse reactions:

CNS: Headache, dizziness, confusion, ***convulsions,*** tremors, psychosis, nervousness, paresthesias, weakness, fatigue, coordination difficulties, change in sleep habits

EENT: Blurred vision, hearing loss, tinnitus

GI: Nausea, vomiting, anorexia, diarrhea, abdominal pain, ***hepatitis,*** dry mouth, peptic ulcer, altered taste, GI bleeding

CV: Hypotension, bradycardia, angina, PVCs, ***heart block, cardiovascular collapse, arrest,*** sinus node slowing, ***left ventricular failure***, syncope, ***cardiogenic shock***

RESP: Dyspnea, ***fibrosis, embolism,*** pneumonia

INTEG: Rash, alopecia, dry skin

HEMA: ***Thrombocytopenia, leukopenia, agranulocytosis, hypoplastic anemia,*** systemic lupus erythematosus syndrome

GU: Urinary hesitancy, decreased libido

MISC: Edema, arthralgia, fever

Contraindications: Hypersensitivity to amides, cardiogenic shock, blood dyscrasias, severe heart block

Precautions: Pregnancy (C), lactation, children, renal disease, liver disease, CHF, respiratory depression, myasthenia gravis

Pharmacokinetics:

PO: Peak 2-3 hr; half-life 12 hr, metabolized by liver, excreted unchanged by kidneys (10%), excreted in breast milk

Interactions:

• Decreased effects: cimetidine

• Decreased levels of mexiletine: phenytoin, phenobarbital, rifampin

• Drug/smoking: decreased drug effect

Lab test interferences:

Increase: CPK

NURSING CONSIDERATIONS

Assess:

• ECG continuously for increased PR or QRS segments; discontinue or reduce rate; watch for increased ventricular ectopic beats; may have to rebolus

• Blood levels (therapeutic level 0.5-2 μg/ml)

• B/P continuously for fluctuations in cardiac rate

• I&O ratio, electrolytes (K, Na, Cl), liver enzymes

• Malignant hyperthermia: tachypnea, tachycardia, changes in B/P, fever

• Respiratory status: rate, rhythm, lung fields for rales, watch for respiratory depression

• CNS effects: dizziness, confusion, psychosis, paresthesias, convulsions; drug should be discontinued

• Lung fields, bilateral rales may occur in CHF patient

• Increased respiration, increased pulse; drug should be discontinued

Evaluate:

• Therapeutic response: decreased dysrhythmias

M

Treatment of overdose: O_2, artificial ventilation, ECG; administer dopamine for circulatory depression, diazepam or thiopental for convulsions, to acidify urine

mezlocillin (℞)

(mez-loe-sill'in)

Mezlin

Func. class.: Broad-spectrum antibiotic

Chem. class.: Extended-spectrum penicillin

Action: Interferes with cell wall replication of susceptible organisms; osmotically unstable cell wall swells, bursts from osmotic pressure

Uses: Effective for gram-positive cocci *(S. aureus, S. viridans, S. faecalis, S. pneumoniae),* gram-negative cocci *(N. gonorrhoeae),* gram-positive bacilli, *C. perfringens, C. tetani,* gram-negative bacilli *(Bacteroides, E. coli, H. influenzae, Klebsiella, P. mirabilis, Peptococcus, Peptostreptococcus, M. morganii, Enterobacter, Serratia, Pseudomonas, P. vulgaris, P. rettgeri, Shigella, Citrobacter, Veillonella)*

Dosage and routes:

- *Adult:* IM/IV 200-300 mg/kg/day in divided doses q4-6h; may give up to 24 g/day for severe infections
- *Child:* IM/IV 50 mg/kg q4-6h
- *Infants >8 days;* >2000 g: 75 mg/kg q6h; <2000 g: 75 mg/kg q8h
- *Infants <8 days:* 75 mg/kg q12h

Available forms: Powder for inj 1, 2, 3, 4 g; INF 2, 3, 4 g

Side effects/adverse reactions:

HEMA: Anemia, increased bleeding time, ***bone marrow depression, granulocytopenia***

GI: Nausea, vomiting, diarrhea, increased AST (SGOT), ALT (SGPT), abdominal pain, glossitis, colitis, abnormal taste

GU: Oliguria, proteinuria, hematuria, (vaginitis, moniliasis), ***glomerulonephritis,*** increased BUN, creatinine

CNS: Lethargy, hallucinations, anxiety, depression, twitching, ***coma, convulsions***

META: Hyperkalemia, hypokalemia, alkalosis, hypernatremia

Contraindications: Hypersensitivity to penicillins

Precautions: Pregnancy (B), lactation, hypersensitivity to cephalosporins, neonates

Pharmacokinetics:

IM: Peak 45 min

IV: Peak 5 min

Half-life 50-55 min; partially metabolized in liver; excreted in urine, bile, breast milk (small amount); crosses placenta

Interactions:

- Decreased effectiveness of aminoglycosides
- Decreased antimicrobial effectiveness of mezlocillin: tetracyclines, erythromycins
- Increased mezlocillin concentrations: aspirin, probenecid
- Incompatible in sol with aminoglycosides, ciprofloxacin, meperidine, verapamil

Lab test interferences:

False positive: Urine glucose, urine protein

NURSING CONSIDERATIONS

Assess:

- I&O ratio; report hematuria, oliguria, since penicillin in high doses is nephrotoxic
- Any patient with compromised renal system, since drug is excreted slowly in poor renal system function; toxicity may occur rapidly
- Liver studies: AST (SGOT), ALT (SGPT)
- Blood studies: WBC, RBC, Hct, Hgb, bleeding time

• Renal studies: urinalysis, protein, blood
• C&S before drug therapy; drug may be given as soon as culture is taken
• Bowel pattern before and during treatment
• Skin eruptions after administration of penicillin to 1 wk after discontinuing drug
• Respiratory status: rate, character, wheezing, and tightness in chest
• Check IV site for thrombophlebitis
• WBC, differential, liver, renal studies periodically for patients on long-term therapy
• Allergies before initiation of treatment, and reaction of each medication; highlight allergies on chart

Administer:
• IV after diluting 1 g or less/10 ml of sterile H_2O, D_5, or 0.9% NaCl for inj; shake, dilute further with D_5W or 0.45 NaCl, and give over 3-5 min; may be given by intermittent inf over ½ hr
• Drug after C&S completed

Perform/provide:
• Adrenalin, suction, tracheostomy set, endotracheal intubation equipment
• Adequate fluid intake (2 L) during diarrhea episodes
• Scratch test to assess allergy after securing order from prescriber; usually done when penicillin is only drug of choice
• Storage at room temp; reconstituted sol is stable for 24 hr refrigerated

Evaluate:
• Therapeutic response: absence of fever, draining wounds

Teach patient/family:
• That culture may be taken after completed course of medication
• To report sore throat, fever, fatigue (may indicate superinfection)
• To wear or carry Medic Alert ID if allergic to penicillins
• To report diarrhea, symptoms of *Candida* vaginitis

Treatment of anaphylaxis: Withdraw drug, maintain airway, administer epinephrine, aminophylline, O_2, IV corticosteroids

miconazole (℞)

(mi-kon'a-zole)
Monistat, Monistat IV
Func. class.: Antifungal
Chem. class.: Imidazole

Action: Alters cell membranes, inhibits fungal enzymes

Uses: Coccidioidomycosis, candidiasis, cryptococcoses, paracoccidioidomycosis, chronic mucocutaneous candidiasis, fungal meningitis; IV for severe infections only

Dosage and routes:
• *Adult:* IV INF 200-3600 mg/day; may be divided in 3 infusions 200-1200 mg/infusion; may have to repeat course; INTRATHECAL 20 mg given simultaneously with IV for fungal meningitis q3-7d
• *Child:* IV 20-40 mg/kg/day, not to exceed 15 mg/kg/day

Available forms: Inj 10 mg/ml; aerosol 2%

Side effects/adverse reactions:
CV: Tachycardia, dysrhythmias (rapid IV)
CNS: Drowsiness, headache, laziness
GI: Nausea, vomiting, anorexia, diarrhea, cramps
GU: Vulvovaginal burning, itching, hyponatremia, pelvic cramps (topical forms)
HEMA: ***Decreased Hct, thrombocytopenia, hyperlipidemia***
INTEG: Pruritus, rash, fever, flushing, ***anaphylaxis,*** hives

M

Contraindications: Hypersensitivity

Precautions: Renal disease, hepatic disease, pregnancy (B)

Pharmacokinetics:

IV: Onset immediate; peak end of inf; half-life triphasic 0.4, 2.1, 24.1 hr; metabolized in liver; excreted in feces, urine (inactive metabolites); >90% protein binding

Interactions:

- Increased action of anticoagulants
- Decreased action of both drugs: amphotericin

Y-site compatibilities: Foscarnet, ondansetron, sargramostim

Lab test interferences:

False positive: Urine glucose, urine protein

NURSING CONSIDERATIONS

Assess:

- Cardiac system: B/P, pulse, ECG; watch for increasing pulse, cardiac dysrhythmias; drug should be discontinued
- Blood studies: WBC, RBC, Hct, Hgb, bleeding time
- Renal studies: urinalysis, protein, blood
- C&S before drug therapy; drug may be given as soon as culture is taken; monitor signs of infection prior to and throughout treatment
- Bowel pattern before and during treatment; diarrhea is common
- Skin eruptions after administration of drug to 1 wk after discontinuing drug
- Respiratory status: rate, character, wheezing, tightness in chest
- IV site for thrombophlebitis
- WBC and differential liver and renal studies periodically for patients on long-term therapy
- Allergies before initiation of treatment, and reaction of each medication; highlight allergies on chart

Administer:

- 200 mg initially to prevent severe hypersensitive reaction
- IV after diluting 1 g or less/10 ml of sterile H_2O, D_5W or 0.45% NaCl; give over 3-5 min; may be given by intermittent INF over ½ hr
- Drug after C&S completed

Perform/provide:

- Adrenalin, suction, tracheostomy set, endotracheal intubation equipment
- Adequate fluid intake (2 L) during diarrhea episodes
- Scratch test to assess allergy after securing order from prescriber; usually done when penicillin is only drug of choice
- Storage at room temp; reconstituted sol stable for 24 hr refrigerated

Evaluate:

- Therapeutic response: absence of fever, draining wounds

Teach patient/family:

- That culture may be taken after completed course of medication
- To report sore throat, fever, fatigue (may indicate superinfection)
- To wear or carry Medic Alert ID if allergic to drug
- To report diarrhea, symptoms of *Candida* vaginitis

Treatment of overdose:

Withdraw drug; maintain airway; administer epinephrine, aminophylline, O_2, IV corticosteroids for anaphylaxis

* Available in Canada only

miconazole nitrate (topical) (OTC, ℞)

(mi-kon'a-zole)

Micatin, miconazole nitrate, Micatin Liquid, Monistat-Derm, Monistat 3, Monistat 7, Monistat Dual-Pak

Func. class.: Local antiinfective

Chem. class.: Antifungal

Action: Interferes with fungal cell membrane, which increases permeability, leaking of nutrients

Uses: Tinea pedis, tinea cruris, tinea corporis, tinea versicolor, vaginal or vulval *Candida albicans*

Dosage and routes:

• *Adult and child:* TOP apply to affected area bid × 2-4 wk

• *Adult:* INTRAVAG give 1 applicator or suppository × 7 days hs

Available forms: Cream, lotion, powder, spray 2%; vag cream 2%; vag supp 100, 200 mg

Side effects/adverse reactions:

GU: Vulvovaginal burning, itching, pelvic cramps

INTEG: Rash, urticaria, stinging, burning, contact dermatitis

Contraindications: Hypersensitivity

Precautions: Child <2 yr, pregnancy (B), lactation

NURSING CONSIDERATIONS

Assess:

• Allergic reaction: burning, stinging, swelling, redness

Administer:

• Enough medication to cover lesions completely

• After cleansing with soap, water before each application; dry well

Perform/provide:

• Storage at room temp in dry place

Evaluate:

• Therapeutic response: decrease in size, number of lesions

Teach patient/family:

• To use medical asepsis (hand washing) before, after each application

• To apply with glove to prevent further infection

• To avoid use of OTC creams, ointments, lotions unless directed by prescriber

• To avoid contact with eyes

• To avoid use of occlusive dressings

• To notify prescriber if no improvement in condition in 4 wk or if symptoms return in 2 mo; pregnancy or a serious medical condition may be the cause

• To use for full prescribed treatment time

microfibrillar collagen hemostat (℞)

Avitene

Func. class.: Hemostatic

Chem. class.: Purified cattle collagen

Action: Platelets adhere to hemostat, cause aggregation to and formation of thrombi

Uses: For hemostasis in surgery when ligature is ineffective/impractical

Dosage and routes:

• *Adult and child:* TOP apply to bleeding area after drying with sponge; compress for 1-5 min; may reapply if needed

Available forms: Fibrous form, nonwoven web form

Side effects/adverse reactions:

INTEG: Rash, abscess, allergic reactions, infection, wound dehiscence

HEMA: Hematoma

Contraindications: Hypersensitivity, closure of skin incision

Precautions: Pregnancy (C)

M

NURSING CONSIDERATIONS

Assess:

• Possible infection: hematoma, abscess

• Allergy: rash, itching

Administer:

• Dry, do not moisten

• Using gloves with forceps; area must be dry for drug to work

• Only new product; do not resterilize

Evaluate:

• Therapeutic response: decreased bleeding in surgery

midazolam (℞)

(mid'ay-zoe-lam)

Versed

Func. class.: Sedative/hypnotic

Chem. class.: Benzodiazepine, short-acting

Controlled Substance Schedule IV

Action: Depresses subcortical levels in CNS; may act on limbic system, reticular formation; may potentiate γ-aminobenzoic acid (GABA) by binding to specific benzodiazepine receptors

Uses: Preoperative sedation, general anesthesia induction, sedation for diagnostic endoscopic procedures, intubation

Dosage and routes:

Preoperative sedation

Adult: IM 0.07-0.08 mg/kg ½-1 hr before general anesthesia

Induction of general anesthesia

Adult: IV (unpremedicated patients) 0.3-0.35 mg/kg over 30 sec, wait 2 min, follow with 25% of initial dose if needed; (premedicated patients) 0.15-0.35 mg/kg over 20-30 sec, allow 2 min for effect

Available forms: Inj 1, 5 mg/ml

Side effects/adverse reactions:

CNS: Retrograde amnesia, euphoria, confusion, headache, anxiety, insomnia, slurred speech, paresthesia, tremors, weakness, chills

RESP: Coughing, ***apnea, bronchospasm, laryngospasm,*** dyspnea

CV: Hypotension, PVCs, tachycardia, bigeminy, nodal rhythm

EENT: Blurred vision, nystagmus, diplopia, blocked ears, loss of balance

GI: Nausea, vomiting, increased salivation, hiccups

INTEG: Urticaria, pain, swelling at injection site, rash, pruritus

Contraindications: Pregnancy (D), hypersensitivity to benzodiazepines, shock, coma, alcohol intoxication, acute narrow-angle glaucoma

Precautions: COPD, CHF, chronic renal failure, chills, elderly, debilitated

Pharmacokinetics:

IM: Onset 15 min, peak ½-1 hr

IV: Onset 3-5 min, onset of anesthesia 1½-2½ min; protein binding 97%; half-life 1.2-12.3 hr

Metabolized in liver; metabolites excreted in urine; crosses placenta, blood-brain barrier

Interactions:

• Prolonged respiratory depression: other CNS depressants, alcohol, barbiturates

• Increased hypnotic effect: fentanyl, narcotic agonists, analgesics, droperidol

Syringe compatibilities: Atropine, benzquinamide, buprenorphine, butorphanol, chlorpromazine, cimetadine, diphenhydramine, droperidol, fentanyl, glycopyrrolate, hydromorphine, hydroxyzine, meperidine, metoclopramide, morphine, nalbuphine, promazine, promethazine, scopolamine, thiethylperazine, trimethobenzamide

Y-site compatibilities: Atracurium, famotidine, fluconazole, pancuronium, vecuronium

NURSING CONSIDERATIONS
Assess:
• Injection site for redness, pain, swelling
• Degree of amnesia in elderly; may be increased
• Anterograde amnesia
• Vital signs for recovery period in obese patient, since half-life may be extended
Administer:
• IV after diluting with D_5W or 0.9% NaCl to 0.25 mg/ml; give over 2 min (conscious sedation) or over 30 sec (anesthesia induction)
• IM deep into large muscle mass
Perform/provide:
• Assistance with ambulation until drowsy period relieved
• Storage at room temp
• Immediate availability of resuscitation equipment, O_2 to support airway; do not give by rapid bolus
Evaluate:
• Therapeutic response: induction of sedation, general anesthesia
Teach patient/family:
• To avoid hazardous activities until drowsiness, weakness subside
• That amnesia occurs; events may not be remembered
Treatment of overdose: O_2, vasopressors, physostigmine, resuscitation

milrinone (℞)

(mill-re′none)
Primacor
Func. class.: Inotropic/vasodilator agent with phosphodiesterase activity
Chem. class.: Bipyridine derivative

Action: Positive inotropic agent with vasodilator properties; reduces preload and afterload by direct relaxation on vascular smooth muscle

Uses: Short-term management of CHF that has not responded to other medication; can be used with digitalis
Dosage and routes:
• *Adult:* IV BOL 50 μg/kg given over 10 min; start infusion of 0.375-0.75 μg/kg/min; reduce dose in renal impairment
Available forms: Inj 1 mg/ml
Side effects/adverse reactions:
HEMA: ***Thrombocytopenia***
MISC: Headache, hypokalemia, tremor
CV: Dysrhythmias, hypotension, chest pain
GI: Nausea, vomiting, anorexia, abdominal pain, ***hepatotoxicity,*** jaundice
Contraindications: Hypersensitivity to this drug, severe aortic disease, severe pulmonic valvular disease, acute myocardial infarction
Precautions: Lactation, pregnancy (C), children, renal disease, hepatic disease, atrial flutter/fibrillation, elderly
Pharmacokinetics:
IV: Onset 2-5 min, peak 10 min, duration variable; half-life 4-6 hr; metabolized in liver; excreted in urine as drug and metabolites 60%-90%
Interactions:
• Excessive hypotension: antihypertensives
Y-site compatibility: Furosemide
NURSING CONSIDERATIONS
Assess:
• B/P and pulse q5min during infusion; if B/P drops 30 mm Hg, stop infusion and call prescriber
• Electrolytes: K, Na, Cl, Ca; renal function studies: BUN, creatinine; blood studies: platelet count
• ALT (SGPT), AST (SGOT), bilirubin qd
• I&O ratio and weight qd; diuresis

M

should increase with continuing therapy
• If platelets are <150,000/mm^3 drug is usually discontinued and another drug started
• Extravasation; change site q48h

Administer:
• Into running dextrose infusion through Y-connector or directly into tubing; dilute with NS to 1-3 mg/ml; do not mix with glucose for long-term infusion
• By infusion pump for doses other than bolus
• K supplements if ordered for K levels <3

Evaluate:
• Therapeutic response: increased cardiac output, decreased PCWP, adequate CVP, decreased dyspnea, fatigue, edema, ECG

Treatment of overdose: Discontinue drug, support circulation

mineral oil (OTC)

Agoral Plain, Fleet Mineral Oil Enema, Kondremul*, Kondremul Plain, Liqui-doss, Lansoyl*, Milkinol, Neo-Cultol, Nujol, Petrogalar Plain, Zymenol

Func. class.: Laxative-lubricant

Chem. class.: Petroleum hydrocarbon

Action: Eases passage of stool by increasing water retention in feces; acts as lubricant

Uses: Constipation, preparation for bowel surgery or exam

Dosage and routes:
• *Adult:* PO 15-30 ml hs; enema 4 oz
• *Child 6-12 yr:* PO 5-15 ml hs; enema 1-2 oz
• *Child 2-11 yr:* Enema 1-2 oz

Available forms: Oil, enema; jelly 55%; susp 1.4, 2.5, 2.75 mg/5 ml

Side effects/adverse reactions:
CNS: Muscle weakness
GI: Nausea, vomiting, anorexia, diarrhea, pruritus ani, hepatic infiltration
META: ***Hypoprothrombinemia***
RESP: Lipid pneumonia

Contraindications: Hypersensitivity, intestinal obstruction, abdominal pain, nausea/vomiting

Precautions: Pregnancy (C)

Pharmacokinetics: Excreted in feces

Interactions:
• Increased effect of oral anticoagulants
• Decreased absorption: fat-soluble vitamins (A, D, E, K) if used for prolonged time

NURSING CONSIDERATIONS

Assess:
• Stool for color, consistency, amount
• Blood, urine electrolytes if drug is used often by patient
• I&O ratio to identify fluid loss
• Cause of constipation; lack of fluids, bulk, exercise
• Cramping, rectal bleeding, nausea, vomiting; drug should be discontinued

Administer:
• Alone for better absorption
• In morning or evening (oral dose)
• Cautiously in elderly to prevent aspiration

Evaluate:
• Therapeutic response: decrease in constipation

Teach patient/family:
• Not to use laxatives for long-term therapy; bowel tone will be lost
• That normal bowel movements do not always occur daily
• Not to use in presence of abdominal pain, nausea, vomiting
• To notify prescriber if constipation unrelieved or if symptoms of electrolyte imbalance occur: muscle

* Available in Canada only

cramps, pain, weakness, dizziness, excessive thirst

- Not to use with food or vitamin preparations; delays digestion and absorption of fat-soluble vitamins

minocycline (℞)

(min-oh-sye'kleen)

Minocin, Minocin IV

Func. class.: Broad-spectrum antiinfective

Chem. class.: Tetracycline

Action: Inhibits protein synthesis, phosphorylation in microorganisms by binding to 30S ribosomal subunits, reversibly binding to 50S ribosomal subunits; bacteriostatic

Uses: Syphilis, chlamydia trachomatis, gonorrhea, lymphogranuloma venereum, rickettsial infections, inflammatory acne, *Neisseria meningitidis, N. gonorrheae, Treponema pallidum, Chlamydia trachomatis, Ureaplasma urealyticum, Mycoplasma pneumoniae, Nocardia*

Dosage and routes:

- *Adult:* PO/IV 200 mg, then 100 mg q12h or 50 mg q6h, not to exceed 400 mg/24h IV
- *Child >8 yr:* PO/IV 4 mg/kg then 4 mg/kg/day PO in divided doses q12h

Gonorrhea

- *Adult:* PO 200 mg, then 100 mg q12h × 4 days

Chlamydia trachomatis

- *Adult:* PO 100 mg bid × 7 days

Syphilis

- *Adult:* PO 200 mg, then 100 mg q12h × 10-15 days

Available forms: Tabs 50, 100 mg; caps 50, 100 mg; oral susp 50 mg/5 ml; powder for inj 100 mg/vial

Side effects/adverse reactions:

CNS: Dizziness, fever, light-headedness, vertigo

HEMA: ***Eosinophilia, neutropenia, thrombocytopenia, hemolytic anemia***

EENT: Dysphagia, glossitis, decreased calcification of deciduous teeth, permanent discoloration of teeth, oral candidiasis

GI: Nausea, abdominal pain, *vomiting, diarrhea,* anorexia, enterocolitis, ***hepatotoxicity,*** flatulence, abdominal cramps, epigastric burning, stomatitis

CV: Pericarditis

GU: Increased BUN, polyuria, polydipsia, ***renal failure, nephrotoxicity***

INTEG: Rash, urticaria, photosensitivity, increased pigmentation, ***exfoliative dermatitis,*** pruritus, angioedema, blue-gray color of skin, mucous membranes

Contraindications: Hypersensitivity to tetracyclines, children <8 yr, pregnancy (D)

Precautions: Hepatic disease, lactation

Pharmacokinetics:

PO: Peak 2-3 hr half-life 11-17 hr; excreted in urine, feces, breast milk; crosses placenta; 55%-88% protein bound

Interactions:

- Decreased effect of minocycline: antacids, $NaHCO_3$, alkali products, iron, kaolin/pectin, cimetidine
- Increased effect of anticoagulants
- Decreased effect of penicillins, oral contraceptives
- Nephrotoxicity: methoxyflurane

Y-site compatibilities: Cyclophosphamide, fludarabine, heparin, hydrocortisone, magnesium sulfate, melphalan, perphenazine, potassium chloride, sargramostim, sodium succinate, vinorelbine, vitamin B with C

Additive compatibilities: Amikacin, cimetidine, clindamycin, gen-

M

tamicin, kanamycin, multivitamins, rifampin, sodium bicarbonate, tobramycin, verapamil, vitamin B complex with C

Syringe compatibility: Heparin

Lab test interferences:

False negative: Urine glucose with Clinistix or Tes-Tape

NURSING CONSIDERATIONS

Assess:

- I&O ratio
- Blood studies: PT, CBC, AST (SGOT), ALT (SGPT), BUN, creatinine
- Signs of anemia: Hct, Hgb, fatigue
- Allergic reactions: rash, itching, pruritus, angioedema
- Nausea, vomiting, diarrhea; administer antiemetic, antacids as ordered
- Overgrowth of infection: fever, malaise, redness, pain, swelling, drainage, perineal itching, diarrhea, changes in cough or sputum, black, furry tongue

Administer:

- IV after diluting 100 mg/5 ml sterile H_2O for inj; further dilute in 500-1000 ml of NaCl, dextrose sol, LR, Ringer's sol; run 100 mg/6 hr
- After C&S obtained
- 2 hr before or after laxative or ferrous products; 3 hr after antacid or kaolin-pectin product (PO)

Perform/provide:

- Storage in air-tight, light-resistant container at room temp

Evaluate:

- Therapeutic response: decreased temp, absence of lesions, negative C&S

Teach patient/family:

- To avoid sunlight; sunscreen does not seem to decrease photosensitivity
- That all prescribed medication must be taken to prevent superinfection
- To take with a full glass of water; may take with food, milk for GI symptoms

---

minoxidil (℞)

(mi-nox'i-dill)

Loniten, Minodyl, minoxidil, Rogaine

Func. class.: Antihypertensive

Chem. class.: Vasodilator—peripheral

Action: Directly relaxes arteriolar smooth muscle, causing vasodilation

Uses: Severe hypertension unresponsive to other therapy (use with diuretic); topically to treat alopecia

Dosage and routes:

- *Adult:* PO 5 mg/day not to exceed 100 mg daily, usual range 10-40 mg/day in single doses
- *Child <12 yr:* (initial) 0.2 mg/kg/day; (effective range) 0.25-1 mg/kg/day; (max) 50 mg/day

Alopecia

- *Adult:* Apply topically, rub into scalp daily

Available forms: Tabs 2.5, 10 mg, top 20 mg/ml

Side effects/adverse reactions:

CV: Severe rebound hypertension, tachycardia, angina, increased T wave, ***CHF, pulmonary edema, pericardial effusion,*** edema, sodium, water retention

CNS: Drowsiness, dizziness, sedation, headache, depression, fatigue

GI: Nausea, vomiting

GU: Gynecomastia, breast tenderness

INTEG: Pruritus, ***Stevens-Johnson syndrome,*** rash, hirsutism

HEMA: Hct, Hgb, erythrocyte count may decrease initially

Contraindications: Acute MI, dissecting aortic aneurysm, hypersensitivity, pheochromocytoma

---

* Available in Canada only

Precautions: Pregnancy (C), lactation, children, renal disease, CAD, CHF

Pharmacokinetics:

PO: Onset 30 min, peak 2-3 hr, duration 75 hr; half-life 4.2 hr; metabolized in liver; metabolites excreted in urine, feces

Interactions:

• Orthostatic hypotension: guanethidine

Lab test interferences:

Increase: Renal function studies

Decrease: Hgb/Hct/RBC

NURSING CONSIDERATIONS

Assess:

• Nausea, edema in feet, legs daily
• Skin turgor, dryness of mucous membranes for hydration status
• Rales, dyspnea, orthopnea

Monitor:

• Electrolytes: K, Na, Cl, CO_2
• Renal function studies: catecholamines, BUN, creatinine
• Hepatic function studies: AST (SGOT), ALT (SGPT), alk phosphatase
• B/P, pulse
• Weight daily, I&O

Administer:

• Topical: 1 ml no matter how much balding has occurred; increasing dosage does not speed growth
• PO: with meals for better absorption, to decrease GI symptoms
• With β-blocker and/or diuretic for hypertension

Perform/provide:

• Storage protected from light and heat

Evaluate:

• Therapeutic response: decreased B/P or increased hair growth

Teach patient/family:

• That body hair will increase but is reversible after discontinuing treatment
• Not to discontinue drug abruptly
• To report pitting edema, dizziness, weight gain >5 lb, shortness of breath, bruising or bleeding, heart rate >20 beats/min over normal, severe indigestion, dizziness, lightheadedness, panting, new or aggravated symptoms of angina
• To take drug exactly as prescribed, or serious side effects may occur
• Topical: treatment must continue long-term or new hair will be lost
• Not to use except on scalp

Treatment of overdose: Administer normal saline IV, vasopressors

misoprostol (℞)

(mye-soe-prost′ole)

Cytotec

Func. class.: Gastric mucosa protectant

Chem. class.: Prostaglandin E_1 analog

Action: Inhibits gastric acid secretion; may protect gastric mucosa; can increase bicarbonate, mucus production

Uses: Prevention of nonsteroidal antiinflammatory drug-induced gastric ulcers

Investigational uses: Used investigationally with methotrexate to produce abortion

Dosage and routes:

• *Adult:* PO 200 μg qid with food for duration of nonsteroidal antiinflammatory therapy; if 200 μg is not tolerated, 100 μg may be given

Available forms: Tabs 100, 200 μg

Side effects/adverse reactions:

GI: Diarrhea, nausea, vomiting, flatulence, constipation, dyspepsia, abdominal pain

GU: Spotting, cramps, hypermenorrhea, menstrual disorders

Contraindications: Hypersensitivity, pregnancy (X)

Precautions: Lactation, children, elderly, renal disease

Pharmacokinetics:

PO: Peak 12 min, plasma steady state achieved within 2 days, excreted in urine

NURSING CONSIDERATIONS

Assess:

• GI symptoms: hematemesis, occult or frank blood in stools, gastric aspirate, cramping, severe diarrhea

• Obtain a negative pregnancy test; miscarriages are common

• Gastric pH (>5 should be maintained)

Administer:

• PO with meals for prolonged drug effect; avoid use of magnesium antacids

Perform/provide:

• Storage at room temp

Evaluate:

• Therapeutic response: absence of pain or GI complaints; prevention of ulcers

Teach patient/family:

• To take only as directed

• Not to take if pregnant (can cause miscarriage) and not to become pregnant while taking this medication; if pregnancy occurs during therapy, discontinue drug, notify prescriber; not to administer to nursing mothers

• Not to give drug to anyone else or take for more than 4 wk unless directed by prescriber

• To avoid OTC preparations: aspirin, cough, cold products; condition may worsen

mitomycin (℞)

(mye-toe-mye'sin)

Mutamycin

Func. class.: Antineoplastic, antibiotic

Action: Inhibits DNA synthesis, primarily; derived from *Streptomyces caespitosus;* appears to cause cross-linking of DNA, a vesicant

Uses: Pancreas, stomach cancer, head and neck or breast cancer

Investigational uses: Palliative treatment of head, neck, colon, breast, biliary, cervical, lung malignancies

Dosage and routes:

• *Adult:* IV 2 mg/m^2/day × 5 days, skip 2 days, then repeat cycle; or 10-20 mg/m^2 as a single dose, repeat cycle in 6-8 wk; stop drug if platelets are <75,000/mm^3 or WBC is <3000/mm^3

Available forms: Inj 5, 20, 40 mg/vial

Side effects/adverse reactions:

HEMA: ***Thrombocytopenia, leukopenia, anemia***

GI: Nausea, vomiting, anorexia, stomatitis, ***hepatotoxicity,*** diarrhea

GU: Urinary retention, ***renal failure,*** edema

INTEG: Rash, alopecia, ***extravasation***

RESP: ***Fibrosis, pulmonary infiltrate,*** dyspnea

CNS: Fever, headache, confusion, drowsiness, syncope, fatigue

EENT: Blurred vision, drowsiness, syncope

Contraindications: Hypersensitivity, pregnancy (1st trimester) (D), as a single agent, thrombocytopenia, coagulation disorders

Precautions: Renal disease, bone marrow depression

Pharmacokinetics: Half-life 1 hr, metabolized in liver, 10% excreted in urine (unchanged)

Interactions:

• Increased toxicity: other antineoplastics (vinca alkaloids), radiation

Syringe compatibilities: Bleomycin, cisplatin, cyclophosphamide, doxorubicin, droperidol, fluorouracil, furosemide, heparin, leucovorin, methotrexate, metoclopramide, vinblastine, vincristine

* Available in Canada only

Y-site compatibilities: Bleomycin, cisplatin, cyclophosphamide, doxorubicin, droperidol, fluorouracil, furosemide, heparin, leucovorin, melphalan, methotrexate, metoclopramide, ondansetron, vinblastine, vincristine

Additive compatibility: Sodium lactate

Solution compatibilities: LR, 0.3% NaCl, 0.5% NaCl

NURSING CONSIDERATIONS

Assess:

- CBC, differential, platelet count weekly; withhold drug if WBC is <4000/mm^3 or platelet count is <75,000/mm^3; notify prescriber
- Pulmonary function tests, chest x-ray before, during therapy; chest x-ray should be obtained q2wk during treatment
- Renal function studies: BUN, serum uric acid, urine CrCl, electrolytes before, during therapy
- I&O ratio; report fall in urine output to <30 ml/hr
- Monitor temp q4h; fever may indicate beginning infection
- Liver function tests before, during therapy: bilirubin, AST (SGOT), ALT (SGPT), alk phosphatase as needed or monthly
- Alkalosis if severe vomiting is present
- Bleeding: hematuria, guaiac, bruising, petechiae, mucosa or orifices q8h
- Dyspnea, rales, unproductive cough, chest pain, tachypnea, fatigue, increased pulse, pallor, lethargy
- Food preferences; list likes, dislikes
- Effects of alopecia on body image; discuss feelings about body changes
- Inflammation of mucosa, breaks in skin
- Yellow skin and sclera, dark urine, clay-colored stools, itchy skin, abdominal pain, fever, diarrhea
- Buccal cavity q8h for dryness, sores, ulceration, white patches, oral pain, bleeding, dysphagia
- Local irritation, pain, burning at injection site
- GI symptoms: frequency of stools, cramping
- Acidosis, signs of dehydration: rapid respirations, poor skin turgor, decreased urine output, dry skin, restlessness, weakness

Administer:

- Apply ice compress for extravasation; stop infusion
- Antiemetic 30-60 min before giving drug to prevent vomiting
- IV after diluting 5 mg/10 ml sterile H_2O for inj; allow to stand, give through Y-tube or 3-way stopcock; give over 5-10 min
- Transfusion for anemia
- Antispasmodic for GI symptoms

Perform/provide:

- Liquid diet: carbonated beverages, gelatin may be added if patient is not nauseated or vomiting
- Rinsing of mouth tid-qid with water; brushing of teeth with baking soda bid-tid with soft brush or cotton tipped applicators for stomatitis; use unwaxed dental floss
- Storage at room temp 1 wk after reconstituting or 2 wk refrigerated

Evaluate:

- Therapeutic response: decreased tumor size, spread of malignancy

Teach patient/family:

- To report any complaints, side effects to nurse or prescriber
- That hair may be lost during treatment and wig or hairpiece may make the patient feel better; tell patient that new hair may be different in color, texture
- To avoid foods with citric acid, hot or rough texture

M

• To report any bleeding, white spots, ulcerations in mouth; tell patient to examine mouth qd
• To avoid crowds, people with infections if granulocyte count is low

mitotane (℞)

(mye'toe-tane)
Lysodren, p'-DDD
Func. class.: Antineoplastic
Chem. class.: Hormone, adrenal cytotoxic agent

Action: Cytotoxic and suppressive activity without cellular destruction in the adrenal cortex
Uses: Adrenocortical carcinoma
Dosage and routes:
• *Adult:* PO 9-10 g/day in divided doses tid or qid; may have to decrease dose for severe reaction
Available forms: Tabs 500 mg
Side effects/adverse reactions:
GI: Nausea, vomiting, anorexia, diarrhea
GU: ***Proteinuria, hematuria***
INTEG: Rash
RESP: ***Fibrosis, pulmonary infiltrate***
CV: Hypertension, orthostatic hypotension
CNS: Light-headedness, flushing, sedation, vertigo
EENT: Lethargy, blurring, retinopathy
Contraindications: Hypersensitivity
Precautions: Lactation, hepatic disease, pregnancy (C)
Pharmacokinetics: Adequately absorbed orally (40%), excreted in urine, bile
Interactions:
• Decreased effects of corticosteroids
Lab test interferences:
Decrease: PBI, urinary 17-OHCS

NURSING CONSIDERATIONS
Assess:
• Adrenal insufficiency: fatigue, orthostatic hypotension, weight loss, weakness, nausea, vomiting, diarrhea
• Pulmonary function tests, chest x-ray films before, during therapy; chest film should be obtained q2wk during treatment
• Renal function studies: BUN, serum uric acid, urine CrCl electrolytes before, during therapy
• I&O ratio
• Urinary 17-OHCS before, during treatment
• Dyspnea, chest pain, tachypnea, fatigue, increased pulse, pallor, lethargy
• Food preferences; list likes, dislikes
• Muscular weakness, fatigue, oliguria, hypoglycemia
• Frequency of stools, characteristics: cramping, acidosis, signs of dehydration (rapid respirations, poor skin turgor, decreased urine output, dry skin, restlessness, weakness)
• Symptoms of severe allergic reactions: rash, pruritus, itching, flushing
• Signs of infection: fever, cough, fatigue, malaise
Administer:
• Antacid before oral agent, give drug after evening meal, before bedtime
• Antiemetic 30-60 min before giving drug to prevent vomiting
• Antispasmodic
Perform/provide:
• Increase fluid intake to 2-3 L/day to prevent dehydration if not contraindicated
• HOB raised to facilitate breathing
• Nutritious diet with iron, vitamin supplements as ordered
• Storage in tight, light-resistant container

* Available in Canada only

Evaluate:
• Therapeutic response: decreased tumor size, spread of malignancy
Teach patient/family:
• To report any complaints, side effects to nurse or prescriber
• To report any changes in breathing, coughing
• To avoid driving, other activities requiring alertness

mitoxantrone (℞)

(mye-toe-zan'trone)
Novantrone
Func. class.: Antineoplastic, antibiotic
Chem. class.: Synthetic anthraquinone

Action: DNA reactive agent, cytocidal effect on both proliferating and nonproliferating cells, suggesting lack of cell cycle phase specificity (vesicant)
Uses: Acute nonlymphocytie leukemia (adult), relapsed leukemia, breast cancer
Investigational uses: Breast and liver malignancies, non-Hodgkin's lymphoma
Dosage and routes:
• *Adult:* IV INF 12 mg/m^2/day on days 1-3, and 100 mg/m^2 cytosine arabinoside × 7 days as a continuous 24hr infusion
Available forms: Inj 2 mg/ml
Side effects/adverse reactions:
GI: Nausea, vomiting, diarrhea, anorexia, mucositis, ***hepatotoxicity***
HEMA: ***Thrombocytopenia, leukopenia, myelosuppression, anemia***
INTEG: Rash, necrosis at injection site, dermatitis, thrombophlebitis at injection site, alopecia
CV: ***CHF, cardiopathy, dysrhythmias***
MISC: Fever
RESP: Cough, dyspnea
Contraindications: Hypersensitivity
Precautions: Myelosuppression, lactation, cardiac disease, children, pregnancy (D), renal, hepatic disease, gout
Pharmacokinetics:
Highly bound to plasma proteins, metabolized in liver, excreted via renal, hepatobiliary systems; half-life 24-72 hr
Interactions:
• Do not mix with heparin; precipitate will form
Y-site compatibilities: Ondansetron, fludarabine, melphalan, sargrasmostin, vinorelbine
Additive compatibilities: Hydrocortisone sodium succinate, cyclophosphamide, cytarabine, fluorouracil, potassium chloride
Solution compatibilities: D_5/0.9 NaCl, D_5W, 0.9% NaCl

NURSING CONSIDERATIONS
Assess:
• CBC, differential, platelet count qwk; withhold drug if WBC is $<4000/mm^3$ or platelet count is $<75,000/mm^3$; notify prescriber of these results
• Liver function test before, during therapy: bilirubin, AST (SGOT), ALT (SGPT), alk phosphatase prn or qmo
• Renal function studies: BUN, serum uric acid, urine CrCl, electrolytes before, during therapy
• Bleeding, hematuria, guaiac, bruising or petechiae, mucosa or orifices q8h
• Food preferences: list likes, dislikes
• Yellow skin and sclera, dark urine, clay-colored stools, itchy skin, abdominal pain, fever, diarrhea
• Acidosis, signs of dehydration: rapid respirations, poor skin turgor, decreased urine output, dry skin, restlessness, weakness

Administer:

• Medications by oral route if possible; avoid IM, SC, IV routes to prevent infections

• Antiemetic 30-60 min before giving drug to prevent vomiting

• IV after diluting with 50 ml or more normal saline or D_5W; give over 3-5 min, running IV of D_5W or NS; may be diluted further in D_5W, NS and run over 15-30 min; check for extravasation

Perform/provide:

• Liquid diet: carbonated beverages, Jell-O; dry toast, crackers may be added if patient is not nauseated or vomiting

• Rinsing of mouth tid-qid with water, club soda, brushing of teeth bid-qid with soft brush or cotton-tipped applicators for stomatitis; use unwaxed dental floss

Evaluate:

• Therapeutic resonse: decreased tumor size, spread of malignancy

Teach patient/family:

• To report side effects to nurse or physician

• To avoid foods with citric acid, rough texture, or hot

• To report any bleeding, white spots, ulcerations in mouth; tell patient to examine mouth qd

mivacurium (℞)

(miv-a-kure′ee-um)

Mivacron

Func. class.: Nondepolarizing neuromuscular blocker

Action: Inhibits transmission of nerve impulses by binding competitively with cholinergic receptor sites, antagonizing action of acetylcholine

Uses: Facilitation of endotracheal intubation, skeletal muscle relaxation during mechanical ventilation, surgery, or general anesthesia

Dosage and routes:

• *Adult:* IV 0.15 mg/kg; maintenance q15min

• *Child:* 2-12 IV 0.2 mg/kg for a 10 min block

Available forms: 5, 10 ml single-use vial (2 mg/ml); premixed infusion in D_5W 50 ml flex container

Side effects/adverse reactions:

CV: Decreased B/P, bradycardia, tachycardia

RESP: ***Prolonged apnea, bronchospasm, wheezing, respiratory depression***

EENT: Diplopia

MS: Weakness, prolonged skeletal muscle relaxation, ***paralysis***

INTEG: Rash, urticaria

Contraindications: Hypersensitivity

Precautions: Pregnancy (C), renal or hepatic disease, lactation, children <3 mo, fluid and electrolyte imbalances, neuromuscular disease, respiratory disease, obesity, elderly

Pharmacokinetics: Rapidly hydrolyzed by plasma cholinesterases, peak 2-3 min, reversal within 15-30 min

Interactions:

• Increased neuromuscular blockade: aminoglycosides, quinidine, local anesthetics, polymyxin antibiotics, enflurane, isoflurane, tetracyclines, halothane, Mg, colistin, procaninamide, bacitracin, lincomycin, clindamycin, lithium

Y-site compatibilities: Alfentanil, droperidol, fentanyl, midazolam, sufentanil

NURSING CONSIDERATIONS

Assess

• For electrolyte imbalances (K, Mg); may lead to increased action of this drug

• Vital signs (B/P, pulse, respirations, airway) until fully recovered;

rate, depth, pattern of respirations, strength of hand grip
- I&O ratio; check for urinary retention, frequency, hesitancy
- Recovery: decresed paralysis of face, diaphragm, leg, arm, rest of body
- Allergic reactions: rash, fever, respiratory distress, pruritus; drug should be discontinued

Administer:
- Using nerve stimulator by anesthesiologist to determine neuromuscular blockade
- Anticholinesterase to reverse neuromuscular blockade
- By slow IV over 1-2 min (only by qualified persons, usually an anesthesiologist)
- Only fresh sol

Perform/provide:
- Storage at room temp; do not freeze
- Reassurance if communication is difficult during recovery from neuromuscular blockade
- Frequent (q2h) instillation of artificial tears and covering eyes to prevent drying of cornea

Evaluate:
- Therapeutic response: paralysis of jaw, eyelid, head, neck, rest of body

Treatment of overdose: Neostigmine, monitor VS; may require mechanical ventilation

---

molindone (℞)

(moe-lin′done)

Moban

Func. class.: Antipsychotic/neuroleptic

Chem. class.: Dihydroindolone

Action: Depresses cerebral cortex, hypothalamus, limbic system, which control activity, aggression; blocks neurotransmission produced by dopamine at synapse; exhibits strong α-adrenergic, anticholinergic blocking action; mechanism for antipsychotic effects is unclear

Uses: Psychotic disorders

Dosage and routes:
- *Adult:* PO 50-75 mg/day increasing to 225 mg/day if needed

Available forms: Tabs 5, 10, 25, 50, 100 mg; conc 20 mg/ml

Side effects/adverse reactions:

RESP: ***Laryngospasm,*** dyspnea, ***respiratory depression***

CNS: EPS: pseudoparkinsonism, akathisia, dystonia, tardive dyskinesia, drowsiness, headache, seizures

HEMA: ***Anemia, leukopenia, leukocytosis, agranulocytosis***

INTEG: Rash, photosensitivity, dermatitis

EENT: Blurred vision, glaucoma

GI: Dry mouth, nausea, vomiting, anorexia, constipation, diarrhea, jaundice, weight gain

GU: Urinary retention, urinary frequency, enuresis, impotence, amenorrhea, gynecomastia

CV: Orthostatic hypotension, hypertension, ***cardiac arrest,*** ECG changes, ***tachycardia***

Contraindications: Hypersensitivity, coma, child

Precautions: Pregnancy (C), lactation, hypertension, hepatic disease, cardiac disease, Parkinson's disease, brain tumor, glaucoma, urinary retention, diabetes mellitus, respiratory disease, prostatic hypertrophy

Pharmacokinetics:

PO: Onset erratic, peak 1½ hr, duration 24-36 hr; metabolized by liver, excreted in urine and feces, may cross placenta, enters breast milk, half-life 1½ hr

Interactions:
- Increased sedation: other CNS depressants

• Increased EPS: other antipsychotics, lithium

Lab test interferences:

Alterations in: BUN, RBC, serum glucose, WBC

Increase: Serum prolactin levels

NURSING CONSIDERATIONS

Assess:

• Mental status before initial administration

• Swallowing of PO medication; check for hoarding or giving of medication to other patients

• I&O ratio; palpate bladder if low urinary output occurs

• Bilirubin, CBC, liver function studies qmo

• Urinalysis is recommended before, during prolonged therapy

• Affect, orientation, LOC, reflexes, gait, coordination, sleep pattern disturbances

• B/P standing and lying; also include pulse, respirations; take these q4h during initial treatment; establish baseline before starting treatment; report drops of 30 mm Hg, watch for ECG changes

• Dizziness, faintness, palpitations, tachycardia on rising

• EPS including akathisia (inability to sit still, no pattern to movements), tardive dyskinesia (bizarre movements of the jaw, mouth, tongue, extremities), pseudoparkinsonism (rigidity, tremors, pill rolling, shuffling gait)

• For neuroleptic malignant syndrome: hyperthermia, increased CPK, altered mental status, muscle rigidity

• Skin turgor daily

• Constipation, urinary retention daily; if these occur, increase bulk and water in diet

Administer:

• Reduced dose in elderly

• Antiparkinsonian agent, after securing order from prescriber for EPS

• Concentrate mixed in orange or grapefruit juice

Perform/provide:

• Decreased sensory input by dimming lights, avoiding loud noises

• Supervised ambulation until stabilized on medication; do not involve in strenuous exercise program because fainting is possible; patient should not stand still for a long time

• Increased fluids to prevent constipation

• Sips of water, candy, gum for dry mouth

• Storage in air-tight, light-resistant container

Evaluate:

• Therapeutic response: decrease in emotional excitement, hallucinations, delusions, paranoia, reorganization of patterns of thought, speech

Teach patient/family:

• That orthostatic hypotension may occur and to rise from sitting or lying position gradually

• To avoid hot tubs, hot showers, tub baths; hypotension may occur

• To avoid abrupt withdrawal of this drug, or EPS may result; drug should be withdrawn slowly

• To avoid OTC preparations (cough, hay fever, cold) unless approved by prescriber, since serious drug interactions may occur; avoid use with alcohol, CNS depressants; increased drowsiness may occur

• To avoid hazardous activities if drowsiness or dizziness occurs

• To use sunscreen during sun exposure to prevent burns

• Regarding compliance with drug regimen

• About necessity for meticulous oral hygiene, since oral candidiasis may occur

* Available in Canada only

• To report impaired vision, jaundice, tremors, muscle twitching
• In hot weather, that heat stroke may occur; take extra precautions to stay cool

Treatment of overdose: Lavage if orally ingested; provide an airway; *do not induce vomiting*

---

moricizine (℞)

(more-i'siz-een)

Ethmozine

Func. class.: Antidysrhythmic, group I

Chem. class.: Phenothiazine

Action: Decreased rate of rise of action potential, prolonging refractory period and shortening the action potential duration; depression of inward influx if sodium mediates the effects; drug may slow atrial and AV nodal conduction

Uses: Symptomatic vertricular and life-threatening dysrhythmias

Dosage and routes:

• *Adult:* PO 10-15 mg/kg/day or 600-900 mg/day in 2-3 divided doses

Available forms: Film-coated tabs 200, 250, 300 mg

Side effects/adverse reactions:

GI: Nausea, abdominal pain, vomiting, diarrhea

CNS: Diziness, headache, fatigue, perioral numbness, euphoria, nervousness, sleep disorders, depression, tinnitus, fatigue

RESP: Dyspnea, hyperventilation, ***apnea,*** asthma, pharyngitis, cough

GU: Sexual dysfunction, difficult urination, dysuria, incontinence

CV: Palpitations, chest pain, ***CHF,*** hypertension, syncope, dysrthmias, bradycardia, ***MI, thrombophlebitis***

MISC: Sweating, musculoskeletal pain

Contraindications: 2nd or 3rd degree AV block, right bundle branch block, cardiogenic shock, hypersensitivity

Precautions: CHF, hypokalemia, hyperkalemia, sick sinus syndrome, pregnancy (B), lactation, children, impaired hepatic and renal function, cardiac dysfunction

Pharmacokinetics: Half-life 1.5-3.5 hr; peak 0.5-2.2 hr; metabolized by the liver; metabolites excreted in feces and urine, protein binding >90%

Interactions:

• Increased plasma levels of moricizine: amantadine
• Digoxin or propranolol may enhance some of cardiac effects of moricizine; moricizine may decrease effects of theophylline

Lab test interferences:

Increase: CPK

NURSING CONSIDERATIONS

Assess:

• GI status: bowel pattern, number of stools
• Cardiac status: rate, rhythm, quality
• Chest x-ray, pulmonary function test during treatment
• I&O ratio; check for decreasing output
• B/P for fluctuations
• Lung fields: bilateral rales may occur in CHF patient
• Increased respiration, increased pulse; drug should be discontinued
• Toxicity: fine tremors, dizziness
• Cardiac rate: respiration, rate, rhythm, character continuously

Evaluate:

• Therapeutic response: absence of dysrhythmias

Teach patient/family:

• To report side effects to prescriber

Treatment of overdose: O_2 artificial ventilation, ECG; administer dopamine for circulatory depression,

M

diazepam or thiopental for convulsions

morphine (℞)

(mor'feen)

Astramorph PF, Duramorph, Epimorph*, Infumorph 200, Infumorph 500, morphine sulfate, Morphitec*, M.O.S.*, M.O.S.-S.R.*, MS Contin, OMS Concentrate, Oramorph SR, RMS, Roxanol, Roxanol 100, Roxanol Rescudose, Roxanol SR

Func. class.: Narcotic analgesic

Chem. class.: Opiate

Combination products: Morphine, Atropine Sulfate Injection: morphine sulfate 16 mg/ml with atropine sulfate 0.4 mg/ml

Controlled Substance Schedule II

Action: Depresses pain impulse transmission at the spinal cord level by interacting with opioid receptors

Uses: Severe pain

Dosage and routes:

• *Adult:* SC/IM 4-15 mg q4h prn; PO 10-30 mg q4h prn; EXT REL q8-12h; REC 10-20 mg q4h prn; IV 4-10 mg diluted in 4-5 ml H_2O for injection, over 5 min

• *Child:* SC 0.1-0.2 mg/kg, not to exceed 15 mg

Available forms: Inj 2, 4, 5, 8, 10, 15 mg/ml; sol tabs 10, 15, 30 mg; oral sol 10, 20 mg/5 ml, 20 mg/10 ml, 20 mg/ml; oral tabs 15, 30 mg; rec supp 5, 10, 20 mg; ext rel tabs 30 mg

Side effects/adverse reactions:

CNS: Drowsiness, dizziness, confusion, headache, sedation, euphoria

CV: Palpitations, bradycardia, change in B/P

EENT: Tinnitus, blurred vision, miosis, diplopia

GI: Nausea, vomiting, anorexia, constipation, cramps, biliary tract pressure

GU: Urinary retention

INTEG: Rash, urticaria, bruising, flushing, diaphoresis, pruritus

RESP: ***Respiratory depression***

Contraindications: Hypersensitivity, addiction (narcotic), hemorrhage, bronchial asthma, increased intracranial pressure

Precautions: Addictive personality, pregnancy (B), lactation, acute MI, severe heart disease, elderly, respiratory depression, hepatic disease, renal disease, child <18 yr

Pharmacokinetics:

PO: Onset variable, peak variable, duration variable

IM: Onset ½ hr peak, ½-1 hr, duration 4-5 hr

SC: Onset 15-20 min, peak 50-90 min, duration 3-5 hr

IV: Peak 20 min

RECT: Peak ½-1 hr, duration 4-5 hr

Intrathecal: Onset rapid, duration up to 24 hr

Metabolized by liver, crosses placenta, excreted in urine, breast milk, half-life 2½-3 hr

Interactions:

• Increased effects with other CNS depressants: alcohol, narcotics, sedative/hypnotics, antipsychotics, skeletal muscle relaxants

Syringe compatibilities: Atropine, benzquinamide, butorphanol, chlorpromazine, cimetidine, dimenhydrinate, diphenhydramine, droperidol, fentanyl, glycopyrrolate, hydroxyzine, metoclopramide, midazolam, perphenazine, promazine, ranitidine, scopolamine

Y-site compatibilities: Acyclovir, aldesleukin, amikacin, aminophylline, ampicillin, ampicillin/sulbactam, atracurium, calcium chloride, cefamandole, cefazolin, cefoperazone, ceforanide, cefotaxime, ce-

* Available in Canada only

fotetan, cefoxitin, ceftizoxime, cefuroxime, cephalothin, cephapirin, chloramphenicol, clindamycin, cotrimoxazole, doxycycline, enalaprilat, erythromycin lactobionate, esmolol, famotidine, foscarnet, gentamicin, heparin, hydrocortisone sodium succinate, insulin, kanamycin, labetalol, magnesium sulfate, melphalan, metronidazole, mezlocillin, moxalactam, nafcillin, ondansetron, oxacillin, oxytocin, paclitaxel, pancuronium, penicillin G potassium, piperacillin, potassium chloride, ranitidine, sodium bicarbonate, ticarcillin, ticarcillin/clavulanate, tobramycin, vancomycin, vecuronium, vinorelbine, vitamin B with C, zidovadine

Additive compatibilities: Dobutamine, succinylcholine, verapamil

Lab test interferences:
Increase: Amylase

NURSING CONSIDERATIONS

Assess:

- Pain: location, type, character; give dose before pain becomes severe
- Bowel status; constipation frequent
- I&O ratio; check for decreasing output; may indicate urinary retention
- B/P, pulse, respirations (character, depth, rate)
- CNS changes: dizziness, drowsiness, hallucinations, euphoria, LOC, pupil reaction
- Allergic reactions: rash, urticaria
- Respiratory dysfunction: depression, character, rate, rhythm; notify prescriber if respirations are <12/min

Administer:

- IV after diluting with 5 ml or more sterile H_2O or NS; give 15 mg or less over 4-5 min; give through Y-tube or 3-way stopcock; may be added to IV sol, each 0.1-1 mg diluted in 1 ml D_5W, $D_{10}W$, 0.9% NaCl, 0.45% NaCl, Ringers, LR, given with inf pump titrated to patient response
- With antiemetic for nausea, vomiting
- When pain is beginning to return; determine dosage interval by response; continuous dosing is more effective than prn
- May be given by patient: controlled analgesia

Perform/provide:

- Storage in light-resistant container at room temp
- Assistance with ambulation
- Safety measures: side rails, nightlight, call bell within easy reach
- Gradual withdrawal after long-term use

Evaluate:

- Therapeutic response; decrease in pain intensity

Teach patient/family:

- To change position slowly; orthostatic hypotension may occur
- To report any symptoms of CNS changes, allergic reactions
- That physical dependency may result from long-term use
- To avoid use of alcohol, CNS depressants
- That withdrawal symptoms may occur: nausea, vomiting, cramps, fever, faintness, anorexia

Treatment of overdose: Naloxone (Narcan) 0.2-0.8 mg IV, O_2, IV fluids, vasopressors

moxalactam (℞)

(mox'a-lak-tam)
Moxam

Func. class.: Antibiotic, broad-spectrum
Chem. class.: Cephalosporin (3rd generation)

Action: Inhibits bacterial cell wall synthesis, rendering cell wall osmotically unstable and leading to cell death

Uses: Gram-negative organisms: *H. influenzae, E. coli, P. mirabilis, Klebsiella, Citrobacter, Salmonella, Shigella, Serratia;* gram-positive organisms: *S. pneumoniae, S. pyogenes, S. aureus;* serious lower respiratory tract, urinary tract, skin, bone infections, septicemia, meningitis, intraabdominal infections

Dosage and routes:

• *Adult:* IM/IV 2-4 g q8-12h

Mild infections

• *Adult:* IM/IV 250-500 mg q8-12h

Severe infections

• *Adult:* IM/IV 2-6 g q8h

• *Child:* IM/IV 50 mg/kg q6-8h

• Dosage reduction indicated even for mild renal impairment (CrCl <80 ml/min)

Available forms: Powder for inj 1, 2, 10 g

Side effects/adverse reactions:

CNS: Headache, dizziness, weakness, paresthesia, fever, chills

GI: Nausea, vomiting, diarrhea, anorexia, pain, glossitis, bleeding, increased AST (SGOT), ALT (SGPT), bilirubin, LDH, alk phosphatase, abdominal pain

GU: ***Proteinuria,*** vaginitis, pruritus, candidiasis, increased BUN, ***nephrotoxicity, renal failure***

HEMA: ***Leukopenia, thrombocytopenia, agranulocytosis, anemia, neutropenia, lymphocytosis, eosinophilia, pancytopenia, hemolytic anemia, bleeding, hypoprothrombinemia***

INTEG: Rash, urticaria, dermatitis, ***anaphylaxis***

RESP: Dyspnea

Contraindications: Hypersensitivity to cephalosporins

Precautions: Hypersensitivity to penicillins, pregnancy (C), lactation, renal disease

Pharmacokinetics:

IV: Peak 5 min

IM: Peak ½-2 hr

Half-life 1½-2½ hr, 25% bound by plasma proteins; 60%-97% eliminated unchanged in urine in 24 hr; crosses placenta, blood-brain barrier; excreted in breast milk; not metabolized

Interactions:

• Incompatible with tetracyclines, erythromycins, aminoglycosides in same parenteral fluid

• Decreased effects of tetracyclines, erythromycins

• Increased toxicity: aminoglycosides, furosemide, probenecid, sulfinpyrazone, colistin, ethacrynic acid, vancomycin, agents affecting platelet function

• Disulfiram reaction: ethanol

Lab test interferences:

Increase (false): Urinary 17-KS

False positive: Urinary protein, direct Coombs' test, urine glucose

Interference: Crossmatching

NURSING CONSIDERATIONS

Assess:

• Nephrotoxicity: increased BUN, creatinine

• I&O daily

• Blood studies: AST (SGOT), ALT (SGPT), CBC, Hct, bilirubin, LDH, alk phosphatase, Coombs' test, protime qmo if patient is on long-term therapy

• Electrolytes: K, Na, Cl qmo during long-term therapy

• Bowel pattern qd; if severe diarrhea occurs, drug should be discontinued; may indicate pseudomembranous colitis

• IV site for extravasation, phlebitis; change site q72h

• Urine output: if decreasing, notify prescriber; may indicate nephrotoxicity

• Allergic reactions: rash, urticaria, pruritus, chills, fever, joint pain, an-

---

gioedema; may occur few days after therapy begins
• Bleeding: ecchymosis, bleeding gums, hematuria, stool guaiac daily
• Overgrowth of infection: perineal itching, fever, malaise, redness, pain, swelling, drainage, rash, diarrhea, change in cough, sputum

Administer:

• For 10-14 days to ensure organism death, prevent superinfection
• IV after diluting 1 g/10 ml sterile H_2O, D_5, 0.9% NaCl; give through Y-tube over 3-5 min; may be further diluted 1 g/20 ml in D_5, 0.9% NaCl, give over ½ hr; may be added 500-1000, give over 6-24 hr
• Vit K for bleeding (10 mg/wk)
• After C&S

Evaluate:

• Therapeutic response: decreased fever, malaise, chills

Teach patient/family:

• To report sore throat, bruising, bleeding, joint pain; may indicate blood dyscrasias (rare)
• Not to drink alcohol while taking this drug

Treatment of overdose: Epinephrine, antihistamines; resuscitate if needed (anaphylaxis)

multivitamins (OTC, ℞)

Adavite, Dayalets, LKV Drops, Multi-75, Multiday, One-A-Day, Optilets, Poly-Vi-sol, Quin tabs, Ru-Lets, Sesame Street Vitamins, Tab-A-Vite, Therabid, Theragram, Unicaps, Vita-Bob, Vita-Kid, many other brands

Func. class.: Vitamins, multiple

Action: Needed for adequate metabolism

Uses: Prevention and treatment of vitamin deficiencies

Dosage and routes:

• *Adult and child:* PO/IV—depends on brand

Available forms: Many

Side effects/adverse reactions: None known at recommended dosage

Precautions: Pregnancy (A)

Y-site compatibilities: Acyclovir, ampicillin, carbenicillin, cefazolin, cephalothin, cephapirin, erythromycin lactobionate, fludarabine, gentamicin, tetracycline

Additive compatibilities: Cefoxitin, isoproterenol, methyldopate, metoclopramide, metronidazole, netilmicin, norepinephrine, sodium bicarbonate, verapamil

NURSING CONSIDERATIONS

Assess:

• Vitamin deficiency: usually more than one vitamin is deficient

Administer:

• Liquid multivitamins diluted or dropped into patient's mouth using dropper provided with some brands
• Chew tabs should be chewed, not swallowed whole
• Give by cont IV inf only after diluting 5-10 ml multivitamins/500-1000 ml of D_5W, $D_{10}W$, $D_{20}W$, LR, D_5/LR, D_5/0.9% NaCl, 0.9% NaCl, 3% NaCl
• Do not use sol with crystals, precipate, or color other than bright yellow

Evaluate:

• Therapeutic response: check each individual vitamin for guidelines

Teach patient/family:

• That adequate nutrition must be maintained to prevent further deficiencies
• Drug interaction that should be avoided
• To comply with regimen

M

• To avoid presenting flavored multivitamins as candy; child may overdose
• To store out of children's reach

mupirocin (℞)

(myoo-peer'oh-sin)
Bactroban, Pseudomonic Acid A
Func. class.: Topical antinfective
Chem. class.: Pseudomonic acid A

Action: Inhibits bacterial protein synthesis, shows no cross-resistance to most antibiotics
Uses: Impetigo caused by *S. aureus,* β-hemolytic *Streptococcus, S. pyogenes,* decreased carrier state of *S. aureus*
Dosage and routes:
Adult: TOP apply small amount to affected area tid; NASAL up to qid
Available forms: Oint 2% (20 mg/g); nasal
Side effects/adverse reactions:
INTEG: Burning, stinging, itching, rash, dry skin, swelling, contact dermatitis, erythema, tenderness, increased exudate
Contraindications: Hypersensitivity
Precautions: Pregnancy (B), lactation
NURSING CONSIDERATIONS
Assess:
• Affected area for continuing infection: increased size, number of lesions
Administer:
• Then cover with 2 × 2 in gauze if needed
Perform/provide:
• Storage at room temp
• Isolation (wound) for hospitalized child (2-5 days)
• Washing of hands after applying ointment
Evaluate:
• Therapeutic response: reduction in size, number of lesions
Teach patient/family:
• To wash hands after applying ointment
• To trim fingernails to prevent scratching
• To report irritation, worsening of rash, itching, pain at site; if no improvement within 3-5 days, report to prescriber

muromonab-CD3 (℞)

(mur-oo-mone'ab)
Orthoclone OKT3
Func. class.: Immunosuppressive
Chem. class.: Murine monoclonal antibody

Action: Reverses graft rejection by blocking T-cell function
Uses: Acute allograft rejection in renal, cardiac/hepatic transplant patients
Dosage and routes:
• *Adult:* IV BOL 5 mg/day × 10-14 days; usually methylprednisolone Na succinate, 1 mg/kg IV is given before muromonab-CD3, 100 mg IV hydrocortisone Na succinate is given ½ hr after muromonab-CD3
Child: IV 100 μg/kg/day × 10-14 days
Cardiac/hepatic allograft rejection, steroid resistant
• *Adult:* IV BOL 5 mg/day × 10-14 days; begin when it is known that rejection has not been reversed by steroids
Available forms: Inj 5 mg/5 ml
Side effects/adverse reactions:
CNS: Pyrexia, chills, tremors

* Available in Canada only

RESP: Dyspnea, wheezing, ***pulmonary edema***
CV: Chest pain
GI: Vomiting, nausea, diarrhea
MISC: Infection
Contraindications: Hypersensitivity to murine origin, fluid overload
Precautions: Pregnancy (C), child <2 yr, fever
Pharmacokinetics:
Trough level steady state 3-14 days
Interactions:
• Incompatible with any drug in syringe or sol

NURSING CONSIDERATIONS
Assess:
• For cytokine release syndrome (CRS): nausea, vomiting, chills, fever, joint pain, weakness, dizziness, diarrhea, tremors, abdominal pain
• For hypersensitivity: dyspnea, bronchospasm, urticaria, tachycardia, angioedema; emergency equipment must be available
• Blood studies: Hgb, WBC, platelets during treatment qmo; if leukocytes are <3000/mm^3, drug should be discontinued
• Liver function studies: alk phosphatase, AST (SGOT), ALT (SGPT), bilirubin
• Hepatotoxicity: dark urine, jaundice, itching, light-colored stools; drug should be discontinued
Administer:
• IV undiluted; withdraw with a 0.2-0.22 low protein-binding μm filter, discard and use new needle for administration; give over 1 min
• For several days before transplant surgery
• All medications PO if possible; avoid IM injection, since infection may occur
Evaluate:
• Therapeutic response: absence of graft rejection
Teach patient/family:
• To report fever, chills, sore throat, fatigue, since serious infection may occur
• To use contraceptive measures during treatment, for 12 wk after ending therapy; possible mutagenic effects

nabumetone (℞)
(na-byoo′me-tone)
Relafen
Func. class.: Nonsteroidal antiinflammatory
Chem. class.: Acetic acid derivative

Action: May inhibit prostaglandin synthesis by decreasing enzyme needed for biosynthesis; analgesic, antiinflammatory, antipyretic
Uses: Osteoarthritis, rheumatoid arthritis, acute or chronic treatment
Dosage and routes:
• *Adult:* PO 1 g as a single dose; may increase to 1.5-2 g/day if needed; may give qd or bid as a divided dose
Available forms: Tabs 500, 750 mg
Side effects/adverse reactions:
CNS: Dizziness, headache, drowsiness, fatigue, tremors, confusion, insomnia, anxiety, depression, nervousness
GU: ***Nephrotoxicity, dysuria, hematuria, oliguria, azotemia,*** cystitis
GI: Nausea, anorexia, vomiting, diarrhea, jaundice, ***cholestatic hepatitis,*** constipation, flatulence, cramps, dry mouth, peptic ulcer, gastritis, ***ulceration, perforation***
CV: Tachycardia, peripheral edema, palpitations, dysrhythmias, ***CHF***
INTEG: Purpura, rash, pruritus, sweating, photosensitivity
HEMA: ***Blood dyscrasias***

N

EENT: Tinnitus, hearing loss, blurred vision
RESP: Dyspnea, pharyngitis, ***bronchospasm***
Contraindications: Hypersensitivity to this drug or aspirin, iodides, NSAIDs, asthma, severe renal disease, severe hepatic disease
Precautions: Pregnancy (B) 1st and 2nd trimester, lactation, children, bleeding disorders, GI disorders, cardiac disorders, renal disorders, hepatic dysfunction, elderly
Pharmacokinetics:
PO: Peak 2½-4 hr, plasma protein binding >90%, half-life 22-30 hr; metabolized in liver to active metabolite; excreted in urine (metabolites), breast milk
Interactions:
- May increase action or toxicity of coumarin, cyclosporine, phenytoin, methotrexate, probenecid
- May decrease effects of nabumetone; salicylates

NURSING CONSIDERATIONS
Assess:
- Renal, liver, blood studies: BUN, creatinine, AST (SGOT), ALT (SGPT), Hgb, before treatment, periodically thereafter
- Audiometric, ophthalmic exam before, during, after treatment
- For eye, ear problems: blurred vision, tinnitus; may indicate toxicity

Administer:
- With food for GI symptoms
- Avoid alcoholic beverages and aspirin

Perform/provide:
- Storage at room temp

Evaluate:
- Therapeutic response: decreased pain and stiffness in joints

Teach patient/family:
- To report blurred vision, ringing, roaring in ears; may indicate toxicity
- To avoid driving, other hazardous activities if dizziness, drowsiness occur
- To report change in urine pattern, increased weight, edema, increased pains in joints, fever, blood in urine; indicates nephrotoxicity
- That therapeutic effects may take up to 1 mo
- To take with a full glass of water to enhance absorption
- To report dark stools; may indicate GI bleeding

---

nadolol (℞)
(nay-doe′lole)
Corgard
Func. class.: Antihypertensive, antianginal
Chem. class.: β-Adrenergic receptor blocker

Action: Long-acting, nonselective β-adrenergic receptor blocking agent; mechanism is similar to that of propranolol
Uses: Chronic stable angina pectoris, mild to moderate hypertension, prophylaxis of migraine headaches
Investigational uses: Tachyarrhythmias, aggression, anxiety, tremors, esophageal varices (rebleeding only)
Dosage and routes:
- *Adult:* PO 40 mg qd, increase by 40-80 mg q3-7d; maintenance 40-240 mg/day for angina, 40-320 mg/day for hypertension

Available forms: Tabs 20, 40, 80, 120, 160 mg
Side effects/adverse reactions:
RESP: Dyspnea, respiratory dysfunction, ***bronchospasm,*** cough, wheezing, nasal stuffiness, pharyngitis, ***laryngospasm***
CV: Bradycardia, hypotension, ***CHF,*** palpitations, ***AV block,*** chest pain, peripheral ischemia, flushing,

edema, vasodilation, conduction disturbances
HEMA: ***Agranulocytosis, thrombocytopenia***
GI: Nausea, vomiting, diarrhea, colitis, constipation, cramps, dry mouth, flatulence, hepatomegaly, ***pancreatitis,*** taste distortion
INTEG: Rash, pruritus, fever
CNS: Depression, hallucinations, dizziness, fatigue, lethargy, paresthesias, headache
EENT: Sore throat
Contraindications: Hypersensitivity to this drug, cardiac failure, cardiogenic shock, 2nd or 3rd degree heart block, bronchospastic disease, sinus bradycardia, CHF, COPD
Precautions: Diabetes mellitus, pregnancy (C), renal disease, lactation, hyperthyroidism, peripheral vascular disease, myasthenia gravis
Pharmacokinetics:
PO: Onset variable, peak 3-4 hr, duration 17-24 hr; half-life 16-20 hr; not metabolized; excreted in urine (unchanged), bile, breast milk
Interactions:
• Increased effects of reserpine, digitalis, ergots, neuromuscular blocking agents, calcium channel blockers
• Increased hypotensive effects: other hypotensive agents, diuretics, phenothiazines
• Decreased effects of norepinephrine, xanthines, isoproterenol, thyroid
Lab test interferences:
Increase: Serum K, serum uric acid, ALT (SGPT)/AST (SGOT), alk phosphatase, LDH, blood glucose, cholesterol
NURSING CONSIDERATIONS
Assess:
• B/P, pulse, respirations during beginning therapy
• Weight qd; report gain of 5 lb
• I&O ratio, CrCl if kidney damage is diagnosed
• Qd, note need to be administered more often
• Pain: duration, time started, activity being performed, character
• Tolerance if taken over long time
• Headache, light-headedness, decreased B/P; may indicate a need for decreased dosage
Administer:
• With 8 oz water
Evaluate:
• Therapeutic response: decreased B/P, symptoms of angina
Teach patient/family:
• That drug may mask signs of hypoglycemia or alter blood glucose in diabetics
• Not to discontinue abruptly
• To avoid OTC drugs unless prescriber approves
• To avoid hazardous activities if dizziness occurs
• To comply with complete medical regimen

nafarelin (℞)

(naf-aa-ree′lin)
Synarel
Func. class.: Gonadotropin
Chem. class.: Analog of gonadotropin-releasing hormone

Action: Stimulates the release of LH and FSH, which increases ovarian steroid production; repeated dosing prevents stimulation of the pituitary gland
Uses: Endometriosis, gonadotropin-dependent precocious puberty
Doses and routes:
• *Adult:* NASAL 400 μg/day as one spray (200 μg) into one nostril in morning and one spray into other nostril in evening; start treatment between days 2 and 4 of menstrual

cycle; may increase to 800 μg/day (one spray into each nostril twice a day); recommended duration of treatment is 6 mo

Available forms: Nasal sol 2 mg/ml

Side effects/adverse reactions:

GU: Decreased libido, vaginal dryness, breast tenderness, increased pubic hair

CNS: Headache, flushing, depression, insomnia, emotional lability, hot flashes

INTEG: Nasal irritation, acne

MISC: Body odor, seborrhea, rhinitis

SENSITIVITY: Shortness of breath, chest pain, urticaria, pruitis

Contraindications: Hypersensitivity, pregnancy (X), lactation, undiagnosed abnormal vaginal bleeding

Precautions: Children

Pharmacokinetics: Rapidly absorbed, peak 10-40 min, half-life 3 hr; 80% bound to plasma proteins

NURSING CONSIDERATIONS

Assess:

- Test results: pituitary/hypothalamus dysfunction (decreased LH); postmenopausal (increased LH)

Administer:

- Repeated doses may be necessary to elevate pituitary gonadotropin reserve

Perform/provide:

- Storage at room temp; protect from light

Evaluate:

- Therapeutic response: decreased symptoms of endometriosis

Teach patient/family

- To use nonhormonal contraception
- On nasal use, one spray in right nostril AM, one in left nostril PM
- Medication may cause hot flashes, decreased libido, vaginal dryness

nafcillin (℞)

(naf-sill'-in)

Nafcil, nafcillin sodium, Nallpen, Unipen

Func. class.: Broad-spectrum antibiotic

Chem. class.: Penicillinase-resistant penicillin

Action: Interferes with cell wall replication of susceptible organisms; osmotically unstable cell wall swells, bursts from osmotic pressure

Uses: Effective for gram-positive cocci *(S. aureus, S. viridans, S. pneumoniae),* infections caused by penicillinase-producing *Staphylococcus*

Dosage and routes:

- *Adult:* IM/IV 2-6 g/day in divided doses q4-6h; PO 2-6 g/day in divided doses q4-6h
- *Child:* IM 25 mg/kg q12h; PO 25-50 mg/kg/day in divided doses q6h
- *Neonates:* IM 10 mg/kg bid

Available forms: Caps 250 mg; tabs 500 mg; powder for oral susp 250 mg/5 ml; powder for inj 500 mg, 1, 2, 10 g; IV 1, 1.5, 2, 4 g

Side effects/adverse reactions:

HEMA: Anemia, increased bleeding time, ***bone marrow depression, granulocytopenia***

GI: Nausea, vomiting, diarrhea, increased AST (SGOT), ALT (SGPT), abdominal pain, glossitis, ***pseudomembranous colitis***

GU: Oliguria, ***proteinuria, hematuria,*** *vaginitis, moniliasis,* ***glomerulonephritis***, interstitial nephritis

CNS: Lethargy, hallucinations, anxiety, depression, twitching, ***coma, convulsions***

Contraindications: Hypersensitivity to penicillins

Precautions: Pregnancy (B), hypersensitivity to cephalosporins, neonates

Pharmacokinetics:

IM/PO: Peak 30-60 min, duration 4-6 hr, half-life 1 hr, metabolized by the liver, excreted in bile, urine

Interactions:

- Decreased antimicrobial effect of nafcillin: tetracyclines, erythromycins
- Increased nafcillin concentrations: aspirin, probenecid

Syringe compatibilities: Cimetidine, heparin

Y-site compatibilities: Acyclovir, atropine, cyclophosphamide, diazepam, enalaprilat, esmolol, famotidine, fentanyl, fluconazole, foscarnet, hydromorphone, magnesium sulfate, morphine perphenazine, zidovudine

Additive compatibilities: Chloramphenicol, chlorothiazide, dexamethasone, diphenhydramine, ephedrine, heparin, hydroxyzine, potassium chloride, prochlorperazine, sodium bicarbonate, sodium lactate

Lab test interferences:

False positive: Urine glucose, urine protein

NURSING CONSIDERATIONS

Assess:

- I&O ratio; report hematuria, oliguria, since penicillin in high doses is nephrotoxic
- Any patient with compromised renal system, since drug is excreted slowly in poor renal system function; toxicity may occur rapidly
- Liver studies: AST (SGOT), ALT (SGPT)
- Blood studies: WBC, RBC, H&H, bleeding time
- Renal studies: urinalysis, protein, blood
- C&S before drug therapy; drug may be given as soon as culture is taken
- Bowel pattern before and during treatment
- Skin eruptions after administration of penicillin to 1 wk after discontinuing drug
- Respiratory status: rate, character, wheezing, and tightness in chest
- Allergies before initiation of treatment and reaction of each medication; highlight allergies on chart, Kardex
- Differential WBC in patients on long-term therapy

Administer:

- IV after diluting 500 mg/1.7 ml of sterile H_2O for inj; further dilute each 500 mg/15-30 ml sterile water or NS sol; give through Y-tube or stopcock 500 mg or less/5-10 min; may be further diluted and run over 24 hr
- IM give deep IM in gluteal muscle
- Drug after C&S has been completed
- Divided oral doses on empty stomach before meals; oral absorption is erratic

Perform/provide:

- Adrenalin, suction, tracheostomy set, endotracheal intubation equipment
- Adequate fluid intake (2 L) during diarrhea episodes
- Scratch test to assess allergy after securing order from prescriber; usually done when penicillin is only drug of choice
- Storage in tight container; refrigerate reconstituted sol

Evaluate:

- Therapeutic response: absence of fever, draining wounds

Teach patient/family:

- Aspects of drug therapy, including need to complete course of medication to ensure organism death (10-14 days); culture may be taken after completed course

N

• To report sore throat, fever, fatigue (may indicate superinfection)
• To wear or carry Medic Alert ID if allergic to penicillins
• To notify nurse of diarrhea

Treatment of anaphylaxis: Withdraw drug; maintain airway; administer epinephrine, aminophylline, O_2, IV corticosteroids

naftifine (℞)

(naf'tee-fin)

Naftin

Func. class.: Topical antifungal

Chem. class.: Synthetic allylamine derivative

Action: Interferes with cell membrane permeability in fungi such as *T. rubrum, T. mentagrophytes, T. tonsurans, E. floccosum, M. canis, M. audouinii, M. gypesum, Candida;* broad-spectrum antifungal

Uses: Tinea cruris, tinea corporis, tinea versicolor

Dosage and routes:
• *Adult:* TOP massage into affected and surrounding area bid (gel); qd (cream) × 7-14 days

Available forms: Cream, gel 1%

Side effects/adverse reactions:
INTEG: Burning, stinging, dryness, itching, local irritation

Contraindications: Hypersensitivity

Precautions: Pregnancy (B), lactation, children

NUSING CONSIDERATIONS

Assess:
• Fon continuing infection: increased size, number of lesions

Administer:
• To affected area, surrounding area; do not cover with occlusive dressings

Perform/provide:
• Storage below 30° C (86° F)

Evaluate:
• Therapeutic response: decrease in size, number of lesions

Teach patient/family:
• To wear cotton clothing
• To use clean towel, dry well
• To avoid contact with mucous membranes
• Not to cover area unless directed by prescriber
• To report excessive itching, burning
• How to apply; massage gel into affected area and surrounding skin in AM, PM, cream AM only; effects observed within 1 wk, continue 1-2 wk after symptoms decrease; wash hands after application

nalbuphine (℞)

(nal'byoo-feen)

Nubain, nalbuphine HCl

Func. class.: Narcotic analgesic

Chem. class.: Synthetic narcotic agonist/antagonist

Controlled Substance Schedule II

Action: Depresses pain impulse transmission at the spinal cord level by interacting with opioid receptors

Uses: Moderate to severe pain

Dosage and routes:

Analgesic
• *Adult:* SC/IM/IV 10-20 mg q3-6h prn, not to exceed 160 mg/day

Balanced anesthesia supplement
• *Adult:* IV 0.3-3 mg/kg given over 10-15 min, may give 0.25-0.5 mg/kg as needed maintenance

Available forms: Inj 10, 20 mg/ml

Side effects/adverse reactions:
CNS: Drowsiness, dizziness, confusion, headache, sedation, euphoria, dysphoria (high doses), hallucinations, dreaming, tolerance, physical, psychological dependency

GI: Nausea, vomiting, anorexia, constipation, cramps
GU: Increased urinary output, dysuria, urinary retention, urgency
INTEG: Rash, urticaria, bruising, flushing, diaphoresis, pruritus
EENT: Tinnitus, blurred vision, miosis, diplopia
CV: Palpitations, bradycardia, change in B/P, orthostatic hypotension
*RESP: **Respiratory depression***

Contraindications: Hypersensitivity, addiction (narcotic)

Precautions: Addictive personality, pregnancy (C), lactation, increased intracranial pressure, MI (acute), severe heart disease, respiratory depression, hepatic disease, renal disease

Pharmacokinetics:
SC/IM/IV: Duration 3-6 hr; metabolized by liver, excreted by kidneys, half-life 5 hr

Interactions:
• Increased effects with other CNS depressants: alcohol, narcotics, sedative/hypnotics, antipsychotics, skeletal muscle relaxants

Y-site compatibilities: Fludarabine, melphalan, paclitaxel, vinorelbine

Syringe compatibilities: Atropine, cimetidine, droperidol, hydroxyzine, lidocaine, midazolam, prochlorperazine, promethazine, ranitidine, scopolamine, trimethobenzamide

Lab test interferences:
Increase: Amylase

NURSING CONSIDERATIONS

Assess:
• I&O ratio; check for decreasing output; may indicate urinary retention
• For withdrawal reactions in narcotic-dependent individuals: pulmonary embolus, vascular occlusion; abscesses, ulcerations, nausea, vomiting, convulsions
• CNS changes: dizziness, drowsiness, hallucinations, euphoria, LOC, pupil reaction
• Allergic reactions: rash, urticaria
• Respiratory dysfunction: respiratory depression, character, rate, rhythm; notify prescriber if respirations are <10/min
• Need for pain medication by pain sedation scoring, physical dependency

Administer:
• IV undiluted 10 mg or less over 3-5 min
• With antiemetic if nausea, vomiting occur
• When pain is beginning to return; determine dosage interval by response
• IM deep in large muscle mass, rotate injection sites

Perform/provide:
• Storage in light-resistant area at room temp
• Assistance with ambulation
• Safety measures: side rails, nightlight, call bell within easy reach

Evaluate:
• Therapeutic response: decrease in pain

Teach patient/family:
• To report any symptoms of CNS changes, allergic reactions
• That physical dependency may result from long-term use
• Withdrawal symptoms may occur: nausea, vomiting, cramps, fever, faintness, anorexia

Treatment of overdose: Naloxone (Narcan) 0.2-0.8 mg IV, O_2, IV fluids, vasopressors

N

nalidixic acid (℞)

(nal-i-dix'ik)

NegGram, NegGram Caplets

Func. class.: Urinary tract anti-infective

Chem. class.: Synthetic naphthyridine derivative

Action: Appears to inhibit DNA polymerization, primary target being single-stranded DNA precursors in late stages of chromosomal replication

Uses: UTIs (acute/chronic) caused by *E. coli, Klebsiella, Enterobacter, P. mirabilis, P. vulgaris, P. morganii*

Dosage and routes:

- *Adult:* PO 1 g qid × 1-2 wk, 2 g/day for long-term treatment
- *Child >3 mo:* PO 55 mg/kg/day in 4 divided doses for 1-2 wk; 33 mg/kg/day in 4 divided doses for long-term treatment

Available forms: Tabs 100, 250, 500 mg, 1 g susp 250 mg/5 ml

Side effects/adverse reactions:

INTEG: Pruritus, rash, urticaria, photosensitivity

CNS: Dizziness, headache, drowsiness, insomnia, ***convulsions***

GI: Nausea, vomiting, abdominal pain, diarrhea

EENT: Sensitivity to light, blurred vision, change in color perception

Contraindications: Hypersensitivity, CNS damage, liver disease, liver failure, infants <3 months

Precautions: Elderly, renal disease, hepatic disease, pregnancy (B), lactation

Pharmacokinetics:

PO: Peak 1-2 hr, metabolized in liver, excreted in urine (unchanged/conjugates), crosses placenta, enters breast milk

Interactions:

- Increased effects of oral coagulants
- Decreased effects of antacids

Lab test interferences:

False positive: Urinary glucose

False increase: 17-OHCS, VMA

NURSING CONSIDERATIONS

Assess:

- Blood count for patients on chronic therapy
- I&O ratio; urine pH <5.5 is ideal
- Renal, hepatic function
- Photosensitivity: drug should be discontinued
- CNS symptoms: insomnia, vertigo, headache, drowsiness, convulsions
- Allergy: fever, flushing, rash, urticaria, pruritus

Administer:

- After clean-catch urine for C&S
- Two daily doses if urine output is high or if patient has diabetes

Perform/provide:

- Limited intake of alkaline foods, drugs: milk, dairy products, peanuts, vegetables, alkaline antacids, sodium bicarbonate
- Protection from freezing

Evaluate:

- Therapeutic response: decreased dysuria, negative culture

Teach patient/family:

- That photosensitivity occurs; that patient should avoid sunlight or use sunscreen to prevent burns
- To take medication with food or milk to decrease GI irritation
- To protect suspension from freezing, shake well before taking
- That drug may cause drowsiness; instruct client to seek aid in walking, other activities; advise client not to drive or operate machinery while on medication
- That diabetics should monitor blood glucose

naloxone (℞)

(nal-oks'one)

naloxone HCl, Narcan

Func. class.: Opioid antagonist

Chem. class.: Thebaine derivative

Action: Competes with narcotics at narcotic receptor sites

Uses: Respiratory depression induced by narcotics, pentazocine, propoxyphene; refractory circulatory shock

Dosage and routes:

Narcotic-induced respiratory depression

• *Adult:* IV/SC/IM 0.4-2 mg; repeat q2-3 min if needed

Postoperative respiratory depression

• *Adult:* IV 0.1-0.2 mg q2-3 min prn

• *Child:* IV/IM/SC 0.01 mg/kg q2-3 min prn

Asphyxia neonatorum

• *Neonates:* IV 0.01 mg/kg given into umbilical vein after delivery; may repeat q2-3 min × 3 doses

Available forms: Inj 0.02, 0.4, 1 mg/ml

Side effects/adverse reactions:

CNS: Drowsiness, nervousness

CV: Rapid pulse, increased systolic B/P (high doses), ventricular tachycardia, fibrillation

GI: Nausea, vomiting

RESP: Hyperpnea

Contraindications: Hypersensitivity, respiratory depression

Precautions: Pregnancy (B), children, cardiovascular disease, opioid dependency, lactation

Pharmacokinetics:

Well absorbed IM, SC; metabolized by liver, crosses placenta, excreted in urine, breast milk, half-life 1 hr

IV: Onset 1 min, duration 45 min

IM/SC: Onset 2-5 min, duration 45-60 min

Interactions:

• Incompatible with alkaline drugs, bisulfites, sulfites

Lab test interferences:

Interferences: Urine VMA, 5-HIAA, urine glucose

NURSING CONSIDERATIONS

Assess:

• Withdrawal: cramping, hypertension, anxiety, vomiting

• VS q3-5 min

• ABGs including Po_2, Pco_2

• Signs of withdrawal in drug-dependent individuals

• Cardiac status: tachycardia, hypertension; monitor ECG

• Respiratory dysfunction: respiratory depression, character, rate, rhythm; if respirations are <10/min, administer naloxone; probably due to opioid overdose; monitor LOC

Administer:

• IV undiluted with sterile H_2O for inj; may be further diluted with NS or D_5 and given as an inf; give 0.4 mg or less over 15 sec or titrate inf to response

• Only with resuscitative equipment, O_2 nearby

• Only sol prepared within 24 hr

Perform/provide:

• Dark storage at room temp

Evaluate:

• Therapeutic response: reversal of respiratory depression; LOC-alert

naltrexone (℞)

(nal-trex'one)

Trexan

Func. class.: Narcotic antagonist

Chem. class.: Thebaine derivative

Action: Competes with narcotics at narcotic receptor sites

N

Uses: Blockage of opioid analgesics, used in treatment of opiate addiction

Dosage and routes:

• *Adult:* PO 25 mg, may give 25 mg after 1 hr if no withdrawal symptoms; 50-150 mg may be given qd depending on need, maintenance 50 mg q24h; 100-150 mg may be given on alternate days or 3 days per wk

Available forms: Tabs 50 mg

Side effects/adverse reactions:

MISC: Increased thirst, chills, fever

MS: Joint and muscle pain

GU: Delayed ejaculation, decreased potency

CNS: Stimulation, drowsiness, dizziness, confusion, ***convulsion,*** headache, flushing, hallucinations, nervousness, irritability

GI: Nausea, vomiting, diarrhea, heartburn, anorexia, ***hepatitis,*** constipation

INTEG: Rash, urticaria, bruising, oily skin, acne, pruritis

EENT: Tinnitus, hearing loss, blurred vision

CV: Rapid pulse, ***pulmonary edema,*** hypertension

RESP: Wheezing, hyperpnea, nasal congestion, rhinorrhea, sneezing, sore throat

Contraindications: Hypersensitivity, opioid dependence, hepatic failure, hepatitis

Precautions: Pregnancy (C), hepatic disease, lacation, child

Pharmacokinetics:

PO: Onset 15-30 min, peak 1-2 hr, duration is dose dependent

Metabolized by liver, excreted by kidneys; crosses placenta, excreted in breast milk; half-life 4 hr; extensive first-pass metabolism

NURSING CONSIDERATIONS

Assess:

• VS q3-5min

• ABGs including Po_2, Pco_2

• Signs of withdrawal in drug-dependent individuals

• Cardiac status: tachycardia, hypertension

• Respiratory dysfunction: respiratory depression, character, rate, rhythm; if respirations are <10/min, respiratory stimulant should be administered

Administer:

• Only if resuscitative equipment is nearby

Perform/provide:

• Storage in tight container

Evaluate:

• Therapeutic response: blocking narcotic ingestion

nandrolone decanoate/nandrolone phenpropionate (℞)

(nan'droe-lone)

Androlone-D 200, Deca-Durabolin, Hybolin Decanoate-50, Hybolin Decanoate-100, nandrolone decanoate, Neo-Durabolic, Durabolin, Hybolin Improved, Nandrobolic, nandrolone phenpropionate

Func. class.: Androgenic anabolic steroid

Chem. class.: Halogenated testosterone derivative

Action: Increases weight by building body tissue, increases potassium, phosphorus, chloride, nitrogen levels, increases bone development

Uses: Tissue building, severe disease, refractory anemias, metastatic breast cancer

Dosage and routes:

Tissue building (possibly effective)

• *Adult:* IM 50-100 mg q3-4wk (decanoate)

* Available in Canada only

• *Child 2-13 yr:* IM 25-50 mg q3-4wk (decanoate)

Severe disease/refractory anemias

• *Adult:* IM 100-200 mg qwk (decanoate)

Breast cancer

• *Adult:* IM 50-100 mg qwk (phenpropionate)

Available forms: Phenpropionate inj 25, 50 mg/ml; decanoate inj 50, 100, 200 mg/ml

Side effects/adverse reactions:

INTEG: Rash, acneiform lesions, oily hair, skin, flushing, sweating, acne vulgaris, alopecia, hirsutism

CNS: Dizziness, headache, fatigue, tremors, paresthesias, flushing, sweating, anxiety, lability, insomnia, carpal tunnel syndrome

MS: Cramps, spasms

CV: Increased B/P

GU: ***Hematuria,*** amenorrhea, vaginitis, decreased libido, decreased breast size, clitoral hypertrophy, testicular atrophy

GI: Nausea, vomiting, constipation, weight gain, ***cholestatic jaundice***

EENT: Conjunctival edema, nasal congestion

ENDO: Abnormal GTT

Contraindications: Severe renal, severe cardiac, severe hepatic disease, hypersensitivity, pregnancy (X), lactation, abnormal genital bleeding, males with cancer of breast, prostate

Precautions: Diabetes mellitus, CV disease, MI

Pharmacokinetics:

IM: Metabolized in liver, crosses placenta, excreted in the breast milk, urine

Interactions:

• Increased effects of oral antidiabetics, oxyphenbutazone
• Increased PT: anticoagulants
• Edema: ACTH, adrenal steroids
• Decreased effects of insulin

Lab test interferences:

Increase: Serum cholesterol, blood glucose, urine glucose

Decrease: Serum Ca, serum K, T_4, T_3, thyroid ^{131}I uptake test, urine 17-OHCS, 17-KS, PBI, BSP

NURSING CONSIDERATIONS

Assess:

• Weight daily; notify prescriber if weekly weight gain is >5 lb
• B/P q4h
• I&O ratio; be alert for decreasing urinary output, increasing edema
• Growth rate in children, since growth rate may be uneven (linear/bone growth) with extended use
• Electrolytes: K, Na, Cl, Ca; cholesterol
• Liver function studies: ALT (SGPT), AST (SGOT), bilirubin
• Edema, hypertension, cardiac symptoms, jaundice
• Mental status: affect, mood, behavioral changes, aggression
• Signs of masculinization in female: increased libido, deepening of voice, decreased breast tissue, enlarged clitoris, menstrual irregularities; male: gynecomastia, impotence, testicular atrophy
• Hypercalcemia: lethargy, polyuria, polydipsia, nausea, vomiting, constipation, drug may have to be decreased
• Hypoglycemia in diabetics, since oral antidiabetic action is increased

Administer:

• Titrated dose; use lowest effective dose

Perform/provide:

• Diet with increased calories, protein; decrease Na if edema occurs

Evaluate:

• Therapeutic response: increased appetite, increased stamina

Teach patient/family:

• That drug must to be combined with complete health plan: diet, rest, exercise

• To notify prescriber if therapeutic response decreases
• Not to discontinue abruptly
• About changes in sex characteristics
• That females should report menstrual irregularities
• That 1-3 mo course is necessary for response in breast cancer
• Procedure for use of buccal tablets: requires 30-60 min to dissolve, change absorption site with each dose; do not eat, drink, chew, or smoke while tablet is in place

---

naphazoline (OTC)

(naff-a-zoe'leen)
Privine
Func. class.: Nasal decongestant
Chem. class.: Sympathomimetic amine

Action: Produces vasoconstriction (rapid, long-acting) of arterioles, thereby decreasing fluid exudation, mucosal engorgement by stimulation of α-adrenergic receptors in vascular smooth muscle
Uses: Nasal congestion
Dosage and routes:
• *Adult:* INSTILL 2 gtt or sprays to nasal mucosa q3-4h
• *Child 6-12 yr:* INSTILL 1-2 gtt or sprays, repeat q3-4h prn, not to exceed 5 days
Available forms: Nasal sol 0.025, 0.05%
Side effects/adverse reactions:
GI: Nausea, vomiting, anorexia
EENT: Irritation, burning, sneezing, stinging, dryness, rebound congestion
INTEG: Contact dermatitis
CNS: Anxiety, restlessness, tremors, weakness, insomnia, dizziness, fever, headache

Contraindications: Hypersensitivity to sympathomimetic amines
Precautions: Child <6 yr, elderly, diabetes, cardiovascular disease, hypertension, hyperthyroidism, increased ICP, prostatic hypertrophy, pregnancy (C), glaucoma
Interactions:
• Hypertension: MAOIs, β-adrenergic blockers
• Hypotension: methyldopa, mecamylamine, reserpine

NURSING CONSIDERATIONS
Assess:
• For systemic absorption: hypertension, tachycardia; notify prescriber
• Redness, swelling, pain in nasal passages
Administer:
• No more than q4h
• For <4 consecutive days
Perform/provide:
• Environmental humidification to decrease nasal congestion, dryness
• Storage in light-resistant containers; do not expose to high temp or let sol come into contact with aluminum
Evaluate:
• Therapeutic response: decreased nasal congestion
Teach patient/family:
• That stinging may occur for several applications; drying of mucosa may be decreased by environmental humidification
• To notify prescriber of irregular pulse, insomnia, dizziness, tremors
• Proper administration to avoid systemic absorption
• To rinse dropper with very hot water to prevent contamination

---

* Available in Canada only

naphazoline (OTC, ℞)

(naf-az'oh-leen)

AK-Con Ophthalmic, Allerest Eye Drops, Albalon Liquifilm Ophthalmic, Clear Eyes, Comfort Eye Drops, Degest 2, Nafazair, naphazoline HCl, Naphcon, Naphcon Forte, Opcon, Vasoclear, Vasocon Regular, Estivin II

Func. class.: Ophthalmic vasoconstrictor

Chem. class.: Direct imidazoline derivative

Action: Vasoconstriction of eye arterioles; decreases eye engorgement by stimulation of α-adrenergic receptors

Uses: Relieves hyperemia, irritation in superficial corneal vascularity

Dosage and routes:

• *Adult:* INSTILL 1-2 gtt q3-4h

Available forms: Oph sol 0.01%, 0.012%, 0.02%, 0.025%, 0.03%, 0.05%

Side effects/adverse reactions:

CNS: Headache, dizziness, sedation, anxiety, weakness, sweating (systemic absorption)

CV: Hypertension, dysrhythmias, tachycardia, ***CV collapse*** (systemic absorption)

EENT: Pupil dilation, increased intraocular pressure, photophobia

Contraindications: Hypersensitivity, glaucoma (narrow-angle)

Precautions: Hypertension, hyperthyroidism, elderly, severe arteriosclerosis, cardiac disease, pregnancy (C)

Pharmacokinetics:

INSTILL: Duration 2-3 hr

Interactions:

• Increased pressor effects: MAOIs, tricyclic antidepressants

NURSING CONSIDERATIONS

Perform/provide:

• Storage in tight, light-resistant container

Evaluate:

• Therapeutic response: vasoconstriction of the eye

Teach patient/family:

• To report change in vision, blurring, or loss of sight; breathing trouble, sweating, flushing, anxiety, weakness

• Method of instillation; tilt head backward, hold dropper over eye, drop medication inside lower lid, using pressure on inside corner of eye hold 1 min, do not touch dropper to eye

• That blurred vision will decrease with repeated use of drug

• To notify prescriber of headache, spots, redness, pain; discontinue use

naproxen (℞, OTC)

(na-prox'en)

Aleve, Anaprox DS, Apo-Napro-Na*, Apo-Naproxen*, Naprosyn Anaprox, Naxen*, Novonaprox*, Novonaprox sodium*, Synflex*

Func. class.: Nonsteroidal antiinflammatory

Chem. class.: Propionic acid derivative

Action: Inhibits prostaglandin synthesis by decreasing an enzyme needed for biosynthesis; analgesic, antiinflammatory, antipyretic

Uses: Mild to moderate pain, osteoarthritis, rheumatoid, gouty arthritis, juvenile arthritis, primary dysmenorrhea

Dosage and routes:

• *Adult:* PO 250-500 mg bid, not to exceed 1 g/day (base); 525 mg, then 275 mg q6-8h prn, not to exceed 1475 mg (sodium)

N

• *Children:* PO 10 mg/kg in 2 divided doses

Available forms: Tabs Naproxen: 250, 375, 500 mg; oral susp 125 mg/5 ml; Naproxen sodium tabs 200, 250, 500 mg; tabs delayed rel 375, 500 mg

Side effects/adverse reactions:

GI: Nausea, anorexia, vomiting, diarrhea, jaundice, ***cholestatic hepatitis,*** constipation, flatulence, cramps, dry mouth, peptic ulcer, ***GI ulceration, bleeding, perforation***

CNS: Dizziness, drowsiness, fatigue, tremors, confusion, insomnia, anxiety, depression

CV: Tachycardia, peripheral edema, palpitations, dysrhythmias

INTEG: Purpura, rash, pruritus, sweating

GU: ***Nephrotoxicity: dysuria, hematuria, oliguria, azotemia***

HEMA: ***Blood dyscrasias***

EENT: Tinnitus, hearing loss, blurred vision

Contraindications: Hypersensitivity, asthma, severe renal disease, severe hepatic disease, ulcer disease

Precautions: Pregnancy (B), lactation, children <2 yr, bleeding disorders, GI disorders, cardiac disorders, hypersensitivity to other antiinflammatory agents, elderly

Pharmacokinetics:

PO: Peak 2-4 hr, half-life 3-3½ hr; metabolized in liver; excreted in urine (metabolites), breast milk; 99% protein binding

Interactions:

• May increase action of heparin
• Increased lithium toxicity: lithium

Lab test interferences:

Increase: BUN, alk phosphatase

False increase: 5-HIAA, 17KGS

NURSING CONSIDERATIONS

Assess:

• Renal, liver, blood studies: BUN, creatinine, AST (SGOT), ALT (SGPT), Hgb before treatment, periodically thereafter
• Audiometric, ophthalmic exam before, during, after treatment
• For eye, ear problems: blurred vision, tinnitus (may indicate toxicity)

Administer:

• With food to decrease GI symptoms; best to take on empty stomach to facilitate absorption

Perform/provide:

• Storage at room temp

Evaluate:

• Therapeutic response: decreased pain, stiffness, swelling in joints, ability to move more easily

Teach patient/family:

• To report blurred vision, ringing, roaring in ears (may indicate toxicity)
• To avoid driving, other hazardous activities if dizziness or drowsiness occurs
• To report change in urine pattern, weight increase, edema (face, lower extremities), pain increase in joints, fever, blood in urine (indicates nephrotoxicity)
• That therapeutic effects may take up to 1 mo
• To avoid ASA, alcohol, steroids

natamycin (ophthalmic) (℞)

(na-ta-mye'sin)

Natacyn

Func. class.: Antiinfective/antifungal

Chem. class.: Tetraene polyene compound

Action: Inhibits transport functions and cell permeability in organism

Uses: Fungal blepharitis, conjunctivitis, keratitis

Dosage and routes:
• *Adult and child:* INSTILL 1 gtt q1-2h × 3-4 days, then decrease to 1 gtt 8 × /day, duration of therapy, 14-21 days
Available forms: Oph susp 5%
Side effects/adverse reactions:
EENT: Temporary visual haze, overgrowth of nonsusceptible organisms
Contraindications: Hypersensitivity
Precautions: Antibiotic hypersensitivity, pregnancy (B); failure of keratitis to improve after 7-10 days suggests infection not caused by susceptible organism
• Allergy: itching, lacrimation, redness, swelling, eye pain

NURSING CONSIDERATIONS
Administer:
• After washing hands; cleanse crusts or discharge from eye before application
Perform/provide:
• Storage at room temp or refrigerate
Evaluate:
• Therapeutic response: absence of redness, inflammation, tearing
Teach patient/family:
• To use drug exactly as prescribed, to shake well before using
• Not to use eye makeup, towels, washcloths, eye medication of others; reinfection may occur
• That drug container tip should not be touched to eye
• To report itching, increased redness, burning, stinging, swelling; drug should be discontinued

nedocromil inhaler (℞)

(ned-o-kroe'mill)
Tilade
Func. class.: Antiasthmatic
Chem. class.: Mast cell stabilizer

Action: Stabilizes the membrane of the sensitized mast cell, preventing release of chemical mediators after an antigen-IgE interaction
Uses: Severe perennial bronchial asthma, exercise-induced bronchospasm (prevention), prevention of acute bronchospasm induced by environmental pollutants; *not* for treatment of acute asthma attacks
Dosage and routes:
Bronchospasm, bronchial asthma
• *Adult and child >12 y;* 2 inhalations 2-4 × a day at regular intervals to provide 14 g/day
Available forms: 1.75 mg nedocromil Na per activation in 16.2 g canisters providing at least 112 metered inhalations
Side effects/adverse reactions:
EENT: Throat irritation, cough, nasal congestion, burning eyes, rhinitis
CNS: Headache, dizziness, neuritis, dysphonia
GI: Nausea, vomiting, anorexia, dry mouth, bitter taste
Contraindications: Hypersensitivity to this drug or lactose, status asthmaticus
Precautions: Pregnancy (B), lactation, children
Pharmacokinetics:
INH: Peak 15 min, duration 4-6 hr; excreted unchanged in urine; half-life 80 min

NURSING CONSIDERATIONS
Assess:
• Eosinophil count during treatment
• Respiratory status: rate, rhythm,

N

characteristics, cough, wheezing, dyspnea

Administer:

- By inhalation only
- Gargle, sip of water to decrease irritation in throat

Evaluate:

- Therapeutic response: decrease in asthmatic symptoms, congested runny nose

Teach patient/family:

- To clear mucus before using
- Proper technique: exhale; using inhaler, inhale deeply with head tipped back to open airway; remove, hold breath, exhale, repeat until all of drug is inhaled
- That therapeutic effect may take up to 4 wk
- That drug is preventive only, not restorative

nefazodone (℞)

(ne-faz′o-done)

Serzone

Func. class.: Antidepressant

Chem. class.: Phenylpiperazine

Action: Selectively inhibits serotonin uptake by brain, potentiates behavorial changes, occupies central S-H_2 receptors

Uses: Major depression

Dosage and routes:

- *Adult:* PO 200 mg/day (100 mg bid); dose may be increased to 300 mg/day (150 mg bid), max 600 mg/day
- *Elderly:* 100 mg/day (50 mg bid)

Available forms: Tabs 100, 150, 200, 250 mg

Side effects/adverse reactions:

CNS: Somnolence, dizziness, ***headache, insomnia***

GI: ***Nausea, constipaion, dry mouth***

GU: ***Urinary frequency, retention, UTI***

CV: ***Postural hypotension***

RESP: ***Pharyngitis, cough***

EENT: Blurred vision, abnormal vision

Contraindications: Hypersensitivity to this drug or phenylpiperazines

Precautions: Pregnancy (C), lactation, children, elderly, cardiovascular disease, seizure disorder

Pharmacokinetics:

Metabolized in liver extensively to metabolites; excreted in urine, breast milk; peak 1-3 hr; half-life triphasic 2-4 hr

Interactions:

- Increased effect: CNS depressants
- ***Fatal reaction:*** antihistamines, nonsedating
- Increased plasma concentrations: benzodiazipines
- Hypertension crisis: MAO inhibitors
- Drug/smoking: increases metabolism, decreases effects

NURSING CONSIDERATIONS

Assess:

- B/P (lying, standing), pulse q4h; if systolic B/P drops 20 mm Hg, hold drug, notify prescriber; take vital signs q4h in patients with cardiovascular disease
- Blood studies: CBC, leukocytes, differential, cardiac enzymes (long-term therapy)
- Hepatic studies: AST (SGOT), ALT (SGPT), bilirubin
- Mental status: mood, sensorium, affect, suicidal tendencies; increase in psychiatric symptoms: depression, panic
- Urinary retention, constipation; constipation is more likely in children, elderly
- For withdrawal symptoms: headache, nausea, vomiting, muscle pain, weakness; unusual unless drug discontinued abruptly
- Alcohol consumption; hold dose until morning

Administer:
- With food, milk for GI symptoms
- Crushed if patient cannot swallow whole
- Storage at room temp; do not freeze

Teach patient/family
- That therapeutic effects may take 3-4 wk
- To use caution in driving, other activities requiring alertness because of drowsiness, dizziness; to avoid rising quickly from sitting to standing, especially elderly
- To avoid alcohol ingestion, other CNS depressants
- Not to discontinue medication quickly after long-term use; may cause nausea, headache, malaise
- To increase bulk in diet for constipation, especially elderly
- To take gum, hard sugarless candy, frequents sips of water for dry mouth

Evaluate:
Therapeutic response: decrease in depression; absence of suicidal thoughts

Treatment of overdose: ECG monitoring; induce emesis; lavage, activated charcoal; administer anticonvulsant

neomycin (℞)

(nee-oh-mye'sin)

Mycifradin Sulfate

Func. class.: Antiinfective

Chem. class.: Aminoglycoside

Action: Inferferes with protein synthesis in bacterial cell by binding to 30S ribosomal subunit, causing inaccurate peptide sequence to form in protein chain, causing bacterial death

Uses: Severe systemic infections of CNS, respiratory, GI, urinary tract, eye, bone, skin, soft tissues caused by *P. aeruginosa, E. coli, Enterobacter, K. pneumoniae, P. vulgaris;* also used for hepatic coma, preoperatively to sterilize bowel, infectious diarrhea caused by enteropathogenic *E. coli*

Dosage and routes:

Severe systemic infections
- *Adult:* IM 15 mg/kg/day in 4 divided doses, not to exceed 1 g/day

Hepatic coma
- *Adult:* PO 4-12 g/day in divided doses × 5-6 days
- *Child:* 50-100 mg/kg/day in divided doses

Preoperative bowel sterilization
- *Adult:* PO on 3rd day of a 3-day regimen, give 1 g early PM, repeat in 1 hr, repeat at hs (given with erythromycin); give saline cathartic before giving this drug

Available forms: Tabs 500 mg; top, inj 500 mg; oral sol 125 mg/5 ml

Side effects/adverse reactions:

GU: ***Oliguria, hematuria, renal damage, azotemia, renal failure, nephrotoxicity***

CNS: Confusion, depression, numbness, tremors, ***convulsions,*** muscle twitching, ***neurotoxicity,*** dizziness, vertigo

EENT: ***Ototoxicity,*** deafness, visual disturbances, tinnitus

HEMA: ***Agranulocytosis, thrombocytopenia,*** leukopenia, eosinophilia, anemia

GI: Nausea, vomiting, anorexia, increased ALT (SGPT), AST (SGOT), bilirubin, hepatomegaly, ***hepatic necrosis,*** splenomegaly

CV: Hypotension, hypertension, palpitation

INTEG: Rash, burning, urticaria, photosensitivity, dermatitis, alopecia

Contraindications: Bowel obstruction (oral use), severe renal disease, hypersensitivity, infants, children

Precautions: Mild renal disease, pregnancy (C), hearing deficits, lactation, myasthenia gravis, Parkinson's disease

Pharmacokinetics:

PO: Onset rapid, peak 1-2 hr

Plasma half-life 2-3 hr; not metabolized, excreted unchanged in feces, crosses placenta

Interactions:

• Increased ototoxicity, neurotoxicity, nephrotoxicity: other aminoglycosides, amphotericin B, polymyxin, vancomycin, ethacrynic acid, furosemide, mannitol, methoxyflurane, cisplatin, cephalosporins, bacitracin

• Do not mix in sol or syringe: carbenicillin, ticarcillin, amphotericin B, cephalothin, erythromycin, heparin

• Increased effects: nondepolarizing muscle relaxants, succinylcholine, oral anticoagulants when given with oral neomycin

• Decreased effects of digoxin, penicillin V when given with oral neomycin

NURSING CONSIDERATIONS

Assess:

• Weight before treatment; calculation of dosage is usually based on ideal body weight, but may be calculated on actual body weight

• I&O ratio, urinalysis qd for proteinuria, cells, casts; report sudden change in urine output

• Urine pH if drug is used for UTI; urine should be kept alkaline

• Renal impairment by securing urine for CrCl testing, BUN, serum creatinine; lower dosage should be given in renal impairment (CrCl <80 ml/min)

• Deafness by audiometric testing, ringing, roaring in ears, vertigo; assess hearing before, during, after treatment

• Dehydration: high specific gravity, decrease in skin turgor, dry mucous membranes, dark urine

• Overgrowth of infection: fever, malaise, redness, pain, swelling, perineal itching, diarrhea, stomatitis, change in cough, sputum

• C&S before starting treatment to identify infecting organism

• Vestibular dysfunction: nausea, vomiting, dizziness, headache; drug should be discontinued if severe

• Injection sites for redness, swelling, abscesses; use warm compresses at site

Administer:

• IM injection in large muscle mass; rotate injection sites

• Drug in evenly spaced doses to maintain blood level

• Bicarbonate to alkalinize urine if ordered in treating UTI, as drug is most active in alkaline environment

Perform/provide:

• Adequate fluids of 2-3 L/day unless contraindicated to prevent irritation of tubules

• Supervised ambulation, other safety measures, with vestibular dysfunction

Evaluate:

• Therapeutic response: absence of fever, draining wounds, negative C&S after treatment

Teach patient/family:

• To report headache, dizziness, symptoms of overgrowth of infection, renal impairment

• To report loss of hearing, ringing, roaring in ears or a feeling of fullness in head

Treatment of overdose: Hemodialysis; monitor serum levels of drug

neomycin (otic) (℞)

(nee-oh-mye'sin)
Drotic, Otocort
Func. class.: Otic antibiotic
Chem. class.: Aminoglycoside

Action: Inhibits protein synthesis in susceptible microorganisms
Uses: Ear infection (external), short-term use
Dosage and routes:
• *Adult and child:* INSTILL 2-5 gtt tid-qid
Available forms: Otic sol in combination with neomycin, hydrocortisone 0.25%, 0.5%
Side effects/adverse reactions:
EENT: Itching, irritation in ear
INTEG: Rash, urticaria
Contraindications: Hypersensitivity, perforated eardrum
Precautions: Pregnancy (C)

NURSING CONSIDERATIONS
Assess:
• For redness, swelling, fever, pain in ear, which indicates superinfection
Administer:
• After removing impacted cerumen by irrigation
• After cleaning stopper with alcohol
• After restraining child if necessary
• Warm solution
Evaluate:
• Therapeutic response: decreased ear pain
Teach patient/family:
• Method of instillation using aseptic technique, including not touching dropper to ear
• That dizziness may occur after instillation

neomycin (topical) (OTC)

(nee-oh-mye'sin)
Myciguent, Neomycin Sulfate
Func. class.: Local antibacterial
Chem. class.: Aminoglycoside

Action: Interferes with bacterial protein synthesis
Uses: Skin infections, minor burns, wounds, skin grafts, primary pyodemas, otitis externa
Dosage and routes:
• *Adult and child:* TOP rub into affected area bid-tid
Available forms: Oint, cream 0.5%
Side effects/adverse reactions:
INTEG: Rash, urticaria, scaling, redness
OTHER: Possible nephrotoxicity, ototoxicity, neuromuscular blockade
Contraindications: Hypersensitivity, large areas, burns, ulcerations
Precautions: Pregnancy (C), lactation, impaired renal function, external ear of perforated eardrum

NURSING CONSIDERATIONS
Assess:
• Allergic reaction: burning, stinging, swelling, redness
• For signs of nephrotoxicity or ototoxicity
Administer:
• Enough medication to cover lesions completely
• After cleansing with soap, water before each application; dry well
• To less than 20% of body surface area when patient has impaired renal function
Perform/provide:
• Storage at room temp in dry place
Evaluate:
• Therapeutic response: decrease in size, number of lesions

N

Teach patient/family:

- To use medical asepsis (hand washing) before, after application
- To apply with glove to prevent further infection
- To avoid use of OTC creams, ointments, lotions unless directed by prescriber
- To notify prescriber if condition worsens
- That prolonged use may lead to overgrowth of susceptible organisms
- Not to use occlusive dressings

neostigmine (℞)

(nee-oh-stig′meen)

neostigmine bromide, neostigmine methylsulfate, Prostigmin

Func. class.: Cholinergic stimulant; anticholinesterase

Chem. class.: Quaternary compound

Action: Inhibits destruction of acetylcholine, which increases concentration at sites where acetylcholine is released; this facilitates transmission of impulses across myoneural junction

Uses: Myasthenia gravis, nondepolarizing neuromuscular blocker, antagonist, bladder distention, postoperative ileus

Dosage and routes:

Myasthenia gravis

- *Adult:* PO 15-375 mg/day; IM/IV 0.5-2 mg q1-3h
- *Child:* PO 2 mg/kg/day q3-4h

Nondepolarizing neuromuscular blocker antagonist

- *Adult:* IV 0.5-2 mg slowly, may repeat if needed (give 0.6-1.2 mg atropine before this drug)

Abdominal distention/postoperative ileus

- *Adult:* IM/SC 0.25-1 mg q4-6h depending on condition

Available forms: Tabs 15 mg; inj 1:1000, 1:2000, 1:4000

Side effects/adverse reactions:

INTEG: Rash, urticaria, flushing

CNS: Dizziness, headache, sweating, weakness, ***convulsions,*** incoordination, ***paralysis,*** drowsiness, loss of consciousness

GI: Nausea, diarrhea, vomiting, cramps, increased peristalsis, salivary and gastric secretions

CV: Tachycardia, dysrhythmias, bradycardia, hypotension, AV block, ECG changes, ***cardiac arrest,*** syncope

GU: Frequency, incontinence, urgency

RESP: ***Respiratory depression, bronchospasm, constriction, laryngospasm, respiratory arrest,*** dyspnea

EENT: Miosis, blurred vision, lacrimation, visual changes

Contraindications: Obstruction of intestine, renal system, pregnancy (C), bromide sensitivity, peritonitis

Precautions: Bradycardia, hypotension, seizure disorders, bronchial asthma, coronary occlusion, hyperthyroidism, dysrhythmias, peptic ulcer, megacolon, poor GI motility, lactation, children

Pharmacokinetics:

PO: Onset 45-75 min, duration 2½-4 hr

IM/SC: Onset 10-30 min, duration 2½-4 hr

IV: Onset 4-8 min; duration 2-4 hr; metabolized in liver, excreted in urine

Interactions:

- Decreased action of gallamine, metocurine, pancuronium, tubocurarine, atropine
- Increased action of decamethonium, succinylcholine
- Decreased action of neostigmine: aminoglycosides, anesthetics, pro-

cainamide, quinidine, mecamylamine, polymyxin, magnesium
Syringe compatibilities: Glycopyrrolate, heparin, pentobarbital, or thiopental
Additive compatibility: Netilmicin

NURSING CONSIDERATIONS
Assess:
- VS, respiration q8h
- I&O ratio; check for urinary retention or incontinence
- For bradycardia, hypotension, bronchospasm, headache, dizziness, convulsions, respiratory depression; drug should be discontinued if toxicity occurs

Administer:
- IV undiluted, give through Y-tube or 3-way stopcock; give 0.5 mg or less over 1 min
- Only with atropine sulfate available for cholinergic crisis
- Only after all other cholinergics have been discontinued
- Increased doses if tolerance occurs
- Larger doses after exercise or fatigue
- On empty stomach for better absorption

Perform/provide:
- Storage at room temp

Evaluate:
- Therapeutic response: increased muscle strength, hand grasp, improved gait, absence of labored breathing (if severe)

Teach patient/family:
- That drug is not a cure; it only relieves symptoms
- To wear Medic Alert ID specifying myasthenia gravis, drugs taken

Treatment of overdose: Respiratory support, atropine 1-4 mg (IV)

netilmicin (℞)
(ne-til-mye'sin)
Netromycin
Func. class.: Antibiotic
Chem. class.: Aminoglycoside

Action: Interferes with protein synthesis in bacterial cell by binding to 30 S ribosomal subunit, causing inaccurate peptide sequence to form in protein chain, causing bacterial death
Uses: Severe systemic infections of CNS, respiratory, GI, urinary tract, bone, skin, soft tissues caused by *P. aeruginosa, E. coli, Enterobacter, Citrobacter, Staphylococcus, K. pneumoniae, P. mirabilis, Serratia, Shigella, Salmonella, Acinetobacter, Neisseria*

Dosage and routes:
Normal renal function
- *Adult and child >12 yr:* IM/IV 3-6.5 mg/kg/day; may give q8-12h for severe infections
- *Child and infant 6 wk-12 yr:* IM/IV 5.5-8 mg/kg/day in divided doses q8-12h
- *Neonate <6 wk:* IM/IV 4-6.5 mg/kg/day in divided doses q12h

Available forms: Inj 10, 25, 100 mg/ml
Side effects/adverse reactions:
GU: ***Oliguria, hematuria, renal damage, azotemia, renal failure, nephrotoxicity***
CNS: Confusion, depression, numbness, tremors, ***convulsions,*** muscle twitching, ***neurotoxicity,*** dizziness, vertigo
EENT: ***Ototoxicity,*** deafness, visual disturbances, tinnitus
HEMA: ***Agranulocytosis, thrombocytopenia, leukopenia, eosinophilia, anemia***
GI: Nausea, vomiting, anorexia, increased ALT (SGPT), AST (SGOT),

bilirubin, hepatomegaly, ***hepatic necrosis,*** splenomegaly
CV: Hypotension, hypertension, palpitations
INTEG: Rash, burning, urticaria, dermatitis
Contraindications: Severe renal disease, hypersensitivity
Precautions: Neonates, mild renal disease, pregnancy (D), children <12 yr, lactation, myasthenia gravis, hearing deficit, Parkinson's disease, severe burns, cystic fibrosis
Pharmacokinetics:
IM: Onset rapid, peak 1-2 hr
IV: Onset immediate, peak 1-2 hr
Plasma half-life 2-3 hr, not metabolized, excreted unchanged in urine, crosses placental barrier
Interactions:
- Increased ototoxicity, neurotoxicity, nephrotoxicity: other aminoglycosides, amphotericin B, polymyxin, vancomycin, ethacrynic acid, furosemide, mannitol, methoxyflurane, cisplatin, cephalosporins, bacitracin
- Increased effects: nondepolarizing muscle relaxants, succinylcholine

Y-site compatibilities: Aminophylline, calcium gluconate, melphalan, vinorelbine

NURSING CONSIDERATIONS
Assess:
- Weight before treatment; calculation of dosage is usually based on ideal body weight, but may be calculated on actual body weight
- Daily I&O ratio, urinalysis for proteinuria, cells, casts; report sudden change in urine output
- VS during infusion, watch for hypotension, change in pulse
- IV site for thrombophlebitis, including pain, redness, swelling q30 min; change site if needed; apply warm compresses to discontinued site
- Serum peak, drawn at 30-60 min after IV infusion or 60 min after IM injection; trough level drawn just before next dose; blood level should be 2-4 times bacteriostatic level; trough = 0.5-2 mEq/ml, peak = 6-10 mEq/ml
- Urine pH if drug is used for UTI; urine should be kept alkaline
- Renal impairment by securing urine for CrCl testing, BUN, serum creatinine; a lower dosage should be given in renal impairment (CrCl <80 ml/min)
- Deafness by audiometric testing, ringing, roaring in ears, vertigo; assess hearing before, during, after treatment
- Dehydration: high specific gravity, decrease in skin turgor, dry mucous membranes, dark urine
- Overgrowth of infection: fever, malaise, redness, pain, swelling, perineal itching, diarrhea, stomatitis, change in cough or sputum
- C&S before starting treatment to identify infecting organism
- Vestibular dysfunction: nausea, vomiting, dizziness, headache; drug should be discontinued if severe
- Injection sites for redness, swelling, abscesses; use warm compresses at site

Administer:
- IM injection in large muscle mass; rotate injection sites
- Drug in evenly spaced doses to maintain blood level
- Bicarbonate to alkalinize urine if ordered in treating UTI, as drug is most active in alkaline environment
- IV diluted in 50-200 ml D_5W, 0.9% NaCl; saline infuse over ½-2 hr

Perform/provide:
- Adequate fluids of 2-3 L/day unless contraindicated to prevent irritation of tubules

• Flush of IV line with NS or D_5W after infusion
• Supervised ambulation, other safety measures, with vestibular dysfunction

Evaluate:
• Therapeutic response: absence of fever, draining wounds, negative C&S after treatment

Teach patient /family:
• To report headache, dizziness, symptoms of overgrowth of infection, renal impairment
• To report loss of hearing, ringing, roaring in ears or feeling of fullness in head

Treatment of overdose: Hemodialysis; monitor serum levels of drug

niacin (vitamin B_3/ nicotinic acid)/niacinamide (nicotinamide) (OTC, ℞)

(nye'a-sin) (nye-a-sin'a-mide)
Nia-Bid, Niac, Niacels, Niacin TD, SpaN Niacin, Niacin TR Niacor, Nico-400, Nicobid, Nicolar, Nicotinex, Nicotinic Acid, Novaniacin*, Slo-Niacin, Tri-B*

Func. class.: Vit B_3
Chem. class.: Water-soluble vitamin

Action: Needed for conversion of fats, protein, carbohydrates, by oxidation reduction; acts directly on vascular smooth muscle, causing vasodilation; high doses decrease serum lipids

Uses: Pellagra, hyperlipidemias, peripheral vascular disease

Dosage and routes:

Adjunct in hyperlipidemia
• *Adult:* PO 500 mg qd in 3 divided doses after meals, may be increased to 2 g/day

Pellagra
• *Adult:* PO 300-500 mg qd in divided doses
Child: PO 100-300 mg qd in divided doses

Peripheral vascular disease
• *Adult:* PO 250-800 mg qd in divided doses

Available forms: Nicotinic acid—tabs 20, 25, 50, 100, 500 mg; caps time release 125, 250, 300, 400, 500 mg; tabs time release 150 mg; elix 50 mg/5 ml; inj 100 mg/ml; nicotinamide—tabs 50, 100, 500 mg; tabs time release 1000 mg

Side effects/adverse reactions:
CNS: Paresthesias, headache, dizziness, anxiety
GI: Nausea, vomiting, anorexia, flatulence, xerostomia, ***jaundice,*** diarrhea, peptic ulcer
GU: Hyperuricemia, ***glycosuria, hypoalbuminemia***
CV: Postural hypotension, vasovagal attacks, dysrhythmias, vasodilation
EENT: Blurred vision, ptosis
INTEG: Flushing, dry skin, rash, pruritus
RESP: Wheezing

Contraindications: Hypersensitivity, peptic ulcer, hepatic disease, lactation, hemorrhage, severe hypotension

Precautions: Glaucoma, cardiovascular disease, CAD, diabetes mellitus, gout, schizophrenia, pregnancy (C)

Pharmacokinetics:
PO: Peak 30-70 min, half-life 45 min; metabolized in liver; 30% excreted unchanged in urine

Interactions:
• Increased action of ganglionic blockers

Additive compatibility: TPN sol

Lab test interferences:
Increase: Bilirubin, alk phosphatase, liver enzymes, LDH, uric acid

N

Decrease: Cholesterol
False increase: Urinary catecholamines
False positive: Urine glucose

NURSING CONSIDERATIONS

Assess:

- Liver function studies: AST (SGOT), ALT (SGPT), bilirubin, alk phosphatase; blood glucose before and during treatment
- Niacin levels
- Cardiac status: rate, rhythm, quality; postural hypotension, dysrhythmias
- Nutritional status: liver, yeast, legumes, organ meat, lean poultry
- Liver dysfunction: clay-colored stools, itching, dark urine, jaundice
- CNS symptoms: headache, paresthesias, blurred vision

Administer:

- With meals for GI symptoms

Evaluate:

- Therapeutic response: decreased lipids, warm extremities, absence of numbness in extremities

Teach patient/family:

- That flushing and increase in feelings of warmth will occur several hours after taking drug (PO); time-release product will minimize flushing
- To remain recumbent if postural hypotension occurs
- To abstain from alcohol if drug is prescribed for hyperlipidemia
- To avoid sunlight if skin lesions are present

nicardipine (℞)

(nye-card'i-peen)
Cardene, Cardene SR
Func. class.: Calcium channel blocker
Chem. class.: Dihydropyridine

Action: Inhibits calcium ion influx across cell membrane during cardiac depolarization; produces relaxation of coronary vascular smooth muscle, peripheral vascular smooth muscle; dilates coronary vascular arteries; increases myocardial oxygen delivery in patients with vasospastic angina

Uses: Chronic stable angina pectoris, hypertension

Dosage and routes:

- *Adult:* PO 20 mg tid initially, may increase after 3 days (range 20-40 mg tid)

Available forms: Caps 20, 30 mg; caps SR 30, 45, 60 mg

Side effects/adverse reactions:

CV: Dysrhythmia, edema, ***CHF,*** bradycardia, hypotension, palpitations, ***MI, pulmonary edema***

GI: Nausea, vomiting, diarrhea, gastric upset, constipation, ***hepatitis,*** abdominal cramps

GU: Nocturia, polyuria, ***acute renal failure***

INTEG: Rash, pruritus, urticaria, photosensitivity, hair loss

CNS: Headache, fatigue, drowsiness, dizziness, anxiety, depression, weakness, insomnia, confusion, paresthesia, somnolence

OTHER: Blurred vision, flushing, nasal congestion, sweating, shortness of breath, gynecomastia, hyperglycemia, sexual difficulties

Contraindications: Sick sinus syndrome, 2nd or 3rd degree heart block, hypotension less than 90 mm Hg systolic, hypersensitivity

Precautions: CHF, hypotension, hepatic injury, pregnancy (C), lactation, children, renal disease, elderly

Pharmacokinetics:

PO: Onset 30 min, peak 1-2 hr, duration 8 hr

PO-SR: onset unknown, peak 2-6 hr, duration 10-12 hr half-life 2-5 hr

Metabolized by liver, excreted in urine (98% as metabolites)
Interactions:
• Increased effects of digitalis, neuromuscular blocking agents, theophylline
• Increased effects of nicardipine: cimetidine
NURSING CONSIDERATIONS
Assess:
• Cardiac status: B/P, pulse, respiration, ECG
Administer:
• ac, hs/on an empty stomach 1 hr ac or 2 or more hr pc
Evaluate:
• Therapeutic response: decreased anginal pain, decreased B/P
Teach patient/family:
• To avoid hazardous activities until stabilized on drug, dizziness is no longer a problem
• To limit caffeine consumption, no alcohol products
• To avoid OTC drugs unless directed by prescriber
• To comply in all areas of medical regimen: diet, exercise, stress reduction, drug therapy
• To notify prescriber of irregular heart beat, shortness of breath, swelling of feet and hands, pronounced dizziness, constipation, nausea, hypotension
Treatment of overdose: Defibrillation, β-agonists, IV Ca, diuretics, atropine for AV block, vasopressor for hypotension

niclosamide (℞)
(ni-kloe'sa-mide)
Niclocide
Func. class.: Anthelmintic
Chem. class.: Salicylanilide derivative

Action: Inhibits synthesis of ATP in mitochondria; leads to destruction in intestine, where worm may be digested, removed in feces; not effective for ova or larval stage
Uses: Regular, dwarf tapeworms
Dosage and routes:
• *Adult:* PO 2 g chewed as a single dose for *T. saginata* and *D. latum;* 2 g × 7 days for *Hymenolepis nana*
• *Child >34 kg:* PO 1.5 g chewed as a single dose for *T. saginata* and *D. latum;* 1.5 g as single dose on day 1 followed by 1 g × 6 days for *H. nana*
• *Child <34 kg:* PO 1 g chewed as a single dose for *T. saginata* and *D. latum;* 1 g on day 1, then 0.5 g × 6 days for *H. nana*
Available forms: Tabs, chewable 500 mg
Side effects/adverse reactions:
INTEG: Rash, pruritus, pruritus ani, alopecia
CNS: Dizziness, headache, drowsiness, restlessness, sweating, fever
EENT: Bad taste, oral irritation
GI: Nausea, vomiting, anorexia, diarrhea, constipation, rectal bleeding
Contraindications: Hypersensitivity
Precautions: Child <2 yr, pregnancy (B), lactation
NURSING CONSIDERATIONS
Assess:
• Stools during entire treatment, 1, 3 mo after treatment; specimens must be sent to lab while still warm
• For allergic reaction: rash, itching in anal area
• For diarrhea during expulsion of worms
• For infection in other family members; infection from person to person is common
Administer:
• May be crushed, mixed with water if unable to swallow whole
• Laxatives if constipated; not needed for drug to work

N

• After breakfast; tab must be chewed, not swallowed whole

Perform/provide:

• Storage in tight, light-resistant container in cool environment; do not freeze

Evaluate:

• Therapeutic response: expulsion of worms, 3 negative stool cultures after completion of treatment

Teach patient/family:

• Proper hygiene after stool, including hand-washing technique; tell patient to avoid putting fingers in mouth

• That infected person should sleep alone; do not shake bed linen; change bed linen qd; wash in hot water

• To clean toilet qd; with disinfectant (green soap solution)

• Need for compliance with dosage schedule, duration of treatment

• To drink fruit juice to remove mucus that intestinal tapeworms burrow in; aids in explusion of worms (dwarf tapeworms only)

Treatment of overdose: Enemas, laxatives; do not induce vomiting

nicotine resin complex (℞)

(nik'o-teen)

Nicorette, Nicorette DS

Func. class.: Smoking deterrent

Chem. class.: Ganglionic cholinergic agonist

Action: Agonist at nicotinic receptors in peripheral, central nervous systems; acts at sympathetic ganglia; on chemoreceptors of aorta, carotid bodies; also affects adrenalin-releasing catecholamines

Uses: Deter cigarette smoking

Dosage and routes:

• *Adult:* Gum 1 piece chewed × ½ hr as needed to abstain from smoking, not to exceed 30/day

Available forms: Gum 2 mg/piece

Side effects/adverse reactions:

RESP: Breathing difficulty, cough, hoarseness, sneezing, wheezing

EENT: Jaw ache, irritation in buccal cavity

CNS: Dizziness, vertigo, insomnia, headache, confusion, convulsions, depression, euphoria, numbness, tinnitus

GI: Nausea, vomiting, anorexia, indigestion, diarrhea, abdominal pain, constipation, eructation

CV: Dysrhythmias, tachycardia, palpitations, edema, flushing, hypertension

Contraindications: Hypersensitivity, immediate post MI recovery period, severe angina pectoris, pregnancy (X)

Precautions: Vasospastic disease, dysrhythmias, diabetes mellitus, children, hyperthyroidism, pheochromocytoma, coronary disease, esophagitis, peptic ulcer, lactation, children, hepatic/renal disease

Pharmacokinetics:

Onset 15-30 min, metabolized in liver, excreted in urine, half-life 2-3 hr, 30-120 hr (terminal)

Interactions:

• Decreased absorption: glutethimide

• Increased absorption: SC insulin

• Decreased metabolism of propoxyphene

• Smoking cessation increases diuretic effects of furosemide

• Increased blood levels with cessation of smoking: caffeine, theophylline, petazocine, imipramine, oxazepam, propranolol, acetaminophen

NURSING CONSIDERATIONS

Assess:

• Adverse reaction: irritation of buccal cavity, dislike of taste, jaw ache

* Available in Canada only

Evaluate:
- Therapeutic response: decrease in urge to smoke, decreased need for gum after 3-6 mo

Teach patient/family:
- To chew gum slowly for 30 min to promote buccal absorption of the drug; do not chew over 45 min
- To begin drug withdrawal after 3 mo use; not to exceed 6 mo
- All aspects of drug; give package insert to patient and explain
- That gum will not stick to dentures, dental appliances
- That gum is as toxic as cigarette; to be used only to deter smoking
- Not to use during pregnancy; birth defects may occur

nicotine transdermal system (℞)

Habitrol, Nicoderm, Nicotrol, Prostep

Func. class.: Smoking deterrent

Chem. class.: Ganglionic cholinergic agonist

Action: Binds to acetylcholine receptors at autonomic ganglia in the adrenal medulla, at neuromuscular junctions, in brain

Uses: Deter cigarette smoking

Dosage and routes:
- *Nicotrol:* 15 mg/day × 12 wk; 10 mg/day × 2 wk; 5 mg/day × 2 wk
- *Prostep:* 22 mg/day × 4-8 wk; 11 mg/day × 2-4 wk

Available forms: Transdermal patch delivering 7, 14, 21 mg, 15 mg, 10 mg, 5 mg, 22 mg, & 11 mg/day depending on product

Side effects/adverse reactions:

RESP: Cough, pharyngitis, sinusitis

MISC: Back pain, chest pain

INTEG: Erythema, pruritus, burning at application site, cutaneous hypersensitivity, sweating, rash

GI: Diarrhea, dyspepsia, constipation, nausea, abdominal pain, vomiting

MS: Arthralgia, myalgia

EENT: Dry mouth, abnormal taste

CNS: Abnormal dreams, insomnia, nervousness, headache, dizziness, paresthesia

Contraindications: Hypersensitivity, children, pregnancy (D), nonsmokers, immediate postmyocardial infarction period, life-threatening dysrhythmias, severe or worsening angina pectoris

Precautions: Skin disease, angina pectoris, MI, renal or hepatic insufficiency, peptic ulcer, accelerated hypertension, serious cardiac dysrhythmias, hyperthyroidism, pheochromocytoma, insulin-dependent diabetes, elderly

Pharmacokinetics:

Half-life 3-4 hr, protein binding <5%, 30% is excreted unchanged in urine

Interactions:
- Decreased absorption: glutethimide
- Decreased dose at cessation of smoking: acetaminophen, caffeine, imipramine, oxazepam, pentazocine, propranolol, theophylline, insulin, adrenergic antagonists
- Increased dose at cessation of smoking: adrenergic agonists
- Decreased metabolism of propoxyphene
- Increased diuretic effects of furosemide
- Increased absorption: SC insulin

NURSING CONSIDERATIONS

Assess:
- Adverse reactions: irritation, pruritus, burning at patch site

Perform/provide:
- Storage below 86° F (30° C)

N

Evaluate:

- Therapeutic response: decrease in urge to smoke, absence of nicotine withdrawal symptoms

Teach patient/family:

- All aspects of drug; give package insert to patient and explain
- That patch is as toxic as cigarettes; to be used only to deter smoking
- Not to use during pregnancy; birth defects may occur
- To keep used and unused system out of reach of children and pets
- To apply once a day to a nonhairy, clean, dry area of skin on upper body or upper outer arm
- To stop smoking immediately on beginning patch treatment
- To apply promptly after removing from protective patch; system may lose strength

nifedipine (℞)

(nye-fed'i-peen)

Adalat, Adalat CC, Adalat P.A.*, Apo-Nifed*, nifedipine, Novo-Nifedin*, Nu N. Sed*, Procardia, Procardia XL

Func. class.: Calcium-channel blocker

Chem. class.: Dihydropyridine

Action: Inhibits calcium ion influx across cell membrane during cardiac depolarization; relaxes coronary vascular smooth muscle; dilates coronary arteries; increases myocardial oxygen delivery in patients with vasospastic angina; dilates peripheral arteries

Uses: Chronic stable angina pectoris, vasospastic angina, hypertension (sus rel only)

Investigational uses: Hypertension (acute), migraines, CHF, Raynaud's disease

Dosage and routes:

- *Adult PO immediate release:* 10 mg tid, increase in 10 mg increments q4-6h, not to exceed 180 mg/24h or single dose of 30 mg
- *Adult PO sus rel:* 30-60 mg/qd, may increase q7-14d, doses >120 mg not recommended

Available forms: Caps 5*, 10, 20 mg; tabs sus rel 30, 60, 90 mg

Side effects/adverse reactions:

CNS: Headache, fatigue, drowsiness, dizziness, anxiety, depression, weakness, insomnia, light-headedness, paresthesia, tinnitus, blurred vision, nervousness

CV: Dysrhythmias, edema, ***CHF,*** hypotension, palpitations, ***MI, pulmonary edema,*** tachycardia

GI: Nausea, vomiting, diarrhea, gastric upset, constipation, increased liver function studies, dry mouth

GU: Nocturia, polyuria

INTEG: Rash, pruritus, flushing, photosensitivity, hair loss

MISC: Flushing, sexual difficulties, cough, fever, chills

Contraindications: Hypersensitivity

Precautions: CHF, hypotension, sick sinus syndrome, 2nd or 3rd degree heart block, hypotension less than 90 mm Hg systolic, hepatic injury, pregnancy (C), lactation, children, renal disease

Pharmacokinetics:

Well absorbed PO

PO-SR: Duration 24 hr

PO: Onset 20 min, peak 0.5-6 hr, duration 6-8 hr, half-life 2-5 hr

Metabolized by liver, excreted in urine (98% as metabolites)

Interactions:

- Increased effects of theophylline, β-blockers, antihypertensives, digitalis
- Increased nifedipine level: cimetidine
- Decreased effects: quinidine

* Available in Canada only

NURSING CONSIDERATIONS
Assess:
• Cardiac status: B/P, pulse, respiration, ECG
Administer:
• SL: Use sterile needle to puncture liquid capsules, squeeze into buccal area
• Before meals, hs
Evaluate:
• Therapeutic response: decreased anginal pain, B/P, activity tolerance
Teach patient/family:
• To avoid hazardous activities until stabilized on drug, dizziness is no longer a problem
• To limit caffeine consumption; no alcohol products
• To avoid OTC drugs unless directed by a prescriber
• To comply with all areas of medical regimen: diet, exercise, stress reduction, drug therapy
• To change position slowly; orthostatic hypotension is common
• Not to chew, divide, or crush sus rel tablets
• To notify prescriber of dyspnea, edema of extremities, nausea, vomiting, severe ataxia
Treatment of overdose: Defibrillation, atropine for AV block, vasopressor for hypotension

nitrofurantoin (℞)

(nye-troe-fyoor'an toyn)
Apo-Nitrofurantoin*, Furadantin, Furalan, Macpac, Macrobid, Macrodantin, Nephronex*, Nitrofuracot, Nitrofurantoin, Novofuran*

Func. class.: Urinary tract anti-infective

Chem. class.: Synthetic nitrofuran derivative

Action: Appears to inhibit bacterial enzymes

Uses: Urinary tract infections caused by *E. coli, Klebsiella, Pseudomonas, P. vulgaris, P. morganii, Serratia, Citrobacter, S. aureus, S. epidermidis, Enterococcus, Salmonella, Shigella*
Dosage and routes:
• *Adult and child >12 yr:* PO 50-100 mg qid pc or 50-100 mg hs for long-term treatment
• *Child 1 mo-3 yr:* PO 5-7 mg/kg/day in 4 divided doses; 1-3 mg/kg/day for long-term treatment
Available forms: Caps 25, 50, 100 mg; tabs 50, 100 mg; susp 25 mg/5 ml; ext rel cap 100 mg; Macrocrystal cap 25, 50, 100 mg
Side effects/adverse reactions:
INTEG: Pruritus, rash, urticaria, angioedema, alopecia, tooth staining
CNS: Dizziness, headache, drowsiness, peripheral neuropathy
GI: Nausea, vomiting, abdominal pain, diarrhea, ***cholestatic jaundice***
Contraindications: Hypersensitivity, anuria, severe renal disease
Precautions: Pregnancy (B), lactation
Pharmacokinetics:
PO: Half-life 20-60 min; crosses blood-brain barrier, placenta; enters breast milk; excreted as inactive metabolites in liver
Interactions:
• Increased levels of nitrofurantoin: probenecid
• Antagonistic effect: nalidixic acid
• Decreased absorption of Mg trisilicate antacid
NURSING CONSIDERATIONS
Assess:
• Blood count during chronic therapy
• I&O ratio; urine pH <5.5 is ideal
• Renal and hepatic function
• CNS symptoms: insomnia, vertigo, headache, drowsiness, convulsions

- Allergy: fever, flushing, rash, urticaria, pruritus

Administer:

- After clean-catch urine for C&S
- Two daily doses if urine output is high or if patient has diabetes

Evaluate:

- Therapeutic response: decreased dysuria, fever

Teach patient/family:

- To take with food or milk
- To protect susp from freezing and shake well before taking
- That drug may cause drowsiness; instruct client to seek aid in walking and other activities; advise client not to drive or operate machinery while on medication
- That diabetics should monitor blood glucose level
- That drug may turn urine rust-yellow to brown

nitrofurazone (topical) (℞)

(nye-troe-fyoor'a-zone)

Furacin, Nitrofurazone

Func. class.: Local antibacterial

Chem. class.: Synthetic nitrofuran

Action: A broad-spectrum, mostly bactericidal agent for aerobic, anaerobic gram-positive organisms; may interfere with enzyme systems needed for carbohydrate metabolism; antibacterial action

Uses: Adjunctive treatment in burns (2nd, 3rd degree), prevention of skin allograft rejection

Dosage and routes:

- *Adult and child:* TOP apply to affected area qd or qod

Available forms: Sol, oint (soluble dressing), cream 0.2%

Side effects/adverse reactions:

INTEG: Rash, urticaria, stinging, burning, superinfections, photosensitivity, local edema

GU: ***Renal toxicity***

Contraindications: Hypersensitivity, G6PD deficiency

Precautions: Pregnancy (C), lactation; superinfection may result in bacterial or fungal overgrowth

NURSING CONSIDERATIONS

Assess:

- Allergic reaction: burning, stinging, swelling, redness

Administer:

- Analgesic before application prn
- Enough medication to cover burns completely
- After cleansing debris from area before each application
- Using sterile technique

Perform/provide:

- Dry storage at room temp

Evaluate:

- Therapeutic response: development of granulation tissue

Teach patient/family:

- That drug may be used until grafting is possible
- To avoid sunlight, ultraviolet light
- To stop drug and notify prescriber if rash or irritation occurs

nitroglycerin (℞)

(nye-troe-gli'ser-in)

Nitro-Bid IV, nitroglycerin, Tridil, Nitrostat, Nitro-Bid Plateau Caps, Nitrocine Timecaps, Nitroglyn, Nitrong, Nitro-Bid, Nitrol, Deponit, Minitran, Nitrodisc, Nitro-Dur, nitroglycerin transdermal, Nitrocine, Transderm-Nitro, Nitrolingual, Nitrogard

Func. class.: Coronary vasodilator, antianginal

Chem. class.: Nitrate

Combination products: Nitrotym-

* Available in Canada only

Plus: nitroglycerin 2.5 mg, butabarbital 48 mg

Action: Decreases preload, afterload, which is responsible for decreasing left ventricular end-diastolic pressure, systemic vascular resistance, dilates coronary arteries, improves blood flow

Uses: Chronic stable angina pectoris, prophylaxis of angina pain, CHF associated with acute MI, controlled hypotension in surgical procedures

Dosage and routes:

• *Adult:* SL dissolve tablet under tongue when pain begins; may repeat q5min until relief occurs; take no more than 3 tabs/15 min; use 1 tab prophylactically 5-10 min before activities; SUS CAP q6-12h on empty stomach; TOP 1-2 in q8h, increase to 4 in q4h as needed; IV 5 μg/min, then increase by 5 μg/min q3-5min; if no response after 20 μg/min, increase by 10-20 μg/min until desired response; trans apply a pad qd to a site free of hair

Available forms: Buccal tabs 1, 2, 3 mg; aero 0.4 mg/meter spray; sus rel caps 2.5, 6.5, 9, 13 mg; tabs sus rel 2.6, 6.5, 9 mg; inj 0.5, 5, mg/ml; SL tabs 0.15, 0.3, 0.4, 0.6 mg; transdermal oint 2%; trans derm syst 0.1, 0.2, 0.3, 0.4, 0.6 mg/24 hr; inj sol 25 mg/250 ml, 50 mg/250 ml, 50 mg/500 ml, 100 mg/500 ml, 200 mg/500 ml

Side effects/adverse reactions:

CV: *Postural hypotension,* tachycardia, ***collapse,*** syncope

GI: Nausea, vomiting

INTEG: Pallor, sweating, rash

CNS: Headache, flushing, dizziness

Contraindications: Hypersensitivity to this drug or nitrites, severe anemia, increased intracranial pressure, cerebral hemorrhage

Precautions: Postural hypotension, pregnancy (C), lactation

Pharmacokinetics:

SUS REL: Onset 20-45 min, duration 3-8 hr

SL: Onset 1-3 min, duration 30 min

TRANS DER: Onset ½-1 hr, duration 12-24 hr

IV: Onset immediate, duration variable

TRANSMUC: Onset 3 min, duration 10-30 min

AEROSOL: Onset 2 min, duration 30-60 min

TOP OINT: Onset 30-60 min, duration 2-12 hr

Metabolized by liver, excreted in urine, half-life 1-4 min

Interactions:

• Increased effects: β-blockers, diuretics, antihypertensives, anticoagulants, alcohol

• Decreased heparin: IV nitroglycerin

Syringe compatibility: Heparin

Y-site compatibilities: Amiodarone, amrinone, atracurium, diltiazem, dobutamine, dopamine, famotidine, haloperidol, lidocaine, nitroprusside, pancuronium, ranitidine, streptokinase, vecuronium

N

NURSING CONSIDERATIONS

Assess:

• Orthostatic B/P, pulse

• Pain: duration, time started, activity being performed, character

• Tolerance if taken over long period of time

• Headache, light-headedness, decreased B/P; may indicate a need for decreased dosage

Administer:

• IV diluted in amount specified D_5 or NS for infusion; use glass infusion bottles, nonpolyvinyl chloride infusion tubing; titrate to patient response; do not use filters

• With 8 oz H_2O on empty stomach (oral tablet) 1 hr before or 2 hr after meals

• Trans tab should be placed between cheek and gum line
• Topical ointment should be measured on papers supplied
• Apply a new TD patch qd and remove after 12-14 hrs to prevent tolerance

Evaluate:
• Therapeutic response: decrease, prevention of anginal pain

Teach patient/family:
• To place buccal tab between lip and gum above incisors or between cheek and gum; sus rel must be swallowed whole, do not chew; SL should be dissolved under tongue, do not swallow; aerosol should be sprayed under tongue, do not inhale
• To use inhaler only when lying down
• Not to inhale spray
• To keep tabs in original container
• If 3 SL tabs in 15 min do not relieve pain, consider MI
• To avoid alcohol
• That drug may cause headache; tolerance usually develops; use nonnarcotic analgesic
• That drug may be taken before stressful activity: exercise, sexual activity
• That SL may sting when drug comes in contact with mucous membranes
• To avoid hazardous activities if dizziness occurs
• To comply with complete medical regimen
• To make position changes slowly to prevent fainting

nitroprusside (℞)

(nye-troe-pruss′ide)
Nitropress, sodium nitroprusside
Func. class.: Antihypertensive
Chem. class.: Peripheral vasodilator

Action: Directly relaxes arteriolar, venous smooth muscle, resulting in reduction in cardiac preload, afterload

Uses: Hypertensive crisis, to decrease bleeding by creating hypotension during surgery, acute CHF

Dosage and routes:
• *Adult:* IV INF dissolve 50 mg in 2-3 ml of D_5W, then dilute in 250-1000 ml of D_5W; run at 0.5-8 μg/kg/min

Available forms: Inj 50 mg

Side effects/adverse reactions:
GI: Nausea, vomiting, abdominal pain
CNS: Dizziness, headache, agitation, twitching, decreased reflexes, ***LOC,*** restlessness
EENT: Tinnitus, blurred vision
GU: Impotence
INTEG: Pain, irritation at injection site, sweating
CV: Palpitation, severe hypotension, dyspnea
MISC: Cyanide, thiocyanate toxicity

Contraindications: Hypersensitivity, hypertension (compensatory)

Precautions: Pregnancy (C), lactation, children, fluid, electrolyte imbalances, hepatic disease, renal disease, hypothyroidism, elderly

Pharmacokinetics:
IV: Onset 1-2 min, duration 1-10 min, half-life 4 days in patients with abnormal renal function; metabolized in liver, excreted in urine

Interactions:
• Severe hypotension: ganglionic

* Available in Canada only

blockers, volatile liquid anesthetics, halothane, enflurane, circulatory depressants

Syringe compatibility: Heparin

Y-site compatibilities: Amrinone, atracurium, dobutamine, dopamine, enalaprilat, famotidine, lidocaine, nitroglycerin, pancuronium, vecuronium

NURSING CONSIDERATIONS

Assess:

- Electrolytes: K, Na, Cl, CO_2, CBC, serum glucose, serum methemoglobin if pulmonary O_2 levels are decreased
- Renal function studies: catecholamines, BUN, creatinine
- Hepatic function studies: AST (SGOT), ALT (SGPT), alk phosphatase
- B/P by direct means if possible; check ECG continuously; pulse, jugular vein distention; PCWP
- Weight qd, I&O
- Thiocyanate, lactate, cyanide levels qd if on long-term treatment
- Nausea, vomiting, diarrhea
- Edema in feet, legs daily; skin turgor, dryness of mucous membranes for hydration status
- Rales, dyspnea, orthopnea q30 min
- For decrease in bicarbonate, Pco_2 blood pH, acidosis

Administer:

- Depending on B/P reading q15 min
- IV after diluting 50 mg/2-3 ml of D_5W, further dilute in 250 ml of D_5W; use an infusion pump only; wrap bottle with aluminum foil to protect from light; observe for color change in the infusion; discard if highly discolored (blue, green, dark red); titrate to patient response

Evaluate:

- Therapeutic response: decreased B/P, absence of bleeding

Teach patient/family:

- To report headache, dizziness, loss of hearing, blurred vision, dyspnea, faintness

Treatment of overdose: Administer amyl nitrite inhalation until 3% sodium nitrate solution can be prepared for IV administration, then inject sodium thiosulfate IV, correct drop in BP with vasopressor

nizatidine

(ni-za'ti-deen)

Axid

Func. class.: H_2-receptor antagonist

Chem. class.: Substituted thiazole

Action: Blocks H_2 receptors thereby reducing gastric acid output

Uses: Benign gastric and duodenal ulceration, prevention of duodenal ulcer recurrence, symptomatic relief of gastro-esophageal reflux

Dosage and routes:

Gastric and duodenal ulcer

- *Adult:* PO 300 mg at night or 150 mg bid for 4-8 weeks; maintenance 150 mg at night for up to 1 yr

Gastro-esophageal reflux

- *Adult:* PO 150-300 mg bid for up to 12 weeks

Available forms: Caps 150 mg, 300 mg

Side effects/adverse reactions:

CNS: Headache, somnolence, confusion, abnormal dreams, dizziness

ENDO: Gynecomastia

HEMA: ***Thrombocytopenia***

INTEG: Pruritus, sweating, urticaria, exfoliative dermatitis

MS: Myalgia

RESP: ***Bronchospasm, laryngeal edema***

METAB: Hyperuricemia

GI: Elevated liver enzymes, hepatitis, jaundice, nausea

N

CV: Cardiac dysrhythmias, ***cardiac arrest***
Contraindications: Hypersensitivity
Precautions: Renal or hepatic impairment (reduce dose in renal impairment), pregnancy (C), lactation
Pharmacokinetics: Partially metabolized by liver, excreted by kidney, plasma half-life 1½ hr, 70% absorbed orally, small amount (0.1% of plasma concentration) enters breast milk, 35% bound to plasma proteins
Assess:
- Gastric pH (>5 should be maintained)
- Fluid balance, I&O

Administer:
- With meals for prolonged drug effect; antacids 1 hr before or 1 hr after drug

Evaluate:
- Mental status, confusion, dizziness, depression, anxiety, weakness, tremors, psychosis, diarrhea, jaundice, report immediately
- For GI symptoms: nausea, vomiting, diarrhea, cramps

Teach patient/family:
- That gynecomastia, impotence may occur, are reversible
- Avoid driving or other hazardous activities until patient is stabilized on this medication; dizziness may occur
- To avoid black pepper, caffeine, alcohol, harsh spices, extremes in temp of food
- To avoid OTC preparations: aspirin, cough, cold preparations

Treatment of overdose: Symptomatic and supportive therapy is recommended; activated charcoal, emesis of lavage may reduce absorption

norepinephrine (℞)
(nor-ep-i-nef'rin)
Levarterenol, Levophed
Func. class.: Adrenergic
Chem. class.: Catecholamine

Action: Causes increased contractility and heart rate by acting on β-receptors in heart; also acts on α-receptors, causing vasoconstriction in blood vessels; B/P is elevated, coronary blood flow improves, cardiac output increases
Uses: Acute hypotension, shock
Dosage and routes:
- *Adult:* IV INF 8-12 μg/min titrated to B/P
- *Child:* IV INF 2 μg/min titrated to B/P

Available forms: Inj 1 mg/ml
Side effects/adverse reactions:
CNS: Headache, anxiety, dizziness, insomnia, restlessness, tremor
CV: Palpitations, tachycardia, hypertension, ectopic beats, angina
GI: Nausea, vomiting
INTEG: Necrosis, tissue sloughing with extravasation, ***gangrene***
RESP: Dyspnea
GU: Decreased urine output
Contraindications: Hypersensitivity, ventricular fibrillation, tachydysrhythmias, pheochromocytoma
Precautions: Lactation, arterial embolism, peripheral vascular disease, hypertension, hyperthyroidism, elderly, heart disease, pregnancy (C)
Pharmacokinetics:
IV: Onset 1-2 min; metabolized in liver; excreted in urine (inactive metabolites); crosses placenta
Interactions:
- Do not use within 2 wk of MAOIs, or hypertensive crisis may result
- Dysrhythmias: general anesthetics

* Available in Canada only

• Decreased action of norepinephrine: α-blockers
• Increased B/P: oxytocics
• Increased pressor effect: tricyclic antidepressant, MAOIs
• Incompatible with alkaline solutions: Na, HCO_3

NURSING CONSIDERATIONS

Assess:

• I&O ratio; notify prescriber if output <30 ml/hr
• ECG during administration continuously; if B/P increases, drug is decreased
• B/P and pulse q2-3min after parenteral route
• CVP or PWP during infusion if possible
• For paresthesias and coldness of extremities; peripheral blood flow may decrease
• Injection site: tissue sloughing; administer phentolamine mixed with 0.9% NaCl

Administer:

• Plasma expanders for hypovolemia
• IV after diluting with 500-1000 ml D_5W or D_5/0.9% NaCl; average dilution is 4 ml/1000 ml diluent; give as infusion 2-3 ml/min; titrate to response
• Using 2-bottle setup so drug may be discontinued while IV is still running; use infusion pump

Perform/provide:

• Storage of reconstituted sol if refrigerated no longer than 24 hr
• Do not use discolored sol

Evaluate:

• Therapeutic response: increased B/P with stabilization

Teach patient/family:

• Reason for drug administration and to report dyspnea, dizziness, chest pain

Treatment of overdose: Administer fluids, electrolyte replacement

norethindrone (℞)

(nor-eth-in′drone)

Micronor, Norlutin, Nor-QD

Func. class.: Progestogen

Chem. class.: Progesterone derivative

Action: Inhibits secretion of pituitary gonadotropins, which prevents follicular maturation, ovulation; stimulates growth of mammary tissue; antineoplastic action against endometrial cancer

Uses: Uterine bleeding (abnormal), amenorrhea, endometriosis

Dosage and routes:

• *Adult:* PO 5-20 mg qd days 5-25 of menstrual cycle

Endometriosis

• *Adult:* PO 10 mg qd × 2 wk, then increased by 5 mg qd × 2 wk, up to 30 mg qd

Available forms: Tabs 5 mg

Side effects/adverse reactions:

CNS: Dizziness, headache, migraines, depression, fatigue

CV: Hypotension, ***thrombophlebitis,*** edema, ***thromboembolism, stroke, pulmonary embolism, MI***

GI: Nausea, vomiting, anorexia, cramps, increased weight, ***cholestatic jaundice***

EENT: Diplopia

GU: Amenorrhea, cervical erosion, breakthrough bleeding, dysmenorrhea, vaginal candidiasis, breast changes, (gynecomastia, testicular atrophy, impotence), endometriosis, ***spontaneous abortion***

INTEG: Rash, urticaria, acne, hirsutism, alopecia, oily skin, seborrhea, purpura, melasma

META: Hyperglycemia

Contraindications: Breast cancer, hypersensitivity, thromboembolic disorders, reproductive cancer, geni-

tal bleeding (abnormal, undiagnosed), pregnancy (X)
Precautions: Lactation, hypertension, asthma, blood dyscrasias, gallbladder disease, CHF, diabetes mellitus, bone disease, depression, migraine headache, convulsive disorders, hepatic disease, renal disease, family history of breast or reproductive tract cancer
Pharmacokinetics:
PO: Duration 24 hr, excreted in urine, feces, metabolized in liver
Lab test interferences:
Increase: Alk phosphatase, nitrogen (urine), pregnanediol, amino acids, factors VII, VIII, IX, X
Decrease: GTT, HDL
NURSING CONSIDERATIONS
Assess:
• Weight qd: notify prescriber of weekly weight gain >5 lb
• B/P at beginning of treatment and periodically
• I&O ratio; be alert for decreasing urinary output, increasing edema
• Liver function studies: ALT (SGPT), AST (SGOT), bilirubin, periodically during long-term therapy
• Edema, hypertension, cardiac symptoms, jaundice
• Mental status: affect, mood, behavioral changes, depression
• Hypercalcemia
Administer:
• Titrated dose; use lowest effective dose
• Oil solution deep in large muscle mass (IM), rotate sites
• In one dose in AM
• With food or milk to decrease GI symptoms
• After warming to dissolve crystals
Perform/provide:
• Storage in dark area
Evaluate:
• Therapeutic response: decreased abnormal uterine bleeding, absence of amenorrhea
Teach patient/family:
• About cushingoid symptoms
• To report breast lumps, vaginal bleeding, edema, jaundice, dark urine, clay-colored stools, dyspnea, headache, blurred vision, abdominal pain, numbness or stiffness in legs, chest pain; male to report impotence or gynecomastia
• To report suspected pregnancy

---

norfloxacin (℞)

(nor-flox'-a-sin)
Chibroxin, Noroxin
Func. class.: Urinary antiinfective
Chem. class.: Fluoroquinolone antibacterial

Action: Interferes with conversion of intermediate DNA fragments into high-molecular-weight DNA in bacteria, inhibits DNA gyrase
Uses: Adult urinary tract infections (including complicated) caused by *E. coli, E. cloacae, P. mirabilis, K. pneumoniae,* group D strep, indole-positive *Proteus, C. freundii, S. aureus;* uncomplicated gonorrhea, ocular infection
Dosage and routes:
Uncomplicated infections
• *Adult:* PO 400 mg bid × 7-10 days 1 hr before or 2 hr after meals
Complicated infections
• *Adult:* PO 400 mg bid × 10-21 days; 400 mg qd × 7-10 days in impaired renal function
Uncomplicated gonorrhea
• *Adult:* PO 800 mg as a single dose
Ocular infection
• *Adult, child:* OPHTH 1 gtt qid, may increase to 1 gtt q2hr for severe infections

* Available in Canada only

Available forms: Tabs 400 mg; ophth sol 3 mg/ml
Side effects/adverse reactions:
CNS: Headache, dizziness, fatigue, somnolence, depression, insomnia
GI: Nausea, constipation, increased ALT (SGPT), AST (SGOT), flatulence, heartburn, vomiting, diarrhea, dry mouth
INTEG: Rash
EENT: Visual disturbances
Contraindications: Hypersensitivity to quinolones
Precautions: Pregnancy (C), lactation, children, renal disease, seizure disorders
Pharmacokinetics:
Peak 1 hr, half-life 3-4 hr; steady state 2 days; excreted in urine as active drug, metabolites
Lab test interferences:
Increase: AST (SGOT), ALT (SGPT), BUN, creatinine, alk phosphatase

NURSING CONSIDERATIONS
Assess:
- Kidney, liver function studies: BUN, creatinine, AST (SGOT), ALT (SGPT)
- I&O ratio, urine pH; <5.5 is ideal
- CNS symptoms: insomnia, vertigo, headache, agitation, confusion
- Allergic reactions: fever, flushing, rash, urticaria, pruritus

Administer:
- After clean-catch urine for C&S
- Two daily doses if urine output is high or if patient has diabetes

Perform/provide:
- Limited intake of alkaline foods, drugs: milk, dairy products, peanuts, vegetables, alkaline antacids, sodium bicarbonate

Evaluate:
- Therapeutic response: decreased pain, frequency, urgency C&S, absence of infection

Teach patient/family:
- Fluid intake must be 3 L/day to avoid crystallization in kidneys
- If dizziness occurs, to walk, perform activities with assistance
- Complete full course of drug therapy
- To contact prescriber if adverse reaction occurs
- To take 1 hr before or 2 hr after meals; not to take antacids with or within 2 hr of this drug; to sip water or use hard candy for dry mouth

norgestrel (℞)
(nor-jess'trel)
Ovrette, Ovral*
Func. class.: Progestogen
Chem. class.: Progesterone derivative

Action: Inhibits secretion of pituitary gonadotropins, which prevents follicular maturation, ovulation, stimulates growth of mammary tissue, antineoplastic action against endometrial cancer
Uses: Female contraception
Dosage and routes:
- *Adult:* PO 1 tablet qd

Available forms: Tabs 0.35, 0.075 mg
Side effects/adverse reactions:
CNS: Dizziness, headache, migraines, depression, fatigue
CV: Hypotension, ***thrombophlebitis,*** edema, ***thromboembolism, stroke, pulmonary embolism, myocardial infarction***
GI: Nausea, vomiting, anorexia, cramps, increased weight, ***cholestatic jaundice***
EENT: Diplopia
GU: Amenorrhea, cervical erosion, breakthrough bleeding, dysmenorrhea, vaginal candidiasis, breast changes, *gynecomastia, testicular at-*

N

rophy, impotence, endometriosis, ***spontaneous abortion***

INTEG: Rash, urticaria, acne, hirsutism, alopecia, oily skin, seborrhea, purpura, melasma

META: Hyperglycemia

Contraindications: Breast cancer, hypersensitivity, thromboembolic disorders, reproductive cancer, genital bleeding (abnormal, undiagnosed), cerebral hemorrhage, pregnancy (X)

Precautions: Lactation, hypertension, asthma, blood dyscrasias, gallbladder disease, CHF, diabetes mellitus, bone disease, depression, migraine headache, convulsive disorders, hepatic disease, renal disease, family history of breast or reproductive tract cancer

Pharmacokinetics:

PO: Duration 24 hr; excreted in urine, feces; metabolized in liver

Lab test interferences:

Increase: Alk phosphatase, nitrogen (urine), pregnanediol, amino acids, factors VII, VIII, IX, X

Decrease: GTT, HDL

NURSING CONSIDERATIONS

Assess:

- Weight qd; notify prescriber of weekly weight gain >5 lb
- B/P at beginning of treatment and periodically
- I&O ratio; be alert for decreasing urinary output, increasing edema
- Liver function studies: ALT (SGPT), AST (SGOT), bilirubin, periodically during long-term therapy
- Edema, hypertension, cardiac symptoms, jaundice
- Mental status: affect, mood, behavioral changes, depression
- Hypercalcemia

Administer:

- Titrated dose; use lowest effective dose
- Oil solution deep in large muscle mass (IM); rotate sites
- In one dose in AM
- With food or milk to decrease GI symptoms
- After warming to dissolve crystals

Perform/provide:

- Storage in dark area

Evaluate:

- Therapeutic response: absence of pregnancy

Teach patient/family:

- About cushingoid symptoms
- To report breast lumps, vaginal bleeding, edema, jaundice, dark urine, clay-colored stools, dyspnea, headache, blurred vision, abdominal pain, numbness or stiffness in legs, chest pain
- To report suspected pregnancy
- To monitor blood sugar if diabetic

nortriptyline (℞)

(nor-trip'ti-leen)

Aventyl, Pamelor

Func. class.: Antidepressant—tricyclic

Chem. class.: Dibenzocycloheptene—secondary amine

Action: Blocks reuptake of norepinephrine, serotonin into nerve endings, increasing action of norepinephrine, serotonin in nerve cells

Uses: Major depression

Investigational uses: Chronic pain management

Dosage and routes:

- *Adult:* PO 25 mg tid or qid; may increase to 150 mg/day; may give daily dose hs

Available forms: Caps 10, 25, 50, 75 mg; sol 10 mg/5 ml

Side effects/adverse reactions:

HEMA: ***Agranulocytosis, thrombocytopenia, eosinophilia, leukopenia***

CNS: Dizziness, drowsiness, confusion, headache, anxiety, tremors, stimulation, weakness, insomnia, nightmares, EPS (elderly), increased psychiatric symptoms
GI: Constipation, dry mouth, nausea, vomiting, ***paralytic ileus,*** increased appetite, cramps, epigastric distress, jaundice, ***hepatitis,*** stomatitis
GU: Retention, ***acute renal failure***
INTEG: Rash, urticaria, sweating, pruritus, photosensitivity
CV: Orthostatic hypotension, ECG changes, tachycardia, ***hypertension,*** palpitations
EENT: Blurred vision, tinnitus, mydriasis

Contraindications: Hypersensitivity to tricyclic antidepressants, recovery phase of MI, convulsive disorders, prostatic hypertrophy

Precautions: Suicidal patients, severe depression, increased intraocular pressure, narrow-angle glaucoma, urinary retention, cardiac disease, hepatic disease, hyperthyroidism, electroshock therapy, elective surgery, pregnancy (C), lactation

Pharmacokinetics:
PO: Steady state 4-19 days; metabolized by liver; excreted by kidneys; crosses placenta; excreted in breast milk; half-life 18-28 hr

Interactions:
- Decreased effects of guanethidine, clonidine, indirect-acting sympathomimetics (ephedrine)
- Increased effects of direct-acting sympathomimetics (epinephrine), alcohol, barbiturates, benzodiazepines, CNS depressants
- Hyperpyretic crisis, convulsions, hypertensive episode: MAOI

Lab test interferences:
Increase: Serum bilirubin, blood glucose, alk phosphatase
False increase: Urinary catecholamines
Decrease: VMA, 5-HIAA

NURSING CONSIDERATIONS

Assess:
- B/P (lying, standing), pulse q4h; if systolic B/P drops 20 mm Hg, hold drug, notify prescriber; take vital signs q4h in patients with cardiovascular disease
- Blood studies: CBC, leukocytes, differential, cardiac enzymes if patient is receiving long-term therapy
- Hepatic studies: AST (SGOT), ALT (SGPT), bilirubin
- Weight qwk; appetite may increase with drug
- ECG for flattening of T wave, bundle branch block, AV block, dysrhythmias in cardiac patients
- EPS primarily in elderly: rigidity, dystonia, akathisia
- Mental status changes: mood, sensorium, affect, suicidal tendencies, increase in psychiatric symptoms, depression, panic
- Urinary retention, constipation; constipation is more likely to occur in children
- Withdrawal symptoms: headache, nausea, vomiting, muscle pain, weakness; do not usually occur unless drug was discontinued abruptly
- Alcohol intake; if alcohol is consumed, hold dose until AM

Administer:
- Increased fluids, bulk in diet if constipation occurs
- With food, milk for GI symptoms
- Dosage hs for oversedation during day; may take entire dose hs; elderly may not tolerate once/day dosing
- Gum, hard candy, frequent sips of water for dry mouth
- Concentrate with fruit juice, water, or milk to disguise taste

Perform/provide:
• Storage in tight, light-resistant container at room temp
• Assistance with ambulation during beginning therapy, since drowsiness/dizziness occurs
• Safety measures including side rails, primarily for elderly
• Checking to see PO medication swallowed

Evaluate:
• Therapeutic response: decreased depression

Teach patient/family:
• That therapeutic effects may take 2-3 wk
• To use caution in driving, other activities requiring alertness because of drowsiness, dizziness, blurred vision
• To avoid alcohol ingestion, other CNS depressants
• Not to discontinue medication quickly after long-term use; may cause nausea, headache, malaise
• To wear sunscreen or large hat, since photosensitivity occurs

Treatment of overdose: ECG monitoring; induce emesis; lavage, activated charcoal; administer anticonvulsant

---

nystatin (℞)

(nye-stat'in)
Mycostatin, Mycostatin Pastilles, Nadostine*, nystatin
Func. class.: Antifungal
Chem. class.: Amphoteric polyene

Action: Interferes with fungal DNA replication; binds sterols in fungal cell membrane, which increases permeability, leaking of cell nutrients

Uses: *Candida* species causing oral, vaginal, intestinal infections

Dosage and routes:

Oral infection
• *Adult:* SUSP 400,000-600,000 U qid
• *Child and infants >3 mo:* SUSP 250,000-500,000 U qid
• *Newborn and premature infants:* SUSP 100,000 U qid

GI infection
• *Adult:* PO 500,000-1,000,000 U tid

Available forms: Tabs 500,000 U; powder 50 million, 150 million, 500 million, 1 billion, 2 billion, 5 billion U; susp 100,000 U

Side effects/adverse reactions:
INTEG: Rash, urticaria (rare)
GI: Nausea, vomiting, anorexia, diarrhea, cramps

Contraindications: Hypersensitivity

Precautions: Pregnancy (B)

Pharmacokinetics:
PO: Little absorption, excreted in feces

NURSING CONSIDERATIONS

Assess:
• For allergic reaction: rash, urticaria; drug may have to be discontinued
• For predisposing factors: antibiotic therapy, pregnancy, diabetes mellitus, sexual partner infection (vaginal infections)

Administer:
• Oral susp dose by placing ½ in each cheek, then swallow
• Topical dose after cleansing area; mouth may be swabbed

Perform/provide:
• Storage in refrigerator for oral susp; tabs in tight, light-resistant containers at room temp

Evaluate:
• Therapeutic response: culture negative for *Candida*

Teach patient/family:
• That long-term therapy may be

---

* Available in Canada only

needed to clear infection; to complete entire course of medication
• Proper hygiene: changing socks if feet are infected; using no commercial mouthwashes for mouth infection
• To avoid getting preparation on hands
• To wear light-day pad for vaginal preparations
• To avoid tight shoes, bandages when using on feet
• To avoid sexual contact during treatment to minimize reinfection
• To notify prescriber of irritation; drug may have to be discontinued
• That relief from itching may occur after 24-72 hr

nystatin (topical) (℞)

(nye-stat'in)
Mycostatin, Nadastine*, Nilstat, Nystatin, Nyoderm*, Nystex, O-V Statin
Func. class.: Local antiinfective
Chem. class.: Antifungal

Action: Interferes with fungal DNA replication; binds sterols in fungal cell membrane, which increases permeability, leaking of cell nutrients
Uses: Cutaneous vulvovaginal candidiasis, vaginal mucocutaneous fungal infections, infant eczema, pruritis ani and vulvae
Dosage and routes:
• *Adult and child:* TOP apply to affected area bid-tid × 14 days; vag 1-2 tabs (100,000 U each) inserted into vagina
Available forms: Cream, oint, powder, spray, vag tabs 100,000 U; vag cream, lotion 2%
Side effects/adverse reactions:
INTEG: Rash, urticaria, stinging, burning
Contraindications: Hypersensitivity
Precautions: Pregnancy (B), lactation

NURSING CONSIDERATIONS
Assess:
• Allergic reaction: burning, stinging, swelling, redness
• For predisposing *Candida* infection; antibiotic therapy, pregnancy, diabetes mellitus, sexual partner infection (vag infection), AIDS
Administer:
• To moist lesions with a swab
• Vaginal tablets by inserting high into vagina with applicator provided
• Enough medication to cover lesions completely
• In gravid client 3-6 wk before term to decrease candidiasis in the newborn
• After cleansing with soap, water before each application; dry well
Perform/provide:
• Storage at room temp; protect from light, air, heat, damp
Evaluate:
• Therapeutic response: decrease in size, number of lesions, decreased itching, white patches on vulva
Teach patient/family:
• To discontinue use and notify prescriber if irritation occurs
• To apply with glove to prevent further infection; drug may stain, pads may protect clothing
• Not to use occlusive dressings
• To avoid use of OTC creams, ointments, lotions unless directed by prescriber
• To use asepsis (hand washing) before, after application
• To complete treatment regimen

ofloxacin (℞)

(o-flox'a-sin)

Floxin, Floxin IV, Occuflox

Func. class.: Antiinfective

Chem. class.: Fluoroquinolone

Action: Interferes with conversion of intermediate DNA fragments into high-molecular-weight DNA in bacteria, inhibits DNA gyrase

Uses: Treatment of lower respiratory tract infections (pneumonia, bronchitis), genitourinary infections (prostatitis, UTIs) caused by *E. coli, K. pneumoniae, C. trachomatis, N. gonorrhoeae;* skin and skin structure infections; conjunctivitis (ophth)

Dosage and routes:

Lower respiratory tract infections/ skin and skin structure infections

• *Adult:* PO, IV 400 mg q12h × 10 days

Cervicitis, urethritis

• *Adult:* PO, IV 300 mg q12h × 7 days

Prostatitis

• *Adult:* PO, IV 300 mg q12h × 6 wk

Acute, uncomplicated gonorrhea

• *Adult:* PO, IV 400 mg as a single dose

Conjunctivitis

• *Adult, child:* OPHTH 1-2 gtt q2-4hr × 2 days, then qid × 5 days

Available forms: Tabs 200, 300, 400 mg; 4 mg/ml (IV); ophth sol 0.3%

Side effects/adverse reactions:

CNS: Dizziness, headache, fatigue, somnolence, depression, insomnia, lethargy, malaise

GI: Diarrhea, nausea, vomiting, anorexia, flatulence, heartburn, dry mouth, increased AST (SGOT), ALT (SGPT), abdominal pain, constipation

INTEG: Rash, pruritus

EENT: Visual disturbances

Contraindications: Hypersensitivity to quinolones

Precautions: Pregnancy (C), lactation, children, elderly, renal disease, seizure disorders, excessive sunlight

Pharmacokinetics:

PO: Peak 1-2 hr, half-life 9 hr, steady state 2 days; excreted in urine as active drug, metabolites; 90%-95%, bioavailability

Interactions:

• Decreased effects of ofloxacin: antacids, nitrofurantoin, sucralfate, iron salts, zinc salts

• Increased ofloxacin levels: probenecid

• Increased effects of warfarin, cyclosporine

NURSING CONSIDERATIONS

Assess:

• Kidney, liver function studies: BUN, creatinine, AST (SGOT), ALT (SGPT)

• I&O ratio; urine pH <5.5 is ideal

• CNS symptoms: insomnia, vertigo, headache, agitation, confusion

• Allergic reactions: rash, flushing, urticaria, pruritus

Administer:

• After clean-catch urine for C&S

Perform/provide:

• Limited intake of alkaline foods, drugs; milk, dairy products, peanuts, vegetables, alkaline antacids, sodium bicarbonate

Evaluate:

• Therapeutic response; negative C&S; absence of redness, swelling (ophth)

Teach patient/family:

• That fluid intake must be 3L/day to avoid crystallization in kidneys

• That if dizziness or light-headedness occurs, ambulate, perform activities with assistance

• To complete full course of therapy

• To notify prescriber of adverse reactions

• To avoid iron- or mineral-containing supplements within 2 hr before or after dose

olsalazine (℞)

(ohl-sal'ah-zeen)

Dipentum

Func. class.: Antiinflammatory

Chem. class.: Salicylate derivative

Action: Bioconverted to 5-aminosalicylic acid, which decreases inflammation

Uses: Maintenance of remission of ulcerative colitis in patients intolerant to sulfasalazine

Dosage and routes:

• *Adult:* PO 1 g/day in 2 divided doses

Available forms: Tabs 250 mg

Side effects/adverse reactions:

EENT: Dry mouth, dry eyes, watery eyes, blurred vision

SYST: ***Anaphylaxis***

GI: Nausea, vomiting, abdominal pain, stomatitis, hepatitis, pancreatitis, diarrhea, bloating

CNS: Headache, insomnia, hallucinations, depression, vertigo, fatigue, drug fever, chills, dizziness, drowsiness, tremors

HEMA: ***Leukopenia, neutropenia, thrombocytopenia, agranulocytosis, anemia***

INTEG: Rash, dermatitis, urticaria, ***Stevens-Johnson syndrome,*** erythema, photosensitivity, alopecia

GU: Frequency, dysuria, hematuria, impotence

CV: Allergic myocarditis, 2nd degree heart block, hypertension, peripheral edema, chest pain, palpitations

RESP: ***Bronchospasm,*** shortness of breath

Contraindications: Hypersensitivity to salicylates

Precautions: Pregnancy (C), child <14 yr, lactation, impaired hepatic renal function, severe allergy, bronchial asthma

Pharmacokinetics:

PO: Partially absorbed, peak 1½ hr, half-life 5-10 hr, excreted in urine as 5-aminosalicylic acid and metabolites, crosses placenta

Lab test interferences:

False positive: Urinary glucose test

NURSING CONSIDERATIONS

Assess:

• I&O ratio: note color, character, pH of urine in treatment for UTIs; output should be 800 ml less than intake; if urine is highly acidic, alkalization may be needed

• Kidney function studies: BUN, creatinine, urinalysis (long-term therapy)

• Blood dyscrasias: skin rash, fever, sore throat, bruising, bleeding, fatigue, joint pain

• Allergic reaction: rash, dermatitis, urticaria, pruritus, dyspnea, bronchospasm

Administer:

• With food in evenly divided doses

• Medication after C&S; repeat C&S after full course of medication

• With resuscitative equipment available; severe allergic reactions may occur

• Total daily dose evenly spaced to minimize GI intolerance

Perform/provide:

• Storage in tight, light-resistant container at room temp

Evaluate:

• Therapeutic response: absence of fever, mucus in stools

omeprazole (℞)

(om-ee-pray'zole)

Losec*, Prilosec

Func. class.: Antisecretory compound

Chem. class.: Benzimidazole

Action: Suppresses gastric secretion by inhibiting hydrogen/potassium ATPase enzyme system in gastric parietal cell; characterized as gastric acid pump inhibitor, since it blocks final step of acid production

Uses: Gastroesophageal reflux disease (GERD), severe erosive esophagitis, poorly responsive systemic GERD, pathologic hypersecretory conditions (Zollinger-Ellison syndrome, systemic mastocytosis, multiple endocrine adenomas); treatment of active duodenal ulcers

Dosage and routes:

Active duodenal ulcers

• *Adults:* PO 20 mg qd × 4-8 wks

Severe erosine esophagitis/poorly responsive GERD

• *Adult:* PO 20 mg qd × 4-8 wk

Pathologic hypersecretory conditions

• *Adult:* PO 60 mg/day; may increase to 120 mg tid; daily doses >80 mg should be divided

Available forms: Cap, delayed rel 10, 20 mg

Side effects/adverse reactions:

CNS: Headache, dizziness, asthenia

GI: Diarrhea, abdominal pain, vomiting, nausea, constipation, flatulence, acid regurgitation, abdominal swelling, anorexia, irritable colon, esophageal candidiasis, dry mouth

RESP: Upper respiratory infections, cough, epistaxis

INTEG: Rash, dry skin, urticaria, pruritus, alopecia

META: Hypoglycemia, increased hepatic enzymes, weight gain

EENT: Tinnitus, taste perversion

CV: Chest pain, angina, tachycardia, bradycardia, palpitations, peripheral edema

GU: UTI, frequency, increased creatinine, ***proteinuria, hematuria,*** testicular pain, glycosuria

HEMA: ***Pancytopenia, thrombocytopenia, neutropenia, leukocytosis,*** anemia

MISC: Back pain, fever, fatigue, malaise

Contraindications: Hypersensitivity

Precautions: Pregnancy (C), lactation, children

Pharmacokinetics:

Peak ½-3½ hr, half-life ½-1 hr, protein binding 95%, eliminated in urine as metabolites and in feces; in elderly elimination rate decreased, bioavailability increased

Interactions:

• Increased serum levels: diazepam, phenytoin

• Possible increased bleeding: warfarin

NURSING CONSIDERATIONS

Assess:

• GI system: bowel sounds q8h, abdomen for pain, swelling, anorexia

• Hepatic enzymes: AST (SGOT), ALT (SGPT), alk phosphatase during treatment

Administer:

• Before eating; swallow capsule whole; do not open, chew, or crush

Evaluate:

• Therapeutic response: absence of epigastric pain, swelling, fullness

Teach patient/family:

• To report severe diarrhea; drug may have to be discontinued

• That diabetic patient should know hypoglycemia may occur

• To avoid hazardous activities; dizziness may occur

* Available in Canada only

• To avoid alcohol, salicylates, ibuprofen; may cause GI irritation

ondansetron (℞)

(on-dan-see'tron)

Zofran

Func. class.: Antiemetic

Chem. class.: 5-HT3 receptor antagonist

Action: Prevents nausea, vomiting by blocking serotonin peripherally, centrally, and in the small intestine

Uses: Prevention of nausea, vomiting associated with cancer chemotherapy, radiotherapy, and prevention of postoperative nausea, vomiting

Dosage and routes:

• *Adult:* IV 0.15 mg/kg infused over 15 min, 30 min before start of cancer chemotherapy; 0.15 mg/kg given 4 hr and 8 hr after first dose; dilute 50 ml of D_5W or 0.9% NaCl before giving

Prevention of nausea/vomiting of cancer chemotherapy

• *Adult:* PO 8 mg tid; give first dose ½ hr before chemotherapy, subsequent doses 4, 8 hr after first dose; give 8 mg tid × 1-2 days after chemotherapy completion

• *Child 4-18 yr:* 0.15 mg/kg

Prevention of postoperative nausea/vomiting

• *Adult:* IV 4 mg undiluted over >30 sec

Available forms: Inj 2 mg/ml, 32 mg/50 ml (premixed); tabs 4, 8 mg

Side effects/adverse reactions:

GI: Diarrhea, constipation, increased AST, ALT

CNS: Headache

MISC: Rash, ***bronchospasm***

Contraindications: Hypersensitivity

Precautions: Pregnancy (B), lactation, children, elderly

Pharmacokinetics:

IV: Mean elimination half-life 3.5-4.7 hr, plasma protein binding 70%-76%; extensively metabolized in the liver

Y-site compatibilities: Amikacin, aztreonam, bleomycin, carboplatin, carmustine, cefazolin, ceforanide, cefotazime, cefoxitin, ceftazidime, ceftizoxime, cefuroxime, chlorpromazine, cimetidine, cisplatin, clindamycin, cyclophosphamide, cytarabine, dacarbazine, dactinomycin, daunorubicin, dexamethasone sodium phosphate, diphenhydramine, doxorubicin, doxycycline, droperidol, etoposide, famotidine, floxuridine, fluconazole, fludarabine, gentamicin, haloperidol, heparin, hydrocortisone sodium succinate, hydromorphone, hydroxyzine, ifosfamide, imipenem/cilastatin, magnesium sulfate, mannitol, mechlorethamine, melphalan, meperidine, mesna, methotrexate, metoclopramide, miconazole, mitomycin, mitoxantrone, morphine, paclitaxel, pentostatin, potassium chloride, prochlorperazine edisylate, ranitidine, streptozocin, teniposide, ticarcillin, ticarcillin/clavulanate, vancomycin, vinblastine, vincristine, vinorelbine, zidovudine

Solution compatibilities: May also be diluted with D_5W, Lactated Ringers, D_5/0.9% NaCl, D_5/0.45% NaCl

NURSING CONSIDERATIONS

Assess:

• For absence of nausea, vomiting during chemotherapy

• Hypersensitivity reaction: rash, bronchospasm

Administer:

• IV after diluting a single dose in 50 ml NS or D_5W, 0.45% or NS and given over 15 min

Perform/provide:
• Storage at room temp 48 hr after dilution

Evaluate:
• Therapeutic response: absence of nausea, vomiting during cancer chemotherapy

Teach patient/family:
• To report diarrhea, constipation, rash, or changes in respirations

opium tincture/ camphorated opium tincture

(oh'pee-um)

Opium Tincture Deodorized, Pantopan, Paregoric, Paregorique*

Func. class.: Antidiarrheal

Chem. class.: Opium/opium and morphine

Combination products: Donnagel-PG: powdered opium 24 mg, Kaolin 6 g, pectin 142.8 mg, hyoscyamine SO_4 0.1037 mg, atropine SO_4 0.0194 mg, scopolamine hydrobromide 0.0065 mg, alcohol 5%/30 ml susp; Opium and Belladonna: powdered opium 60 mg with belladonna extract 15 mg (equivalent to belladonna alkaloids 0.2 mg); Parepectolin: opium 15 mg, kaolin 5.85 g, pectin 162 mg, alcohol 0.69%/30 ml susp; Pathibamate-200: meprobamate 400 mg/tridihexethyl 25 mg

Controlled Substance Schedule III/II (depending on amount of opium)

Action: Antiperistaltic activity

Uses: Diarrhea (cause undetermined); withdrawal symptoms in infants born to addicted mothers

Dosage and routes:
• *Adult:* PO 0.3-1 ml qid, not to exceed 6 ml/day (tincture) or 5-10 ml qd-qid (camphorated)
• *Child:* PO 0.25-0.5 ml/kg qd-qid (camphorated)

Withdrawal
• *Neonates:* PO 1:25 dilution, 3-6 gtt q3-6hr (tincture), dosage adjustment to control symptoms

Available forms: Liq 2 mg morphine equivalent per 5 ml

Side effects/adverse reactions:
CNS: Dizziness, drowsiness, fainting, flushing, physical dependency, ***CNS depression***
GI: Nausea, vomiting, constipation, abdominal pain

Contraindications: Hypersensitivity, severe ulcerative colitis, pseudomembranous colitis

Precautions: Liver disease, addiction proneness, prostatic hypertrophy (severe), pregnancy (B)

Pharmacokinetics:
PO: Duration 4 hr, half-life 2-3 hr; metabolized in liver; excreted in urine

Interactions:
• Increased action of both drugs: other CNS depressants
• Increased CNS toxicity: cimetidine

NURSING CONSIDERATIONS

Assess:
• Electrolytes (K, Na, Cl) if on long-term therapy
• Skin turgor q8h if dehydration is suspected
• Bowel pattern before; for rebound constipation
• Response after 48 hr; if no response, drug should be discontinued
• Dehydration in children
• Abdominal distention; toxic megacolon may occur in ulcerative colitis

Administer:
• Undiluted with water
• For 48 hr only

* Available in Canada only

Evaluate:
- Therapeutic response: decreased diarrhea

Teach patient/family:
- To avoid OTC products (cough, cold, hay fever preparations) unless directed by prescriber
- Not to exceed recommended dose
- That drug may be habit-forming
- To avoid hazardous activities; drowsiness may occur

oral contraceptives (℞)

Func. class.: Hormone

Chem. class.: Estrogen/progestin combinations

Action: Prevents ovulation by suppressing FSH, LH; *monophasic:* estrogen/progestin (fixed dose) used during a 21-day cycle; ovulation is inhibited by suppression of FSH and LH; thickness of cervical mucus and endometrial lining prevents pregnancy; *biphasic:* ovulation is inhibited by suppression of FSH and LH; alteration of cervical mucus, endometrial lining prevents pregnancy; *triphasic:* ovulation is inhibited by suppression of FSH and LH; change of cervical mucus, endometrial lining prevents pregnancy, variable doses of estrogen/progestin combinations may be similar to natural hormonal fluctuations; *progestin-only pill and implant:* change of cervical mucus and endometrial lining prevents pregnancy; ovulation may be suppressed

Uses: To prevent pregnancy, endometriosis, hypermenorrhea

Dosage and routes:
- *Adult:* PO 1 qd starting on day 5 of menstrual cycle; day 1 is 1st day of period

20/21 tablet packs
- *Adult:* PO 1 qd starting on day 7 of menstrual cycle; day 1 is 1st day of period, then on 20 or 21 days, off 7 days

28 tablet packs
- *Adult:* PO 1 qd continuously

Biphasic
- *Adult:* 1 qd × 10 days, then next color 1 qd × 11 days

Triphasic
- *Adult:* 1 qd; check package insert

Endometriosis
- *Adult:* PO 1 qd × 20 days from day 5 to 24 of cycle
- *Adult:* PO 1 qd; check package insert for specific instructions

Available forms: Check specific brand

Side effects/adverse reactions:

GI: Nausea, vomiting, cramps, diarrhea, bloating, constipation, change in appetite, ***cholestatic jaundice***

INTEG: Chloasma, melasma, acne, rash, urticaria, erythema, pruritus, hirsutism, alopecia, photosensitivity

CV: Increased B/P, thromboembolic conditions, fluid retention, edema

ENDO: Decreased glucose tolerance, increased TBG, PBI, T_4, T_3

GU: Breakthrough bleeding, amenorrhea, spotting, dysmenorrhea, galactorrhea, endocervical hyperplasia, vaginitis, cystitis-like syndrome, breast change

CNS: Depression, fatigue, dizziness, nervousness, anxiety, headache

EENT: Optic neuritis, retinal thrombosis, cataracts

HEMA: Increased fibrinogen, clotting factor

Contraindications: Pregnancy (X), lactation, reproductive cancer, thrombophlebitis, MI, hepatic tumors, hepatic disease, CAD, women 40 and over, CVA

Precautions: Depression, hypertension, renal disease, seizure disorders, lupus erythematosus, rheumatic disease, migraine headache, amenorrhea, irregular menses, breast cancer (fibrocystic), gallbladder disease, diabetes mellitus, heavy smoking, acute mononucleosis, sickle cell disease

Pharmacokinetics: Excreted in breast milk

Interactions:

• Decreased effectiveness of oral contraceptives: anticonvulsants, rifampin, analgesics, antibiotics, antihistamines, chenodiol, griseofulvin

• Decreased action of oral anticoagulants

• Increased clotting: aminocaproic acid

Lab test interferences:

Increase: Pro-time, clotting factors VII, VIII, IX, X, TBG, PBI, T_4, platelet aggregability, BSP, triglycerides, bilirubin, AST (SGOT), ALT (SGPT)

Decrease: T_3, antithrombin III, folate, metyrapone test, GTT, 17-OHCS

NURSING CONSIDERATIONS

Assess:

• Glucose, thyroid function, liver function tests

• Reproductive changes: change in breasts, tumors, positive Pap smear; drug should be discontinued

Administer:

• PO with food for GI symptoms; give at same time each day

• Subdermal implant of 6 caps effective for 5 yr; then should be removed

• IM deep in large muscle mass after shaking suspension; ensure patient not pregnant if injections are 2 wk or more apart

Evaluate:

• Therapeutic response: absence of pregnancy, endometriosis, hypermenorrhea

Teach patient/family:

• About detection of clots using Homan's sign

• To use sunscreen or avoid sunlight; photosensitivity can occur

• To take at same time each day to ensure equal drug level

• To report GI symptoms that occur after 4 mo

• To use another birth control method during 1st week of oral contraceptive use

• To take another tablet as soon as possible if one is missed

• That after drug is discontinued, pregnancy may not occur for several months

• To report abdominal pain, change in vision, shortness of breath, change in menstrual flow, spotting, breakthrough bleeding, breast lumps, swelling, headache, severe leg pain

• That continuing medical care is needed: Pap smear and gynecologic examinations q6mo

• To notify physicians and dentist of oral contraceptive use

orphenadrine (℞)

(or-fen'a-dreen)

Banflex, Flexoject, Flexon, Marflex, Myolin, Neocyten, Norflex, O-Flex, Orphenadrine Citrate, Orphenate

Func. class.: Skeletal muscle relaxant, central acting; anticholinergic

Chem. class.: Tertiary amine

Combination products: Norgesic: orphenadrine citrate 25 mg, aspirin 385 mg, caffeine 30 mg; Norgesic Forte: orphenadrine citrate 50 mg, aspirin 770 mg, caffeine 60 mg

Action: Acts centrally on skeletal muscle to relax, inhibit muscle spasm

* Available in Canada only

Uses: Pain in musculoskeletal disorders

Dosage and routes:

- *Adult:* PO 100 mg bid; IM/IV 60 mg q12h

Available forms: Tabs 100 mg; tabs sus rel 100 mg; inj IM, IV 30 mg/ml

Side effects/adverse reactions:

HEMA: ***Aplastic anemia***

CNS: *Dizziness, weakness, fatigue, drowsiness,* headache, disorientation, insomnia, stimulation, hallucination, agitation

EENT: Nasal congestion, blurred vision, increased intraocular pressure, mydriasis

CV: Orthostatic hypotension, tachycardia

GI: *Nausea,* vomiting, constipation, dry mouth

GU: Urinary frequency, hesitancy, retention

INTEG: Rash, pruritus, urticaria

Contraindications: Hypersensitivity, narrow-angle glaucoma, GI obstruction, myasthenia gravis, stenosing peptic ulcer, bladder neck obstruction, cardiospasm

Precautions: Pregnancy (C), children, cardiac disease, tachycardia

Pharmacokinetics:

PO: Peak 2 hr, duration 4-6 hr, half-life 14 hr; metabolized in liver, excreted in urine (unchanged)

Interactions:

- Increased CNS effects: propoxyphene, other anticholinergics, oral contraceptives
- Incompatibility unknown

NURSING CONSIDERATIONS

Assess:

- Monitor vital signs q10-15min during administration
- Blood studies: CBC, WBC, differential; blood dyscrasias may occur (rare)
- I&O ratio; check for urinary retention, frequency, hesitancy
- Dosage: even slight overdose can cause toxicity
- Allergic reactions: rash, fever, respiratory distress
- Blood dyscrasias: fever, bleeding, fatigue (rare)
- CNS symptoms: dizziness, drowsiness, psychiatric symptoms

Administer:

- With meals for GI symptoms
- IV undiluted, or diluted in 5-10 ml sterile H_2O for inj; give 60 mg or less over 5 min
- When giving IV, may cause paradoxic initial bradycardia; usually disappears in 2 min

Perform/provide:

- Assistance with ambulation if dizziness/drowsiness occurs

Evaluate:

- Therapeutic response: decreased rigidity, spasms

Teach patient/family:

- Not to discontinue medication quickly; insomnia, nausea, headache will occur
- Not to take with alcohol, other CNS depressants
- To avoid altering activities while taking this drug
- To avoid hazardous activities if drowsiness/dizziness occurs
- To avoid using OTC medication: cough preparations, antihistamines, unless directed by prescriber
- To use gum, frequent sips of water for dry mouth

oxacillin (℞)

(ox-a-sill'in)

Bactocill, oxacillin sodium, Prostaphilin

Func. class.: Broad-spectrum antiinfective

Chem. class.: Penicillinase-resistant penicillin

Action: Interferes with cell wall replication of susceptible organisms; osmotically unstable cell wall swells, bursts from osmotic pressure

Uses: Effective for gram-positive cocci *(S. aureus, S. pneumoniae),* infections caused by penicillinase-producing *Staphylococcus*

Dosage and routes:

• *Adult:* PO 2-6 g/day in divided doses q4-6h; IM/IV 2-12 g/day in divided doses q4-6h

• *Child:* PO 50-100 mg/kg/day in divided doses q6h; IM/IV 50-100 mg/kg/day in divided doses q4-6h

Available forms: Caps 250, 500 mg; powder for oral susp 250 mg/5 ml; powder for inj 250, 500 mg, 1, 2, 4, 10 g; inf 1, 2 g

Side effects/adverse reactions:

HEMA: Anemia, increased bleeding time, ***bone marrow depression, granulocytopenia***

GI: Nausea, vomiting, diarrhea, increased AST (SGOT), ALT (SGPT), abdominal pain, glossitis, colitis

GU: ***Oliguria, proteinuria, hematuria,*** *vaginitis, moniliasis,* ***glomerulonephritis***

CNS: Lethargy, hallucinations, anxiety, depression, twitching, ***coma, convulsions***

Contraindications: Hypersensitivity to penicillins

Precautions: Pregnancy (B), hypersensitivity to cephalosporins, neonates

Pharmacokinetics:

PO/IM: Peak 30-60 min, duration 4-6 hr

IV: Peak 5 min, duration 4-6 hr, half-life 30-60 min

Metabolized in the liver, excreted in urine, bile, breast milk, crosses placenta

Interactions:

• Decreased antimicrobial effectiveness of oxacillin: tetracyclines, erythromycins

• Increased oxacillin concentrations: aspirin, probenecid

Y-site compatibilities: Acyclovir, cyclophosphamide, famotidine, fluconazole, foscarnet, heparin, hydrocortisone sodium succinate, hydromorphone, labetalol, magnesium sulfate, meperidine, morphine, perphenazine, potassium chloride, vitamin B with C, zidovudine

Additive compatibilities: Cephapirin, chloramphenicol, dopamine, potassium chloride, sodium bicarbonate

Lab test interferences:

False positive: Urine glucose, urine protein

NURSING CONSIDERATIONS

Assess:

• I&O ratio; report hematuria, oliguria, since penicillin in high doses is nephrotoxic

• Any patient with compromised renal system, since drug is excreted slowly in poor renal system function; toxicity may occur rapidly

• Liver studies: AST (SGOT), ALT (SGPT)

• Blood studies: WBC, RBC, Hct/Hgb, bleeding time

• Renal studies: urinalysis, protein, blood

• C&S before therapy; drug may be given as soon as culture is taken

• Bowel pattern before and during treatment

• Skin eruptions after administration of penicillin to 1 wk after discontinuing drug

• Respiratory status: rate, character, wheezing, tightness in chest

• Allergies before initiation of treatment, and reaction of each medication; highlight allergies on chart

Administer:

• IV after diluting 500 mg or less/5 ml sterile H_2O or NaCl for inj; may dilute further in D_5W, NS, LR and

* Available in Canada only

give 1 g/10 min; may be given as infusion over 6 hr
• Drug after C&S completed
• PO with full glass of water 1 hr before or 2 hr after meals
• IM deep in gluteal muscle
Perform/provide:
• Adrenalin, suction, tracheostomy set, endotracheal intubation equipment
• Scratch test to assess allergy, after securing order from prescriber; usually done when penicillin is only drug of choice
• Storage in air-tight container; refrigerate reconstituted sol up to 2 wk
Evaluate:
• Therapeutic response: absence of fever, draining wounds
Teach patient/family:
• Aspects of drug therapy, including need to complete course of medication to ensure organism death (10-14 days); culture may be taken after completed course
• To report sore throat, fever, fatigue (may indicate superinfection)
• To wear or carry Medic Alert ID if allergic to penicillins
• To take on empty stomach with a full glass of water
Treatment of anaphylaxis: Withdraw drug, maintain airway, administer epinephrine, aminophylline, O_2, IV corticosteroids

oxamniquine (℞)
(ox-am′ni-kwin)
Vansil
Func. class.: Anthelmintic
Chem. class.: Tetrahydroquinone derivative

Action: Causes paralysis, contraction, leading to dislodgement of suckers; they are carried to liver, where phagocytosis takes place
Uses: Schistosomiasis
Dosage and routes:
• *Adult, child >30 kg:* PO 12-15 mg/kg as single dose
• *Child <30 kg:* PO 20 mg/kg in 2 divided doses q2-8h
Available forms: Caps 250 mg
Side effects/adverse reactions:
INTEG: Rash, pruritus, urticaria
CNS: Dizziness, headache, drowsiness, insomnia, ***convulsions,*** hallucination, personality changes, stimulation
EENT: Bad taste, oral irritation
GI: Nausea, vomiting, anorexia, abdominal pain
HEMA: Increased sed rate, reticulocyte count, increase or decrease in leukocytes
Contraindications: Hypersensitivity
Precautions: Pregnancy (C), lactation, seizure disorders
Pharmacokinetics:
PO: Peak 1-1½ hr, half-life 1 2½ hr; excreted in urine (unchanged/metabolites)
Lab test interferences:
Interferences: Urinalysis

NURSING CONSIDERATIONS
Assess:
• Stools during entire treatment, 1, 3 mo after treatment; specimens must be sent to lab while still warm
• For allergic reaction: rash, itching, urticaria
• For infection in other family members, since infection from person to person is common
Administer:
• PO after meals to avoid GI symptoms
Perform/provide:
• Storage in tight container, cool environment

Evaluate:
- Therapeutic response: expulsion of worms, 3 negative stool cultures after completion of treatment

Teach patient/family:
- Proper hygiene after stool, including hand-washing technique; tell patient not to put fingers in mouth
- That infected person should sleep alone; not to shake bed linen; change bed linen daily; wash in hot water
- To clean toilet qd with disinfectant (green soap)
- Need for compliance with dosage schedule, duration of treatment
- That urine may turn orange or red
- To avoid hazardous activities since drowsiness occurs
- That seizures may recur in patient who is controlled on medication

oxandrolone (℞)

(ox-an′droe-lone)

Oxandrin, oxandrolone

Func. class.: Androgenic anabolic steroid

Chem. class.: Halogenated testosterone derivative

Action: Increases weight by building body tissue, increases potassium, phosphorus, chloride, nitrogen levels, increases bone development

Uses: Tissue building after steroid therapy, osteoporosis, prolonged immobility

Dosage and routes:
- *Adult:* PO 2.5 mg bid-qid, not to exceed 20 mg qd × 2-3 wk
- *Child:* PO 0.25 mg/kg/day × 2-4 wk, not to exceed 3 mo

Available forms: Tabs 2.5 mg

Side effects/adverse reactions:

INTEG: Rash, acneiform lesions, oily hair, skin, flushing, sweating, acne vulgaris, alopecia, hirsutism

CNS: Dizziness, headache, fatigue, tremors, paresthesias, flushing, sweating, anxiety, lability, insomnia

MS: Cramps, spasms

CV: Increased B/P

GU: ***Hematuria,*** amenorrhea, vaginitis, decreased libido, decreased breast size, clitoral hypertrophy, testicular atrophy

GI: Nausea, vomiting, constipation, weight gain, ***cholestatic jaundice***

EENT: Carpal tunnel syndrome, conjunctional edema, nasal congestion

ENDO: Abnormal GT

Contraindications: Severe renal, severe cardiac, severe hepatic disease, hypersensitivity, pregnancy (X), lactation, genital bleeding (abnormal)

Precautions: Diabetes mellitus, CV disease, MI

Pharmacokinetics:

PO: Metabolized in liver, excreted in urine, breast milk, crosses placenta

Interactions:
- Increased effects of oral antidiabetics, oxyphenbutazone
- Increased PT: anticoagulants
- Edema: ACTH, adrenal steroids
- Decreased effects of insulin

Lab test interferences:

Increase: Serum cholesterol, blood glucose, urine glucose

Decrease: Serum Ca, serum K, T_4, T_3, thyroid ^{131}I uptake test, urine 17-OHCS, 17-KS, PBI, BSP

NURSING CONSIDERATIONS

Assess:
- Weight qd; notify prescriber if weekly weight gain is >5 lb
- B/P q4h
- I&O ratio; be alert for decreasing urinary output, increasing edema
- Growth rate in children, since growth rate may be uneven (linear/bone growth) in long-term use

• Electrolytes: K, Na, Cl, Ca; cholesterol
• Liver function studies: ALT (SGPT), AST (SGOT), bilirubin
• Edema, hypertension, cardiac symptoms, jaundice
• Mental status: affect, mood, behavioral changes, aggression
• Signs of masculinization in female: increased libido, deepening of voice, decreased breast tissue, enlarged clitoris, menstrual irregularities; male: gynecomastia, impotence, testicular atrophy
• Hypercalcemia: lethargy, polyuria, polydipsia, nausea, vomiting, constipation; drug may have to be decreased
• Hypoglycemia in diabetics, since oral anticoagulant action is decreased

Administer:
• Titrated dose, use lowest effective dose

Perform/provide:
• Diet with increased calories and protein; decrease Na for edema

Evaluate:
• Therapeutic response: occurs in 4-6 wk in osteoporosis

Teach patient/family:
• That drug must be combined with complete health plan: diet, rest, exercise
• To notify prescriber if therapeutic response decreases
• Not to discontinue abruptly
• About change in sex characteristics
• Women to report menstrual irregularities
• That 1-3 mo course is necessary for response in breast cancer
• Procedure for use of buccal tablets (requires 30-60 min to dissolve, change absorption site with each dose; do not eat, drink, chew, or smoke while tablet is in place)

oxaprozin (℞)

(ox-a-proe′zin)
Daypro
Func. class.: Nonsteroidal antiinflammatory
Chem. class.: Propionic acid derivative

Action: May inhibit prostaglandin synthesis by decreasing enzyme needed for biosynthesis; analgesic, antiinflammatory, antipyretic
Uses: Acute and long-term management of osteoarthritis, rheumatoid arthritis
Dosage and routes:
• *Adult:* PO 1200 mg qd; maximum dose 1800 mg/day or 26 mg/kg, whichever is lower
Available forms: Caplets 600 mg
Side effects/adverse reactions:
GI: Nausea, anorexia, vomiting, diarrhea, jaundice, ***cholestatic hepatitis***, constipation, flatulence, cramps, dry mouth, peptic ulcer
CNS: Dizziness, headache, drowsiness, fatigue, tremors, confusion, insomnia, anxiety, depression
CV: Tachycardia, peripheral edema, palpitations, dysrhythmias
INTEG: Purpura, rash, pruritus, sweating
GU: ***Nephrotoxicity: dysuria, hematuria, oliguria, azotemia***
HEMA: ***Blood dyscrasias***
EENT: Tinnitus, hearing loss, blurred vision
Contraindications: Hypersensitivity, asthma, patients in whom aspirin and iodides have induced symptoms of allergic reactions or asthma
Precautions: Pregnancy (B) 1st and 2nd trimester, lactation, children, bleeding disorders, GI disorders, cardiac disorders, hypersensitivity to other antiinflammatory agents, se-

vere renal and hepatic disease, elderly
Pharmacokinetics:
PO: Onset 1 wk, peak unknown, duration unknown, half-life 10-20 hr; metabolized in liver; excreted in urine (metabolites), breast milk; 99% plasma protein binding
Interactions:
• Oxaprozin may decrease effects of loop diuretics and β-blockers
• May increase the action or toxicity of coumarin, phenytoin, lithium, methotrexate
• May increase effects of oxaprozin: phenobarbital, probenecid
• Salicylates may decrease plasma levels of oxaprozin
NURSING CONSIDERATIONS
Assess:
• Renal, liver, blood studies: BUN, creatinine, AST (SGOT), ALT (SGPT), Hgb, before treatment, periodically thereafter
• Audiometric: ophthalmic exam before, during, after treatment
• For eye, ear problems: blurred vision, tinnitus; may indicate toxicity
Administer:
• With food to decrease GI symptoms
Perform/provide:
• Storage at room temp
Evaluate:
• Therapeutic response: decreased pain, stiffness in joints, decreased swelling in joints, ability to move more easily
Teach patient/family:
• To report blurred vision, ringing, roaring in ears; may indicate toxicity
• To avoid driving, other hazardous activities if dizziness/drowsiness occurs
• To report change in urine pattern, increased weight, edema, increased pain in joints, fever, blood in urine; indicates nephrotoxicity
• That therapeutic effects may take up to 1 mo
• To take with a full glass of water to enhance absorption

oxazepam (℞)

(ox-a'ze-pam)
Apo-Oxazepam*, Novoxapam*, oxazepam, Ox-Pam*, Serax, Zapex*
Func. class.: Sedative/hypnotic; antianxiety
Chem. class.: Benzodiazepine

Controlled Substance Schedule IV
Action: Potentiates the actions of GABA, especially in limbic system and reticular formation
Uses: Anxiety, alcohol withdrawal
Dosage and routes:
Anxiety
• *Adult:* PO 10-30 mg tid-qid
Alcohol withdrawal
• *Adult:* PO 15-30 mg tid-qid
Available forms: Caps 10, 15, 30 mg; tabs 10, 15, 30 mg
Side effects/adverse reactions:
CNS: Dizziness, drowsiness, confusion, headache, anxiety, tremors, fatigue, depression, insomnia, hallucinations, paradoxical excitement, transient amnesia
GI: Nausea, vomiting, anorexia
INTEG: Rash, dermatitis, itching
CV: Orthostatic hypotension, ***ECG changes, tachycardia,*** hypotension
EENT: Blurred vision, tinnitus, mydriasis
Contraindications: Hypersensitivity to benzodiazepines, narrow-angle glaucoma, psychosis, pregnancy (D), lactation, child <12 yr
Precautions: Elderly, debilitated, hepatic disease, renal disease
Pharmacokinetics:
PO: Peak 2-4 hr, metabolized by

* Available in Canada only

liver, excreted by kidneys, half-life 5-15 hr

Interactions:

- Decreased effects of oxazepam: oral contraceptives, valproic acid
- Increased effects of oxazepam: CNS depressants, alcohol, disulfiram, oral contraceptives

Lab test interferences:

Increase: AST (SGOT), ALT (SGPT), serum bilirubin
Decrease: RAIU
False increase: 17-OHCS

NURSING CONSIDERATIONS

Assess:

- B/P (lying, standing), pulse; if systolic B/P drops 20 mm Hg, hold drug, notify prescriber
- Blood studies: CBC during long-term therapy; blood dyscrasias have occurred rarely
- Hepatic studies: AST (SGOT), ALT (SGPT), bilirubin, creatinine, LDH, alk phosphatase
- Mental status: mood, sensorium, affect, sleeping pattern, drowsiness, dizziness
- Physical dependency, withdrawal symptoms: headache, nausea, vomiting, muscle pain, weakness, tremors, ***convulsions*** (long-term use)
- Suicidal tendencies

Administer:

- With food, milk for GI symptoms
- Sugarless gum, hard candy, frequent sips of water for dry mouth

Perform/provide:

- Assistance with ambulation during beginning therapy; drowsiness/dizziness occurs
- Safety measures, including side rails
- Check to see PO medication has been swallowed

Evaluate:

- Therapeutic response: decreased anxiety, restlessness, insomnia

Teach patient/family:

- That the drug may be taken with food
- Not to be used for everyday stress or used longer than 4 mo unless directed by prescriber; not to take more than prescribed dose; may be habit forming
- To avoid OTC preparations (cough, cold, hay fever) unless approved by prescriber
- To avoid driving, activities that require alertness, since drowsiness may occur
- To avoid alcohol ingestion, other psychotropic medications unles directed by prescriber
- Not to discontinue medication abruptly after long-term use
- To rise slowly, or fainting may occur, especially elderly
- That drowsiness may worsen at beginning of treatment

Treatment of overdose: Lavage, VS, supportive care, flumazenil

oxidized cellulose (℞)

Oxycel, Surgicel

Func. class.: Hemostatic
Chem. class.: Cellulose product

Action: Absorbs blood, acts as an artificial clot

Uses: Hemostasis in surgery, oral surgery, exodontia

Dosage and routes:

- *Adult and child:* TOP apply using sterile technique as needed, remove after bleeding stops, if possible, or leave in place if needed

Available forms: TOP knitted fabric as strips, pads, pledgets

Side effects/adverse reactions:

EENT: Sneezing, burning in epistaxis
INTEG: Burning, stinging, encapsulation of fluid, foreign bodies
CNS: Headache in epistaxis

Contraindications: Hypersensitivity, large artery hemorrhage, oozing surfaces, implantation in bone deficit, placement around optic nerve, and chiasm

NURSING CONSIDERATIONS

Assess:

• Allergy: fever, rash, itching, burning, stinging

Administer:

• Dry; use only amount needed to control bleeding

• Loosely; remove excess before closure in surgery; irrigate first, then remove using sterile technique

• Using sterile technique; cannot be resterilized

Evaluate:

• Therapeutic response: decreased bleeding in surgery

---

oxtriphylline (℞)

(ox-trye'fi-lin)

Apo-Oxtriphylline*, Choledyl, Choledyl SA, Novotriphyl*, oxtriphylline

Func. class.: Bronchodilator, spasmolytic

Chem. class.: Choline salt of theophylline

Action: Relaxes smooth muscle of respiratory system by blocking phosphodiesterase, which increases cyclic AMP; 64% theophylline

Uses: Acute bronchial asthma, reversible bronchospasm in chronic bronchitis and COPD

Dosage and routes:

• *Adult and child >12 yr:* PO 200 mg qid or sus action q12hr

• *Child 2-12 yr:* PO 4 mg/kg q6h; may be increased to desired response, therapeutic level

Available forms: Elix 100 mg/5 ml; syr 50 mg/5 ml; tabs 100, 200, 400, 600 mg; sus action tabs 400, 600 mg

Side effects/adverse reactions:

CNS: Anxiety, restlessness, insomnia, diziness, ***convulsions,*** headache, light-headedness

CV: Palpitations, sinus tachycardia, hypotension

GI: Nausea, vomiting, anorexia, diarrhea, bitter taste, dyspepsia

RESP: Increased rate

INTEG: Flushing, urticaria, alopecia

Contraindications: Hypersensitivity to xanthines, tachydysrhythmias

Precautions: Elderly, CHF, cor pulmonale, hepatic disease, active peptic ulcer disease, diabetes mellitus, hyperthyroidism, hypertension, children, pregnancy (C), glaucoma, prostatic hypertrophy

Pharmacokinetics:

ELIXIR: Peak 1 hr

PO-SA: Peak 4-7 hr, duration 8-12 hr

Metabolized in liver; excreted in urine, breast milk; crosses placenta

Interactions:

• Increased action of oxtriphylline: cimetidine, erythromycin, troleandomycin, oral contraceptive, propranolol

• May increase effects of anticoagulants, coffee (caffeine items)

• Cardiotoxicity: β-blockers

• Decreased effect of lithium

• Decreased theophylline level: rifampin, phenytoin

NURSING CONSIDERATIONS

Assess:

• Therapeutic blood levels; toxicity may occur with small increase above therapeutic level

• Therapeutic theophylline levels: 11-20 μg/ml

• Smoking reduces effects of theophyllines, requiring larger doses

• Respiratory rate, rhythm, depth; auscultate lung fields bilaterally; notify prescriber of abnormalities

• Allergic reactions: rash, urticaria; drug should be discontinued

---

* Available in Canada only

Administer:
• PO after meals to decrease GI symptoms; absorption may be affected
• After meals, hs

Perform/provide:
• Storage in closed container away from heat; protect elixir from light

Evaluate:
• Therapeutic response: absence of dyspnea, wheezing

Teach patient/family:
• Tablets should not be chewed or crushed
• To check OTC medications, prescription medications for ephedrine, which will increase stimulation
• To avoid hazardous activities; dizziness may occur
• If GI upset occurs, to take drug with 8 oz water; avoid food; absorption may be decreased
• To notify prescriber of toxicity: nausea, vomiting, anxiety, convulsions, insomnia, rapid pulse
• To notify prescriber of change in smoking habit; may need to change dose; encourage not to smoke

oxybutynin (℞)

(ox-i-byoo'ti-nin)

Ditropan, oxybutynin chloride

Func. class.: Spasmolytic

Chem. class.: Synthetic tertiary amine

Action: Relaxes smooth muscles in urinary tract by inhibiting acetylcholine at postganglionic sites

Uses: Antispasmodic for neurogenic bladder

Dosage and routes:
• *Adult:* PO 5 mg bid-tid, not to exceed 5 mg qid
• *Child >5 yr:* PO 5 mg bid, not to exceed 5 mg tid

Available forms: Syrup 5 mg/5 ml; tabs 5 mg

Side effects/adverse reactions:

HEMA: ***Leukopenia, eosinophilia***

CNS: Anxiety, restlessness, dizziness, ***convulsions,*** headache, drowsiness, confusion

CV: Palpitations, sinus tachycardia, hypotension

GI: Nausea, vomiting, anorexia, abdominal pain, constipation

GU: Dysuria, retention, hesitancy

INTEG: Urticaria, dermatitis

EENT: Blurred vision, increased intraocular tension, dry mouth, throat

Contraindications: Hypersensitivity, GI obstruction, GI hemorrhage, GU obstruction, glaucoma, severe colitis, myasthenia gravis, unstable CV status in acute hemorrhage

Precautions: Pregnancy (C), lactation, suspected glaucoma, children <12 yr

Pharmacokinetics: Onset ½-1 hr, peak 3-4 hr, duration 6-10 hr; metabolized by liver, excreted in urine

NURSING CONSIDERATIONS

Assess:
• Urinary patterns: distention, nocturia, frequency, urgency, incontinence
• Allergic reactions: rash, urticaria; if these occur, drug should be discontinued

Evaluate:
• Urinary status: dysuria, frequency, nocturia, incontinence

Teach patient/family:
• To avoid hazardous activities; dizziness may occur
• To avoid OTC medications with alcohol, other CNS depressants
• To prevent photophobia by wearing sunglasses

O

oxycodone (℞)

(ox-i-koe'done)

Supeudol*, Roxicodone, Oxycodone/Aspirin Endodan*, Oxycodan*, Percodan, Percodan-Demi, Roxiprin Oxycodone/Acetaminophen Endocet*, Oxycocet*, Percocet, Roxicet, Roxilox, Tylox

Func. class.: Narcotic analgesic

Chem. class.: Opiate, semisynthetic derivative

Combination products: Codoxy, Percodan, Roxiprin: oxycodone HCl 4.5 mg, oxycodone terephthalate 0.38 mg with aspirin 325 mg; Roxicet: oxycodone HCl 5 mg/5 ml, acetaminophen 325 mg/5 ml

Controlled Substance Schedule II

Action: Inhibits ascending pain pathways in CNS, increases pain threshold, alters pain perception

Uses: Moderate to severe pain

Dosage and routes:

• *Adult:* PO 5 mg q4-6 hr or 10 mg tid or qid prn

Available forms: Oxycodone supp 10, 20 mg; tabs 5 mg; oral sol conc 20 mg/ml; oxycodone with acetaminophen tabs 5 mg/325 mg; cap 5 mg/500 mg; oral sol 5 mg/325 mg/5 ml; oxycodone with aspirin 2.44 mg/325 mg, 4.88/325 mg

Side effects/adverse reactions:

CNS: Drowsiness, dizziness, confusion, headache, sedation, euphoria

GI: Nausea, vomiting, anorexia, constipation, cramps

GU: Increased urinary output, dysuria, urinary retention

INTEG: Rash, urticaria, bruising, flushing, diaphoresis, pruritus

EENT: Tinitus, blurred vision, miosis, diplopia

CV: Palpitations, bradycardia, change in B/P

RESP: Respiratory depression

Contraindications: Hypersensitivity, addiction (narcotic)

Precautions: Addictive personality, pregnancy (B), lactation, increased intracranial pressure, MI (acute), severe heart disease, respiratory depression, hepatic disease, renal disease, child <18 yr

Pharmacokinetics:

PO: Onset 10-15 min, peak ½-1 hr, duration 4-5 hr; detoxified by liver, excreted in urine, crosses placenta, excreted in breast milk

Interactions:

• Increased effects with other CNS depressants: alcohol, narcotics, sedative/hypnotics, antipsychotics, skeletal muscle relaxants

Lab test interferences:

Increase: Amylase

NURSING CONSIDERATIONS

Assess:

• I&O ratio; check for decreasing output; may indicate urinary retention

• CNS changes: dizziness, drowsiness, hallucinations, euphoria, LOC, pupil reaction

• Allergic reactions: rash, urticaria

• Respiratory dysfunction: respiratory depression, character, rate, rhythm; notify prescriber if respirations are <10/min

• Need for pain medication by pain, sedation scoring; physical dependence

Administer:

• With antiemetic if nausea, vomiting occur

• When pain is beginning to return; determine dosage interval by response

Perform/provide:

• Storage in light-resistant area at room temp

• Assistance with ambulation

• Safety measures: side rails, nightlight, call bell within easy reach

* Available in Canada only

Evaluate:
- Therapeutic response: decrease in pain

Teach patient/family:
- To report any symptoms of CNS changes, allergic reactions
- That physical dependency may result from extended use
- That withdrawal symptoms may occur: nausea, vomiting, cramps, fever, faintness, anorexia

Treatment of overdose: Naloxone (Narcan) 0.2-0.8 mg IV, O_2, IV fluids, vasopressors

oxymetazoline (nasal) (OTC)

(ox-i-met-az'oh-leen)

Afrin, Afrin Children's Nose Drops, Allerest 12-Hour Nasal, Chlorphed-LA, Coricidin Nasal Mist, Dristan Long Lasting, Duramist Plus, Duration, Genasal, NTZ Long-Acting Nasal, Nafrine*, Neo-Synephrine 12 Hour, Nōstrilla, oxymetazoline HCl, Sinarest 12-Hour, Sinex Long-Acting, Twice-A-Day Nasal, 4-Way Long Acting Nasal

Func. class.: Nasal decongestant

Chem. class.: Sympathomimetic amine

Action: Produces vasoconstriction (rapid, long-acting) of arterioles, thereby decreasing fluid exudation, mucosal engorgement

Uses: Nasal congestion

Dosage and routes:
- *Adult, child >6 yr:* INSTILL 2-3 gtt or sprays to each nostril bid
- *Child 2-6 yr:* INSTILL 2-3 gtt or sprays 0.025% sol bid, not to exceed 3 days

Available forms: Nasal sol 0.025%, 0.05%

Side effects/adverse reactions:

GI: Nausea, vomiting, anorexia

EENT: Irritation, burning, sneezing, stinging, dryness, rebound congestion

INTEG: Contact dermatitis

CNS: Anxiety, restlessness, tremors, weakness, insomnia, dizziness, fever, headache

Contraindications: Hypersensitivity to sympathomimetic amines

Precautions: Child <6 year, elderly, diabetes, cardiovascular disease, hypertension, hyperthyroidism, increased ICP, prostatic hypertrophy, pregnancy (C), glaucoma

Interactions:
- Hypertension: MAOIs, β-adrenergic blockers
- Hypotension: methyldopa, mecamylamine, reserpine

NURSING CONSIDERATIONS

Assess:
- For redness, swelling, pain in nasal passages

Administer:
- No more than q4h
- For <3 consecutive days

Perform/provide:
- Environmental humidification to decrease nasal congestion, dryness
- Store in light resistant container; do not expose to heat

Evaluate:
- Therapeutic response: decreased nasal congestion

Teach patient/family:
- That stinging may occur for a few applications; drying of mucosa may be decreased by environmental humidification
- To notify prescriber of irregular pulse, insomnia, sizziness, tremors
- Proper administration to avoid systemic absorption

O

oxymetholone (℞)

(ox-i-meth′oh-lone)

Anadrol-50, Anapolon 50*

Func. class.: Androgenic anabolic steroid

Chem. class.: Halogenated testosterone derivative

Action: Increases weight by building body tissue, increases potassium, phosphorus, chloride, and nitrogen levels, increases bone development

Uses: Tissue building after steroid therapy, osteoporosis, aplastic anemia, anemias caused by deficient RBC production

Dosage and routes:

Aplastic anemia

• *Adult and child:* PO 1-5 mg/kg/day, titrated to patient response, not to exceed 3 mo

Osteoporosis/tissue building (possible indication)

• *Adult:* PO 5-15 mg/day, not to exceed 30 mg/day or 3 mo

• *Child >6 yr:* PO up to 10 mg/day, not to exceed 1 mo

• *Child <6 yr:* PO 1.25 mg qd-qid, not to exceed 1 mo

Available forms: Tabs 50 mg

Side effects/adverse reactions:

INTEG: Rash, acneiform lesions, oily hair, skin, flushing, sweating, acne vulgaris, alopecia, hirsutism

CNS: Dizziness, headache, fatigue, tremors, paresthesias, flushing, sweating, anxiety, lability, insomnia

MS: Cramps, spasms

CV: Increased B/P

GU: ***Hematuria,*** amenorrhea, vaginitis, decreased libido, decreased breast size, clitoral hypertrophy, testicular atrophy

GI: Nausea, vomiting, constipation, weight gain, ***cholestatic jaundice***

EENT: Carpal tunnel syndrome, conjunctival edema, nasal congestion

ENDO: Abnormal GTT

Contraindications: Severe renal, severe cardiac, severe hepatic disease, hypersensitivity, pregnancy (X), lactation, genital bleeding (abnormal)

Precautions: Diabetes mellitus, CV disease, MI

Pharmacokinetics:

PO: Metabolized in liver, excreted in urine, crosses placenta, excreted in breast milk

Interactions:

• Increased effects of oral antidiabetics, oxyphenbutazone

• Increased PT: anticoagulants

• Edema: ACTH, adrenal steroids

• Decreased effects of insulin

Lab test interferences:

Increase: Serum cholesterol, blood glucose, urine glucose

Decrease: Serum Ca, serum K, T_4, T_3, thyroid ^{131}I uptake test, urine 17-OHCS, 17-KS, PBI, BSP

NURSING CONSIDERATIONS

Assess:

• Weight qd, notify prescriber of weekly weight gain >5 lb

• B/P q4h

• I&O ratio; be alert for decreasing urinary output, increasing edema

• Growth rate in children, since growth rate may be uneven (linear/bone growth) with extended use

• Electrolytes: K, Na, Cl, Ca; cholesterol

• Liver function studies: ALT (SGPT), AST (SGOT), bilirubin

• Edema, hypertension, cardiac symptoms, jaundice

• Mental status: affect, mood, behavioral changes, aggression

• Signs of masculinization in female: increased libido, deepening of voice, breast tissue, enlarged clitoris, menstrual irregularities; male:

* Available in Canada only

gynecomastia, impotence, testicular atrophy
• Hypercalcemia: lethargy, polyuria, polydipsia, nausea, vomiting, constipation; drug may have to be decreased
• Hypoglycemia in diabetics; oral antidiabetic action is increased

Administer:
• Titrated dose; use lowest effective dose

Perform/provide:
• Diet with increased calories, protein; decreased Na for edema

Evaluate:
• Therapeutic response: occurs in 4-6 wk in osteoporosis

Teach patient/family:
• That drug must be combined with complete health plan: diet, rest, exercise
• To notify prescriber if therapeutic response decreases
• Not to discontinue abruptly
• About changes in sex characteristics
• That women should report menstrual irregularities
• That 1-3 mo course is necessary for response in breast cancer
• Procedure for use of buccal tablets (requires 30-60 min to dissolve; change absorption site with each dose; do not eat, drink, chew, or smoke while tablet is in place)

oxymorphone (℞)

(ox-i-mor′fone)
Numorphan
Func. class.: Narcotic analgesic
Chem. class.: Opiate, semisynthetic phenanthrene derivative

Controlled Substance Schedule II
Action: Inhibits ascending pain pathways in CNS, increases pain threshold, alters pain perception

Uses: Moderate to severe pain

Dosage and routes:
• *Adult:* IM/SC 1-1.5 mg q4-6h prn; IV 0.5 mg q4-6h prn; REC 2.5-5 mg q4-6h prn

Labor analgesia
• *Adult:* IM: 0.5-1 mg

Available forms: Inj 1, 1.5 mg/ml; supp 5 mg

Side effects/adverse reactions:
CNS: Drowsiness, dizziness, confusion, headache, sedation, euphoria
GI: Nausea, vomiting, anorexia, constipation, cramps
GU: Increased urinary output, dysuria, urinary retention
INTEG: Rash, urticaria, bruising, flushing, diaphoresis, pruritus
EENT: Tinnitus, blurred vision, miosis, diplopia
CV: Palpitations, bradycardia, change in B/P
RESP: ***Respiratory depression***

Contraindications: Hypersensitivity, addiction (narcotic)

Precautions: Addictive personality, pregnancy (B), lactation, increased intracranial pressure, MI (acute), severe heart disease, respiratory depression, hepatic disease, renal disease, child <18 yr

Pharmacokinetics:
SC/IM: Onset 10-15 min, peak 1½ hr, duration, 2-6 hr
IV: Onset 5-10 min, peak 15-30 min, duration 3-6 hr
REC: Onset 15-30 min, duration 3-6 hr
Metabolized by liver, excreted in urine, crosses placenta

Interactions:
• Increased effects with other CNS depressants: alcohol, narcotics, sedative/hypnotics, antipsychotics, skeletal muscle relaxants

Y-site compatibilities: Glycopyrrolate, hydroxyzine, ranitidine

O

Lab test interferences:
Increase: Amylase

NURSING CONSIDERATIONS

Assess:

- I&O ratio for decreasing output; may indicate urinary retention
- CNS changes: dizziness, drowsiness, hallucinations, euphoria, LOC, pupil reaction
- Allergic reactions: rash, urticaria
- Respiratory dysfunction: respiratory depression, character, rate, rhythm; notify prescriber if respirations are <10/min
- Need for pain medication, physical dependence

Administer:

- IV after diluting with 5 ml sterile H_2O or NS for inj; give over 2-5 min through Y-tube or 3-way stopcock
- With antiemetic for nausea, vomiting
- When pain is beginning to return; determine interval by response

Perform/provide:

- Storage in light-resistant area at room temp
- Assistance with ambulation
- Safety measures: side rails, nightlight, call bell within easy reach

Evaluate:

- Therapeutic response: decrease in pain

Teach patient/family:

- To report any symptoms of CNS changes, allergic reactions
- That physical dependency may result from extended use
- That withdrawal symptoms may occur: nausea, vomiting, cramps, fever, faintness, anorexia

Treatment of overdose: Naloxone (Narcan) 0.2-0.8 mg IV, O_2, IV fluids, vasopressors

oxyphenbutazone (℞)

(ox-i-fen-byoo′ta-zone)
Oxybutazone*, oxyphenbutazone

Func. class.: Nonsteroidal antiinflammatory

Chem. class.: Pyrazolone derivative

Action: Inhibits prostaglandin synthesis by decreasing an enzyme needed for biosynthesis; analgesic, antiinflammatory, antipyretic

Uses: Mild to moderate pain, osteoarthritis, rheumatoid arthritis

Dosage and routes:

Pain

- *Adult:* PO 100-200 mg tid-qid

Acute arthritis

- *Adult:* PO 400 mg, then 100 mg q4h × 4 days or until desired response

Available forms: Tabs 100 mg

Side effects/adverse reactions:

GI: Nausea, anorexia, vomiting, diarrhea, jaundice, ***cholestatic hepatitis,*** constipation, flatulence, cramps, dry mouth, peptic ulcer

CNS: Dizziness, drowsiness, fatigue, tremors, confusion, insomnia, anxiety, depression

CV: Tachycardia, peripheral edema, palpitations, dysrhythmias, hypertension, cardiac decompensation

INTEG: Purpura, rash, pruritus, sweating

GU: ***Nephrotoxicity: dysuria, hematuria, oliguria, azotemia***

HEMA: ***Blood dyscrasias,*** bone marrow suppression

EENT: Tinnitus, hearing loss, blurred vision

Contraindications: Hypersensitivity, asthma, severe renal disease, severe hepatic disease, pregnancy (D), children <14 yr, ulcer disease

* Available in Canada only

Precautions: Lactation, children, bleeding disorders, GI disorders, cardiac disorders, hypersensitivity to other antiinflammatory agents

Pharmacokinetics:
PO: Peak 2 hr, half-life 3-3½ hr, metabolized in liver, excreted in urine (metabolites), breast milk

Interactions:
• Increased action of coumarin, phenytoin, sulfonamides

NURSING CONSIDERATIONS

Assess:
• Renal, liver, blood studies: BUN, creatinine, AST (SGOT), ALT (SGPT), Hgb before treatment, periodically thereafter
• Audiometric, ophthalmic exam before, during, after treatment
• For eye, ear problems: blurred vision, tinnitus (may indicate toxicity)

Administer:
• With food to decrease GI symptoms; best to take on empty stomach to facilitate absorption

Perform/provide:
• Storage at room temp

Evaluate:
• Therapeutic response: decreased pain, stiffness, swelling in joints, ability to move more easily

Teach patient/family:
• To report blurred vision, ringing, roaring in ears (may indicate toxicity)
• To avoid driving, other hazardous activities if dizzy or drowsy
• To report change in urine pattern, weight increase, edema, pain increase in joints, fever, blood in urine (indicates nephrotoxicity)
• That therapeutic effects may take up to 1 mo

oxytetracycline (℞)

(ox-i-tet-ra-sye′kleen)
Oxytetracycline HCl, Terramycin, Terramycin IM, Uri-Tet
Func. class.: Broad-spectrum antibiotic/antiinfective
Chem. class.: Tetracycline

Combination products: Terramycin Intramuscular Solution: oxytetracycline 125 mg/ml with lidocaine 2%; Urobiotic-250: oxytetracycline HCl 250 mg (of oxytetracycline) with phenazopyridine HCl 50 mg, sulfamethizole 250 mg

Action: Inhibits protein synthesis, phosphorylation in microorganisms by binding to 30S ribosomal subunits, reversibly binding to 50S ribosomal subunits; bacteriostatic artificial clot

Uses: Syphilis, chlamydia trachomatis, gonorrhea, lymphogranuloma venereum, uncommon gram-positive/negative organisms, rickettsial infections

Dosage and routes:
• *Adult:* PO 250-500 mg q6h; IM 100 mg q8h or 150 mg q12h; IV 250-500 mg q12h, 250 mg q24h
• *Child >8 yr:* PO 25-50 mg/kg day in divided doses q6h; IM 15-25 mg/kg/day in divided doses q8-12h; IV 10-20 mg/kg/day in divided doses q12h

Gonorrhea
• *Adult:* PO 1.5 g, then 500 mg qid for a total of 9 g

Chlamydia trachomatis
• *Adult:* PO 500 mg qid × 7 days

Syphilis
• *Adult:* PO 2-3 g in divided doses × 10-15 days up to 30-40 g total
• Dosage adjustment necessary in renal impairment

O

Available forms: Tabs 250 mg; caps 125, 250 mg; powder for inj IV 250, 500 mg; inj IM 50, 125 mg/ml

Side effects/adverse reactions:

CNS: Fever

HEMA: ***Eosinophilia, neutropenia, thrombocytopenia, leukocytosis, hemolytic anemia***

EENT: Dysphagia, glossitis, decreased calcification of deciduous teeth, oral candidiasis

GI: Nausea, abdominal pain, *vomiting, diarrhea,* anorexia, enterocolitis, ***hepatotoxicity,*** flatulence, abdominal cramps, epigastric burning, stomatitis

CV: Pericarditis

GU: Increased BUN

INTEG: Rash, urticaria, photosensitivity, increased pigmentation, ***exfoliative dermatitis,*** pruritus, angioedema, pain at injection site

Contraindications: Hypersensitivity to tetracyclines, children <8 yr, pregnancy (D)

Precautions: Renal disease, hepatic disease, lactation

Pharmacokinetics:

PO: Peak 2-4 hr, half-life 6-12 hr; excreted in urine, bile, feces in active form; crosses placenta; 20%-40% protein bound

Interactions:

- Decreased effect of oxytetracycline: antacids, $NaHCO_3$, dairy products, alkali products, iron, kaolin/pectin, cimetidine
- Increased effect: anticoagulants
- Decreased effect: penicillins, oral contraceptives
- Nephrotoxicity: methoxyflurane
- Do not mix with other drugs

Lab test interferences:

False negative: Urine glucose with Clinistix or Tes-Tape

False increase: Urinary catecholamines

NURSING CONSIDERATIONS

Assess:

- I&O ratio
- Blood studies: PT, CBC, AST (SGOT), ALT (SGPT), BUN, creatinine
- Signs of anemia: Hct, Hgb, fatigue
- Allergic reactions: rash, itching, pruritus, angioedema
- Nausea, vomiting, diarrhea; administer antiemetic, antacids as ordered
- Overgrowth of infection: fever, malaise, redness, pain, swelling, drainage, perineal itching, diarrhea, changes in cough or sputum

Administer:

- PO with a full glass of water
- IM, deep only
- IV after diluting 250 mg or less/10 ml of sterile H_2O for inj; further dilute with at least 100 ml of D_5W or NS for inj; give 100 mg or less/5 min or more; use within 12 hr, decrease rate or increase vol of diluent if vein irritation occurs; do not give SC
- After C&S obtained
- 2 hr before or after laxative or ferrous products, 3 hr after antacid

Perform/provide:

- Storage in tight, light-resistant container at room temp

Evaluate:

- Therapeutic response: decreased temp, absence of lesions, negative C&S

Teach patient/family:

- To avoid sunlight; sunscreen does not seem to decrease photosensitivity
- If diabetic use blood glucose testing
- That all prescribed medication must be taken to prevent superinfection
- To avoid milk products, to take with a full glass of water

oxytocin, synthetic injection (℞)

(ox-i-toe'sin)

Pitocin, Syntocinon

Func. class.: Oxytocic

Chem. class.: Hormone

Action: Acts directly on myofibrils, producing uterine contraction; stimulates milk ejection by the breast

Uses: Stimulation, induction of labor; missed or incomplete abortion; postpartum bleeding

Dosage and routes:

Postpartum hemorrhage

• *Adult:* IV 10 U infused at 20-40 μU/min

• *Adult:* IM 10 U after delivery of placenta

Fetal stress test

• *Adult:* IV 0.5 μU/min, increase q20min until 3 contractions within 10 min

Stimulation of labor

• *Adult:* IV 0.5-2 μU/min, increase by 1-2 μU q15-60 min until contractions occur; then decrease dose

Incomplete abortion

• *Adult:* IV INF 10 U/500 ml D_5W or 0.9% NaCl at 20-40 mU/min

Available forms: Inj 10 U/ml

Side effects/adverse reactions:

CNS: Hypertension, ***convulsions, tetanic contractions***

CV: Hypotension, dysrhythmias, increased pulse, bradycardia, tachycardia, PVC

FETUS: Dysrhythmias, jaundice, hypoxia, ***intracranial hemorrhage***

GI: Anorexia, nausea, vomiting, constipation

GU: ***Abruptio placentae, decreased uterine blood flow***

HEMA: Increased hyperbilirubinemia

INTEG: Rash

RESP: ***Asphyxia***

Contraindications: Hypersensitivity, serum toxemia, cephalopelvic disproportion, fetal distress, hypertonic uterus

Precautions: Cervical/uterine surgery, uterine sepsis, primipara >35 yr, 1st, 2nd stage of labor

Pharmacokinetics:

IM: Onset 3-7 min, duration 1 hr, half-life 12-17 min

IV: Onset 1 min, duration 30 min, half-life 12-17 min

Interactions:

• Hypertension: vasopressors

Additive compatibilities: Chloramphenicol, metaraminol, netilmicin, sodium bicarbonate, tetracycline, thiopental, verapamil

Y-site compatibilities: Heparin, insulin hydrocortisone, meperidine, morphine, potassium chloride, vitamin B with C

NURSING CONSIDERATIONS

Assess:

• I&O ratio

• Respiration

• B/P, pulse; watch for changes that may indicate hemorrhage

• Respiratory rate, rhythm, depth; notify prescriber of abnormalities

• Length, intensity, duration of contraction; notify prescriber of contractions lasting over 1 min or absence of contractions; turn patient on her side

• FHTs, fetal distress; watch for acceleration, deceleration; notify prescriber if problems occur; fetal presentation, pelvic dimensions; turn patient on left side if FHT change in rate

• For signs and symptoms of water intoxication; confusion, anuria, drowsiness, headache

Administer:

Labor induction

• IV after diluting 10 U/L of 0.9% NS or D_5 NS run at 1-2 mU/min at

15-30 min intervals to begin normal labor; dilute 10-40 mU/min, titrate to control postpartum bleeding; dilute 10 U/500 ml sol; run 10 U-20 mU/ml; administer by only 1 route at a time; use inf pump; rotate inf to provide mixing; do not shake

Control of postpartum bleeding
- IV: Dilute 10-40 U/1 L of sol, run at 10-20 mU min; adjust rate as needed
- With crash cart available on unit (Mg^+SO_4 at bedside)

Evaluate:
- Therapeutic response: stimulation of labor, control of postpartum bleeding

Teach patient/family:
- To report increased blood loss, abdominal cramps, fever, foul-smelling lochia
- That contractions will be similar to menstrual cramps, gradually increasing in intensity

oxytocin, synthetic nasal (℞)

(ox-i-toe'sin)

Func. class.: Oxytocic hormone

Action: Acts directly on myofibrils, producing uterine contraction; stimulates milk ejection by the breast

Uses: Postpartum breast engorgement, initial milk letdown

Dosage and routes:
- *Adult:* NAS SPRAY 1 spray into one or both nostrils q2-3 min before breast-feeding; NAS DROPS 3 gtt into one or both nostrils q2-3 min before breast-feeding

Available forms: Nas spray 40 U/ml; nas drops

Side effects/adverse reactions:
None

Pharmacokinetics:
Onset 5-10 min, half-life 1 min

Interactions:
- Hypertension: vasopressors

NURSING CONSIDERATIONS

Assess:
- I&O ratio
- Environment conducive to letdown reflex

Evaluate
- Therapeutic response: stimulation of milk ejection

Teach patient/family:
- To blow nose before administering; not to touch dropper to inside of nares
- To rinse dropper with warm water after each use
- Not to overuse

paclitaxel (℞)

(pa-kli-tax'el)

Taxol

Func. class.: Misc. antineoplastic

Chem. class.: Natural diterpene

Action: Inhibits reorganization of microtubule network needed for interphase and mitotic cellular functions; also causes abnormal bundles of microtubules during cell cycle and multiple esters of microtubules during mitosis

Uses: Metastatic carcinoma of the ovary

Dosage and routes:
- *Adult:* IV INF 135 mg/m^2 given over 24 hr q3wk

Available forms: Inj 30 mg/5 ml vial

Side effects/adverse reactions:

HEMA: ***Neutropenia, leukopenia, thrombocytopenia, anemia,*** bleeding, infections

SYST: Hypersensitivity reactions, ***anaphylaxis***

CV: Bradycardia, *hypotension,* abnormal ECG
NEURO: Peripheral neuropathy
MS: Arthralgia, myalgia
GI: Nausea, vomiting, diarrhea, mucositis, increased bilirubin, alk phosphatase, AST (SGOT)
INTEG: Alopecia
Contraindications: Hypersensitivity to paclitaxel or other drugs with polyoxyethylated castor oil, neutropenia of <1500/mm^3, pregnancy (D)
Precautions: Children, lactation, hepatic, cardiovascular disease, CNS disorder
Pharmacokinetics: 89%-98% of drug is serum protein bound, metabolized in liver, excreted in bile and urine; terminal half-life 5.3-17.4 hr
Interactions:
• Increased myelosuppression: cisplatin
• Decreased metabolism of paclitaxel: ketoconazole

NURSING CONSIDERATIONS
Assess:
• CBC, differential, platelet count qwk; withhold drug if WBC is <4000 or platelet count is 100,000, neutrophil is <1500/mm^3; notify prescriber
• Monitor temp q4h (may indicate beginning infection)
• Liver function tests before, during therapy (bilirubin, AST [SGOT], alk phosphatase) prn or qmo
• VS during 1st hr of infusion, check IV site for signs of infiltration
• Hypersensitive reactions including hypotension, dyspnea, angioedema, generalized urticaria; discontinue infusion immediately
• Bleeding: hematuria, guaiac, bruising or petechiae, mucosa or orifices q8h; obtain prescription for viscous lidocaine (Xylocaine)
• Food preferences; list likes, dislikes
• Effects of alopecia on body image; discuss feelings about body changes
Administer:
• IV after diluting in 0.9% NaCl, D_5, D_5 and 0.9% NaCl, D_5LR to a concentration of 0.3-1.2 mg/ml
• Using an in-line filter <0.22 μm
• After premedicating with dexamethasone 20 mg PO 12 hr and 6 hr before paclitaxel or diphenhydramine 50 mg IV ½-1 hr before paclitaxel and cimetidine 300 mg or ranitidine 50 mg IV ½-1 hr before paclitaxel
• Using only glass bottles, polypropylene, polyolefin bags and administration sets; do not use PVC infusion bags or sets
• Using gloves and cytotoxic handling precautions
• Antiemetic 30-60 min before giving drug and prn
• Antibiotics for prophylaxis of infection
Perform/provide:
• Confirmation that dexamethasone was given 12 hr and 6 hr before infusion begins
• Storage of prepared sol up to 27 hr in refrigeration
Evaluate:
• Therapeutic response: decreased tumor size, spread of malignancy
Teach patient/family:
• To report signs of infection: fever, sore throat, flu symptoms
• To report signs of anemia: fatigue, headache, faintness, shortness of breath, irritability
• To report bleeding; avoid use of razors, commercial mouthwash
• To avoid use of aspirin, ibuprofen
• To report any complaints or side effects to nurse or prescriber
• That hair may be lost during treatment; a wig or hairpiece may make

P

patient feel better; new hair may be different in color, texture
• About side effects and what to do about them
• That pain in muscles and joints 2-5 days after infusion is common

pamidronate (℞)

(pam-i-drone′ate)
Aredia
Func. class.: Bone-resorption inhibitor
Chem. class.: Bisphosphonate

Action: Absorbs calcium phosphate crystals in bone and may directly block dissolution of hydroxyappetite crystals of bone; inhibits bone resorption, apparently without inhibiting bone formation and mineralization
Uses: Moderate to severe hypercalcemia associated with malignancy with or without bone metastases
Dosage and routes:
• *Adult:* IV INF 60-90 mg in moderate hypercalcemia, 90 mg in severe hypercalcemia over 24 hr
Available forms: Inj 30 mg pamidronate disodium and 470 mg of mannitol
Side effects/adverse reactions:
INTEG: Redness, swelling, induration, pain on palpitation at site of catheter insertion
META: Anemia, hypokalemia, hypomagnesemia, hypophosphatemia
GI: Abdominal pain, anorexia, constipation, nausea, vomiting
MS: Bone pain
CV: Hypertension
GU: UTI, fluid overload
Contraindications: Hypersensitivity to biphosphonates
Precautions: Children, nursing mothers, pregnancy (C), renal dysfunction
Pharmacokinetics: Rapidly cleared from circulation and taken up mainly by bones, eliminated primarily by kidneys
Interactions:
• Do not mix with Ca-containing infusion sol such as Ringer's sol
NURSING CONSIDERATIONS
Assess:
• Renal studies and Ca, P, Mg, K
• For hypercalcemia: paresthesia, twitching, laryngospasm, Chvostek's, Trousseau's signs
Administer:
• After reconstituting by adding 10 ml of sterile water for inj to each vial, then adding to 1000 ml of sterile 0.45%, 0.9% NaCl, D_5W, run over 24 hr
Perform/provide:
• Storage of infusion sol up to 24 hr at room temp
• Reconstituted sol with sterile water may be stored under refrigeration for up to 24 hr
Evaluate:
• Therapeutic response: decreased Ca levels

pancreatin (℞)

(pan′kree-a-tin)
Elzyme 303 Enseals
Func. class.: Digestant
Chem. class.: Pancreatic enzyme concentrate—bovine/porcine

Action: Pancreatic enzyme needed for proper pancreatic functioning
Uses: Exocrine pancreatic secretion insufficiency, cystic fibrosis (digestive aid)
Dosage and routes:
• *Adult:* PO 8000-24,000 USP U with meals
Available forms: Tab 650, 2000, 12,000 U

* Available in Canada only

Side effects/adverse reactions:
GI: Anorexia, nausea, vomiting, diarrhea, glossitis, anal soreness
GU: Hyperuricuria, hyperuricemia
INTEG: Rash, hypersensitivity
EENT: Buccal soreness
Contraindications: Hypersensitivity to pork, chronic pancreatic disease
Precautions: Pregnancy (C), lactation
Interactions:
• Decreased absorption: cimetidine, antacids, oral iron
NURSING CONSIDERATIONS
Assess:
• I&O ratio; watch for increasing urinary output
• Fecal fat, nitrogen, pro-time, Ca during treatment
• For polyuria, polydipsia, polyphagia (may indicate diabetes mellitus)
Administer:
• After antacid or H_2 blockers; decreased pH inactivates drug
• Whole; not to be crushed, chewed (enteric coated)
• Low-fat diet for GI symptoms
Perform/provide:
• Storage in tight container at room temp
Evaluate:
• For allergy to pork

pancrelipase (℞)
(pan-kre-li'pase)
Catozym, Cotazym Capsules, Cotazym-S Capsules, Creon Capsules, Festal II Tablets, Ilozyme, Ku-Zyme HP Capsules, Pancrease Capsules, Pancrease MT 4, Pancrease MT 10, Pancrease MT 16, Ultrase MT 12, Ultrase MT 20, Ultrase MT 24, Viokase Powder, Viokase Tablets, Zymase

Func. class.: Digestant
Chem. class.: Pancreatic enzyme—bovine/porcine

Action: Pancreatic enzyme needed for proper pancreatic functioning
Uses: Exocrine pancreatic secretion insufficiency, cystic fibrosis (digestive aid), steatorrhea, pancreatic enzyme deficiency
Dosage and routes:
• *Adult and child:* PO 1-3 caps/tabs ac or with meals, or 1 cap/tab with snack or 1-2 pdr pkt ac
Available forms: Tabs 8000, 11,000, 30,000 U; caps 8000, 30,000 U; enteric coated caps 4000, 5000, 20,000, 25,000 U; powd 16,800 U
Side effects/adverse reactions:
GI: Anorexia, nausea, vomiting, diarrhea
GU: Hyperuricuria, hyperuricemia
Contraindications: Allergy to pork, chronic pancreatic disease
Precautions: Pregnancy (C)
Interactions:
• Decreased absorption: cimetidine, antacids, oral iron
NURSING CONSIDERATIONS
Assess:
• For appropriate height, weight development; may be delayed
• I&O ratio; watch for increasing urinary output

P

• Fecal fat, nitrogen, pro-time during treatment
• For polyuria, polydipsia, polyphagia (may indicate diabetes mellitus)

Administer:
• After antacid or cimetidine; decreased pH inactivates drug
• Powder mixed in prepared fruit for infants, children
• Whole, not crushed or chewed (enteric coated)
• Low-fat diet for GI symptoms
• Powder mixed with pureed fruit; take tabs with or before food

Perform/provide:
• Storage in tight container at room temp

Teach patient/family:
• To take with 8 oz water or more, not to allow to sit in mouth, have patient sit up during administration
• To notify prescriber of allergic reactions, abdominal pain, cramping or blood in the urine

Evaluate:
• Therapeutic response: improved digestion of carbohydrates, protein, fat; absence of steatorrhea

pancuronium (℞)

(pan-kyoo-roe′nee-um)
pancuronium Bromide, Pavulon

Func. class.: Neuromuscular blocker (nondepolarizing)

Chem. class.: Synthetic curariform

Action: Inhibits transmission of nerve impulses by binding with cholinergic receptor sites, antagonizing action of acetylcholine

Uses: Facilitation of endotracheal intubation, skeletal muscle relaxation during mechanical ventilation, surgery, or general anesthesia

Dosage and routes:
• *Adult:* IV 0.04-0.1 mg/kg, then 0.01 mg/kg q½-1hr
• *Child >10 yr:* IV 0.04-0.1 mg/kg, then ⅕ initial dose q½-1hr

Available forms: Inj 1, 2 mg/ml

Side effects/adverse reactions:
CV: Bradycardia; tachycardia; increased, decreased B/P; ventricular extra systoles
RESP: ***Prolonged apnea, bronchospasm, cyanosis, respiratory depression***
EENT: Increased secretions
MS: Weakness to prolonged skeletal muscle relaxation
INTEG: Rash, flushing, pruritus, urticaria, sweating, salivation

Contraindications: Hypersensitivity to bromide ion

Precautions: Pregnancy (C), renal disease, cardiac disease, lactation, children <2 yr, electrolyte imbalances, dehydration, neuromuscular disease, respiratory disease

Pharmacokinetics:
IV: Onset 30-45 sec, peak 3-5 min; metabolized (small amounts), excreted in urine (unchanged), crosses placenta

Interactions:
• Increased neuromuscular blockade: aminoglycosides, clindamycin, lincomycin, quinidine, local anesthetics, polymyxin antibiotics, lithium, narcotic analgesics, thiazides, enflurane, isoflurane
• Dysrhythmias: theophylline

Syringe compatibility: Heparin

Y-site compatibilities: Aminophylline, cefazolin, cefuroxime, cimetidine, cotrimoxazole, dobutamine, dopamine, epinephrine, esmolol, fentanyl, gentaamicin, heparin, hydrocortisone sodium succinate, isoproterenol, lorazepam, midazolam, morphine, nitroglycerin, ranitidine,

sodium nitroprusside, sulfamethoxazole/trimethoprim, vancomycin
Additive compatibility: Verapamil
Lab test interferences:
Decrease: Cholinesterase

NURSING CONSIDERATIONS

Assess:

• For electrolyte imbalances (K, Mg); may lead to increased action of this drug
• Vital signs (B/P, pulse, respirations, airway) until fully recovered; rate, depth, pattern of respirations, strength of hand grip
• I&O ratio; check for urinary retention, frequency, hesitancy
• Recovery: decreased paralysis of face, diaphragm, leg, arm, rest of body; allow to recover fully before neuro assessment
• Allergic reactions: rash, fever, respiratory distress, pruritus; drug should be discontinued

Administer:

• With diazepam or morphine when used for therapeutic paralysis; this drug provides no sedation
• Using nerve stimulator by anesthesiologist to determine neuromuscular blockade
• Atropine to counteract muscarinic effects
• After succinylcholine effects subside
• Anticholinesterase to reverse neuromuscular blockade
• IV undiluted, give over 1-2 min (only by qualified persons)

Perform/provide:

• Storage in refrigerator; do not store in plastic; use only fresh sol
• Reassurance if communication is difficult during recovery from neuromuscular blockade
• Frequent (q2h) instillation of artificial tears and covering eyes to prevent drying of cornea

Evaluate:

• Therapeutic response: paralysis of jaw, eyelid, head, neck, rest of body

Treatment of overdose: Edrophonium or neostigmine, atropine, monitor VS; may require mechanical ventilation

papaverine (℞)

(pa-pav'er-een)
Cerespan, Genabid, papaverine HCl, Pavabid HP Capsulets, Pavabid Plateau Caps, Pavarine Spancaps, Pavased, Pavatine, Pavatym, Paverolan Lanacaps

Func. class.: Peripheral vasodilator

Chem. class.: Opium alkaloid (no narcotic activity)

Action: Relaxes all smooth muscle; inhibits cyclic nucleotide phosphodiesterase, which increases intracellular cAMP, causing vasodilation
Uses: Arterial spasm resulting in cerebral and peripheral ischemia; myocardial ischemia associated with vascular spasm or dysrhythmias; angina pectoris; peripheral pulmonary embolism; visceral spasm as in ureteral, biliary, GI colic PVD
Investigational uses: Male impotence caused by organic condition
Dosage and routes:
• *Adult:* PO 100-300 mg 3-5 × day; SUS REL 150-300 mg q8-12h; IM/IV 30-120 mg q3h prn
Available forms: Cap time-release 150, 200, 300 mg; tabs 30, 60, 100, 150, 200, 300 mg; inj 30 mg/ml
Side effects/adverse reactions:
CV: ***Tachycardia,*** increased B/P
RESP: Increased depth of respirations
CNS: Headache, dizziness, drowsiness, sedation, vertigo, malaise

GI: Nausea, anorexia, abdominal pain, constipation, diarrhea, jaundice, altered liver enzymes, ***hepatotoxicity***
INTEG: Flushing, sweating, rash
Contraindications: Hypersensitivity, complete AV heart block
Precautions: Cardiac dysrhythmias, glaucoma, pregnancy (C), lactation, drug dependency, child
Pharmacokinetics:
PO: Onset 30 sec, peak 1-2 hr, duration 3-4 hr
SUS REL: Onset erratic, duration 3 hr
90% bound to plasma proteins, metabolized in liver, excreted in urine (inactive metabolites)
Interactions:
• Decreased effect of levodopa
• Increased hypotension: antihypertensives, vasodilators, diazoxide, alcohol
Syringe compatibility: Phentolamine
Solution/additive compatibilities: 0.9% NaCl, 0.45% NaCl, D_5W, $D_{10}W$, D_5/0.9% NaCl, D_5/0.45% NaCl, D_5/0.25% NaCl, Ringer's inj, phentolamine

NURSING CONSIDERATIONS
Assess:
• B/P, pulse, respiratory rate, rhythm, character during treatment until stable; take B/P lying, standing; orthostatic hypotension is common
• Hepatic tests: AST (SGOT), ALT (SGPT), bilirubin; liver enzymes may increase
• Hepatic hypersensitivity reaction: nausea, vomiting, jaundice; drug should be discontinued
Administer:
• With meals to reduce GI upset
• An ordered analgesic if headache develops
• IV undiluted or dluted in equal amount of sterile H_2O; give 30 mg or less/2 min through Y-tube or 3-way stopcock
Perform/provide:
• Storage at room temp
Evaluate:
• Therapeutic response: ability to walk without pain, increased pulse volume, increased temp in extremities; orientation, long- and short-term memory
Teach patient/family:
• That medication is not cure, may have to be taken continuously depending on condition; therapeutic response may not be evident for 2-3 mo
• That must quit smoking to prevent excessive vasoconstriction
• To avoid hazardous activities until stabilized on medication; dizziness may occur
• To notify prescriber of nausea, flushing, sweating, headache, or jaundice
Treatment of overdose: Discontinue medication

paraldehyde (℞)
(par-al'de-hyde)
Paral, Paraldehyde
Func. class.: Anticonvulsant
Chem. class.: Cyclic ether

Controlled Substance Schedule IV
Action: CNS depressant; exact mechanism of action is unknown
Uses: Refractory seizures, status epilepticus, sedation, insomnia, alcohol withdrawal, tetanus, eclampsia
Dosage and routes:
Seizures
• *Adult:* IM 5-10 ml; divide 10 ml into 2 inj; IV 0.2-0.4 ml/kg in NS inj
• *Child:* IM 0.15 ml/kg; REC 0.3 ml/kg q4-6h or 1 ml/yr of age, not to exceed 5 ml; may repeat in 1 hr

prn; IV 5 ml/90 ml NS inj; begin infusion at 5 ml/hr; titrate to patient response

Alcohol withdrawal

• *Adult:* PO/REC 5-10 ml, not to exceed 60 ml; IM 5 ml q4-6h × 24 hr, then q6h on following days, not to exceed 30 ml

Sedation

• *Adult:* PO/REC 4-10 ml; IM 5 ml; IV 3-5 ml in emergency only

• *Child:* PO/REC/IM 0.15 ml/kg

Tetanus

• *Adult:* IV 4-5 ml or 12 ml by gastric tube q4h diluted with water; IM 5-10 ml prn

Available forms: Inj IM, IV; oral and rectal liquid

Side effects/adverse reactions:

HEMA: ***Thrombocytopenia, agranulocytosis, leukopenia, neutropenia, hemolytic anemia,*** increased protime

CNS: Stimulation, drowsiness, dizziness, confusion, ***convulsion,*** headache, flushing, hallucinations, coma

GI: Foul breath, irritation

GU: Nephrosis

INTEG: Rash, erythema, local pain, sloughing fat necrosis

CV: Pulmonary edema, ***pulmonary hemnorrhage, circulatory collapse, respiratory depression***

Contraindications: Hypersensitivity, gastroenteritis with ulceration

Precautions: Asthma, hepatic disease, pulmonary disease, pregnancy (C)

Pharmacokinetics:

PO: 10-15 min, peak 1-2 hr, duration 6-8 hr

REC: Onset slow, duration 4-6 hr

Metabolized by liver; excreted by kidneys, lungs; crosses placenta; half-life 7.5 hr

Interactions:

• Increased blood levels of paraldehyde: alcohol, CNS depressants, general anesthetics, disulfiram

• Increase crystallization in kidneys: sulfonamides

• Incompatible with chlorpromazine, prochlorperazine, plastics; do not mix in syringe or sol with any drug

Lab test interferences:

False positive: Urinary serum ketones, interference, 17-OHCS

NURSING CONSIDERATIONS

Assess:

• VS q30min after parenteral route

• Blood studies: Hct, Hgb, RBCs, serum folate, Vit D if on long-term therapy

• Hepatic studies: AST (SGOT), ALT (SGPT), bilirubin, creatinine, failure

• For signs of jaundice, hepatitis

• Mental status: mood, sensorium, affect, memory (long, short)

• Respiratory dysfunction; respiratory depression, character, rate, rhythm; hold drug if respirations <10/min or pupils dilated

Administer:

• IV after diluting 1 ml/20 ml of NaCl for inj; give 21 ml or less over 3-5 min

• IM inj deep in large muscle mass; use Z-track method to prevent tissue sloughing; max of 5 ml at any one site

• After conservative measures have been tried for insomnia

• Rectal after diluting in cottonseed or olive oil as retention enema or 200 ml NS for enema

• Keep patient's room well ventilated to remove exhaled drug

• Orally with juice or milk to cover taste/smell, decrease GI symptoms

• Using fresh supply; don't expose to air, don't use if brown or if odor is vinegary or if container opened >24 hr

• Using glass container only; reacts with plastic

Perform/provide:
- Ventilation of room

Evaluate:
- Therapeutic response: increased sedation, decreased seizures

Teach patient/family:
- That physical dependency may result from extended use
- To avoid driving, other activities that require alertness
- Not to discontinue medication quickly after long-term use; taper over several weeks

---

paramethadione (℞)

(par-a-meth-a-dye′one)

Paradione

Func. class.: Anticonvulsant

Chem. class.: Oxazolidinedione

Action: Increases seizure threshold in cortex and basal ganglia; decreases synaptic stimulation to low-frequency impulses

Uses: Refractory absence (petit mal) seizures

Dosage and routes:
- *Adult:* PO 300 mg tid; may increase by 300 mg/wk, not to exceed 600 mg qid
- *Child >6 yr:* PO 0.9 g/day in divided doses tid or qid
- *Child 2-6 yr:* PO 0.6 g/day in divided doses tid or qid
- *Child <2 yr:* PO 0.3 g/day in divided doses tid or qid

Available forms: Caps 150, 300 mg; sol 300 mg/ml

Side effects/adverse reactions:

HEMA: ***Thrombocytopenia, agranulocytosis, leukopenia, neutropenia, hemolytic anemia,*** increased protime

CNS: Drowsiness, dizziness, fatigue, paresthesia, irritability, headache

GU/GYN: Vaginal bleeding, albuminuria, nephrosis

GI: Nausea, vomiting, abdominal pain, weight loss, bleeding gums, abnormal liver function tests

INTEG: ***Exfoliative dermatitis,*** rash, alopecia, petechiae, erythema

EENT: Photophobia, diplopia, epistaxis, retinal hemorrhage

CV: Hypertension, hypotension

Contraindications: Hypersensitivity, blood dyscrasias, pregnancy (D), lactation

Precautions: Hepatic disease, renal disease, retinal or optic nerve damage

Pharmacokinetics:

PO: Onset 15-30 min, peak 1-2 hr, duration 4-6 hr

REC: Onset slow, duration 4-6 hr

Metabolized by liver, excreted by kidneys, crosses placenta, excreted in breast milk, half-life 1-3½ hr

NURSING CONSIDERATIONS

Assess:
- Blood studies: Hct, Hgb, RBCs, serum folate, Vit D if on long-term therapy; discontinue drug if neutrophil count falls below 2500/mm^3
- Hepatic studies: ALT (SGPT), AST (SGOT), bilirubin
- Skin rash; withhold drug
- Mental status: mood, sensorium, affect, memory (long, short)

Administer:
- After diluting oral sol with water
- Oral with juice or milk to cover taste/smell, to decrease GI symptoms

Perform/provide:
- Ventilation of room

Evaluate:
- Therapeutic response: decreased seizures

Teach patient/family:
- To avoid driving, other activities that require alertness
- Not to discontinue medication quickly after long-term use; convulsions may result

---

* Available in Canada only

• To obtain liver function tests and urinalysis qmo
• To notify prescriber of sore throat, fever, malaise, bruises, petechiae, or epistaxis
• To wear dark glasses if photosensitivity occurs
• To take drug with food, milk to decrease GI symptoms

paramethasone (℞)

(par-a-meth'a-sone)
Haldrone
Func. class.: Corticosteroid
Chem. class.: Glucocorticoid, long acting

Action: Decreases inflammation by suppression of migration of polymorphonuclear leukocytes, fibroblasts, reversal to increase capillary permeability and lysosomal stabilization
Uses: Severe inflammation, collagen disorders, respiratory, dermatologic disorders, adrenal insufficiency
Dosage and routes:
• *Adult:* PO 0.5-6 mg tid-qid
• *Child:* PO 58-800 μg/kg/day in divided doses tid-qid
Available forms: Tabs 2 mg
Side effects/adverse reactions:
INTEG: Acne, poor wound healing, ecchymosis, petechiae
CNS: Depression, flushing, sweating, headache, mood changes
CV: Hypertension, ***circulatory collapse, thrombophlebitis, embolism,*** tachycardia, edema
HEMA: ***Thrombocytopenia***
MS: Fractures, osteoporosis, weakness
GI: Diarrhea, nausea, abdominal distention, ***GI hemorrhage,*** increased appetite, ***pancreatitis***
EENT: Fungal infections, increased intraocular pressure, blurred vision

Contraindications: Psychosis, hypersensitivity, idiopathic thrombocytopenia, acute glomerulonephritis, amebiasis, fungal infections, nonasthmatic bronchial disease, child <2 yr, AIDS, TB
Precautions: Pregnancy (C), diabetes mellitus, glaucoma, osteoporosis, seizure disorders, ulcerative colitis, CHF, myasthenia gravis, renal disease, esophagitis, peptic ulcer
Pharmacokinetics:
PO: Peak 1-2 hr, duration 2 days
IM: Peak 3-4.5 hr
Interactions:
• Decreased action of paramethasone: cholestyramine, colestipol, barbiturates, rifampin, ephedrine, phenytoin, theophylline
• Decreased effects of anticoagulants, anticonvulsants, antidiabetics, ambenonium, neostigmine, isoniazid, toxoids, vaccines
• Increased side effects: alcohol, salicylates, indomethacin, amphotericin B, digitalis preparations
• Increased action of paramethasone: salicylates, estrogens, indomethacin
Lab test interferences:
Increase: Cholesterol, Na, blood glucose, uric acid, Ca, urine glucose
Decrease: Ca, K, T_4, T_3, thyroid ^{131}I uptake test, urine 17-OHCS, 17-KS, PBI
False negative: Skin allergy tests

NURSING CONSIDERATIONS

Assess:
• K, blood sugar, urine glucose while on long-term therapy; hypokalemia and hyperglycemia
• Weight qd; notify prescriber of weekly gain >5 lb
• B/P q4h, pulse; notify prescriber of chest pain
• I&O ratio for decreasing urinary output, increasing edema
• Plasma cortisol levels during long-term therapy (normal level: 138-

P

635 nmol/L SI units when drawn at 8 AM)
• Infection: increased temp, WBC, even after withdrawal, drug masks symptoms of infection
• K, depletion: paresthesias, fatigue, nausea, vomiting, depression, polyuria, dysrhythmias, weakness
• Edema, hypertension, cardiac symptoms
• Mental status: affect, mood, behavioral changes, aggression

Administer:
• Titrated dose; use lowest effective dose
• In one dose in AM to prevent adrenal suppression; avoid SC administration; may damage tissue
• With food or milk to decrease GI symptoms

Perform/provide:
• Assistance with ambulation in patient with bone tissue disease to prevent fractures

Evaluate:
• Therapeutic response: ease of respirations, decreased inflammation

Teach patient/family:
• That ID as steroid user should be carried
• To notify prescriber if therapeutic response decreases; dosage adjustment may be needed
• Not to discontinue abruptly or adrenal crisis can result
• To avoid OTC products: salicylates, alcohol in cough products, cold preparations unless directed by prescriber
• About cushingoid symptoms
• Symptoms of adrenal insufficiency: nausea, anorexia, fatigue, dizziness, dyspnea, weakness, joint pain

paromomycin (℞)

(par-oh-moe-mye'sin)
Humatin
Func. class.: Amebicide
Chem. class.: Aminoglycoside antibiotic

Action: Direct action in intestinal lumen
Uses: Intestinal amebiasis, adjunt in hepatic coma
Dosage and routes:
Intestinal amebiasis
• *Adult and child:* PO 25-35 mg/kg/day in 3 divided doses × 5-10 days pc
Hepatic coma
• *Adult:* 4 g qd in divided doses × 5-6 days
Available forms: Caps 250 mg
Side effects/adverse reactions:
EENT: Ototoxicity
GI: Nausea, vomiting, diarrhea, epigastric distress, anorexia, steatorrhea, pruritus ani, hypocholesterolemia
GU: ***Nephrotoxicity, hematuria***
Contraindications: Hypersensitivity, renal disease, GI obstruction
Precautions: GI ulcerations, pregnancy (C), children, lactation
Pharmacokinetics:
PO: Excreted in feces, urine, slowly
Lab test interferences:
Decrease: Serum cholesterol

NURSING CONSIDERATIONS

Assess:
• Stools during entire treatment; should be clear at end of therapy: stools should be free of parasite for 1 yr before patient is considered cured
• I&O, stools for number, frequency, character
• Allergic reaction: rash, itching; drug should be discontinued
• Diarrhea for 2-3 days

* Available in Canada only

Administer:
- Cleansing enema if ordered before beginning treatment
- PO after meals to avoid GI symptoms

Perform/provide:
- Storage in tight container

Evaluate:
- Therapeutic response: decreased diarrhea, stools clear on culture

Teach patient/family:
- Proper hygiene after BM: handwashing technique
- Avoid contact of drug with eyes, mouth, nose, other mucous membranes
- Need for compliance with dosage schedule, duration of treatment

---

paroxetine (℞)

(par-ox′e-teen)

Paxil

Func. class.: Antidepressant, serotonin reuptake inhibitor

Chem. class.: Phenylpiperidine derivative

Action: Inhibits CNS neuron uptake of serotonin but not of norepinephrine or dopamine

Uses: Major depressive disorder

Dosage and routes:
- *Adult:* PO 20 mg qd in AM; after 4 wk if no clinical improvement is noted, dose may be increased by 10 mg/day qwk to desired response, not to exceed 50 mg/day

Available forms: Tabs 20, 30 mg

Side effects/adverse reactions:

CNS: Headache, nervousness, insomnia, drowsiness, anxiety, tremor, dizziness, fatigue, sedation, abnormal dreams, agitation, apathy, euphoria, hallucinations, delusions, psychosis

GI: Nausea, diarrhea, dry mouth, anorexia, dyspepsia, constipation, cramps, vomiting, taste changes, flatulence, decreased appetite

INTEG: Sweating, rash

RESP: Infection, pharyngitis, nasal congestion, sinus headache, sinusitis, cough, dyspnea

CV: Vasodilation, postural hypotension, palpitations

MS: Pain, arthritis, myalgia, myopathy, myosthenia

GU: Dysmenorrhea, decreased libido, urinary frequency, UTI, amenorrhea, cystitis, impotence, abnormal ejaculation

EENT: Visual changes

SYST: Asthenia, fever

Contraindications: Hypersensitivity, patients taking MAOIs

Precautions: Pregnancy (B), lactation, children, elderly, seizure history, patients with history of mania, renal and hepatic disease

Pharmacokinetics:

PO: Peak 6-8 hr; metabolized in liver, unchanged drugs and metabolites excreted in feces and urine; half-life 2-7 days

Interactions:
- When used with warfarin: increased bleeding
- Do not use with MAOIs
- Cimetidine increases paroxetine plasma levels
- Increased agitation: L-tryptophan
- Phenobarbital and phenytoin decrease paroxetine levels
- Increased side effects: highly protein-bound drugs
- Paroxetine may increase digoxin levels

Lab test interferences:
- *Increase:* Serum bilirubin, blood glucose, alk phosphatase
- *Decrease:* VMA, 5-HIAA
- *False increase:* Urinary catecholamines

NURSING CONSIDERATIONS

Assess:
- Mental status: mood, sensorium,

P

affect, suicidal tendencies, increase in psychiatric symptoms, depression, panic
• B/P (lying/standing), pulse q4h; if systolic B/P drops 20 mm Hg, hold drug, notify prescriber; take vital signs q4h in patients with cardiovascular disease
• Blood studies: CBC, leukocytes, differential, cardiac enzymes if patient is receiving long-term therapy
• Hepatic studies: AST (SGOT), ALT (SGPT), bilirubin, creatinine
• Weight qwk; appetite may decrease with drug
• ECG for flattening of T wave, bundle branch, AV block, dysrhythmias in cardiac patients
• EPS primarily in elderly, rigidity, dystonia, akathisia
• Urinary retention, constipation
• Withdrawal symptoms: headache, nausea, vomiting, muscle pain, weakness; not usual unless drug discontinued abruptly
• Alcohol intake; if alcohol is consumed, hold dose until morning

Administer:
• Increased fluids, bulk in diet for constipation, urinary retention
• With food, milk for GI symptoms
• Crushed if patient is unable to swallow medication whole
• Dosage hs for oversedation during day; may take entire dose hs; elderly may not tolerate once/day dosing
• Gum, hard candy, frequent sips of water for dry mouth

Perform/provide:
• Storage at room temp; do not freeze
• Assistance with ambulation during therapy, since drowsiness, dizziness occur
• Safety measures including side rails, primarily in elderly
• Checking to see PO medication swallowed

Evaluate:
• Therapeutic response: decreased depression

Teach patient/family:
• That therapeutic effect may take 1-4 wk
• To use caution in driving, other activities requiring alertness because of drowsiness, dizziness, blurred vision
• Not to discontinue medication quickly after long-term use; may cause nausea, headache, malaise
• To avoid alcohol ingestion, other CNS depressants

pegaspargase (℞)

(peg-as′per-gase)
Elspar, Oncaspar
Func. class.: Antineoplastic
Chem. class.: E. coli enzyme

Action: Indirectly inhibits protein synthesis in tumor cells; without amino acid, DNA, RNA synthesis is halted; asparagine, protein synthesis is halted; G_1 phase; cell cycle specific; a nonvesicant a modified version of L-asparginase

Uses: Acute lymphocytic leukemia in combination with other antineoplastics

Dosage and routes:
In combination
• *Adult:* IV/IM 2500 IU q14 days, run IV over 2 hrs in 100 ml of NaCl or D_5 through a running IV, IM should be no more than 2 ml in one inj site
Sole induction
• *Adult:* 2500 IU/m^2 q14 days

Available forms: Inj 750 IU/ml in a phosphate buffered saline sol

Side effects/adverse reactions:
SYST: ***Anaphylaxis, hypersensitivity***

* Available in Canada only

HEMA: ***Thrombocytopenia, leukopenia, myelosuppression, anemia, decreased clotting factors, pancytopenia***
GI: Nausea, vomiting, anorexia, cramps, stomatitis, ***hepatotoxicity, pancreatitis,*** *diarrhea*
GU: Urinary retention, ***renal failure,*** glycosuria, polyuria, azotemia, uric acid neuropathy
INTEG: Rash, urticaria, chills, fever
ENDO: Hyperglycemia
RESP: ***Fibrosis, pulmonary infiltrate, severe bronchospasm***
CV: Chest pain, ***hypertension***
CNS: Neuritis, dizziness, headache, ***coma,*** depression, fatigue, confusion, hallucinations, seizures

Contraindications: Hypersensitivity, infant, pregnancy (D), lactation, pancreatitis

Precautions: Renal disease, hepatic disease, pregnancy (C), CNS disease

Pharmacokinetics: Unknown

Interactions:

- Decreased action of methotrexate
- Do not use with radiation
- Coagulation factor imbalances: heparin, warfarin, aspirin, nonsteroidal antiinflammatories
- Considered incompatible with other drugs in syringe or sol

NURSING CONSIDERATIONS

Assess:

- For signs and symptoms of pancreatitis (nausea, vomiting, severe abdominal pain), anaphylaxis (bronchospasm, dyspnea), cyanosis
- CBC, differential, platelet count qwk; withhold drug if WBC count is <4000 or platelet count is <75,000; notify prescriber of results
- Pulmonary function tests, chest x-ray studies before and during therapy; chest x-ray film should be obtained q2wk during treatment, watch for severe bronchospasm, fibrosis, pulmonary infiltrate
- Renal function studies: BUN, serum uric acid, ammonia urine CrCl, electrolytes before and during therapy
- I&O ratio; report fall in urine output of 30 ml/hr, may indicate renal failure
- Temp q4h (may indicate beginning infection)
- Liver function tests before and during therapy (bilirubin, AST [SGOT], ALT [SGPT], LDH) as needed or monthly, hepatotoxicity can occur
- RBC, Hct, Hgb; may be decreased
- Serum, urine glucose levels, glycosuria can occur
- Bleeding: hematuria, stool guaiac, bruising or petechiae, mucosa or orifices q8h
- Dyspnea, rales, nonproductive cough, chest pain, tachypnea, fatigue, increased pulse, pallor, lethargy, swelling around eyes or lips; anaphylaxis may occur
- B/P, since hypertension can occur
- Food preferences; list likes, dislikes
- Yellow skin, sclera, dark urine, clay-colored stools, itchy skin, abdominal pain, fever, diarrhea
- Local irritation, pain, burning, discoloration at injection site
- Symptoms of severe allergic reaction: rash, pruritus, urticaria, purpuric skin lesions, itching, flushing, dyspnea
- Frequency of stools, characteristics; cramping, acidosis; signs of dehydration: rapid respirations, poor skin turgor, decreased urine output, dry skin, restlessness, weakness

Administer:

- Allopurinol or sodium bicarbonate to reduce uric acid levels, alkalinization of urine
- IV infusion using 21, 23, 25G needle; administer by slow IV infusion via Y-tube or 3-way stop cock

P

of flowing D_5W or NS infusion over 2 hr after diluting
• Transfusion for severe anemia
• Antispasmodic if GI symptoms occur

Perform/provide:
• Deep-breathing exercises with patient tid-qid; place in semi-Fowler's position
• Increase fluid intake to 2-3 L/day to prevent urate deposits, calculi formation
• Diet low in purines: no organ meats (kidney, liver), dried beans, peas to maintain alkaline urine
• Rinsing of mouth tid-qid with water, club soda
• Brushing of teeth bid-tid with soft brush or cotton-tipped applicators for stomatitis; use unwaxed dental floss
• Warm compresses at injection site for inflammation
• Nutritious diet with iron, vitamin supplements
• HOB raised to facilitate breathing

Evaluate:
• Therapeutic response: decreased exacerbations in acute lymphocytic leukemia

Teach patient/family
• To report any complaints or side effects to nurse or prescriber
• To report any changes in breathing or coughing

Treatment of anaphylaxis: Administer epinephrine, diphenhydramine, IV corticosteroids

pemoline (℞)

(pem'oh-leen)
Cylert, Cylert Chewable
Func. class.: Cerebral stimulant
Chem. class.: Oxazolidinone derivative

Controlled Substance Schedule IV
Action: Exact mechanism unknown; may act through dopaminergic mechanisms; produces CNS stimulation and a paradoxic effect in ADHD
Uses: Attention deficit hyperactivity disorder
Investigational uses: Schizophrenia, fatigue, depression
Dosage and routes:
• *Child >6 yr:* 37.5 mg in AM, increasing by 18.75 mg/wk, not to exceed 112.5 mg/day
Available forms: Tabs 18.75, 37.5, 75 mg; chewable tabs 37.5 mg
Side effects/adverse reactions:
MISC: Rashes, growth suppression in children
CNS: Hyperactivity, insomnia, restlessness, dizziness, depression, headache, stimulation, irritability, aggressiveness, hallucinations, ***seizures, Gilles de la Tourette's disorder,*** drowsiness, dyskinetic movements
GI: Nausea, anorexia, diarrhea, abdominal pain, increased liver enzymes, hepatitis, jaundice, weight loss
CV: Tachycardia
Contraindications: Hypersensitivity, hepatic insufficiency
Precautions: Renal disease, pregnancy (B), lactation, drug abuse, child <6 yr, psychosis, tics, seizure disorder
Pharmacokinetics:
PO: Peak 2-4 hr, duration 8 hr, metabolized (50%) by liver, excreted (40%) by kidneys, half-life 10-30 hr

* Available in Canada only

NURSING CONSIDERATIONS
Assess:
• Hepatic function studies: ALT (SGOT), AST (SGOT), bilirubin, creatinine
• Child for growth retardation
• Mental status: mood, sensorium, affect, stimulation, insomnia, aggressiveness
Administer:
• At least 6 hr before hs
Evaluate:
• Therapeutic response: decreased hyperactivity
Teach patient/family:
• To decrease caffeine consumption (coffee, tea, cola, chocolate); may increase irritability, stimulation
• To avoid OTC preparations unless approved by prescriber
• To withdraw over several weeks
• To avoid alcohol ingestion
• To avoid hazardous activities until patient is stabilized
• That therapeutic effect may take 2-4 wk

penicillin G benzathine (℞)

(pen-i-sill'in)
Bicillin L-A, Megacillin*, Permapen, Bicillin C-R, Bicillin C-R 900/300
Func. class.: Broad-spectrum antiinfective
Chem. class.: Natural penicillin

Combination products: Bicillin C-R: 150,000 units (of penicillin G) per ml with penicillin G benzathine 150,000 units (of penicillin G) per ml; Bicillin C-R: penicillin G procaine 300,000 units (of penicillin G) per ml with penicillin G benzathine 300,000 units (of penicillin G) per ml; Bicillin C-R 900/300: penicillin G procaine 150,000 units (of penicillin G) per ml with penicillin G benzathine 450,000 units (of penicillin G) per ml

Action: Interferes with cell wall replication of susceptible organisms; osmotically unstable cell wall swells, bursts from osmotic pressure
Uses: Respiratory infections, scarlet fever, erysipelas, otitis media, pneumonia, skin and soft tissue infections, gonorrhea; effective for gram-positive cocci *(Staphylococcus, S. pyogenes, S. viridans, S. faecalis, S. bovis, S. pneumoniae)*, gram-negative cocci *(N. gonorrhoeae)*, gram-positive bacilli *(B. anthracis, C. perfringens, C. tetani, C. diphtheriae, L. monocytogenes)*, gram-negative bacilli *(E. coli, P. mirabilis, Salmonella, Shigella, Enterobacter, S. moniliformis)*, spirochetes *(T. pallidum), Actinomyces*
Dosage and routes:
Early syphilis
• *Adult:* IM 2.4 million U in single dose
Congenital syphilis
• *Child <2 yr:* IM 50,000 U/kg in single dose
Prophylaxis of rheumatic fever, glomerulonephritis
• *Adult and child >60 lb:* IM 1.2 million U in single dose qmo or 600,000 U q2wk
• *Child <60 lb:* IM 600,000 U in single dose
Upper respiratory infections (group A streptococcal)
• *Adult:* IM 1.2 million U in single dose, PO 400,000-600,000 U q4-6h
• *Child >27 kg:* IM 900,000 U in single dose
• *Child <27 kg:* IM 50,000 U/kg in single dose
Available forms: Inj 300,000, 600,000 U/ml; tabs 200,000 U

P

Side effects/adverse reactions:
HEMA: Anemia, increased bleeding time, ***bone marrow depression, granulocytopenia***
GI: Nausea, vomiting, diarrhea, increased AST (SGOT), ALT (SGPT), abdominal pain, glossitis, colitis
GU: ***Oliguria, proteinuria, hematuria,*** *vaginitis, moniliasis,* ***glomerulonephritis***
CNS: Lethargy, hallucinations, anxiety, depression, twitching, ***coma, convulsions***
META: Hyperkalemia, hypokalemia, alkalosis, hypernatremia
MISC: Local pain, tenderness and fever with IM injection
Contraindications: Hypersensitivity to penicillins; neonates
Precautions: Hypersensitivity to cephalosporins, pregnancy (B), lactation
Pharmacokinetics:
IM: Very slow absorption, duration 21-28 days, half-life 30-60 min; excreted in urine, feces, breast milk; crosses placenta
Interactions:
• Decreased antimicrobial effect of penicillin: tetracyclines, erythromycins
• Increased penicillin concentrations: aspirin, probenecid
Lab test interferences:
False positive: Urine glucose, urine protein

NURSING CONSIDERATIONS
Assess:
• I&O ratio; report hematuria, oliguria, since penicillin in high doses is nephrotoxic
• Any patient with compromised renal system, since drug is excreted slowly in poor renal system function; toxicity may occur rapidly
• Liver studies: AST (SGOT), ALT (SGPT)
• Blood studies: WBC, RBC, H&H, bleeding time
• Renal studies: urinalysis, protein, blood
• C&S before therapy; drug may be given as soon as culture is taken
• Bowel pattern before and during treatment
• Skin eruptions after administration of penicillin to 1 wk after discontinuing drug
• Respiratory status: rate, character, wheezing, tightness in chest
• Allergies before initiation of treatment, reaction of each medication; highlight allergies on chart; because of prolonged action, allergic reaction may be prolonged and severe
Administer:
• Orally on an empty stomach for best absorption
• Drug after C&S completed
• After shaking well, deep IM inj in large muscle masses; avoid intravascular inj, aspirate
Perform/provide:
• Adrenalin, suction, tracheostomy set, endotracheal intubation equipment
• Adequate fluid intake (2 L) during diarrhea episodes
• Scratch test to assess allergy after securing order from prescriber; usually done when penicillin is only drug of choice
• Storage in tight container; refrigerate injection
Evaluate:
• Therapeutic response: absence of fever, purulent drainage, redness, inflammation
Teach patient/family:
• To take oral penicillin on empty stomach with full glass of water
• That culture may be taken after completed course of medication
• To report sore throat, fever, fatigue; may indicate superinfection

• To wear or carry Medic Alert ID if allergic to penicillins
• To notify nurse of diarrhea

Treatment of hypersensitivity: Withdraw drug; maintain airway; administer epinephrine, aminophylline, O_2, IV corticosteroids

penicillin G potassium (℞)

Acrocillin, Burcillin-G, Deltapen, Megacillin*, Novopen G*, Pentids, Pfizerpen

Func. class.: Broad-spectrum antibiotic—penicillin

Chem. class.: Natural penicillin

Action: Interferes with cell wall replication of susceptible organisms; osmotically unstable cell wall swells, bursts from osmotic pressure

Uses: Empyema, gangrene, anthrax, gonorrhea, mastoiditis, meningitis, osteomyelitis, pneumonia, tetanus, UTI, prophylactically in rheumatic fever; effective for non-penicillinase-producing gram-positive cocci *(S. aureus, S. pyogenes, S. viridans, S. faecalis, S. bovis, S. pneumoniae),* gram-negative cocci *(N. gonorrhoeae, N. meningitidis),* gram positive bacilli *(B. anthracis, C. perfringens, C. tetani, C. diphtheriae, L. monocytogenes),* gram-negative bacilli *(Bacteroides, F. nucleatum, P. multocida, S. minor, S. moniliformis),* spirochetes *(T. pallidum, T. pertenue, B. recurrentis, L. icterohaemorrhagiae), Actinomyces*

Dosage and routes:

Pneumococcal/streptococcal infections (mild to moderate)

• *Adult:* PO 400,000-500,000 U q6-8h × 10 days (streptococcal infections) or afebrile × 2 days (pneumococcal infections); IM/IV 1.2-24 million U in divided doses q4hr
• *Child <12 yr:* PO 25,000-90,000 U/kg/day in 3-6 divided doses

Prevention of recurrence of rheumatic fever

• *Adult:* PO 200,000-250,000 U bid continuously
• *Child <12 yr:* PO 25,000-90,000 U/kg/day in 3-6 divided doses

Vincent's gingivitis/pharyngitis

• *Adult:* PO 400,000-500,000 U q6-8h

Available forms: Tabs 200,000, 250,000, 400,000, 500,000, 800,000 U; powder for oral sol 200,000, 400,000 U/5 ml; inj

Side effects/adverse reactions:

CNS: Lethargy, hallucinations, anxiety, depression, twitching, ***coma, convulsions***

GI: Nausea, vomiting, diarrhea, increased AST (SGOT) ALT (SGPT), abdominal pain, glossitis, colitis

HEMA: Anemia, ***increased bleeding time, bone marrow depression, granulocytopenia***

META: ***Hyperkalemia, hypokalemia, alkalosis, hypernatremia***

Contraindications: Hypersensitivity to penicillins; neonates

Precautions: Hypersensitivity to cephalosporins, pregnancy (B), lactation

Pharmacokinetics:

IV: Peak immediate
IM: Peak ¼-½ hr
PO: Peak 1 hr, duration 6 hr

Excreted in urine unchanged, excreted in breast milk, crosses placenta

Interactions:

• Decreased antimicrobial effectiveness of penicillin: tetracyclines, erythromycins
• Decreased absorption: cholestyramine, colestipol
• Increased penicillin concentrations: aspirin, probenecid

Syringe compatibility: Heparin

Additive compatibilities: Ascorbic

acid, calcium chloride, calcium gluconate, cephapirin, chloramphenicol, cimetidine, clindamycin, colistimethate, corticotropin, dimenhydrinate, diphenhydramine, ephedrine, erythromycin, furosemide, hydrocortisone sodium succinate, kanamycin, lidocaine, magnesium sulfate, methicillin, methylprednisolone sodium succinate, metronidazole, polymyxin B, prednisolone sodium phosphate, potassium chloride, procaine, prochlorperazine edisylate, verapamil

Y-site compatibilities: Acyclovir, amiodarone, cyclophosphamide, enalaprilat, esmolol, fluconazole, foscarnet, heparin, hydromorphone, labetalol, magnesium sulfate, meperidine, morphine, perphenazine, potassium chloride, verapamil, vitamin B with C

Lab test interferences:

Decrease: Uric acid

False positive: Urine glucose, urine protein

NURSING CONSIDERATIONS

Assess:

- I&O ratio; report hematuria, oliguria, since penicillin in high doses is nephrotoxic
- For infection: draining wounds, color of sputum, condition of urine, VS, cough
- Any patient with compromised renal system, since drug is excreted slowly in poor renal system function; toxicity may occur rapidly
- Liver studies: AST (SGOT), ALT (SGPT); liver enzyme may increase
- Blood studies: WBC, RBC, Hgb, Hct, bleeding time
- Renal studies: urinalysis, protein, blood
- C&S before therapy; drug may be given as soon as culture is taken
- Bowel pattern before and during treatment
- Skin eruptions after administration of penicillin to 1 wk after discontinuing drug; rash, pruritus, wheezing, laryngeal spasm
- Respiratory status: rate, character, wheezing, tightness in chest

Administer:

- Orally on an empty stomach for best absorption; avoid acidic or carbonated beverages for 1 hr before and after taking PO form
- Drug after C&S

Perform/provide:

- Adrenalin, suction, tracheostomy set, endotracheal intubation equipment
- Adequate fluid intake (2 L) during diarrhea episodes
- Scratch test to assess allergy after securing order from prescriber; usually done when penicillin is only drug of choice
- Storage in dry, tight container; oral susp refrigerated 2 wk, 1 wk at room temp

Evaluate:

- Therapeutic response: absence of fever, draining wounds
- Allergies before initiation of treatment, reaction of each medication; highlight allergies on chart; hypersensitivity reaction may be delayed

Teach patient/family:

- Aspects of drug therapy, including need to complete course of medication to ensure organism death (10-14 days); culture may be taken after completed course
- To report sore throat, fever, fatigue; may indicate superinfection
- To wear or carry Medic Alert ID if allergic to penicillins
- To report diarrhea, prevent dehydration

Treatment of anaphylaxis: Withdraw drug, maintain airway, administer epinephrine, aminophylline, O_2, IV corticosteroids

* Available in Canada only

penicillin G procaine (℞)

Crysticillin A.S., Duracillin A.S., Wycillin, Pfizerpen-AS

Func. class.: Broad-spectrum long-acting antiinfective

Chem. class.: Natural penicillin

Action: Interferes with cell wall replication of susceptible organisms; osmotically unstable cell wall swells, bursts from osmotic pressure

Uses: Empyema, gangrene, anthrax, gonorrhea, mastoiditis, meningitis, osteomyelitis, pneumonia, tetanus, UTIs, prophylactically in rheumatic fever; effective for gram-positive cocci *(S. aureus, S. pyogenes, S. viridans, S. faecalis, S. bovis, S. pneumoniae),* gram-negative cocci *(N. gonorrhoeae, N. meningitidis),* gram-positive bacilli *(B. anthracis, C. perfringens, C. tetani, C. diphtheriae, L. monocytogenes),* gram-negative bacilli *(Bacteroides, F. nucleatum, P. multocida, S. minor, S. moniliformis),* spirochetes *(T. pallidum, T. pertenue, B. recurrentis, L. icterohaemorrhagiae), Actinomyces*

Dosage and routes:

Moderate to severe infections

• *Adult and child:* IM 600,000-1.2 million U in one or two doses/day for 10 days to 2 wk

• *Newborn:* 50,000 U/kg IM once daily

Gonorrhea

• *Adult and child >12 yr:* IM 4.8 million units in two injections given 30 min after probenecid 1 g

Pneumonia (pneumococcal)

• *Adult and child >12 yr:* IM 300,000-600,000 U q6-12h

Available forms: Inj 300,000, 500,000, 600,000 U/ml, 600,000 U/1.2 ml, 1,200,000 U/dose, 2,400,000 U/dose

Side effects/adverse reactions:

HEMA: Anemia, increased bleeding time, ***bone marrow depression, granulocytopenia***

GI: Nausea, vomiting, diarrhea, increased AST (SGOT), ALT (SGPT), abdominal pain, glossitis, colitis

GU: ***Oliguria, proteinuria, hematuria,*** *vaginitis, moniliasis,* ***glomerulonephritis***

CNS: Lethargy, hallucinations, anxiety, depression, twitching, ***coma, convulsions***

META: Hyperkalemia, hypokalemia, alkalosis, hypernatremia

Contraindications: Hypersensitivity to penicillins, procaine

Precautions: Hypersensitivity to cephalosporins, pregnancy (B)

Pharmacokinetics:

IM: Peak 1-4 hr, duration 15 hr, excreted in urine

Interactions:

• Decreased antimicrobial effect of penicillin: tetracyclines, erythromycins

• Increased penicillin concentrations: aspirin, probenecid

Lab test interferences:

False positive: Urine glucose, urine protein

NURSING CONSIDERATIONS

Assess:

• I&O ratio; report hematuria, oliguria, since penicillin in high doses is nephrotoxic

• Any patient with compromised renal system, since drug is excreted slowly in poor renal system function; toxicity may occur rapidly

• Liver studies: AST (SGOT), ALT (SGPT)

• Blood studies: WBC, RBC, Hgb, Hct, bleeding time

• Renal studies: urinalysis, protein, blood

P

• C&S before therapy; drug may be given as soon as culture is taken
• Bowel pattern before and during treatment
• Skin eruptions after administration of penicillin to 1 wk after discontinuing drug
• Respiratory status: rate, character, wheezing, tightness in chest
• Allergies before initiation of treatment, reaction of each medication; highlight allergies on chart
• For transient toxic reaction to procaine, which may occur immediately and subside after 15-30 min

Administer:
• Drug after C&S
• Deep IM, avoid intravascular inj, aspirate

Perform/provide:
• Adrenalin, suction, tracheostomy set, endotracheal intubation equipment
• Adequate fluid intake (2 L) during diarrhea episodes
• Scratch test to assess allergy after securing order from prescriber; usually done when penicillin is only drug of choice
• Storage in refrigerator

Evaluate:
• Therapeutic response: absence of fever, purulent drainage, redness, inflammation

Teach patient/family:
• That culture may be taken after completed course of medication
• To report sore throat, fever, fatigue; may indicate superinfection
• To wear or carry Medic Alert ID if allergic to penicillins; allergic reaction may be prolonged because of drug's long duration
• To notify nurse of diarrhea

Treatment of hypersensitivity: Withdraw drug; maintain airway; administer epinephrine, aminophylline, O_2, IV corticosteroids

penicillin G sodium (℞)

Crystapen*, Pfizerpen

Func. class.: Broad-spectrum antiinfective

Chem. class.: Natural penicillin

Action: Acts by interfering with cell wall replication of susceptible organisms; osmotically unstable cell wall swells and bursts from osmotic pressure

Uses: Empyema, gangrene, anthrax, gonorrhea, mastoiditis, meningitis, osteomyelitis, pneumonia, tetanus, UTI, prophylactically in rheumatic fever; effective for non-penicillinase-producing gram-positive cocci *(S. aureus, S. pyogenes, S. viridans, S. faecalis, S. bovis, S. pneumoniae),* gram-negative cocci *(N. gonorrhoeae, N. meningitidis),* gram-positive bacilli *(B. anthracis, C. perfringens, C. tetani, C. diphtheriae, L. monocytogenes),* gram-negative bacilli *(Bacteroides, E. nucleatum, P. multocida, S. minor, S. moniliformis),* spirochetes *(T. pallidum, T. pertenue, B. recurrentis, L. icterohaemorrhagiae), Actinomyces*

Dosage and routes:

Moderate to severe infections
• *Adult:* IM/IV 12 million-30 million U/day in divided doses q4h
• *Child:* IM/IV 25,000-300,000 U/day in divided doses q4-12h

Dental surgery prophylaxis for endocarditis
• *Adult:* IM/IV 2 million U ½-1 hr before procedure, then 1 million U 6 hr after procedure

Available forms: Inj 1 million, 5 million, 20 million U

Side effects/adverse reactions:
HEMA: Anemia, increased bleeding time, ***bone marrow depression, granulocytopenia***

* Available in Canada only

GI: Nausea, vomiting, diarrhea, increased AST (SGOT), ALT (SGPT), abdominal pain, glossitis, colitis
GU: ***Oliguria, proteinuria, hematuria,*** vaginitis, moniliasis, ***glomerulonephritis***
CNS: Lethargy, hallucinations, anxiety, depression, twitching, ***convulsions***
META: Hyperkalemia, hypokalemia, alkalosis, hypernatremia
Contraindications: Hypersensitivity to penicillins; neonates
Precautions: CHF caused by Na retention, pregnancy (B)
Pharmacokinetics:
IM: Peak 1-3 hr, duration 6 hr; excreted in urine
Interactions:
• Decreased antimicrobial effect of penicillin: tetracyclines, erythromycins
• Increased penicillin concentrations: aspirin, probenecid
• Decreases bacterial action when mixed with acids, alkalis, aminophylline, amphotericin B, cephalothin, chlorpromazine, dopamine, heparin, lincomycin, pentobarbital, phenytoin, prochlorperazine, promazine, promethazine, tetracycline, thiopental, trifluoperazine, vancomycin, Vit C, Vit B with C
• Drug/food: decreased absorption: food, carbonated drink, citrus fruit juices
Syringe compatibilities: Aminoglycosides, chloramphenicol, cimetidine, colistimethate, gentamicin, heparin, kanamycin, lincomycin, polymyxin B, streptomycin
Additive compatibilities: Calcium chloride, calcium gluconate, chloramphenicol, clindamycin, colistimethate, diphenhydramine, erythromycin, furosemide, gentamicin, hydrocortisone sodium succinate, kanamycin, methicillin, polymyxin B, prednisolone, procaine, ranitidine, verapamil, vitamin B with C
Lab test interferences:
False positive: Urine glucose, urine protein

NURSING CONSIDERATIONS

Assess:
• I&O ratio; report hematuria, oliguria, since penicillin in high doses is nephrotoxic
• Any patient with a compromised renal system, since drug is excreted slowly in poor renal system function; toxicity may occur rapidly
• Liver studies: AST (SGOT), ALT (SGPT)
• Blood studies: WBC, RBC, Hgb, Hct, bleeding time
• Renal studies: urinalysis, protein, blood
• C&S before therapy; drug may be given as soon as culture is taken
• Bowel pattern before, during treatment
• Skin eruptions after administration of penicillin to 1 wk after discontinuing drug
• Respiratory status: rate, character, wheezing, tightness in chest
• Allergies before initiation of treatment, reaction of each medication; highlight allergies on chart; hypersensitivity reaction may be delayed

Administer:
• IV after diluting with sterile H_2O; shake; follow manufacturer's instructions for dilution; may be added to 0.9% NaCl; give by continuous inf, usually over 12 hr
• Drug after C&S

Perform/provide:
• Adrenalin, suction, tracheostomy set, endotracheal intubation equipment
• Adequate fluid intake (2 L) during diarrhea episodes
• Scratch test to assess allergy after securing order from prescriber; usu-

P

ally done when penicillin is only drug of choice

• Storage of sterile sol in refrigerator for 1 wk, IV sol at room temp for 24 hr

Evaluate:

• Therapeutic response: absence of fever, purulent drainage, redness, inflammation

Teach patient family:

• That culture may be taken after completed course of medication

• To report sore throat, fever, fatigue; may indicate superinfection

• To wear or carry Medic Alert ID if allergic to penicillins

• To notify nurse of diarrhea

Treatment of anaphylaxis: Withdraw drug, maintain airway, administer epinephrine, aminophylline, O_2, IV corticosteroids

penicillin V potassium (℞)

Pen-Vee K*, Deltapen-VK, V-Cillin K, Veetids, PVFK*, Apo-Pen-VK*, Novopen-VK*, Ledercillin-VK, Uticillin-VK, Betapen-VK, Penapar-VK, Robicillin-VK

Func. class.: Broad-spectrum antiinfective

Chem. class.: Natural penicillin

Action: Interferes with cell wall replication of susceptible organisms; osmotically unstable cell wall swells, bursts from osmotic pressure.

Uses: Effective for gram-positive cocci *(S. aureus, S. pyogenes, S. viridans, S. faecalis, S. bovis, S. pneumoniae),* gram-negative cocci *(N. gonorrhoeae, N. meningitidis),* gram-positive bacilli *(B. anthracis, C. perfringens, C. tetani, C. diphtheriae, L. monocytogenes),* gram-negative bacilli *(S. moniliformis),* spirochetes *(T. pallidum), Actinomyces*

Dosage and routes:

Pneumococcal/staphylococcal infections

• *Adult:* PO 250-500 mg g6h

• *Child <12 yr:* PO 15-50 mg/kg/day in divided doses q6-8hr

Streptococcal infections

• *Adult:* PO 125-250 mg q6-8h × 10 days

Prevention of recurrence of rheumatic fever/chorea

• *Adult:* PO 125-250 mg bid continuously

Vincent's infection of oropharynx

• *Adult:* PO 500 mg q6h

Available forms: Tabs 125, 250, 500 mg; film-coated tabs 250, 500 mg; powder for oral susp 125, 250 mg/5 ml

Side effects/adverse reactions:

HEMA: Anemia, increased bleeding time, ***bone marrow depression, granulocytopenia***

GI: Nausea, vomiting, diarrhea, increased AST (SGOT), ALT (SGPT), abdominal pain, glossitis, colitis

GU: ***Oliguria, proteinuria, hematuria,*** *vaginitis, moniliasis,* ***glomerulonephritis***

CNS: Lethargy, hallucinations, anxiety, ***depression,*** twitching, ***coma, convulsions***

META: Hyperkalemia, hypokalemia, alkalosis

Contraindications: Hypersensitivity to penicillins; neonates

Precautions: Hypersensitivity to cephalosporins, pregnancy (B)

Pharmacokinetics:

PO: Peak 30-60 min, duration 6-8 hr, half-life 30 min, excreted in urine, breast milk

Interactions:

• Decreased antimicrobial effectiveness of penicillin: tetracyclines, erythromycins

* Available in Canada only

• Increased penicillin concentrations: aspirin, probenecid
• Drug/food: decreased absorption: food, carbonated drinks, citrus fruit juices

Lab test interferences:
False positive: Urine glucose, urine protein

NURSING CONSIDERATIONS

Assess:
• I&O ratio; report hematuria, oliguria, since penicillin in high doses is nephrotoxic
• Any patient with compromised renal system, since drug is excreted slowly in poor renal system function; toxicity may occur rapidly
• Liver studies: AST (SGOT), ALT (SGPT)
• Blood studies: WBC, RBC, Hgb, Hct, bleeding time
• Renal studies: urinalysis, protein, blood
• C&S before therapy; drug may be given as soon as culture is taken
• Bowel pattern before and during treatment
• Skin eruptions after administration of penicillin to 1 wk after discontinuing drug
• Respiratory status: rate, character, wheezing, tightness in chest
• Allergies before initiation of treatment, reaction of each medication; highlight allergies on chart

Administer:
• Orally on empty stomach for best absorption
• Drug after C&S

Perform/provide:
• Adrenalin, suction, tracheostomy set, endotracheal intubation equipment
• Adequate fluid intake (2 L) during diarrhea episodes
• Scratch test to assess allergy after securing order from prescriber; usually done when penicillin is only drug of choice
• Storage in tight container; after reconstituting, refrigerate for up to 2 wk

Evaluate:
• Therapeutic response: absence of fever, draining wounds

Teach patient/family:
• Aspects of drug therapy, including need to complete entire course of medication to ensure organism death (10-14 days); culture may be taken after completed course
• To report sore throat, fever, fatigue; may indicate superinfection
• To wear or carry Medic Alert ID if allergic to penicillins
• To notify nurse of diarrhea

Treatment of anaphylaxis: Withdraw drug, maintain airway, administer epinephrine, aminophylline, O_2, IV corticosteroids

pentaerythritol (℞)

(pen-ta-er-ith'ri-tole)

Duotrate, Duotrate 45, P.E.T.N., Pentylan, Peritrate, Peritrate SA

Func. class.: Vasodilatory, coronary

Chem. class.: Nitrate

Combination products: Dimycor: pentaerythritol tetranitrate 10 mg, phenobarbital 15 mg; Bitrate: pentaerythritol tetranitrate 15 mg, phenobarbital 20 mg; Perbuzem: pentaerythritol tetranitrate 10 mg, butabarbital 15 mg

Action: Decreases preload, afterload, which is responsible for decreasing left ventricular end-diastolic pressure, systemic vascular resistance

Uses: Chronic stable angina pectoris, prophylaxis of angina pain

Dosage and routes:
• *Adult:* PO 10-20 mg tid or qid, max 40 mg qid; sus rel 30-80 mg q12h
Available forms: Caps ext rel 30, 45, 80 mg; tabs 10, 20, 40, 80 mg; tabs ext rel 80 mg
Side effects/adverse reactions:
CV: Postural hypotension, palpitations, tachycardia, ***collapse,*** syncope
GI: Nausea, vomiting, abdominal pain
INTEG: Pallor, sweating, rash
CNS: Headache, flushing, dizziness, restlessness, weakness, faintness
MISC: Muscle twitching, ***hemolytic anemia, methemoglobinemia***
Contraindications: Hypersensitivity to this drug or nitrates, severe anemia, increased intracranial pressure, cerebral hemorrhage, acute MI
Precautions: Postural hypotension, pregnancy (C), lactation, children
Pharmacokinetics:
PO: Onset 30 min, duration 4-5 hr
SUS REL: Onset 30 min, duration 12 hr
Metabolized by liver, excreted in urine, half-life 10 min
Interactions:
• Increased effects: β-blockers, diuretics, antihypertensives, alcohol
NURSING CONSIDERATIONS
Assess:
• B/P, pulse, respirations during beginning therapy
• Pain: duration, time started, activity being performed, character
• Tolerance if taken over long period of time
• Headache, light-headedness, decreased B/P; may indicate a need for decreased dosage
Administer:
• With 8 oz of water on empty stomach
Evaluate:
• Therapeutic response: decrease, prevention of anginal pain
Teach patient/family:
• To keep tabs in original container; not to crush or chew sus rel preparations
• To avoid alcohol products
• That drug may cause headache; tolerance usually develops
• That drug may be taken before stressful activity: exercise, sexual activity
• To avoid hazardous activities if dizziness occurs
• To comply with complete medical regimen
• To make position changes slowly to prevent fainting

pentamidine (℞)
(pen-tam'i-deen)
Nebupent, Pentam 300, Pentacarinat*, Pneumopent*
Func. class.: Antiprotozoal
Chem. class.: Aromatic diamide derivative

Action: Interferes with DNA/RNA synthesis in protozoa
Uses: *P. carinii* infections
Dosage and routes:
• *Adult and child:* IV/IM 4 mg/kg/day × 2 wk: NEB 600 mg/6ml NS via specific nebulizer given q4wk for prevention
Available forms: Inj IV, IM; aerosol 300 mg/vial
Side effects/adverse reactions:
CV: Hypotension, ventricular tachycardia, ECG abnormalities
HEMA: Anemia, ***leukopenia, thrombocytopenia***
INTEG: Sterile abscess, pain at injection site, pruritus, urticaria, rash
GU: ***Acute renal failure, increased serum creatinine, renal toxicity***

* Available in Canada only

GI: Nausea, vomiting, anorexia, increased AST (SGOT), ALT (SGPT), ***acute pancreatitis***, metallic taste
CNS: Disorientation, hallucinations, dizziness, confusion
RESP: Cough, shortness of breath, ***bronchospasm*** (with aerosol)
MISC: Fatigue, chills, night sweats
META: Hyperkalemia, hypocalcemia, hypoglycemia
Precautions: Blood dyscrasias, hepatic disease, renal disease, diabetes mellitus, cardiac disease, hypocalcemia, pregnancy (C), hypertension, hypotension, lactation, children
Pharmacokinetics: Excreted unchanged in urine (66%)
Interactions:
• Nephrotoxicity: aminoglycosides, amphotericin B, colistin, cisplatin, methoxyflurane, polymyxin B, vancomycin
Y-site compatibility: Zidovudine
NURSING CONSIDERATIONS
Assess:
• Blood studies, blood glucose, CBC, platelets
• I&O ratio; report hematuria, oliguria
• ECG for cardiac dysrhythmias
• Patient should be lying down when receiving drug; severe hypotension may develop; monitor BP during administration and until BP stable
• Any patient with compromised renal system; drug is excreted slowly in poor renal system function; toxicity may occur rapidly
• Liver studies: AST (SGOT), ALT (SGPT)
• Renal studies: urinalysis, BUN, creatinine; nephrotoxicity may occur
• Signs of infection, anemia
• Bowel pattern before, during treatment
• Sterile abscess, pain at injection site
• Respiratory status: rate, character, wheezing, dyspnea
• Dizziness, confusion, hallucination
• Allergies before treatment, reaction of each medication; place allergies on chart in bright red letters; notify all people giving drugs
Administer:
• IV by intermittent inf over 60 min
• Inhalation through nebulizer; mix contents in 6 ml of sterile H_2O; do not use low pressure (<20 psi); flow rate should be 5-7 L/min (40-50 psi) air or O_2 source over 30-45 min until chamber is empty
• IM diluted in 3 ml sterile H_2O; give deep IM; painful by this route
Perform/provide:
• Storage in refrigerator protected from light
Evaluate:
• Therapeutic response: decreased temperature, ability to breathe
Teach patient/family:
• To report sore throat, fever, fatigue; may indicate superinfection

pentazocine (℞)

(pen-taz'oh seen)
Talwin, Talwin NX
Func. class.: Narcotic analgesic, antagonist
Chem. class.: Synthetic benzomorphan

Combination products: Talacen: pentazocine HCl 25 mg (of pentazocine) with acetaminophen 650 mg

Controlled Substance Schedule IV
Action: Inhibits ascending pain pathways in CNS, increases pain threshold, alters pain perception
Uses: Moderate to severe pain
Dosage and routes:
• *Adult:* PO 50-100 mg q3-4h prn, not to exceed 600 mg/day; IV/

IM/SC 30 mg q3-4h prn, not to exceed 360 mg/day

Available forms: Inj 30 mg/ml; tabs 50 mg

Side effects/adverse reactions:

CNS: Drowsiness, dizziness, confusion, headache, sedation, euphoria, hallucinations, dreaming

GI: Nausea, vomiting, anorexia, constipation, *cramps*

GU: Increased urinary output, dysuria, retention

INTEG: Rash, urticaria, bruising, flushing, diaphoresis, pruritus, severe irritation at injection sites

EENT: Tinnitus, blurred vision, miosis, diplopia

CV: Palpitations, bradycardia, change in B/P, tachycardia, increased B/P (high doses)

RESP: ***Respiratory depression***

Contraindications: Hypersensitivity, addiction (narcotic)

Precautions: Addictive personality, pregnancy (C), lactation, increased intracranial pressure, MI (acute), severe heart disease, respiratory depression, hepatic disease, renal disease, seizure disorder, child <18 yr

Pharmacokinetics:

SC/IM: Onset 15-30 min, peak 1-2 hr, duration 2-4 hr

IV: Onset 2-3 min, duration 4-6 hr

Metabolized by liver, excreted by kidneys, crosses placenta, half-life 2-3 hr, extensive first-pass metabolism with less than 20% entering circulation

Interactions:

• Increased effects: CNS depressants; alcohol, sedative/hypnotics, antipsychotics, skeletal muscle relaxants

• Decreased effects: narcotics

Syringe compatibilities: Atropine, benzquinamide, butorphanol, chlorpromazine, cimetidine, dimenhydrinate, diphenhydramine, droperidol, fentanyl, hydromorphone, hydroxyzine, meperidine, metoclopramide, morphine, perphenazine, prochlorperazine edisylate, promazine, promethazine, rantidine, scopolamine

Y-site compatibilities: Heparin, hydrocortisone sodium succinate, potassium chloride, vitamin B with C

Lab test interferences:

Increase: Amylase

NURSING CONSIDERATIONS

Assess:

• I&O ratio; check for decreasing output; may indicate urinary retention

• For withdrawal symptoms in narcotic-dependent patients

• Pulmonary embolism, abscesses, ulcerations, vascular occlusion, WBC

• CNS changes: dizziness, drowsiness, hallucinations, euphoria, LOC, pupil reaction

• Allergic reactions: rash, urticaria

• Respiratory dysfunction: respiratory depression, character, rate, rhythm; notify prescriber if respirations are <10/min

• Need for pain medication, physical dependence

Administer:

• IV undiluted or diluted 5 mg/ml of sterile H_2O for inj; give 5 mg or less over 1 min

• With antiemetic if nausea, vomiting occur

• When pain is beginning to return; determine dosage interval by patient response

Perform/provide:

• Storage in light-resistant area at room temp

• Assistance with ambulation

• Safety measures: side rails, nightlight, call bell within easy reach

Evaluate:

• Therapeutic response: decrease in pain

* Available in Canada only

Teach patient/family:
- To report any symptoms of CNS changes, allergic reactions
- That physical dependency may result from extended use
- That withdrawal symptoms may occur: nausea, vomiting, cramps, fever, faintness, anorexia

Treatment of overdose: Naloxone (Narcan) 0.2-0.8 mg IV, O_2, IV fluids, vasopressors

---

pentobarbital (℞)

(pen-toe-bar′bi-tal)

Nembutal, Nembutal Sodium, Nembutal Sodium Solution, Nova-Rectal*, pentobarbital sodium, Pentogen*

Func. class.: Sedative/hypnotic barbiturate

Chem. class.: Barbitone, short acting

Controlled Substance Schedule II (USA), Schedule G (Canada)

Action: Depresses activity in brain cells, primarily in reticular activating system in brain stem; selectively depresses neurons in posterior hypothalamus, limbic structures

Uses: Insomnia, sedation, preoperative medication, increased intracranial pressure, dental anesthetic

Dosage and routes:
- *Adult:* PO 100-200 mg hs; IM 150-200 mg hs; IV 100 mg initially, then up to 500 mg; REC 120-200 mg hs
- *Child:* IM 3-5 mg, not to exceed 100 mg
- *Child 2 mo-1 yr:* REC 30 mg
- *Child 1-4 yr:* REC 30-60 mg
- *Child 5-12 yr:* REC 60 mg
- *Child 12-14 yr:* REC 60-120 mg

Available forms: Caps 50, 100 mg; elix 18.2 mg/5 ml; powder, rec supp 30, 60, 120, 200 mg; inj 50 mg/ml

Side effects/adverse reactions:

CNS: Lethargy, drowsiness, hangover, dizziness, paradoxical stimulation in elderly and children, lightheadedness, dependence, ***CNS depression,*** mental depression, slurred speech

GI: Nausea, vomiting, diarrhea, constipation

INTEG: Rash, urticaria, pain, abscesses at injection site, angioedema, thrombophlebitis, ***Stevens-Johnson syndrome***

CV: Hypotension, bradycardia

RESP: ***Respiratory, depression, apnea, laryngospasm, bronchospasm***

HEMA: ***Agranulocytosis, thrombocytopenia, megaloblastic anemia*** (long-term treatment)

Contraindications: Hypersensitivity to barbiturates, respiratory depression, addiction to barbiturates, severe liver, renal impairment, porphyria, uncontrolled pain

Precautions: Anemia, pregnancy (D), lactation, hepatic disease, renal disease, hypertension, elderly, acute/chronic pain

Pharmacokinetics:

PO: Onset 15-30 min, duration 4-6 hr

REC: Onset slow, duration 4-6 hr

Metabolized by liver, excreted by kidneys (metabolites); half-life 15-48 hr

Interactions:
- Increased CNS depression: alcohol, MAOIs, sedatives, narcotics
- Decreased effect of oral anticoagulants, corticosteroids, griseofulvin, quinidine
- Increased half-life of doxycycline

Syringe compatibilities: Aminophylline, ephedrine, hydromorphone, neostigmine, scopolamine, sodium bicarbonate, thiopental

Y-site compatibilities: Acyclovir, regular insulin

P

Additive compatibilities: Amikacin, aminophylline, calcium chloride, cephapirin, chloramphenicol, dimenhydrinate, erythromycin lactobionate, lidocaine, thiopental, verapamil

Lab test interferences:

False increase: Sulfobromophthalein

NURSING CONSIDERATIONS

Assess:

• VS q30min after parenteral route for 2 hr

• Blood studies: Hct, Hgb, RBCs, serum folate, vit D (long-term therapy); pro-time in patients receiving anticoagulants

• Hepatic studies: AST (SGOT), ALT (SGPT), bilirubin; if increased, drug is usually discontinued

• Mental status: mood, sensorium, affect, memory (long, short)

• Physical dependency: more frequent requests for medication, shakes, anxiety

• Barbiturate toxicity: hypotension; pupillary constriction; cold, clammy skin; cyanosis of lips; insomnia; nausea; vomiting; hallucinations; delirium; weakness; coma; mild symptoms may occur in 8-12 hr without drug

• Respiratory dysfunction: respiratory depression, character, rate, rhythm; hold drug if respirations are <10/min or if pupils are dilated

• Blood dyscrasias: fever, sore throat, bruising, rash, jaundice, epistaxis

Administer:

• After removal of cigarettes to prevent fires

• IM injection deep in large muscle mass to prevent tissue sloughing and abscesses; do not inject more than 5 ml in one site

• After trying conservative measures for insomnia

• After mixing with sterile H_2O for injection, inject within 30 min of preparation

• IV undiluted or dilute in sterile H_2O, LR, NaCl, give 50 mg or less/min; titrate to patient response; use only clear sol; avoid extravasation

• IV only with resuscitative equipment available; administer at <100 mg/min (only by qualified personnel)

• ½-1 hr before hs for sleeplessness

• On empty stomach for best absorption

• For <14 days, since not effective after that; tolerance develops

• Crushed or whole

• Alone; do not mix with other drugs or inject if there is precipitate

Perform/provide:

• Assistance with ambulation after receiving dose

• Safety measure: side rails, nightlight, call bell within easy reach

• Checking to see PO medication has been swallowed

• Storage of suppositories in refrigerator; do not use aqueous solutions that contain precipitate

Evaluate:

• Therapeutic response: ability to sleep at night, less early morning awakening if taking drug for insomnia, or decrease in number, severity of seizures if taking drug for seizure disorder

Teach patient/family:

• That hangover is common

• That drug is indicated only for short-term treatment of insomnia; probably ineffective after 2 wk

• That physical dependency may result from extended use (45-90 days depending on dose)

• To avoid driving, other activities requiring alertness

• To avoid alcohol ingestion, CNS depressants; serious CNS depression may result

---

* Available in Canada only

• Not to discontinue medication quickly after long-term use; drug should be tapered over 1-2 wk
• To tell all prescribers that a barbiturate is being taken
• That withdrawal insomnia may occur after short-term use; not to start using drug again; insomnia will improve in 1-3 nights
• That effects may take 2 nights for benefits to be noticed
• Alternative measures to improve sleep (reading, exercise several hours before hs, warm bath, warm milk, TV, self-hypnosis, deep breathing)

Treatment of overdose: Lavage, activated charcoal, warming blanket, vital signs, hemodialysis, I&O ratio

pentostatin (℞)

(pen'toe-sta-tin)
Nipent

Func. class.: Antineoplastic, enzyme inhibitor
Chem. class.: Streptomyces antibioticus derivative

Action: Inhibits the enzyme adenosine deaminase (ADA), which is able to block DNA synthesis and some RNA synthesis

Uses: α-Interferon-refractory hairy cell leukemia

Dosage and routes:

• *Adult:* IV 4 mg/m^2 every other week; may be given IV BOL, or diluted in a larger volume and given over 20-30 min

Available forms: Inj 10 mg/vial

Side effects/adverse reactions:

CNS: Headache, anxiety, confusion, depression, dizziness, insomnia, nervousness, paresthesia

RESP: Cough, upper respiratory infection, bronchitis, dyspnea, epistaxis, pneumonia, pharyngitis, rhinitis, sinusitis

SYST: Fever, infection, fatigue, pain, allergic reaction, chills, ***death, sepsis,*** chest pain, flu syndrome

HEMA: ***Leukopenia, anemia, thrombocytopenia, ecchymosis, lymphadenopathy,*** petechial

GI: Nausea, vomiting, anorexia, diarrhea, constipation, flatulence, stomatitis, elevated liver function tests

INTEG: Rash, eczema, dry skin, pruritus, sweating, herpes simplex/zoster

GU: ***Hematuria,*** dysuria, increased BUN/creatinine

Contraindications: Hypersensitivity to this drug or mannitol

Precautions: Renal disease, pregnancy (C), lactation, children, bone marrow depression

Pharmacokinetics:

IV: Elimination half-life 5.7 hr, low protein binding, 90% excreted in urine unchanged or as metabolites

Interactions:

• Fatal pulmonary toxicity: fludarabine
• Increased adverse reactions: vidarabine

Y-site compatibilities: Melphalan, ondansetron, paclitaxel, sargramostim

Solution compatibilities: D_5W, 0.9% NaCl, Ringer's inj

Lab test interferences:

Increase: Uric acid

NURSING CONSIDERATIONS

Assess:

• CBC, differential, platelet count qwk; withhold drug if WBC is 4000/mm^3 or platelet count is <75,000/mm^3; notify prescriber
• Renal function studies; BUN, serum uric acid, urine CrCl, electrolytes before, during therapy
• I&O ratio; report fall in urine output to <30 ml/hr
• Monitor temp q4h; fever may indicate beginning infection

• Liver function tests before, during therapy: bilirubin, AST (SGOT), ALT, (SGPT) alk phosphatase, prn or qmo
• Bleeding: hematuria, guaiac stools, bruising, petechiae, mucosa or orifices q8h
• Effects of alopecia on body image; discuss feelings about body changes
• Inflammation of mucosa, breaks in skin
• Yellow skin and sclera, dark urine, clay-colored stools, itchy skin, abdominal pain, fever, diarrhea
• Buccal cavity q8h for dryness, sores, ulceration, white patches, oral pain, bleeding, dysphagia
• Local irritation, pain, burning at injection site
• Symptoms of severe allergic reaction: rash, pruritus, urticaria, purpuric skin lesions, itching, flushing
• GI symptoms: frequency of stools, cramping
• Acidosis, signs of dehydration; rapid respiration, poor skin turgor, decreased urine output, dry skin, restlessness, weakness

Administer:
• Antiemetic 30-60 min before giving drug to prevent vomiting
• Antibiotics as ordered for prophylaxis of infection
• After diluting, use with 5 ml sterile H_2O for injection and mix thoroughly (2 mg/ml); may be given by bolus or diluted in 25-50 ml 5% dextrose, or 0.9% NaCl (0.33 or 0.18 mg/ml)

Perform/provide:
• Hydrocortisone, sodium thiosulfate to infiltration area, and ice compress after stopping infusion
• Strict hand-washing technique, gloves, protective covering
• Liquid diet: carbonated beverages; gelatin may be added if patient is not nauseated or vomiting
• Rinsing of mouth tid-qid with water, club soda; brushing of teeth bid-qid with soft brush or cotton-tipped applicators for stomatitis; use unwaxed dental floss
• Storage in refrigerator; reconstituted or diluted sol may be stored at room temp up to 8 hr

Evaluate:
• Therapeutic response: decrease in tumor size, spread of malignancy

Teach patient/family:
• To report any complaints, side effects to nurse or prescriber
• That hair may be lost during treatment and wig or hairpiece may make patient feel better; tell patient that new hair may be different in color, texture
• To avoid foods with citric acid, hot or rough texture
• To report any bleeding, white spots, ulcerations in mouth to physician; tell patient to examine mouth qd
• To avoid crowds and sources of infection when granulocyte count is low

pentoxifylline (℞)

(pen-tox-if′i-lin)

Trental

Func. class.: Hemorrheologic agent

Chem. class.: Dimethylxanthine derivative

Action: Decreases blood viscosity, stimulates prostacyclin formation, increases blood flow by increasing flexibility of RBCs; decreases RBC hyperaggregation; reduces platelet aggregation, decreases fibrinogin concentration

Uses: Intermittent claudication related to chronic occlusive vascular disease

* Available in Canada only

Dosage and routes:
• *Adult:* PO 400 mg tid with meals
Available forms: Tabs, controlled-release 400 mg
Side effects/adverse reactions:
MISC: Epistaxis, flulike symptoms, laryngitis, nasal congestion, ***leukopenia,*** malaise, weight changes
EENT: Blurred vision, earache, increased salivation, sore throat, conjunctivitis
CNS: Headache, anxiety, *tremors,* confusion, *dizziness*
GI: Dyspepsia, nausea, vomiting, anorexia, bloating, belching, constipation, cholecystitis, dry mouth, thirst, bad taste
INTEG: Rash, pruritus, urticaria, brittle fingernails
CV: Angina, dysrhythmias, palpitation, hypotension, chest pain, dyspnea, edema
Contraindications: Hypersensitivity to this drug or xanthines
Precautions: Pregnancy (C), angina pectoris, cardiac disease, lactation, children, impaired renal function
Pharmacokinetics:
PO: Peak 1 hr, half life ½ 1 hr, degradation in liver, excreted in urine
Interactions:
Increased bleeding: warfarin, aspirin, heparin, cefamandole, cefoperazone, cefotetan, plicamycin, valproic acid
NURSING CONSIDERATIONS
Assess:
• B/P, respirations of patient taking antihypertensives also
Administer:
• With meals to prevent GI upset
Evaluate:
• Therapeutic response: decreased pain, cramping, increased ambulation
Teach patient/family:
• That therapeutic response may take 2-4 wk
• That decreased fats, increased cholesterol, increased exercise, decreased smoking are necessary to correct condition
• To observe feet for arterial insufficiency
• To use cotton socks, well-fitted shoes; not to go barefoot
• To watch for bleeding, bruises, petechiae, epistaxis

perindopril (℞)
(per-in-doe′pril)
Aceon
Func. class.: Diuretic; carbonic anhydrase inhibitor
Chem. class.: Sulfonamide derivative

Action: Inhibits carbonic anhydrase activity in proximal renal tubules to decrease reabsorption of water, sodium, potassium, bicarbonate; decreases carbonic anhydrase in CNS, increasing seizure threshold
Uses: Essential hypertension
Dosage and routes:
• *Adult:* PO 4 mg qd, max 16 mg/day
Available forms: Tabs 2, 4, 8 mg
Side effects/adverse reactions:
CNS: Drowsiness, paresthesia, anxiety, depression, headache, dizziness, confusion, stimulation, fatigue, ***convulsions,*** sedation, nervousness
EENT: Myopia, tinnitus
ENDO: Hyperglycemia
GI: Nausea, vomiting, anorexia, constipation, diarrhea, melena, weight loss, ***hepatic insufficiency,*** taste alterations
GU: Frequency, hypokalemia, polyuria, ***uremia,*** glucosuria, hematuria, dysuria, crystalluria, renal calculi
HEMA: ***Aplastic anemia, hemolytic anemia, leukopenia, agranulocytosis, thrombocytopenia, purpura, pancytopenia***

P

INTEG: Rash, pruritus, urticaria, fever, ***Stevens-Johnson syndrome,*** photosensitivity

Contraindications: Hypersensitivity to sulfonamides, severe renal disease, severe hepatic disease, electrolyte imbalances (hyponatremia, hypokalemia), hyperchloremic acidosis, Addison's disease, COPD

Precautions: Hypercalciuria, pregnancy (C)

Pharmacokinetics: Unknown

Interactions:
- Increased action of amphetamines, procainamide, quinidine, tricyclics, flecainide, ephedrine, pseudoephedrine
- Increased excretion of barbiturates, ASA, lithium
- Toxicity: salicylates
- Hypokalemia: with other diuretics, corticosteroids, amphotericin B
- IV compatibility: cimetidine, D_5W, $D_{10}W$, NaCl, LR, Ringer's sol

NURSING CONSIDERATIONS

Assess:
- Weight daily, I&O daily to determine fluid loss; effect of drug may be decreased if used qd
- Rate, depth, rhythm of respiration, effect of exertion
- B/P lying, standing; postural hypotension may occur
- Electrolytes: K, Na, Cl; include BUN, blood sugar, CBC, serum creatinine, blood pH, ABGs, liver function tests

Administer:
- In AM to avoid interference with sleep if using drug as diuretic
- K replacement if K level <3
- With food if nausea occurs; absorption may be decreased slightly

Perform/provide:
- Storage in dark, cool area; use reconstituted sol within 24 hr

Evaluate:
- Therapeutic response: improvement in B/P
- Signs of metabolic acidosis: drowsiness, restlessness
- Signs of hypokalemia: postural hypotension, malaise, fatigue, tachycardia, leg cramps, weakness
- Rashes, fever qd
- Confusion, especially in elderly; take safety precautions if needed

Teach patient/family:
- To notify prescriber of sore throat, unusual bleeding, bruising, paresthesias, tremors, flank pain, skin rash
- To avoid hazardous activities if drowsiness occurs

Treatment of overdose: Lavage if taken orally; monitor electrolytes; administer dextrose in saline; monitor hydration, CV, renal status

permethrin (OTC, ℞)

(per-meth'ren)

Elimite, Nix, Nix Dermal Cream

Func. class.: Pediculicide

Chem. class.: Synthetic pyrethroid

Action: Acts by disrupting sodium channel current in parasite's nerve cell; delayed repolarization, paralysis of lice

Uses: Lice, nits, ticks, flea nits

Dosage and routes:

Lice (Head)
- *Adult and child:* Wash hair, towel dry; apply liberally to hair, leave on 10 min, rinse with water

Scabies
- *Adult and child:* Top 5% cream applied and massaged into all skin surfaces; leave cream on 8-14 hr, then wash

Available forms: Liq 1%, cream 5%

Side effects/adverse reactions:

INTEG: Pruritus, burning, stinging, rash, tingling, numbness, edema

Contraindications: Hypersensitivity

* Available in Canada only

Precautions: Head rash, children, lactation, pregnancy (B)
Pharmacokinetics:
Metabolized in liver to inactive metabolites, excreted in urine
NURSING CONSIDERATIONS
Administer:
- To body area, scalp only; do not apply to face, lips, mouth, eyes, any mucous membranes, anus, or meatus
- Topical corticosteroids as ordered to decrease contact dermatitis
- Lotions of menthol or phenol to control itching
- Topical antibiotics for infection

Perform/provide:
- Isolation until areas on skin, scalp have cleared and treatment is complete
- Removal of nits with a fine-tooth comb rinsed in vinegar after treatment

Evaluate:
- Therapeutic response: decreased crusts, nits, itching, papules in skin folds

Teach patient/family:
- To wash all inhabitants' clothing, bed linen using insecticide; preventive treatment may be required of all persons living in same house, using lotion or shampoo to decrease spread of infection
- That itching may continue for 4-6 wk
- That drug must be reapplied if accidentally washed off, or treatment will be ineffective
- Not to apply to face; apply from neck down for body lice
- To treat sexual partners simultaneously

Treatment of ingestion: Gastric lavage, saline laxatives, IV diazepam for convulsions

perphenazine (℞)
(per-fen'a-zeen)
Apo-Perphenazine*, perphenazine, Phenazine, PMS Perphenazine*, Trilafon
Func. class.: Antipsychotic/neuroleptic
Chem. class.: Phenothiazine piperidine

Combination products: Etrafon 2-10: perphenazine 2 mg, amitriptyline HCl 10 mg; Etrafon: perphenazine 2 mg, amitriptyline HCl 10 mg; Etrafon-A: perphenazine 4 mg, amitriptyline HCl 10 mg; Etrafon-Forte: perphenazine 4 mg, amitriptyline HCl 25 mg; Triavil 2-10, Triavil 4-10, Triavil 2-25, Triavil 4-25 (see Etrafon—same products); Triavil 4-50: perphenazine 4 mg, amitriptyline HCl 50 mg

Action: Depresses cerebral cortex, hypothalamus, limbic system, which control activity, aggression; blocks neurotransmission produced by dopamine at synapse; exhibits strong α-adrenergic, anticholinergic blocking action; as antiemetic inhibits medullary chemoreceptor trigger zone; mechanism for antipsychotic effects is unclear
Uses: Psychotic disorders, schizophrenia, nausea, vomiting, alcoholism
Dosage and routes:
Nausea/vomiting/alcoholism
- *Adult, child >12 yr:* IM 5-10 mg prn, max 15 mg in ambulatory patients, 30 mg in hospitalized patients; PO 8-16 mg/day in divided doses, up to 24 mg; IV not to exceed 5 mg, give diluted or slow IV drip

Psychiatric use in hospitalized patients
- *Adults:* PO 8-16 mg bid-qid, gradu-

ally increased to desired dose, not to exceed 64 mg/day; IM 5 mg q6h, not to exceed 30 mg/day

• *Child >12 yr:* PO 6-12 mg in divided doses

Nonhospitalized patients

• *Adult:* PO 4-8 mg tid or 8-32 mg repeat-action bid; IM 5 mg q6h

Available forms: Tabs 2, 4, 8, 16 mg; oral sol 16 mg/5ml; inj 5 mg/ml

Side effects/adverse reactions:

RESP: ***Laryngospasm,*** dyspnea, ***respiratory depression***

CNS: EPS: pseudoparkinsonism, akathisia, dystonia, tardive dyskinesia, ***seizures,*** *headache*

HEMA: Anemia, ***leukopenia, leukocytosis, agranulocytosis***

INTEG: Rash, photosensitivity, dermatitis

EENT: Blurred vision, glaucoma

GI: Dry mouth, nausea, vomiting, anorexia, constipation, diarrhea, jaundice, weight gain

GU: Urinary retention, urinary frequency, enuresis, impotence, amenorrhea, gynecomastia

CV: Orthostatic hypotension, ***cardiac arrest,*** ECG changes, ***tachycardia***

Contraindications: Hypersensitivity, blood dyscrasias, coma, child <12 yr, brain damage, bone marrow depression

Precautions: Pregnancy (C), lactation, seizure disorders, hypertension, hepatic disease, cardiac disease

Pharmacokinetics:

PO: Onset erratic, peak 2-4 hr

IM: Onset 10 min, peak 1-2 hr, duration 6 hr, occasionally 12-24 hr

Metabolized by liver, excreted in urine, breast milk, crosses placenta

Interactions:

• Oversedation: other CNS depressants, alcohol, barbiturate anesthetics

• Toxicity: epinephrine

• Decreased absorption: aluminum hydroxide or magnesium hydroxide antacids

• Decreased effects of lithium, levodopa

• Increased effects of both drugs: β-adrenergic blockers, alcohol

• Increased anticholinergic effects: anticholinergics

Syringe compatibilities: Atropine, butorphanol, chlorpromazine, cimetidine, dimenhydrinate, diphenhydramine, droperidol, fentanyl, meperidine, metoclopramide, morphine, pentazocine, prochlorperazine, promethazine, scopolamine

Y-site compatibilities: Acyclovir, amikacin, ampicillin, azlocillin, cefamandole, cefazolin, ceforanide, cefotaxime, cefoxitin, cefuroxime, cephalothin, cephapirin, chloramphenicol, clindamycin, cotrimoxazole, doxycycline, erythromycin lactobionate, famotidine, gentamicin, kanamycin, metronidazole, mezlocillin, minocycline, moxalactam, nafcillin, oxacillin, penicillin G potassium, piperacillin, tetracycline, ticarcillin, tacarcillin/clavulanate, tobramycin, vancomycin

Additive compatibilities: Ascorbic acid, ethacrynate, netilmicin

Lab test interferences:

Increase: Liver function tests, cardiac enzymes, cholesterol, blood glucose, prolactin, bilirubin, PBI, cholinesterase, ^{131}I

Decrease: Hormones (blood, urine)

False positive: Pregnancy tests, PKU

False negative: Urinary steroids, 17-OHCS

NURSING CONSIDERATIONS

Assess:

• Mental status before initial administration

• Swallowing of PO medication; check for hoarding or giving of medication to other patients

* Available in Canada only

- I&O ratio; palpate bladder if urinary output is low
- Bilirubin, CBC, liver function studies qmo
- Urinalysis is recommended before and during prolonged therapy
- Affect, orientation, LOC, reflexes, gait, coordination, sleep pattern disturbances
- B/P standing and lying; also include pulse, respirations q4h during initial treatment; establish baseline before starting treatment; report drops of 30 mm Hg
- Dizziness, faintness, palpitations, tachycardia on rising
- EPS including akathisia (inability to sit still, no pattern to movements), tardive dyskinesia (bizarre movements of jaw, mouth, tongue, extremities), pseudoparkinsonism (rigidity, tremors, pill rolling, shuffling gait)
- Skin turgor daily
- For neuroleptic malignant syndrome: hyperthermia, altered mental status, increased CPK, muscle rigidity
- Constipation, urinary retention daily; increase bulk, water in diet

Administer:

- IV after diluting each 5 mg/9 ml of NaCl, shake, give 0.5 mg or less (1ml = 0.5 mg) over 1 min; may be further diluted and infused
- Antiparkinsonian agent on order from prescriber for EPS
- Concentrate mixed in water, orange, pineapple, apricot, prune, tomato, grapefruit juice; do not mix with caffeine beverages (coffee, cola), tannics (tea), or pectinates (apple juice), since incompatibility may result; use 60 ml diluent for each 5 ml of concentrate
- Repeat-action tablets whole; do not crush or chew
- IM inj into large muscle mass

Perform/provide:

- Decreased sensory input by dimming lights, avoiding loud noises
- Supervised ambulation until stabilized on medication; do not involve in strenuous exercise program because fainting is possible; patient should not stand still for long periods
- Increased fluids to prevent constipation
- Sips of water, candy, gum for dry mouth
- Storage in tight, light-resistant container

Evaluate:

- Therapeutic response: decrease in emotional excitement, hallucinations, delusions, paranoia, reorganization of patterns of thought, speech

Teach patient/family:

- That orthostatic hypotension occurs frequently and to rise from sitting or lying position gradually; to avoid hazardous activities until stabilized on medication
- To remain lying down after IM inj for at least 30 min
- To avoid hot tubs, hot showers, tub baths, since hypotension may occur
- To avoid abrupt withdrawal of this drug, or EPS may result; drug should be withdrawn slowly
- To avoid OTC preparations (cough, hay fever, cold) unless approved by prescriber, since serious drug interactions may occur; avoid use with alcohol or CNS depressants; increased drowsiness may occur
- To use a sunscreen
- Regarding compliance with drug regimen
- About necessity for meticulous oral hygiene, since oral candidiasis may occur

P

• To report sore throat, malaise, fever, bleeding, mouth sores; if these occur, CBC should be drawn and drug discontinued
• In hot weather, that heat stroke may occur; to take extra precautions to stay cool
Treatment of overdose: Lavage if orally ingested; provide an airway; *do not induce vomiting*

phenacemide (℞)

(fe-nass′e-mide)
Phenurone
Func. class.: Anticonvulsant
Chem. class.: Hydantoin

Action: Increases seizure threshold in cortex
Uses: Refractory, generalized tonic-clonic (grand mal), complex-partial (psychomotor), absence (petit mal), atypical seizures
Dosage and routes:
• *Adult:* PO 500 mg tid, may increase by 500 mg/wk, not to exceed 5 g/day
• *Child 5-10 yr:* PO 250 mg tid, may increase by 250 mg/wk, not to exceed 1.5 g/day prn
Available forms: Tabs 500 mg
Side effects/adverse reactions:
HEMA: ***Agranulocytosis, leukopenia, aplastic anemia***
CNS: Drowsiness, dizziness, insomnia, paresthesias, depression, suicidal tendencies, aggression, headache
GI: Anorexia, weight loss, ***hepatitis,*** jaundice, nausea
GU: ***Nephritis, albuminuria***
INTEG: Rash
Contraindications: Hypersensitivity, psychiatric condition, pregnancy (D)
Precautions: Allergies, hepatic disease, renal disease
Pharmacokinetics:
PO: Duration 5 hr, metabolized by liver, excreted by kidneys
Interactions:
• Paranoid signs and symptoms: ethotoin
NURSING CONSIDERATIONS
Assess:
• Blood, liver function, renal function studies
• Drug level: drug is highly toxic
• Mental status: mood, sensorium, affect, memory (long, short); psychosis is common
• Respiratory depression: respirations <10/min, shallow
• Blood dyscrasias: fever, sore throat, bruising, rash, jaundice
Administer:
• With food for GI symptoms
Evaluate:
• Therapeutic response: decreased seizures
Teach patient/family:
• To notify prescriber of sore throat, fever, rash, fatigue, bleeding, bruising (blood dyscrasia)
• To notify prescriber of dark urine, jaundice, yellow sclerae, itching (liver dysfunction)
• To avoid hazardous activities until stabilized on drug
• Never to withdraw abruptly
• To report personality changes

phenazopyridine (℞)

(fen-az-eh-peer′i-deen)
Azo-Standard, Baridium, Eridium, Geridium, Phenazo*, Phenazodine, phenazopyridine HCl, Pyridiate, Pyridium, Urodine, Urogesic, Viridium
Func. class.: Nonnarcotic analgesic
Chem. class.: Azodye

Action: Exerts analgesic, anesthetic action on the urinary tract mucosa

* Available in Canada only

Uses: Urinary tract irritation, infection used with a urinary antiinfective

Dosage and routes:

- *Adult:* PO 100-200 mg tid
- *Child 6-12 yr:* PO 12 mg/kg/24 hr in divided doses × 2 days

Available forms: Tabs 95, 100, 200 mg

Side effects/adverse reactions:

HEMA: ***Thrombocytopenia, agranulocytosis, leukopenia, neutropenia, hemolytic anemia, methemoglobinemia***

CNS: Headache, vertigo

GI: Nausea, vomiting, GI bleeding, diarrhea, heartburn, anorexia, ***hepatic toxicity***

INTEG: Rash, urticaria, skin pigmentation

GU: ***Renal toxicity,*** *orange-red urine*

Contraindications: Hypersensitivity, hepatic disease

Precautions: Pregnancy (B), renal disease

Pharmacokinetics: Metabolized by liver, excreted by kidneys, crosses placenta, duration 6-8 hr

Lab test interferences:

Interference: Bilirubin, urinary glucose tests, urinalysis, PSP excretion, urinary ketones, steroids, proteins

False positive: Clinitest

NURSING CONSIDERATIONS

Assess:

- Urinary status: burning, pain, itching, urgency, frequency, hematuria, before and after completion of treatment
- Liver function studies: AST (SGOT), ALT (SGPT), bilirubin if patient is on long-term therapy
- Hepatotoxicity: dark urine, clay-colored stools, yellow skin and sclera, itching, abdominal pain, fever, diarrhea if patient is on long-term therapy
- Allergic reactions: rash, urticaria; drug may have to be discontinued

Administer:

- To patient crushed or whole; chewable tablets may be chewed
- With food or milk to decrease gastric symptoms

Evaluate:

- Therapeutic response: decrease in pain

Teach patient/family:

- To report any symptoms of hepatotoxicity
- Not to exceed recommended dosage and to take with meals
- To read label on other OTC drugs; many contain aspirin
- To discontinue after pain is relieved but continue to take concurrent prescribed antibiotic until finished
- That urine may turn red-orange, may stain clothing

Treatment of overdose: Methylene blue 1-2 mg/kg IV or 100-200 mg vit C PO

phendimetrazine (℞)

(fen-dye-me'tra-zeen)

Adipost, Anorex, Bacarate, Bontril PDM, Bontril Slow-Release, Ditall, Dyrexan-OD, Melfiat-105 Unicelles, Metra, Phenazine-35, Phenzine, Obalan, Obeval, Plegine, phendimetrazine tartrate, Prelu-2, Sprx-105, Slyn-LL, Trimstat, TrimTabs, Weh-Less, Wehless Timecelles, X-Trozine, X-Trozine LA, Weightrol

Func. class.: Anorexiant

Chem. class.: Morpholine derivative

Controlled Substance Schedule IV

Action: Increases release of norepinephrine, dopamine in cerebral cortex to reticular activating system

P

Uses: Exogenous obesity

Dosage and routes:

Adult: PO 35 mg bid-tid 1 hr ac, not to exceed 70 mg tid, SUS REL 105 mg qd ac AM

Available forms: Tabs 35 mg; caps 35 mg; sus rel cap 105 mg

Side effects/adverse reactions:

HEMA: ***Bone marrow depression, leukopenia, agranulocytosis***

CNS: Hyperactivity, insomnia, restlessness, dizziness, tremor headache, fatigue, malaise, euphoria, depression, confusion

INTEG: Urticaria, rash, erythema

GI: Nausea, anorexia, dry mouth, diarrhea, constipation, cramps, vomiting

GU: Dysuria, impotence, menstrual irregularities, change in libido, urinary frequency

CV: Palpitations, tachycardia, hypertension

EENT: Blurred vision, mydriasis, eye irritation

Contraindications: Hypersensitivity, hyperthyroidism, hypertension, glaucoma, severe arteriosclerosis, severe cardiovascular disease, children <12 yr, agitated states, drug abuse

Precautions: Drug abuse, anxiety, pregnancy (C), lactation, convulsive disorders

Pharmacokinetics:

PO: Onset 30 min, peak 1-3 hr, duration 4-20 hr; metabolized by liver; crosses placenta; excreted in urine, breast milk; half-life 2-10 hr

Interactions:

- Hypertensive crisis: MAOIs or within 14 days of MAOIs, furazolidone
- Decreased effect of phendimetrazine: tricyclics, phenothiazides, haloperidol
- Decreased effect of guanethidine

NURSING CONSIDERATIONS

Assess:

- VS, B/P, since this drug may reverse antihypertensives; check patients with cardiac disease often
- CBC, urinalysis; in diabetes: blood sugar, urine sugar; insulin changes may have to be made, since eating will decrease
- Height, growth rate in children; growth rate may decrease

Administer:

- At least 6 hr before hs to avoid sleeplessness
- For obesity only if patient is on weight reduction program, including dietary changes, exercise; patient will develop tolerance; loss of weight requires additional methods; give 1 hr before meals
- Gum, hard candy, frequent sips of water for dry mouth

Teach patient/family:

- Not to crush or chew sus rel preps or to take more than prescribed amount
- To decrease caffeine consumption (coffee, tea, cola, chocolate), which may increase irritability, stimulation
- To avoid OTC preparations unless approved by prescriber
- To taper off drug over several weeks, or depression, increased sleeping, lethargy will ensue
- To avoid alcohol ingestion
- To avoid hazardous activities until stabilized on medication
- To get needed rest; patients will feel more tired at end of day

Treatment of overdose: Administer fluids, hemodialysis or peritoneal dialysis; antihypertensive for increased B/P; ammonium Cl for increased excretion

phenelzine (℞)

(fen'el-zeen)

Nardil

Func. class.: Antidepressant MAOI

Chem. class.: Hydrazine

Action: Increases concentrations of endogenous epinephrine, norepinephrine, serotonin, dopamine in storage sites in CNS by inhibition of MAO; increased concentration reduces depression

Uses: Depression, when uncontrolled by other means

Dosage and routes:

- *Adult:* PO 45 mg/day in divided doses; may increase to 60 mg/day; dose should be reduced to 15 mg/day, not to exceed 90 mg/day

Available forms: Tabs 15 mg

Side effects/adverse reactions:

HEMA: ***Anemia***

CNS: Dizziness, drowsiness, confusion, headache, anxiety, tremors, stimulation, weakness, hyperreflexia, mania, insomnia, fatigue, weight gain

GI: Constipation, dry mouth, nausea, vomiting, *anorexia,* diarrhea, weight gain

GU: Change in libido, frequency

INTEG: Rash, flushing, increased perspiration

CV: Orthostatic hypotension, hypertension, dysrhythmias, ***hypertensive crisis***

EENT: Blurred vision

ENDO: ***SIADH-like syndrome***

Contraindications: Hypersensitivity to MAOIs, elderly, hypertension, CHF, severe hepatic disease, pheochromocytoma, severe renal disease, severe cardiac disease

Precautions: Suicidal patients, convulsive disorders, severe depression, schizophrenia, hyperactivity, diabetes mellitus, pregnancy (C)

Pharmacokinetics:

Metabolized by liver, excreted by kidneys

Interactions:

- Increased pressor effects: guanethidine, clonidine, indirect acting sympathomimetics (ephedrine)
- Increased effects of direct-acting sympathomimetics (epinephrine), alcohol, barbiturates, benzodiazepines, CNS depressants, levodopa
- Hyperpyretic crisis, convulsions, hypertensive episode: tricyclic antidepressants, meperidine
- Increased hypoglycemic effect: insulin

NURSING CONSIDERATIONS

Assess:

- B/P (lying, standing), pulse; if systolic B/P drops 20 mm Hg, hold drug, notify prescriber
- Blood studies: CBC, leukocytes, cardiac enzymes (long-term therapy)
- Hepatic studies: ALT (SGPT), AST (SGOT), bilirubin; hepatotoxicity may occur
- Toxicity: increased headache, palpitation; discontinue drug immediately; prodromal signs of hypertensive crisis
- Mental status changes: mood, sensorium, affect, memory (long, short); increase in psychiatric symptoms
- Urinary retention, constipation, edema; take weight qwk
- Withdrawal symptoms: headache, nausea, vomiting, muscle pain, weakness

Administer:

- Increased fluids, bulk in diet for constipation
- With food, milk for GI symptoms
- Crushed if patient cannot swallow medication whole
- Dosage hs for oversedation during day

P

- Gum, hard candy, or frequent sips of water for dry mouth
- Phentolamine for severe hypertension

Perform/provide:
- Storage in tight container in cool environment
- Assistance with ambulation during beginning therapy, since drowsiness/dizziness occurs, especially elderly
- Safety measures including side rails
- Checking to see PO medication swallowed

Evaluate:
- Therapeutic response: decreased depression

Teach patient/family:
- That therapeutic effects may take 1-4 wk
- To avoid driving, other activities requiring alertness
- To avoid alcohol ingestion, CNS depressants, OTC medications: cold, weight loss, hay fever, cough syrup
- Not to discontinue medication quickly after long-term use
- To avoid high-tyramine foods: cheese (aged), sour cream, beer, wine, pickled products, liver, raisins, bananas, figs, avocados, meat tenderizers, chocolate, yogurt; increased caffeine
- To report headache, palpitation, neck stiffness

Treatment of overdose: Lavage, activated charcoal, monitor electrolytes, vital signs, diazepam IV, $NaHCO_3$

phenobarbital (℞)

(fee-noe-bar'bi-tal)

Barbita, Phenobarbital, Phenobarbital Sodium, Solfoton

Func. class.: Anticonvulsant

Chem. class.: Barbiturate

Combination products: Tri-Barb Capsules: phenobarbital 32 mg, butabarbital sodium 32 mg, secobarbital sodium 32 mg

Controlled Substance Schedule IV

Action: Decreases impulse transmission; increases seizure threshold at cerebral cortex level

Uses: All forms of epilepsy, status epilepticus, febrile seizures in children, sedation, insomnia

Investigational uses: Hyperbilirubinemia, chronic cholestasis

Dosage and routes:

Seizures
- *Adult:* PO 100-200 mg/day in divided doses tid or total dose hs
- *Child:* PO 4-6 mg/kg/day in divided doses q12h; may be given as single dose

Status epilepticus
- *Adult:* IV INF 10 mg/kg; run no faster than 50/mg/min; may give up to 20 mg/kg
- *Child:* IV INF 5-10 mg/kg; may repeat q10-15min up to 20 mg/kg; run no faster than 50 mg/min

Insomnia
- *Adult:* PO/IM 100-320 mg
- *Child:* PO/IM 3-6 mg/kg

Sedation
- *Adult:* PO 30-120 mg/day in 2-3 divided doses
- *Child:* PO 6 mg/kg/day in 3 divided doses

Preoperative sedation
- *Adult:* IM 100-200 mg 1-1½ hr before surgery

• *Child:* PO 6 mg/kg/day in 3 divided doses

Hyperbilirubinemia

• *Neonate:* PO 7 mg/kg/day on days 1-5 after birth; IM 5 mg/kg/day on day 1, then PO on days 2-7 after birth

Chronic cholestasis

• *Adult:* PO 90-180 mg/day in 2-3 divided doses

• *Child <12 yr:* PO 3-12 mg/kg/day in 2-3 divided doses

Available forms: Caps 16 mg; elix 15, 20 mg/5 ml; tabs 8, 15, 16, 30, 32, 60, 65, 100 mg; inj 30, 60, 65, 130 mg/ml

Side effects/adverse reactions:

CNS: Paradoxic excitement (elderly), drowsiness, lethargy, hangover headache, flushing, hallucinations, ***coma***

GI: Nausea, vomiting

INTEG: Rash, urticaria, ***Stevens-Johnson syndrome, angioedema,*** local pain, swelling, necrosis, ***thrombophlebitis***

Contraindications: Hypersensitivity to barbiturates, porphyria, hepatic disease, respiratory disease, nephritis, hyperthyroidism, diabetes mellitus, elderly, lactation, pregnancy (D)

Precautions: Anemia

Pharmacokinetics:

IV: Onset 5 min, peak 30 min, duration 4-6 hr

IM/SC: Onset 10-30 min, duration 4-6 hr

PO: Onset 20-60 min, peak 8-12 hr, duration 6-10 hr

Metabolized by liver; crosses placenta; excreted in urine, breast milk; half-life 53-118 hr

Interactions:

• Increased effects: CNS depression, alcohol, chloramphenicol, valproic acid, disulfiram, nondepolarizing skeletal muscle relaxants, sulfonamides

• Decreased effects: theophylline, oral anticoagulants, corticosteroids, OCs, metronidazole, doxycycline, quinidine

• Increased orthostatic hypotension: furosemide

Syringe compatibility: Heparin

Solution compatibilities: D_5W, $D_{10}W$, 0.45% NaCl, 0.9% NaCl, Ringer's, dextrose/saline combinations, dextrose/Ringer's, dextrose/LR combinations, sodium lactate

Additive compatibilities: Amikacin, aminophylline, calcium chloride, calcium gluceptate, cephapirin, colistimethate, dimenhydrinate, polymyxin B, sodium bicarbonate, thiopental, verapamil

NURSING CONSIDERATIONS

Assess:

• Mental status: mood, sensorium, affect, memory (long, short)

• Respiratory depression

• Blood dyscrasias: fever, sore throat, bruising, rash, jaundice

• Convulsion activity: type, duration, precipitating factors

• Blood studies, liver function tests during long-term treatment

• Therapeutic blood level periodically: 15-40 mg/ml

• Respiratory status: rate, rhythm, depth

Administer:

• IV after slow dilution with at least 10 ml sterile H_2O for inj regardless of dose; give 65 mg or less/min; titrate to patient response

• Give IM inj deep in large muscle mass to prevent tissue sloughing; use <5 ml in each site

Perform/provide:

• Supervision of ambulation for dizziness, drowsiness

Evaluate:

• Therapeutic response: decreased seizures, increased sedation

Teach patient/family:

• To use exactly as ordered

• To avoid other CNS depressants, including alcohol
• To avoid hazardous activities until stabilized on drug; drowsiness may occur
• Never to withdraw drug abruptly; withdrawal symptoms may occur
• That therapeutic effects (PO) may not be seen for 2-3 wk

Treatment of overdose: Calcium gluconate IV

---

phenolphthalein

(OTC)

(fee-nol-thay'leen)

Alophen, Correctol, Espotabs, Evac-U-Gen, Evac-U-Lax, Ex-Lax, Feen-A-Mint, Lax-Pills, Medilax, Modane, Phenolax, Prulet

Func. class.: Laxative, stimulant/irritant

Chem. class.: Diphenylmethane

Action: Directly acts on intestinal smooth muscle by increasing motor activity; thought to irritate colonic intramural plexus; action requires presence of bile

Uses: Constipation, preparation for bowel surgery or examination

Dosage and routes:
• *Adult:* PO 60-270 mg hs
• *Child >6 yr:* 30-60 mg/day
• *Child 2-5 yr:* 15-20 mg/day

Available forms: Tabs 60, 90, 97.2, 130 mg; chew tab 65, 90, 97.2 mg; chew gum 97.2 mg; wafers 64.8 mg; chew wafers 80 mg

Side effects/adverse reactions:

INTEG: Rash, urticaria, ***Stevens-Johnson syndrome***

GI: Nausea, vomiting, anorexia, diarrhea, abdominal cramps, rectal burning

META: Hypokalemia, electrolyte, fluid imbalances

Contraindications: Hypersensitivity, GI obstructions, abdominal pain, nausea/vomiting, fecal impaction, rectal fissures, hemorrhoids (ulcerated)

Precautions: Pregnancy (C), lactation

Pharmacokinetics:

PO: Onset 6-8 hr; excreted in feces

Lab test interferences:

Increase: BSP test

NURSING CONSIDERATIONS

Assess:
• Stool for color, consistency, amount
• Blood, urine electrolytes if drug is used often by patient
• I&O ratio to identify fluid loss
• Cause of constipation; missing fluids, bulk, exercise
• Cramping, rectal bleeding, nausea, vomiting; drug should be discontinued

Administer:
• Alone for better absorption
• In morning or evening (oral dose)

Evaluate:
• Therapeutic response: decrease in constipation

Teach patient/family:
• To keep out of children's reach; some is fruit or chocolate flavored
• To swallow tabs whole; not to chew
• Not to use laxatives for long-term therapy; bowel tone will be lost
• That normal bowel movements do not always occur daily
• Not to use in presence of abdominal pain, nausea, vomiting
• To notify prescriber if constipation unrelieved, of symptoms of electrolyte imbalance: muscle cramps, pain, weakness, dizziness
• That urine, feces may turn pink to yellow-brown

---

phenoxybenzamine (℞)

(fen-ox-ee-ben'za-meen)
Dibenzyline
Func. class.: Antihypertensive
Chem. class.: α-Adrenergic blocker

Action: α-Adrenergic blocker that binds to α-adrenergic receptors, dilating peripheral blood vessels, lowers peripheral resistance, lowers blood pressure
Uses: Pheochromocytoma
Investigational uses: Peripheral vascular disease
Dosage and routes:
• *Adult:* PO 10 mg qd, increase by 10 mg qod, usual range: 20-40 mg bid-tid
• *Child:* PO 0.2 mg/kg or 6 mg/m^2/day, max 10 mg; may increase q4d; maintenance dose 0.4-1.2 mg/kg/day or 12-36 mg/m^2/day divided doses tid or qid
Available forms: Caps 10 mg
Side effects/adverse reactions:
GI: Dry mouth, nausea, vomiting, diarrhea
CV: Postural hypotension, tachycardia, palpitations
CNS: Dizziness, flushing, drowsiness, sedation, weakness, confusion, headache, malaise
GU: Inhibition of ejaculation
EENT: Nasal congestion, dry mouth, miosis
INTEG: Allergic contact dermatitis
Contraindications: Hypersensitivity, CHF, angina, cerebral vascular insufficiency, coronary arteriosclerosis
Precautions: Severe renal disease, severe pulmonary disease, pregnancy (C)
Pharmacokinetics:
PO: Onset 2 hr, peak 4-6 hr, duration 3-4 days; half-life 24 hr, metabolized in liver, excreted in urine, bile
Interactions:
• Hypotensive response: epinephrine, antihypertensives
NURSING CONSIDERATIONS
Assess:
• Electrolytes: K, Na, Cl, CO_2
• Weight qd, I&O
• B/P lying, standing before starting treatment, q4h after
• Nausea, vomiting, diarrhea
• Skin turgor, dryness of mucous membranes for hydration status
Administer:
• Starting with low dose, gradually increasing to prevent side effects
• Gum, frequent rinsing of mouth or hard candy for dry mouth
• With food or milk for GI symptoms
Evaluate:
• Therapeutic response: decreased B/P, increased peripheral pulses
Teach patient/family:
• To avoid alcoholic beverages
• To report dizziness, palpitations, fainting
• To change position slowly, or fainting may occur
• To take drug exactly as prescribed
• To avoid all OTC products: cough, cold, allergy, unless directed by prescriber
Treatment of overdose: Administer IV saline, norepinephrine, elevate legs, discontinue drug

phensuximide (℞)

(fen-sux'i-mide)
Kapseals, Milontin
Func. class.: Anticonvulsant
Chem. class.: Succinimide

Action: Inhibits spike, wave formation in absence seizures (petit mal), decreases amplitude, frequency, duration

Uses: Absence (petit mal) seizures

Dosage and routes:

• *Adult and child:* PO 500 mg-1 g bid or tid

Available forms: Caps 500 mg

Side effects/adverse reactions:

HEMA: ***Agranulocytosis, aplastic anemia, thrombocytopenia, leukocytosis, eosinophilia, pancytopenia***

CNS: Drowsiness, dizziness, fatigue, euphoria, lethargy, anxiety, depression, irritability, insomnia, aggressiveness, weakness, headache

GI: Nausea, vomiting, heartburn, anorexia, diarrhea, abdominal pain, cramps, constipation

GU: Vaginal bleeding, ***hematuria, renal damage,*** urinary frequency

INTEG: Urticaria, pruritic erythema, hirsutism, ***Stevens-Johnson syndrome***

EENT: Myopia, gum hypertrophy, tongue swelling, blurred vision

Contraindications: Hypersensitivity to succinimide derivatives

Precautions: Lactation, hepatic disease, pregnancy (D), renal disease

Pharmacokinetics:

PO: Peak 1-4 hr, metabolized by liver, excreted by kidneys, half-life 5-12 hr

Interactions:

• Antagonist effect: tricyclic antidepressants (imipramine, doxepin)

• Decreased effects of: estrogens, oral contraceptives

Lab test interferences:

Increase: Coombs' test

NURSING CONSIDERATIONS

Assess:

• Renal studies: urinalysis, BUN, urine creatinine q6mo

• Blood studies: CBC, Hct, Hgb, reticulocyte counts q3mo

• Hepatic studies: AST (SGOT), ALT (SGPT), bilirubin, creatinine q6mo

• Drug levels during initial treatment, therapeutic range (40-80 μg/ml)

• Mental status: mood, sensorium, affect, behavioral changes; if mental status changes, notify prescriber

• Eye problems; need for ophthalmic exam before, during, after treatment (slit lamp, fundoscopy, tonometry)

• Allergic reaction: red raised rash; drug should be discontinued

• Blood dyscrasias: fever, sore throat, bruising, rash, jaundice

• Toxicity: bone marrow depression, nausea, vomiting, ataxia, diplopia

Administer:

• With food, milk for GI symptoms

Perform/provide:

• Hard candy, frequent rinsing of mouth, gum for dry mouth

• Assistance with ambulation during early part of treatment; dizziness occurs

Evaluate:

• Therapeutic response: decreased seizures

Teach patient/family:

• To carry ID card or Medic Alert bracelet stating drugs taken, condition, prescriber's name, phone number

• To avoid driving, other activities that require alertness

• To avoid alcohol ingestion, CNS depressants; increased sedation may occur

• Not to discontinue medication quickly after long-term use

• To call prescriber if sore throat, fever, malaise, bruises, epistaxis occur

• That drug may color urine pink or red

Treatment of overdose: Lavage, activated charcoal, monitor electrolytes, VS; do not induce vomiting

phentermine (℞)

(fen'ter-meen)

Adipex-P, Fastin, Ionamin, Obephen, Obe-Nix, Phentermine Resin, phentermine HCl, Phentrol

Func. class.: Cerebral stimulant

Chem. class.: Sympathomimetic amine

Controlled Substance Schedule IV

Action: Stimulates satiety center by action on adrenergic pathways

Uses: Exogenous obesity

Dosage and routes:

- *Adult:* PO 8 mg tid 30 min before meals or 15-37.5 mg qd before breakfast

Available forms: Tabs 8, 15, 30, 37.5 mg; caps 15, 18.75, 30, 37.5 mg; caps time rel 15, 30 mg

Side effects/adverse reactions:

CNS: Hyperactivity, insomnia, restlessness, dizziness, tremor, headache

GI: Nausea, anorexia, dry mouth, constipation, unpleasant taste

GU: Impotence, change in libido

CV: Palpitations, tachycardia, hypertension

INTEG: Urticaria

EENT: Blurred vision

Contraindications: Hypersensitivity, hyperthyroidism, hypertension, glaucoma, severe arteriosclerosis, angina pectoris, cardiovascular disease, pregnancy (C), child <12 yr

Precautions: Pregnancy (C), lactation, drug abuse, anxiety

Pharmacokinetics:

CON REL: Duration 10-14 hr; metabolized by liver, excreted by kidneys

Interactions:

- Hypertensive crisis: MAOIs or within 14 days of MAOIs
- Increased effect of phentermine: acetazolamide, antacids, sodium bicarbonate
- Decreased effect of phentermine: tricyclics, ascorbic acid, ammonium chloride
- Decreased effect of guanethidine, other antihypertensives
- Decreased insulin requirements: diabetes mellitus

NURSING CONSIDERATIONS

Assess:

- VS, B/P, since drug may reverse antihypertensives; check patients with cardiac disease often
- CBC, urinalysis, in diabetes: blood sugar, urine sugar; insulin changes may have to be made, since eating will decrease
- Height and growth rate in children; growth rate may be decreased
- Mental status: mood, sensorium, affect, stimulation, insomnia, aggressiveness
- Physical dependency: should not be used for extended periods; dose should be discontinued gradually; tolerance occurs with long-term use
- Withdrawal symptoms: headache, nausea, vomiting, muscle pain, weakness

Administer:

- At least 6 hr before hs to avoid sleeplessness
- For obesity only if patient is on weight reduction program including dietary changes, exercise; patient will develop tolerance, and loss of weight won't occur without additional methods; give 30 min before meals
- Gum, hard candy, frequent sips of water for dry mouth

Perform/provide:

- Check to see PO medication has been swallowed

Evaluate:

- Therapeutic response: decreased weight

Teach patient/family:

- To decrease caffeine consumption (coffee, tea, cola, chocolate), which may increase irritability, stimulation
- To avoid OTC preparations unless approved by prescriber
- To taper off drug over several weeks, or depression, increased sleeping, lethargy may ensue
- To avoid alcohol ingestion
- To avoid hazardous activities until stabilized on medication
- To get needed rest; patients will feel more tired at end of day

Treatment of overdose: Administer fluids; hemodialysis or peritoneal dialysis; antihypertensive for increased B/P; ammonium Cl for increased excretion

---

phentolamine (℞)

(fen-tole'a-meen)

Regitine, Rogitine*

Func. class.: Antihypertensive

Chem. class.: α-Adrenergic blocker

Action: α-Adrenergic blocker, binds to α-adrenergic receptors, dilating peripheral blood vessels, lowering peripheral resistances, lowering blood pressure

Uses: Hypertension, pheochromocytoma, prevention, treatment of dermal necrosis following extravasation of norepinephrine or dopamine

Dosage and routes:

Treatment of hypertensive episodes in pheochromocytoma

- *Adult:* IV/IM, 5 mg repeat if necessary
- *Child:* IV/IM, 1 mg repeat if necessary
- *Adult:* IV 2.5 mg, if negative repeat with 5 mg IV
- *Child:* IV 0.5 mg, if negative repeat with 1 mg IV

Prevention, treatment of necrosis

- *Adult:* 5-10 mg/10 ml NS injected into area of norepinephrine extravasation within 12 hr

Impotence (adjunct)

Adult: Intracavernosal 0.5-1 mg with 30 mg papaverine given 1, 2, or 3 treatments/wk

Available forms: Inj 5 mg/ml; tabs 25, 50 mg (only injectable form available in US)

Side effects/adverse reactions:

GI: Dry mouth, nausea, vomiting, diarrhea, abdominal pain

CV: Hypotension, tachycardia, angina, dysrhythmias, ***MI***

CNS: Dizziness, flushing, weakness

EENT: Nasal congestion

Contraindications: Hypersensitivity, MI, coronary insufficiency, angina

Precautions: Pregnancy (C), lactation

Pharmacokinetics:

IV: Peak 2 min, duration 10-15 min

IM: Peak 15-20 min, duration 3-4 hr

Metabolized in liver, excreted in urine

Interactions:

- Increased effects of epinephrine, antihypertensives

Y-site compatibility: Amiodarone

Syringe compatibility: Papaverine

Additive compatibilities: Dobutamine, verapamil

NURSING CONSIDERATIONS

Assess:

- Electrolytes: K, Na, Cl, CO_2
- Weight qd, I&O
- B/P lying, standing before starting treatment, q4h after
- Nausea, vomiting, diarrhea, edema in feet, legs daily; skin turgor, dryness of mucous membranes for hydration status, postural hypotension, cardiac system: pulse, ECG

---

* Available in Canada only

Administer:

- IV after diluting 5 mg/1 ml sterile H_2O for inj; may be further diluted with 5-10 ml sterile H_2O for inj; give 5 mg or less/min
- Gum, frequent rinsing of mouth or hard candy for dry mouth
- With vasopressor available
- After discontinuing all medication for 24 hr
- 10 mg/L may be added to norepinephrine in IV sol for prevention of dermal necrosis

Evaluate:

- Therapeutic response: decreased B/P

Teach patient/family:

- That bed rest is required during treatment, 1 hr after

Treatment of overdose: Administer norepinephrine; discontinue drug

phenylbutazone (℞)

(fen-ill-byoo′ta-zone)

Butazolidin, phenylbutazone

Func. class.: Nonsteroidal antiinflammatory

Chem. class.: Pyrazolone derivative

Action: Inhibits prostaglandin synthesis by decreasing an enzyme needed for biosynthesis; analgesic, antiinflammatory, antipyretic

Uses: Mild to moderate pain, osteoarthritis, rheumatoid arthritis, acute gouty arthritis

Dosage and routes:

Pain

- *Adult:* PO 100-200 mg tid-qid, then after desired response 100 mg tid-qid, not to exceed 600 mg/day

Acute arthritis

- *Adult:* PO 400 mg, then 100 mg q4h × 4 days or until desired response

Available forms: Tabs 100 mg; caps 100 mg

Side effects/adverse reactions:

GI: Nausea, anorexia, vomiting, diarrhea, jaundice, ***cholestatic hepatitis,*** constipation, flatulence, cramps, dry mouth, peptic ulcer

CNS: Dizziness, drowsiness, fatigue, tremors, confusion, insomnia, anxiety, depression

CV: Tachycardia, peripheral edema, palpitations, dysrhythmias, pericarditis, myocarditis, cardiac decompensation

INTEG: Purpura, rash, pruritus, sweating

GU: ***Nephrotoxicity: dysuria, hematuria, oliguria, azotemia***

HEMA: ***Bone marrow suppression***

EENT: Tinnitus, hearing loss, blurred vision

Contraindications: Hypersensitivity, asthma, severe renal disease, severe hepatic disease, pregnancy (D), children <14 yr, ulcer disease

Precautions: Lactation, children, bleeding disorders, GI disorders, cardiac disorders, hypersensitivity to other antiinflammatory agents

Pharmacokinetics:

PO: Peak 2 hr, half-life 3-3½ hr; metabolized in liver; excreted in urine (metabolites), breast milk; 98% protein binding

Interactions:

- Increased action of coumarin, phenytoin, sulfonamides

NURSING CONSIDERATIONS

Assess:

- Renal, liver, blood studies: BUN, creatinine, AST (SGOT), ALT (SGPT), Hgb, before treatment, periodically thereafter
- Record weight, I&O qd
- Audiometric, ophthalmic exam before, during, after treatment
- For history of peptic ulcer disease

P

- For eye, ear problems: blurred vision, tinnitus (may indicate toxicity)

Administer:

- With food to decrease GI symptoms; best to take on empty stomach to facilitate absorption

Perform/provide:

- Storage at room temp

Evaluate:

- Therapeutic response: decreased pain, stiffness, swelling in joints, ability to move more easily

Teach patient/family:

- To report blurred vision or ringing, roaring in ears (may indicate toxicity)
- To avoid driving, other hazardous activities if dizziness or drowsiness occurs
- To report change in urine pattern, weight increase, edema, pain increase in joints, fever, blood in urine (indicates nephrotoxicity)
- That therapeutic effects may take up to 1 mo
- To report black, tarry stools or unusual bleeding, bruising
- To take with full glass of water

phenylephrine (℞)

(fen-ill-ef′rin)

Neo-Synephrine

Func. class.: Adrenergic, direct acting

Chem. class.: Substituted phenylethylamine

Action: Powerful and selective (α_1) receptor agonist causing contraction of blood vessels

Uses: Hypotension, paroxysmal supraventricular tachycardia, shock, maintain B/P during spinal anesthesia

Dosage and routes:

Hypotension

- *Adult:* SC/IM 2-5 mg, may repeat q10-15min if needed; IV 0.1-0.5 mg, may repeat q10-15min if needed

PVCs

- *Adult:* IV BOL 0.5 mg given rapidly, not to exceed prior dose by >0.1 mg; total dose >1 mg

Shock

- *Adult:* IV INF 10 mg/500 ml D_5W given 100-180 gtts/min, then 40-60 gtts/min titrated to B/P

Available forms: Inj 1% (10 mg/ml)

Side effects/adverse reactions:

CNS: Headache, anxiety, tremor, insomnia, dizziness

CV: Palpitations, tachycardia, hypertension, ectopic beats, angina, reflex bradycardia

GI: Nausea, vomiting

INTEG: Necrosis, tissue sloughing with extravasation, ***gangrene***

Contraindications: Hypersensitivity, ventricular fibrillation, tachydysrhythmias, pheochromocytoma, narrow-angle glaucoma

Precautions: Pregnancy (C), lactation, arterial embolism, peripheral vascular disease, elderly, hyperthyroidism, bradycardia, myocardial disease, severe arteriosclerosis

Pharmacokinetics:

IV: Duration 20-30 min

IM/SC: Duration 45-60 min

Interactions:

- Do not use within 2 wk of MAOIs, or hypertensive crisis may result
- Dysrhythmias: general anesthetics, bretylium
- Decreased action of phenylephrine: α-blockers
- Increase in B/P: oxytocics
- Increased pressor effect: tricyclic antidepressant, MAOIs, guanethidine

Y-site compatibilities: Amrinone, famotidine, zidovudine

Additive compatibilities: Chloramphenicol, dobutamine, lidocaine, potassium chloride, sodium bicarbonate

NURSING CONSIDERATIONS

Assess:

- I&O ratio; notify prescriber if output <30 ml/hr
- ECG during administration continuously; if B/P increases, drug is decreased
- B/P and pulse q5min after parenteral route
- CVP or PWP during inf if possible
- For paresthesias and coldness of extremities; peripheral blood flow may decrease

Administer:

- Plasma expanders for hypovolemia
- IV after diluting 1 mg/9 ml sterile H_2O for inj; give dose over ½-1 min; may be diluted 10 mg/500 ml of D_5W or NS; titrate to response (normal B/P); check for extravasation, check site for infiltration, use infusion pump

Perform/provide:

- Storage of reconstituted sol if refrigerated for no longer than 24 hr
- Discard discolored sol

Evaluate:

- Therapeutic response: increased B/P with stabilization

Teach patient/family:

- Reason for administration
- To report pain at infusion site immediately

Treatment of overdose: Administer an α-blocker

phenylephrine (nasal) (OTC)

(fen-ill-ef′rin)

Alconefrin, Alconefrin-25, Alconefrin-50, Duration, Neo-Synephrine, Nōstril, Rhinall-10, Sinex, St. Joseph Measured Dose

Func. class.: Nasal decongestant

Chem. class.: Sympathomimetic amine

Action: Produces vasoconstriction (rapid, long-acting) of arterioles, thereby decreasing fluid exudation, mucosal engorgement

Uses: Nasal congestion

Dosage and routes:

- *Adult:* INSTILL 2-3 gtt or sprays to nasal mucosa bid (0.25%-1%); TOP apply to nasal mucosa q3-4h prn
- *Child 6-12 yr:* INSTILL 1-2 gtt or sprays (0.25%) q3-4h prn
- *Child <6 yr:* INSTILL 2-3 gtt or sprays (0.125%) q3-4h prn

Available forms: Sol 0.125%, 0.16%, 0.2%, 0.25%, 0.5%, 1%; jelly 0.5%

Side effects/adverse reactions:

GI: Nausea, vomiting, anorexia

EENT: Irritation, burning, sneezing, stinging, dryness, rebound congestion

INTEG: Contact dermatitis

CNS: Anxiety, restlessness, tremors, weakness, insomnia, dizziness, fever, headache

Contraindications: Hypersensitivity to sympathomimetic amines

Precautions: Child <6 yr, elderly, diabetes, cardiovascular disease, hypertension, hyperthyroidism, increased ICP, prostatic hypertrophy, pregnancy (C), glaucoma

P

Interactions:

• Hypertension: MAOIs, β-adrenergic blockers

• Hypotension: methyldopa, mecamylamine, reserpine

NURSING CONSIDERATIONS

Assess:

• Redness, swelling, pain in nasal passages

Administer:

• No more than q4h

• For <4 consecutive days

Perform/provide:

• Environmental humidification to decrease nasal congestion, dryness

• Storage in light-resistant containers; do not expose to heat

Evaluate:

• Therapeutic response: decreased nasal congestion

Teach patient/family:

• That stinging may occur for a few applications; drying of mucosa may be decreased by environmental humidification

• To notify prescriber of irregular pulse, insomnia, dizziness, tremors

• Proper administration to avoid systemic absorption

phenylephrine (optic) (OTC)

(fen-ill-ef′rin)

AK-Dilate Ophthalmic, AK-Nefrin Ophthalmic, Isopto Frin, Neo-Synephrine 2.5%, Neo-Synephrine 10% Plain, Neo-Synephrine Viscous, Phenylephrine HCl, 2.5% Mydfrin Ophthalmic, Phenoptic, Relief, Prefrin

Func. class.: Ophthalmic vasoconstrictor

Chem. class.: Direct sympathomimetic amine (α-agonist)

Action: Vasoconstriction of eye arterioles; decreases eye engorgement by stimulation of α-adrenergic receptors

Uses: Topical ocular vasoconstrictor in uveitis, open-angle glaucoma, prior to surgery, diagnostic procedures, refraction without cycloplegia

Dosage and routes:

Eye irritation

• *Adult:* INSTILL 2 gtt 0.12% sol; may repeat q3-4h

Refraction/ophthalmoscopic exam

• *Adult:* INSTILL 1 gtt 2.5% sol

Uveitis/glaucoma/surgery

• *Adult, child:* INSTILL 1 gtt of 2.5% or 10% sol in upper surface of cornea

Available forms: Sol 10%, 2.5%, 0.12%

Side effects/adverse reactions:

CNS: Headache, dizziness, weakness

CV: Bradycardia, hypertension, dysrhythmias, ***tachycardia, CV collapse,*** palpitation

EENT: Stinging, lacrimation, blurred vision, conjunctival allergy

Contraindications: Hypersensitivity, narrow-angle glaucoma

Precautions: Severe hypertension, diabetes, hyperthyroidism, elderly, severe arteriosclerosis, cardiac disease, infants, pregnancy (C)

Pharmacokinetics:

INSTILL: Peak 1 hr, duration 0.5-7 hr depending on strength

Interactions:

• Increased pressor effects: MAOIs, tricyclic antidepressants, H_1 antihistamines, guanethedine

NURSING CONSIDERATIONS

Assess:

• B/P, pulse; systemic absorption does occur

Perform/provide:

• Storage in tight, light-resistant container; do not use discolored sol

Evaluate:
- Therapeutic response: decreased eye irritation

Teach patient/family:
- To report change in vision, blurring, loss of sight; breathing trouble, sweating, flushing
- Method of instillation: tilt head backward, hold dropper over eye, drop medication inside lower lid, using pressure on inside corner of eye hold 1 min, do not touch dropper to eye
- That blurred vision will decrease with repeated use of drug
- To notify prescriber of headache, spots, redness, pain; discontinue use
- To use sunglasses for photophobia
- To use exactly as prescribed

phenytoin (℞)

(fen′i-toy-in)

Dilantin, Dilantin Capsules, Di-Phen, diphenylhydantoin, Diphenylan, phenytoin oral suspension

Func. class.: Anticonvulsant; antidysrhythmic (IB)

Chem. class.: Hydantoin

Combination products: Dilantin with Phenobarbital: phenytoin sodium 100 mg, phenobarbital 32 mg; Dilantin with Phenobarbital: phenobarbital 16 mg, phenytoin sodium 100 mg

Action: Inhibits spread of seizure activity in motor cortex by altering ion transport; increases AV conduction

Uses: Generalized tonic-clonic seizures; status epilepticus; nonepileptic seizures associated with Reye's syndrome or after head trauma; migraines, trigeminal neuralgia, Bell's palsy, ventricular dysrhythmias uncontrolled by antidysrhythmics

Dosage and routes:

Seizures
- *Adult:* IV loading dose 900 mg-1.5 g run at 50 mg/min; if patient has received phenytoin, 100-300 mg run at 50 mg/min; PO loading dose 900 mg-1.5 g divided tid, then 300 mg/day (extended) or divided tid (extended/prompt)
- *Child:* IV loading dose 15 mg/kg run at 50 mg/min; if patient has received phenytoin, 5-7 mg/kg run at 50 mg/min; may repeat in 30 min; PO loading dose of 15 mg/kg divided q8-12h, then 5-7 mg/kg in divided doses q12h

Status epilepticus
- *Adult:* IV 15-20 mg/kg, max 25-50 mg/min, may give 100 mg q6-8hr thereafter
- *Child:* IV 15-20 mg/kg given 1-3 mg/kg/min

Neuritic pain
- *Adult:* PO 200-400 mg/day

Ventricular dysrhythmias
- *Adult:* PO loading dose 1 g divided over 24 hr, then 500 mg/day × 2 days; IV 250 mg over 5 min until dysrhythmias subside or until 1 g is given, or 100 mg q15min until dysrhythmias subside or until 1 g given
- *Child:* PO 3-8 mg/kg or 250 mg/m^2/day as single dose or 2 divided doses; IV 3-8 mg/kg over several min, or 250 mg/m^2/day as single dose or 2 divided doses

Available forms: Susp 30, 125 mg/5 ml; tabs, chewable 50 mg; inj 50 mg/ml; caps ext rel 30, 100 mg; caps prompt 30, 100 mg

Side effects/adverse reactions:

CNS: Drowsiness, dizziness, insomnia, paresthesias, depression, suicidal tendencies, aggression, headache, confusion, slurred speech

CV: Hypotension, ***ventricular fibrillation***
EENT: Nystagmus, diplopia, blurred vision
GI: Nausea, vomiting, constipation, anorexia, weight loss, ***hepatitis,*** jaundice, gingival hyperplasia
GU: ***Nephritis,*** urine discoloration
HEMA: ***Agranulocytosis, leukopenia, aplastic anemia, thrombocytopenia, megaloblastic anemia***
INTEG: Rash, ***lupus erythematosus, Stevens-Johnson syndrome,*** hirsutism
SYST: Hypocalcemia

Contraindications: Hypersensitivity, psychiatric condition, pregnancy (D), bradycardia, SA and AV block, Stokes-Adams syndrome

Precautions: Allergies, hepatic disease, renal disease

Pharmacokinetics:
PO-ER: Onset 2-24 hr, peak 4-12 hr, duration 12-36 hr
IV: Onset 1-2 hr, duration 12-24 hr
PO: Onset 2-24 hr, peak 1½-2½ hr, duration 6-12 hr
Metabolized by liver, excreted by kidneys

Interactions:
- Decreased effects of phenytoin: alcohol (chronic use), antihistamines, antacids, antineoplastics, CNS depressants, rifampin, folic acid

Y-site compatibilities: Esmolol, famotodine, foscarnet

Lab test interferences:
Decrease: Dexamethasone, metyrapone test serum, PBI, urinary steroids
Increase: Glucose, alk phosphatase, BSP

NURSING CONSIDERATIONS

Assess:
- Drug level: toxic level 30-50 μg/ml
- Blood studies: CBC, platelets q2wk until stabilized, then qmo × 12, then q3mo; discontinue drug if neutrophils <1600/mm^3
- Mental status: mood, sensorium, affect, memory (long, short)
- Respiratory depression; rate, depth, character
- Blood dyscrasias: fever, sore throat, bruising, rash, jaundice

Administer:
- IV after diluting with diluent provided (2.2 ml/100 mg, 5.2 ml/250 mg) (1 ml/50 mg); shake; place vial in warm water to dissolve powder; give through Y-tube or 3-way stopcock; inject slowly <50 mg/min; clear IV tubing first with NS sol; use in-line filter; discard 4 hr after preparation; inject into large veins to prevent purple glove syndrome

Evaluate:
- Therapeutic response; decrease in severity of seizures, ventricular dysrhythmias

Teach patient/family:
- To take PO doses divided with or after meals to decrease adverse effects
- That if diabetic, urine glucose should be monitored
- That urine may turn pink
- Not to discontinue drug abruptly; seizures may occur
- Proper brushing of teeth using a soft toothbrush, flossing to prevent gingival hyperplasia; need to see dentist frequently
- To avoid hazardous activities until stabilized on drug
- To carry Medic Alert ID stating drug use
- That heavy use of alcohol may diminish effect of drug; to avoid OTC medications
- Not to change brands or forms once stabilized on therapy; brands may vary

physostigmine (ophthalmic) (℞)

(fi-zoe-stig'meen)

Isopto Eserine Solution/Eserine Sulfate Ointment, Fisostin

Func. class.: Miotic

Chem. class.: Cholinesterase inhibitor

Action: Increases concentration of acetylcholine at cholinergic transmission sites, causing prolonged, exaggerated action; produces constriction of ciliary muscles, iris sphincter, causing iris to be pulled away from anterior chamber angle, aiding in aqueous humor drainage

Uses: Wide-angle glaucoma

Dosage and routes:

• *Adult and child:* INSTILL OINT ¼ inch strip of 0.25% oint in conjunctival sac; INSTILL SOL 1-2 gtt 0.25%-0.5% sol in conjunctival sac qd-qid

Available forms: Oint 0.25% (sulfate); sol 0.25% (salicylate)

Side effects/adverse reactions:

CNS: ***Convulsions,*** headache

CV: Hypertension, hypotension, bradycardia, irregular pulse

GI: Nausea, vomiting, abdominal cramps

RESP: ***Bronchospasm,*** dyspnea, ***pulmonary edema***

EENT: Blurred vision, conjunctivitis, allergic reactions, rhinorrhea, salivation, eye, brow pain, lacrimation, twitching of eyelids

Contraindications: Hypersensitivity, inflammatory disease of iris or ciliary body

Precautions: Epilepsy, parkinsonism, bradycardia, pregnancy (C), asthma, bronchitis, diabetes mellitus, CV disease

Interactions:

• Benzalkonium chloride in sol or syringe

Pharmacokinetics:

Miosis: Onset 20-30 min, duration 12-36 hr

Intraocular pressure: Peak 2-6 hrs, duration 12-36 hrs

NURSING CONSIDERATIONS

Administer:

• Topically to conjunctival sac

• Immediately after reconstituting; discard unused portion

Perform/provide:

• Only clear sol, never pink or brown

Evaluate

• Therapeutic response: decreased intraocular pressure

Teach patient/family:

• To report change in vision, blurring or loss of sight, trouble breathing, sweating, flushing

• Method of instillation, including pressure on lacrimal sac for 1 min, not to touch dropper to eye

• That long-term therapy may be required

• That blurred vision will decrease with repeated use of drug

• That drug is often irritating to eye, rarely tolerated for prolonged periods

• That drug may be prescribed for bedtime use to prevent nocturnal rise in ocular tension

• That maximal effect of topical application is reached in 30 min, may last 12-36 hr

• To observe eyes for irritation, development of cataracts

physostigmine (℞)

(fi-zoe-stig'meen)

Antilirium

Func. class.: Antidote, reversible anticholinesterase

Chem. class.: Tertiary amine

Action: Increases acetylcholine at cholinergic nerve terminals; reverses central, peripheral anticholinergic effects

Uses: To reverse CNS effects of diazepam; anticholinergic, tricyclic antidepressant, Alzheimer's disease, hereditary ataxia

Dosage and routes:

Overdose of anticholinergics

• *Adult:* IM/IV 2 mg; give no more than 1 mg/min; may repeat

• *Pediatric:* IM/IV inj 0.02 mg/kg, not more than 0.5 mg/min; may repeat at 5-10 min intervals until max dose of 2 mg

Postanesthesia

• *Adult:* IM/IV 0.5-1 mg; give no more than 1 mg/min (IV); can repeat at 10 to 30 min intervals

Available forms: Inj IM, IV 1 mg/ml

Side effects/adverse reactions:

INTEG: Rash, urticaria

CNS: Dizziness, headache, sweating, weakness, ***convulsions,*** incoordination, ***paralysis,*** hallucination, delirium, drowsiness

GI: Nausea, diarrhea, vomiting, cramps, increased salivary and gastric secretions

CV: Bradycardia, hypotension, syncope

GU: Frequency, incontinence, urgency

RESP: ***Respiratory depression, bronchospasm, constriction***, dyspnea

EENT: Miosis, blurred vision, lacrimation

Contraindications: Hypotension, obstruction of intestine or renal system, asthma, gangrene, CV disease, choline esters, depolarizing neuromuscular blocking agents, diabetes

Precautions: Seizure disorders, bronchial asthma, coronary occlusion, hyperthyroidism, dysrhythmias, peptic ulcer, megacolon, poor GI motility, pregnancy (C), Parkinson's disease, bradycardia, lactation

Pharmacokinetics:

IM/IV: Peak 5 min, duration 45-60 min; crosses blood-brain barrier, excreted in urine

Interactions:

• Decreased action of gallamine, metocurine, pancuronium, tubocurarine, atropine

• Increased action of decamethonium, succinylcholine

• Decreased action of physostigmine: aminoglycosides, anesthetics, procainamide, quinidine

• Considered incompatible with any drug in sol or syringe

NURSING CONSIDERATIONS

Assess:

• VS; respiration q8h

• I&O ratio; check for urinary retention or incontinence

• Toxicity; drug should be discontinued

Administer:

• IV undiluted, give through Y-tube or 3-way stopcock; give 1 mg or less/1-3 min or 0.5 mg or less over 1 min or more (child)

• Only with atropine sulfate available for cholinergic crisis

• Only after all other cholinergics have been discontinued

• Increased doses for tolerance

Perform/provide:

• Storage at room temp

Evaluate:

• Therapeutic response: LOC—alert

Treatment of overdose: Can cause cholinergic crisis; atropine is an antagonist

phytonadione (vit K_1) (℞)

(fye-toe-na-dye'one)

AquaMEPHYTON, Konakion, Mephyton

Func. class.: Vit K_1, fat-soluble vitamin

Action: Needed for adequate blood clotting (factors II, VII, IX, X)

Uses: Vit K malabsorption, hypoprothrombinemia, prevention of hypoprothrombinemia caused by oral anticoagulants, prevention of hemorrhagic disease of newborn

Dosage and routes:

Hypoprothrombinemia caused by vit K malabsorption

- *Adult:* PO/IM 2-25 mg, may repeat or increase to 50 mg
- *Child:* PO/IM 5-10 mg
- *Infants:* PO/IM 2 mg

Prevention of hemorrhagic disease of the newborn

- *Neonate:* SC/IM 0.5-1 mg after birth, repeat in 6-8 hr if required

Hypoprothrombinemia caused by oral anticoagulants

- *Adult:* PO/SC/IM 2.5-10 mg, may repeat 12-48 hr after PO dose or 6-8 hr after SC/IM dose, based on PT

Available forms: Tabs 5 mg; inj 2 mg, 10 mg/ml aqueous colloidal (IM, IV); inj aqueous dispersion 2, 10 mg/ml, (IM)

Side effects/adverse reactions:

CNS: Headache, ***brain damage*** (large doses)

GI: Nausea, decreased liver function tests

HEMA: ***Hemolytic anemia, hemoglobinuria, hyperbilirubinemia***

INTEG: Rash, urticaria

Contraindications: Hypersensitivity, severe hepatic disease, last few weeks of pregnancy

Precautions: Pregnancy (C), neonates

Pharmacokinetics:

PO/Inj: Metabolized, crosses placenta

Interactions:

- Decreased action of phytonadione: cholestyramine, mineral oil
- Decreased action of oral anticoagulants
- Incompatible with vits C and B_{12}, dextran, pentobarbital, phenobarbital, phenytoin, vancomycin, warfarin

NURSING CONSIDERATIONS

Assess:

- Pro-time during treatment (2-sec deviation from control time, bleeding time, and clotting time); monitor for bleeding, pulse, and BP
- Nutritional status: liver (beef), spinach, tomatoes, coffee, asparagus, broccoli, cabbage, lettuce, greens

Administer:

- IV after diluting with D_5 NS 10 ml or more; give 1 mg/min or more
- IV only when other routes not possible (deaths have occurred)

Perform/provide:

- Storage in tight, light-resistant container

Evaluate:

- Therapeutic response: decreased bleeding tendencies, decreased protime, decreased clotting time

Teach patient/family:

- Not to take other supplements unless directed by prescriber
- Necessary foods for diet
- To avoid IM injections, use soft toothbrush, don't floss, use electric razor until coagulation defect corrected
- To report symptoms of bleeding
- Not to use OTC medications unless approved by prescriber

• Emphasize importance of frequent lab tests to monitor coagulation factors

pilocarpine (℞)

(pye-loe-kar′peen)

Adsorbocarpine, Akarpine, Isopto Carpine, Ocu-Carpine Ocusert Pilo, Pilagan, Pilocar, pilocarpine HCl, Pilopine HS, Piloptic-1, Piloptic-2, Pilostat, Pilopto-Carpine

Func. class.: Direct-acting miotic

Chem. class.: Cholinergic agonist

Action: Acts directly on cholinergic receptor sites; induces miosis, spasm of accommodation, fall in intraocular pressure, caused by stimulation of ciliary, pupillary sphincter muscles, which leads to pulling away of iris from filtration angle, resulting in increased outflow of aqueous humor

Uses: Primary glaucoma, early stages of wide-angle glaucoma (less useful in advanced stages), chronic open-angle glaucoma, acute narrow-angle glaucoma before emergency surgery; also neutralizes mydriatics used during eye exam; may be used alternately with mydriatics to break adhesions between iris and lens

Dosage and routes:

• *Adult and child:* INSTILL SOL 1-2 gtt of 1% or 2% sol in eye q6-8h; INSTILL 20-40 μg/hr (Ocusert) in cul-de-sac of eye

Available forms: Oph sol 0.25%, 0.5%, 1%, 2%, 3%, 4%, 6%, 8%, 10%; Ocusert Pilo 20 μg/hr, 40 μg/hr system; 4% gel

Side effects/adverse reactions:

CV: Hypotension, tachycardia

RESP: ***Bronchospasm***

GI: Nausea, vomiting, abdominal cramps, diarrhea

GU: Bladder tightness

EENT: Blurred vision, browache, twitching of eyelids, eye pain with change in focus

Contraindications: Hypersensitivity

Precautions: Bronchial asthma, hypertension, pregnancy (C), bradycardia, hyperthyroidism, coronary artery disease, obstruction of GI/urinary tracts (or if strength of walls of these structures in question, peptic ulcers), epilepsy, parkinsonism, asthma

NURSING CONSIDERATIONS

Assess:

• Heart rate, respiratory status, B/P

• Replacement of ocular systems qwk; check system each hs, AM

Administer:

• After shaking vial to mix drug to clear sol; push stopper to mix sterile water with powder

• After cleaning stopper with alcohol

• Wipe away excess sol promptly to prevent flow into lacrimal system, producing systemic symptoms

• With atropine readily available as antidote

• Immediately after reconstituting; discard unused portion

Perform/provide:

• Protect sol from light

• Store Ocusert systems and sol at 36°-46° F (2°-8° C), 46°-86° F (8°-30° C); refrigerate gel until dispensed; discard unused sol after 8wk

Evaluate:

• Therapeutic response: decreased intraocular pressure

Teach patient/family:

• To report change in vision, blurring or loss of sight, trouble breathing, sweating, flushing

* Available in Canada only

• Method of instillation, including pressure on lacrimal sac for 1 min, not to touch dropper to eye
• That long-term therapy may be required
• That blurred vision will decrease with repeated use of drug
• To discontinue use if local hypersensitivity reaction occurs
• That acuity in dim light will be reduced
• Not to drive while using drug

pinacidil (℞)

(pye-na'si-dil)
Pindac

Func. class.: Antihypertensive
Chem. class.: Vasodilator—peripheral

Action: Directly relaxes arteriolar smooth muscle, causing vasodilation

Uses: Severe hypertension not responsive to other therapy; topically to treat alopecia

Dosage and routes:

• *Adult:* PO 12.5-25 mg bid

Available forms: Tabs 12.5, 25 mg

Side effects/adverse reactions:

CV: Severe rebound hypertension, tachycardia, angina, increased T wave, ***CHF, pulmonary edema,*** edema, sodium, water retention

CNS: Drowsiness, dizziness, sedation, headache, depression

GI: Nausea, vomiting, diarrhea, constipation, dry mouth

GU: Gynecomastia, breast tenderness

INTEG: Pruritus, ***Stevens-Johnson syndrome***, rash, hirsutism

Contraindications: Acute MI, dissecting aortic aneurysm, hypersensitivity, pheochromocytoma

Precautions: Pregnancy (C), lactation, children, renal disease, CAD, post MI

Pharmacokinetics:

Peak 1 hr, 60% protein bound; metabolized in the liver; excreted in urine, feces (active metabolites); half-life 1½-3 hr

Interactions:

• Orthostatic hypotension: guanethidine
• Reduced effect of pinacidil: nonsteroidal antiinflammatory drugs

Lab test interferences:

Increase: Renal function studies
Decrease: Hgb/Hct/RBC

NURSING CONSIDERATIONS

Assess:

• Electrolytes: K, Na, Cl; CO_2
• Renal function studies: AST, ALT, alk phosphatase
• B/P, pulse
• Weight qd, I&O, nausea
• Edema in feet, legs qd
• Skin turgor, dryness of mucous membranes for hydration status
• Rales, dyspnea, orthopnea

Administer:

• With meals for better absorption, to decrease GI symptoms
• With β-blocker and/or diuretic

Evaluate:

• Therapeutic response: decreased B/P or increased hair growth

Teach patient/family:

• That body hair will increase but is reversible after treatment is discontinued
• Not to discontinue drug abruptly
• To report pitting edema, dizziness, weight gain >5 lb, shortness of breath, bruising or bleeding, heart rate >20 beats/min over normal, severe indigestion, dizziness, lightheadedness, panting, new or aggravated symptoms of angina
• To take drug exactly as prescribed or serious side effects may occur

Treatment of overdose: Administer normal saline IV, phenylephrine, angiotensin II, vasopressor; dopamine may reverse hypotension

pindolol (℞)

(pin′doe-lole)

Visken

Func. class.: Antihypertensive

Chem. class.: Nonselective β-blocker

Action: Competitively blocks stimulation of β-adrenergic receptor within vascular smooth muscle; produces chronotropic, inotropic activity (decreases rate of SA node discharge, increases recovery time), slows conduction of AV node, decreases heart rate, which decreases O_2 consumption in myocardium; also decreases renin-aldosterone-angiotensin system, at high doses inhibits β-2 receptors in bronchial system

Uses: Mild to moderate hypertension

Investigational uses: Mitral valve prolapse, hypertrophic cardiomyopathy, angina pectoris

Dosage and routes:

• *Adult:* PO 5 mg bid, usual dose 15 mg/day (5 mg tid), may increase by 10 mg/day q3-4wk to a max of 60 mg/day

Available forms: Tabs 5, 10 mg

Side effects/adverse reactions:

CV: Hypotension, bradycardia, ***CHF,*** edema, chest pain, palpitation, claudication, tachycardia, ***AV block***

CNS: Insomnia, dizziness, hallucinations, anxiety, fatigue

GI: Nausea, vomiting, ***ischemic colitis,*** diarrhea, *abdominal pain,* ***mesenteric arterial thrombosis***

INTEG: Rash, alopecia, pruritus, fever

HEMA: ***Agranulocytosis, thrombocytopenia, purpura***

EENT: Visual changes, sore throat, *double vision,* dry burning eyes

GU: Impotence, urinary frequency

RESP: ***Bronchospasm,*** *dyspnea,* cough, rales

MISC: Joint pain, muscle pain

Contraindications: Hypersensitivity to β-blockers, cardiogenic shock, 2nd, 3rd degree heart block, sinus bradycardia, CHF, cardiac failure, bronchial asthma

Precautions: Major surgery, pregnancy (B), lactation, diabetes mellitus, renal disease, thyroid disease, COPD, well-compensated heart failure, CAD, nonallergic bronchospasm

Pharmacokinetics:

PO: Peak 2-4 wk; half-life 3-4 hr, excreted 30%-45% unchanged; 60%-65% metabolized by liver; excreted in breast milk

Interactions:

• Increased hypotension, bradycardia: reserpine, hydralazine, methyldopa, prazosin, anticholinergics

• Decreased antihypertensive effects: indomethacin, sympathomimetics

• Increased hypoglycemic effect: insulin

• Decreased bronchodilation: theophyllines, $β_2$ agonists

Lab test interferences:

Increase: Liver function tests, renal function tests

NURSING CONSIDERATIONS

Assess:

• I&O, weight qd

• B/P during initial treatment, periodically thereafter; pulse q4h, note rate, rhythm, quality

• Apical, radial pulse before administration; notify prescriber of any significant changes

• Baselines in renal, liver function tests before therapy begins

* Available in Canada only

• Edema in feet, legs qd
• Skin turgor, dryness of mucous membranes for hydration status

Administer:
• PO ac, hs; tablet may be crushed or swallowed whole
• Reduced dosage in renal dysfunction

Perform/provide:
• Storage in dry area at room temp; do not freeze

Evaluate:
• Therapeutic response: decreased B/P after 1-2 wk

Teach patient/family:
• To take with or immediately after meals
• Not to discontinue drug abruptly; taper over 2 wk; may cause precipitate angina
• Not to use OTC products containing α-adrenergic stimulants (nasal decongestants, OTC cold preparations) unless directed by prescriber
• To report bradycardia, dizziness, confusion, depression, fever, sore throat, shortness of breath to prescriber
• To take pulse at home; advise when to notify prescriber
• To avoid alcohol, smoking, Na
• To comply with weight control, dietary adjustments, modified exercise program
• To carry Medic Alert ID to identify drug, allergies
• To avoid hazardous activities if dizziness is present
• To report symptoms of CHF: difficult breathing, especially on exertion or when lying down, night cough, swelling of extremities
• To take medication at bedtime to prevent orthostatic hypotension
• To wear support hose to minimize effects of orthostatic hypotension

Treatment of overdose: Lavage, IV atropine for bradycardia, IV theophylline for bronchospasm, digitalis, O_2, diuretic for cardiac failure, hemodialysis, hypotension; give vasopressor (norepinephrine)

pipecuronium (℞)

(pip-e-kyoor′oh-nee-um)
Arduran

Func. class.: Neuromuscular blocker (nondepolarizing)
Chem. class.: Synthetic curariform

Action: Inhibits transmission of nerve impulses by binding with cholinergic receptor sites, antagonizing action of acetylcholine

Uses: Facilitation of endotracheal intubation, skeletal muscle relaxation during mechanical ventilation, surgery, or general anesthesia

Dosage and routes:
• *Adult:* IV dosage is individualized; in patients with normal renal function who are not obese, initial dose is 70-85 μg/kg; maintenance dose ranges from 10-15 μg/kg
• *Child 1-14 yr:* IV 57 μg/kg
• *Child 3 mo-1 yr:* IV 40 μg/kg

Available forms: Inj 10-mg vials

Side effects/adverse reactions:

CV: Bradycardia, tachycardia, increased or decreased B/P, ventricular extrasystole, ***myocardial ischemia, cardiovascular accident, thrombosis, atrial fibrillation***

RESP: ***Prolonged apnea, bronchospasm, cyanosis, respiratory depression***

GU: ***Anuria***

EENT: Increased secretions

CNS: Hypesthesia, CNS depression

MS: Weakness to prolonged skeletal muscle relaxation

INTEG: Rash, urticaria

META: Hypoglycemia, hyperkalemia, increased creatinine

Contraindications: Hypersensitivity to bromide ion

Precautions: Pregnancy (C), renal disease, cardiac disease, lactation, children <3 mo, fluid and electrolyte imbalances, neuromuscular diseases, respiratory disease, obesity

Pharmacokinetics:

IV: Onset 30-45 sec, peak 3-5 min: metabolized (small amounts), excreted in urine (unchanged), crosses placenta

Interactions:

- Increased neuromuscular blockade: aminoglycosides, quinidine, local anesthetics, polymyxin antibiotics, enflurane, isoflurane, tetracyclines, halothane, magnesium, colistin

NURSING CONSIDERATIONS

Assess:

- For electrolyte imbalances (K, Mg); may lead to increased action of this drug
- Vital signs (B/P, pulse, respirations, airway) until fully recovered: rate, depth, pattern of respirations, strength of hand grip
- I&O ratio; check for urinary retention, frequency, hesitancy
- Recovery: decreased paralysis of face, diaphragm, leg, arm, rest of body
- Allergic reactions: rash, fever, respiratory distress, pruritus; drug should be discontinued

Administer:

- Using nerve stimulator by anesthesiologist to determine neuromuscular blockade
- Atropine to counteract muscarinic effects
- After succinylcholine effects subside
- Anticholinesterase to reverse neuromuscular blockade
- By slow IV over 1-2 min (only by qualified persons, usually an anesthesiologist)
- Only fresh sol

Perform/provide:

- Storage in refrigerator; do not store in plastic container or syringe
- Reassurance if communication is difficult during recovery from neuromuscular blockade
- Use of reconstituted sol within 24 hr or discard
- Frequent (q2h) instillation of artificial tears and covering eyes to prevent drying of cornea

Evaluate:

- Therapeutic response: paralysis of jaw, eyelid, head, neck, rest of body

Treatment of overdose: Neostigmine, atropine; monitor VS; may require mechanical ventilation

piperacillin (℞)

(pi-per′a-sill-in)

Pipracil

Func. class.: Broad-spectrum antiiinfective

Chem. class.: Extended-spectrum penicillin

Action: Interferes with cell wall replication of susceptible organisms; osmotically unstable cell wall swells and bursts from osmotic pressure

Uses: Respiratory, skin, urinary tract, bone infections; gonorrhea; pneumonia; effective for gram-positive cocci *(S. aureus, S. pyogenes, S. viridans, S. faecalis, S. bovis, S. pneumoniae),* gram-negative cocci *(N. gonorrhoeae, N. meningitidis),* gram-positive bacilli *(C. perfringens, C. tetani),* gram-negative bacilli *(Bacteroides, F. nucleatum, E. coli, Klebsiella, P. mirabilis, M. morganii, P. vulgaris, P. rehgesii, Enterobacter, Citrobacter, P. aeruginosa, Serratia, Acinetobacter, Peptococcus, Peptostreptococcus, Eubacterium)*

Dosage and routes:
Systemic infections
• *Adult, child >12 yr:* IM/IV 100-300 mg/kg/day in divided doses q4-6h
Prophylaxis of surgical infections
• *Adult:* IV 2g ½-1 hr before procedure; may be repeated during surgery or after surgery
Available forms: Inj 2, 3, 4, 40 g; Inf 2, 3, 4 g
Side effects/adverse reactions:
HEMA: Anemia, increased bleeding time, ***bone marrow depression***
GI: Nausea, vomiting, diarrhea, increased AST (SGOT), ALT (SGPT), abdominal pain, glossitis, colitis
GU: ***Oliguria, proteinuria, hematuria,*** *vaginitis, moniliasis,* ***glomerulonephritis***
CNS: Lethargy, hallucinations, anxiety, depression, twitching, ***coma, convulsions***
META: Hypokalemia, hypernatremia
Contraindications: Hypersensitivity to penicillins; neonates
Precautions: Pregnancy (B), lactation, hypersensitivity to cephalosporins; CHF
Pharmacokinetics:
IM: Peak 30-50 min
IV: Peak 20-30 min
Half-life 0.7-1.33 hr; excreted in urine, bile, breast milk; crosses placenta
Interactions:
• Decreased antimicrobial effect of piperacillin: tetracyclines, erythromycins, aminoglycosides IV
• Increased piperacillin concentrations: aspirin, probenecid
• Drug/food: decreased absorption: food, carbonated drinks, citrus fruit juices
Syringe compatibility: Heparin
Y-site compatibilities: Acyclovir, aldesleukin, ciprofloxacin, cyclophosphamide, enalaprilat, esmolol, famotidine, fludarabine, foscarnet, hydromorphone, labetalol, magnesium sulfate, melphalan, merperidine, morphine, perphenazine, verapamil, zidovudine
Additive compatibilities: Ciprofloxacin, clindamycin, hydrocortisone sodium succinate, potassium chloride, verapamil
Lab test interferences:
False positive: Urine glucose, urine protein, Coombs' test

NURSING CONSIDERATIONS

Assess:
• I&O ratio; report hematuria, oliguria, since penicillin in high doses is nephrotoxic
• Any patient with compromised renal system, since drug is excreted slowly in poor renal system function; toxicity may occur rapidly
• Liver studies: AST (SGOT), ALT (SGPT)
• Blood studies: WBC, RBC, Hgb, Hct, bleeding time
• Renal studies: urinalysis, protein, blood
• C&S before drug therapy; drug may be taken as soon as culture is taken
• Bowel pattern before and during treatment
• Skin eruptions after administration of penicillin to 1 wk after discontinuing drug
• Respiratory status: rate, character, wheezing, tightness in chest
• Allergies before initiation of treatment, reaction of each medication; highlight allergies on chart
Administer:
• IV after diluting 1 g or less/5 ml or more sterile H_2O or 0.9% NaCl; shake; give dose over 3-5 min; may further dilute to 50-100 ml with D_5W, 0.9% NS, and give over ½ hr; discontinue primary IV
• Drug after C&S completed

Perform/provide:

- Adrenalin, suction, tracheostomy set, endotracheal intubation equipment on unit
- Adequate intake of fluids (2 L) during diarrhea episodes
- Scratch test to assess allergy after securing order from physician; usually done when penicillin is only drug of choice
- Storage of reconstituted sol 24 hr at room temp or 7 days refrigerated

Evaluate:

- Therapeutic response: absence of fever, purulent drainage, redness, inflammation

Teach patient/family:

- That culture may be taken after completed course of medication
- To report sore throat, fever, fatigue; may indicate superinfection
- To wear or carry Medic Alert ID if allergic to penicillins
- To notify nurse of diarrhea

Treatment of anaphylaxis: Withdraw drug, maintain airway, administer epinephrine, aminophylline, O_2, IV corticosteroids

piperacillin and tazobactam (℞)

(pi-per'a-sill-in)
Zosyn

Func. class.: Broad-spectrum antibiotic

Chem. class.: Extended-spectrum penicillin/β-lactamase inhibitor

Action: Interferes with cell wall replication of susceptible organisms; osmotically unstable cell wall swells and bursts from osmotic pressure

Uses: Moderate to severe infections: piperacillin-resistant, β-lactamase producing strains causing infections in respiratory, skin, urinary tract, bone, gonorrhea, pneumonia; effective for resistant *S. aureus,* resistant *E. coli, B. fragilis, B. ovatus, B. thetaiotaomicron, B. vulgatus*

Dosage and routes:

- *Adult:* IV INF 12-15 g day given 3.375 g q6h over 30 min × 7-10 days

Available forms: Powder for inj IV 2 g piperacillin/0.25 g tazobactam, 3 g piperacillin/0.375 g tazobactam, 4 g piperacillin/0.5 g tazobactam

Side effects/adverse reactions:

CNS: Lethargy, hallucinations, anxiety, depression, twitching, ***coma, convulsions***

GI: Nausea, vomiting, diarrhea, increased AST (SGOT), ALT (SGPT), abdominal pain, glossitis, colitis

GU: ***Oliguria, proteinuria, hematuria,*** *vaginitis, moniliasis,* ***glomerulonephritis***

HEMA: Anemia, increased bleeding time, ***bone marrow depression***

META: Hypokalemia, hypernatremia

Contraindications: Hypersensitivity to penicillins, neonates

Precautions: Pregnancy (B), lactation, hypersensitivity to cephalosporins, CHF

Pharmacokinetics:

IV: Peak completion of IV, duration 6 hr

Half-life 0.7-1.2 hr; excreted in urine, bile, breast milk; crosses placenta; 33% bound to plasma proteins

Interactions:

- Decreased antimicrobial effect of piperacillin: tetracyclines, erythromycins, aminoglycosides IV
- Increased piperacillin concentrations: aspirin, probenecid

Syringe compatibility: Heparin

Y-site compatibilities: Acyclovir, aldesleukin, ciprofloxacin, cyclophosphamide, enalaprilat, esmolol, famotidine, fludarabine, foscarnet, hydromorphone, labetalol, magnesium sulfate, melphalan, merperidine, morphine, perphenazine, verapamil, zidovudine

Additive compatibilities: Ciprofloxacin, clindamycin, hydrocortisone sodium succinate, potassium chloride, verapamil

Lab test interferences:

False positive: Urine glucose, urine protein, Coombs' test

Decreased: Hct, Hgb, electrolytes

Increased: Platelet count, eosinophilia, neutropenia, leukopenia, serum creatine, PTT, AST (SGOT), ALT (SGPT), alk phosphatase, bilirubin, BUN, electrolytes

NURSING CONSIDERATIONS

Assess:

- I&O ratio; report hematuria, oliguria, since penicillin in high doses is nephrotoxic
- Any patient with compromised renal system, since drug is excreted slowly in poor renal system function; toxicity may occur rapidly
- Liver studies: AST (SGOT), ALT (SGPT)
- Blood studies: WBC, RBC, Hct, Hgb, bleeding time
- Renal studies: urinalysis, protein, blood
- C&S before drug therapy; drug may be given as soon as culture is taken
- Bowel pattern before and during treatment
- Skin eruptions after administration of penicillin to 1 wk after discontinuing drug
- Respiratory status: rate, character, wheezing, tightness in chest
- Allergies before initiation of treatment, reaction of each medication; highlight allergies on chart

Administer:

- IV after diluting 5 ml 0.9% NaCl for injection or sterile H_2O for injection, dextran 6% in NS, dextrose 5%, KCl 40 mEq, bacteriostatic saline/parabens, bacteriostatic saline/benzyl alcohol, bacteriostatic H_2O/benzyl alcohol per 1 g piperacillin; shake well; further dilute in at least 50 ml compatible IV sol and run as int inf over at least 30 min
- Drug after C&S is complete

Perform/provide:

- Adrenalin, suction, tracheostomy set, endotracheal intubation equipment on unit
- Adequate intake of fluids (2 L) during diarrhea episodes
- Scratch test to assess allergy on order from prescriber; usual when penicillin is only drug of choice
- Discard after 24 hr if stored at room temp or after 48 hr if refrigerated; use single-dose vials immediately after reconstitution; stable in ambulatory IV pump for 12 hr

Evaluate:

- Therapeutic response: absence of fever, purulent drainage, redness, inflammation; culture shows decreased organisms

Teach patient/family:

- That culture may be taken after completed course of medication
- To report sore throat, fever, fatigue; may indicate superinfection
- To wear or carry Medic Alert ID if allergic to penicillins
- To notify nurse of diarrhea

Treatment of overdose: Withdraw drug, maintain airway, administer epinephrine, aminophylline, O_2, IV corticosteroids for anaphylaxis

piperazine (℞)

(pi'per-a-zeen)

Piperazine

Func. class.: Anthelmintic

Action: Causes paralysis in worm, leading to expulsion by normal peristalsis

P

Uses: Pinworm, roundworm
Dosage and routes:
Pinworm
• *Adult, child:* PO 65 mg/kg × 7-8 days, not to exceed 2.5 g/day
Roundworm
• *Adult:* PO 3.5 g in single dose × 2 days
• *Child:* PO 75 mg/kg/day in a single dose × 2 days
Available forms: Tabs 250; syr 500 mg/5 ml
Side effects/adverse reactions:
HEMA: ***Hemolytic anemia***
INTEG: Rash, urticaria, photosensitivity
RESP: ***Bronchospasm***
CNS: Dizziness, headache, paresthesia, ***convulsions,*** fever, headache, ataxia
EENT: Blurred vision, nystagmus, strabismus, cataracts, rhinorrhea
GI: Nausea, vomiting, anorexia, diarrhea, abdominal cramps
Contraindications: Hypersensitivity, renal disease, hepatic disease, seizures
Precautions: Severe malnutrition, seizure disorders, anemia, pregnancy (B)
Pharmacokinetics:
PO: Excreted in urine (unchanged)
Interactions:
• Increased EPS: phenothiazines
Lab test interferences:
Decrease: Serum uric acid

NURSING CONSIDERATIONS
Assess:
• Stools during entire treatment, 1, 3 mo after treatment; specimens must be sent to lab while still warm
• For allergic reaction: rash, itching, urticaria
• For infection in other family members, since infection from person to person is common
Administer:
• Powder for oral suspension in 57 ml H_2O, milk, or fruit juice
• May be crushed or chewed if unable to swallow whole
• Laxatives if constipated; not needed for drug to work
• Second course after 1 wk off drug if infection is severe
Perform/provide:
• Storage in tight container at room temp
Evaluate:
• Therapeutic response: expulsion of worms, 3 negative stool cultures after completion of treatment
Teach patient/family:
• Proper hygiene after BM, including hand-washing technique, tell patient not to put fingers in mouth
• That infected person should sleep alone; not to shake bed linen; change bed linen qd, wash in hot water; change and wash undergarments qd
• To clean toilet qd with disinfectant (green soap solution)
• Need for compliance with dosage schedule and duration of treatment
• That urine may turn orange or red
• To avoid hazardous activities, since drowsiness occurs
• That seizures may recur in patient who is controlled on medication

pirbuterol (℞)

(peer-byoo'ter-ole)
Maxair
Func. class.: Bronchodilator
Chem. class.: β-Adrenergic agonist

Action: Causes bronchodilation with little effect on heart rate by action on β-receptors, causing increased cAMP and relaxation of smooth muscle
Uses: Reversible bronchospasm (prevention, treatment) including asthma; may be given with theophylline or steroids

* Available in Canada only

Dosage and routes:
• *Adult and child >12 yr:* AEROSOL 1-2 inh (0.4 mg) q4-6h; do not exceed 12 INH/day
Available forms: Aerosol delivers 0.2 mg pirbuterol/actuation
Side effects/adverse reactions:
CNS: Tremors, anxiety, insomnia, headache, dizziness, stimulation, restlessness, hallucinations, drowsiness, irritability
EENT: Dry nose and mouth, irritation of nose, throat
CV: Palpitations, tachycardia, hypertension, angina, hypotension, dysrhythmias
GI: Gastritis, nausea, vomiting, anorexia
MS: Muscle cramps
RESP: ***Bronchospasm,*** dyspnea, coughing
Contraindications: Hypersensitivity to sympathomimetics, tachycardia
Precautions: Lactation, pregnancy (C), cardiac disorders, hyperthyroidism, diabetes mellitus, prostatic hypertrophy
Pharmacokinetics:
INH: Onset 3 min, peak ½-1 hr, duration 5 hr
Interactions:
• Increased action of other aerosol bronchodilators
• Increased action of pirbuterol: tricyclic antidepressants, antihistamines, sodium levothyroxine
• Decreased action of pirbuterol: β-blockers
• Increased dysrhythmias: halogenated hydrocarbon anesthetics
NURSING CONSIDERATIONS
Assess:
• Respiratory function: vital capacity, forced expiratory volume, ABGs, B/P
Administer:
• After shaking; exhale, place mouthpiece in mouth, inhale slowly, hold breath, remove, exhale slowly
• Gum, sips of water for dry mouth
Perform/provide:
• Storage in light-resistant container; do not expose to temps over 86° F (30° C)
Evaluate:
• Therapeutic response: absence of dyspnea, wheezing over 1 hr
Teach patient/family:
• Not to use OTC medications; extra stimulation may occur
• Use of inhaler; review package insert with patient
• To avoid getting aerosol in eyes
• To wash inhaler in warm water and dry qd, rinse mouth after use; if used with inhalers containing glucocorticosteroids, wait 5 min before using steroid inhaler
• About all aspects of drug; avoid smoking, smoke-filled rooms, persons with respiratory infections
• To keep fluid intake >2 L/day to liquefy thick secretions
Treatment of overdose: Administer a β-adrenergic blocker

P

piroxicam (℞)
(peer-ox'i-kam)
Apo-Piroxicam*, Feldene, novopirocam*
Func. class.: Nonsteroidal antiinflammatory
Chem. class.: Oxicam derivative

Action: Inhibits prostaglandin synthesis by decreasing an enzyme needed for biosynthesis; has analgesic, antiinflammatory, antipyretic properties
Uses: Mild to moderate pain, osteoarthritis, rheumatoid arthritis

Dosage and routes:
• *Adult:* PO 20 mg qd or 10 mg bid
Available forms: Caps 10, 20 mg
Side effects/adverse reactions:
GI: Nausea, anorexia, vomiting, diarrhea, jaundice, ***cholestatic hepatitis,*** constipation, flatulence, cramps, dry mouth, peptic ulcer, ***bleeding, ulceration, perforation***
CNS: Dizziness, *drowsiness,* fatigue, tremors, confusion, insomnia, anxiety, depression, *headache*
CV: Tachycardia, peripheral edema, palpitations, dysrhythmias
INTEG: Purpura, rash, pruritus, sweating, photosensitivity
GU: ***Nephrotoxicity: dysuria, hematuria, oliguria, azotemia***
HEMA: ***Blood dyscrasias***
EENT: Tinnitus, hearing loss, blurred vision
Contraindications: Hypersensitivity, asthma, severe renal disease, severe hepatic disease, ulcer disease, cardiac disease
Precautions: Pregnancy (C), lactation, children, bleeding disorders, GI disorders, cardiac disorders, hypersensitivity to other antiinflammatory agents
Pharmacokinetics:
PO: Peak 2 hr, half-life 50 hr; metabolized in liver; excreted in urine (metabolites), breast milk; 99% protein binding
Interactions:
• Increased action of coumarin, phenytoin, sulfonamides

NURSING CONSIDERATIONS
Assess:
• Renal, liver, blood studies: BUN, creatinine, AST (SGOT), ALT (SGPT), Hgb, before treatment, periodically thereafter
• Audiometric, ophthalmic exam before, during, after treatment
• For eye, ear problems: blurred vision, tinnitus (may indicate toxicity)
Administer:
• With food to decrease GI symptoms; best to take on empty stomach to facilitate absorption; take drug same time qd
Perform/provide:
• Storage at room temp
Evaluate:
• Therapeutic response: decreased pain, stiffness, swelling in joints; ability to move more easily
Teach patient/family:
• To report blurred vision or ringing, roaring in ears (may indicate toxicity)
• To avoid driving, other hazardous activities if dizzy or drowsy
• Patient should drink at least 6-8 glasses of water/day
• To report change in urine pattern, weight increase, edema, pain increase in joints, fever, blood in urine (indicates nephrotoxicity)
• That therapeutic effects may take up to 1 mo
• To avoid ASA, other OTC meds, alcohol; advise patient to use sunscreen

plasma protein fraction (℞)

Plasmanate, Plasma Plex, Plasmatein, PPF Protenate
Func. class.: Blood derivative
Chem. class.: Human plasma in NaCl

Action: Exerts similar oncotic pressure as human plasma, expands blood volume
Uses: Hypovolemic shock, hypoproteinemia, ARDS, preoperative cardiopulmonary bypass, acute liver failure, nephrotic syndrome

* Available in Canada only

Dosage and routes:
Hypovolemia
• *Adult:* IV INF 250-500 ml (12.5-25 g protein), not to exceed 10 ml/min
• *Child:* IV INF 22-33 ml/kg at 5-10 ml/min
Hypoproteinemia
• *Adult:* IV INF 1000-1500 ml qd, not to exceed 8 ml/min
Available forms: Inj 50 mg/ml
Side effects/adverse reactions:
GI: Nausea, vomiting, increased salivation
INTEG: Rash, urticaria, cyanosis
CNS: Fever, chills, headache, paresthesias, flushing
RESP: Altered respirations, dyspnea, ***pulmonary edema***
CV: ***Fluid overload,*** hypotension, erratic pulse
Contraindications: Hypersensitivity, CHF, severe anemia, renal insufficiency
Precautions: Decreased salt intake, decreased cardiac reserve, lack of albumin deficiency, hepatic disease, renal disease, pregnancy (C)
Pharmacokinetics:
Metabolized as a protein/energy source
Additive compatibilities: Carbohydrate and electrolyte sol, whole blood, packed red blood cells, chloramphenicil, tetracycline
Lab test interferences:
False increase: Alk phosphatase
NURSING CONSIDERATIONS
Assess:
• Blood studies: Hct, Hgb, electrolytes, serum protein; if serum protein declines, dyspnea, hypoxemia can result
• B/P (decreased), pulse (erratic), respiration during infusion
• I&O ratio; urinary output may decrease
• CVP, pulmonary wedge pressure (increases if overload occurs)
• Allergy: fever, rash, itching, chills, flushing, urticaria, nausea, vomiting, or hypotension requires discontinuation of infusion; use new lot if therapy reinstituted
• Increased CVP reading: distended neck veins indicate circulatory overload; SOB, anxiety, insomnia, expiratory rales, frothy blood-tinged cough, cyanosis indicate pulmonary overload
Administer:
• No dilution required; use infusion pump, use large-gauge needle (≥20G), discard unused portion, infuse slowly
• Within 4 hr of opening
Perform/provide:
• Adequate hydration before administration
• Storage—check type of albumin, date; may have to refrigerate
Evaluate:
• Therapeutic repsonse: increased B/P, decreased edema, increased serum albumin

---

plicamycin (℞)
(plik-a-mi′cin)
mithramycin, Mithracin
Func. class.: Antineoplastic, antibiotic; hypocalcemic
Chem. class.: Crystalline aglycone

Action: Inhibits DNA, RNA, protein synthesis; derived from *Streptomyces plicatus;* replication is decreased by binding to DNA; demonstrates calcium-lowering effect not related to its tumoricidal activity; also acts on osteoclasts and blocks action of parathyroid hormone; a vesicant
Uses: Testicular cancer, hypercalcemia, hypercalciuria, symptomatic treatment of advanced neoplasms

Dosage and routes:
Testicular tumors
• *Adult:* IV 25-30 μg/kg/day × 8-10 days, not to exceed 30 μg/kg/day
Hypercalcemia/hypercalciuria
• *Adult:* IV 25 μg/kg/day × 3-4 days, repeat at intervals of 1 wk
Available forms: Inj 2.5 mg/vial powder
Side effects/adverse reactions:
META: Decreased serum Ca, P, K
HEMA: ***Hemorrhage, thrombocytopenia,*** decreased pro-time, WBC count
GI: Nausea, vomiting, anorexia, diarrhea, stomatitis, increased liver enzymes
GU: Increased BUN, creatinine, ***proteinuria***
INTEG: Rash, cellulitis, ***extravasation,*** facial flushing
CNS: Drowsiness, weakness, lethargy, headache, flushing, fever, depression
Contraindications: Hypersensitivity, thrombocytopenia, bone marrow depression, bleeding disorders, pregnancy (X), lactation
Precautions: Renal disease, hepatic disease, electrolyte imbalances
Pharmacokinetics: Crosses blood-brain barrier, excreted in urine; little known about pharmacokinetics
Interactions:
• Increased toxicity: other antineoplastics or radiation
• Considered incompatible with any drugs in sol or syringe
NURSING CONSIDERATIONS
Assess:
• CBC, differential, platelet count qwk; withhold drug if WBC is $<4000/mm^3$ or platelet count is $<50,000/mm^3$; notify prescriber
• Renal function studies: BUN, serum uric acid, urine CrCl, electrolytes before, during therapy
• I&O ratio; report urine output <30 ml/hr
• Monitor temp q4h; fever may indicate beginning infection
• Liver function tests before, during therapy: bilirubin, AST (SGOT), ALT (SGPT), alk phosphatase prn or qmo
• Alkalosis if severe vomiting is present
• Toxicity: facial flushing, epistaxis, increased pro-time, thrombocytopenia; drug should be discontinued
• Bleeding: hematuria, guaiac stools, bruising or petechiae, mucosa or orifices q8h
• Food preferences; list likes, dislikes
• Inflammation of mucosa, breaks in skin
• Yellow skin, sclera, dark urine, clay-colored stools, itchy skin, abdominal pain, fever, diarrhea
• Buccal cavity q8h for dryness, sores, ulceration, white patches, oral pain, bleeding, dysphagia
• Local irritation, pain, burning at injection site
• Frequency of stools, characteristics, cramping
• Acidosis, signs of dehydration: rapid respirations, poor skin turgor, decreased urine output, dry skin, restlessness, weakness
Administer:
• IV direct over 30 min
• IV dilute 2.5 mg/4.9 ml of sterile H_2O; (1 ml = 500 μg) dilute single dose in 1000 ml of D_5W run over 4-6 hr
• EDTA for extravasation, apply ice compress
• Antiemetic 30-60 min before giving drug and 4-10 hr after treatment to prevent vomiting
• Slow IV infusion using 20G, 21G needle
• Transfusion for anemia
• Antispasmodic for diarrhea, phenothiazine for nausea and vomiting

* Available in Canada only

Perform/provide:

- Liquid diet: carbonated beverages; gelatin may be added if patient is not nauseated or vomiting
- Rinsing of mouth tid-qid with water; brushing of teeth with baking soda bid-tid with soft brush or cotton-tipped applicators for stomatitis; unwaxed dental floss
- Usage immediately after mixing

Evaluate:

- Therapeutic response: decreased tumor size, spread of malignancy

Teach patient/family:

- To report any complaints or side effects to nurse or prescriber
- To avoid foods with citric acid, hot or rough texture
- To report to prescriber any bleeding, white spots, ulcerations in the mouth; tell patient to examine mouth qd
- To avoid driving, activities requiring alertness; drowsiness may occur
- To report leg cramps, tingling of fingertips, weakness; may indicate hypocalcemia
- To avoid crowds, persons with infections when granulocyte count is low

podophyllum resin (℞)

(poe doe-fil'um)

Pod-Ben-25, Podocon-25, Podofilm*, Podofin

Func. class.: Keratolytic

Chem. class.: Podophyllum derivative

Action: Arrests mitosis by binding to tubulin, protein subunit of spindle microtubules; also interferes with movements of chromosomes

Uses: Venereal warts, keratoses, multiple superficial epitheliomatoses

Dosage and routes:

Warts

- *Adult:* TOP cover wart, cover with wax paper, bandage for 1-4 hr, wash, may repeat qwk if needed

Keratoses/epitheliomatoses

- *Adult:* TOP apply qd with applicator, let dry, remove tissue, may reapply if needed

Available forms: Sol 11.5%, 25%

Side effects/adverse reactions:

HEMA: ***Thrombocytopenia, leukopenia***

INTEG: Irritation of unaffected areas

CNS: Peripheral neuropathy

MISC: Paresthesia, nausea, vomiting, diarrhea, abdominal pain, confusion, dizziness, ***stupor, convulsions, coma, death***

Contraindications: Hypersensitivity, pregnancy (X), bleeding, warts, lactation, poor blood circulation, diabetes

Interactions:

- Necrosis of skin: when used with other keratolytic

NURSING CONSIDERATIONS

Assess:

- Platelets, WBC if systemic absorption occurs
- Allergic reactions: irritation, redness, itching, stinging, burning; drug should be discontinued
- Blood dyscrasias if systemic absorption is suspected: decrease platelets
- CNS toxicity: peripheral neuropathy; drug should be discontinued

Administer:

- Only to affected area; cover normal skin with petrolatum for protection; do not apply to broken or inflamed skin; applied only by prescriber; not dispensed to patient
- Only to small areas or for short periods, or absorption (systemic) may occur

P

Evaluate:
• Therapeutic response: decrease in size, number of lesions
Teach patient/family:
• That discomfort will begin after 24 hr, subside in 2-4 days
• To use soap and water to clean area and remove drug

poliovirus vaccine, live, oral, trivalent (℞)

Orimune
Func. class.: Vaccine

Action: Produces specific antibodies for poliomyelitis
Uses: Prevention of polio
Dosage and routes:
• *Adult and child >2 yr:* PO 0.5 ml, given q8wk × 2 doses, then 0.5 ml ½-1 yr after dose 2
• *Infant:* PO 0.5 ml at 2, 4, 18 mo
Available forms: Oral vaccine
Side effects/adverse reactions:
SYST: ***Paralysis***
Contraindications: Hypersensitivity, active infection, allergy to neomycin/streptomycin, immunosuppression, vomiting or diarrhea
Precautions: Pregnancy
Interactions:
• Do not use TB skin test or other live virus vaccines within 6 wk of vaccine
• Do not use within 3 mo of transfusion of whole blood, plasma, or use with immune serum globulin
NURSING CONSIDERATIONS
Assess:
• For anaphylaxis: inability to breathe, bronchospasm
Administer:
• Only PO
• Do not administer within 1 mo of other live virus vaccines
Perform/Provide:
• Storage at 7° F (−13° C)
• Written record of immunization
Evaluate:
• For history of allergies, skin conditions (eczema, psoriasis, dermatitis), reactions to vaccinations

polymyxin B (℞)

(pol-ee-mix'in)
Aerosporin, polymyxin B Sulfate
Func. class.: Antiinfective
Chem. class.: Polymyxin

Combination products: Neosporin G.U. Irrigant: polymyxin B sulfate 200,000 units (of polymyxin B)

Action: Interferes with phospholipids, penetrates cell wall; immediately changes bacterial membrane, causing leakage of essential metabolites
Uses: Serious *P. aeruginosa, E. aerogenes, K. pneumoniae, E. coli, H. influenzae* infections or when other antibiotics cannot be used; septicemia, meningitis, UTIs
Dosage and routes:
• *Adult and child:* IV INF 15,000-25,000 U/kg/day in divided doses q12h, or 25,000 U/kg/day in divided doses q4-8h
P. aeruginosa/H. influenzae
• *Adult and child >2 yr:* INTRATHECAL 50,000 U/day × 3-4 days, then 50,000 U/qod × 2 wk after CSF negative, glucose normal
• *Child <2 yr:* INTRATHECAL 20,000 U/day × 3-4 days, then 25,000 U qod × 2 wk after CSF negative
Available forms: Inj 500,000 U
Side effects/adverse reactions:
INTEG: Urticaria, pain at inj site, phlebitis, flushing
CNS: Dizziness, confusion, weakness, drowsiness, paresthesia, slurred speech, ***coma, seizures,*** headache, stiff neck

* Available in Canada only

RESP: ***Paralysis***
GU: ***Proteinuria, hematuria, azotemia, leukocyturia***
SYST: ***Anaphylaxis,*** superinfection
Contraindications: Hypersensitivity, severe renal disease
Precautions: Pregnancy (B)
Pharmacokinetics:
IM: Peak 2 hr, half-life 4½-6 hr, excreted in urine unchanged (60%)
IV: Data not available
Interactions:
• Increased skeletal muscle relaxation: anesthetics, neuromuscular blockers (tubocurarine decamethonium, succinylcholine, gallamine)
• Increased nephrotoxicity, neurotoxicity: aminoglycosides
Y-site compatibility: Esmolol
Additive compatibilities: Amikacin, colistimethate, diphenhydramine, erythromycin lactobionate, hydrocortisone sodium succinate, kanamycin, methicillin, penicillin G potassium, sodium

NURSING CONSIDERATIONS
Assess:
• I&O ratio; report hematuria, oliguria
• Any patient with compromised renal system; drug is excreted slowly in poor renal system function; toxicity may occur rapidly; monitor BUN, creatinine
• Renal studies: urinalysis, protein, blood
• C&S before drug therapy; drug may be given as soon as culture is taken; C&S may be done after completion of therapy
• Skin eruptions, itching; drug should be discontinued
• Respiratory status: rate, character, dyspnea, symptoms of neuromuscular blockade, tightness in chest; discontinue drug
• Allergies before initiation of treatment, reaction of each medication; place allergies on chart in bright red letters; notify all people giving drugs
• For flushing of face, dizziness, disorientation, weakness, paresthesia, blurred vision, slurred speech, restlessness, irritability; indicate neurotoxicity
• For headache, fever, stiff neck; after intrathecal administration, indicate meningeal irritation
Administer:
• IV after diluting 500,000 U/5 ml sterile H_2O or NS for inj (100,000 U/ml), then dilute each dose with 300-500 ml D_5W as cont inf over 60-90 min
• Intrathecal after reconstituting with 10 ml NS to yield 50,000 U/ml
Perform/provide:
• Storage in dark area at room temp
• Do not use procaine HCl in intrathecal injection
• Adrenalin, suction, tracheostomy set, endotracheal intubation equipment on unit
Evaluate:
• Therapeutic response: absence of fever, purulent drainage, C&S negative
Teach patient/family:
• To report sore throat, fever, fatigue; may indicate superinfection
Treatment of overdose: Withdraw drug, maintain airway, administer epinephrine, aminophylline, O_2, IV corticosteroids

polymyxin B (ophthalmic) (℞)
(pol-ee-mix'in)

Func. class.: Antiinfective (ophthalmic)

Action: Inhibits cell wall permeability in susceptible organisms
Uses: Superficial external ocular infections

P

Dosage and routes:
• *Adult and child:* INSTILL 1-2 gtt bid-qid × 7-10 days
Available forms: Powder for sol; 500,000 U
Side effects/adverse reactions:
EENT: Poor corneal wound healing, temporary visual haze, overgrowth of nonsusceptible organisms
Contraindications: Hypersensitivity
Precautions: Antibiotic hypersensitivity, pregnancy (B), varicella, vaccinia, mycobacterial, or fungal infections

NURSING CONSIDERATIONS
Assess:
• Allergy: itching, lacrimation, redness, swelling
Administer:
• After washing hands; cleanse crusts or discharge from eye before application
• After reconstituting powder to 20-50 ml
Perform/provide:
• Storage in refrigerator
Evaluate:
• Therapeutic response: absence of redness, inflammation, tearing
Teach patient/family:
• To use drug exactly as prescribed
• Not to use eye makeup, towels, washcloths, eye medication of others; reinfection may occur
• That drug container tip should not be touched to eye
• To report itching, increased redness, burning, stinging, swelling; drug should be discontinued

potassium bicarbonate/potassium acetate/ potassium chloride/ potassium gluconate/ potassium phosphate (℞, OTC)

Effer-K, K-Lyte, K-Lyte DS, Klorvess, Tri-K, Twin-K, Cena-K, Gen-K, K^+10, K-Tab, K-Norm, K-Dur 10, K-Dur 20, K-Lyte/Cl, K-Lease, K^+ Care, Kaon-Cl, Kaon-Cl-10, Kaochlor, Kaochlor S-F, Kato, Kay Ciel, Klor, Klor-Con, Klor-Con 8, Klor-Con 10, Klor-Con/25, Klortrix, Klorvess, Micro-K, Micro KLS, Potachlor, Potage, Potasalan, potassium chloride, Rum-K, Slow-K, Ten-K, Urocit-K, Kao-Nor, Kaylixir, K-G Elixir, My-K Elixir, Potassium Gluconate

Func. class.: Electrolyte
Chem. class.: Potassium

Action: Needed for adequate transmission of nerve impulses and cardiac contraction, renal function, intracellular ion maintenance
Uses: Prevention and treatment of hypokalemia
Dosage and routes:
Potassium bicarbonate
• *Adult:* PO dissolve 25-50 mEq in water qd-qid
Potassium acetate—hypokalemia
• *Adult and child:* PO 40-100 mEq/day in divided doses 2-4 days
Hypokalemia (prevention)
• *Adult and child:* PO 20 mEq/day in 2-4 divided doses
Potassium chloride
• *Adult:* PO 40-100 mEq in divided doses tid-qid; IV 20 mEq/hr when diluted as 40 mEq/1000 ml, not to exceed 150 mEq/day

Potassium gluconate
• *Adult:* PO 40-100 mEq in divided doses tid-qid
Potassium phosphate
• *Adult:* IV 1 mEq/hr in sol of 60 mEq/L, not to exceed 150 mEq/day; PO 40-100 mEq/day in divided doses
Available forms: Tabs for sol 6.5, 25 mEq; caps ext rel 8, 10 mEq; powder for sol 3.3, 5, 6.7, 10, 13.3 mEq/5 ml; tabs 2, 4, 5, 13.4 mEq; tabs ext rel 6.7, 8, 10 mEq; elix 6.7 mEq/5 ml; oral sol 2.375 mEq/5 ml; inj for prep of IV 1.5, 2, 2.4, 3, 3.2, 4.4, 4.7 mEq/ml
Side effects/adverse reactions:
CNS: Confusion
CV: Bradycardia, ***cardiac depression, dysrhythmias, arrest, peaking T waves, lowered R and depressed RST, prolonged P-R interval, widened QRS complex***
GI: Nausea, vomiting, cramps, pain, *diarrhea,* ulceration of small bowel
GU: Oliguria
INTEG: Cold extremities, rash
Contraindications: Renal disease (severe), severe hemolytic disease, Addison's disease, hyperkalemia, acute dehydration, extensive tissue breakdown
Precautions: Cardiac disease, K-sparing diuretic therapy, systemic acidosis, pregnancy (A)
Interactions:
• Hyperkalemia: potassium phosphate IV and products containing Ca or Mg; K-sparing, diuretic, or other K products
• Incompatible with amikacin, amphotericin B, dobutamine, fat emulsion, penicillin G sodium
Pharmacokinetics:
PO: Excreted by kidneys and in feces; onset of action ≈ 30 min
IV: Immediate onset of action

NURSING CONSIDERATIONS
Assess:
• ECG for peaking T waves, lowered R, depressed RST, prolonged P-R interval, widening QRS complex, hyperkalemia; drug should be reduced or discontinued
• K level during treatment (3.5-5 mg/dl is normal level)
• I&O ratio; watch for decreased urinary output; notify prescriber immediately
• Cardiac status: rate, rhythm, CVP, PWP, PAWP, if being monitored directly
Administer:
• Through large-bore needle to decrease vein inflammation; check for extravasation
• In large vein, avoiding scalp vein in child (IV)
• IV after diluting in large volume of IV sol and give as an inf, slowly by IV Inf to prevent toxicity; never give IV bolus or IM
• PO, with or pc meal; dissolve effervescent tabs, powder in 8 oz cold water or juice; do not give IM, SC
Perform/provide:
• Storage at room temp
Evaluate:
• Therapeutic response: absence of fatigue, muscle weakness; decreased thirst and urinary output; cardiac changes
Teach patient/family:
• To add potassium-rich foods to diet: bananas, orange juice, avocados; whole grains, broccoli, carrots, prunes, cocoa after this medication is discontinued
• To avoid OTC products: antacids, salt substitutes, analgesics, vitamin preparations, unless specifically directed by prescriber
• To report hyperkalemia symptoms (lethargy, confusion, diarrhea, nausea, vomiting, fainting, decreased output) or continued hypokalemia

P

symptoms (fatigue, weakness, polyuria, polydipsia, cardiac changes)
• To take capsules with full glass of liquid
• To dissolve powder or tablet completely in at least 120 ml water or juice
• Not to chew time-release or extended-release preparations
• Emphasize importance of regular follow-up

potassium iodide (℞)

Pima, potassium iodide solution, SSKI, Thyro-Block

Func. class.: Thyroid hormone antagonist

Chem. class.: Iodine product

Action: Inhibits secretion of thyroid hormone, fosters colloid accumulation in thyroid follicles, decreases vascularity of gland

Uses: Preparation for thyroidectomy, thyrotoxic crisis, neonatal thyrotoxicosis, radiation protectant, thyroid storm

Dosage and routes:

Thyrotoxic crisis
• *Adult and child:* PO 1 ml in water tid after meals (strong iodine sol)

Preparation for thyroidectomy
• *Adult and child:* PO 0.1-0.3 ml tid (strong iodine sol) or 5 gtt in water tid pc × 2-3 wk before surgery (potassium iodide sol)

Available forms: Sol 5%, 10%, 21 mg/gtt; tabs 130, 300 mg; inj 10%, 20%; oral syrup 325 mg/5 ml; tabs 130 mg*

Side effects/adverse reactions:

ENDO: Hypothyroidism, hyperthyroid adenoma

INTEG: Rash, urticaria, ***angineurotic edema,*** acne, mucosal hemorrhage, fever

CNS: Headache, confusion, paresthesias

GI: Nausea, diarrhea, vomiting, small-bowel lesions, upper gastric pain

MS: Myalgia, arthralgia, weakness

EENT: Metallic taste, stomatitis, salivation, periorbital edema, sore teeth and gums, cold symptoms

Contraindications: Hypersensitivity to iodine, pulmonary edema, pulmonary TB, pregnancy (D)

Precautions: Lactation, children

Pharmacokinetics:

PO: Onset 24-48 hr, peak 10-15 days after continuous therapy, uptake by thyroid gland or excreted in urine; crosses placenta

Interactions:
• Hypothyroidism: lithium, other antithyroid agents

Lab test interferences:

Interferes: Urinary 17-OHCS

NURSING CONSIDERATIONS

Assess:
• Pulse, B/P, temp
• I&O ratio; check for edema: puffy hands, feet, periorbit; indicate hypothyroidism
• Weight qd; same clothing, scale, time of day
• T_3, T_4, which is increased; serum TSH, which is decreased; free thyroxine index, which is increased if dosage is too low; discontinue drug 3-4 wk before RAIU
• Overdose: peripheral edema, heat intolerance, diaphoresis, palpitations, dysrhythmias, severe tachycardia, fever delirium, CNS irritability
• Hypersensitivity: rash; enlarged cervical lymph nodes may indicate drug should be discontinued
• Hypoprothrombinemia: bleeding, petechiae, ecchymosis
• Clinical response: after 3 wk should include increased weight, pulse; decreased T_4

* Available in Canada only

Administer:

- Strong iodine solution after diluting with water or juice to improve taste
- Through straw to prevent tooth discoloration
- With meals to decrease GI upset
- At same time each day to maintain drug level
- Lowest dose that relieves symptoms, discontinue before RAIU

Perform/provide:

- Fluids to 3-4 L/day, unless contraindicated

Evaluate:

- Therapeutic response: weight gain, decreased pulse, T_4, size of thyroid gland

Teach patient/family:

- To abstain from breast-feeding after delivery
- To keep graph of weight, pulse, mood
- To avoid OTC products that contain iodine
- That seafood, other iodine products may be restricted
- Not to discontinue this medication abruptly; thyroid crisis may occur; stress response
- That response may take several months if thyroid is large
- To discontinue drug, notify prescriber of fever, rash, metallic taste, swelling of throat, burning of mouth, throat, sore gums, teeth, severe GI distress, enlargement of thyroid, cold symptoms

---

potassium iodide (SSKI) (℞)

Pima, Iosat, Thyro-Block

Func. class.: Expectorant

Action: Increases respiratory tract fluid by decreasing surface tension, adhesiveness, which increases removal of mucus

Uses: Bronchial asthma, emphysema, bronchitis, nuclear radiation protection

Dosage and routes:

- *Adult:* PO 0.3-0.6 ml q4-6h
- *Child:* PO 0.25-1 ml saturated sol bid-qid

Radiation protection:

- *Adult:* PO 0.13 ml SSKI before or after initial exposure
- *Infant <1 yr:* Half adult dose

Available forms: Sol 1 g/ml

Side effects/adverse reactions:

EENT: Burning mouth, throat, eye irritation, swelling of eyelids

GI: Gastric irritation

ENDO: Iodism, goiter, myxedema

RESP: ***Pulmonary edema***

INTEG: ***Angioedema,*** rash

CNS: Frontal headache, ***CNS depression,*** fever, parkinsonism

Contraindications: Hypersensitivity to iodides, pulmonary TB, pregnancy (D), hyperthyroidism, hyperkalemia, acute bronchitis

Precautions: Hypothyroidism, cystic fibrosis, lactation

Pharmacokinetics: Excreted in urine

Interactions:

- Increased hypothyroid effects: lithium, antithyroid drugs
- Dysrhythmias, hyperkalemia: K-sparing diuretics, K-containing medication

NURSING CONSIDERATIONS

Assess:

- Cough: type, frequency, character including sputum

Administer:

- Decreased dose to elderly patients; excretion may be slowed
- Diluted water or fruit juice to improve taste, decrease nausea

Perform/provide:

- Storage at room temp in tight container
- Increased fluids to liquefy secretions

P

Evaluate:
• Therapeutic response: absence of cough

Teach patient/family:
• Not to use if pregnant
• Symptoms of iodism: eruptions, burning of oral cavity, eye irritation
• Symptoms of hyperthyroidism: CNS depression, fever, glomerulonephritis
• To discontinue, notify prescriber if fever, rash, metallic taste occur

povidone iodine (OTC)

(poe'vi-done)

Acu-Dyne, Betadine, Biodine Topical 1%, Efo-Dine, Iodex Regular, Mallisol, Operand Povidone-Iodine, Pharmadine, Polydine, Proviodine*

Func. class.: Disinfectant

Chem. class.: Iodophor

Action: Destroys a wide variety of microorganisms by local irritation, germicidal action

Uses: Cleansing wounds, disinfection, preoperative skin preparation

Dosage and routes:
• *Adult and child:* Use SOL as needed, topical only

Available forms: Top sol 1.5%, 3%

Side effects/adverse reactions:

GU: ***Renal damage***

META: ***Metabolic acidosis***

INTEG: Irritation

Contraindications: Hypersensitivity to iodine, pregnancy (vaginal antiseptic) (D)

Precautions: Extensive burns

Interactions:
• Do not use with alcohol or hydrogen peroxide

NURSING CONSIDERATIONS

Assess:
• For allergies to seafood; drug should not be used

Perform/provide:
• Storage in tight, light-resistant container
• Bandaging of areas if needed

Evaluate:
• Area of the body involved: irritation, rash, breaks, dryness, scales

Teach patient/family:
• To discontinue use if rash, irritation, or redness occurs

pralidoxime (℞)

(pra-li-dox'eem)

Protopam Chloride

Func. class.: Cholinesterase reactivator

Chem. class.: Quaternary ammonium oxide

Action: Reactivated enzyme metabolizes and inactivates acetylcholine at both muscarinic and nicotinic sites in the periphery

Uses: Cholinergic crisis in myasthenia gravis, organophosphate poisoning antidote (early) relief of paralysis of respiratory muscles; used as an adjunct to systemic atropine administration

Dosage and routes:

Anticholinesterase overdose
• *Adult:* IV 1-2 g, then 250 mg q5min until desired response

Organophosphate poisoning
• *Adult:* IV INF 1-2 g/100 ml 0.9% NaCl over 15-30 min; may repeat in 1 hr; PO 1-3 g q5h
• *Child:* IV INF 20-40 mg/kg/dose diluted in 100 ml 0.9% NaCl over 15-30 min

Available forms: Inj 600 mg/2 ml; tabs 500 mg; emergency kit 1 g/20-ml vial

Side effects/adverse reactions:

CNS: Dizziness, headache, drowsiness, blurred vision, diplopia, impaired accommodation

* Available in Canada only

GI: Nausea
MS: Weakness, muscle rigidity
CV: Tachycardia
RESP: Hyperventilation, ***laryngospasm***
Contraindications: Hypersensitivity, carbamate insecticide poisoning
Precautions: Myasthenia gravis, pregnancy (C), renal insufficiency, children, lactation
Pharmacokinetics:
PO: Peak 2-3 hr
IV: Peak 5-15 min
IM: Peak 10-20 min
Half-life 1½ hr, metabolized in liver, excreted in urine (unchanged)
Interactions:
- Avoid use with aminophylline, morphine, phenothiazines, reserpine, succinylcholine, theophylline in organophosphate poisoning
- Incompatible with any drug in sol or syringe

NURSING CONSIDERATIONS
Assess:
- Liver function studies: AST (SGOT), ALT (SGPT), CPK; return to normal in 10-14 days
- Insecticide ingested, amount, time
- Neurologic, muscular effects: weakness, pale skin, hypertension, tachycardia, muscle cramping, twitching
- For 48-72 hr after poisoning
- B/P, VS, I&O ratio; observe for decreased urinary output for 48-72 hr after poisoning to determine atropine toxicity
- Respiratory status: rate, rhythm, characteristics

Administer:
- Only with emergency equipment available
- As soon as possible after poisoning; within 4 hr
- IV after diluting 1 g/20 ml sterile H_2O for inj; further dilute/100 ml NS and give 1 g or less/5 min; may be given as an inf over 15-30 min
- Slowly (IV) after dilution with sterile water
- Concurrent atropine 2-4 mg IV or IM if cyanosis is present, to block accumulated acetylcholine in respiratory center; repeat q5-10min until toxicity occurs: dry mouth, flushing, tachycardia, delirium, hallucinations
- Only with edrophonium (Tensilon) on unit for myasthenia gravis patient

Evaluate:
Therapeutic response: decreased effects of organophosphate poisoning, anticholesterase overdose

pramoxine (topical) (OTC)

(pra-mox'een)
Heet Relief, Prax, ProctoFoam, Tronolane, Tronothane
Func. class.: Topical anesthetic

Action: Inhibits nerve impulses from sensory nerves, which produces anesthesia
Uses: Pruritus, sunburn, toothache, sore throat, cold sores, oral pain, rectal pain and irritation
Dosage and routes:
- *Adult and child:* TOP apply q3-4h; REC apply 1 full applicator bid-tid and after each BM

Available forms: Cream 1%; rec oint 1%; rec, aerofoam, cream supp, 1%
Side effects/adverse reactions:
INTEG: Rash, irritation, sensitization
Contraindications: Hypersensitivity, infants <1 yr, application to large areas
Precautions: Child <6 yr, sepsis, pregnancy (C), denuded skin
NURSING CONSIDERATIONS
Assess:
- Allergy: rash, irritation, reddening, swelling

• Infection: if affected area is infected, do not apply

Administer:

• After cleansing and drying affected area

• Rectal aerosol using applicator or tissue

• Directly, using gauze

Evaluate:

• Therapeutic response: absence of pain, itching of affected area

Teach patient/family:

• To report rash, irritation, redness, swelling

• How to apply

• Not for long-term use; consult prescriber after 4 wk of use

pravastatin (℞)

(pra'va-sta-tin)

Pravachol

Func. class.: Antilipidemic

Action: Inhibits HMG-CoA reductase enzyme, which reduces cholesterol synthesis

Uses: As an adjunct in primary hypercholesterolemia (types IIa, IIb)

Dosage and routes:

• *Adult:* PO 10-20 mg qd at hs (range 10-40 mg qd); elderly may require lowest dose

Available forms: Tabs 10, 20 mg

Side effects/adverse reactions:

INTEG: Rash, pruritus

GI: Nausea, constipation, diarrhea, dyspepsia, flatus, abdominal pain, heartburn, ***liver dysfunction,*** pancreatitis, ***hepatitis***

EENT: Lens opacities, common cold, rhinitis, cough

MS: Muscle cramps, myalgia, ***myositis, rhabdomyolysis***

CNS: Headache, dizziness, psychic disturbances

Contraindications: Hypersensitivity, pregnancy (X), lactation, active liver disease

Precautions: Past liver disease, alcoholism, severe acute infections, trauma, hypotension, uncontrolled seizure disorders, severe metabolic disorders, electrolyte imbalances

Pharmacokinetics: Peak 1-1½ hr; metabolized by the liver, highly protein bound; excreted in urine, feces, breast milk; crosses placenta

Interactions:

• Increased effects of coumadin

• Decreased bioavailability of pravastatin: bile acid sequestrants

Lab test interferences:

Increase: CPK, liver function tests

NURSING CONSIDERATIONS

Assess:

• Cholesterol levels periodically during treatment

• Liver function studies: baseline, q6wk during the first 3 mo, q8wk for remainder of yr, then q6mo; AST, ALT, liver function tests may increase

• Renal studies in patients with compromised renal system: BUN, I&O ratio, creatinine

Administer:

• Without regard to meals, hs

Perform/provide:

• Storage in cool environment in tight container protected from light

Evaluate:

• Therapeutic response: decrease in cholesterol to desired level after 8 wk

Teach patient/family:

• That treatment will take several years

• That blood work will be necessary during treatment

• To report blurred vision, severe GI symptoms, dizziness, headache

• That regimen will continue: low-cholesterol diet, exercise program

prazepam (℞)

(pra'ze-pam)

Centrax

Func. class.: Sedative/hypnotic; antianxiety

Chem. class.: Benzodiazepine

Controlled Substance Schedule IV

Action: Potentiates the actions of GABA, especially in limbic system and reticular formation

Uses: Anxiety, sedation

Dosage and routes:

• *Adult:* PO 20-60 mg in divided doses or 20 mg at hs

• *Elderly:* PO 10-15 mg/day in divided doses

Available forms: Caps 5, 10, 20 mg; tabs 10 mg

Side effects/adverse reactions:

CNS: Dizziness, drowsiness, confusion, headache, anxiety, tremors, stimulation, fatigue, insomnia, weakness

GI: Constipation, dry mouth, nausea, vomiting, anorexia, diarrhea

INTEG: Rash, dermatitis, itching

CV: Orthostatic hypotension, ***ECG changes, tachycardia,*** hypotension, palpitations, syncope

EENT: Blurred vision, tinnitus, mydriasis

Contraindications: Hypersensitivity to benzodiazepines, narrow-angle glaucoma, psychosis, pregnancy (D), lactation, child <18 yr

Precautions: Elderly, debilitated, hepatic disease, renal disease

Pharmacokinetics:

PO: Peak 6 hr, duration up to 48 hr; metabolized by liver; excreted in urine, breast milk; crosses placenta; half-life 30-100 hr

Interactions:

• Decreased effects of prazepam: oral contraceptives, valproic acid

• Increased effects of prazepam: CNS depressants, alcohol, disulfiram, oral contraceptives, cimetidine

Lab test interferences:

Increase: AST (SGOT), ALT (SGPT), serum bilirubin, LDH

Decrease: RAIU

False increase: 17-OHCS

NURSING CONSIDERATIONS

Assess:

• B/P (lying, standing), pulse; if systolic B/P drops 20 mm Hg, hold drug, notify prescriber

• Blood studies: CBC

• Hepatic studies: AST (SGOT), ALT (SGPT), bilirubin, CrCl

• Mental status: mood, sensorium, affect

• Physical dependency, withdrawal symptoms: headache, nausea, vomiting, muscle pain, weakness, tremors, ***convulsions*** after long-term use

• Check to see PO medication has been swallowed

Administer:

• With food or milk for GI symptoms

• Crushed if patient cannot swallow whole

• Gum, hard candy, frequent sips of water for dry mouth

Perform/provide:

• Assistance with ambulation during beginning therapy, since drowsiness, dizziness occur

• Safety measures including side rails

Evaluate:

• Therapeutic response: decreased anxiety

Teach patient/family:

• Not to be used for everyday stress or longer than 4 mo; not to use more than prescribed amount; may be habit forming

• To avoid OTC preparations (cough, cold, hay fever) unless approved by prescriber

P

• To avoid driving, other activities that require alertness
• To avoid alcohol ingestion, other psychotropic medications
• Not to discontinue medication quickly after long-term use
• To rise slowly or fainting may occur, especially elderly

Treatment of overdose: Lavage, VS, supportive care, flumazenil

praziquantel (℞)

(pray-zi-kwon'tel)
Biltricide
Func. class.: Anthelmintic
Chem. class.: Pyrazinoisoquiolone derivative

Action: Causes contraction, paralysis, leading to dislodgement of suckers; they are carried to liver, where phagocytosis takes place

Uses: Schistosomiasis, liver flukes, lung flukes, intestinal flukes, tapeworms

Dosage and routes:

• *Adult and child >4 yr:* PO 20 mg/kg q4-6h × 1 day

Available forms: Tabs 600 mg

Side effects/adverse reactions:

INTEG: Rash, pruritus, urticaria, internal hypertension

CNS: Dizziness, headache, drowsiness, malaise, increased seizure activity, fever, sweating

GI: Nausea, vomiting, anorexia, diarrhea, abdominal pain, increased liver enzymes

Contraindications: Hypersensitivity, lactation

Precautions: Child <4 yr, seizure disorders, pregnancy (B)

Pharmacokinetics:

PO: Peak 1-3 hr, half-life 48-90 min; metabolized by liver (metabolites); excreted in urine, breast milk, CSF

NURSING CONSIDERATIONS

Assess:

• Liver function test: AST (SGOT), ALT (SGPT); watch for increase
• Stools during entire treatment, 1, 3 mo after treatment; specimens must be sent to lab while still warm
• For allergic reaction: rash, urticaria, pruritus
• For diarrhea during expulsion of worms
• For CSF reaction: headache, high fever; drug should be discontinued, prescriber notified

Administer:

• Corticosteroids as ordered to reduce CNS effects (cerebral cysticercosis)
• Laxatives before treatment to cleanse bowel
• PO with liquids during meals to avoid GI symptoms; not to be chewed

Perform/provide:

• Storage in tight container in cool environment

Evaluate:

• Therapeutic response: expulsion of worms, 3 negative stool cultures after completion of treatment

Teach patient/family:

• To avoid driving, hazardous activities on day of treatment and day after treatment
• Proper hygiene after BM, including hand-washing technique; tell patient not to put fingers in mouth
• Tablets taste very bitter; keeping in mouth too long may cause gagging/vomiting
• Need for compliance with dosage schedule, duration of treatment
• To refrain from breast-feeding on day of treatment, 72 hr after

Treatment of overdose: Fast-acting laxative

* Available in Canada only

prazosin (℞)

(pra'zoe-sin)
Minipress, Prazosin
Func. class.: Antihypertensive
Chem. class.: α_1-Adrenergic blocker

Combination products: Minizide 1: prazosin HCl 1 mg (of prazosin) with polythiazide 0.5 mg; Minizide 2: prazosin HCl 2 mg (of prazosin) with polythiazide 0.5 mg; Minizide 5: prazosin HCl 5 mg (of prazosin) with polythiazide 0.5 mg

Action: Peripheral blood vessels dilate, peripheral resistance drops; reduction in blood pressure results from α-adrenergic receptors being blocked

Uses: Hypertension, refractory CHF, Raynaud's vasospasm

Investigational uses: Benign prostatic hypertrophy to decrease urine outflow obstruction

Dosage and routes:
- *Adult:* PO 1 mg bid or tid, increasing to 20 mg qd in divided doses if required; usual range 6-15 mg/day, not to exceed 1 mg initially; max 20-40 mg/day

Available forms: Caps 1, 2, 5 mg

Side effects/adverse reactions:

CV: Palpitations, orthostatic hypotension, tachycardia, edema, rebound hypertension

CNS: Dizziness, headache, drowsiness, anxiety, depression, vertigo, weakness, fatigue

GI: Nausea, vomiting, diarrhea, constipation, abdominal pain

GU: Urinary frequency, incontinence, impotence, priapism, H_2O, sodium retention

EENT: Blurred vision, epistaxis, tinnitus, dry mouth, red sclera

Contraindications: Hypersensitivity

Precautions: Pregnancy (C), children

Pharmacokinetics:
PO: Onset 2 hr, peak 1-3 hr, duration 6-12 hr; half-life 2-3 hr, metabolized in liver, excreted via bile, feces (>90%), in urine (<10%)

Interactions:
- Increased hypotensive effects: β-blockers, nitroglycerin
- Decreased effect: indomethacin

Lab test interferences:
Increase: Urinary norepinephrine, VMA

NURSING CONSIDERATIONS

Assess:
- B/P during initial treatment, periodically thereafter
- Pulse, jugular venous distention q4h
- BUN, uric acid if on long-term therapy
- Weight qd, I&O
- Edema in feet, legs qd
- Skin turgor, dryness of mucous membranes for hydration status
- Rales, dyspnea, orthopnea q30min

Perform/provide:
- Storage in tight container in cool environment

Evaluate:
- Therapeutic response: decreased B/P

Teach patient/family:
- Fainting occasionally occurs after 1st dose; do not drive or operate machinery for 4 hr after 1st dose, or take 1st dose at bedtime

Treatment of overdose: Administer volume expanders or vasopressors, discontinue drug, place in supine position

P

prednicarbate (℞)

(pred-ni-car′bate)

Dermatop

Func. class.: Topical corticosteroid

Action: Antipruritic, antiinflamatory

Uses: Psoriasis, eczema, contact dermatitis, pruritus

Dosage and routes:

- *Adult and child:* Apply to affected area bid-qid

Available forms: Cream 0.1%

Side effects/adverse reactions:

INTEG: Burning, dryness, itching, irritation, acne, folliculitis, hypertrichosis, perioral dermatitis, hypopigmentation, atrophy, striae, miliaria, allergic contact dermatitis, secondary infection

Contraindications: Hypersensitivity to corticosteroids; fungal, bacterial, viral infections

Precautions: Hepatic disease, pregnancy, lactation

NURSING CONSIDERATIONS

Assess:

- Temp; if fever develops, drug should be discontinued

Administer:

- Only to affected areas; do not get in eyes
- Medication; cover with occlusive dressing if prescribed, seal to normal skin, change q12h; use occlusive dressing with extreme caution (group II potency); systemic absorption may occur
- Only to dermatoses; do not use on weeping, denuded, or infected areas

Perform/provide:

- Cleansing before application; apply to slightly moist skin; use gloves, cotton-tipped applicator
- Treatment for a few days after area has cleared
- Storage at room temp

Evaluate:

- Therapeutic response: absence of severe itching, patches on skin, flaking
- For systemic absorption: fever, inflammation, irritation

Teach patient/family:

- To avoid sunlight on affected area; burns may occur

prednisolone/prednisolone acetate/prednosolone phosphate/prednisolone tebutate (℞)

(pred-niss′oh-lone)

Articulose-50, Delta-Cortef, Prednisolone, Prelone, Key-Pred 25, Key-Pred 50, Predaject-50, Predalone 50, Predcor-25, Predcor-50, Prednisolone Acetate, Hydeltrasol, Key-Pred-SP, Pediapred, Hydeltra-T.B.A., Predalone-T.B.A., Prednisol TBA

Func. class.: Corticosteroid

Chem. class.: Glucocorticoid, immediate acting

Action: Decreases inflammation by suppression of migration of polymorphonuclear leukocytes, fibroblasts; reversal to increase capillary permeability and lysosomal stabilization

Uses: Severe inflammation, immunosuppression, neoplasms

Dosage and routes:

- *Adult:* PO 2.5-15 mg bid-qid; IM 2-30 mg (acetate, phosphate) q12h; IV 2-30 mg (phosphate) q12h; 2-30 mg in joint or soft tissue (phosphate), 4-40 mg in joint of lesion (tebutate), 0.25-1 ml qwk in joints (acetate-phosphate)

* Available in Canada only

Available forms: Tabs 5 mg; inj 25, 50, 100 mg/ml acetate; inj 20 mg/ml terbutate; inj 20 mg/ml phosphate; inj 80 mg/ml acetate/phosphate

Side effects/adverse reactions:

INTEG: Acne, poor wound healing, ecchymosis, petechiae

CNS: ***Depression,*** flushing, sweating, headache, mood changes

CV: Hypertension, ***circulatory collapse, thrombophlebitis, embolism,*** tachycardia

HEMA: ***Thrombocytopenia***

MS: Fractures, osteoporosis, weakness

GI: Diarrhea, nausea, abdominal distention, ***GI hemorrhage,*** increased appetite, ***pancreatitis***

EENT: Fungal infections, increased intraocular pressure, blurred vision

Contraindications: Psychosis, hypersensitivity, idiopathic thrombocytopenia, acute glomerulonephritis, amebiasis, fungal infections, nonasthmatic bronchial disease, child <2 yr

Precautions: Pregnancy (C), diabetes mellitus, glaucoma, osteoporosis, seizure disorders, ulcerative colitis, CHF, myasthenia gravis

Pharmacokinetics:

PO: Peak 1-2 hr, duration 2 days

IM: Peak 3-45 hr

Interactions:

- Decreased action of prednisolone: cholestyramine, colestipol, barbiturates, rifampin, ephedrine, phenytoin, theophylline
- Decreased effects of anticoagulants, anticonvulsants, antidiabetics, ambenonium, neostigmine, isoniazid, toxoids, vaccines, anticholinesterases, salicylates, somatrem
- Increased side effects: alcohol, salicylates, indomethacin, amphotericin B, digitalis, cyclosporine, diuretics
- Increased action of prednisolone: salicylates, estrogens, indomethacin, oral contraceptives, ketoconazole, macrolide antibiotics

Y-site compatibilities: Potassium chloride, vitamin B with C

Additive compatibilities: Ascorbic acid, cephalothin, cytarabine, erythromycin lactobionate, fluorouracil, heparin, methicillin, penicillin G potassium, penicillin G sodium, vitamin B with C

Lab test interferences:

Increase: Cholesterol, Na, blood glucose, uric acid, Ca, urine glucose

Decrease: Ca, K, T_4, T_3, thyroid ^{131}I uptake test, urine 17-OHCS, 17-KS, PBI

False negative: Skin allergy tests

NURSING CONSIDERATIONS

Assess:

- K, blood sugar, urine glucose while on long-term therapy; hypokalemia and hyperglycemia
- Weight qd; notify prescriber if weekly gain of >5 lb
- B/P q4h, pulse; notify prescriber if chest pain occurs
- I&O ratio; be alert for decreasing urinary output, increasing edema
- Plasma cortisol levels (long-term therapy) (normal level: 138-635 nmol/L SI units when drawn at 8 AM)
- Infection: increased temp, WBC, even after withdrawal of medication; drug masks infection
- K depletion: paresthesias, fatigue, nausea, vomiting, depression, polyuria, dysrhythmias, weakness
- Edema, hypertension, cardiac symptoms
- Mental status: affect, mood, behavioral changes, aggression

Administer:

- IV undiluted or added to NaCl or D_5 and given by IV Inf; give 10 mg or less/1 min; decrease rate if burning occurs

P

• After shaking suspension (parenteral)
• Titrated dose; use lowest effective dose
• IM inj deeply in large muscle mass; rotate sites; avoid deltoid; use 21G needle
• In one dose in AM to prevent adrenal suppression; avoid SC administration; may damage tissue
• With food or milk to decrease GI symptoms

Perform/provide:
• Assistance with ambulation to patient with bone tissue disease to prevent fractures

Evaluate:
• Therapeutic response: ease of respirations, decreased inflammation

Teach patient/family:
• That ID as steroid user should be carried
• To notify prescriber if therapeutic response decreases; dosage adjustment may be needed
• Not to discontinue abruptly; adrenal crisis can result
• To avoid OTC products: salicylates, alcohol in cough products, cold preparations unless directed by prescriber
• About cushingoid symptoms
• Symptoms of adrenal insufficiency: nausea, anorexia, fatigue, dizziness, dyspnea, weakness, joint pain

prednisolone acetate (suspension)/prednisolone sodium phosphate (solution) (℞)

(pred-niss'oh-lone)

Econopred, Econopred Plus, Pred-Forte, Pred-Mild, AK-Pred, Inflamase Forte, Inflamase Mild Ophthalmic, Metreton Ophthalmic

Func. class.: Ophthalmic antiinflammatory

Chem. class.: Analog of hydrocortisone

Action: Decreases inflammation, resulting in decreases in pain, photophobia, hyperemia, cellular infiltration

Uses: Inflammation of eye, lids, conjunctiva, cornea, uveitis, iridocyclitis, allergic condition, burns, foreign bodies

Dosage and routes:
• *Adult and child:* INSTILL 1-2 gtt into conjunctival sac q1h × 2 days, if needed, then bid-qid

Available forms: Susp 0.12%, 0.125%, 1%; sol 0.125%, 0.5%, 1%

Side effects/adverse reactions:

EENT: ***Increased intraocular pressure,*** poor corneal wound healing, increased possibility of corneal infections, glaucoma exacerbation, ***optic nerve damage,*** decreased acuity, visual field

Contraindications: Hypersensitivity, acute superficial herpes simplex, fungal/viral diseases of eye or conjunctiva, active diabetes mellitus, ocular TB, infections of the eye

Precautions: Corneal abrasions, glaucoma, pregnancy (C), lactation, children

NURSING CONSIDERATIONS

Administer:
• After shaking, suspension

Perform/provide:
- Storage in tight, light-resistant container

Evaluate:
- Therapeutic response: absence of swelling, redness, exudate

Teach patient/family:
- Instillation method: pressure on lacrimal duct for 1 min
- Not to share eye medications
- Not to use if purulent drainage is present
- Not to discontinue abruptly; taper over 1-2 wk

prednisone (℞)

(pred'ni-sone)

Apo-Prednisone*, Deltasone, Liquid Pred, Meticorten, Orasone, Panasol-S, Prednicen-M, Prednisone, Sterapred, Winpred

Func. class.: Corticosteroid

Chem. class.: Intermediate-acting glucocorticoid

Action: Decreases inflammation by suppression of migration of polymorphonuclear leukocytes, fibroblasts, reversal to increase capillary permeability, and lysosomal stabilization

Uses: Severe inflammation, immunosuppression, neoplasms, multiple sclerosis, collagen disorders, dermatologic disorders

Dosage and routes:
- *Adult:* PO 1.5-2.5 mg bid-qid, then qd or qod; maintenance up to 250 mg/day

Nephrosis
- *Child 18 mo-4 yr:* 7.5-10 mg qid initially
- *Child 4-10 yr:* 15 mg qid initially
- *Child >10 yr:* 20 mg qid initially

Multiple sclerosis
- *Adult:* PO 200 mg/day × 1 wk, then 80 mg qod × 1 mo

Available forms: Tabs 1, 2.5, 5, 10, 20, 25, 50 mg; oral sol 5 mg/5 ml; syr 5 mg/5 ml

Side effects/adverse reactions:

CNS: Depression, flushing, sweating, headache, mood changes

CV: Hypertension, ***circulatory collapse, thrombophlebitis, embolism,*** tachycardia

EENT: Fungal infections, increased intraocular pressure, blurred vision

GI: Diarrhea, nausea, abdominal distention, ***GI hemorrhage,*** increased appetite, pancreatitis

HEMA: ***Thrombocytopenia***

INTEG: Acne, poor wound healing, ecchymosis, petechiae

MS: Fractures, osteoporosis, weakness

Contraindications: Psychosis, hypersensitivity, idiopathic thrombocytopenia, acute glomerulonephritis, amebiasis, fungal infections, nonasthmatic bronchial disease, child <2 yr, AIDS, TB

Precautions: Pregnancy (C), diabetes mellitus, glaucoma, osteoporosis, seizure disorders, ulcerative colitis, CHF, myasthenia gravis, renal disease, esophagitis, peptic ulcer

Pharmacokinetics:
Well absorbed PO

PO: Peak 1-2 hr, duration 1-1½ days, half-life 3½-4 hr

Crosses placenta, enters breast milk, metabolized by the liver after conversion

Interactions:
- Decreased action of prednisone: cholestyramine, colestipol, barbiturates, rifampin, ephedrine, phenytoin, theophylline
- Decreased effects of anticoagulants, anticonvulsants, antidiabetics, ambenonium, neostigmine, isoniazid, toxoids, vaccines, anticho-

P

linesterases, salicylates, somatrem
• Increased side effects: alcohol, salicylates, indomethacin, amphotericin B, digitalis, cyclosporine, diuretics
• Increased action of prednisone: salicylates, estrogens, indomethacin, oral contraceptives, ketoconazole, macrolide antibiotics

Lab test interferences:
Increase: Cholesterol, Na, blood glucose, uric acid, Ca, urine glucose
Decrease: Ca, K, T_4, T_3, thyroid ^{131}I uptake test, urine 17-OHCS, 17-KS, PBI
False negative: Skin allergy tests

NURSING CONSIDERATIONS

Assess:
• Adrenal insufficiency: nausea, vomiting, anorexia, confusion, hypotension
• K, blood sugar, urine glucose while on long-term therapy; hypokalemia and hyperglycemia
• Weight qd; notify prescriber of weekly gain >5 lb
• B/P q4h, pulse; notify prescriber of chest pain; monitor for rales, crackles, dyspnea if edema is present
• I&O ratio; be alert for decreasing urinary output, increasing edema
• Plasma cortisol (long-term therapy) (normal: 138-635 nmol/L SI units drawn at 8 AM)
• Infection: increased temp, WBC, even after withdrawal of medication; drug masks infection
• K depletion: paresthesias, fatigue, nausea, vomiting, depression, polyuria, dysrhythmias, weakness
• Edema, hypertension, cardiac symptoms
• Mental status: affect, mood, behavioral changes, aggression

Administer:
• Titrated dose; use lowest effective dose
• With food or milk to decrease GI symptoms

Perform/provide:
• Assistance with ambulation to patient with bone tissue disease to prevent fractures

Evaluate:
• Therapeutic response: ease of respirations, decreased inflammation

Teach patient/family:
• That ID as steroid user should be carried; information on drug being taken and condition
• To notify prescriber if therapeutic response decreases; dosage adjustment may be needed
• To avoid vaccinations
• Not to discontinue abruptly, or adrenal crisis can result
• To avoid OTC products: salicylates, alcohol in cough products, cold preparations unless directed by prescriber
• About cushingoid symptoms: moon face, weight gain
• That drug causes immunosuppression; to report any symptoms of infection (fever, sore throat, cough)
• Symptoms of adrenal insufficiency; nausea, anorexia, fatigue, dizziness, dyspnea, weakness, joint pain

---

primaquine (℞)

(prim'a-kween)

Func. class.: Antimalarial
Chem. class.: Synthetic 8-aminoquinolone

Action: Unknown; thought to destroy exoerythrocytic forms by gametocidal action
Uses: Malaria caused by *P. vivax*
Dosage and routes:
• *Adult:* PO 15 mg (base) qd × 2 wk; 26.3-mg tab is 15-mg base
• *Child:* PO 0.3 mg/kg × 2 wk
Available forms: Tabs 26.3 mg

---

* Available in Canada only

Side effects/adverse reactions:
INTEG: Pruritus, skin eruptions
CNS: Headache
EENT: Blurred vision, difficulty focusing
GI: Nausea, vomiting, anorexia, cramps
CV: Hypertension
HEMA: ***Agranulocytosis, granulocytopenia, leukopenia, hemolytic anemia, leukocytosis,*** mild anemia, ***methemoglobinemia***

Contraindications: Hypersensitivity, anemia, lupus erythematosus, methemoglobinemia, porphyria, rheumatoid arthritis, methemoglobin reductase deficiency, G6PD deficiency

Precautions: Pregnancy (C)

Pharmacokinetics:
PO: Metabolized by liver (metabolites), half-life 3.7-9.6 hr

Interactions:
- Toxicity: quinacrine

NURSING CONSIDERATIONS

Assess:
- Ophthalmic test if long-term treatment or drug dosage >150 mg/day
- Liver studies qwk: AST, ALT, bilirubin, if on long-term therapy
- Blood studies: CBC; blood dyscrasias occur
- Allergic reactions: pruritus, rash, urticaria
- Blood dyscrasias: malaise, fever, bruising, bleeding (rare)
- For renal status: dark urine, hematuria, decreased output
- For hemolytic reaction: chills, fever, chest pain, cyanosis; drug should be discontinued immediately

Administer:
- Before or after meals at same time each day to maintain drug level

Evaluate:
- Therapeutic response: decreased symptoms of malaria

Teach patient/family:
- To report visual problems, fever, fatigue, dark urine, bruising, bleeding; may indicate blood dyscrasias

primidone (℞)

(pri'mi-done)
Apo-Primidone*, myidone, Mysoline, primidone, Sertan*
Func. class.: Anticonvulsant
Chem. class.: Barbiturate derivative

Action: Raises seizure threshold by conversion of drug to phenobarbital, decreases neuron firing

Uses: Generalized tonic-clonic (grand mal), complex-partial psychomotor seizures

Dosage and routes:
- *Adult and child >8 yr:* PO 250 mg/day; may increase by 250 mg/wk, not to exceed 2 g/day in divided doses qid
- *Child <8 yr:* PO 125 mg/day; may increase by 125 mg/wk, not to exceed 1 g/day in divided doses qid

Available forms: Tabs 50, 250 mg; susp 250 mg/5 ml; chew tab 125 mg

Side effects/adverse reactions:
HEMA: ***Thrombocytopenia, leukopenia, neutropenia, eosinophilia, megaloblastic anemia,*** decreased serum folate level, lymphadenopathy
CNS: Stimulation, drowsiness, dizziness, confusion, sedation, headache, flushing, hallucinations, coma, psychosis, ataxia, vertigo
GI: Nausea, vomiting, anorexia, hepatitis
INTEG: Rash, edema, alopecia, lupuslike syndrome
EENT: Diplopia, nystagmus, edema of eyelids
GU: Impotence, polyuria

Contraindications: Hypersensitivity, porphyria, pregnancy (D)

Precautions: COPD, hepatic disease, renal disease, hyperactive children

Pharmacokinetics:

PO: Peak 4 hr; excreted by kidneys, in breast milk; half-life 3-24 hr

Interactions:

• Increased blood levels: alcohol, heparin, CNS depressants, isoniazid, phenytoin, phenobarbital

NURSING CONSIDERATIONS

Assess:

• For seizures, folic acid deficiency
• Drug level: therapeutic level 5-12 μg/ml; CBC should be done q6mo
• Mental status: mood, sensorium, affect, memory (long, short)
• Respiratory depression, wheezing
• Blood dyscrasias: fever, sore throat, bruising, rash, jaundice

Administer:

• Shake liquid susp well
• With food for GI upset
• Crush tablets, mix with food or fluid for swallowing difficulties

Evaluate:

• Therapeutic response: decreased seizures

Teach patient/family:

• Not to withdraw drug quickly; withdrawal symptoms may occur
• To avoid hazardous activities until stabilized on drug
• To carry ID with condition and medication
• Signs of blood dyscrasias, when to notify prescriber
• To avoid alcohol, CNS depressants

probenecid (℞)

(proe-ben'e-sid)

Benemid, Benuryl*, Probalan, probenecid

Func. class.: Uricosuric

Chem. class.: Sulfonamide derivative

Action: Inhibits tubular reabsorption of urates, with increased excretion of uric acids

Uses: Gonorrhea, hyperuricemia in gout, gouty arthritis, adjunct to cephalosporin or penicillin treatment

Dosage and routes:

Gonorrhea

• *Adult:* PO 1 g with 3.5 g ampicillin or 1 g ½ hr before 4.8 million U of aqueous penicillin G procaine injected into 2 sites IM

Gout/gouty arthritis

• *Adult:* PO 250 mg bid for 1 wk, then 500 mg bid, not to exceed 2 g/day; maintenance: 500 mg/day × 6 mo

Adjunct in penicillin/cephalosporin treatment

• *Adult and child >50 kg:* PO 500 mg qid
• *Child <50 kg:* PO 25 mg/kg, then 40 mg/kg in divided doses qid

Available forms: Tabs 0.5 g

Side effects/adverse reactions:

CNS: Drowsiness, headache

CV: Bradycardia

GU: Glycosuria, thirst, frequency, ***nephrotic syndrome***

GI: Gastric irritation, nausea, vomiting, anorexia, ***hepatic necrosis***

INTEG: Rash, dermatitis, pruritus, fever

META: Acidosis, hypokalemia, hyperchloremia, hyperglycemia

RESP: ***Apnea,*** irregular respirations

Contraindications: Hypersensitivity, severe hepatic disease, blood dyscrasias, severe renal disease, CrC

* Available in Canada only

<50 mg/min, history of uric acid calculus

Precautions: Pregnancy (B), severe respiratory disease, lactation, cardiac edema, child <2 yr

Pharmacokinetics:

PO: Peak 2-4 hr, duration 8 hr, half-life 8-10 hr; metabolized by liver; excreted in urine; crosses placenta

Interactions:

- Increased activity of oral anticoagulants
- Increased toxicity: sulfa drugs, dapsone, clofibrate, PAS, indomethacin, rifampin, naproxen, methotrexate, pantothenic acid, oral hypoglycemics
- Decreased action of probenecid: alcohol, salicylates, nitrofurantoin, diazoxides, diuretics
- Decreased action of: oral hypoglycemics

Lab test interferences:

False positive: Urine glucose with copper sulfate test (Clinitest)
False positive: Theophylline levels
Increase: BSP/urinary PSP
Decrease: Urinary 17-KS

NURSING CONSIDERATIONS

Assess:

- Uric acid levels (3-7 mg/dl); mobility, joint pain, swelling
- Respiratory rate, rhythm, depth; notify prescriber of abnormalities
- Electrolytes, CO_2 before, during treatment
- Urine pH, output, glucose during beginning treatment
- For CNS symptoms: confusion, twitching, hyperreflexia, stimulation, headache; may indicate overdose

Administer:

- After meals or with milk if GI symptoms occur
- Increase fluid intake to 2-3 L/day to prevent urinary calculi

Perform/provide:

- Low purine diet restricting organ meats, anchovies, sardines, meat gravy, dried beans, meat extracts if prescribed

Evaluate:

- Therapeutic response: absence of pain, stiffness in joints

Teach patient/family

- To avoid high-purine foods, alcohol; urinary calculi may form
- To avoid OTC preparations (aspirin) unless directed by prescriber

---

probucol (℞)

(proe′byoo-kole)
Lorelco
Func. class.: Antilipemic

Action: Increases bile acid excretion, catabolism of LDL-cholesterol; increases HDL reverse cholesterol transport and blocks oxidation of LDL-cholesterol

Uses: Severe hypercholesterolemia when other treatment unsuccessful

Dosage and routes:

Adult: PO 500 mg bid with breakfast, supper

Available forms: Tabs 250, 500 mg

Side effects/adverse reactions:

GI: Nausea, vomiting, diarrhea, flatulence, anorexia
CV: Palpitations, dysrhythmias, ***MI,*** prolonged QT interval
EENT: Visual disturbances, ptosis, tinnitus
CNS: Insomnia, dizziness, palpitations, paresthesias, syncope

Contraindications: Hypersensitivity

Precautions: Dysrhythmias, pregnancy (B), lactation, children

Pharmacokinetics:

PO: Excreted in bile, feces

Interactions:

- Do not use with clofibrate

P

Lab test interferences:
Increase: Liver function studies, CPK, blood glucose, uric acid, BUN

NURSING CONSIDERATIONS

Assess:
- Hepatic function (long-term therapy)
- Bowel pattern qd; increase bulk, water in diet if constipation develops

Administer:
- With meals for GI symptoms

Evaluate:
- Therapeutic response: decreased cholesterol levels, (hyperlipidemia), diarrhea, pruritus (excess bile area)

Teach patient/family:
- That compliance is necessary, since toxicity may result if doses are missed
- That risk factors should be decreased: high fat diet, smoking, alcohol consumption, absence of exercise
- Birth control should be practiced while on this drug

procainamide (℞)

(proe-kane-ah'mide)
Procan SR, Promine, procainamide, Pronestyl, Pronestyl-SR, Rhythmin

Func. class.: Antidysrhythmic (Class IA)

Chem. class.: Procaine HCl amide analog

Action: Depresses excitability of cardiac muscle to electrical stimulation and slows conduction in atrium, bundle of His, and ventricle

Uses: PVCs, atrial fibrillation, PAT, ventricular tachycardia, atrial dysrhythmias, ventricular tachycardia

Dosage and routes:

Atrial fibrillation/PAT
- *Adult:* PO 1-1.25 g, may give another 750 mg if needed; if no response, 500 mg-1g q2h until desired response; maintenance 50 mg/kg in divided doses q6h

Ventricular tachycardia
- *Adult:* PO 1g; maintenance 50 mg/kg/day given in 3 hr intervals; SUS REL TABS 500 mg-1.25 g q6h

Other dysrhythmias
- *Adult:* IV BOL 100 mg q5min, given 25-50 mg/min, not to exceed 500 mg; or 17 mg/kg total then IV INF 2-6 mg/min

Available forms: Caps 250, 375, 500 mg; tabs 250, 375, 500 mg; tabs sus rel 250, 500, 750, 1000 mg; inj 100, 500 mg/ml

Side effects/adverse reactions:
CNS: Headache, dizziness, confusion, psychosis, restlessness, irritability, weakness
GI: Nausea, vomiting, anorexia, diarrhea, hepatomegaly
CV: Hypotension, ***heart block, cardiovascular collapse, arrest***
HEMA: SLE syndrome, ***agranulocytosis, thrombocytopenia, neutropenia, hemolytic anemia***
INTEG: Rash, urticaria, edema, swelling (rare), pruritus

Contraindications: Hypersensitivity, myasthenia gravis, severe heart block

Precautions: Pregnancy (C), lactation, children, renal disease, liver disease, CHF, respiratory depression

Pharmacokinetics:
PO: Peak 1-2 hr, duration 3 hr (8 hr extended)
IM: Peak 10-60 min, duration 3 hr; half-life 3 hr
Metabolized in liver to active metabolites, excreted unchanged by kidneys (60%)

Interactions:
- Increased effects of neuromuscular blockers, anticholinergics, antihypertensives

* Available in Canada only

• Increased procainamide effects: cimetidine
• Decreased effects of procainamide: barbiturates
• Increased toxicity: other antidysrhythmics

Y-site compatibilities: Amiodarone, famotidine, heparin, hydrocortisone sodium succinate, potassium chloride, ranitidine, vitamin B with C
Additive compatibilities: Amiodarone, dobutamine, lidocaine, netilmicin, verapamil
Solution compatibilities: D_5W, D_5/0.9% NaCl, 0.45% NaCl, 0.9% NaCl, water for inj

NURSING CONSIDERATIONS

Assess:
• ECG continuously to determine increased PR or QRS segments; discontinue immediately; watch for increased ventricular ectopic beats, maximum need to rebolus
• Blood levels, 3-10 μg/ml
• B/P continuously for fluctuations
• I&O ratio; electrolytes (K, Na, Cl)
• Malignant hyperthermia: tachypnea, tachycardia, changes in B/P, fever
• Cardiac rate, rhythm, character
• Respiratory status: rate, rhythm, character, lung fields; bilateral rales may occur in CHF patient; watch for respiratory depression
• CNS effects: dizziness, confusion, psychosis, paresthesias, convulsions; drug should be discontinued
• Increased respiration, increased pulse; drug should be discontinued

Administer:
• IV after diluting 100 mg/ml of D_5W or sterile H_2O for inj; give 20 mg or less/1 min; may dilute 1 g/250-500 ml D_5W, run at 2-6 mg/min
• IM injection in deltoid; aspirate to avoid intravascular administration; check IV site q8h for infiltration or extravasation

Evaluate:
• Therapeutic response: decreased dysrhythmias

procaine (℞)

(proe'kane)
Novocain, Unicaine
Func. class.: Local anesthetic
Chem. class.: Ester

Action: Competes with calcium for sites in nerve membrane that control sodium transport across cell membrane; decreases rise of depolarization phase of action potential
Uses: Spinal anesthesia, epidural, peripheral nerve block, perineum, lower extremities, infiltration
Dosage and routes:
Vary by route of anesthesia
Available forms: Inj 1%, 2%, 10%
Side effects/adverse reactions:
CNS: Anxiety, restlessness, ***convulsions, loss of consciousness,*** drowsiness, disorientation, tremors, shivering
CV: ***Myocardial depression, cardiac arrest, dysrhythmias,*** bradycardia, hypotension, hypertension, fetal bradycardia
GI: Nausea, vomiting
EENT: Blurred vision, tinnitus, pupil constriction
INTEG: Rash, urticaria, allergic reactions, edema, burning, skin discoloration at injection site, tissue necrosis
RESP: ***Status asthmaticus, respiratory arrest, anaphylaxis***
Contraindications: Hypersensitivity, child <12 yr, elderly, severe liver disease
Precautions: Elderly, severe drug allergies, pregnancy (C)
Pharmacokinetics:
Onset 2-5 min, duration 1 hr; me-

P

tabolized by liver, excreted in urine (metabolites)

Interactions:

- Dysrhythmias: epinephrine, halothane, enflurane
- Hypertension: MAOIs, tricyclic antidepressants, phenothiazines
- Decreased action of procaine: chloroprocaine

NURSING CONSIDERATIONS

Assess:

- B/P, pulse, respiration during treatment
- Fetal heart tones if drug is used during labor
- Allergic reactions: rash, urticaria, itching
- Cardiac status: ECG for dysrhythmias, pulse, B/P during anesthesia

Administer:

- Only drugs that are not cloudy, do not contain precipitate
- Only with crash cart, resuscitative equipment nearby
- Only drugs without preservatives for epidural or caudal anesthesia

Perform/provide:

- Use of new sol; discard unused portions

Evaluate:

- Therapeutic response: anesthesia necessary for procedure

Treatment of overdose: Airway, O_2, vasopressor, IV fluids, anticonvulsants for seizures

procarbazine (℞)

(proe-kar'ba-zeen)

Matulane, Natulan*

Func. class.: Antineoplastic, alkylating agent

Chem. class.: Hydrazine derivative

Action: Inhibits DNA, RNA, protein synthesis; has multiple sites of action; a nonvesicant

Uses: Lymphoma, Hodgkin's disease, cancers resistant to other therapy

Investigational uses: Brain, lung malignancies, other lymphomas, multiple myeloma, malignant melanoma, polycythemia vera

Dosage and routes:

- *Adult:* PO 2-4 mg/kg/day for first wk; maintain dosage of 4-6 mg/kg/day until platelets and WBC fall; after recovery, 1-2 mg/kg/day
- *Child:* PO 50 mg/day for 7 days, then 100 mg/m^2 until desired response, leukopenia, or thrombocytopenia occurs; 50 mg/day is maintenance after bone marrow recovery

Available forms: Caps 50 mg

Side effects/adverse reactions:

HEMA: ***Thrombocytopenia, anemia, leukopenia, myelosuppression, bleeding tendencies,*** purpura, petechiae, epistaxis

GI: Nausea, vomiting, anorexia, diarrhea, constipation, dry mouth, stomatitis

EENT: Retinal hemorrhage, nystagmus, photophobia, diplopia

INTEG: Rash, pruritus, dermatitis, alopecia, herpes, hyperpigmentation

CNS: Headache, dizziness, insomnia, hallucinations, confusion, coma, pain, chills, fever, sweating, paresthesias

RESP: Cough, pneumonitis

MS: Arthralgias, myalgias

GU: Azoospermia, cessation of menses

Contraindications: Hypersensitivity, thrombocytopenia, bone marrow depression

Precautions: Renal disease, hepatic disease, pregnancy (D), radiation therapy

Pharmacokinetics: Half-life 1 hr; concentrates in liver, kidney, skin;

* Available in Canada only

metabolized in liver, excreted in urine

Interactions:

• Increased CNS depression: barbiturates, antihistamines, narcotics, hypotensive agents, phenothiazines
• Disulfiram-like reaction: ethyl alcohol, MAOIs, tricyclic antidepressants, tyramine foods, sympathomimetic drugs
• Hypertension: guanethidine, levodopa, methyldopa, reserpine
• Increased hypoglycemia: insulin, oral hypoglycemics

NURSING CONSIDERATIONS

Assess:

• CBC, differential, platelet count qwk; withhold drug if WBC is <4000/mm^3 or platelet count is <100,000/mm^3; notify prescriber
• Renal function studies: BUN, serum uric acid, urine CrCl, electrolytes before, during therapy
• I&O ratio, report fall in urine output to <30 ml/hr
• Monitor temp q4h; fever may indicate beginning infection
• Liver function tests before, during therapy: bilirubin, AST, ALT, alk phosphatase prn or qmo
• CNS changes: confusion, paresthesias, neuropathies, drug should be discontinued
• Toxicity: facial flushing, epistaxis, increased pro-time, thrombocytopenia; drug should be discontinued
• Bleeding: hematuria, guaiac stools, bruising or petechiae, mucosa or orifices q8h
• Food preferences; list likes, dislikes
• Effects of alopecia on body image; discuss feelings about body changes
• Inflammation of mucosa, breaks in skin
• Yellow skin, sclera, dark urine, clay-colored stools, itchy skin, abdominal pain, fever, diarrhea
• Buccal cavity q8h for dryness, sores or ulceration, white patches, oral pain, bleeding, dysphagia
• Alkalosis if vomiting is severe
• GI symptoms: frequency of stools, cramping
• Acidosis, signs of dehydration: rapid respirations, poor skin turgor, decreased urine output, dry skin, restlessness, weakness

Administer:

• In divided doses and at hs to minimize nausea and vomiting
• Nonphenothiazine antiemetic 30-60 min before giving drug and 4-10 hr after treatment to prevent vomiting
• Transfusion for anemia
• Antispasmodic for GI symptoms

Perform/provide:

• Liquid diet: carbonated beverages; gelatin may be added if patient is not nauseated or vomiting
• Storage in tight, light-resistant container in cool environment

Evaluate:

• Therapeutic response: decreased tumor size, spread of malignancy

Teach patient/family:

• To report any complaints, side effects to nurse or prescriber; cough, shortness of breath, fever, chills, sore throat, bleeding, bruising, vomiting blood, black tarry stools
• That hair may be lost during treatment and wig or hairpiece may make patient feel better; tell patient that new hair may be different in color, texture
• To avoid foods with citric acid, hot or rough texture
• To report any bleeding, white spots, ulcerations in mouth to prescriber; tell patient to examine mouth qd
• To avoid driving, activities requiring alertness; dizziness may occur
• That contraceptive measures are recommended during therapy

P

• To avoid ingestion of alcohol, tyramine-containing foods; cold, hay fever, weight-reducing products may cause serious drug interactions
• To avoid crowds, persons with infections if granulocytes are low

prochlorperazine (℞)

(proe-klor-pair'a-zeen)
Chlorpazine, Compa-Z, Compazine, Contranzine, Provacin*, Stemetil*, Ultrazine

Func. class.: Antiemetic

Chem. class.: Phenothiazine, piperazine derivative

Action: Acts centrally by blocking chemoreceptor trigger zone, which in turn acts on vomiting center

Uses: Nausea, vomiting

Dosage and routes:

Postoperative nausea/vomiting

• *Adult:* IM 5-10 mg 1-2 hr before anesthesia; may repeat in 30 min; IV 5-10 mg 15-30 min before anesthesia; IV INF 20 mg/L D_5W or NS 15-30 min before anesthesia, not to exceed 40 mg/day

Severe nausea/vomiting

• *Adult:* PO 5-10 mg tid-qid; SUST REL 15 mg qd in AM or 10 mg q12h; REC 25 mg/bid; IM 5-10 mg; may repeat q4h, not to exceed 40 mg/day
• *Child 18-39 kg:* PO 2.5 mg tid or 5 mg bid, not to exceed 15 mg/day; IM 0.132 mg/kg
• *Child 14-17 kg:* PO/REC 2.5 mg bid-tid, not to exceed 10 mg/day; IM 0.132 mg/kg
• *Child 9-13 kg:* PO/REC 2.5 mg qd-bid, not to exceed 7.5 mg/day; IM 0.132 mg/kg

Available forms: Syrup 5 mg/ml; inj 5 mg/ml; tabs 5, 10, 25 mg; caps sus rel 10, 15, 30 mg; supp 2.5, 5, 25 mg

Side effects/adverse reactions:

CNS: *Euphoria,* ***depression, EPS,*** restlessness, tremor, dizziness

GI: Nausea, vomiting, anorexia, dry mouth, diarrhea, constipation, weight loss, metallic taste, cramps

CV: ***Circulatory failure, tachycardia***

RESP: ***Respiratory depression***

Contraindications: Hypersensitivity to phenothiazines, coma, seizure, encephalopathy, bone marrow depression

Precautions: Children <2 yr, pregnancy (C), elderly, lactation

Pharmacokinetics:

PO: Onset 30-40 min, duration 3-4 hr

SUS REL: Onset 30-40 min, duration 10-12 hr

REC: Onset 60 min, duration 3-4 hr

IM: Onset 10-20 min, duration 12 hr; metabolized by liver; excreted in urine, breast milk; crosses placenta

Interactions:

• Decreased effect of prochlorperazine: barbiturates, antacids
• Increased anticholinergic action: anticholinergics, antiparkinson drugs, antidepressants

Syringe compatibilities: Atropine, butorphanol, chlorpromazine, cimetidine, diamorphine, diphenhydramine, droperidol, fentanyl, glycopyrrolate, hydroxyzine, meperidine, metoclopramide, nalbuphine, pentazocine, perphenazine, prochlorperazine, promazine, promethazine, ranitidine, scopolamine

Y-site compatibilities: Amsacrine, fluconazole, fludarabine, gentamicin, heparin, hydrocortisone, kanamycin, melphalan, metronidazole, mezlocillin, minocycline, moxalactam, nafcillin, ondansetron, oxacillin, paclitaxel, penicillin G potassium, piperacillin, potassium chloride, sargramostim, tetracycline,

* Available in Canada only

ticarcillin, ticarcillin/clavulanate, tobramycin, vancomycin, vinorelbine, vitamin B with C
Additive compatibilities: Amikacin, ascorbic acid, dexamethasone, dimenhydrinate, erythromycin, ethacrynate, lidocaine, nafcillin, netilmicin, sodium bicarbonate, vitamin B with C
Lab test interferences:
Increase: Liver function tests, cardiac enzymes, cholesterol, blood glucose, prolactin, bilirubin, PBI, ^{131}I, alk phosphatase, leukocytes, granulocytes, platelets
Decrease: Hormones (blood and urine)
False positive: Pregnancy tests, PKU, urine bilirubin
False negative: Urinary steroids, 17-OHCS, pregnancy tests
NURSING CONSIDERATIONS
Assess:
• VS, B/P; check patients with cardiac disease more often
• Respiratory status before, during, after administration of emetic; check rate, rhythm, character; respiratory depression can occur rapidly with elderly or debilitated patients
Administer:
• IM injection in large muscle mass; aspirate to avoid IV administration
• Keep patient recumbent for ½ hour
• IV after diluting 5 mg/9 ml of NaCl for inj (1 ml = 0.5 mg); give 5 mg or less/min; may dilute 10-20 mg/L NaCl and give as infusion; can cause contact dermatitis
Evaluate:
• Therapeutic response: absence of nausea, vomiting
Teach patient/family:
• To avoid hazardous activities, activities requiring alertness; dizziness may occur
• To avoid alcohol
• Not to double or skip doses
• That urine may be pink to reddish brown
• To report dark urine, clay-colored stools, bleeding, bruising, rash, blurred vision

procyclidine (℞)
(proe-sye'kli-deen)
Kemadrin, Procyclid*
Func. class.: Cholinergic blocker
Chem. class.: Tertiary amine

Action: Centrally acting anticholinergic
Uses: Parkinson symptoms, extrapyramidal disorders
Dosage and routes:
• *Adult:* PO 2.5 mg tid pc, titrated to patient response
Available forms: Tabs 5 mg
Side effects/adverse reactions:
MS: Weakness, cramping
INTEG: Rash, urticaria, dermatoses
MISC: Fever, flushing, decreased sweating, hyperthermia, ***heat stroke,*** numbness of fingers
CNS: Confusion, anxiety, restlessness, irritability, delusions, hallucinations, headache, sedation, depression, incoherence, dizziness, lightheadedness, memory loss
EENT: Blurred vision, photophobia, dilated pupils, difficulty swallowing, mydriasis, increased intraocular tension, angle-closure glaucoma
CV: Palpitations, tachycardia, postural hypotension, bradycardia
GI: Dryness of mouth, constipation, nausea, vomiting, abdominal distress, ***paralytic ileus,*** *epigastric distress*
GU: Hesitancy, retention, dysuria
Contraindications: Hypersensitivity, narrow-angle glaucoma, myasthenia gravis, GI/GU obstruction, child <3 yr, megacolon, stenosing peptic ulcer, prostatic hypertrophy

P

Precautions: Pregnancy (C), elderly, lactation, tachycardia, children, kidney, liver disease, drug abuse, hypotension, hypertension, psychiatric patients, prostatic hypertrophy

Pharmacokinetics:

PO: Onset 30-45 min, duration 4-6 hr

Interactions:

- Decreased action of haloperidol, levodopa
- Increased anticholinergic effect: antihistamines, MAOIs, phenothiazines, amantadine

NURSING CONSIDERATIONS

Assess:

- I&O ratio; retention commonly causes decreased urinary output
- Heart rate, rhythm, B/P
- Parkinsonism: shuffling gait, muscle rigidity, involuntary movements
- Urinary hesitancy, retention; palpate bladder if retention occurs
- Constipation, especially elderly; increase fluids, bulk, exercise; if this occurs, palpate abdomen
- For tolerance over long-term therapy; dose may have to be increased or changed
- Mental status: affect, mood, CNS depression, worsening of mental symptoms during early therapy

Administer:

- With or after meals for GI upset; may give with fluids other than water
- At hs to avoid daytime drowsiness in patient with parkinsonism

Perform/provide:

- Storage at room temp in tight container
- Hard candy, frequent drinks, sugarless gum to relieve dry mouth

Evaluate:

- Therapeutic response: decreased involuntary movements

Teach patient/family:

- Not to discontinue this drug abruptly; to taper off over 1 wk
- To avoid driving, other hazardous activities; drowsiness may occur
- To avoid OTC medication: cough, cold preparations with alcohol, antihistamines unless directed by prescriber
- To avoid alcohol

---

progesterone (℞)

(proe-jess'ter-one)

Femotrone, Gesterol 50, Progestasert, progesterone, Progesterone in Oil, Progestillin*

Func. class.: Progestogen

Chem. class.: Progesterone derivative

Action: Inhibits secretion of pituitary gonadotropins, which prevents follicular maturation, ovulation; stimulates growth of mammary tissue; antineoplastic action against endometrial cancer

Uses: Contraception, amenorrhea, premenstrual syndrome, abnormal uterine bleeding

Dosage and routes:

Amenorrhea/uterine bleeding

- *Adult:* IM 5-10 mg qd × 6-8 doses

Contraception

- *Adult:* INSERT 1 in uterine cavity, active for 1 yr

PMS

- *Adult:* REC SUPP/VAG SUPP 200-400 mg

Available forms: Inj 25, 50, 100 mg/ml; IU system 38 mg, rec supp, vag supp

Side effects/adverse reactions:

CNS: Dizziness, headache, migraines, depression, fatigue

CV: Hypotension, ***thrombophlebitis,*** edema, ***thromboembolism, stroke, pulmonary embolism, MI***

---

* Available in Canada only

GI: Nausea, vomiting, anorexia, cramps, increased weight, ***cholestatic jaundice***
EENT: Diplopia
GU: Amenorrhea, cervical erosion, breakthrough bleeding, dysmenorrhea, vaginal candidiasis, breast changes, *gynecomastia, testicular atrophy, impotence,* endometriosis, ***spontaneous abortion***
INTEG: Rash, urticaria, acne, hirsutism, alopecia, oily skin, seborrhea, purpura, melasma
META: Hyperglycemia
Contraindications: Breast cancer, hypersensitivity, thromboembolic disorders, reproductive cancer, genital bleeding (abnormal, undiagnosed), cerebral hemorrhage, pregnancy (X)
Precautions: Lactation, hypertension, asthma, blood dyscrasias, gallbladder disease, CHF, diabetes mellitus, bone disease, depression, migraine headache, convulsive disorders, hepatic disease, renal disease, family history of breast or reproductive tract cancer
Pharmacokinetics:
IM, Rec, Vag: Duration 24 hr
Excreted in urine, feces; metabolized in liver
Lab test interferences:
Increase: Alk phosphatase, nitrogen (urine), pregnanediol, amino acids, factors VII, VIII, IX, X
Decrease: GTT, HDL
NURSING CONSIDERATIONS
Assess:
• Weight qd; notify prescriber of weekly weight gain >5 lb
• B/P at beginning of treatment and periodically
• I&O ratio; be alert for decreasing urinary output, increasing edema
• Liver function studies: ALT (SGPT), AST (SGOT), bilirubin periodically during long-term therapy
• Edema, hypertension, cardiac symptoms, jaundice
• Mental status: affect, mood, behavioral changes, depression
• Hypercalcemia
Administer:
• Titrated dose; use lowest effective dose
• Oil solution deep in large muscle mass IM; rotate sites
• After warming to dissolve crystals
• In one dose in AM
• With food or milk to decrease GI symptoms
Perform/provide:
• Storage in dark area
Evaluate:
• Therapeutic response: decreased abnormal uterine bleeding, absence of amenorrhea
Teach patient/family:
• To report breast lumps, vaginal bleeding, edema, jaundice, dark urine, clay-colored stools, dyspnea, headache, blurred vision, abdominal pain, numbness or stiffness in legs, chest pain
• To report suspected pregnancy
• To monitor blood sugar if diabetic

promazine (℞)

(proe'ma-zeen)
Promanyl, promazine, Prozine, Sparine
Func. class.: Antipsychotic/neuroleptic
Chem. class.: Phenothiazine, aliphatic

Action: Depresses cerebral cortex, hypothalamus, limbic system, which control activity, aggression; blocks neurotransmission produced by dopamine at synapse; exhibits a strong α-adrenergic, anticholinergic blocking action; as antiemetic, inhibits medullary chemoreceptor trigger zone; mechanism for antipsychotic effects is unclear

Uses: Psychotic disorders, schizophrenia, nausea, vomiting, alcohol withdrawal

Dosage and routes:

Psychosis

- *Adult:* PO 10-200 mg q4-6h, max dose 1 g/day; IM 50-150 mg, followed in 30 min with additional dose up to a total dose of 300 mg
- *Child >12 yr:* PO 10-25 mg q4-6h

Nausea/vomiting

- *Adult:* PO 25-50 mg q4-6h; IM 50 mg; IV not recommended, but may use in concentrations of <25 mg/ml

Available forms: Tabs 25, 50, 100 mg; inj 25, 50 mg/ml

Side effects/adverse reactions:

RESP: ***Laryngospasm,*** dyspnea, ***respiratory depression***

CNS: EPS: pseudoparkinsonism, akathisia, dystonia, tardive dyskinesia, drowsiness, headache, ***seizures***

HEMA: Anemia, ***leukopenia, leukocytosis, agranulocytosis***

INTEG: Rash, photosensitivity, dermatitis

EENT: Blurred vision, glaucoma, dry eyes

GI: Dry mouth, nausea, vomiting, anorexia, constipation, diarrhea, jaundice, weight gain

GU: Urinary retention, urinary frequency, enuresis, impotence, amenorrhea, gynecomastia

CV: Orthostatic hypotension, ***cardiac arrest,*** ECG changes, ***tachycardia***

Contraindications: Hypersensitivity, blood dyscrasias, coma, child <12 yr, brain damage, bone marrow depression, glaucoma

Precautions: Pregnancy (C), lactation, seizure disorders, hypertension, hepatic or cardiac disease

Pharmacokinetics:

PO: Onset erratic, peak 2-4 hr

IM: Onset 15 min, peak 1 hr, duration 4-6 hr; metabolized by liver; excreted in urine, breast milk; crosses placenta

Interactions:

- Oversedation: other CNS depressants, alcohol, barbiturate anesthetics
- Toxicity: epinephrine
- Decreased absorption: aluminum hydroxide, magnesium hydroxide antacids
- Decreased effects of lithium, levodopa
- Increased effects of both drugs: β-adrenergic blockers, alcohol
- Increased anticholinergic effects: anticholinergics
- Incompatible with aminophylline, amobarbital, ampicillin, atropine, chloramphenicol, chlorothiazide, dimenhydrinate, epinephrine, heparin, hydrocortisone, methicillin, methohexital, nafcillin, penicillin G, pentobarbital, phenobarbital, phenytoin, prednisolone, thiopental, warfarin, $NaCO_3$

Lab test interferences:

Increase: Liver function tests, cardiac enzymes, cholesterol, blood glucose, prolactin, bilirubin, PBI, cholinesterase, ^{131}I

Decrease: Hormones (blood and urine)

False positive: Pregnancy tests, PKU

False negative: Urinary steroids, 17-OHCS, pregnancy tests

NURSING CONSIDERATIONS

Assess:

- Mental status before initial administration
- Swallowing of PO medication; check for hoarding or giving of medication to other patients
- I&O ratio; palpate bladder if urinary output is low

* Available in Canada only

• Bilirubin, CBC, liver function studies qmo
• Urinalysis is recommended before and during prolonged therapy
• Affect, orientation, LOC, reflexes, gait, coordination, sleep pattern disturbances
• B/P standing and lying; also include pulse, respirations, q4h during initial treatment; establish baseline before starting treatment; report drops of 30 mm Hg
• Dizziness, faintness, palpitations, tachycardia on rising
• EPS including akathisia (inability to sit still, no pattern to movements), tardive dyskinesia (bizarre movements of jaw, mouth, tongue, extremities), pseudoparkinsonism (rigidity, tremors, pill rolling, shuffling gait)
• For neuroleptic malignant syndrome: muscle rigidity, altered mental status, hyperthermia, increased CPK
• Skin turgor qd
• Constipation, urinary retention qd; increase bulk, water in diet

Administer:
• Reduced dose in elderly
• IV undiluted; give at 25 mg/min or less over 1 min; may dilute 25-60 mg/9 ml NaCl for inj
• Antiparkinsonian agent on order from prescriber for EPS
• Syrup mixed in citrus- or chocolate-flavored drinks
• IM inj into large muscle mass

Perform/provide:
• Decreased sensory input by dimming lights, avoiding loud noises
• Supervised ambulation until stabilized on medication; do not involve in strenuous exercise program because fainting is possible; patient should not stand still for long periods
• Increased fluids to prevent constipation
• Sips of water, candy, gum for dry mouth
• Storage in air-tight, light-resistant container; avoid contact with hands

Evaluate:
• Therapeutic response: decrease in emotional excitement, hallucinations, delusions, paranoia; reorganization of patterns of thought, speech

Teach patient/family:
• That orthostatic hypotension occurs frequently and to rise from sitting or lying position gradually, to avoid hazardous activities until stabilized on medication
• To remain lying down for at least 30 min after IM injection
• To avoid hot tubs, hot showers, tub baths; hypotension may occur
• To avoid abrupt withdrawal of this drug, or EPS may result; drug should be withdrawn slowly
• To avoid OTC preparations (cough, hay fever, cold) unless approved by prescriber, since serious drug interactions may occur; avoid use with alcohol, CNS depressants; increased drowsiness may occur
• To use a sunscreen
• Regarding compliance with drug regimen
• About EPS and necessity for meticulous oral hygiene, since oral candidiasis may occur
• To report sore throat, malaise, fever, bleeding, mouth sores; CBC should be drawn and drug discontinued
• That in hot weather, heat stroke may occur; take extra precautions to stay cool

Treatment of overdose: Lavage if orally ingested; provide an airway; *do not induce vomiting*

promethazine (℞)

(proe-meth'a-zeen)

Anergan 25, Anergan 50, Histanil*, Mallergan Pentazine, Phenameth, Phenazine 25, Phenazine 50, Phenergan, Phenergan Fortis, Phenergan Plain, Phenoject-50, PMS Promethazine*, Pro 50, Prometh-50, promethazine HCl, Prorex 25, Prorex 50, Prothazine Plain, Remsed, V-Gan 25, V-Gan 50

Func. class.: Antihistamine, H_1-receptor antagonist

Chem. class.: Phenothiazine derivative

Combination products: Phenergan: promethazine HCl 6.25 mg/5 ml with phenylephrine HCl 5 mg/5 ml; Phenergan-D: promethazine HCl 6.25 mg with pseudoephedrine HCl 60 mg; Phenergan VC Syrup, Promethazine HCl VC: promethazine HCl 6.25 mg/5 ml with phenylephrine HCl 5 mg/5 ml

Action: Acts on blood vessels, GI, respiratory system by competing with histamine for H_1-receptor site; decreases allergic response by blocking histamine

Uses: Motion sickness, rhinitis, allergy symptoms, sedation, nausea, preoperative and postoperative sedation

Dosage and routes:

Nausea

• *Adult:* PO/IM/IV 10-25 mg; may repeat 12.5-25 mg q4-6h

• *Child >2 yr:* PO/IM 0.25-0.5 mg/kg q4-6h

Motion sickness

• *Adult:* PO 25 mg bid, give ½-1 hr before departure

• *Child >2 yr:* PO/IM/REC 12.5-25 mg bid, give ½-1 hr before departure

Allergy/rhinitis

• *Adult:* PO 12.5 mg qid, or 25 mg hs

• *Child >2 yr:* PO 6.25-12.5 mg tid or 25 mg hs

Sedation

• *Adult:* PO/IM 25-50 mg hs

• *Child >2 yr:* PO/IM/REC 12.5-25 mg hs

Sedation (preoperative/postoperative)

• *Adult:* PO/IM/IV 25-50 mg

• *Child >2 yr:* PO/IM/IV 12.5-25 mg

Available forms: Tabs 12.5, 25, 50 mg; supp 12.5, 25, 50 mg; inj 25, 50 mg/ml

Side effects/adverse reactions:

CNS: Dizziness, drowsiness, poor coordination, fatigue, anxiety, euphoria, confusion, paresthesia, neuritis

CV: Hypotension, palpitations, tachycardia

RESP: Increased thick secretions, wheezing, chest tightness

HEMA: ***Thrombocytopenia, agranulocytosis, hemolytic anemia***

GI: Constipation, dry mouth, nausea, vomiting, anorexia, diarrhea

INTEG: Rash, urticaria, photosensitivity

GU: Retention, dysuria, frequency

EENT: Blurred vision, dilated pupils, tinnitus, nasal stuffiness, dry nose, throat, mouth, photosensitivity

Contraindications: Hypersensitivity to H_1-receptor antagonist, acute asthma attack, lower respiratory tract disease

Precautions: Increased intraocular pressure, renal disease, cardiac disease, hypertension, bronchial asthma, seizure disorder, stenosed peptic ulcers, hyperthyroidism, prostatic hypertrophy, bladder neck obstruction, pregnancy (C)

* Available in Canada only

Pharmacokinetics:
PO: Onset 20 min, duration 4-6 hr; metabolized in liver; excreted by kidneys, GI tract (inactive metabolites)
Interactions:
• Increased CNS depression: barbiturates, narcotics, hypnotics, tricyclic antidepressants, alcohol
• Decreased effect of oral anticoagulants, heparin
• Increased effect of promethazine: MAOIs
Syringe compatibilities: Atropine, butorphanol, chlorpromazine, cimetidine, diphenhydramine, droperidol, fentanyl, glycopyrrolate, hydromorphone, hydroxyzine, meperidine, metoclopromide, midazolam, morphine, pentazocine, perphenazine, prochlorperazine, promazine, ranitidine, scopolamine
Y-site compatibilities: Amsacrine, fluconazole, fludarabine, melphalan, ondansetron, sargramostim, vinorelbine
Additive compatibilities: Amikacin, ascorbic acid, netilmicin, vitamin B with C
Lab test interferences:
False negative: Skin allergy test
False positive: Urine pregnancy test

NURSING CONSIDERATIONS
Assess:
• I&O ratio; be alert for urinary retention, frequency, dysuria; drug should be discontinued
• CBC during long-term therapy; blood dyscrasias
• Respiratory status: rate, rhythm, increase in bronchial secretions, wheezing, chest tightness
• Cardiac status: palpitations, increased pulse, hypotension
Administer:
• IV after diluting each 25-50 mg/9 ml of NaCl for inj; give 25 mg or less/2 min
• With meals for GI symptoms; absorption may slightly decrease
• Deep IM in large muscle; rotate site
• When used for motion sickness, 30 min before travel
Perform/provide:
• Hard candy, gum, frequent rinsing of mouth for dryness
• Storage in tight, light-resistant container
Evaluate:
• Therapeutic response: absence of running, congested nose, rashes, absence of motion sickness, nausea; sedation
Teach patient/family:
• That drug may cause photosensitivity; to avoid prolonged sunlight
• To notify prescriber of confusion, sedation, hypotension
• To avoid driving, other hazardous activity if drowsy
• To avoid concurrent use of alcohol, other CNS depressants
Treatment of overdose: Administer ipecac syrup or lavage, diazepam, vasopressors, barbiturates (short-acting)

P

propafenone (℞)
(proe-paff'e-nown)
Rythmol
Func. class.: Antidysrhythmic, (Class IC)

Action: Slows conduction velocity; reduces membrane responsiveness; inhibits automaticity; increases ratio of effective refractory period to action potential duration; β-blocking activity
Uses: Life-threatening dysrhythmias, sustained ventricular tachycardia
Dosage and routes:
• *Adult:* PO 300-900 mg/day in divided doses, 150 mg q8h; allow a

3-4 day interval before increasing dose

Available forms: Tabs 150, 300 mg

Side effects/adverse reactions:

INTEG: Rash

CV: Dysrhythmias, palpitations, AV block, intraventricular conduction delay, AV dissociation, ***CHF, sudden death, atrial flutter***

HEMA: ***Leukopenia, agranulocytosis, granulocytopenia, thrombocytopenia,*** anemia

CNS: Headache, dizziness, abnormal dreams, syncope, confusion, ***seizures***

GI: Nausea, vomiting, constipation, dyspepsia, cholestasis, ***hepatitis,*** abnormal liver function studies, dry mouth

RESP: Dyspnea

EENT: Blurred vision, altered taste, tinnitus

Contraindications: 2nd or 3rd degree AV block, right bundle branch block, cardiogenic shock, hypersensitivity, bradycardia, uncontrolled CHF, sick-sinus node syndrome, marked hypotension, bronchospastic disorders

Precautions: CHF, hypokalemia, hyperkalemia, recent MI, nonallergic bronchospasm, pregnancy (C), lactation, children, hepatic or renal disease

Pharmacokinetics:

Peak 3-5 hr, half-life 2-10 hr; metabolized in liver; excreted in urine (metabolite)

Interactions:

- Increased effect of propafenone: cimetidine, quinidine
- Increased anticoagulation: warfarin
- Increased digoxin level: digoxin
- Increased β-blocker effect: propranolol, metoprolol

Lab test interferences:

Increase: CPK

NURSING CONSIDERATIONS

Assess:

- GI status: bowel pattern, number of stools
- Cardiac status: rate, rhythm, quality
- Chest x-ray film, pulmonary function test during treatment
- I&O ratio; check for decreasing output
- B/P for fluctuations
- Lung fields; bilateral rales may occur in CHF patient
- Increased respiration, increased pulse; drug should be discontinued
- Toxicity: fine tremors, dizziness
- Cardiac function: respiratory rate, rhythm, character continuously

Evaluate:

- Therapeutic response: absence of dysrhythmias

Treatment of overdose: O_2, artificial ventilation, ECG; administer dopamine for circulatory depression, diazepam or thiopental for convulsions

propantheline (℞)

(proe-pan'the-leen)

Norpanth, Pro-Banthine, Propanthel*, propantheline bromide

Func. class.: GI anticholinergic

Chem. class.: Synthetic quaternary ammonium compound

Action: Inhibits muscarinic actions of acetylcholine at postganglionic parasympathetic neuroeffector sites

Uses: Treatment of peptic ulcer disease, irritable bowel syndrome, duodenography, urinary incontinence

Investigational uses: Antispasmodic uses

Dosage and routes:

- *Adult:* PO 15 mg tid ac, 30 mg hs
- *Elderly:* PO 7.5 mg tid ac

* Available in Canada only

Available forms: Tabs 7.5, 15 mg
Side effects/adverse reactions:
CNS: Confusion, stimulation in elderly, headache, insomnia, dizziness, drowsiness, anxiety, weakness, hallucinations
GI: Dry mouth, constipation, ***paralytic ileus,*** heartburn, nausea, vomiting, dysphagia, absence of taste
GU: Hesitancy, retention, impotence
CV: Palpitations, tachycardia
EENT: Blurred vision, photophobia, mydriasis, cycloplegia, increased ocular tension
INTEG: Urticaria, rash, pruritus, anhidrosis, fever, allergic reactions
Contraindications: Hypersensitivity to anticholinergics, narrow-angle glaucoma, GI obstruction, myasthenia gravis, paralytic ileus, GI atony, toxic megacolon
Precautions: Hyperthyroidism, coronary artery disease, dysrhythmias, CHF, ulcerative colitis, hypertension, hiatal hernia, hepatic disease, renal disease, pregnancy (C), urinary retention, prostatic hypertrophy
Pharmacokinetics:
PO: Onset 30-45 min, duration 6 hr; metabolized by liver, GI system, excreted in urine, bile
Interactions:
• Increased anticholinergic effect: amantadine, tricyclic antidepressants, MAOIs, H_1 antihistamines
• Decreased effect of phenothiazines, levodopa, ketoconazole

NURSING CONSIDERATIONS
Assess:
• VS, cardiac status: checking for dysrhythmias, increased rate, palpitations
• I&O ratio; check for urinary retention or hesitancy
• GI complaints: pain, bleeding (frank or occult), nausea, vomiting, anorexia

Administer:
• ½-1 hr ac for better absorption
• Decreased dose to elderly patients; metabolism may be slowed
• Gum, hard candy, frequent rinsing for dry mouth

Perform/provide:
• Storage in tight container protected from light
• Increased fluids, bulk, exercise to decrease constipation

Evaluate:
• Therapeutic response: absence of epigastric pain, bleeding, nausea, vomiting

Teach patient/family:
• To avoid driving, other hazardous activities until stabilized on medication; may cause blurred vision
• To avoid alcohol, other CNS depressants; will enhance sedating properties of this drug
• To drink plenty of fluids
• To report dysphagia

---

propofol (℞)
(proe-po'fol)
Diprivan, Disoprofol
Func. class.: General anesthetic

Action: Produces dose-dependent CNS depression; action is unknown
Uses: Induction or maintenance of anesthesia as part of balanced anesthetic technique; sedation in mechanically ventilated patients
Dosage and routes:
Induction
• *Adult:* IV 2-2.5 mg/kg, approximately 40 mg q10sec until induction onset
• *Elderly:* 1-1.5 mg/kg, approximately 20 mg q10sec until induction onset
Maintenance
• *Adult:* 0.1-0.2 mg/kg/min (6-12 mg/kg/hr)

• *Elderly:* 0.05-0.1 mg/kg/min (3-6 mg/kg/hr)

Intermittent bolus

• *Adult:* Increments of 25-50 mg as needed

Critical care sedatives

• *Adult:* IV 5 mg/kg over 5 min; may give 5-10 mg/kg/min over 5-10 min until desired response

Available forms: Inj 10 mg/ml in 20 ml amp, 50 cc and 100 cc vials

Side effects/adverse reactions:

CNS: Movement, headache, jerking, fever, dizziness, shivering, tremor, confusion, somnolence, paresthesia, agitation, abnormal dreams, euphoria, fatigue

GI: Nausea, vomiting, abdominal cramping, dry mouth, swallowing, hypersalivation

MS: Myalgia

GU: Urine retention, green urine

EENT: Blurred vision, tinnitus, eye pain, strange taste

CV: Bradycardia, hypotension, hypertension, PVC, PAC, tachycardia, abnormal ECG, ST segment depression, ***asystole***

RESP: ***Apnea,*** *cough, hiccups,* dyspnea, hypoventilation, sneezing, wheezing, tachypnea, hypoxia

INTEG: Flushing, phlebitis, hives, burning/stinging at injection site

Contraindications: Hypersensitivity, hyperlipidemia

Precautions: Elderly, respiratory depression, severe respiratory disorders, cardiac dysrhythmias, pregnancy (B), labor and delivery, lactation, children

Pharmacokinetics:

Onset 40 sec, rapid distribution, half-life 1-8 min, terminal elimination half-life 5-10 hr; 70% excreted in urine; metabolized in liver by conjugation to inactivate metabolites

Interactions:

• Increased CNS depression: alcohol, narcotics, sedative/hypnotics, antipsychotics, skeletal muscle relaxants, inhalational anesthetics

• Do not administer with other drugs

NURSING CONSIDERATIONS

Assess:

• Injection site: phlebitis, burning, stinging

• ECG for changes: PVC, PAC, ST segment changes

• CNS changes: movement, jerking, tremors, dizziness, LOC, pupil reaction

• Allergic reactions: hives

• Respiratory dysfunction: respiratory depression, character, rate, rhythm; notify prescriber if respirations are <10/min

Administer:

• After diluting with D_5W mixed in lipid base; use only glass containers when mixing, not stable in plastic

• By IV infusion only

• Alone; do not mix with other agents before using

• Only with resuscitative equipment available

• Only by qualified persons trained in anesthesia

Perform/provide:

• Storage in light-resistant area at room temperature

• Safety measures: side rails, night-light, call bell within reach

Evaluate:

• Therapeutic response: induction of anesthesia

Treatment of overdose: Discontinue drug; administer vasopressor agents or anticholinergics, artificial ventilation

* Available in Canada only

propoxyphene (℞)

(proe-pox'i-feen)

Darvon, Darvon-N, Dolene, Doraphen, Doxaphene, Novapropoxyn*, Profene, Pro-Pox, Propoxycon, propoxyphene HCl; propoxyphene/acetaminophen Darvocet-N, Dolane AP, Doxapap-N, D-Rex, E-Lor, Genagesic, Pancet Propacet, Pro-Pox with APAP, Propoxyphene with APAP, Wygesic; propoxyphene/aspirin/caffeine, Benophene, Cotanal, Darvon Compound-65, Darvon-N Compound*, Doraphen Compound, Margesic A-C, Novopropoxy Compound*, Pro-Pox Plus

Func. class.: Narcotic analgesic
Chem. class.: Synthetic opiate

Combination products: Darvocet-N 50, Propoxyphene Napsylate with Acetaminophen Tablets: acetaminophen 325 mg with propoxyphene napsylate 50 mg; Darvocet-N 100, Doxapap-N, Propacet 100: propoxyphene napsylate 100 mg with acetaminophen 650 mg; 65, Dolene Compound-65, Doxaphene Compound, Propoxyphene AC, Propoxyphene Compound-65: propoxyphene HCl 65 mg with aspirin 389 mg, caffeine 32.4 mg

Controlled Substance Schedule IV
Action: Depresses pain impulse transmission at the spinal cord level by interacting with opioid receptors
Uses: Mild to moderate pain
Dosage and routes:
• *Adult:* PO 65 mg q4h prn (HCl)
• *Adult:* PO 100 mg q4h prn (napsylate)
Available forms: Propoxyphene HCl Cap 65 mg, tabs 65 mg*; propoxyphene napslylate Tabs 50, 100 mg; cap 100 mg*, oral susp 50 mg/5 ml propoxyphene HCl, acetaminophen tabs 65 mg/650 mg; propoxyphene napsylate/acetaminophen tabs 50 mg/325 mg, 100 mg/650 mg; propoxyphene/aspirin/caffeine cap 65 mg/389 mg/32.4 mg
Side effects/adverse reactions:
CNS: Drowsiness, dizziness, confusion, headache, sedation, euphoria, ***convulsions, hyperthermia***
GI: Nausea, vomiting, anorexia, constipation, cramps
GU: Urinary retention, dysuria
INTEG: Rash, urticaria, bruising, flushing, diaphoresis, pruritus
EENT: Tinnitus, blurred vision, miosis, diplopia
CV: Palpitations, bradycardia, change in B/P, ***dysrhythmias***
RESP: ***Respiratory depression***
Contraindications: Hypersensitivity to ASA products (some preparations), addiction (narcotic)
Precautions: Addictive personality, pregnancy (C), lactation, increased intracranial pressure, MI (acute), severe heart disease, respiratory depression, hepatic disease, renal disease, child <18 yr
Pharmacokinetics:
PO: Onset 15-30 min, peak 2-3 hr, duration 4-6 hr
REC: Onset slow; duration 4-6 hr
Metabolized by liver, excreted by kidneys (as metabolites), crosses placenta, excreted in breast milk, half-life 12 hr (metabolites)
Interactions:
• Increased effects with other CNS depressants: alcohol, narcotics, sedative/hypnotics, antipsychotics, skeletal muscle relaxants
Lab test interferences:
Increase: Amylase

NURSING CONSIDERATIONS
Assess:
• I&O ratio; check for decreasing output; may indicate retention

P

• CNS changes: dizziness, drowsiness, hallucinations, euphoria, loss of consciousness, pupil reaction
• Allergic reactions: rash, urticaria
• Respiratory dysfunction: respiratory depression, character, rate, rhythm; notify prescriber if respirations are <10/min
• Need for pain medication; physical dependence

Administer:
• With antiemetic for nausea, vomiting
• When pain is beginning to return; determine dosage interval by response

Perform/provide:
• Storage in light-resistant area at room temp
• Assistance with ambulation
• Safety measures: side rails, nightlight, call bell within easy reach

Evaluate:
• Therapeutic response: decrease in pain

Teach patient/family:
• To report any symptoms of CNS changes, allergic reactions
• That physical dependency may result when used for extended periods; not to exceed dose
• That withdrawal symptoms may occur: nausea, vomiting, cramps, fever, faintness, anorexia

Treatment of overdose: Naloxone (Narcan) 0.2-0.8 mg IV, O_2, IV fluids, vasopressors

propranolol (℞)

(proe-pran'oh-lole)
Apo-Propanolol*, Detensol*, Inderal, Inderal LA, Inderal 10, Inderal 20, Inderal 40, Inderal 60, Inderal 80, propranolol HCl, Propranolol Intensol, Novo-Pranol*

Func. class.: Antihypertensive, antianginal
Chem. class.: β-Adrenergic blocker

Combination products: Inderide 40/25, Propranolol HCl, Hydrochlorothiazide Tablets 40/25: propranolol HCl 40 mg with hydrochlorothiazide 25mg; Inderide 80/25, Propranolol HCl, Hydrochlorothiazide Tablets 80/25: propranolol HCl 80 mg with hydrochlorothiazide 25 mg; Inderide LA 80/50: propranolol HCl 80 mg with hydrochlorothiazide 50 mg

Action: Nonselective β-blocker with negative inotropic, chronotropic, dromotropic properties

Uses: Chronic stable angina pectoris, hypertension, supraventricular dysrhythmias, migraine, prophylaxis, MI, pheochromocytoma, essential tremor, tetralogy of Fallot, cyanotic spells

Investigational uses: Mitral valve prolapse, anxiety, dysrhythmias associated with thyrotoxicosis

Dosage and routes:

Dysrhythmias
• *Adult:* PO 10-30 mg tid-qid; IV BOL 0.5-3 mg over 1 mg/min; may repeat in 2 min, may repeat q4h thereafter

Hypertension
• *Adult:* PO 40 mg bid or 80 mg qd (EXT REL) initially; usual dose 120-

* Available in Canada only

240 mg/day bid-tid or 120-160 mg qd (EXT REL)

Angina

• *Adult:* PO 80-320 mg in divided doses bid-qid or 80 mg qd (EXT REL); usual dose 160 mg qd (EXT REL)

MI prophylaxis

• *Adult:* PO 180-240 mg/day tid-qid starting 5 day to 2 wk after MI

Pheochromocytoma

• *Adult:* PO 60 mg/day × 3 days preoperatively in divided doses or 30 mg/day in divided doses (inoperable tumor)

Migraine

• *Adult:* PO 80 mg/day (EXT REL) or in divided doses; may increase to 160-240 mg/day in divided doses

Essential tremor

• *Adult:* PO 40 mg bid; usual dose 120 mg/day

Available forms: Caps ext rel 60, 80, 120, 160 mg; tabs 10, 20, 40, 60, 80, 90 mg; inj 1 mg/ml; oral sol 4 mg, 8 mg/ml; conc oral sol 80 mg/ml

Side effects/adverse reactions:

RESP: Dyspnea, respiratory dysfunction, *bronchospasm*

CV: Bradycardia, hypotension, ***CHF,*** palpitations, AV block, peripheral vascular insufficiency, vasodilation

HEMA: ***Agranulocytosis, thrombocytopenia***

GI: Nausea, vomiting, diarrhea, colitis, constipation, cramps, dry mouth, hepatomegaly, gastric pain, acute pancreatitis

GU: Impotence, decreased libido, UTIs

MS: Joint pain, arthralgia, muscle cramps, pain

MISC: Facial swelling, weight change, Raynaud's phenomenon

INTEG: Rash, pruritus, fever

CNS: Depression, hallucinations, dizziness, fatigue, lethargy, paresthesias, bizarre dreams, disorientation

EENT: Sore throat, ***laryngospasm,*** blurred vision, dry eyes

META: Hyperglycemia, hypoglycemia

Contraindications: Hypersensitivity to this drug, cardiac failure, cardiogenic shock, 2nd or 3rd degree heart block, bronchospastic disease, sinus bradycardia, CHF

Precautions: Diabetes mellitus, pregnancy (C), renal disease, lactation, hyperthyroidism, COPD, hepatic disease, children, myasthenia gravis, peripheral vascular disease, hypotension, CHF

Pharmacokinetics:

PO: Onset 30 min, peak 1-1½ hr, duration 6-12 hr

PO-ER: Peak 6 hr, duration 24 hr

IV: Onset 2 min, peak 15 min, duration 3-6 hr; immediate rel half-life 3-5 hr; ext rel half-life 8-11 hr; metabolized by liver; crosses placenta, blood-brain barrier; excreted in breast milk

Interactions:

• AV block: digitalis, calcium channel blockers

• Increased negative inotropic effects: verapamil, disopyramide

• Increased effects of reserpine, digitalis, neuromuscular blocking agents

• Decreased β-blocking effects: norepinephrine, isoproterenol, barbiturates, rifampin, dopamine, dobutamine, smoking

• Increased β-blocking effect: cimetidine

• Increased hypotension: quinidine, haloperidol, hydralazine

Syringe compatibilities: Amrione, benzquinamide, milrinone

Y-site compatibilities: Amrione, heparin, hydrocortisone sodium succinate, meperidine, milrinone, morphine, potassium chloride, vitamin B with C

P

Additive compatibilities: Dobutamine, verapamil

Solution compatibilities: 0.9% NaCl, 0.45 NaCl, Ringer's, D_5W, D_5/0.9% NaCl, D_5/0.45% NaCl

Lab test interferences:

Increase: Serum K, serum uric acid, ALT (SGPT)/AST (SGOT), alk phosphatase, LDH

Decrease: Blood glucose

NURSING CONSIDERATIONS

Assess:

- B/P, pulse, respirations during beginning therapy
- Weight qd; report gain of 5 lb
- I&O ratio, CrCl if kidney damage is diagnosed
- ECG if using as antidysrhythmic
- Hepatic enzymes: AST (SGOT), ALT (SGPT), bilirubin
- Pain: duration, time started, activity being performed, character
- Tolerance (long-term use)
- Headache, light-headedness, decreased B/P; may indicate a need for decreased dosage

Administer:

- Do not give with aluminum-containing antacid; may decrease GI absorption
- IV undiluted or diluted 10 ml D_5W for inj; give 1 mg or less/min; may be diluted in 50 ml NaCl and run 1 mg over 10-15 min
- With 8 oz water on empty stomach

Perform/provide:

- Protection from light (injection)

Evaluate:

- Therapeutic response: decreased B/P, dysrhythmias

Teach patient/family:

- Not to discontinue abruptly, to take drug at same time each day
- To avoid OTC drugs unless approved by prescriber
- To avoid hazardous activities if dizzy
- Stress importance of compliance with complete medical regimen
- To make position changes slowly to prevent fainting
- To decrease dosage over 2 wk to prevent cardiac damage

propylthiouracil (℞)

(proe-pill-thye-oh-yoor'a-sill)

propylthiouracil, Propyl-Thyracil*, PTU

Func. class.: Thyroid hormone antagonist (antithyroid)

Chem. class.: Thioamide

Action: Blocks synthesis peripherally of T_3, T_4 (triiodothyronine, thyroxine), inhibits organification of iodine

Uses: Preparation for thyroidectomy, thyrotoxic crisis, hyperthyroidism, thyroid storm

Dosage and routes:

Thyrotoxic crisis

- *Adult and child:* PO same as hyperthyroidism with iodine and propranolol

Preparation for thyroidectomy

- *Adult*: 600-1200 mg/day
- *Child*: 10 mg/kg/day in divided doses

Hyperthyroidism

- *Adult:* PO 100 mg tid increasing to 300 mg q8h if condition is severe; continue to euthyroid state, then 100 mg qd-tid
- *Child >10 yr:* PO 100 mg tid; continue to euthyroid state, then 25 mg tid to 100 mg bid
- *Child 6-10 yr:* PO 50-150 mg in divided doses q8h
- *Neonates:* PO 10 mg/kg/day in divided doses

Available forms: Tabs 50 mg

Side effects/adverse reactions:

INTEG: Rash, urticaria, pruritus, alopecia, hyperpigmentation, lupus-like syndrome

* Available in Canada only

GU: ***Nephritis***
CNS: Drowsiness, headache, vertigo, fever, paresthesias, neuritis
HEMA: ***Agranulocytosis, leukopenia, thrombocytopenia, hypothrombinemia, lymphadenopathy,*** bleeding, vasculitis, periarteritis
GI: Nausea, diarrhea, vomiting, ***jaundice, hepatitis,*** loss of taste
MS: Myalgia, arthralgia, nocturnal muscle cramps, osteoporosis

Contraindications: Hypersensitivity, pregnancy (D), lactation

Precautions: Infection, bone marrow depression, hepatic disease

Pharmacokinetics:
PO: Onset up to 3 wk, peak 6-10 wk, duration 1 wk to 1 mo half-life 1-2 hr; excreted in urine, bile, breast milk; crosses placenta; concentration in thyroid gland

Interactions:
- Increased anticoagulant effect: heparin, oral anticoagulants

Lab test interferences:
Increases: Pro-time, AST (SGOT), ALT (SGPT), alk phosphatase

NURSING CONSIDERATIONS

Assess:
- Pulse, B/P, temp
- I&O ratio; check for edema: puffy hands, feet, periorbits; indicates hypothyroidism
- Weight qd; same clothing, scale, time of day
- T_3, T_4, which are increased; serum TSH, which is decreased; free thyroxine index, which is increased if dosage is too low; discontinue drug 3-4 wk before RAIU
- Blood work: CBC for blood dyscrasias: leukopenia, thrombocytopenia, agranulocytosis; LFTs
- Overdose: peripheral edema, heat intolerance, diaphoresis, palpitations, dysrhythmias, severe tachycardia, increased temperature, delirium, CNS irritability
- Hypersensitivity: rash, enlarged cervical lymph nodes; drug may have to be discontinued
- Hypoprothrombinemia: bleeding, petechiae, ecchymosis
- Clinical response: after 3 wk should include increased weight, pulse; decreased T_4
- Bone marrow depression: sore throat, fever, fatigue

Administer:
- With meals to decrease GI upset
- At same time each day to maintain drug level
- Lowest dose that relieves symptoms

Perform/provide:
- Storage in light-resistant container
- Fluids to 3-4 L/day, unless contraindicated

Evaluate:
- Therapeutic response: weight gain, decreased pulse, decreased T_4, decreased B/P

Teach patient/family:
- To abstain from breast-feeding after delivery
- To take pulse qd
- To report redness, swelling, sore throat, mouth lesions, which indicate blood dyscrasias
- To keep graph of weight, pulse, mood
- To avoid OTC products that contain iodine
- That seafood, other iodine products may be restricted
- Not to discontinue this medication abruptly; thyroid crisis may occur; stress response
- That response may take several months if thyroid is large
- Symptoms/signs of overdose: periorbital edema, cold intolerance, mental depression
- Symptoms of inadequate dose: tachycardia, diarrhea, fever, irritability

P

• To take medication as prescribed; not to skip or double dose; missed doses should be taken when remembered up to 1 hr before next dose
• To carry ID listing condition, medication

protamine (℞)

(proe'ta-meen)

Func. class.: Heparin antagonist

Chem. class.: Low-molecular-weight protein

Action: Binds heparin, making it ineffective

Uses: Heparin overdose

Dosage and routes:

• *Adult, child:* IV 1 mg of protamine/ 90-115 U heparin given; administer slowly 1-3 min; give undiluted to 1%, not to exceed 50 mg/10 min

Available forms: Inj 10 mg/ml

Side effects/adverse reactions:

CV: Hypotension, bradycardia, ***circulatory collapse***

GI: Nausea, vomiting, anorexia

INTEG: Rash, dermatitis, urticaria

CNS: Lassitude

HEMA: Bleeding, ***anaphylaxis***

RESP: Dyspnea, ***pulmonary edema, severe respiratory distress***

Contraindications: Hypersensitivity

Precautions: Pregnancy (C), lactation, children, allergy to fish

Pharmacokinetics:

IV: Onset 5 min, duration 2 hr

Additive compatibilities: Cimetidine, verapamil

NURSING CONSIDERATIONS

Assess:

• Blood studies (Hct, platelets, occult blood in stools) q3mo
• Coagulation tests (APTT, ACT) 15 min after dose, then in several hours
• VS, B/P, pulse of 30 min; plus 3 hr after dose
• Skin rash, urticaria, dermatitis
• Allergy to fish; use with caution

Administer:

• IV after diluting 50 mg/5 ml sterile bacteriostatic H_2O for inj; shake, give 20 mg or less over 1-3 min; may further dilute with equal volume of NaCl or D_5W and run over 2-3 hr; titrate to APTT, ACT; use infusion pump

Perform/provide:

• Storage at 36°-46° F (2°-8° C)

Evaluate:

• Therapeutic response: reversal of heparin overdose

protriptyline (℞)

(proe-trip'te-leen)

Triptil*, Vivactil

Func. class.: Tricyclic antidepressant

Chem. class.: Dibenzocycloheptene—secondary amine

Action: Blocks reuptake of norepinephrine, serotonin into nerve endings, increasing action of norepinephrine, serotonin in nerve cells

Uses: Depression

Dosage and routes:

• *Adult:* PO 15-40 mg/day in divided doses; may increase to 60 mg/day

Available forms: Tabs 5, 10 mg

Side effects/adverse reactions:

HEMA: ***Agranulocytosis, thrombocytopenia, eosinophilia, leukopenia***

CNS: Dizziness, drowsiness, confusion, headache, anxiety, tremors, stimulation, weakness, insomnia, nightmares, EPS (elderly), increased psychiatric symptoms, paresthesia, seizures

* Available in Canada only

GI: Diarrhea, dry mouth, nausea, vomiting, ***paralytic ileus,*** increased appetite, cramps, epigastric distress, jaundice, ***hepatitis,*** stomatitis, constipation
GU: Retention, ***acute renal failure***
INTEG: Rash, urticaria, sweating, pruritus, photosensitivity
CV: Orthostatic hypotension, ECG changes, tachycardia, ***hypertension,*** palpitations
EENT: Blurred vision, tinnitus, mydriasis
Contraindications: Hypersensitivity to tricyclic antidepressants, recovery phase of MI, convulsive disorders, prostatic hypertrophy
Precautions: Suicidal patients, severe depression, increased intraocular pressure, narrow-angle glaucoma, urinary retention, cardiac disease, hepatic disease, hyperthyroidism, electroshock therapy, elective surgery, pregnancy (C)
Pharmacokinetics:
PO: Onset 15-30 min, peak 24-30 hr, duration 4-6 hr; therapeutic effect 2-3 wk; metabolized by liver, excreted by kidneys, crosses placenta, half-life 54-98 hr
Interactions:
• Decreased effects of guanethidine, clonidine, indirect-acting sympathomimetics (ephedrine)
• Increased effects of direct-acting sympathomimetics (epinephrine), alcohol, barbiturates, benzodiazepines, CNS depressants
• Hyperpyretic crisis, convulsions, hypertensive episode: MAOI (pargyline [Eutonyl])
Lab test interferences:
Increase: Serum bilirubin, blood glucose, alk phosphatase
False increase: Urinary catecholamines
Decrease: VMA, 5-HIAA

NURSING CONSIDERATIONS
Assess:
• B/P (lying, standing), pulse q4h; if systolic B/P drops 20 mm Hg, hold drug, notify prescriber; take vital signs q4h in patients with cardiovascular disease
• Blood studies: CBC, leukocytes, differential, cardiac enzymes (long-term therapy)
• Hepatic studies: AST (SGOT), ALT (SGPT), bilirubin
• Weight qwk; appetite may increase with drug
• ECG for flattening of T wave, bundle branch block, AV block, dysrhythmias in cardiac patients
• EPS primarily in elderly: rigidity, dystonia, akathisia
• Mental status changes: mood, sensorium, affect, suicidal tendencies, increase in psychiatric symptoms: depression, panic
• Urinary retention, constipation; constipation most likely in children
• Withdrawal symptoms: headache, nausea, vomiting, muscle pain, weakness; not usual unless discontinued abruptly
• Alcohol consumption; hold dose until morning
Administer:
• Increased fluids, bulk in diet if constipation occurs
• With food, milk for GI symptoms
• Dosage hs if oversedation occurs during day; may take entire dose hs; elderly may not tolerate once/day dosing
• Gum, hard candy, or frequent sips of water for dry mouth
Perform/provide:
• Storage in tight, light-resistant container at room temp
• Assistance with ambulation during beginning therapy for drowsiness/dizziness
• Safety measures including side rails, primarily in elderly

• Checking to see PO medication swallowed

Evaluate:

• Therapeutic response: decreased depression

Teach patient/family:

• That therapeutic effects may take 2-3 wk
• To use caution in driving, other activities requiring alertness because of drowsiness, dizziness, blurred vision
• To avoid alcohol ingestion, other CNS depressants
• Not to discontinue medication quickly after long-term use; may cause nausea, headache, malaise
• To wear sunscreen or large hat

Treatment of overdose: ECG monitoring; induce emesis; lavage, activated charcoal; administer anticonvulsant

pseudoephedrine (OTC)

(soo-doe-e-fed'rin)

Allerid, Children's Sudafed, Decofed Syrup, DeFed-60, Dorcol Children's Decongestant, Drixoral Non-Drowsy Formula, Eltor*, Efidac/24, Genaphed, Halofed, Myfedrine, Novafed, Pedia Care Infant's Decongestant, pseudoephedrine HCl, Pseudogest Decongestant, Pseudo Syrup, Sinustat, Sudafed, Sudafed 12 hour, Sudrin

Func. class.: Adrenergic

Chem. class.: Substituted phenylethylamine

Combination products: Bayer Select Head Cold Caplets, Bayer Select Maximum Strength Sinus Pain Relief Caplets, Dristan Cold Caplets, Maximum Strength Dynafed Tablets, Maximum Strength Ornex Caplets, Maximum Strength Sine-Aid Tablets, Gelcaps, Caplets, No Drowsiness Sinarest Tablets, Sinus Excedrin Extra Strength Tablets and Caplets: Pseudoephedrine 30 mg, acetaminophen 500 mg; Dristan Sinus, Advil Cold and Sinus, Dimetapp Sinus, Motrin IB Sinus, Sine-Aid IB: pseudoephedrine 30 mg, Ibuprofen 200 mg; Kronofed-A Jr., Duri-Tap/PD, Rescon Jr, Atrohist Pediaetric: pseudoephedrine 60 mg, chlorpheniramine 4 mg; Bromfed PD, Dallergy-JR, ULTRAbrom PD: pseudoephedrine 60 mg, bromopheniramine 6 mg

Action: Primary activity through α-effects on respiratory mucosal membranes reducing congestion hyperemia, edema; minimal bronchodilation secondary to β-effects

Uses: Nasal decongestant, adjunct in otitis media; with antihistamines

Dosage and routes:

• *Adult:* PO 60 mg q6h; EXT REL 60-120 mg q12h or q24h
• *Child 6-12 yr:* PO 30 mg q6h, not to exceed 120 mg/day
• *Child 2-6 yr:* PO 15 mg q6h, not to exceed 60 mg/day

Available forms: Caps ext rel 120, 240 mg; oral sol 15 mg, 30 mg/5 ml; drops 7.5 mg/0.8 ml; tabs 30, 60 mg; caps 60 mg; tabs ext rel 120 mg

Side effects/adverse reactions:

CNS: Tremors, anxiety, insomnia, headache, dizziness, hallucinations, ***seizures***

EENT: Dry nose, irritation of nose and throat

CV: Palpitations, tachycardia, hypertension, chest pain, ***dysrhythmias***

GI: Anorexia, nausea, vomiting, dry mouth

GU: Dysuria

* Available in Canada only

Contraindications: Hypersensitivity to sympathomimetics, narrow-angle glaucoma
Precautions: Pregnancy (C), cardiac disorders, hyperthyroidism, diabetes mellitus, prostatic hypertrophy, lactation
Pharmacokinetics:
PO: Onset 15-30 min, duration 4-6 hr, 8-12 hr (ext rel); metabolized in liver, excreted in feces and breast milk
Interactions:
• Do not use with MAOIs or tricyclic antidepressants; hypertensive crisis may occur
• Decreased effect of this drug: methyldopa, urinary acidifiers, rauwolfia alkaloids
• Increased effect of this drug: urinary alkalizers

NURSING CONSIDERATIONS
Assess:
• For nasal congestion; auscultate lung sounds; check for tenacious bronchial secretions
• B/P, pulse throughout treatment
Perform/provide:
• Storage at room temp
Evaluate:
• Therapeutic response: Decreased nasal congestion
Teach patient/family:
• Reason for drug administration
• Not to use continuously, or more than recommended dose; rebound congestion may occur
• To check with prescriber before using other drugs, as drug interactions may occur
• To avoid taking near hs; stimulation can occur
• Not to use if stimulation, restlessness, or tremors occur

psyllium (OTC)
(sill'i-um)
Cillium, Effer-Syllium, Fiberall, Fiberall Natural Flavor and Orange Flavor, Hydrocil Instant Powder, Karacil*, Konsyl-D, Metamucil, Metamucil Instant Mix Lemon Lime, Metamucil Instant Mix Orange, Metamucil Orange Flavor, Metamucil Sugar Free, Metamucil Sugar Free Orange Flavor, Modane Bulk, Natural Vegetable Reguloid, Perdiem, Pro-Lax, Prodiem Plain*, Reguloid Natural, Reguloid Orange, Reguloid Sugar Free Orange, Reguloid Sugar Free Regular, Serutan, Siblin, Syllact, V-Lax
Func. class.: Bulk laxative
Chem. class.: Psyllium colloid

Action: Bulk-forming laxative
Uses: Chronic constipation, ulcerative colitis, irritable bowel syndrome
Dosage and routes:
• *Adult:* PO 1-2 tsp in 8 oz H_2O bid or tid, then 8 oz H_2O or 1 premeasured packet in 8 oz H_2O bid or tid, then 8 oz H_2O
• *Child >6 yr:* 1 tsp in 4 oz H_2O hs
Available forms: Chew pieces 1.7 g/piece; pdr 309, 390, 430, 450, 486, 500, 600, 630, 654, 672, 791, 919, 950 mg/g, 1 g/g; granules 2.5 g/dose
Side effects/adverse reactions:
GI: Nausea, vomiting, anorexia, diarrhea, cramps
Contraindications: Hypersensitivity, intestinal obstruction, abdominal pain, nausea/vomiting, fecal impaction
Precautions: Pregnancy (C)
Pharmacokinetics: Excreted in feces, not absorbed in GI tract

P

NURSING CONSIDERATIONS

Assess:

• Blood, urine electrolytes if used often

• I&O ratio to identify fluid loss

• Cause of constipation; fluids, bulk, exercise missing

• Cramping, rectal bleeding, nausea, vomiting; drug should be discontinued

Administer:

• Alone for better absorption

• In morning or evening (oral dose)

• After mixing with H_2O immediately before use

• With 8 oz H_2O or juice followed by another 8 oz of fluid

Evaluate:

• Therapeutic response: decrease in constipation or decreased diarrhea in colitis

Teach patient/family:

• To maintain adequate fluid consumption

• That normal bowel movements do not always occur daily

• Not to use in presence of abdominal pain, nausea, vomiting

• To notify prescriber if constipation unrelieved or if symptoms of electrolyte imbalance occur: muscle cramps, pain, weakness, dizziness, excessive thirst

---

pyrantel (℞)

(pi-ran′tel)

Antiminth, Combantrin*, Pin-X, Reese's Pinworm

Func. class.: Anthelmintic

Chem. class.: Pyrimidine derivative

Action: Causes paralysis in worm by neuroblockade, caused by stimulation of ganglionic receptors; worms expelled by normal peristalsis

Uses: Pinworms, roundworms

Dosage and routes:

• *Adult and child >2 yr:* PO 11 mg/kg as single dose, not to exceed 1 g; repeat in 2 wk for pinworms

Available forms: Oral susp 250 mg/5 ml

Side effects/adverse reactions:

INTEG: Rash

CNS: Dizziness, headache, drowsiness, insomnia, fever, weakness

GI: Nausea, vomiting, anorexia, diarrhea, distention

Contraindications: Hypersensitivity

Precautions: Seizure disorders, hepatic disease, dehydration, anemia, child <2 yr, pregnancy (C)

Pharmacokinetics:

PO: Peak 1-3 hr; metabolized in liver; excreted in feces, urine (unchanged/metabolites)

Interactions:

• Antagonizes effect of pyrantel: piperazine

NURSING CONSIDERATIONS

Assess:

• Stools during entire treatment; specimens must be sent to lab while still warm

• For allergic reaction: rash

• For diarrhea during expulsion of worms

Administer:

• PO after meals to avoid GI symptoms

• After shaking suspension

Perform/provide:

• Storage in tight, light-resistant container in cool environment

Evaluate:

• Therapeutic response: expulsion of worms, 3 negative stool cultures after completion of treatment

Teach patient/family:

• Proper hygiene after BM, including hand washing technique; tell patient not to put fingers in mouth

---

* Available in Canada only

• That infected person should sleep alone; not to shake bed linen; change bed linen qd, wash in hot water
• To clean toilet qd with disinfectant (green soap solution)
• Need for compliance with dosage schedule, duration of treatment
• To drink fruit juice to help expel worms
• To wear shoes, wash all fruits, vegetables well before eating

pyrazinamide (℞)

(peer-a-zin′a-mide)
PMS Pyrazinamide*, pyrazinamide, Tebrazid*
Func. class.: Antitubercular agent
Chem. class.: Pyrazinoic acid amine/nicoturimide analog

Action: Bactericidal interference with lipid, nucleic acid biosynthesis
Uses: Tuberculosis, as an adjunct when other drugs are not feasible
Dosage and routes:
• *Adult:* PO 20-35 mg/kg/day qd or in divided dose not to exceed 3 g/day
• *Child:* PO 15-30 mg/kg/day qd or divided bid, max 1.5 g/day
Available forms: Tabs 500 mg
Side effects/adverse reactions:
INTEG: Photosensitivity, urticaria
CNS: Headache
GI: ***Hepatotoxicity,*** abnormal liver function tests, peptic ulcer
GU: Urinary difficulty, increased uric acid
HEMA: ***Hemolytic anemia***
Contraindications: Hypersensitivity
Precautions: Pregnancy (C), child <13 yr
Pharmacokinetics:
PO: Peak 2 hr, half-life 9-10 hr; metabolized in liver, excreted in urine (metabolites/unchanged drug)
Lab test interferences:
Increase: PBI
Decrease: 17-KS
NURSING CONSIDERATIONS
Assess:
• Signs of anemia: Hct, Hgb, fatigue
• Temp; if >101° F (38° C), drug should be reduced
• Liver studies qwk: ALT (SGPT), AST (SGOT), bilirubin
• Renal status before, qmo: BUN, creatinine, output, sp gr, urinalysis
• Hepatic status: decreased appetite, jaundice, dark urine, fatigue
Administer:
• With meals for GI symptoms
• After C&S is completed; qmo to detect resistance
Evaluate:
• Therapeutic response: decreased symptoms of TB, culture negative
Teach patient/family:
• That compliance with dosage schedule, length is necessary
• To avoid alcohol

pyrethrins (℞)

(peer′e-thrins)
A-200 Pyrinate, Barc, Pyrinyl, RID, TISIT, Triple X
Func. class.: Pediculocide
Chem. class.: Pyrethrin/piperonyl butoxide/petroleum distillate

Action: Causes paralysis, death of organism by acting as a contact poison
Uses: Head, body, pubic lice; nits; scabies
Dosage and routes:
• *Adult and child:* Apply undiluted to infested area; allow application to remain no longer than 10 min, wash thoroughly with warm water, soap, or shampoo; remove dead lice,

eggs with fine-toothed comb; do not exceed 2 consecutive applications within 24 hr; may repeat in 7-10 days
• *Adult and child:* CREAM/LOTION wash area with soap, water; remove visible crusts, apply to skin surfaces, remove with soap, water in 8-12 hr; may reapply in 1 wk if needed; SHAMPOO using 30 ml, work into lather, rub for 5 min, rinse, dry with towel
Available forms: Gel, liq, shampoo, cream, lotion
Side effects/adverse reactions:
INTEG: Irritation, pruritus, urticaria, eczema
Contraindications: Hypersensitivity, inflammation of skin, abrasions, or breaks in skin
Precautions: Child/infant, ragweed sensitivity, pregnancy (C)
NURSING CONSIDERATIONS
Administer:
• To body areas, scalp only; do not apply to face, lips, mouth, eyes, any mucous membrane, anus, or meatus; apply from neck down for body lice
• Topical corticosteroids as ordered to decrease contact dermatitis
• Lotions of menthol or phenol to control itching
• Topical antibiotics for infection
Perform/provide:
• Storage in tight container
• Isolation until areas on skin, scalp have cleared and treatment is complete
• Removal of nits by using a fine-toothed comb rinsed in vinegar after treatment
Evaluate:
• Therapeutic response: decreased nits, crusts
Teach patient/family:
• To discontinue use, notify prescriber of irritation or infection
• To flush with water in case of contact with eyes
• To wash all inhabitants' clothing, bed linen using insecticide; preventive treatment may be required of all persons living in same house, using lotion or shampoo to decrease spread of infection
• That itching may continue 4-6 wk
• That drug must be reapplied if accidentally washed off, or treatment will be ineffective
• To use externally only
• To treat sexual partners simultaneously

pyridostigmine (℞)

(peer-id-oh-stig′meen)
Mestinon, Mestinon SR*, Mestinon Timespan, Regonol
Func. class.: Cholinergic; anticholinesterase
Chem. class.: Tertiary amine carbamate

Action: Inhibits destruction of acetylcholine, which increases concentration at sites where acetylcholine is released; this facilitates transmission of impulses across myoneural junction
Uses: Nondepolarizing muscle relaxant antagonist, myasthenia gravis
Dosage and routes:
Myasthenia gravis
• *Adult:* PO 60-180 mg bid-qid, not to exceed 1.5 g/day; IM/IV 1/30 of PO dose; SUS REL 180-540 mg qd or bid at intervals of at least 6 hr
Nondepolarizing neuromuscular blocker antagonist
• *Adult:* 0.6-1.2 mg IV atropine, then 10-30 mg
Available forms: Tabs 60 mg; tabs sus rel 180 mg; syr 60 mg/5 ml; inj 5 mg/ml

* Available in Canada only

Side effects/adverse reactions:
INTEG: Rash, urticaria, flushing
CNS: Dizziness, headache, sweating, weakness, ***convulsions,*** incoordination, paralysis, drowsiness, LOC
GI: Nausea, diarrhea, vomiting, cramps, increased salivary and gastric secretions, peristalsis
CV: Tachycardia, dysrhythmias, bradycardia, AV block, hypotension, ECG changes, ***cardiac arrest,*** syncope
GU: Frequency, incontinence, urgency
RESP: ***Respiratory depression, bronchospasm, constriction, laryngospasm, respiratory arrest***
EENT: Miosis, blurred vision, lacrimation, visual changes

Contraindications: Bradycardia; hypotension; obstruction of intestine, renal system; bromide sensitivity

Precautions: Seizure disorders, bronchial asthma, coronary occlusion, hyperthyroidism, dysrhythmias, peptic ulcer, megacolon, poor GI motility, pregnancy (C)

Pharmacokinetics:
PO: Onset 20-30 min, duration 3-6 hr
IM/IV/SC: Onset 2-15 min, duration 2½-4 hr; metabolized in liver, excreted in urine

Interactions:
- Decreased action: gallamine, metocurine, pancuronium, tubocurarine, atropine
- Increased action: decamethonium, succinylcholine
- Decreased action of pyridostigmine: aminoglycosides, anesthetics, procainamide, quinidine, mecamylamine, polymyxin, magnesium, corticosteroids, antidysrhythmics

Syringe compatibility: Glycopyrrolate

Y-site compatibilities: Heparin, hydrocortisone sodium succinate, potassium chloride, vitamin B with C

NURSING CONSIDERATIONS

Assess:
- VS, respiration q8h
- I&O ratio; check for urinary retention or incontinence
- Bradycardia, hypotension, bronchospasm, headache, dizziness, convulsions, respiratory depression; drug should be discontinued if toxicity occurs

Administer:
- IV undiluted, give through Y-tube or 3-way stopcock, give 0.5 mg or less/min
- Only with atropine sulfate available for cholinergic crisis
- Only after all other cholinergics have been discontinued
- Increased doses for tolerance
- Larger doses after exercise or fatigue
- On empty stomach for better absorption

Perform/provide:
- Storage at room temp

Evaluate:
- Therapeutic response: increased muscle strength, hand grasp, improved gait, absence of labored breathing (if severe)

Teach patient/family:
- Not to crush or chew sus rel prep
- That drug is not a cure, only relieves symptoms
- To wear Medic Alert ID specifying myasthenia gravis, drugs taken

Treatment of overdose:
Discontinue drug, atropine 1-4 mg IV

P

pyridoxine (vit B_6)
(PO-OTC, IM/IV-℞)
(peer-i-dox'een)
Beesix, Nestrex, Pyridoxine HCl, Vitamin B_6, Rodex TD, Hexa-Betalin
Func. class.: Vit B_6, water soluble

Action: Needed for fat, protein, carbohydrate metabolism; enhances glycogen release from liver and muscle tissue; needed as coenzyme for metabolic transformations of a variety of amino acids
Uses: Vit B_6 deficiency of inborn errors of metabolism, seizures, isoniazid therapy, oral contraceptives, alcoholic polyneuritis
Dosage and routes:
Vit B_6 deficiency
• *Adult:* PO/IM/IV 2.5-10 mg until corrected, then 2-5 mg qd
• *Child:* PO/IM/IV 100 mg until desired response
Inborn errors of metabolism
• *Adult:* IM/IV/PO 600 mg or less qd, then 50 mg qd for life
• *Child:* IM/PO/IV 100 mg, then 2-10 mg IM or 10-100 mg PO qd
Deficiency caused by isoniazid
• *Adult:* PO 100 mg qd × 3 wk, then 50 mg qd
• *Child:* PO dose titrated to response
Prevention of deficiency caused by isoniazid
• *Adult:* PO 10-50 mg qd
• *Child:* PO 0.5-1.5 mg qd
• *Infant:* PO 0.1-0.5 mg qd
Available forms: Tabs 10, 25, 50, 100, 200, 250, 500 mg; tabs time rel 500 mg; inj IM-IV 100 mg/ml; oral cap 500 mg
Side effects/adverse reactions:
CNS: Paresthesia, flushing, warmth, lethargy (rare with normal renal function)
INTEG: Pain at injection site
Contraindications: Hypersensitivity
Precautions: Pregnancy (A), lactation, child, Parkinson's disease
Pharmacokinetics:
PO/Inj: Half-life 2-3 wk, metabolized in liver, excreted in urine
Interactions:
• Decreased effects of levodopa
• Decreased effects of pyridoxine: oral contraceptives, INH, cycloserine, hydralazine, penicillamine
• Incompatible with alkaline sol, iron salts

NURSING CONSIDERATIONS
Assess:
• Pyridoxine levels throughout treatment
• Nutritional status: yeast, liver, legumes, bananas, green vegetables, whole grains
Administer:
• IV undiluted or added to most IV sol; give 50 mg or less/1 min if undiluted
• IM rotate sites; burning or stinging at site may occur
• Z-track to minimize pain
Perform/provide:
• Storage in tight, light-resistant container
Evaluate:
• Therapeutic response: absence of nausea, vomiting, anorexia, skin lesions, glossitis, stomatitis, edema, convulsions, restlessness, paresthesia
Teach patient/family:
• To avoid vitamin supplements unless directed by prescriber
• To keep out of children's reach
• To increase meat, bananas, potatoes, lima beans, whole grain cereals
• To discuss birth control status with prescriber

pyrimethamine (℞)

(peer-i-meth'a-meen)

Daraprim, Fansidar (with sulfadoxine)

Func. class.: Antimalarial

Chem. class.: Folic acid antagonist

Action: Inhibits folic acid metabolism in parasite, prevents transmission by stopping growth of fertilized gametes

Uses: Malaria prophylaxis, *P. vivax*

Investigational uses: *Pneumocystis carinii* pneumonia as an adjunct

Dosage and routes:

Prophylaxis of malaria

- *Adult:* PO 1 tab qwk or 2 tabs q2wk (Fansidar)
- *Child 9-14 yr:* PO ¾ tab qwk or 1½ tabs q2wk (Fansidar)
- *Child >10 yr:* PO 25 mg qwk
- *Child 4-10 yr:* PO 12.5 mg qwk
- *Child 4-8 yr:* PO ½ tab qwk or 1 tab q2wk (Fansidar)
- *Child <4 yr:* PO ¼ tab qwk or ½ tab q2wk (Fansidar)
- *Child <4 yr:* PO 6.25 mg qwk

Acute attacks of malaria

- *Adult:* PO 2-3 tabs as a single dose (Fansidar) alone or with quinine or primaquine
- *Child 9-14 yr:* 2 tabs
- *Child 4-8 yr:* 1 tab
- *Child <4 yr:* ½ tab

Toxoplasmosis

- *Adult:* PO 100 mg, then 25 mg qd × 4-5 wk, with 1 g sulfadiazine q6h
- *Child:* PO 1 mg/kg, then 0.25 mg/kg qd × 4-5 wk, with sulfadiazine 100 mg/kg/day in divided doses q6h

Available forms: Tabs 25 mg; combo tabs 500 mg sulfadoxine/25 mg pyrimethamine

Side effects/adverse reactions:

RESP: ***Respiratory failure***

INTEG: Skin eruptions, photosensitivity

CNS: Stimulation, irritability, ***convulsions,*** tremors, ataxia, fatigue

GI: Nausea, vomiting, cramps, anorexia, diarrhea, atrophic glossitis, gastritis

HEMA: ***Thrombocytopenia, leukopenia, pancytopenia, megaloblastic anemia,*** decreased folic acid, ***agranulocytosis***

Contraindications: Hypersensitivity, chloroquine-resistant malaria, megaloblastic anemia caused by folate deficiency

Precautions: Blood dyscrasias, seizure disorder, pregnancy (C), lactation, G6PD disease, renal, hepatic disease

Pharmacokinetics:

PO: Peak 2 hr, half-life 111 hr; metabolized in liver, highly protein bound, excreted in urine (metabolites)

Interactions:

- Synergestic action: paraaminobenzoic acid or folic acid
- Increased bone marrow suppression: antibiotics

NURSING CONSIDERATIONS

Assess:

- Folic acid level; megaloblastic anemia occurs
- Blood studies, CBC, platelets, since blood dyscrasias occur; twice weekly if dosage is increased
- For toxicity: vomiting, anorexia, seizure, blood dyscrasia, glossitis; drug should be discontinued immediately

Administer:

- Leucovorin IM 3-9 mg/day × 3 days if folic acid deficiency occurs
- Before or after meals at same time each day to maintain drug level, to decrease GI symptoms

P

Perform/provide:
• Storage in tight, light-resistant container

Evaluate:
• Therapeutic response: decreased symptoms of malaria

Teach patient/family:
• To report visual problems, fever, fatigue, bruising, bleeding; may indicate blood dyscrasias

Treatment of overdose: Gastric lavage, short-acting barbiturate, leucovorin, respiratory support if needed

quazepam (℞)

(kway′ze-pam)

Doral

Func. class.: Sedative-hypnotic

Chem. class.: Benzodiazepine derivative

Controlled Substance Schedule IV (USA)

Action: Produces CNS depression at the limbic, thalamic, hypothalamic levels of CNS; may be mediated by neurotransmitter γ-aminobutyric acid (GABA); results are sedation, hypnosis, skeletal muscle relaxation, anticonvulsant activity, anxiolytic action

Uses: Insomnia

Dosage and routes:
• *Adult:* PO 15 mg hs; then 7.5-15 mg hs
• *Elderly:* PO 15 mg hs × 2 days, then 7.5 mg hs

Available forms: Tabs 7.5, 15 mg

Side effects/adverse reactions:

HEMA: ***Leukopenia, granulocytopenia*** (rare)

CNS: Lethargy, drowsiness, daytime sedation, dizziness, confusion, lightheadedness, headache, anxiety, irritability, weakness, tremor, depression

GI: Nausea, vomiting, diarrhea, heartburn, abdominal pain, constipation, anorexia, taste alteration

CV: Chest pain, pulse changes, palpitations, tachycardia

MISC: Joint pain, congestion, dermatitis, sweating

Contraindications: Hypersensitivity to benzodiazepines, pregnancy (X), lactation

Precautions: Hepatic or renal disease, suicidal individuals, drug abuse, elderly, psychosis, child <18 yr, depression, pulmonary insufficiency

Pharmacokinetics:

PO: Onset 15-45 min, duration 7-8 hr; metabolized by liver, excreted by kidneys (inactive/active metabolites), crosses placenta, excreted in breast milk

Interactions:
• Increased effects of quazepam: cimetidine, disulfiram, OC
• Decreased effects: smoking, rifampin, theophylline with increased levels of phenytoin and digoxin
• Increased CNS depression: alcohol, CNS depressants
• Decreased effect of quazepam: antacids

Lab test interferences:

Increase: AST (SGOT), ALT (SGPT), serum bilirubin

Decrease: RAI uptake

NURSING CONSIDERATIONS

Assess:
• Blood studies: Hct, Hgb, RBCs (if on long-term therapy)
• Hepatic studies: AST (SGOT), ALT (SGPT), bilirubin
• Mental status: mood, sensorium, affect, memory (long, short)
• Blood dyscrasias: fever, sore throat, bruising, rash, jaundice, epistaxis (rare)
• Type of sleep problem: falling asleep, staying asleep

* Available in Canada only

Administer:

- After removal of cigarettes to prevent fires
- After trying conservative measures for insomnia
- ½-1 hr before hs for sleeplessness
- On empty stomach for fast onset, but may be taken with food if GI symptoms occur

Perform/provide:

- Assistance with ambulation after receiving dose
- Safety measure: side rails, night-light, call bell within easy reach
- Checking to see PO medication has been swallowed
- Storage in tight container in cool environment

Evaluate:

- Therapeutic response: ability to sleep at night, decreased amount of early morning awakening

Teach patient/family:

- To avoid driving or other activities requiring alertness until drug is stabilized
- To avoid alcohol ingestion, CNS depressants; serious CNS depression may result
- That effects may take two nights for benefits to be noticed
- Alternative measures to improve sleep: reading, exercise several hours before hs, warm bath, warm milk, TV, self-hypnosis, deep breathing
- That hangover is common in elderly but less common than with barbiturates

Treatment of overdose: Lavage, activated charcoal; monitor electrolytes, vital signs

quinacrine (℞)

(kwin'a-kreen)

Atabrine HCl

Func. class.: Anthelmintic

Chem. class.: Acridine dye derivative

Action: Causes worm scolex to detach from GI tract; inhibits DNA synthesis in susceptible parasites

Uses: Giardiasis, tapeworms (cestodiasis), malaria

Dosage and routes:

- *Adult:* PO 100 mg tid × 5-7 days
- *Child:* PO 7 mg/kg/day in 3 divided doses pc × 5 days, not to exceed 300 mg/day; may repeat in 2 wk if needed; administer 1-3 mo for malaria

Tapeworm

- *Adults and children >14 yr:* 4 doses of 200 mg PO given 10 min apart (800 mg total)
- *Children 11-14 yr:* 200 mg PO 10 min apart × 3 (600 mg total)

Available forms: Tabs 100 mg

Side effects/adverse reactions:

INTEG: Rash, dermatitis, yellow pigmentation of skin, urticaria

CNS: Dizziness, headache, insomnia, restlessness, confusion, behavioral changes, psychosis, ***convulsions,*** nightmares

EENT: Bad taste, oral irritation, corneal deposits, retinopathy

GI: Nausea, vomiting, anorexia, diarrhea, cramps, ***hepatitis***

GU: Yellow discoloration of urine

HEMA: ***Aplastic anemia, agranulocytosis***

Contraindications: Hypersensitivity, porphyria, psoriasis

Precautions: Seizure disorders, elderly, psychosis, alcoholism, hepatic disease, depression, child <12 yr, G6PD deficiency, pregnancy (C), hepatic disease

Q

Pharmacokinetics:

PO: Peak 8 hr, metabolized by the liver (slowly), excreted primarily in urine, crosses placenta, high protein bindings

Interactions:

- Increased toxicity: primaquine, hepatotoxic drugs
- Disulfiram-like reaction: alcohol

Lab test interferences:

False positive: Adrenal function tests
Increase: 17-OHCS (Mattingly method)

NURSING CONSIDERATIONS

Assess:

- Stools during entire treatment, collect entire stools × 48 hr, pass through sieve, check for scolex (yellow tapeworms)
- CBC, ophthalmic exam (long-term treatment)
- Stools 2 wk after last dose for giardiasis
- For allergic reaction (rash), visual problems (halos, blurring, inability to focus)
- For infection in family members; infection from person to person is common
- Mental status: affect, mood, behavioral changes

Administer:

- By duodenal tube for pork tapeworm; prevents vomiting, transportation of parasites into stomach
- Bland liquid diet, no fat, no residue 24-48 hr before beginning therapy; patient should be fasting night before, given saline enemas, cleansing enema before beginning therapy (tapeworms only)
- Laxatives before treatment to cleanse bowel; $NaCO_3$ with each dose for nausea and vomiting
- After meals with fluids for giardiasis, malaria
- In jam or honey to disguise bitter taste of pulverized tablets (children)

Perform/provide:

- Storage in tight container

Evaluate:

- Therapeutic response: expulsion of worms, 3 negative stool cultures after completion of treatment

Teach patient/family:

- Proper hygiene after BM, including hand-washing technique; tell patient not to put fingers in mouth
- To clean toilet qd with disinfectant (green soap solution)
- Need for compliance with dosage schedule, duration of treatment
- That skin, urine may turn deep yellow
- To report any visual changes
- Not to drink alcohol

Treatment of overdose: Induce vomiting

quinapril (℞)

(kwin′a-pril)

Accupril

Func. class.: Antihypertensive
Chem. class.: Angiotensin-converting enzyme (ACE) inhibitor

Action: Selectively suppresses renin-angiotensin-aldosterone system; inhibits ACE, prevents conversion of angiotensin I to angiotensin II; results in dilation of arterial, venous vessels

Uses: Hypertension, alone or in combination with thiazide diuretics

Dosage and routes:

Hypertension

- *Adult:* PO 10 mg qd initially, then 20-80 mg/day divided bid or qd

Congestive heart failure

- *Adult:* PO 2.5 mg initially, then 5-40 mg/day maintenance qd or in 2 divided doses

Available forms: Tabs 5, 10, 20, 40 mg

Side effects/adverse reactions:
CV: Hypotension, postural hypotension, syncope, palpitations, angina pectoris, MI, tachycardia, vasodilation
GU: Increased BUN, creatinine, decreased libido, impotence, urinary tract infection
HEMA: ***Thrombocytopenia, agranulocytosis***
INTEG: ***Angioedema,*** rash, sweating, photosensitivity, pruritus
RESP: Cough, bronchitis
META: Hyperkalemia
GI: Nausea, constipation, vomiting, gastritis, GI hemorrhage, dry mouth
CNS: Headache, dizziness, fatigue, somnolence, depression, malaise, nervousness, vertigo
MISC: Back pain, amblyopia, pharyngitis
MS: Arthralgia, arthritis, myalgia

Contraindications: Hypersensitivity to ACE inhibitors, pregnancy (D), children

Precautions: Impaired renal, liver function, dialysis patients, hypovolemia, blood dyscrasias, COPD, asthma, elderly, lactation

Pharmacokinetics:
PO: Peak ½-1 hr, serum protein binding, 97%, half-life 2 hr, metabolized by liver (metabolites), metabolites excreted in urine

Interactions:
- Increased hypotension: diuretics, other antihypertensives, ganglionic blockers, adrenergic blockers, phenothiazines
- Use caution with vasodilators, hydralazine, prazosin, potassium-sparing diuretics, sympathomimetics, K supplements
- Decreased absorption of tetracycline
- Reduced hypotensive effect of quinipril: indomethacin
- Increased toxicity: lithium, digoxin

Lab test interferences:
False positive: Urine acetone

NURSING CONSIDERATIONS

Assess:
- Blood studies: neutrophils, decreased platelets
- B/P, orthostatic hypotension, syncope
- Renal studies: protein, BUN, creatinine; watch for increased levels; may indicate nephrotic syndrome
- Baselines in renal, liver function tests before therapy begins
- K levels; hyperkalemia is rare
- Dipstick of urine for protein qd in first morning specimen; if protein is increased, a 24-hr urinary protein should be collected
- Edema in feet, legs qd
- Allergic reactions: rash, fever, pruritus, urticaria; drug should be discontinued if antihistamines fail to help
- Renal symptoms: polyuria, oliguria, frequency, dysuria

Administer:
- IV infusion of 0.9% NaCl (as ordered) to expand fluid volume if severe hypotension occurs

Perform/provide:
- Supine or Trendelenburg position for severe hypotension

Evaluate:
- Therapeutic response: decrease in B/P

Teach patient/family:
- To take 1 hr before meals; not to take antacids within 1-2 hr of quinapril
- Not to discontinue drug abruptly
- Not to use OTC products (cough, cold, allergy); not to use salt substitutes containing potassium unless directed by prescriber
- To comply with dosage schedule, even if feeling better
- To rise slowly to sitting or standing position to minimize orthostatic hypotension

• To notify prescriber of mouth sores, sore throat, fever, swelling of hands or feet, irregular heartbeat, chest pain, persistent dry cough
• To report excessive perspiration, dehydration, vomiting, diarrhea; may lead to fall in B/P
• That drug may cause dizziness, fainting, light-headedness; may occur during 1st few days of therapy
• That drug may cause skin rash or impaired taste perception
• How to take B/P, and normal readings for age group

Treatment of overdose: 0.9% NaCl IV Inf, hemodialysis

quinestrol (℞)

(kwin-ess'trole)
Estrovis
Func. class.: Estrogen
Chem. class.: Nonsteroidal synthetic estrogen

Action: Needed for adequate functioning of female reproductive system; affects release of pituitary gonadotropins, inhibits ovulation, promotes adequate calcium use in bone structures

Uses: Menopause, atrophic vaginitis, kraurosis vulvae, female castration, female hypogonadism, primary ovarian failure

Dosage and routes:
• *Adult:* PO 100 μg qd × 1 wk, then 100 μg qwk starting 2 wk after beginning treatment; may increase to 200 μg/wk

Available forms: Tabs 100 μg

Side effects/adverse reactions:
CNS: Dizziness, headache, migraine, depression
CV: Hypotension, thrombophlebitis, edema, ***thromboembolism, stroke, pulmonary embolism, MI***
GI: Nausea, vomiting, diarrhea, anorexia, ***pancreatitis,*** cramps, constipation, increased appetite, increased weight, ***cholestatic jaundice***
EENT: Contact lens intolerance, increased myopia, astigmatism
GU: Amenorrhea, cervical erosion, breakthrough bleeding, dysmenorrhea, vaginal candidiasis, breast changes, *gynecomastia, testicular atrophy, impotence*
INTEG: Rash, urticaria, acne, hirsutism, alopecia, oily skin, seborrhea, purpura, melasma
META: Folic acid deficiency, hypercalcemia, hyperglycemia

Contraindications: Breast cancer, thromboembolic disorders, reproductive cancer, genital bleeding (abnormal, undiagnosed), pregnancy (X), lactation

Precautions: Hypertension, asthma, blood dyscrasias, gallbladder disease, CHF, diabetes mellitus, bone disease, depression, migraine headache, convulsive disorders, hepatic desease, renal disease, family history of cancer of breast or reproductive tract

Pharmacokinetics:
PO: Degraded in liver; excreted in urine, breast milk; crosses placenta

Interactions:
• Decreased action of anticoagulants, oral hypoglycemics
• Toxicity: tricyclic antidepressants
• Decreased action of quinestrol: anticonvulsants, barbiturates, phenylbutazone, rifampin
• Increased action of corticosteroids

NURSING CONSIDERATIONS

Assess:
• Uring glucose in patient with diabetes; urine glucose may rise
• Weight qd; notify prescriber of weekly gain >5 lb; if increase, diuretic may be ordered
• B/P q4h; watch for increase caused by H_2O, Na retention

* Available in Canada only

• I&O ratio; be alert for decreasing urinary output, increasing edema
• Liver function studies, including AST, ALT, bilirubin, alk phosphatase
• Edema, hypertension, cardiac symptoms, jaundice, calcemia
• Mental status: affet mood, behavioral changes, aggression

Administer:
• Titrated dose; use lowest effective dose
• With food or milk to decrease GI symptoms

Evaluate:
• Therapeutic response: reversal of menopause or decrease in tumor size in prostatic cancer

Teach patient/family:
• To weigh qwk, report gain >5 lb
• To report breast lumps, vaginal bleeding, edema, jaundice, dark urine, clay-colored stools, dyspnea, headache, blurred vision, abdominal pain, numbness or stiffness in legs, chest pain; male to report impotence or gynecomastia

quinidine (℞)

(kwin'i-deen)

Quinaglute, Quinalan, quinidine gluconate; Cardioquin; Quinidex Extentabs, quinidine sulfate, Quinora, Apo Quinidine*, Cin-Quin, Novoquinidin*

Func. class.: Antidysrhythmic (Class IA)

Chem. class.: Quinine dextro isomer

Action: Prolongs duration of action potential and effective refractory period, thus decreasing myocardial excitability; anticholinergic properties

Uses: PVCs, atrial fibrillation, PAT, ventricular tachycardia, atrial dysrhythmias

Investigational uses: Malaria/IV quinidine gluconate

Dosage and routes:

Quinidine sulfate

Atrial fibrillation/flutter
• *Adult:* PO 200 mg q2-3h × 5-8 doses; may increase qd until sinus rhythm is restored; max 4 g/day given only after digitalization

Paroxysmal supraventricular tachycardia
• *Adult:* PO 400-600 mg q2-3h, then 200-300 mg q6-8h or 300-600 mg q8-12h (SUS REL)

Premature atrial/ventricular contraction
• *Adult:* PO 200-300 mg q6-8h or 300-600 mg (SUS REL) q8-12h; max 4 g/day
• *Child:* PO 6 mg/kg or 180 mg/m^2 5× /day

Quinidine gluconate
• *Adult:* PO 324-660 mg q6-12h (sus rel); IM 600 mg, then 400 mg q2h; IV give 16 mg/min

Quinidine polygalacturonate
• *Adult:* PO 275-825 mg q3-4h × 4 doses, then increase by 137.5-275 mg; repeat up to 4× until dysrhythmias decreased
• *Child:* PO 8.25 mg/kg (247.5 mg/m^2) 5× /day

Available forms: Gluconate tabs sus rel 324, 330 mg; inj gluconate 80 mg/ml; sulfate tabs 200, 300 mg; tabs sus rel 300 mg; polygalacturonate tabs 275 mg

Side effects/adverse reactions:

CNS: Headache, dizziness, involuntary movement, confusion, psychosis, restlessness, irritability, syncope, excitement

EENT: Cinchonism: tinnitus, blurred vision, hearing loss, mydriasis, disturbed color vision

GI: Nausea, vomiting, anorexia, *diarrhea,* ***hepatotoxicity***

Q

CV: Hypotension, bradycardia, PVCs, ***heart block, cardiovascular collapse, arrest***
HEMA: ***Thrombocytopenia,*** hemolytic anemia, agranulocytosis, hypoprothrombinemia
RESP: Dyspnea, ***respiratory depression***
INTEG: Rash, urticaria, angioedema, swelling, photosensitivity
Contraindications: Hypersensitivity, blood dyscrasias, severe heart block, myasthenia gravis
Precautions: Pregnancy (C), lactation, children, renal disease, K imbalance, liver disease, CHF, respiratory depression
Pharmacokinetics:
PO: Peak 0.5-6 hr, duration 6-8 hr; half-life 6-7 hr, metabolized in liver, excreted unchanged by kidneys
Interactions:
- Increased effects of neuromuscular blockers, digoxin, coumadin
- Increased effects of quinidine: cimetidine, propranolol, thiazides, sodium bicarbonate, carbonic anhydrase inhibitors, antacids, hydroxide suspensions
- May decrease effects of quinidine: barbiturates, phenytoin, rifampin, nifedipine
- Additive vagolytic effect: anticholinergic blockers
- Additive cardiac depression: other antidysrhythmics, phenothiazines, reserpine

Y-site compatibilities: Diazepam, milrinone
Additive compatibilities: Bretylium, cimetidine, milrinone, verapamil
Lab test interferences:
Increase: CPK
NURSING CONSIDERATIONS
Assess:
- ECG continuously to determine increased PR or QRS segments; discontinue or reduce dose
- Blood levels (therapeutic level 2-6 μg/ml)
- B/P continuously for fluctuations
- Cinchonism: tinnitus, headache, nausea, dizziness, fever, vertigo, tremor; may lead to hearing loss
- Cardiac rate, respiration: rate, rhythm, character, continuously
- Respiratory status: rate, rhythm, lung fields for rales; increased respiration, increased pulse; drug should be discontinued
- CNS effects: dizziness, confusion, psychosis, paresthesias, convulsions; drug should be discontinued

Administer:
- IV after diluting 800 mg/40 ml or more D_5; give 16 mg or less over 1 min as inf; use inf pump
- IM inj in deltoid; aspirate to avoid intravascular administration
- AV node blocker (digoxin, verapamil) before starting quinidine to avoid increased ventricular rate

Evaluate:
- Therapeutic response: decreased dysrhythmias

Treatment of overdose: O_2, artificial ventilation, ECG, administer dopamine for circulatory depression, diazepam or thiopental for convulsions

---

quinine (℞, OTC)
(kwye'nine)
Formula Q, Legatrin, M-Kya, Novoquine*, Quinamm, Quinine Sulfate, Quiphile, Q-Vel
Func. class.: Antimalarial
Chem. class.: Cinchona tree alkaloid

Action: Inhibits parasite replications, transcription of DNA to RNA by forming complexes with DNA of parasite

* Available in Canada only

Uses: *Plasmodium falciparum* malaria, nocturnal leg cramps

Dosage and routes:

• *Adult:* PO 650 mg q8h × 10 days, given with pyrimethamine 25 mg q12h × 3 days, with sulfadiazine 500 mg qid × 5 days

Available forms: Caps 130, 195, 200, 300, 325 mg; tabs 260, 325 mg

Side effects/adverse reactions:

RESP: Dyspnea

INTEG: Pruritus, pigmentary changes, skin eruptions, lichen planuslike eruptions, flushing, facial edema, sweating

HEMA: ***Thrombocytopenia, purpura, hypothrombinemia, hemolysis***

CNS: Headache, stimulation, fatigue, irritability, ***convulsion,*** bad dreams, dizziness, fever, confusion, anxiety

EENT: Blurred vision, corneal changes, retinal changes, difficulty focusing, tinnitus, vertigo, deafness, photophobia, diplopia, night blindness

GU: Renal tubular damage, ***anuria***

GI: Nausea, vomiting, anorexia, diarrhea, epigastric pain

CV: Angina, dysrhythmias, tachycardia, hypotension, ***acute circulatory failure***

ENDO: Hypoglycemia

Contraindications: Hypersensitivity, G6PD deficiency, retinal field changes, pregnancy (X)

Precautions: Blood dyscrasias, severe GI disease, neurologic disease, severe hepatic disease, psoriasis, cardiac dysrhythmias, tinnitus

Pharmacokinetics:

PO: Peak 1-3 hr, metabolized in liver, excreted in urine, half-life 4-5 hr

Interactions:

• Toxicity: $NaHCO_3$, acetazolamide

• Decreased absorption: magnesium or aluminum salts

• Increase levels of digoxin, digitoxin, neuromuscular blockers, other anticoagulants

Lab test interferences:

Increase: 17-KS

Interference: 17-OHCS

NURSING CONSIDERATIONS

Assess:

• B/P, pulse, watch for hypotension, tachycardia

• Liver studies qwk: ALT (SGPT), AST (SGOT), bilirubin

• Blood studies, CBC, since blood dyscrasias occur

• For cinchonism: nausea, blurred vision, tinnitus, headache, difficulty focusing

Administer:

• Before or after meals at same time each day to maintain level

Perform/provide:

• Storage in tight, light-resistant container

Evaluate:

• Therapeutic response: decreased symptoms of malaria

Teach patient/family:

• To avoid OTC preparations: cold preparations, tonic water

rabies immune globulin, human (℞)

Hyperab, Imogam

Func. class.: Immune serum

Chem. class.: IgG

Action: Provides passive immunity; given with HDCV; may be used regardless of time of bite, treatment

Uses: Exposure to rabies

Dosage and routes:

• *Adult and child:* IM 20 IU/kg given at same time as 1st rabies vaccine; infiltrate wound with ½ dose, then administer rest IM, 1 ml dose on each of days 3, 7, 14, 28 after 1st dose

R

Available forms: Inj IM 125 IU/ml

Side effects/adverse reactions:

INTEG: Pain at injection site, rash, pruritus

MS: Arthralgia

SYST: Lymphadenopathy, ***anaphylaxis***, fever

CNS: Headache, fatigue, malaise

GI: Abdominal pain

Contraindications: Hypersensitivity to equine products and thimerosal

Interactions:

• Decreased action of rabies immune globulin: corticosteroids, immunosuppressants

NURSING CONSIDERATIONS

Administer:

• Test dose: dilute drug either with 1:100 or 1:1000 0.9% NaCl for inj, inj 0.1 ml 0.9% NaCl in other arm intradermally, check for wheal ≥10 mm after 10 min; if present, drug should not be used

• Only with epinephrine 1:1000, resuscitative equipment available

• As soon as possible after exposure

Perform/provide:

• Storage at 36°-46°F (2°-8°C)

Evaluate:

• Allergic reactions: dyspnea, rash, pruritus, eruptions

Teach patient/family:

• That pain, swelling, itching may occur at injection site

• To take acetaminophen to alleviate headache, fever, and pain

---

radioactive iodine (sodium iodide) ^{131}I (℞)

Func. class.: Antithyroid

Chem. class.: Radiopharmaceutical

Action: Converted to protein-bound iodine by thyroid gland for use when needed

Uses:

High dose: Thyroid cancer, hyperthyroidism

Low dose: Visualization to determine thyroid cancer, diagnostic aid in thyroid function studies

Dosage and routes:

Thyroid cancer

• *Adult:* PO 50-150 mCi, may repeat depending on clinical status

Hyperthyroidism

• *Adult:* PO 4-10 mCi, depending on serum thyroxine level

Available forms: Caps 1-50, 0.8-100 mCi; oral sol 7.05 mCi/ml, 3.5-150 mCi/vial

Side effects/adverse reactions:

ENDO: Hypothyroidism, ***hyperthyroid adenoma,*** transient thyroiditis

INTEG: Alopecia

HEMA: ***Eosinophilia, lymphedema, leukemia, bone marrow depression, leukopenia,*** anemia

GI: Nausea, diarrhea, vomiting

EENT: Sore throat, cough

Contraindications: Recent MI, lactation, large nodular goiter, pregnancy (X), age <30 yr, vomiting/diarrhea, acute hyperthyroidism, use of thyroid drugs, lactation

Pharmacokinetics:

PO: Onset 3-6 days; excreted in urine, sweat, feces, breast milk; crosses placenta; excreted in 56 days

Interactions:

• Hypothyroidism: lithium

• Decreased uptake if recent intake of stable iodine, thyroid, antithyroid drugs

NURSING CONSIDERATIONS

Assess:

• Weight qd in same clothing, scale, time of day

• Blood work, including CBC for blood dyscrasias (leukopenia, thrombocytopenia, agranulocytosis)

• Overdose: peripheral edema, heat intolerance, diaphoresis, palpitations, dysrhythmias, severe tachycardia, increased temp, delirium, CNS irritability
• Hypersensitivity: rash, enlarged cervical lymph nodes; drug may have to be discontinued
• Hypoprothrombinemia: bleeding, petechiae, ecchymosis
• Clinical response: after 3 wk should include increased weight, pulse; decreased T_4
• Bone marrow depression: sore throat, fever, fatigue

Administer:
• Only after discontinuing all other antithyroid agents × 5-7 days
• After NPO overnight, food delays action
• During or within 10 days after menstruation

Perform/provide:
• Limited contact with patient ½ hr/day for each person
• Adequate rest after treatment
• Fluids to 3-4 L/day for 48 hr to remove agent from body

Evaluate:
• Therapeutic response: weight gain, decreased pulse, decreased T_4, B/P

Teach patient/family:
• To empty bladder often during treatment; avoids irradiation of gonads
• To report redness, swelling, sore throat, mouth lesions; indicate blood dyscrasias
• To avoid extended contact with children, spouse for 1 wk
• That bathroom may be used by entire family
• Not to take antithyroid agents but propranolol, which decreases hyperthyroid symptoms, until total effects of taking ^{131}I has occurred (about 6 wk)
• To avoid coughing, expectorating for 24 hr (saliva and vomitus are highly radioactive for 6-8 hr)

ramipril (℞)

(ra-mi'pril)
Altace
Func. class.: Antihypertensive
Chem. class.: Angiotensin-converting enzyme (ACE) inhibitor

Action: Selectively suppresses renin-angiotensin-aldosterone system; inhibits ACE, prevents conversion of angiotensin I to angiotensin II; results in dilation of arterial, venous vessels

Uses: Hypertension, alone or in combination with thiazide diuretics

Dosage and routes:
• *Adult:* PO 2.5 mg qd initially, then 2.5-20 mg/day divided bid or qd; renal impairment: 1.25 mg qd with CrCl <40 ml/min/1.73 m^2, increase as needed to max or 5 mg/day

Available forms: Caps 1.25, 2.5, 5, 10 mg

Side effects/adverse reactions:
CV: Hypotension, chest pain, palpitations, angina, syncope, dysrhythmia
GU: ***Proteinuria,*** increased BUN, creatinine, impotence
HEMA: Decreased Hct, Hgb, ***eosinophilia, leukopenia***
INTEG: ***Angioedema,*** rash, sweating, photosensitivity, pruritus
RESP: Cough, dyspnea
META: Hyperkalemia
GI: Nausea, constipation, vomiting, dyspepsia, dysphagia, anorexia, diarrhea, abdominal pain
CNS: Headache, dizziness, anxiety, insomnia, paresthesia, fatigue, depression, malaise, vertigo, ***convulsions,*** hearing loss
MS: Arthralgia, arthritis, myalgia

R

Contraindications: Hypersensitivity to ACE inhibitors, pregnancy (D), lactation, children

Precautions: Impaired renal, liver function, dialysis patients, hypovolemia, blood dyscrasias, CHF, COPD, asthma, elderly

Pharmacokinetics:

PO: Peak ½-1 hr, serum protein binding 97%, half-life 1-2 hr, metabolized by liver (metabolites excreted in urine, feces)

Interactions:

• Increased hypotension: diuretics, other antihypertensives, ganglionic blockers, adrenergic blockers

• Increased toxicity: vasodilators, hydralazine, prazosin, K-sparing diuretics, sympathomimetics, K supplements

• Decreased absorption: antacids

• Decreased antihypertensive effect: indomethacin

• Increased serum levels of digoxin, lithium

• Increased hypersensitivity: allopurinol

Lab test interferences:

False positive: Urine acetone

NURSING CONSIDERATIONS

Assess:

• Blood studies: neutrophils, decreased platelets

• B/P, orthostatic hypotension, syncope

• Renal studies: protein, BUN, creatinine; increased levels may indicate nephrotic syndrome

• Baselines in renal, liver function tests before therapy begins

• K levels, although hyperkalemia rarely occurs

• Dipstick of urine for protein qd in first morning specimen; if protein is increased, a 24-hr urinary protein should be collected

• Edema in feet, legs qd

• Allergic reactions: rash, fever, pruritus, urticaria; drug should be discontinued if antihistamines fail to help

• Renal symptoms: polyuria, oliguria, frequency, dysuria

Administer:

• IV inf 0.9% NaCl (as ordered) to expand fluid volume if severe hypotension occurs

Perform/provide:

• Storage in tight container at 48° F (30° C) or less

• Supine or Trendelenburg position for severe hypotension

Evaluate:

• Therapeutic response: decrease in B/P

Teach patient/family:

• Not to discontinue drug abruptly

• Not to use OTC products (cough, cold, allergy) unless directed by prescriber; not to use salt substitutes containing potassium without consulting prescriber

• To comply with dosage schedule, even if feeling better

• To rise slowly to sitting or standing position to minimize orthostatic hypotension

• To notify prescriber of mouth sores, sore throat, fever, swelling of hands or feet, irregular heartbeat, chest pain

• To report excessive perspiration, dehydration, vomiting, diarrhea; may lead to fall in B/P

• That drug may cause dizziness, fainting, light-headedness; may occur during 1st few days of therapy

• That drug may cause skin rash or impaired perspiration

• How to take B/P, and normal readings for age group

Treatment of overdose: 0.9% NaCl IV Inf, hemodialysis

ranitidine (℞)

(ra-nit′i-deen)

Apo-Ranitidine*, Zantac, Zantac C*, Zantac EFFERdose

Func. class.: H_2-histamine receptor antagonist

Action: Inhibits histamine at H_2 receptor site in parietal cells, which inhibits gastric acid secretion

Uses: Duodenal ulcer, Zollinger-Ellison syndrome, gastric ulcers, hypersecretory conditions, gastroesophageal reflux disease, stress ulcers, erosive esophagitis (maintenance)

Investigational uses: Prevention of aspiration pneumonitis, stress ulcers, upper GI bleeding

Dosage and routes:

• *Adult:* PO 150 mg bid, 300 mg hs; IM 50 mg q6-8h; IV BOL 50 mg diluted to 20 ml over 5 min q6-8h; IV INT INF 50 mg/100 ml D_5 over 15-20 min, q6-8h

Available forms: Tabs 150, 300 mg; tabs, effervescent 150 mg; inj 0.5, 25 mg/ml; caps 150, 300 mg; syr 15 mg/ml; granules, effervescent 150 mg

Side effects/adverse reactions:

CNS: Headache, sleeplessness, dizziness, confusion, agitation, depression, hallucination

GI: Constipation, abdominal pain, diarrhea, nausea, vomiting, ***hepatotoxicity***

GU: Impotence, gynecomastia

CV: Tachycardia, bradycardia, PVCs

EENT: Blurred vision, increased ocular pressure

INTEG: Urticaria, rash, fever

Contraindications: Hypersensitivity

Precautions: Pregnancy (B), lactation, child <12 yr, hepatic disease, renal disease

Pharmacokinetics:

PO: Peak 2-3 hr, duration 8-12 hr; metabolized by liver; excreted in urine, breast milk; half-life 2-3 hr

Interactions:

• Increased absorption, toxicity: anticoagulants, sufonylureas, procainamide

• Decreased absorption of ranitidine: antacids, diazepam, anticholinergics, metoclopramide

Syringe compatibilities: Atropine, cyclizine, dexamethasone, dimenhydrinate, diphenhydramine, fentanyl, glycopyrrolate, hydromorphone, meperidine, metoclopramide, morphine, nalbuphine, oxymorphone, pentazocine, perphenizine, prochlorperazine, promethazine, scopolamine, thiethyl perazine

Y-site compatibilities: Acyclovir, aminophylline, atracurium, bretylium, dobutamine, dopamine, enalaprilat, esmolol, fludarabine, foscarnet, heparin, labetalol, meperidine, morphine, nitroglycerin, ondansetron, pancuronium, procainamide, sargramostim, vecuronium, zidovudine

Additive compatibilities: Amikacin, chloramphenicol, doxycycline, furosemide, gentamicin, heparin, lidocaine, penicillin G sodium, potassium chloride, ticarcillin, tobramycin, vancomycin

Lab test interferences:

Increase: AST (SGOT), ALT (SGPT), alk phosphatase, creatinine, LDH, bilirubin

False positive: Urine protein

NURSING CONSIDERATIONS

Assess:

• Gastric pH (>5 should be maintained)

• I&O ratio, BUN, creatinine

• Mental status: confusion, dizziness, depression, anxiety, weakness, tremors, psychosis, diarrhea, ab-

R

dominal discomfort, jaundice; report immediately
• GI complaints: nausea, vomiting, diarrhea, cramps

Administer:
• With meals for prolonged effect
• Antacids 1 hr before or 1 hr after ranitidine
• IV after diluting 50 mg/20 ml NS, D_5W, $D_{10}W$, LR, $NaCO_3$ 5% and give 50 mg or less/5 min or more; may dilute 50 mg/50-100 ml of 0.9% NaCl, D_5W, $D_{10}W$, LR, $NaCO_3$ 5% and give over 15-20 min

Perform/provide:
• Storage at room temp

Evaluate:
• Therapeutic response: decreased abdominal pain

Teach patient/family:
• That gynecomastia, impotence may occur but are reversible
• To avoid driving, other hazardous activities until stabilized on this medication
• To avoid black pepper, caffeine, alcohol, harsh spices, extremes in temp of food
• That drug must be continued for prescribed time to be effective

reserpine (℞)

(re-ser′peen)

Novoreserpine*, Reserfia*, reserpine, Serpasil

Func. class.: Antihypertensive

Chem. class.: Antiadrenergic agent, peripheral action

Combination products: Chloroserp-250, Chloroserpine-250, Diupres-250: reserpine 0.125 mg with chlorothiazide 250 mg; Chloroserp-500, Chloroserpine-500, Diupres-500: reserpine 0.125 mg with chlorothiazide 500 mg; Hydromox R: quinethazone 50 mg with reserpine 0.125 mg; Hydropres-25, Hydro-Reserpine-25, Hydroserp, Hydroserpine No. 1, Hydrosine 25 mg, Mallopress: reserpine 0.125 mg with hydrochlorothiazide 25 mg; Hydropres-50, Hydro-Reserpine-50, Hydroserp, Hydroserpine No. 2, Hydrosine 50 mg, Hydrotensin, Hydorserpalan: reserpine 0.125 mg with hydrochlorothiazide 50 mg; Regroton: reserpine 0.25 mg, chlorthalidone 50 mg; Renese-R: reserpine 0.25 mg, polythiazide 2 mg; Serpasil-Esidrix No. 1: reserpine 0.1 mg, hydrochlorothiazide 25 mg; Serpasil-Esidrix No. 2: reserpine 0.1 mg, hydrochlorothiazide 50 mg

Action: Inhibits norepinephrine release, depleting norepinephrine stores in adrenergic nerve endings

Uses: Hypertension

Dosage and routes:

Hypertension
• *Adult:* PO 0.25-0.5 mg qd × 1-2 wk, then 0.1-0.25 mg qd maintenance

Available forms: Tabs 0.1, 0.25

Side effects/adverse reactions:

CV: Bradycardia, chest pain, dysrhythmias, prolonged bleeding time, ***thrombocytopenia,*** purpura

CNS: Drowsiness, fatigue, lethargy, dizziness, depression, anxiety, headache, increased dreaming, nightmares, convulsions, parkinsonism, EPS (high doses)

GI: Nausea, vomiting, cramps, peptic ulcer, dry mouth, increased appetite, anorexia

INTEG: Rash, purpura, alopecia, flushing, warm feeling, pruritus, ecchymosis

EENT: Lacrimation, miosis, blurred vision, ptosis, dry mouth, epistaxis

GU: Impotence, dysuria, nocturia, Na and H_2O retention, edema, breast engorgement, galactorrhea, gynecomastia

* Available in Canada only

RESP: ***Bronchospasm,*** dyspnea, cough, rales

Contraindications: Hypersensitivity, depression, suicidal patients, active peptic ulcer disease, ulcerative colitis, pregnancy (D), Parkinson's disease

Precautions: Lactation, seizure disorders, renal disease

Pharmacokinetics:

PO: Peak 4 hr, duration 2-6 wk; half-life 50-100 hr; metabolized by liver; excreted in urine, feces, breast milk; crosses placenta; blood-brain barrier

Interactions:

- Increased hypotension: diuretics, hypotension, β-blockers, methotrimeprazine
- Dysrhythmias: cardiac glycosides
- Increased cardiac depression: quinidine, procainamide
- Excitation, hypertension: MAOIs, avoid use
- Increased CNS depression: barbiturates, alcohol, narcotics
- Increased pressor effects: epinephrine, isoproterenol, norepinephrine
- Decreased pressor effects: ephedrine, amphetamine

Lab test interferences:

Increase: VMA excretion, 5-HIAA excretion

Interferences: 17-OHCS, 17-KS

NURSING CONSIDERATIONS

Assess:

- Renal function studies in renal impairment (BUN, creatinine)
- Bleeding time; check for ecchymosis, thrombocytopenia, purpura
- I&O in renal disease patient
- Cardiac status: B/P, pulse; watch for hypotension, bradycardia
- Edema in feet, legs qd; take weight qd
- Skin turgor, dryness of mucous membranes for hydration status
- Symptoms of CHF: edema, dyspnea, wet rales

Evaluate:

- Therapeutic response: decreased hypertension

Teach patient/family:

- To avoid driving, hazardous activities if drowsiness occurs
- Not to discontinue drug abruptly
- Not to use OTC products (cough, cold preparations) unless directed by prescriber
- To report bradycardia, dizziness, confusion, depression, fever, sore throat
- That impotence, gynecomastia may occur but are reversible
- To rise slowly to sitting or standing position to minimize orthostatic hypotension
- That therapeutic effect may take 2-4 wk

Treatment of overdose: Lavage, IV atropine for bradycardia, supportive therapy

RH_o(D) immune globulin, human (℞)

HypoRho D, MICRhoGAM, Mini-Gamulin RH, Hydro Rho D Mini-Dose, Gamulin Rh, Rhesonatre Rho-Gam

Func. class.: Immunizing agent

Chem. class.: IgG

Action: Suppresses immune response of nonsensitized Rh_o (D or D^u)-negative patients who are exposed to Rh_o (D or D^u)-positive blood

Uses: Prevention of isoimmunization in Rh-negative women given Rh-positive blood after abortions, miscarriages, amniocentesis

Dosage and routes:

Prior delivery

- *Adult:* IM 1 vial (standard dose) at 26-28 wk, 1 vial (standard dose) 72 hr after delivery

R

Pregnancy termination <13 wk
• *Adult:* IM 1 vial (microdose) within 72 hr
Following delivery
• *Adult:* IM 1 vial if fetal packed RBCs <15 ml, or 2 vials if fetal packed RBCs >15 ml; given within 72 hr of delivery or miscarriage
Transfusion error
• *Adult:* IM give within 72 hr
Available forms: Inj single-dose vial (50 µg/vial-microdose; 300 µg/vial-standard)
Side effects/adverse reactions:
INTEG: Irritation at inj site, fever
CNS: Lethargy
MS: Myalgia
Contraindications: Previous immunization with this drug, Rh_o (O)-positive/D^u-positive patient
NURSING CONSIDERATIONS
Assess:
• Allergies, reactions to immunizations; previous immunization with this drug
Administer:
• After sending newborn's cord blood to lab after delivery for cross-match, type; infant must be Rh-positive, with Rh-negative mother
• IM in deltoid; aspirate
• Only equal lot numbers of drug, cross-match
• Only MICRhoGAM for abortions or miscarriages <12 wk unless fetus or father is Rh^-; unless patient is Rh_o (D)-positive, D^u-positive, Rh antibodies are present
Evaluate:
• Rho (D) sensitivity in transfusion error, prevention of erythroblastosis fetalis
Perform/provide:
• Storage in refrigerator
Teach patient/family:
• How drug works; that drug must be given after subsequent deliveries if subsequent babies are Rh positive

riboflavin (vit B_2) (OTC)
(rye'boo-flay-vin)
Func. class.: Vit B_2, water soluble

Action: Needed for respiratory reactions by catalyzing proteins and for normal vision
Uses: Vit B_2 deficiency or polyneuritis; cheilosis adjunct with thiamine
Dosage and routes:
• *Adult and child >12 yr:* PO 5-50 mg qd in divided doses
• *Child <12 yr:* PO 2-10 mg qd, then 0.6 mg/1000 calories ingested
Available forms: Tabs 10, 25, 50, 100 mg
Side effects/adverse reactions:
GU: Yellow discoloration of urine (large doses)
Contraindications: Child <12 yr
Precautions: Pregnancy (A)
Pharmacokinetics:
PO: Half-life 65-85 min, 60% protein-bound, unused amounts excreted in urine (unchanged)
Interactions:
• Decreased action of tetracyclines
Lab test interferences:
• May cause false elevations of urinary catecholamines
NURSING CONSIDERATIONS
Assess:
• Nutritional status: liver, eggs, dairy products, yeast, whole grain, green vegetables
Administer:
• With food for better absorption
Perform/provide:
• Storage in air-tight, light-resistant container
Evaluate:
• Therapeutic response: absence of headache, GI problems, cheilosis,

skin lesions, depression, burning, itchy eyes, anemia

Teach patient/family:

- That urine may turn bright yellow
- About addition of needed foods that are rich in riboflavin
- To avoid alcohol

rifabutin (℞)

(riff'a-byoo-ten)

Mycobutin

Func. class.: Antimycobacterial agent

Chem. class.: Rifamycin S derivative

Action: Inhibits DNA-dependent RNA polymerase in susceptible strains of *E. coli* and *B. subtilis;* mechanism of action against *M. avium* unknown

Uses: Prevention of *M. avium* complex in patients with advanced HIV infection

Dosage and routes:

- *Adult:* 300 mg qd (may take as 150 mg bid)

Available forms: Caps 150 mg

Side effects/adverse reactions:

INTEG: Rash

MS: Asthenia, arthralgia, myalgia

MISC: Flulike syndrome, shortness of breath, chest pressure

GI: Nausea, vomiting, anorexia, diarrhea, heartburn, hepatitis

GU: Hematuria

CNS: Headache, fatigue, anxiety, confusion, insomnia

HEMA: ***Hemolytic anemia, eosinophilia, thrombocytopenia, leukopenia***

Contraindications: Hypersensitivity, active TB

Precautions: Pregnancy (B), lactation, hepatic disease, blood dyscrasias, children

Pharmacokinetics:

PO: Peak 2-3 hr, duration >24 hr, half-life 3 hr; metabolized in liver (active/inactive metabolites), excreted in urine primarily as metabolites

Interactions:

- Decreased action: barbiturates, clofibrate, corticosteroids, dapsone, anticoagulants, sulfonylureas, estrogens, digitoxin and digoxin, oral contraceptives, theophylline, β-blockers
- Rifabutin does not appear to alter the acetylation of INH

Lab test interferences:

Interference: Folate level, Vit B_{12}, BSP, gallbladder studies

NURSING CONSIDERATIONS

Assess:

- CBC for neutropenia, thrombocytopenia, eosinophilia
- For acute TB: chest x-ray, sputum culture, blood culture, biopsy of lymph nodes, PPD; drug should not be given for acute TB
- Signs of anemia: Hct, Hgb, fatigue
- Liver studies qwk: ALT (SGPT), AST (SGOT), bilirubin
- Renal status before, qmo: BUN, creatinine, output, specific gravity, urinalysis
- Hepatic studies: decreased appetite, jaundice, dark urine, fatigue

Administer:

- With food if GI upset occurs; better to take on empty stomach 1 hr ac or 2 hr pc, fat foods slow absorption
- Antiemetic if vomiting occurs
- After C&S is completed; qmo to detect resistance

Evaluate:

- Therapeutic response: not used for active TB because of risk of development of resistance to rifampin; culture negative

Teach patient/family:

- That patients using oral contraceptives should consider using non-

R

hormonal methods of birth control, since rifabutin may decrease their efficacy

• That compliance with dosage schedule, duration is necessary

• That scheduled appointments must be kept; relapse may occur

• That urine, feces, saliva, sputum, sweat, tears may be colored red-orange; soft contact lenses may be permanently stained

• To report flulike symptoms: excessive fatigue, anorexia, vomiting, sore throat; unusual bleeding, yellowish discoloration of skin, eyes

rifampin (℞)

(rif′am-pin)

Rifadin, Rifampicin, Rimactane, Rofact*

Func. class.: Antitubercular

Chem. class.: Rifamycin B derivative

Action: Inhibits DNA-dependent polymerase, decreases tubercle bacilli replication

Uses: Pulmonary tuberculosis, meningococcal carriers (prevention)

Dosage and routes:

Tuberculosis

• *Adult:* PO/IV 600 mg/day as single dose 1 hr ac or 2 hr pc or 10 mg/kg/day

• *Child >5 yr:* PO/IV 10-20 mg/kg/day as single dose 1 hr ac or 2 hr pc, not to exceed 600 mg/day, with other antituberculars

Meningococcal carriers

• *Adult:* PO/IV 600 mg bid × 2 days

• *Child >5 yr:* PO/IV 10 mg/kg bid × 2 days, not to exceed 600 mg/dose

• *Infant 3 mo-1 yr:* 5 mg/kg PO bid for 2 days

Available forms: Caps 150, 300 mg; inj 600 mg/vial

Side effects/adverse reactions:

INTEG: Rash, pruritus, urticaria

EENT: Visual disturbances

MS: Atoxia, weakness

MISC: Flulike syndrome, menstrual disturbances, edema, shortness of breath

GI: Nausea, vomiting, anorexia, diarrhea, ***pseudomembranous colitis,*** *heartburn,* sore mouth and tongue, ***pancreatitis***

GU: ***Hematuria, acute renal failure, hemoglobinuria***

CNS: Headache, fatigue, anxiety, drowsiness, confusion

HEMA: ***Hemolytic anemia, eosinophilia, thrombocytopenia, leukopenia***

Contraindications: Hypersensitivity

Precautions: Pregnancy (C), lactation, hepatic disease, blood dyscrasias

Pharmacokinetics:

PO: Peak 2-3 hr, duration >24 hr, half-life 3 hr; metabolized in liver (active/inactive metabolites), excreted in urine as free drug (30% crosses placenta), excreted in breast milk

Interactions:

• Decreased action: barbiturates, clofibrate, corticosteroids, dapsone, anticoagulants, antidiabetics, hormones, digoxin, PAS, alcohol, oral contraceptives

• Hepatotoxicity: INH

• Incompatible with sodium lactate

Lab test interferences:

Interference: Folate level, vit B_{12}, BSP, gallbladder studies

NURSING CONSIDERATIONS

Assess:

• For infection: sputum culture, lung sounds

• Signs of anemia: Hct, Hgb, fatigue

• Liver studies qwk: ALT (SGPT), AST (SGOT), bilirubin

* Available in Canada only

• Renal status before, qmo: BUN, creatinine, output, specific gravity, urinalysis
• Hepatic status: decreased appetite, jaundice, dark urine, fatigue

Administer:
• IV after diluting each 600 mg/10 ml of sterile water for inj (60 mg/ml), agitate, withdraw dose and dilute in 100 ml or 500 ml of D_5W or 0.9% NaCl given as an inf over 3 hr, or if diluted in 100 ml, give over ½ hr
• PO on empty stomach, 1 hr ac or 2 hr pc
• Antiemetic if vomiting occurs
• After C&S is completed; qmo to detect resistance

Evaluate:
• Therapeutic response: decreased symptoms of TB, culture negative

Teach patient/family:
• That compliance with dosage schedule, duration is necessary
• That scheduled appointments must be kept; relapse may occur
• To avoid alcohol
• That urine, feces, saliva, sputum, sweat, tears may be colored red-orange; soft contact lenses may be permanently stained
• To report flulike symptoms: excessive fatigue, anorexia, vomiting, sore throat; unusual bleeding, yellowish discoloration of skin, eyes

rimantadine (℞)

(ri-man′ti-deen)

Flumadine

Func. class.: Synthetic antiviral
Chem. class.: Tricyclic amine

Action: Prevents uncoating of nucleic acid in viral cell, preventing penetration of virus to host; causes release of dopamine from neurons

Uses: Prophylaxis or treatment of influenza type A

Dosage and routes:
Influenza type A
Prophylaxis
• *Adult:* PO 100 mg bid; in renal hepatic disease, lower dose to 100 mg/day
• *Child <10 yr:* PO 5 mg/kg/day, not to exceed 150 mg

Treatment
• *Adult:* PO 100 mg bid; in renal or hepatic disease, lower dose to 100 mg/day; start treatment at onset of symptoms, continue for at least 1 wk

Available forms: Tabs 100 mg; syrup 50 mg/5 ml

Side effects/adverse reactions:
CNS: Headache, dizziness, fatigue, depression, hallucinations, tremors, ***convulsions,*** insomnia, poor concentration, asthenia, gait abnormalities
CV: Pallor, palpitations, hypertension
EENT: Tinnitus, taste abnormality, eye pain
GI: Nausea, vomiting, constipation, dry mouth, anorexia, abdominal pain, diarrhea, dyspepsia
INTEG: Rash

Contraindications: Hypersensitivity, lactation, child <1 yr, pregnancy (C)

Precautions: Epilepsy, hepatic disease, renal disease

Pharmacokinetics:
PO: Peak 6 hr, elimination half-life 25½ hr, plasma protein binding (40%)

Interactions:
• Decreased peak concentration of rimantadine: acetaminophen, aspirin

NURSING CONSIDERATIONS

Assess:
• I&O ratio; report frequency, hesitancy in renal disease
• Bowel pattern before, during treatment

R

• Skin eruptions, photosensitivity after administration of drug
• Respiratory status: rate, character, wheezing, tightness in chest
• Allergies before initiation of treatment, reaction of each medication; list allergies on chart in bright red letters
• Signs of infection

Administer:
• Before exposure to influenza; continue for 10 days after contact
• At least 4 hr before hs to prevent insomnia
• After meals for better absorption, to decrease GI symptoms
• In divided doses to prevent CNS disturbances: headache, dizziness, fatigue, drowsiness

Perform/provide:
• Storage in tight, dry container

Evaluate:
• Therapeutic response: absence of fever, malaise, cough, dyspnea in infection

Teach patient/family:
• About aspects of drug therapy: need to report dyspnea, dizziness, poor concentration, behavioral changes
• To avoid hazardous activities if dizziness occurs

Treatment of overdose:
Withdraw drug, maintain airway, administer epinephrine, aminophylline, O_2, IV corticosteroids, physostigmine

rimexolone (℞)

(ri-mex'a-lone)
Vexol
Func. class.: Ophthalmic corticosteroid

Action: Reduces inflammation, resulting in decreased pain, photophobia, hyperemia, cellular infiltration

Uses: Postoperative inflammation after ocular surgery; treatment of anterior uveitis

Dosage and routes:
Post operative inflammation
• *Adult:* INSTILL 1-2 gtts in the conjunctival sac qid; begin treatment 24 hrs after surgery, continue treatment 14 days post op
Anterior uveitis
• *Adult:* INSTILL 1-2 gtts in the conjunctival sac qh while awake × 7 days, then 1 gtt × 7 days, then taper

Available forms: Ophth susp 1%

Side effects/adverse reactions:
EENT: Increased intraocular pressure, poor corneal wound healing, increased possibility of corneal infection, glaucoma exacerbation, *optic nerve damage,* decreased acuity, visual field, cataracts

Contraindications: Hypersensitivity, acute superficial herpes simplex, fungal, viral diseases of eye or conjunctiva, active diabetes mellitus, ocular TB, eye infections

Precautions: Corneal abrasions, glaucoma, pregnancy (C)

NURSING CONSIDERATIONS

Perform/provide:
• Store in light-resistant container

Evaluate:
• Therapeutic response: absence of swelling, redness, exudate

Teach patient/family:
• Instillation method: pressure on lacrimal duct for 1 min, to shake before using, not to discontinue abruptly, taper over 1-2 wk
• Not to share eye medications
• Not to use if purulent drainage is present

risperidone (℞)

(res-pare'a-done)
Risperdal
Func. class.: Antipsychotic/ neuroleptic
Chem. class.: Benzisoxazole derivative

Action: Unknown; may be mediated through both dopamine type 2 (D_2) and serotonin type 2 ($5\text{-}HT_2$) antagonism

Uses: Psychotic disorders

Dosage and routes:

• *Adult:* PO 1 mg bid, with incremental increases of 1 mg bid on days 2 and 3 to a dose of 3 mg bid by day 3; then do not increase dose for at least 1 wk

Available forms: Tabs 1, 2, 3, 4 mg

Side effects/adverse reactions:

CNS: EPS, pseudoparkinsonism, akathisia, dystonia, tardive dyskinesia; drowsiness, insomnia, agitation, anxiety, headache, seizures, ***neuroleptic malignant syndrome***

CV: Orthostatic hypotension, ***tachycardia***

EENT: Blurred vision

GI: Nausea, vomiting, *anorexia, constipation,* jaundice, weight gain

RESP: Rhinitis

Contraindications: Hypersensitivity, lactation, seizure disorders

Precautions: Children, renal disease, pregnancy (C), hepatic disease, elderly, breast cancer

Pharmacokinetics:

PO: Extensively metabolized by liver to a major active metabolite, plasma protein binding 90%

Interactions:

• Increased sedation: other CNS depressants, alcohol

• Increased EPS: other antipsychotics, lithium

Lab test interferences:
Not known

NURSING CONSIDERATIONS

Assess:

• Mental status before initial administration

• Swallowing of PO medication; check for hoarding or giving of medication to other patients

• I&O ratio; palpate bladder if urinary output is low

• Bilirubin, CBC, liver function studies qmo

• Urinalysis before, during prolonged therapy

• Affect, orientation, LOC, reflexes, gait, coordination, sleep pattern disturbances

• B/P standing and lying; also pulse, respirations; take these q4h during initial treatment; establish baseline before starting treatment; report drops of 30 mm Hg; watch for ECG changes

• Dizziness, faintness, palpitations, tachycardia on rising

• EPS, including akathisia (inability to sit still, no pattern to movements), tardive dyskinesia (bizarre movements of the jaw, mouth, tongue, extremities), pseudoparkinsonism (rigidity, tremors, pill rolling, shuffling gait)

• For neuroleptic malignant syndrome: hyperthermia, increased CPK, altered mental status, muscle rigidity

• Skin turgor qd

• Constipation, urinary retention qd; if these occur, increase bulk and water in diet

Administer:

• Reduced dose in elderly

• Antiparkinsonian agent on order from prescriber, to be used for EPS

Perform/provide:

• Decreased stimulus by dimming lights, avoiding loud noises

• Supervised ambulation until patient is stabilized on medication; do not involve in strenuous exercise program because fainting is possible; patient should not stand still for a long time
• Increased fluids to prevent constipation
• Sips of water, candy, gum for dry mouth
• Storage in tight, light-resistant container

Evaluate:
• Therapeutic response: decrease in emotional excitement, hallucinations, delusions, paranoia; reorganization of patterns of thought, speech

Teach patient/family:
• That orthostatic hypotension may occur and to rise from sitting or lying position gradually
• To avoid hot tubs, hot showers, tub baths; hypotension may occur
• To avoid abrupt withdrawal of this drug; EPS may result; drug should be withdrawn slowly
• To avoid OTC preparations (cough, hay fever, cold) unless approved by prescriber, since serious drug interactions may occur; avoid use with alcohol, CNS depressants; increased drowsiness may occur
• To avoid hazardous activities if drowsy or dizzy
• Compliance with drug regimen
• To report impaired vision, tremors, muscle twitching
• In hot weather, that heat stroke may occur; take extra precautions to stay cool

Treatment of overdose: Lavage if orally ingested; provide airway; *do not induce vomiting*

ritodrine (℞)

(ri′toe-dreen)
ritodrine, Yutopar
Func. class.: Tocolytic, uterine relaxant
Chem. class.: β_2-adrenergic agonist

Action: Reduces frequency, intensity of uterine contractions by stimulation of the β_2 receptors in uterine smooth muscle

Uses: Management of preterm labor

Dosage and routes:
• Adult: IV INF 150 mg/500 ml (0.3 mg/ml) given 0.1 mg/min, increased gradually by 0.05 mg/min q10min until desired response

Available forms: Inj 10 mg/ml, 15 mg/ml

Side effects/adverse reactions:
MISC: Erythema, rash, dyspnea, hyperventilation, glycosuria, ***lactic acidosis***
META: Hyperglycemia, hypokalemia
CNS: Headache, restlessness, anxiety, nervousness, sweating, chills, drowsiness, tremor
GI: Nausea, vomiting, anorexia, malaise, bloating, constipation, diarrhea
CV: Altered maternal, fetal heart rate, B/P, dysrhythmias, palpitation, chest pain, maternal pulmonary edema

Contraindications: Hypersensitivity, eclampsia, hypertension, dysrhythmias, thyrotoxicosis, before 20th wk of pregnancy, antepartum hemorrhage, intrauterine fetal death, maternal cardiac disease, pulmonary hypertension, uncontrolled diabetes, pheochromocytoma, bronchial asthma

* Available in Canada only

Precautions: Migraine, sulfite sensitivity, pregnancy-induced hypertension, diabetes

Pharmacokinetics:

IV: Immediate, distribution half-life 6 min, 2nd phase 1½-2½ hr, elimination phase >10 hr; metabolized in liver; 90% excreted in urine; crosses placenta

Interactions:

- Pulmonary edema: corticosteroids
- Increased CV effects of ritodrine: magnesium sulfate, diazoxide, meperidine, potent general anesthetics
- Increased effects of sympathomimetic amines
- Systemic hypertension: atropine
- Decreased action of ritodrine: β-blockers
- Considered incompatible with any drug in sol or syringe

Lab test interferences:

Increase: Blood glucose, free fatty acids, insulin, GTT

Decrease: K

NURSING CONSIDERATIONS

Assess:

- Maternal, fetal heart tones during infusion
- Intensity, length of uterine contractions
- Fluid intake to prevent fluid overload; discontinue if this occurs
- Blood glucose in diabetics

Administer:

- Only clear sol
- After dilution: 150 mg/500 ml D_5W or NS, give at 0.3 mg/ml
- Using infusion pump

Perform/provide:

- Positioning of patient in left lateral recumbent position to decrease hypotension, increase renal blood flow

Evaluate:

- Therapeutic response: decreased intensity, length of contraction, absence of preterm labor, decreased B/P

Teach patient/family:

- To remain in bed during infusion

rocuronium (℞)

(ro-kyů(ə)r-roe′nium)

Zemuron

Func. class.: Neuromuscular blocker (nondepolarizing)

Chem. class.: Biquaternary ammonium ester

Action: Inhibits transmission of nerve impulses by binding with cholinergic receptor sites, antagonizing action of acetylcholine

Uses: Facilitation of endotracheal intubation, skeletal muscle relaxation during mechanical ventilation, surgery, or general anesthesia

Dosage and routes:

Intubation

- *Adult:* IV 0.6 mg/kg

Available forms: Inj IV 10 mg/ml

Side effects/adverse reactions:

CV: Bradycardia, tachycardia, change in B/P

RESP: ***Prolonged apnea, bronchospasm, cyanosis, respiratory depression***

GI: Nausea, vomiting

INTEG: Rash, flushing, pruritus, urticaria

Contraindications: Hypersensitivity

Precautions: Pregnancy (C), cardiac disease, lactation, child <2 yr, electrolyte imbalances, dehydration, neuromuscular disease, respiratory disease

Pharmacokinetics: Half-life 71-203 min, duration ½ hr

Interactions:

- Blocked action of rocuronium: phenylephrine

• Increased effect of rocuronium: anesthetics

NURSING CONSIDERATIONS

Assess:

• For electrolyte imbalances (K, Mg), before drug is used; electrolyte imbalances may lead to increased action of this drug

• Vital signs (B/P, pulse, respirations, airway) until fully recovered; rate, depth, pattern of respirations, strength of hand grip; patient should be intubated before use

• Recovery: decreased paralysis of face, diaphragm, leg, arm, rest of body; residual weakness and respiratory problems may occur during recovery

• Allergic reactions: rash, fever, respiratory distress, pruritus; drug should be discontinued

Administer:

• Using peripheral nerve stimulator by anesthesiologist to determine neuromuscular blockade; deep tendon reflexes should be monitored during extended use

• Undiluted direct IV over 2 min (only by qualified person, usually anesthesiologist); do not administer IM

• Maintenance q20-45min after 1st dose; titrate to response

Perform/provide:

• Storage in light-resistant area

• Reassurance if communication is difficult during recovery from neuromuscular blockade

Teach patient/family

• About all procedures or treatments; patient will remain conscious if anesthesia is not given also

Evaluate:

Therapeutic response: paralysis of jaw, eyelid, head, neck, rest of body as evaluated by peripheral nerve stimulator

Treatment of overdose: Edrophonium or neostigmine, atropine, monitor VS; may require mechanical ventilation

salicylic acid (OTC)

Calicylic Creme, Clear Away, Clear Away Plantar, Compound W, Duofilm, Freezone, Gordofilm, Hydrisalic, Keralyt, Lactisol, Lactisol Forte, Mediplast, Mosco, Occlusal, Occlusal HP, Off-Ezy Wart Remover, Panscol, Paplex Ultra, Pediapatch, Sal-Acid, Salacid 25%, Salacid 60%, Salactic Film, Salicylic Acid Creme 60%, Sal Plant, Trans-Ver-Sal, Trans-Plantar, Vergogel Duoplant for Feet, Verukan HP Paplex, Viranol Gel Ultra, Viranol, Wart-Off, Wart Remover

Func. class.: Keratolytic

Action: Corrects abnormal keratinization and causes peeling of skin

Uses: Dandruff, seborrheic dermatitis, psoriasis, multiple superficial epitheliomatoses

Dosage and routes:

• *Adult:* TOP apply as needed, cover at night

Available forms: Powder, cream 2%, 2.5%, 10%; gel 6%, 17%; oint 3%, 25%, 60%; plaster 40%; pledgets 0.5%; shampoo 2%, 4%; sol 13.6%, 17%; stick 2%; susp 2%, liquid 12%, 16.7%, 17%, 20%, 26%

Side effects/adverse reactions:

INTEG: Irritation, drying

CNS: ***Salicylism: hearing loss, tinnitus, dizziness, confusion, headache, hyperventilation***

Contraindications: Hypersensitivity, diabetes, impaired circulation, use on moles, genital or facial warts

Precautions: Pregnancy (C), diabetes

* Available in Canada only

NURSING CONSIDERATIONS
Assess:
• Platelets, WBC if systemic absorption occurs
• Salicylism: tinnitus, hearing loss, dizziness, confusion, headache, hyperventilation
• Allergic reactions: irritation, redness
Administer:
• Only to intact skin; do not use on inflamed, denuded skin
• After wetting skin; wash thoroughly each AM after treatment
• With occlusive dressing to increase absorption; apply more often to areas where occlusion is impossible
Evaluate:
• Therapeutic response: decrease in dandruff, size of lesions
Teach patient/family:
• To avoid contact with eyes, mucous membranes
• To apply lotion if drying occurs
• To avoid applying to large areas; salicylate toxicity may occur

---

salmeterol (℞)

(sal-met'er-ole)
Serevent
Func. class.: Adrenergic β_2 agonist

Action: Causes bronchodilation by action on β_2 (pulmonary) receptors by increasing levels of cAMP, which relaxes smooth muscle; with very little effect on heart rate, maintains improvement in FEV from 3 to 12 hr; prevents nocturnal asthma symptoms
Uses: Prevention of exercise-induced asthma, bronchospasm
Dosage and routes:
• *Adult:* INH 2 puffs bid (AM and PM)
Available forms: Aerosol

Side effects/adverse reactions:
CNS: Tremors, anxiety, insomnia, headache, dizziness, stimulation, restlessness, hallucinations, flushing, irritability
CV: Palpitations, tachycardia, hypertension, angina, hypotension, dysrhythmias
EENT: Dry nose, irritation of nose and throat
GI: Heartburn, nausea, vomiting
MS: Muscle cramps
RESP: ***Bronchospasm***
Contraindications: Hypersensitivity to sympathomimetics, tachydysrhythmias, severe cardiac disease
Precautions: Lactation, pregnancy (C), cardiac disorders, hyperthyroidism, diabetes mellitus, hypertension, prostatic hypertrophy, narrow-angle glaucoma, seizures
Pharmacokinetics:
Inh: Onset 5-15 min, peak 4 hr, duration 12 hr, metabolized in liver, excreted in urine, breast milk; crosses placenta; blood-brain barrier
Interactions:
• Increased action of aerosol bronchodilators
• Increased action of salmeterol: tricyclic antidepressants, MAOIs
• May inhibit action of salmeterol: other β-blockers

NURSING CONSIDERATIONS
Assess:
• Respiratory function: vital capacity, forced expiratory volume, ABGs, lung sounds, heart rate and rhythm
Administer:
• After shaking; exhale, place mouthpiece in mouth, inhale slowly, hold breath, remove, exhale slowly
• Gum, sips of water for dry mouth
Perform/provide:
• Storage in light-resistant container; do not expose to temps over 86° F (30° C)

S

Evaluate:
- Therapeutic response: absence of dyspnea, wheezing

Teach patient/family:
- Not to use OTC medications; extra stimulation may occur
- Use of inhaler; review package insert with patient
- To avoid getting aerosol in eyes
- To wash inhaler in warm water qd and dry
- To avoid smoking, smoke-filled rooms, persons with respiratory infections

Treatment of overdose: β_2-Adrenergic blocker

salsalate (℞)

(sal-sa'late)

Amigesic, Argesic-SA, Arthra-G, Disalcid, Mono-Gesic, Salflex, salsalate, Salsitab

Func. class.: Nonnarcotic analgesic, nonsteroidal antiinflammatory

Chem. class.: Salicylate

Action: Blocks formation of peripheral prostaglandins, which cause pain and inflammation; antipyretic action results from inhibition of hypothalamic heat-regulating center; does not inhibit platelet aggregation

Uses: Mild to moderate pain or fever, including arthritis, juvenile rheumatoid arthritis

Dosage and routes:
- *Adult:* PO 3 g/day in divided doses

Available forms: Caps 500 mg; tabs 500, 750 mg

Side effects/adverse reactions:

HEMA: ***Thrombocytopenia, agranulocytosis, leukopenia, neutropenia, hemolytic anemia,*** increased pro-time

CNS: Stimulation, drowsiness, dizziness, confusion, ***convulsions,*** headache, flushing, hallucinations, coma

GI: Nausea, vomiting, GI bleeding, diarrhea, heartburn, anorexia, ***hepatotoxicity***

INTEG: Rash, urticaria, bruising

EENT: Tinnitus, hearing loss

CV: Rapid pulse, ***pulmonary edema***

RESP: Wheezing, hyperpnea

ENDO: Hypoglycemia, hyponatremia, hypokalemia, alteration in acid-base balance

Contraindications: Hypersensitivity to salicylates, NSAIDs, GI bleeding, bleeding disorders, children <3 yr, vit K deficiency

Precautions: Anemia, hepatic disease, renal disease, Hodgkin's disease, pregnancy (C), lactation

Pharmacokinetics: Metabolized by liver; excreted by kidneys; half-life 1 hr; highly protein bound; crosses blood-brain barrier and placenta slowly

Interactions:
- Decreased effects of salsalate: antacids, steroids, urinary alkalizers
- Increased blood loss: alcohol, heparin, ibuprofen, warfarin
- Increased effects of anticoagulants, insulin, methotrexate, probenecid
- Decreased effects of spironolactone, sulfinpyrazone, sulfonylmides, loop diuretics
- Toxic effects: PABA
- Decreased blood sugar levels: salicylates

Lab test interferences:

Increase: Coagulation studies, liver function studies, serum uric acid, amylase, CO_2, urinary protein

Decrease: Serum K, PBI, cholesterol, blood glucose

Interference: Urine catecholamines, pregnancy test

* Available in Canada only

NURSING CONSIDERATIONS

Assess:

- Liver function studies: AST, ALT, bilirubin (long-term therapy)
- Renal function studies: BUN, urine creatinine (long-term therapy)
- Blood studies: CBC, Hct, Hgb, pro-time (long-term therapy)
- I&O ratio; decreasing output may indicate renal failure (long-term therapy)
- Hepatotoxicity: dark urine, clay-colored stools, yellow skin, sclera, itching, abdominal pain, fever, diarrhea (long-term therapy)
- Allergic reactions: rash, urticaria; drug may have to be discontinued
- Ototoxicity: tinnitus, ringing, roaring in ears; audiometric testing is needed before, after long-term therapy
- Visual changes: blurring, halos, corneal and retinal damage
- Edema in feet, ankles, legs
- Drug history; many interactions

Administer:

- To patient crushed or whole; chewable tablets may be chewed
- With food or milk to decrease gastric symptoms; give 30 min before or 2 hr after meals
- With full glass of water

Evaluate:

- Therapeutic response: decreased pain, fever

Teach patient/family:

- To report any symptoms of hepatotoxicity, renal toxicity, visual changes, ototoxicity, allergic reactions (long-term therapy)
- Not to exceed recommended dosage; acute poisoning may result
- To read label on other OTC drugs; many contain aspirin
- That therapeutic response takes 2 wk (arthritis)
- To avoid alcohol ingestion; GI bleeding may occur

Treatment of overdose: Lavage, activated charcoal, monitor electrolytes, VS

sargramostim (℞)

(sar-gram'oh-stim)

Leukine, Prokine, rhu GM-CSF, recombinant human

Func. class.: Biologic modifier

Action: Stimulates proliferation and differentiation of hematopoietic progenitor cells (granulocytes, macrophages)

Uses: Acceleration of myeloid recovery in patients with non-Hodgkin's lymphoma, acute lymphoblastic leukemia, autologous bone marrow transplantation in Hodgkin's disease; bone marrow transplantation failure or engraftment delay

Dosage and routes:

Myeloid reconstitution after autologous bone marrow transplantation

- *Adult:* IV 250 $\mu g/m^2$/day × 3 wks; give over 2 hr, 2-4 hr after autologous bone marrow infusion, not less than 24 hr after last dose of antineoplastics and 12 hr after last dose of radiotherapy, bone marrow transplantation failure, or engraftment delay

Acceleration of myeloid recovery

- *Adult:* IV 250 $\mu g/m^2$/day × 14 days; give over 2 hr; may repeat in 7 days, may repeat 500 $\mu g/m^2$/day × 14 days after another 7 days if no improvement

Available forms: Powder for inj lyophilized 250, 500 µg

Side effects/adverse reactions:

CNS: Fever, malaise, CNS disorder, weakness, chills

GI: Nausea, vomiting, diarrhea, anorexia, ***GI hemorrhage,*** stomatitis, ***liver damage***

HEMA: ***Blood dyscrasias, hemorrhage***
INTEG: Alopecia, rash, peripheral edema
GU: Urinary tract disorder, abnormal kidney function
RESP: Dyspnea
CV: ***Supraventricular tachycardia,*** peripheral edema, ***pericardial effusion***

Contraindications: Hypersensitivity to GM-CSF, yeast products; excessive leukemic myeloid blast in bone marrow, peripheral blood

Precautions: Pregnancy (C), lactation, child; renal, hepatic, lung disease; cardiac disease; pleural, pericardial effusions

Pharmacokinetics: Half-life 2 hr, detected within 5 min after administration, peak 2 hr

Interactions:

- Do not use this drug concomitantly with antineoplastics
- Increased myeloproliferation: lithium, corticosteroids

Y-site compatibilities: Amikacin, aminophylline, aztreonam, bleomycin, butorphanol, calcium gluconate, carboplatin, carmustine, cefazolin, ceforanide, cefotaxime, cefotetan, ceftizoxime, ceftriaxone, cefuroxime, cimetidine, cisplatin, clindamycin, cyclophosphamide, cytarabine, dacarbazine, dactinomycin, dexamethasone sodium phosphate, diphenhydramine, doxorubicin, doxycycline, droperidol, etoposide, famotidine, floxuridine, fluconazole, fluorouracil, furosemide, gentamicin, heparin, ifosfamide, magnesium sulfate, mannitol, mechlorethamine, meperidine, mesna, methotrexate, metoclopramide, metronidazole, mezlocillin, miconazole, minocycline, mitoxantrone, netilmicin, pentostatin, potassium chloride, prochlorperazine, promethazine, ranitidine, teniposide, ticarcillin, ticarcillin/clavulanate, trimethoprim/sulfamethoxazole, vancomycin, vinblastine, vincristine, zidovudine

NURSING CONSIDERATIONS

Assess:

- Blood studies: CBC, differential count before treatment and twice weekly; leukocytosis may occur (WBC >50,000 cells/mm^3, ANC >20,000 cells/mm^3)
- Renal and hepatic studies before treatment: BUN, creatinine, urinalysis; AST (SGOT), ALT (SGPT), alk phosphatase; twice weekly monitoring is needed in renal, hepatic disease
- For hypersensitivity, rashes, local inj site reactions; usually transient
- For increased fluid retention in cardiac disease

Administer:

- After reconstituting with 1 ml sterile water for inj without preservative; do not reenter vial; discard unused portion; direct reconstitution sol at side of vial; rotate contents; do not shake
- Dilute in 0.9% NaCl inj to prepare IV inf; if final concentration is <10 µg/ml, add human albumin to make a final concentration of 0.1% to NaCl before adding sargramostim to prevent adsorption; for a final concentration of 0.1% albumin, add 1 mg human albumin/1 ml 0.9% NaCl inj run over 2 hr; give within 6 hr after reconstitution

Perform/provide:

- Storage in refrigerator; do not freeze

Evaluate:

- Therapeutic response: WBC and differential recovery

scopolamine (℞)

(skoe-pol'a-meen)

Func. class.: Cholinergic blocker

Chem. class.: Belladonna alkaloid

Combination products: Murocoll-2: scopolamine 0.3%, phenylephrine 10%

Action: Inhibits acetylcholine at receptor sites in autonomic nervous system, which controls secretions, free acids in stomach; blocks central muscarinic receptors, which decreases involuntary movements

Uses: Reduction of secretions before surgery, calm delirium, motion sickness, parkinsonian symptoms

Dosage and routes:

Parkinsonian symptoms

• *Adult:* IM/SC/IV 0.3-0.6 mg tid-qid using dilution provided

• *Child:* SC 0.006 mg/kg tid-qid or 0.2 mg/m^2

Preoperatively

• *Adult:* SC 0.4-0.6 mg

Available forms: Inj 0.3, 0.4, 0.86, 1 mg/ml

Side effects/adverse reactions:

CNS: Confusion, anxiety, restlessness, irritability, delusions, hallucinations, headache, sedation, depression, incoherence, dizziness, excitement, delirium, flushing, weakness

INTEG: Urticaria

MISC: Suppression of lactation, nasal congestion, decreased sweating

EENT: Blurred vision, photophobia, dilated pupils, difficulty swallowing, mydriasis, cycloplegia

CV: Palpitations, tachycardia, postural hypotension, paradoxic bradycardia

GI: Dryness of mouth, constipation, nausea, vomiting, abdominal distress, ***paralytic ileus***

GU: Hesitancy, retention

Contraindications: Hypersensitivity, narrow-angle glaucoma, myasthenia gravis, GI/GU obstruction, hypersensitivity to belladonna, barbiturates

Precautions: Pregnancy (C), elderly, lactation, prostatic hypertrophy, CHF, hypertension, dysrhythmia, children, gastric ulcer

Pharmacokinetics:

SC/IM: Peak 30-45 min, duration 7 hr

IV: Peak 10-15 min, duration 4 hr

Excreted in urine, bile, feces (unchanged)

Interactions:

• Increased anticholinergic effect: alcohol, narcotics, antihistamines, phenothiazines, tricyclics

Syringe compatibilities: Benzaquinamide, butorphanol, chlorpromazine, cimetidine, dimenhydrinate, diphenhydramine, droperidol, fentanyl, hydromorphone, hydroxyzine, meperidine, metoclopramide, midazolam, morphine, nalbuphine, pentazocine, pentobarbital, perphenazine, prochlorperazine, promazine, promethazine, ranitidine, thiopental

Y-site compatibilities: Heparin, hydrocortisone sodium succinate, potassium chloride, vitamin B with C

NURSING CONSIDERATIONS

Assess:

• I&O ratio; retention commonly causes decreased urinary output

• Parkinsonism, EPS: shuffling gait, muscle rigidity, involuntary movements

• Urinary hesitancy, retention; palpate bladder if retention occurs

• Constipation; increase fluids, bulk, exercise if this occurs

• For tolerance over long-term therapy; dose may have to be increased or changed

• Mental status: affect, mood, CNS

depression, worsening of mental symptoms during early therapy

Administer:

- Parenteral dose with patient recumbent to prevent postural hypotension
- With or after meals for GI upset; may give with fluids other than H_2O
- At hs to avoid daytime drowsiness in patient with parkinsonism
- Parenteral dose slowly; keep in bed for at least 1 hr after dose
- With analgesic to avoid behavioral changes when given as a preop

Perform/provide:

- Storage at room temp in light-resistant container
- Hard candy, frequent drinks, sugarless gum to relieve dry mouth

Evaluate:

- Therapeutic response: decreased secretions

Teach patient/family:

- Not to discontinue this drug abruptly; to taper off over 1 wk
- To avoid driving, other hazardous activities; drowsiness may occur
- To avoid OTC medication: cough, cold preparations with alcohol, antihistamines unless directed by prescriber

scopolamine (optic) (℞)

(skoe-pol'a-meen)

Isopto-Hyoscine

Func. class.: Mydriatic

Chem. class.: Synthetic alkaloid

Action: Blocks response of iris sphincter muscle, muscle of accommodation of ciliary body to cholinergic stimulation, resulting in dilation, paralysis of accommodation

Uses: Uveitis, iritis, cycloplegia, mydriasis

Dosage and routes:

- *Adult:* INSTILL 1-2 gtt before refraction or 1-2 gtt qd-tid for iritis or uveitis
- *Child:* INSTILL 1 gtt bid × 2 days before refraction

Available forms: Sol 0.25%

Side effects/adverse reactions:

CV: Tachycardia

CNS: Confusion, somnolence, flushing, fever

EENT: Blurred vision, photophobia, increased intraocular pressure, irritation, edema

Contraindications: Hypersensitivity, children <6 yr, narrow-angle glaucoma, increased intraocular pressure, infants

Precautions: Children, elderly, hypertension, hyperthyroidism, diabetes, pregnancy (C), lactation, Down syndrome

Pharmacokinetics:

Instill: Peak 20-30 min, duration 3-7 days

NURSING CONSIDERATIONS

Assess:

- Eye pain; discontinue use

Evaluate:

- Therapeutic response: decrease in inflammation, cycloplegic refraction

Teach patient/family:

- To report change in vision; blurring or loss of sight; trouble breathing; inhibition of sweating; flushing
- Method of instillation: pressure on lacrimal sac for 1 min; not to touch dropper to eye
- That blurred vision will decrease with repeated use of drug
- Not to engage in hazardous activities until able to see
- Wait 5 min to use other drops
- Do not blink more than usual

* Available in Canada only

scopolamine (transdermal) (℞)

(skoe-pol'-a-meen)

Transderm-Scop

Func. class.: Antiemetic, anticholinergic

Chem. class.: Belladonna alkaloid

Action: Competitive antagonism of acetylcholine at receptor site in eye, smooth muscle, cardiac muscle, glandular cells; inhibition of vestibular input to the CNS, resulting in inhibition of vomiting reflex

Uses: Prevention of motion sickness

Dosage and routes:

• *Adult:* PATCH 1 placed behind ear 4-5 hr before travel

• Not recommended for children

Available forms: Patch, 0.5 mg delivered in 72 hr

Side effects/adverse reactions:

INTEG: Rash, erythema

GU: Difficult urination

CNS: *Dizziness, drowsiness,* confusion, disorientation, memory disturbances, hallucinations

EENT: *Blurred vision,* altered depth perception, *dilated pupils,* photophobia, *dry mouth;* dry, itchy, red eyes; acute narrow-angle glaucoma

Contraindications: Hypersensitivity, glaucoma

Precautions: Children, elderly, pregnancy (C); pyloric, urinary, bladder neck, intestinal obstruction; liver, kidney disease

Pharmacokinetics:

Patch: Onset 4-5 hr, duration 72 hr

Interactions:

• Increased anticholinergic effects: antihistamines, antidepressants

NURSING CONSIDERATIONS

Teach patient/family:

• To avoid hazardous activities, activities requiring alertness; dizziness may occur

• To wash, dry hands before and after applying to surface behind ear

• To change patch q72h

• To apply at least 4 hr before traveling

• If blurred vision, severe dizziness, drowsiness occurs, to discontinue use, use another type of antiemetic

• To read label of all OTC medications; if any scopolamine is found in product, avoid use

• To keep out of children's reach

secobarbital (℞)

(see-koe-bar'bi-tal)

Secobarbital Sodium, Secogen Sodium*, Seconal Sodium, Seconal Sodium Pulvules, Seral*, Secretin-Ferring

Func. class.: Sedative/hypnotic-barbiturate

Chem. class.: Barbitone (short acting)

Controlled Substance Schedule II (USA), Schedule G (Canada)

Action: Depresses activity in brain cells primarily in reticular activating system in brain stem; selectively depresses neurons in posterior hypothalamus, limbic structures; decreases seizure activity by inhibition of epileptic activity in CNS

Uses: Insomnia, sedation, preoperative medication, status epilepticus, acute tetanus convulsions

Dosage and routes:

Insomnia

• *Adult:* PO/IM 100-200 mg hs

• *Child:* IM 3-5 mg/kg, not to exceed 100 mg, not to inject >5 ml in one site; REC 4-5 mg/kg

Sedation/preoperatively

• *Adult:* PO 200-300 mg 1-2 hr preoperatively

• *Child:* PO 50-100 mg 1-2 hr preoperatively; REC 4-5 mg/kg 1-2 hr preoperatively

Status epilepticus

• *Adult, child:* IM/IV 250-350 mg

Acute psychotic agitation

• *Adult, child:* IM/IV 5.5 mg/kg q3-4h

Available forms: Caps 50, 100 mg; tabs 100 mg; inj 50 mg/ml; powder, rec supp 200 mg

Side effects/adverse reactions:

CNS: Lethargy, drowsiness, hangover, dizziness, paradoxical stimulation in elderly and children, lightheadedness, dependency, CNS depression, mental depression, slurred speech

GI: Nausea, vomiting, diarrhea, constipation

INTEG: Rash, urticaria, pain, abscesses at injection site, angioedema, thrombophlebitis, ***Stevens-Johnson syndrome***

CV: Hypotension, bradycardia

RESP: Depression, ***apnea, laryngospasm, bronchospasm***

HEMA: ***Agranulocytosis, thrombocytopenia, megaloblastic anemia*** (long-term treatment)

Contraindications: Hypersensitivity to barbiturates, respiratory depression, addiction to barbiturates, severe liver impairment, porphyria, uncontrolled severe pain

Precautions: Anemia, pregnancy (D), lactation, hepatic disease, renal disease, hypertension, elderly, acute/chronic pain

Pharmacokinetics:

IM: Onset 10-15 min, duration 4-6 hr

REC: Onset slow, duration 3-6 hr; metabolized by liver, excreted by kidneys (metabolites); half-life 15-40 hr

Interactions:

• Do not mix with other drugs in sol or syringe

• Increased CNS depression: alcohol, MAOIs, sedatives, narcotics

• Decreased effect of oral anticoagulants, corticosteroids, griseofulvin, quinidine

• Decreased half-life of doxycycline

Syringe compatibilities: Heparin

Solution compatibilities: D_5W, $D_{10}W$, 0.45% NaCl, 0.9% NaCl, Ringer's sol, dextrose/saline combinations, dextrose/Ringer's or dextrose/lactated Ringer's combinations

Additive compatibilities: Amikacin, aminophylline, calcium chloride, calcium gluceptate, cephapirin, colistimethate, dimenhydrinate, polymyxin B, sodium bicarbonate, thiopental, verapamil

Lab test interferences:

False increase: Sulfobromophthalein

NURSING CONSIDERATIONS

Assess:

• VS q30min after parenteral route for 2 hr

• Blood studies: Hct, Hgb, RBCs, serum folate, vit D (if on long-term therapy); pro-time in patients receiving anticoagulants

• Hepatic studies: AST, ALT, bilirubin; if increased, drug is usually discontinued

• Unresolved pain; drug may cause severe stimulation if pain is present

• Mental status: mood, sensorium, affect, memory (long, short)

• Physical dependency: frequent requests for medication, shakes, anxiety

• Barbiturate toxicity: hypotension; pulmonary constriction; cold, clammy skin; cyanosis of lips; insomnia; nausea; vomiting; hallucinations; delirium; weakness; mild symptoms may occur in 8-12 hr without drug

• Respiratory dysfunction: depression, character, rate, rhythm; hold drug if respirations <10/min or if pupils dilated
• Blood dyscrasias: fever, sore throat, bruising, rash, jaundice, epistaxis
• Perianal irritation if rectal forms used

Administer:
• IV after diluting with sterile H_2O for inj; rotate; give 50 mg or less over 1 min; titrate to response
• After removal of cigarettes to prevent fires
• IM inj deep in large muscle mass to prevent tissue sloughing and abscesses
• After conservative measures for insomnia have been tried
• Within 30 min of mixing with sterile water for inj; reconstitute after rotating ampule; do not shake; do not use cloudy sol; may be given directly or indirectly
• IV only with resuscitative equipment available; administer at <100 mg/min (only by qualified personnel)
• ½-1 hr before hs for sleeplessness
• On empty stomach for best absorption
• For <14 days, since drug is not effective after that; tolerance develops
• Crushed or whole
• Alone; do not mix with other drugs or inject if there is precipitate
• After cleansing enema if given rectally preoperatively in children

Perform/provide:
• Assistance with ambulation after receiving dose
• Safety measure: side rails, nightlight, call bell within easy reach
• Checking to see PO medication has been swallowed
• Storage of suppositories in refrigerator; do not use aqueous sol containing precipitate

Evaluate:
• Therapeutic response: ability to sleep at night, decreased early morning awakening if taking drug for insomnia, or decrease in number, severity of seizures if taking drug for seizure disorder

Teach patient/family:
• That morning hangover is common
• That drug is indicated only for short-term treatment of insomnia, probably ineffective after 2 wk
• That physical dependency may result when used for extended periods (45-90 days depending on dose)
• To avoid driving, other activities requiring alertness
• To avoid alcohol ingestion, CNS depressants; serious CNS depression may result
• Not to discontinue medication quickly after long-term use; drug should be tapered over 1-2 wk
• To tell all prescribers that barbiturate is being taken
• That withdrawal insomnia may occur after short-term use; not to start using drug again; insomnia will improve in 1-3 nights; may experience increased dreaming
• That effects may take 2 nights for benefits to be noticed
• Alternative measures to improve sleep (reading, exercise several hours before hs, warm bath, warm milk, TV, self-hypnosis, deep breathing)

Treatment of overdose: Lavage, activated charcoal, warming blanket, vital signs, hemodialysis, I&O ratio

S

selegiline (℞)

(se-le'ji-leen)
Eldepryl, SD-Deprenyl
Func. class.: Antiparkinson agent
Chem. class.: Levorotatory acetylenic derivative of phenethylamine

Action: Increased dopaminergic activity by inhibition of MAO type B activity; not fully understood
Uses: Adjunct management of Parkinson's disease in patients being treated with levodopa/carbidopa who had poor response to therapy
Dosage and routes:
• *Adult:* PO 10 mg/day in divided doses 5 mg at breakfast and lunch; after 2-3 days begin to reduce dose of levodopa/carbidopa 10%-30%
Available forms: Tabs 5 mg
Side effects/adverse reactions:
CNS: Increased tremors, chorea, restlessness, blepharospasm, increased bradykinesia, grimacing, tardive dyskinesia, dystonic symptoms, involuntary movements, increased apraxia, hallucinations, dizziness, mood changes, nightmares, delusions, lethargy, apathy, overstimulation, sleep disturbances, headache, migraine, numbness, muscle cramps, confusion, anxiety, tiredness, vertigo, personality change, back/leg pain
CV: Orthostatic hypotension, hypertension, dysrhythmia, palpitations, angina pectoris, hypotension, tachycardia, edema, sinus bradycardia, syncope
GI: Nausea, vomiting, constipation, weight loss, anorexia, diarrhea, heartburn, rectal bleeding, poor appetite, dysphagia
GU: Slow urination, nocturia, prostatic hypertrophy, hesitation, retention, frequency, sexual dysfunction
INTEG: Increased sweating, alopecia, hematoma, rash, photosensitivity, facial hair
RESP: Asthma, shortness of breath
EENT: Diplopia, dry mouth, blurred vision, tinnitus
Contraindications: Hypersensitivity
Precautions: Pregnancy (C), lactation, children
Pharmacokinetics:
Rapidly absorbed, peak ½-2 hr; rapidly metabolized (active metabolites: N-desmethyldeprenyl, amphetamine, methamphetamine), metabolites excreted in urine
Interactions:
• ***Fatal interaction:*** Opioids (especially meperidine); do not administer together
Lab test interferences:
False positive: Urine ketones, urine glucose
False negative: Urine glucose (glucose oxidase)
False increase: Uric acid, urine protein
Decrease: VMA

NURSING CONSIDERATIONS

Assess:
• Decreased parkinsonian symptoms: rigidity, unsteady gait, weakness, tremors
• B/P, respiration throughout treatment
• Mental status: affect, mood behavioral changes, depression; perform suicide assessment
Administer:
• Drug until NPO before surgery
• Adjusting dosage to response
• With meals; limit protein taken with drug
• At doses <10 mg/day because of risks associated with nonselective inhibition of MAO

* Available in Canada only

Perform/provide:
• Assistance with ambulation during beginning therapy
Evaluate:
• Therapeutic response: decrease in akathisia, improved mood
Teach patient/family:
• To change positions slowly to prevent orthostatic hypotension
• To report side effects: twitching, eye spasms; indicate overdose
• To use drug exactly as prescribed; if discontinued abruptly, parkinsonian crisis may occur
• To avoid foods high in tyramine: cheese, pickled products, wine, beer, large amounts of caffeine
• Not to exceed recommended dose of 10 mg; might precipitate hypertensive crisis; report severe headache, other unusual symptoms
Treatment of overdose: IV fluids for hypertension, IV dilute pressure agent for B/P titration

selenium (OTC)

(see-leen'ee-um)
Exsel, Head and Shoulders Intensive Treatment, Selenium Sulfide, Selsun, Selsun Blue
Func. class.: Local antiseborrheic, antifungal

Action: Appears to have cytostatic effect on epidural cells and reduces corneocyte production
Uses: Dandruff, seborrhea; dermatitis of the scalp, versicolor
Dosage and routes:
• *Adult and child:* TOP wash hair with 1-2 tsp, leave on 2-3 min; rinse, repeat; use 2 applications/wk × 2 wk, then q3-4 wk or as needed
Available forms: Shampoo; lotion 1%, 2.5%
Side effects/adverse reactions:
INTEG: Oiliness of hair, scalp, alopecia, discoloration of hair, skin irritation
Contraindications: Hypersensitivity to sulfur, inflamed skin
Precautions: Infants, pregnancy (C)
NURSING CONSIDERATIONS
Assess:
• Area of body involved, including time involved, what helps or aggravates condition
Perform/provide:
• Thorough hair rinsing after use
• Storage at room temp in tight container
Evaluate:
• Toxicity: tremors, perspiration, pain in abdomen, weakness, anorexia
Teach patient/family:
• To avoid contact with eyes, genital area
• To discontinue use if rash or irritation occurs
• That drug may damage jewelry; remove before application
• That drug is not to be taken internally

senna (OTC)

(sen'na)
Black Draught, Dr. Caldwell Senna Laxative, Fletcher's Castoria, Gentlax, Senexon, Senna-Gen, Senokot, Senokotxtra, Senolax
Func. class.: Laxative-stimulant
Chem. class.: Anthraquinone

Action: Stimulates peristalsis by action on Auerbach's plexus; softens feces by increasing water, electrolytes in large intestine
Uses: Acute constipation; bowel preparation for surgery or examination
Dosage and routes:
• *Adult:* PO 1-8 tabs (Senokot)/day or ½ to 4 tsp of granules (1 tsp-4 ml)

S

added to water or juice; REC SUPP 1-2 hs; SYR 1-4 tsp hs, 7.5-15 ml; (Black Draught) ¾ oz dissolved in 2.5 oz liquid given between 2-4 PM the day before procedure (X-Prep)
• *Child >27 kg:* ½ adult dose; do not use Black Draught for children
• *Child 1 mo-1 yr:* SYR 1.25-2.5 ml (Senokot) hs

Available forms: Supp 625 mg, 30 mg sennosides; powder 662 mg/g, 6, 15 mg sennosides/3g; tabs 8.6 sennosides, 180 mg

Side effects/adverse reactions:
GI: Nausea, vomiting, anorexia, cramps, diarrhea, flatulence
META: Hypocalcemia, enteropathy, alkalosis, hypokalemia, ***tetany***
GU: Pink, red or brown, black urine

Contraindications: Hypersensitivity, GI bleeding, obstruction, CHF, lactation, abdominal pain, nausea/vomiting, appendicitis, acute surgical abdomen

Precautions: Pregnancy (C)

Pharmacokinetics:
PO: Onset 6-24 hr; metabolized by liver, excreted in feces

Interactions:
• Do not use with disulfiram (Antabuse)

NURSING CONSIDERATIONS

Assess:
• Stool: color, consistency, amount
• Blood, urine electrolytes if drug is used often
• I&O ratio to identify fluid loss
• Cause of constipation; fluids, bulk, exercise missing
• Cramping, rectal bleeding, nausea, vomiting; drug should be discontinued

Administer:
• In morning or evening (oral dose) with full glass of water
• Dissolve granules in water or juice before administration
• On empty stomach for more rapid results
• Shake oral sol before giving

Evaluate:
• Therapeutic response: decrease in constipation

Teach patient/family:
• That urine, feces may turn yellow-brown to red
• Not to use laxatives for long-term therapy; bowel tone will be lost
• That normal bowel movements do not always occur daily
• Not to use in presence of abdominal pain, nausea, vomiting
• To notify prescriber if constipation unrelieved or of symptoms of electrolyte imbalance: muscle cramps, pain, weakness, dizziness, excessive thirst

sertraline (℞)

(ser′tra-leen)
Zoloft
Func. class.: Antidepressant

Action: Inhibits serotonin reuptake in CNS; increases action of serotonin; does not affect dopamine, norepinephrine

Uses: Major depression

Dosage and routes:
• *Adult:* PO 50 mg qd; may increase to max of 200 mg/day; do not change dose at intervals of <1 wk; administer qd in AM or PM

Available forms: Tabs 50, 100 mg

Side effects/adverse reactions:
CNS: Insomnia, agitation, somnolence, dizziness, headache, tremor, fatigue, paresthesia, twitching, confusion, ataxia
GU: Male sexual dysfunction, micturition disorder
GI: Diarrhea, nausea, constipation, anorexia, *dry mouth,* dyspepsia, *vomiting,* flatulence
CV: Palpitations, chest pain, hypotension
EENT: Vision abnormalities

* Available in Canada only

INTEG: Increased sweating, rash, hot flashes

Contraindications: Hypersensitivity

Precautions: Pregnancy (B), lactation, elderly, hepatic, renal disease, epilepsy

Pharmacokinetics:

PO: Peak 6-10 hr, plasma protein binding 99%, elimination half-life 25 hr, extensively metabolized, metabolite excreted in urine

Interactions:

- Increased effects of alcohol, diazepam, tolbutamide, warfarin
- Fatal reactions: MAOIs
- Altered lithium levels: lithium

Lab test interferences:

Increase: Serum bilirubin, blood glucose, alk phosphatase

Decrease: VMA, 5-HIAA

False increase: Urinary catecholamines

NURSING CONSIDERATIONS

Assess:

- Mental status: mood sensorium, affect, suicidal tendencies, increase in psychiatric symptoms, depression, panic
- B/P (lying/standing), pulse q4h; if systolic B/P drops 20 mm Hg, hold drug, notify prescriber; take vital signs q4h in patients with cardiovascular disease
- Weight qwk; appetite may decrease with drug
- Urinary retention, constipation, especially in elderly
- Withdrawal symptoms: headache, nausea, vomiting, muscle pain, weakness; not usual unless discontinued abruptly
- Alcohol consumption; hold dose until morning

Administer:

- Increased fluids, bulk in diet for constipation, urinary retention
- With food, milk for GI symptoms
- Crushed if patient is unable to swallow medication whole
- Gum, hard candy, frequent sips of water for dry mouth

Perform/provide:

- Storage at room temp; do not freeze
- Assistance with ambulation during therapy, since drowsiness, dizziness occur
- Safety measures, including side rails, primarily for elderly
- Checking to see that PO medication is swallowed

Evaluate:

- Therapeutic response: significant improvement in depression

Teach patient/family:

- That therapeutic effect may take 2-3 wk
- To use caution in driving, other activities requiring alertness; drowsiness, dizziness, blurred vision may occur
- Not to discontinue medication quickly after long-term use; may cause nausea, headache, malaise
- To avoid alcohol, other CNS depressants
- To notify prescriber if pregnant or plan to become pregnant or breastfeed

silver nitrate (℞)

Func. class.: Keratolytic

Action: Antiinfective, astringent, caustic

Uses: Cauterization of lesions, warts, burns (low concentrations)

Dosage and routes:

- *Adult and child:* TOP apply to area to be treated
- ***Available forms:*** Sticks, sol 10%, 25%, 50%

Side effects/adverse reactions:

INTEG: Skin discoloration

Contraindications: Hypersensitivity

Interactions:

• Not to be used with alkalies, phosphates, thimerosal, benzalkonium chloride, halogenated acids

NURSING CONSIDERATIONS

Administer:

• After moistening stick with water

• To burns using a wet dressing (low concentrations 0.125%)

Evaluate:

• Therapeutic response: absence of lesions, healing of burned areas

Perform/provide:

• Storage in cool area

Teach patient/family:

• To avoid contact with clothing, unaffected areas; discoloration may occur

silver nitrate 1% (ophthalmic) (℞)

Func. class.: Antiinfective

Action: Inhibits metabolic actions in susceptible organisms

Uses: Prevention, treatment of gonorrheal ophthalmia neonatorum

Dosage and routes:

• *Neonate:* INSTILL 2 gtt 1% sol into each eye

• *Available forms:* Sol

Side effects/adverse reactions:

EENT: Redness, discharge, edema, swelling

Contraindications: Hypersensitivity

Precautions: Antibiotic hypersensitivity, pregnancy (C)

NURSING CONSIDERATIONS

Administer:

• After washing hands

Perform/provide:

• Storage at room temp in tight, light-resistant container

Evaluate:

• Allergy: itching, lacrimation, redness, swelling

silver protein, mild (℞, OTC)

Argyrol S.S. 10%, Argyrol S.S. 20%

Func. class.: Disinfectant

Chem. class.: Silver colloidal compound

Action: Destroys gram-positive, gram-negative organisms

Uses: Eye, nose, throat, swelling, infection

Dosage and routes:

• *Adult and child:* TOP sol use as needed

Available forms: Top sol 5%, 10%, 25%; eyedrops 20%

Side effects/adverse reactions:

INTEG: Irritation, discolored tissue

Contraindications: Hypersensitivity

Precautions: Pregnancy (C)

NURSING CONSIDERATIONS

Administer:

• To area to be treated only; do not apply to healthy skin

Perform/provide:

• Storage in tight container

Evaluate:

• Area of body involved: irritation, rash, breaks, dryness, scales

silver sulfadiazine (topical) (℞)

(sul-fa-dye'a-zeen)

Flamazine*, Silvadene, SSD, SSD AF, Thermazene

Func. class.: Local antiinfective

Chem. class.: Sulfonamide

Action: Interferes with bacterial cell wall synthesis, broad-spectrum

Uses: Burns (2nd, 3rd degree); prevention of wound sepsis

Dosage and routes:

• *Adult and child:* TOP apply 1%

cream qd-bid 1.5 mm thick to all burned areas
Available forms: Cream 10 mg/g
Side effects/adverse reactions:
INTEG: Rash, urticaria, stinging, burning, itching, pain, skin necrosis, erythema
HEMA: Reversible leukopenia
Contraindications: Hypersensitivity, child <2 mo
Precautions: Impaired renal function, pregnancy (C), impaired hepatic function, lactation
NURSING CONSIDERATIONS
Assess:
• For infection/sepsis in all burned areas: drainage, fever, increased WBCs, odor; culture should be done
• Allergic reaction: burning, stinging, swelling, redness, itching
• Renal function studies; check for crystalluria; CBC should be completed to identify leukopenia
Administer:
• After cleansing debris before each application; bathe qd
• Analgesic before application if needed; pain may be severe
• Using aseptic technique, use sterile gloves
• Enough medication to cover burns completely; keep covered with medication at all times
Perform/provide:
• Storage at room temp in dry place
Evaluate:
• Therapeutic response: relief or prevention of infection
Teach patient/family:
• That drug may be continued until graft can be done

simethicone (OTC)

(si-meth'i-kone)
Extra Strength Gas-X, Flatulex Gas Relief, Gas-X, Major Con, Mylanta Gas, Mylicon, Mylicon 80, Ovol*, Phazyme, Phazyme 95, Phazyme 125
Func. class.: Antiflatulent

Action: Disperses, prevents gas pockets in GI system; does not decrease gas production
Uses: Flatulence
Dosage and routes:
• *Adult, child >12 yr:* PO 40-100 mg pc, hs
Available forms: Chew tabs 40, 80 mg; tabs 50, 60, 95, 125 mg; drops 40 mg/0.6 ml; cap 125 mg
Side effects/adverse reactions:
GI: Belching, rectal flatus
Contraindications: Hypersensitivity
Precautions: Pregnancy (C)
NURSING CONSIDERATIONS
Assess:
• Reason for excess gas production, decreased bowel sounds, recent surgery, other GI conditions
Administer:
• After meals, HS; shake susp well before giving; chew tabs should be chewed
Evaluate:
• Therapeutic response: absence of flatulence
Teach patient/family:
• That tablets must be chewed
• To shake suspension well before pouring

S

simvastatin (℞)

(sem-va-sta'tin)
Zocor
Func. class.: Antihyperlipidemic
Chem. class.: Synthetically derived fermentation product

Action: Inhibits HMG-CoA reductase enzyme, which reduces cholesterol synthesis
Uses: As an adjunct in primary hypercholesterolemia (types IIa, IIb)
Dosage and routes:
• *Adult:* PO 5-10 mg qd in PM initially; usual range 5-40 mg/day qd in PM, not to exceed 40 mg/day; dosage adjustments may be made in 4-wk intervals or more
Available forms: Tabs 5, 10, 20, 40 mg
Side effects/adverse reactions:
INTEG: Rash, pruritus, alopecia
GI: Nausea, constipation, diarrhea, dyspepsia, flatus, abdominal pain, heartburn, ***liver dysfunction,*** pancreatitis
EENT: Lens opacities
MS: Muscle cramps, myalgia, ***myositis, rhabdomyolysis***
CNS: Headache, tremor, vertigo, peripheral neuropathy
Contraindications: Hypersensitivity, pregnancy (X), lactation, active liver disease
Precautions: Past liver disease, alcoholism, severe acute infections, trauma, hypotension, uncontrolled seizure disorders, severe metabolic disorders, electrolyte imbalances
Pharmacokinetics: Peak 1-2½ hr, metabolized in liver (active metabolites), highly protein bound, excreted primarily in bile, feces
Interactions:
• Increased effects of coumadin
• Increased myalgia, myositis: cyclosporine, gemfibrozil, niacin, erthyromycin
• Increased serum level of digoxin
Lab test interferences:
Increase: CPK, liver function tests
NURSING CONSIDERATIONS
Assess:
• Cholesterol levels periodically during treatment
• Liver function studies q1-2mo during the first 1½ yr of treatment; AST (SGOT), ALT (SGPT), liver function tests may increase
• Renal studies in patients with compromised renal system: BUN, I&O ratio, creatinine
• Eyes with slit lamp before, 1 mo after treatment begins, annually; lens opacities may occur
Administer:
• Total daily dose in evening
Perform/provide:
• Storage in cool environment in tight container protected from light
Evaluate:
• Therapeutic response: decrease in cholesterol to desired level after 8 wk
Teach patient/family:
• That treatment will take several years
• That blood work and eye exam will be necessary during treatment
• To report blurred vision, severe GI symptoms, dizziness, headache
• That previously prescribed regimen will continue: low-cholesterol diet, exercise program

sodium bicarbonate (OTC)

Arm & Hammer Pure Baking Soda, Bellans, Citrocarbonate, Soda Mint

Func. class.: Alkalinizer

Chem. class.: $NaHCO_3$

Action: Orally neutralizes gastric acid, which forms water, NaCl, CO_2; increases plasma bicarbonate, which buffers H^+ ion concentration; reverses acidosis IV

Uses: Acidosis (metabolic), cardiac arrest, alkalinization (systemic/urinary) antacid

Dosage and routes:

Acidosis, metabolic

• *Adult and child:* IV INF 2-5 mEq/kg over 4-8 hr depending on CO_2, pH

Cardiac arrest

• *Adult, child:* IV BOL 1 mEq/kg, then 0.5 mEq/kg q10 min, then doses based on ABGs

• *Infant:* IV INF not to exceed 8 mEq/kg/day based on ABGs (4.2% sol)

Alkalinization of urine

• *Adult:* PO 325 mg-2 g qid or 48 mEq (4g), then 12-24 mEq q4h

• *Child:* PO 12-120 mg/kg/day (1-10 mEq/kg)

Antacid

• *Adult:* PO 300 mg-2 g chewed, taken with H_2O qd-qid

Available forms: Tabs 300, 325, 600, 650 mg; inj 4%, 4.2%, 5%, 7.5%, 8.4%

Side effects/adverse reactions:

CNS: Irritability, headache, confusion, stimulation, tremors, *twitching, hyperreflexia,* ***tetany,*** weakness, ***convulsions*** of alkalosis

CV: Irregular pulse, ***cardiac arrest,*** water retention, edema, weight gain

GI: Flatulence, *belching, distention,* ***paralytic ileus,*** acid rebound

META: Alkalosis

GU: Calculi

RESP: Shallow, slow respirations, cyanosis, ***apnea***

Contraindications: Hypertension, peptic ulcer, renal disease, hypocalcemia

Precautions: CHF, cirrhosis, toxemia, renal disease, pregnancy (C)

Pharmacokinetics:

PO: Onset 2 min, duration 10 min

IV: Onset 15 min, duration 1-2 hr, excreted in urine

Interactions:

• Increased effects: amphetamines, mecamylamine, quinine, quinidine, pseudoephedrine, flecainide, anorexiants

• Decreased effects: lithium, chlorpropamide, barbiturates, salicylates, benzodiazepines

• Increased Na and decreased K: corticosteroids

Syringe compatibilities: Milrinone, pentobarbital

Y-site compatibilities: Acyclovir, famotidine, fludarabine, indomethacin sodium trihydrate, insulin, melphan, morphine, paclitaxel, potassium chloride, tolazoline, vitamin B with C

Additive compatibilities: Amikacin, aminophylline, amobarbital, amphotericin B, atropine, bretylium, calcium chloride, calcium gluceptate, carbenicillin, cefoxitin, ceftazine, cephalothin, cephapirin, chloramphenicol, chlorothiazide, cimetidine, clindamycin, cytarabine, droperidol/fentanyl, ergonovine maleate, erythromycin, floxacillin, furosemide, heparin, hyaluronidase, hydrocortisone sodium succinate, kanamycin, lidocaine, metaraminol, methotrexate, methyldopate, multivitamins, nafcillin, netilmicin, nizatidine, oxacillin, oxytocin, phenobarbital, phenylephrine, phenytoin, phytonadione, potassium chloride, prochlorperazine, sodium iodide, thiopental, verapamil

Lab test interferences:
Increase: Urinary urobilinogen
False positive: Urinary protein, blood lactate

NURSING CONSIDERATIONS

Assess:

- Respiratory and pulse rate, rhythm, depth, lung sounds; notify prescriber of abnormalities
- Fluid balance (I&O, weight qd, edema); notify prescriber of fluid overload
- Electrolytes, blood pH, PO_2, HCO_3, during treatment; ABGs frequently during emergencies
- Urine pH, urinary output, during beginning treatment
- Extravasation with IV administration (tissue sloughing, ulceration, and necrosis)
- Weight qd with initial therapy
- Alkalosis: irritability, confusion, twitching, hyperreflexia stimulation, slow respirations, cyanosis, irregular pulse
- Milk-alkali syndrome: confusion, headache, nausea, vomiting, anorexia, urinary stones, hypercalcemia

Administer:

- IV in prepared sol or diluted in an equal amount of compatible sol given 2-5mEq/kg over 4-8 hr, not to exceed 50mEq/hr; slower rate in children

Evaluate:

- Therapeutic response: ABGs, electrolytes, blood pH, HCO_3 WNL

Teach patient/family:

- To chew antacid tablets and drink 8 oz water
- Not to take antacid with milk, or milk-alkali syndrome may result
- Not to use antacid for more than 2 wk
- To notify prescriber if indigestion is accompanied by chest pain, dyspnea, diarrhea, dark, tarry stools
- About sodium-restricted diet; to avoid use of baking soda for indigestion

sodium biphosphate/ sodium phosphate (OTC)

Fleet Enema, Phospho-Soda

Func. class.: Laxative, saline

Action: Increases water absorption in the small intestine by osmotic action, laxative effect occurs by increased peristalsis and water retention

Uses: Constipation, bowel or rectal preparation for surgery, exam

Dosage and routes:

- *Adult:* PO 20-30 ml (Phospho-Soda)
- *Child:* PO 5-15 ml (Phospho-Soda)
- *Adult, child >12 yr:* REC 1 enema (118 ml)
- *Child 2-12 yrs:* REC ½ enema (59 ml)

Available forms: enema 7 g phosphate/19 g biphosphate/118 ml; oral sol 18 g phosphate/48 g biphosphate/100 ml

Side effects/adverse reactions:
GI: Nausea, cramps, diarrhea
META: Electrolyte, fluid imbalances

Contraindications: Hypersensitivity, rectal fissures, abdominal pain, nausea/vomiting, appendicitis, acute surgical abdomen, ulcerated hemorrhoids, Na-restricted diets (Sal-Hepatica, PhosphoSoda)

Precautions: Pregnancy (C)

Pharmacokinetics: Excreted in feces

* Available in Canada only

NURSING CONSIDERATIONS
Assess:
- Stools: color, amount, consistency
- Bowel pattern, bowel sounds, flatulence, distention, fever, dietary patterns, exercise
- Blood, urine electrolytes if drug is used often by patient
- Cramping, rectal bleeding, nausea, vomiting; if these symptoms occur, drug should be discontinued

Administer:
- Alone for better absorption; do not take within 1 hr of other drugs

Evaluate:
- Therapeutic response: decrease in constipation

Teach patient/family:
- Not to use laxatives for long-term therapy; bowel tone will be lost
- That normal bowel movements do not always occur daily
- Not to use in presence of abdominal pain, nausea, vomiting
- To notify prescriber if constipation unrelieved or if symptoms of electrolyte imbalance occur: muscle cramps, pain, weakness, dizziness, excessive thirst
- To maintain adequate fluid consumption

sodium chloride, hypertonic

Adsorbonac Ophthalmic Solution, AK-NaCl, Dey-Pak Sodium Chloride 3% and 10%, Muro-128 Ophthalmic, Muroptic-S

Func. class.: Miscellaneous ophthalmic agent

Chem. class.: Hyperosmolar ophthalmic

Action: Reduces corneal edema by osmosis of water through corneal epithelium, which is semipermeable

Uses: Reduces corneal edema

Dosage and routes:
- *Adult:* INSTILL 1-2 gtt q3-4h or ointment hs

Available forms: Sol 2%, 5%; oint 5%

Side effects/adverse reactions:
EENT: Stinging

Contraindications: Hypersensitivity

NURSING CONSIDERATIONS
Perform/provide:
- Storage in tight container

Evaluate:
- Therapeutic response: decreased corneal edema

Teach patient/family:
- Method of instillation, including pressure on lacrimal sac for 1 min, and not to touch dropper to eye
- That blurred vision is common with oint
- To report double vision, rapid change in vision, appearance of floating spots, acute redness of eyes

sodium polystyrene sulfonate (℞)

(po-lee-stye'reen)

Kayexalate, SPS Suspension

Func. class.: Potassium-removing resin

Chem. class.: Cation exchange resin

Action: Removes potassium by exchanging sodium for potassium in body primarily in large intestine

Uses: Hyperkalemia in conjunction with other measures

Dosage and routes:
- *Adult:* PO 15 g qd-qid; REC enema 30-50 g/100 ml of sorbitol warmed to body temp q6h
- *Child:* PO/REC 1 mEq of K exchanged/g of resin, approximate dose 1g/kg q6h

Available forms: Susp, 15 g polystyrene sulfonate, 21.5 ml sorbitol, 15 g (65 mEq) Na/60 ml; powder 15 g/4 level tsp

Side effects/adverse reactions:
GI: Constipation, anorexia, nausea, vomiting, diarrhea (sorbitol), fecal impaction, gastric irritation
META: Hypocalcemia, hypokalemia, hypomagnesemia, Na retention

Precautions: Pregnancy (C), renal failure, CHF, severe edema, severe hypertension

Interactions:
- Decreased effect of sodium polystyrene: antacids, laxatives

NURSING CONSIDERATIONS

Assess:
- Bowel function qd
- Hypotension: confusion, irritability, muscular pain, weakness
- Serum K, Ca, Mg, Na, acid-base balance

Administer:
- Oral dose as susp mixed with H_2O or syr (20-100 ml)
- Mild laxative as ordered to prevent constipation, fecal impaction
- Sorbitol as ordered to prevent constipation
- Retention enema after mixing with warm water; introduce by gravity, continue stirring, flush with 100 ml of fluid, clamp, and leave in place

Perform/provide:
- Retention of enema for at least ½-1 hr
- Irrigation of colon after enema with 1-2 qt nonsodium sol, drain
- Storage of freshly prepared sol 24 hr at room temp

Evaluate:
- Therapeutic response: K level WNL

sodium thiosalicylate (℞)

Rexolate, Tusal

Func. class.: Nonnarcotic analgesic

Chem. class.: Salicylate

Action: Blocks pain impulses in CNS that occur in response to inhibition of prostaglandin synthesis; antipyretic action results from inhibition of hypothalamic heat-regulating center

Uses: Mild to moderate pain (rheumatic fever, acute gout)

Dosage and routes:

Pain
- *Adult:* IM 50-100 mg qd or qod

Rheumatic fever
- *Adult:* IM 100-150 mg q4-6h × 3 days, then 100 mg bid

Arthritis
- *Adult:* IM 100 mg/day

Available forms: Inj IM 50 mg/ml

Side effects/adverse reactions:
HEMA: ***Thrombocytopenia, agranulocytosis, leukopenia, neutropenia, hemolytic anemia,*** increased protime
CNS: Stimulation, drowsiness, dizziness, confusion, ***convulsions,*** headache, flushing, hallucinations, coma
GI: Nausea, vomiting, GI bleeding, diarrhea, heartburn, anorexia, ***hepatitis***
INTEG: Rash, urticaria, bruising
EENT: Tinnitus, hearing loss
CV: Rapid pulse, ***pulmonary edema***
RESP: Wheezing, hyperpnea
ENDO: Hypoglycemia, hyponatremia, hypokalemia

Contraindications: Hypersensitivity to salicylates, GI bleeding, bleeding disorders, children <3 yr, vit K deficiency, peptic ulcer

* Available in Canada only

Precautions: Anemia, hepatic disease, renal disease, Hodgkin's disease, pregnancy (C), lactation

Pharmacokinetics:

PO: Onset 15-30 min, peak 1-2 hr, duration 4-6 hr

REC: Onset slow, duration 4-6 hr, metabolized by liver, excreted by kidneys, crosses placenta, excreted in breast milk, half-life 1-3½ hr

Interactions:

• Decreased effects of sodium thiosalicylate: antacids, steroids, urinary alkalizers

• Increased blood loss: alcohol, heparin

• Increased effects of anticoagulants, insulin, methotrexate

• Decreased effects of probenecid, spironolactone, sulfinpyrazone, sulfonylmides

• Toxic effects: PABA

Lab test interferences:

Increase: Coagulation studies, liver function studies, serum uric acid, amylase, CO_2, urinary protein

Decrease: Serum K, PBI, cholesterol, blood glucose

Interfere: Urine catecholamines, pregnancy test

NURSING CONSIDERATIONS

Assess:

• Liver function studies: ALT, AST, bilirubin (long-term therapy)

• Renal function studies: BUN, urine creatinine (long-term therapy)

• Blood studies: CBC, Hct, Hgb, pro-time (long-term therapy)

• I&O ratio; decreasing output may indicate renal failure (long-term therapy)

• Hepatotoxicity: dark urine, clay-colored stools, yellow skin, sclera, itching, abdominal pain, fever, diarrhea (long-term therapy)

• Allergic reactions: rash, urticaria; drug may have to be discontinued

• Renal dysfunction: decreased urine output

• Ototoxicity: tinnitus, ringing, roaring in ears; audiometric testing is needed before, after long-term therapy

• Visual changes: blurring, halos, corneal, retinal damage

• Edema in feet, ankles, legs

• Prior drug history; many drug interactions

Evaluate:

• Therapeutic response: less pain

Teach patient/family:

• To report any symptoms of hepatotoxicity, renal toxicity, visual changes, ototoxicity, allergic reactions (long-term therapy)

• Not to exceed recommended dosage; acute poisoning may result

• To read label on other OTC drugs; many contain aspirin

• That therapeutic response takes 2 wk (arthritis)

• To avoid alcohol ingestion; GI bleeding may occur

Treatment of overdose: Lavage, activated charcoal, monitor electrolytes, VS

somatotropin (℞)

(soe-ma-toe-troe′pin)

Humatrope, Nutropin

Func. class.: Pituitary hormone

Chem. class.: Growth hormone

Action: Stimulates growth; somatotropin similar to natural growth hormone; both preparations developed by recombinant DNA

Uses: Pituitary growth hormone deficiency (hypopituitary dwarfism)

Dosage and routes:

• *Child:* SC/IM 2 IU 3 × /wk, less than 48 hr between doses, may give 4 IU if growth is <1 inch/6 mo

Available forms: Inj 5 mg (13 IU)/vial, 10 mg (26 IU)/vial

Side effects/adverse reactions:
GU: Hypercalciuria
INTEG: Rash, urticaria, pain, inflammation at injection site
CNS: Headache, growth of intracranial tumor
ENDO: ***Hyperglycemia, ketosis, hypothyroidism***
SYST: ***Antibodies to growth hormone***
Contraindications: Hypersensitivity to benzyl alcohol, closed epiphyses, intracranial lesions
Precautions: Diabetes mellitus, hypothyroidism, pregnancy (C)
Pharmacokinetics:
Half-life 15-60 min, duration 7 days; metabolized in liver
Interactions:
• Decreased growth: glucocorticosteroids
• Epiphyseal closure: androgens, thyroid hormones

NURSING CONSIDERATIONS
Assess:
• Growth hormone antibodies if patient fails to respond to therapy
• Thyroid function tests: T_3, T_4, T_7, TSH to identify hypothyroidism
• Allergic reaction: rash, itching, fever, nausea, wheezing
• Hypercalciuria: urinary stones; groin, flank pain; nausea, vomiting, frequency, hematuria, chills
• Growth rate of child at intervals during treatment
Administer:
• IM; rotate injection site
• Nutropin: after reconstituting 10 IU/5 ml bacteriostatic H_2O for injection, do not shake
• Humetrope: 5 mg/1.5-5 ml diluent, do not shake
Perform/provide:
• Storage in refrigerator for <1 mo if reconstituted <1 wk; do not use discolored or cloudy sol
Evaluate:
• Therapeutic response: growth in children

sotalol (℞)
(soe-ta'lole)
Betapace, Sotacar*
Func. class.: Antidysrhythmic group II, III
Chem. class.: Nonselective β-blocker

Action: Blockade of β_1 and β_2 receptors leads to antidysrhythmic effect
Uses: Life-threatening ventricular dysrhythmias
Dosage and routes:
• *Adult:* PO initial 80 mg bid, may increase to 240-320 mg/day
Available forms: Tabs 80, 160, 240 mg
Side effects/adverse reactions:
CV: Orthostatic hypotension, bradycardia, CHF, chest pain, ventricular dysrhythmias, AV block, peripheral vascular insufficiency, palpitations
CNS: Dizziness, mental changes, drowsiness, fatigue, headache, catatonia, depression, anxiety, nightmares, paresthesia, lethargy, insomnia, decreased concentration
GI: Nausea, vomiting, diarrhea, dry mouth, flatulence, constipation, anorexia
INTEG: Rash, alopecia, urticaria, pruritus, fever
HEMA: ***Agranulocytosis, thrombocytopenic purpura (rare), thrombocytopenia, leukopenia***
EENT: Tinnitus, visual changes, sore throat, double vision, dry burning eyes
GU: Impotence, dysuria, ejaculatory failure, urinary retention
RESP: ***Bronchospasm***, dyspnea, wheezing, nasal stuffiness, pharyngitis

* Available in Canada only

MS: Joint pain, arthralgia, muscle cramps, pain
OTHER: Facial swelling, decreased exercise tolerance, weight change, Raynaud's disease
Contraindications: Hypersensitivity to β-blockers, cardiogenic shock, heart block (2nd or 3rd degree), sinus bradycardia, CHF, bronchial asthma, congenital or acquired long QT syndrome
Precautions: Major surgery, pregnancy (B), lactation, diabetes mellitus, renal disease, thyroid disease, COPD, well-compensated heart failure, CAD, nonallergic bronchospasm, electrolyte disturbances, bradycardia, cardiac dysrhythmias, peripheral vascular disease
Pharmacokinetics:
PO: Onset 1-2 hr, peak 2-4 hr, duration 8-12 hr, half-life 12 hr; metabolized by liver (metabolites inactive), excreted unchanged in urine, crosses placenta, excreted in breast milk
Interactions:
• Increased hypotension: diuretics, other antihypertensives, nitroglycerin, prazosin
• Decreased β-blocker effects: sympathomimetics, nonsteroidal antiinflammatory agents, salicylates
• Increased hypoglycemia effect: insulin
• Increased effects of lidocaine
• Decreased bronchodilating effects of theophylline
• Decreased hypoglycemic effects of sulfonylureas
Lab test interferences:
• *False increase:* Urinary catecholamines
• *Interference:* Glucose, insulin tolerance tests
NURSING CONSIDERATIONS
Assess:
• I&O, weight qd
• B/P, pulse q4h; note rate, rhythm, quality
• Apical/radial pulse before administration: notify prescriber of any significant changes
• Baselines in renal, liver function tests before therapy begins
• Edema in feet, legs qd
• Skin turgor, dryness of mucous membranes for hydration status
Administer:
• PO: ac, hs; tablet may be crushed or swallowed whole
• Reduced dosage in renal dysfunction
Perform/provide:
• Storage in dry area at room temp; do not freeze
Evaluate:
• Therapeutic response: absence of life-threatening dysrhythmias
Teach patient/family:
• Not to discontinue drug abruptly; taper over 2 wk or may precipitate angina
• Not to use OTC products containing α-adrenergic stimulants (nasal decongestants, OTC cold preparations) unless directed by prescriber
• To report bradycardia, dizziness, confusion, depression, fever
• To take pulse at home; advise when to notify prescriber
• To avoid alcohol, smoking, sodium intake
• To carry Medic Alert ID to identify drug being taken, allergies
• To avoid hazardous activities if dizziness is present
• To report symptoms of CHF including: difficulty in breathing, especially on exertion or when lying down; night cough, swelling of extremities
• To take medication to minimize orthostatic hypotension
• To wear support hose to minimize effects of orthostatic hypotension

Treatment of overdose: Lavage, IV atropine for bradycardia, IV theophylline for bronchospasm, digitalis, O_2, diuretic for cardiac failure; hemodialysis is useful for removal; administer vasopressor (norepinephrine) for hypotension, isoproterenol for heart block

spectinomycin (℞)

(spek-ti-noe-mye'sin)

Trobicin

Func. class.: Antibiotic

Chem. class.: Aminocyclitol

Action: Inhibits bacterial synthesis by binding to 30S subunit on ribosomes

Uses: Gonorrhea

Dosage and routes:

• *Adult:* IM 2-4 g as single dose

Available forms: Inj IM 2, 4 g

Side effects/adverse reactions:

CNS: Dizziness, chills, fever, insomnia, headache, anxiety

HEMA: Anemia

GI: Nausea, vomiting, increased BUN

GU: Decreased urine output

INTEG: Pain at injection site, urticaria, rash, pruritus, fever

Contraindications: Hypersensitivity, syphilis

Precautions: Pregnancy (B), infants, children

Pharmacokinetics:

IM: Peak 1-2 hr, duration >8 hr, half-life 1-3 hr, excreted in urine (active form)

NURSING CONSIDERATIONS

Assess:

• Gonorrhea culture after treatment

• I&O ratio; report decreased output

• Liver studies: AST (SGOT), ALT (SGPT), serum alk phosphatase following multiple doses

• Blood studies: Hct, Hgb, BUN if multiple diagnoses given

• Serologic test for gonorrhea 3 mo after treatment

• Allergies before treatment, reaction of each medication

Administer:

• After shaking vial

• IM in deep muscle mass

• With 20G needle; no more than 5 ml per site

Perform/provide:

• Storage at room temp; discard reconstituted sol after 24 hr

• Treatment of partner; report infection

Evaluate:

• Therapeutic response: negative gonorrhea culture after treatment

spirapril (℞)

(spir'a-pril)

Renormax

Func. class.: Antihypertensive

Chem. class.: Angiotensin-converting enzyme (ACE) inhibitor

Action: Selectively suppresses renin-angiotensin-aldosterone system; inhibits ACE, prevents conversion of angiotensin I to angiotensin II; results in dilation of arterial, venous vessels

Uses: Hypertension

Dosage and routes:

Unknown at this time

Available forms: Not available at this time

Side effects/adverse reactions:

• Possible side effects, adverse reactions

CV: Hypotension, postural hypotension, syncope, palpitations, angina

GU: Increased BUN, creatinine, decreased libido, impotence, urinary tract infection

* Available in Canada only

HEMA: ***Neutropenia, agranulocytosis***
INTEG: ***Angioedema,*** *rash,* flushing, sweating
RESP: *Cough,* asthma, bronchitis, dyspnea, sinusitis
META: Hyperkalemia, hyponatremia
GI: *Nausea, diarrhea,* vomiting, gastritis, melena
CNS: Anxiety, hypertonia, insomnia, paresthesia, headache, dizziness, fatigue
MS: Arthralgia, arthritis, myalgia

Contraindications: Hypersensitivity to ACE inhibitors

Precautions: Impaired renal, liver function, dialysis patients, hypovolemia, blood dyscrasias, CHF, COPD, asthma, elderly, bilateral renal artery, stenosis, pregnancy, lactation, children

Pharmacokinetics:
Biphasic half-life 2 hrs, 35 hrs, metabolized by liver

Interactions:
- Possible interactions
- Increased hypotension: diuretics, other antihypertensives, ganglionic blockers, adrenergic blockers
- Increased toxicity: vasodilators, hydralazine, prazosin, potassium-sparing diuretics, sympathomimetics, potassium supplements
- Decreased absorption: antacids

Lab test interferences:
False positive: Urine acetone

NURSING CONSIDERATIONS
Assess:
- Blood studies: neutrophils, decreased platelets
- B/P, check for orthostatic hypotension, syncope
- Renal studies: protein, BUN, creatinine; rise may indicate nephrotic syndrome
- Baselines in renal, liver function tests before therapy
- Potassium throughout treatment, although hyperkalemia rare
- Dipstick of urine for protein qd in first morning specimen; if protein is increased, 24 hr urinary protein should be collected
- Edema in feet, legs daily
- Allergic reactions: rash, fever, pruritus, urticaria; drug should be discontinued if antihistamines fail to help
- Renal symptoms: polyuria, oliguria, frequencey, dysuria

Administer:
- IV infusion of 0.9% NaCl (as ordered) to expand fluid volume if severe hypotension occurs

Perform/provide:
- Storage in air-tight container below 86° F (30° C)
- Supine or Trendelenburg position for severe hypotension

Evaluate:
- Therapeutic response: decrease in B/P

Teach patient/family:
- Not to discontinue drug abruptly
- Not to use OTC products (cough, cold, allergy) unless directed by prescriber
- Not to use salt substitutes containing potassium without consulting prescriber
- Importance of complying with dosage schedule, even if feeling better
- To rise slowly to sitting or standing position to minimize orthostatic hypotension
- To notify prescriber of mouth sores, sore throat, fever, swelling of hands or feet, irregular heartbeat, chest pain
- To report excessive perspiration, dehydration, vomiting, diarrhea; may lead to fall in B/P

• That drug may cause dizziness, fainting, light-headedness during 1st few days of therapy
• That drug may cause skin rash or impaired perspiration
• How to take B/P, and normal readings for age group

Treatment of overdose: 0.9% NaCl IV infusion, hemodialysis

spironolactone (℞)

(speer'on-oh-lak'tone)
Aldactone, Novospiroton, Sincomen

Func. class.: Potassium-sparing diuretic

Chem. class.: Aldosterone antagonist

Action: Competes with aldosterone at receptor sites in distal tubule, resulting in excretion of sodium chloride, water, retention of potassium, phosphate

Uses: Edema, hypertension, diuretic-induced hypokalemia, primary hyperaldosteronism (diagnosis, short-term treatment, long-term treatment), nephrotic syndrome, cirrhosis of the liver with ascites

Dosage and routes:

Edema/hypertension
• *Adult:* PO 25-200 mg/qd in single or divided doses
• *Child:* PO 3.3 mg/kg/day in single or divided doses

Hypokalemia
• *Adult:* PO 25-100 mg/day; if PO, K supplements must not be used

Primary hyperaldosteronism diagnosis
• *Adult:* PO 400 mg/day × 4 days or 4 wk depending on test, then 100-400 mg/day maintenance

Available forms: Tab 25, 50, 100 mg

Side effects/adverse reactions:
CNS: Headache, confusion, drowsiness, lethargy, ataxia
GI: Diarrhea, cramps, ***bleeding,*** gastritis, *vomiting,* anorexia, nausea
CV: Dysrythmias
INTEG: Rash, pruritus, urticaria
ENDO: Impotence, gynecomastia, irregular menses, amenorrhea, postmenopausal bleeding, hirsutism, deepening voice
HEMA: Decreased WBCs, platelets
ELECT: Hyperchloremic metabolic acidosis, ***hyperkalemia,*** hyponatremia

Contraindications: Hypersensitivity, anuria, severe renal disease, hyperkalemia, pregnancy (D)

Precautions: Dehydration, hepatic disease, lactation

Pharmacokinetics:
PO: Onset 24-48 hr, peak 48-72 hr; metabolized in liver, excreted in urine, crosses placenta

Interactions:
• Increased action of antihypertensives, digitalis, lithium
• Increased hyperkalemia: K-sparing diuretics, K products, ACE inhibitors, salt substitutes
• Decreased effect of spironolactone: ASA

Lab test interferences:
Interference: 17-OHCS, 17-KS, radioimmunoassay, digoxin assay

NURSING CONSIDERATIONS

Assess:
• Electrolytes: Na, Cl, K, BUN, serum creatinine, ABGs, CBC
• Weight, I&O qd to determine fluid loss; effect of drug may be decreased if used qd; ECG periodically (long-term therapy)
• Signs of metabolic acidosis: drowsiness, restlessness
• Rashes, temperature qd
• Confusion, especially in elderly; take safety precautions if needed

• Hydration: skin turgor, thirst, dry mucous membranes

Administer:

• In AM to avoid interference with sleep

• With food; if nausea occurs, absorption may be decreased slightly

Evaluate:

• Therapeutic response: improvement in edema of feet, legs, sacral area qd if medication is being used in CHF

Teach patient/family:

• To avoid foods with high K^+ content: oranges, bananas, salt substitutes, dried apricots, dates

• That drowsiness, ataxia, mental confusion may occur; observe caution in driving

• To notify prescriber of cramps, diarrhea, lethargy, thirst, headache, skin rash, menstrual abnormalities, deepening voice, breast enlargement

Treatment of overdose: Lavage if taken orally; monitor electrolytes, administer IV fluids, monitor hydration, renal, CV status

stanozolol (℞)

(stan-oh'zoe'lole)

Winstrol

Func. class.: Androgenic anabolic steroid

Chem. class.: Halogenated testosterone derivative

Action: Increases weight by building body tissue; increases potassium, phosphorus, chloride, and nitrogen levels; increases bone development

Uses: Prevention of hereditary angioedema, aplastic anemia to increase hemoglobin

Dosage and routes:

Aplastic anemia (possibly effective)

• *Adult:* PO 2 mg tid

• *Child 6-12 yr:* PO up to 2 mg tid

• *Child <6 yr:* PO 1 mg bid

Angioedema

• *Adult:* PO 2 mg tid, then decrease q1-3 mo, down to 2 mg qd or q2d

Available forms: Tabs 2 mg

Side effects/adverse reactions:

INTEG: Rash, acneiform lesions, oily hair, skin, flushing, sweating, acne vulgaris, alopecia, hirsutism

CNS: Dizziness, headache, fatigue, tremors, paresthesias, flushing, sweating, anxiety, lability, insomnia, carpal tunnel syndrome

MS: Cramps, spasms

CV: Increased B/P

GU: ***Hematuria,*** amenorrhea, vaginitis, decreased libido, decreased breast size, clitoral hypertrophy, testicular atrophy

GI: Nausea, vomiting, constipation, weight gain, ***cholestatic jaundice***

EENT: Conjunctional edema, nasal congestion

ENDO: Abnormal GTT

Contraindications: Severe renal, severe cardiac, severe hepatic disease, hypersensitivity, pregnancy (X), lactation, genital bleeding (abnormal)

Precautions: Diabetes mellitus, CV disease, MI

Pharmacokinetics:

PO: Metabolized in liver, excreted in urine, crosses placenta, excreted in breast milk

Interactions:

• Increased effects of oral antidiabetics, oxyphenbutazone

• Increased PT: anticoagulants

• Edema: ACTH, adrenal steroids

• Decreased effects of insulin

Lab test interferences:

Increase: Serum cholesterol, blood glucose, urine glucose

S

Decrease: Serum Ca, serum K, T_4, T_3, thyroid ^{131}I uptake test, urine 17-OHCS

NURSING CONSIDERATIONS

Assess:

- Weight qd, notify prescriber if weekly weight gain is >5 lb
- B/P q4h
- I&O ratio; be alert for decreasing urinary output, increasing edema
- Growth rate in children; growth rate may be uneven (linear/bone growth) (extended use)
- Electrolytes: K, Na, Cl, Ca; cholesterol
- Liver function studies: ALT (SGPT), AST (SGOT), bilirubin
- Edema, hypertension, cardiac symptoms, jaundice
- Mental status: affect, mood, behavioral changes, aggression
- Signs of masculinization in female: increased libido, deepening of voice, breast tissue, enlarged clitoris, menstrual irregularities; male: gynecomastia, impotence, testicular atrophy
- Hypercalcemia: lethargy, polyuria, polydipsia, nausea, vomiting, constipation; dosage may have to be decreased
- Hypoglycemia in diabetics, since oral antidiabetic action is increased

Administer:

- Titrated dose; use lowest effective dose

Perform/provide:

- Diet with increased calories and protein; decrease Na for edema
- Supportive drug of anemia

Evaluate:

- Therapeutic response: 4-6 wk in osteoporosis

Teach patient/family:

- That drug must be combined with complete health plan: diet, rest, exercise
- To notify prescriber if therapeutic response decreases
- Not to discontinue abruptly
- About change in sex characteristics
- Women to report menstrual irregularities
- That 1-3-mo course is necessary for response in breast cancer
- Procedure for use of buccal tablets (requires 30-60 min to dissolve; change absorption site with each dose; do not eat, drink, chew, or smoke while tablet is in place)

---

stavudine (℞)

(sta'vu-deen)

Zerit

Func. class.: Antiviral

Chem. class.: Thymidine nucleoside

Action: Prevents replication of HIV by the inhibition of the enzyme reverse transcriptase, causes DNA chain termination

Uses: Treatment of advanced HIV infection not responsive to other antivirals

Dosage and routes:

- *Adult >60 kg:* PO 40 mg q12h up to 2 mg/kg/day
- *Adult <60 kg:* 30 mg q12hr

Available forms: Caps 15, 20, 30, 40 mg

Side effects/adverse reactions:

HEMA: ***Bone marrow suppression***

CNS: Peripheral neuropathy, insomnia, anxiety, neuropathy, depression, dizziness, confusion

GI: ***Hepatotoxicity,*** diarrhea, nausea, vomiting, anorexia, dyspepsia, constipation, stomatitis

MS: Myalgia, arthralgia

CV: Chest pain, vasodilation, hypertension

RESP: Dyspnea, pneumonia, asthma

INTEG: Rash, sweating, pruritis, benign neoplasms

---

* Available in Canada only

EENT: Conjunctivitis, abnormal vision
Contraindications: Hypersensitivity to this drug or zidovudine, didanosine, zalcitabine; severe peripheral neuropathy
Precautions: Advanced HIV infection, pregnancy (C), lactation, bone marrow suppression, renal, liver disease
Interactions:
• Increased myelosuppression: other myelosuppressants
Pharmacokinetics: Excreted in urine, breast milk; peak 1 hr; half-life: elimination: 1-1.6 hr, intracellular: 3-3.5 hr

NURSING CONSIDERATIONS
Assess:
• Liver studies: AST (SGOT), ALT (SGPT)
• Blood studies: WBC, diff, RBC, Hct, Hgb, platelets
• Renal studies: urinalysis, protein, blood
• C&S before drug therapy; drug may be given as soon as culture is taken
• Bowel pattern before, during treatment
• Weakness, tremors, confusion, dizziness; drug may have to be decreased or discontinued
Administer:
• With or without meals; absorption does not appear to be lowered when taken with food
Teach patient/family:
• Signs of peripheral neuropathy: burning, weakness, pain, pricking feeling in the extremities
• Drug should not be given with antineoplastics
• Not cure for AIDS, but will control symptoms
• To call prescriber if sore throat, swollen lymph nodes, malaise, fever occur; other drugs may be needed to prevent other infections
• Even with this drug, patient may pass AIDS virus to others
• Follow-up visits necessary; serious toxicity may occur; blood counts must be done q2wk
• To take q12h around clock
• Serious drug interactions may occur if OTC products are ingested; see prescriber before taking aspirin, acetaminophen, indomethacin
• May cause fainting or dizziness
Evaluate:
Therapeutic response: decreased symptoms of HIV

streptokinase (℞)
(strep-toe-kye′nase)
Kabikinase, Streptase
Func. class.: Thrombolytic enzyme
Chem. class.: β-Hemolytic streptococcus filtrate (purified)

Action: Activates conversion of plasminogen to plasmin (fibrinolysin): plasmin breaks down clots (fibrin), fibrinogen, factors V, VII; occlusion of venous access lines
Uses: Deep vein thrombosis, pulmonary embolism, arterial thrombosis, arterial embolism, arteriovenous cannula occlusion, lysis of coronary artery thrombi after MI, acute evolving transmural MI
Dosage and routes:
Lysis of coronary artery thrombi
• *Adult:* IC 20,000 IU, then 2000 IU/min over 1 hr as IV INF
Arteriovenous cannula occlusion
• *Adult:* IV INF 250,000 IU/2 ml sol into occluded limb of cannula run over ½ hr; clamp for 2 hr; aspirate contents; flush with NaCl sol and reconnect
Thrombosis/embolism
• *Adult:* IV INF 250,000 IU over ½ hr, then 100,000 IU/hr for 72 hr for

S

deep thrombosis; 100,000 IU/hr over 24-72 hr for pulmonary embolism
Acute evolving transmural MI
• *Adult:* IV INF 1,500,000 IU diluted to a volume of 45 ml; give within 1 hr
Available forms: Inj IV 250,000, 600,000, 750,000 IU
Side effects/adverse reactions:
CNS: Headache, fever
EENT: Periorbital edema
GI: Nausea
HEMA: Decreased Hct, ***bleeding***
INTEG: Rash, urticaria, phlebitis at IV inf site, itching, flushing
MS: Low back pain
RESP: Altered respirations, SOB, ***bronchospasm***
SYST: ***GI, GU, intracranial retroperitoneal bleeding, surface bleeding, anaphylaxis***
Contraindications: Hypersensitivity, active bleeding, intraspinal surgery, CNS neoplasms, ulcerative colitis, enteritis, severe hypertension, severe renal disease, hepatic disease, hypocoagulation, COPD, subacute bacterial endocarditis, rheumatic valvular disease, cerebral embolism/thrombosis/hemorrhage, intraarterial diagnostic procedure or surgery (10 days), recent major surgery
Precautions: Arterial emboli from left side of heart, pregnancy (C)
Pharmacokinetics:
IV: Onset immediate, duration <12 hr; excreted in bile, urine, half-life <20 min
Interactions:
• Bleeding potential: aspirin, indomethacin, phenylbutazone, anticoagulants
Y-site compatibility: Lidocaine
Lab test interferences:
Increase: PT, APTT, TT
NURSING CONSIDERATIONS
Assess:
• Allergy: fever, rash, itching, chills; mild reaction may be treated with antihistamines
• For bleeding during 1st hr of treatment; hematuria, hematemesis, bleeding from mucous membranes, epistaxis, ecchymosis
• Blood studies (Hct, platelets, PTT, PT, TT, APTT) before starting therapy; PT or APTT must be less than ×2 control before starting therapy; PTT or PT q3-4h during treatment
• For hypersensitive reactions: fever, rash, dyspnea; drug should be discontinued
• VS, B/P, pulse, respirations, neuro signs, temp at least q4h; temp >104° F (40° C) indicates internal bleeding, cardiac rhythm following intracoronary administration; systolic pressure increase >25 mm Hg should be reported to prescriber
• For neurologic changes that may indicate intracranial bleeding
• Retroperitoneal bleeding: back pain, leg weakness, diminished pulses
• For streptokinase reactions previously
Administer:
• As soon as thrombi identified; not useful for thrombi over 1 wk old
• Cryoprecipitate or fresh frozen plasma if bleeding occurs
• Loading dose at beginning of therapy; may require increased loading doses
• Heparin after fibrinogen level >100 mg/dl; heparin infusion to increase PTT to 1.5-2 × baseline for 3-7 days
• After reconstituting with 5 ml NS or D_5W; do not shake; further dilute to total volume of 45 ml; may be diluted to 500 ml in 45 ml increments; may dilute vial in 15 ml NS, further dilute 750,000 IU/50 ml NS or D_5W; further dilute 1,500,000 IU dose/100 ml or more

* Available in Canada only

• About 10% patients have high streptococcal antibody titers requiring increased loading doses
• IV therapy using 0.8 μm filter

Perform/provide:
• Storage of reconstituted sol in refrigerator; discard after 24 hr
• Bed rest during entire course of treatment
• Avoidance of venous or arterial puncture, inj, rectal temp; any invasive treatment
• Treatment of fever with acetaminophen or aspirin
• Pressure for 30 sec to minor bleeding sites; inform prescriber if this does not attain hemostasis; apply pressure dressing

Evaluate:
• Therapeutic response: resolution of thrombosis, embolism

---

streptomycin (℞)

(strep-toe-mye'sin)

Func. class.: Antiinfective/antitubercular

Chem. class.: Aminoglycoside

Action: Interferes with protein synthesis in bacterial cell by binding to ribosomal subunit, causing inaccurate peptide sequence to form in protein chain, causing bacterial death

Uses: Sensitive strains of *M. tuberculosis,* nontuberculous infections caused by sensitive strains of *Y. pestis, Brucella, H. influenzae, K. pneumoniae, E. coli, E. aerogenes, S. viridans, F. tularensis, Proteus*

Dosage and routes:

Tuberculosis
• *Adult:* IM 1g qd × 2-3 mo, then 1 g 2-3 × /week with other antitubercular drugs
• *Child:* IM 20-40 mg/kg/day in divided doses with other antitubercular drugs; max 15 mg/kg/day

Streptococcal endocarditis
• *Adult:* IM 1 g q12h × 1 wk with penicillin, then 500 mg bid × 1 wk

Enterococcal endocarditis
• *Adult:* IM 1 g q12h × 2 wk, then 500 mg q12h × 4 wk with penicillin, max 15 mg/kg/day

Available forms: Inj 1, 5 g: 400 mg/ml

Side effects/adverse reactions:

GU: ***Oliguria, hematuria, renal damage, azotemia, renal failure, nephrotoxicity***

CNS: Confusion, depression, numbness, tremors, ***convulsions,*** muscle twitching, ***neurotoxicity***

EENT: ***Ototoxicity,*** deafness, visual disturbances

HEMA: ***Agranulocytosis, thrombocytopenia, leukopenia, eosinophilia, anemia***

GI: Nausea, vomiting, anorexia, increased ALT (SGPT), AST (SGOT), bilirubin, hepatomegaly, ***hepatic necrosis,*** splenomegaly

CV: Hypotension, myocarditis, palpitations

INTEG: Rash, burning, urticaria, dermatitis, alopecia

Contraindications: Severe renal disease, hypersensitivity

Precautions: Neonates, mild renal disease, pregnancy (B), myasthenia gravis, lactation, hearing deficit, elderly, Parkinson's disease

Pharmacokinetics:

IM: Onset rapid, peak 1-2 hr; plasma half-life 2-2½ hr; not metabolized, excreted unchanged in urine, crosses placental barrier

Interactions:
• Increased ototoxicity, neurotoxicity, nephrotoxicity: other aminoglycosides, amphotericin B, polymyxin, vancomycin, ethacrynic acid, furosemide, mannitol, methoxyflurane, cisplatin, cephalosporins, bacitracin

• Do not mix in sol or syringe: carbenicillin, ticarcillin, amphotericin B, cephalothin, erythromycin, heparin
• Increased effects: nondepolarizing muscle relaxants, succinylcholine, warfarin

NURSING CONSIDERATIONS
Assess:
• Weight before treatment; calculation of dosage is usually based on ideal body weight, but may be calculated on actual body weight
• I&O ratio, urinalysis qd for proteinuria, cells, casts; report sudden change in urine output
• Serum peak 20-30 min after IM injection, trough level drawn 8 hr
• Urine pH if drug is used for UTI; urine should be kept alkaline
• Renal impairment by collecting urine for CrCl testing, BUN, serum creatinine; lower dosage should be given in renal impairment (CrCl <80 ml/min)
• Deafness by audiometric testing, ringing, roaring in ears, vertigo; assess hearing before, during, after treatment
• Dehydration: high specific gravity, decrease in skin turgor, dry mucous membranes, dark urine
• Overgrowth of infection: fever, malaise, redness, pain, swelling, perineal itching, diarrhea, stomatitis, change in cough, sputum
• C&S before starting treatment to identify infecting organism
• Vestibular dysfunction: nausea, vomiting, dizziness, headache; drug should be discontinued if severe
• Inj sites for redness, swelling, abscesses; use warm compresses at site

Administer:
• IM inj in large muscle mass; rotate inj sites
• Drug in evenly spaced doses to maintain blood level

Perform/provide:
• Adequate fluids of 2-3 L/day unless contraindicated to prevent irritation of tubules
• Supervised ambulation, other safety measures with vestibular dysfunction

Evaluate:
• Therapeutic effect: absence of fever, draining wounds, negative C&S after treatment

Teach patient/family:
• To report headache, dizziness, symptoms of overgrowth of infection, renal impairment
• To report loss of hearing, ringing, roaring in ears, fullness in head

Treatment of overdose: Hemodialysis; monitor serum levels of drug

streptozocin (℞)
(strep-toe-zoe'sin)
Zanosar
Func. class.: Antineoplastic alkylating agent
Chem. class.: Nitrosourea

Action: Alkylates DNA, RNA; inhibits enzymes that allow synthesis of amino acids in proteins; is also responsible for cross-linking DNA strands; activity is not cell cycle phase specific
Uses: Metastatic islet cell carcinoma of pancreas
Investigational uses: Prevention of spread of Hodgkin's disease, metastatic carcinoid tumor, pancreatic adenocarcinoma colon malignancies
Dosage and routes:
• *Adult:* IV 500 mg/m^2 × 5 days q6wk until desired response; alternate with 1 g/m^2 qwk × 2 wk, not to exceed 1.5 g/m^2 in 1 dose
Available forms: Inj 1 g
Side effects/adverse reactions:
HEMA: ***Thrombocytopenia, leukopenia, pancytopenia***

* Available in Canada only

CNS: Confusion, depression, lethargy
GI: Nausea, vomiting, diarrhea, weight loss, ***hepatotoxicity***
GU: ***Azotemia, anuria,*** hypophosphatemia, glycosuria, renal tubular acidosis, ***renal toxicity***
Contraindications: Hypersensitivity
Precautions: Radiation therapy, children, lactation, pregnancy (C), hepatic disease, renal disease
Pharmacokinctics:
IV: Metabolized by liver, excreted in urine, half-life 5 min, terminal 35-40 min
Interactions:
- Increased toxicity: neurotoxic agents, other antineoplastics
- Increased action of doxorubicin
- Decreased effect of streptozocin: phenytoin
- Considered incompatible in sol or syringe with any other drug

NURSING CONSIDERATIONS
Assess:
- CBC, differential, platelet count qwk; withhold drug if WBC is <4000 or platelet count is <75,000; notify prescriber
- Renal function studies: BUN, serum uric acid, phosphate urine CrCl before, during therapy
- I&O ratio; report fall in urine output of 30 ml/hr
- Monitor temp q4h (may indicate beginning infection)
- Liver function tests before, during therapy (bilirubin, AST [SGOT], ALT [SGPT], LDH) as needed or qmo, blood sugar levels qd and observe for hypoglycemia
- Bleeding: hematuria, guaiac, bruising or petechiae, mucosa or orifices q8h
- Food preferences; list likes, dislikes
- Inflammation of mucosa, breaks in skin
- Yellow skin, sclera, dark urine, clay-colored stools, itchy skin, abdominal pain, fever, diarrhea
- Local irritation, pain, burning, discoloration at injection site
- Symptoms indicating severe allergic reaction: rash, urticaria, itching, flushing

Administer:
- Antiemetic 30-60 min before giving drug to prevent vomiting
- Antibiotics for prophylaxis of infection
- IV after diluting 1 g/9.5 ml 0.9% NaCl or D_5; may be further diluted in 50-250 mg; may be given directly over 5-15 min
- Using 21G, 23G, 25G needle
- Topical or systemic analgesics for pain
- Local or systemic drugs for infection

Perform/provide:
- Storage protected from light; refrigerate reconstituted sol; stable for 48 hr at room temp
- Strict medical asepsis, protective isolation if WBC levels are low
- Special skin care
- Warm compresses at inj site for inflammation
- Adequate hydration that may reduce renal toxicity

Evaluate:
- Therapeutic response: decreased tumor size, spread of malignancy

Teach patient/family:
- About protective isolation
- To report signs of infection: fever, sore throat, flu symptoms
- To report signs of anemia: fatigue, headache, faintness, shortness of breath, irritability
- To avoid use of razors, commercial mouthwash
- To avoid use of aspirin products, ibuprofen

S

succimer (℞)

(sux'i-mer)
Chemet
Func. class.: Heavy metal antagonist
Chem. class.: Chelating agent

Action: Binds with ions of lead to form a water-soluble complex excreted by kidneys
Uses: Lead poisoning in children with lead levels above 45 μg/dl; may be beneficial in mercury, arsenic poisoning
Dosage and routes:
• *Child:* PO 10 mg/kg or 350 mg/m^2 q8h × 5 days, then 10 mg/kg or 350 mg/m^2 q12h × 2 wk; another course may be required depending on lead levels; allow 2 wk between courses
Available forms: Caps 100 mg
Side effects/adverse reactions:
SYST: Back, stomach, head, rib flank pain, abdominal cramps, chills, fever, flulike symptoms, head cold, headache
HEMA: ***Increased platelets, intermittent eosinophilia***
GU: ***Proteinuria,*** decreased urination, voiding difficulties
INTEG: Rash, urticaria, pruritus
META: Increased AST (SGOT), ALT (SGOT), alk phosphatase, cholesterol
GI: Nausea, vomiting, diarrhea, metallic taste, anorexia
CNS: Drowsiness, dizziness, paresthesia, sensorimotor neuropathy
EENT: Otitis media, watery eyes, film in eyes, plugged ears
RESP: Sore throat, rhinorrhea, nasal congestion, cough
Contraindications: Hypersensitivity
Precautions: Pregnancy (C), lactation, children <1 yr
Pharmacokinetics:
PO: Peak 1-2 hr, 49% excreted as 39% in feces, 9% urine, 1% as CO_2 from the lungs
Interactions:
• Not recommended concurrently with other chelating agents
NURSING CONSIDERATIONS
Assess:
• Hepatic, renal studies: ALT (SGPT), AST (SGOT), alk phosphatase, BUN, creatinine, serum lead level
• I&O
• For lead sources in home, school
• Allergic reactions: rash, pruritus, urticaria; drug should be discontinued if antihistamines fail to help
Administer:
• To children who cannot swallow capsule by separating the capsule and sprinkling content on food or in a spoon followed by a drink
Perform/provide:
• Adequate fluids; check hydration status qd
Evaluate:
• Therapeutic response: decrease in serum lead level
Teach patient/family:
• That therapeutic effect may take 1-3 mo
• To report urticaria, rash

succinylcholine (℞)

(suk-sin-ill-koe'leen)
Anectine, Anectine Flo-Pack, Quelicin, succinylcholine chloride, Sucostrin, Suxamethonium
Func. class.: Neuromuscular blocker (depolarizing-ultra short)

Action: Inhibits transmission of nerve impulses by binding with cholinergic receptor sites, antagonizing action of acetylcholine; causes release of histamine

* Available in Canada only

Uses: Facilitation of endotracheal intubation, skeletal muscle relaxation during orthopedic manipulations

Dosage and routes:

- *Adult:* IV 25-75 mg, then 2.5 mg/min as needed; IM 2.5 mg/kg, not to exceed 150 mg
- *Child:* IV/IM 1-2 mg/kg, not to exceed 150 mg IM

Available forms: Inj 20, 50, 100 mg/ml; powder for inj 100, 500 mg/vial, 1 g/vial

Side effects/adverse reactions:

CV: Bradycardia, tachycardia; increased, decreased B/P, ***sinus arrest, dysrhythmias***

RESP: ***Prolonged apnea, bronchospasm, cyanosis, respiratory depression***

EENT: Increased secretions, increased intraocular pressure

MS: Weakness, muscle pain, fasciculations, prolonged relaxation

HEMA: ***Myoglobulinemia***

INTEG: Rash, flushing, pruritus, urticaria

Contraindications: Hypersensitivity, malignant hyperthermia, decreased plasma pseudocholinesterase, penetrating eye injuries, acute narrow-angle glaucoma

Precautions: Pregnancy (C), cardiac disease, severe burns, fractures—fasciculations may increase damage—lactation, children <2 yr, electrolyte imbalances, dehydration, neuromuscular disease, respiratory disease, collagen diseases, glaucoma, eye surgery, elderly or debilitated patients

Pharmacokinetics:

IV: Onset 1 min, peak 2-3 min, duration 6-10 min

IM: Onset 2-3 min

Hydrolyzed in urine (active/inactive metabolites)

Interactions:

- Increased neuromuscular blockade: aminoglycosides, clindamycin, lincomycin, quinidine, local anesthetics, polymyxin antibiotics, lithium, narcotic analgesics, thiazides, enflurane, isoflurane, Mg salts, oxytocin
- Dysrhythmias: theophylline

Syringe compatibility: Heparin

Y-site compatibilities: Potassium chloride, vitamin B with C

Additive compatibilities: Amikacin, cephapirin, isoproterenol, meperidine, methyldopate, morphine, norepinephrine, scopolamine

NURSING CONSIDERATIONS

Assess:

- For electrolyte imbalances (K, Mg); may lead to increased action of this drug
- Vital signs (B/P, pulse, respirations, airway) until fully recovered; rate, depth, pattern of respirations, strength of hand grip
- I&O ratio; check for urinary retention, frequency, hesitancy
- Recovery: decreased paralysis of face, diaphragm, leg, arm, rest of body
- Allergic reactions: rash, fever, respiratory distress, pruritus; drug should be discontinued

Administer:

- Using nerve stimulator by anesthesiologist to determine neuromuscular blockade
- Anticholinesterase to reverse neuromuscular blockade
- IV inf; dilute 1-2 mg/ml in D_5, isotonic saline sol, give 0.5-10 mg/min, titrate to response; may be given directly over 1 min
- Deep IM, preferably high in deltoid muscle

Perform/provide:

- Storage in refrigerator, powder at room temp; close tightly

• Reassurance if communication is difficult during recovery from neuromuscular blockade; postoperative stiffness is normal, soon subsides

Evaluate:

• Therapeutic response: paralysis of jaw, eyelid, head, neck, rest of body

Treatment of overdose: Edrophonium or neostigmine, atropine, monitor VS; may require mechanical ventilation

sucralfate (℞)

(soo-kral'fate)

Carafate, Sulcrate*

Func. class.: Protectant

Chem. class.: Aluminum hydroxide/sulfated sucrose

Action: Forms a complex that adheres to ulcer site, adsorbs pepsin

Uses: Duodenal ulcer

Investigational uses: Gastric ulcers, gastroesophageal reflux

Dosage and routes:

• *Adult:* PO 1 g qid 1 hr ac, hs

Available forms: Tabs 1 g; oral susp 500 mg/5 ml

Side effects/adverse reactions:

CNS: Drowsiness, dizziness

GI: Dry mouth, constipation, nausea, gastric pain, vomiting

INTEG: Urticaria, rash, pruritus

Contraindications: Hypersensitivity

Precautions: Pregnancy (B), lactation, children

Pharmacokinetics:

PO: Duration up to 5 hr

Interactions:

• Decreased action of tetracyclines, phenytoin, fat-soluble vitamins

NURSING CONSIDERATIONS

Assess:

• Gastric pH (>5 should be maintained)

Administer:

• On an empty stomach, 1 hr before meals and HS

Perform/provide:

• Storage at room temp

Evaluate:

• Therapeutic response: absence of pain, GI complaints

Teach patient/family:

• To avoid black pepper, caffeine, alcohol, harsh spices, extremes in temp of food

• To take on empty stomach

• To take full course of therapy

• To avoid antacids within ½ hr of drug

sufentanil (℞)

(soo-fen'ta-nil)

Sufenta

Func. class.: Narcotic analgesic

Chem. class.: Opiate, synthetic

Controlled Substance Schedule II

Action: Inhibits ascending pain pathways in CNS, increases pain threshold, alters pain perception

Uses: Primary anesthetic, adjunct to general anesthetic

Dosage and routes:

Primary anesthetic

• *Adult:* IV 8-30 μg/kg given with 100% O_2, a muscle relaxant

Adjunct

• *Adult:* IV 1-8 μg/kg given with nitrous oxide/O_2

Available forms: Inj 50 μg/ml

Side effects/adverse reactions:

CNS: Drowsiness, dizziness, confusion, headache, sedation, euphoria

GI: Nausea, vomiting, anorexia, constipation, cramps

GU: Increased urinary output, dysuria, urinary retention

INTEG: Rash, urticaria, bruising, flushing, diaphoresis, pruritus

* Available in Canada only

EENT: Tinnitus, blurred vision, miosis, diplopia
CV: Palpitations, bradycardia, change in B/P
RESP: ***Respiratory depression***
Contraindications: Hypersensitivity, addiction (narcotic)
Precautions: Addictive personality, pregnancy (C), lactation, increased intracranial pressure, MI (acute), severe heart disease, respiratory depression, hepatic disease, renal disease, child <18 yr
Pharmacokinetics:
Half-life 1-2 hr
Interactions:
• Increased effects with other CNS depressants: alcohol, narcotics, sedative/hypnotics, antipsychotics, skeletal muscle relaxants
Lab test interferences:
Increase: Amylase
NURSING CONSIDERATIONS
Assess:
• I&O ratio; decreasing output may indicate urinary retention
• CNS changes: dizziness, drowsiness, hallucinations, euphoria, LOC, pupil reaction
• Allergic reactions: rash, urticaria
• Respiratory dysfunction: respiratory depression, character, rate, rhythm; notify prescriber if respirations are <10/min
• Need for pain medication, physical dependence
Administer:
• IV undiluted over 1-2 min or give as inf
• With antiemetic if nausea, vomiting occur
Perform/provide:
• Storage in light-resistant area at room temp
• Safety measures: side rails, nightlight, call bell within easy reach
Evaluate:
• Therapeutic response: maintenance of anesthesia
Teach patient/family:
• To report any symptoms of CNS changes, allergic reactions
Treatment of overdose: Naloxone (Narcan) 0.2-0.8 mg IV, O_2, IV fluids, vasopressors

sulfacetamide (ophthalmic) (℞)

(sul-fa-seet'a-mide)
AK-Sulf, Bleph-10 Liquifilm, Bleph-10 S.O.P., Isopto Cetamide, Ophthacet, Sodium Sulamyd, sodium sulfacetamide 10%, sodium sulfacetamide 15%, sodium sulfacetamide 30%, SOSS-10, Sulfair 15
Func. class.: Antiinfective, ophthalmic
Chem. class.: Sulfonamide

Action: Inhibits folic acid synthesis by preventing PABA use, which is necessary for bacterial growth
Uses: Conjunctivitis, superficial eye infections, corneal ulcers, adjunct to systemic sulfonamide therapy in treatment of trachoma
Dosage and routes:
• *Adult and child:* INSTILL 1-2 gtt q2-3h; TOP apply ½-1 inch oint into conjunctival sac qid-tid and at bedtime
Available forms: Ophth sol 10%, 15%, 30%; ophth oint 10%
Side effects/adverse reactions:
EENT: Burning, stinging, swelling
Contraindications: Hypersensitivity, infants <2 mo, varicella, vaccinia, viral disease, mycobacterial/fungal infection of the eye, epithelial herpes simplex, keratitis
Precautions: Antibiotic hypersensitivity, pregnancy (C), lactation, children, dry eye

Interactions:
- Incompatible with silver preparations

NURSING CONSIDERATIONS

Assess:
- Allergy: itching, lacrimation, redness, swelling

Administer:
- After washing hands; cleanse crusts or discharge from eye before application

Perform/provide:
- Storage at room temp

Evaluate:
- Therapeutic response: absence of redness, inflammation, tearing

Teach patient/family:
- To use drug exactly as prescribed
- Not to use eye makeup, towels, washcloths, eye medication of others; reinfection may occur
- That drug container tip should not be touched to eye
- To report itching, increased redness, burning, stinging; drug should be discontinued
- That drug may cause blurred vision when ointment is applied; may cause sensitivity to bright light

sulfadiazine (℞)

(sul-fa-dye'a-zeen)

Func. class.: Antibiotic

Chem. class.: Sulfonamide, intermediate acting

Action: Interferes with bacterial biosynthesis of proteins by competitive antagonism of PABA

Uses: UTIs, rheumatic fever prophylaxis, adjunctive in toxoplasmosis

Dosage and routes:

UTIs
- *Adult:* PO 2-4 g, then 1-2 g q6h × 10 days
- *Child:* PO 75 mg/kg or 2 g/m^2, then 150 mg/kg/day or 4 g/m^2 in 4-6 divided doses, max 6 g/day

Rheumatic fever prophylaxis
- *Child >30 kg:* PO 1 g qd
- *Child <30 kg:* PO 500 mg qd

Available forms: Tabs 500 mg

Side effects/adverse reactions:

SYST: ***Anaphylaxis***

GI: Nausea, vomiting, abdominal pain, stomatitis, ***hepatitis,*** glossitis, pancreatitis, diarrhea, ***enterocolitis,*** anorexia

CNS: Headache, insomnia, hallucinations, depression, vertigo, fatigue, anxiety, ***convulsions,*** drug fever, chills, drowsiness

HEMA: ***Leukopenia, thrombocytopenia, agranulocytosis, hemolytic anemia, aplastic anemia***

INTEG: Rash, dermatitis, urticaria, ***Stevens-Johnson syndrome,*** erythema, photosensitivity, alopecia

GU: ***Renal failure, toxic nephrosis,*** increased BUN, creatinine, crystalluria, hematuria, proteinuria

CV: ***Allergic myocarditis***

Contraindications: Hypersensitivity to sulfonamides, sulfonylureas, thiazide and loop diuretics, salicylates, pregnancy at term

Precautions: Pregnancy (C), lactation, impaired hepatic function, severe allergy, bronchial asthma, renal dysfunction

Pharmacokinetics:

PO: Rapidly absorbed, onset ½ hr; peak 3-6 hr, 30%-50% bound to plasma proteins, half-life 8-10 hr; excreted in urine, breast milk; crosses placenta, metabolized in liver

Interactions:
- Decreased effectiveness: oral contraceptives
- Increased hypoglycemic response: sulfonylurea agents
- Increased anticoagulant effects: oral anticoagulants

• Decreased renal excretion of: methotrexate
• Decreased hepatic clearance of: phenytoin

Lab test interferences:
False positive: Urinary glucose test (Benedict's method)

NURSING CONSIDERATIONS

Assess:
• I&O ratio; note color, character, pH of urine if drug administered for UTIs; output should be 800 ml less than intake; if urine is highly acidic, alkalization may be needed
• Kidney function studies: BUN, creatinine, urinalysis (long-term therapy)
• Blood dyscrasias: skin rash, fever, sore throat, bruising, bleeding, fatigue, joint pain
• Allergic reaction: rash, dermatitis, urticaria, pruritus, dyspnea, bronchospasm

Administer:
• With full glass of H_2O to maintain adequate hydration; increase fluids to 2 L/day to decrease crystallization in kidneys
• Medication after C&S; repeat C&S after full course of medication
• With resuscitative equipment available; severe allergic reaction may occur

Perform/provide:
• Storage in tight, light-resistant container at room temp

Evaluate:
• Therapeutic response: absence of pain, fever, C&S negative

Teach patient/family:
• To take each oral dose with full glass of water to prevent crystalluria
• To complete full course of treatment to prevent superinfection
• To avoid sunlight or use sunscreen to prevent burns
• To avoid OTC medication (aspirin, vit C) unless directed by prescriber
• To use alternative contraceptive measures; decreased effectiveness of oral contraceptives may result
• To notify prescriber of skin rash, sore throat, fever, mouth sores, unusual bruising, bleeding

sulfamethizole (℞)

(sul-fa-meth'i-zole)
Sulfasol, Thiosulfil
Func. class.: Antibiotic
Chem. class.: Sulfonamide, short acting

Action: Interferes with bacterial biosynthesis of proteins by competitive antagonism of PABA

Uses: UTIs

Dosage and routes:
• *Adult:* PO 0.5-1 g tid-qid
• *Child >2 mo:* PO 30-45 mg/kg/day in divided doses q6h

Available forms: Tabs 250, 500 mg

Side effects/adverse reactions:
SYST: ***Anaphylaxis***
GI: Nausea, vomiting, abdominal pain, stomatitis, ***hepatitis,*** glossitis, pancreatitis, diarrhea, ***enterocolitis***
CNS: Headache, confusion, insomnia, hallucinations, depression, vertigo, fatigue, anxiety, ***convulsions,*** drug fever, chills
HEMA: ***Leukopenia, neutropenia, thrombocytopenia, agranulocytosis, hemolytic anemia***
INTEG: Rash, dermatitis, urticaria, ***Stevens-Johnson syndrome,*** erythema, photosensitivity
GU: ***Renal failure, toxic nephrosis,*** increased BUN, creatinine, crystalluria
CV: ***Allergic myocarditis***

Contraindications: Hypersensitivity to sulfonamides, pregnancy at term

S

Precautions: Pregnancy (C), lactation, impaired hepatic function, severe allergy, bronchial asthma

Pharmacokinetics:

PO: Rapidly absorbed, peak 2 hr, 90% bound to plasma proteins, excreted in urine, breast milk, crosses placenta

Interactions:

- Decreased absorption of digoxin
- Decreased effectiveness: oral contraceptives
- Increased hypoglycemic response: sulfonylurea agents
- Increased anticoagulant effects: oral anticoagulants
- Decreased renal excretion of methotrexate
- Decreased hepatic clearance of phenytoin

Lab test interferences:

False positive: Urinary glucose test (Benedict's method)

NURSING CONSIDERATIONS

Assess:

- I&O ratio; note color, character, pH of urine if drug administered for UTIs; output should be 800 ml less than intake; if urine is highly acidic, alkalization may be needed
- Kidney function studies: BUN, creatinine, urinalysis if on long-term therapy
- Blood dyscrasias: skin rash, fever, sore throat, bruising, bleeding, fatigue, joint pain
- Allergic reaction: rash, dermatitis, urticaria, pruritus, dyspnea, bronchospasm

Administer:

- With full glass of H_2O to maintain adequate hydration; increase fluids to 2 L/day to decrease crystallization in kidneys
- Medication after C&S; repeat C&S after full course of medication
- With resuscitative equipment available; severe allergic reactions may occur

Perform/provide:

- Storage in tight, light-resistant container at room temp

Evaluate:

- Therapeutic response: absence of pain, fever, C&S negative

Teach patient/family:

- To take each oral dose with full glass of H_2O to prevent crystalluria
- To complete full course of treatment to prevent superinfection
- To avoid sunlight or use sunscreen to prevent burns
- To avoid OTC medication (aspirin, vit C) unless directed by prescriber
- To use alternative contraceptive measures; decreased effectiveness of oral contraceptives may result
- To notify prescriber of skin rash, sore throat, fever, mouth sores, unusual bruising, bleeding

sulfamethoxazole (℞)

(sul-fa-meth-ox'a-zole)

Apo-Sulfamethoxazole*, Gantanol, Gantanol DS

Func. class.: Antiinfective

Chem. class.: Sulfonamide, intermediate acting

Combination products: Azo Gantanol, Azo Sulfamethoxazole, Uro Gantanol: sulfamethoxazole 500 mg, phenazopyridine 100 mg

Action: Interferes with bacterial biosynthesis of proteins by competitive antagonism of PABA

Uses: UTIs, lymphogranuloma venereum, systemic infections

Dosage and routes:

- *Adult:* PO 2 g, then 1 g bid or tid for 7-10 days
- *Child >2 mo:* PO 50-60 mg/kg then 25-30 mg/kg bid, not to exceed 75 mg/kg/day

* Available in Canada only

Lymphogranuloma venereum
• *Adult:* PO 1 g bid × 14 days
Available forms: Tabs 500 mg; oral susp 500 mg/5 ml
Side effects/adverse reactions:
SYST: ***Anaphylaxis***
GI: Nausea, vomiting, abdominal pain, stomatitis, ***hepatitis,*** glossitis, pancreatitis, diarrhea, ***enterocolitis,*** anorexia
CNS: Headache, insomnia, hallucinations, depression, vertigo, fatigue, anxiety, convulsions, drug fever, chills, drowsiness
HEMA: ***Leukopenia, thrombocytopenia, agranulocytosis, hemolytic anemia, aplastic anemia***
INTEG: Rash, dermatitis, urticaria, ***Stevens-Johnson syndrome,*** erythema, photosensitivity, alopecia
GU: ***Renal failure, toxic nephrosis,*** increased BUN, creatinine, crystalluria, hematuria, proteinuria
CV: ***Allergic myocarditis***
Contraindications: Hypersensitivity to sulfonamides, sulfonylureas, thiazide and loop diuretics, salicylates, pregnancy at term
Precautions: Pregnancy (C), lactation, impaired hepatic function, severe allergy, bronchial asthma
Pharmacokinetics:
PO: Poorly absorbed, peak 3-4 hr, 50%-70% bound to plasma proteins, half-life 7-12 hr; excreted in urine (unchanged 90%), breast milk; crosses placenta
Interactions:
• Decreased effectiveness: oral contraceptives
• Increased hypoglycemic response: sulfonylurea agents
• Increased anticoagulant effects: oral anticoagulants
• Decreased renal excretion of methotrexate
• Decreased hepatic clearance of phenytoin
Lab test interferences:
False positive: Urinary glucose test (Benedict's method)

NURSING CONSIDERATIONS
Assess:
• I&O ratio; note color, character, pH of urine if drug administered for UTIs; output should be 800 ml less than intake; if urine is highly acidic, alkalization may be needed
• Kidney function studies: BUN, creatinine, urinalysis (long-term therapy)
• Blood dyscrasias: skin rash, fever, sore throat, bruising, bleeding, fatigue, joint pain
• Allergic reaction: rash, dermatitis, urticaria, pruritus, dyspnea, bronchospasm
Administer:
• With full glass of H_2O to maintain adequate hydration; increase fluids to 2 L/day to decrease crystallization in kidneys
• Medication after C&S; repeat C&S after full course of medication
• With resuscitative equipment available; severe allergic reaction may occur
Perform/provide:
• Storage in tight, light-resistant container at room temp
Evaluate:
• Therapeutic response: absence of pain, fever, C&S negative
Teach patient/family:
• To take each oral dose with full glass of H_2O to prevent crystalluria
• To complete full course of treatment to prevent superinfection
• To avoid sunlight or use sunscreen to prevent burns
• To avoid OTC medication (aspirin, vit C) unless directed by prescriber
• To use alternative contraceptive measures; decreased effectiveness of oral contraceptives may result

• To notify prescriber of skin rash, sore throat, fever, mouth sores, unusual bruising, bleeding

sulfamethoxazole and trimethoprim (℞)

(sul-fa-meth-ox'a-zole/ trye-meth'oh-prim)

Apo-Sulfatrim*, Bactrim, Cotrim, Comoxol, Septra, Sulfatrim, Bethaprim

Func. class.: Antibiotic

Chem. class.: Miscellaneous sulfonamide

Action: Sulfamethoxazole (SMZ) interferes with bacterial biosynthesis of proteins by competitive antagonism of PABA when adequate levels are maintained; trimethoprim (TMP) blocks synthesis of tetrahydrofolic acid; combination blocks 2 consecutive steps in bacterial synthesis of essential nucleic acids, protein

Uses: UTI, otitis media, acute and chronic prostatitis, shigellosis, *P. carinii* pneumonitis, chronic bronchitis, chancroid, traveler's diarrhea

Dosage and routes:

UTI

• *Adult:* PO 160 mg TMP/800 mg SMZ q12h × 10-14 days

• *Child:* PO 8 mg/kg TMP/40 mg/kg SMZ qd in 2 divided doses q12h

Otitis media

• *Child:* PO 8 mg/kg TMP/40 mg/kg SMZ qd in 2 divided doses q12h × 10 days

Chronic bronchitis

• *Adult:* PO 160 mg TMP/800 mg SMZ q12h × 14 days

Pneumocystis carinii pneumonitis

• *Adult and child:* PO 20 mg/kg TMP/100 mg/kg SMZ qd in 4 divided doses q6h × 14 days; IV 15-20 mg/kg/day (based on TMP) in 3-4 divided doses for up to 14 days

• Dosage reduction necessary in moderate to severe renal impairment (CrCl <30 ml/min)

Available forms: Tabs 80 mg trimethoprim (TMP)/400 mg sulfamethoxazole (SMZ), 160 mg trimethoprim/800 mg sulfamethoxazole; susp 40 mg/200 mg/5 ml; IV inj 16 mg/80 mg/ml

Side effects/adverse reactions:

CNS: Headache, insomnia, hallucinations, depression, vertigo, fatigue, anxiety, convulsions, drug fever, chills, aseptic meningitis

CV: ***Allergic myocarditis***

GI: Nausea, vomiting, abdominal pain, stomatitis, ***hepatitis,*** glossitis, pancreatitis, diarrhea, ***enterocolitis***, anorexia

GU: ***Renal failure, toxic nephrosis;*** increased BUN, creatinine, crystalluria

HEMA: ***Leukopenia, neutropenia, thrombocytopenia, agranulocytosis, hemolytic anemia, hypoprothrombinemia, Henoch-Schönlein purpura, methemoglobinemia, eosinophilia I***

INTEG: Rash, dermatitis, urticaria, ***Stevens-Johnson syndrome,*** erythema, photosensitivity, pain, inflammation at injection site

RESP: Cough, shortness of breath

SYST: ***Anaphylaxis, SLE***

Contraindications: Hypersensitivity to trimethoprim or sulfonamides, pregnancy at term, megaloblastic anemia, infants <2 mo, CrCl <15 ml/min, lactation

Precautions: Pregnancy (C), renal disease, elderly, G6PD deficiency, impaired hepatic function, possible folate deficiency, severe allergy, bronchial asthma

Pharmacokinetics:

PO: Rapidly absorbed, peak 1-4 hr; half-life 8-13 hr, excreted in urine

* Available in Canada only

(metabolites and unchanged), breast milk; crosses placenta; highly bound to plasma proteins; TMP achieves high levels in prostatic tissue and fluid

Interactions:

• Increased hypoglycemic response: sulfonylurea agents

• Increased anticoagulant effects: oral anticoagulants

• Decreased hepatic clearance of phenytoin

• Increased nephrotoxicity: cyclosporine

• Increased bone marrow depressant effects: methotrexate

• Thrombocytopenia: thiazide diuretics

Lab test interferences:

Increase: Alk phosphatase, creatinine, bilirubin

False positive: Urinary glucose test

NURSING CONSIDERATIONS

Assess:

• Allergic reactions: rash, fever (AIDS patients more susceptible)

• I&O ratio; note color, character, pH of urine if drug administered for UTI; output should be 800 ml less than intake; if urine is highly acidic, alkalization may be needed

• Kidney function studies: BUN, creatinine, urinalysis (long-term therapy)

• Type of infection; obtain C&S before starting therapy

• Blood dyscrasias, skin rash, fever, sore throat, bruising, bleeding, fatigue, joint pain

• Allergic reaction: rash, dermatitis, urticaria, pruritus, dyspnea, bronchospasm

Administer:

• With full glass of water to maintain adequate hydration; increase fluids to 2 L/day to decrease crystallization in kidneys

• Medication after C&S; repeat C&S after full course of medication

• After diluting 5 ml of drug/125 ml D_5W, run over 1-1½ hr

• With resuscitative equipment, epinephrine available; severe allergic reactions may occur

Perform/provide:

• Storage in tight, light-resistant container at room temp

Evaluate:

• Therapeutic response: absence of pain, fever, C&S negative

Teach patient/family:

• To take each oral dose with full glass of water to prevent crystalluria; drink 8-10 glasses of water/day

• To complete course of full treatment to prevent superinfection

• To avoid sunlight or use sunscreen to prevent burns

• To avoid OTC medications (aspirin, vit C) unless directed by prescriber

• If diabetic, to use Clinistix or Tes-Tape

• To use alternative contraceptive measures; decreased effectiveness of oral contraceptives may result

• To notify prescriber if skin rash, sore throat, fever, mouth sores, unusual bruising, bleeding occur

sulfasalazine (℞)

(sul-fa-sal'a-zeen)

Azulfidine, Azulfidine EN-Tabs, Salazopyrin*, sulfasalazine

Func. class.: Antiinflammatory

Chem. class.: Sulfonamide

Action: Prodrug to deliver sulfapyridine and 5-aminosalicylic acid to colon

Uses: Ulcerative colitis

Dosage and routes:

• *Adult:* PO 3-4 g/day in divided doses; maintenance 1.5-2 g/day in divided doses q6h

• *Child >2 yr:* PO 40-60 mg/kg/day in 4-6 divided doses, then 20-30 mg/kg/day in 4 doses, max 2 g/day
Available forms: Tabs 500 mg; oral susp 250 mg/5ml; enteric-coated tabs 500 mg
Side effects/adverse reactions:
SYST: ***Anaphylaxis***
GI: Nausea, vomiting, abdominal pain, stomatitis, ***hepatitis,*** glossitis, pancreatitis, diarrhea
CNS: Headache, confusion, insomnia, hallucinations, depression, vertigo, fatigue, anxiety, ***convulsions,*** drug fever, chills
HEMA: ***Leukopenia, neutropenia, thrombocytopenia, agranulocytosis, hemolytic anemia***
INTEG: Rash, dermatitis, urticaria, ***Stevens-Johnson syndrome,*** erythema, photosensitivity
GU: ***Renal failure, toxic nephrosis,*** increased BUN, creatinine, crystalluria
CV: ***Allergic myocarditis***
Contraindications: Hypersensitivity to sulfonamides or salicylates, pregnancy at term, child <2 yr, intestinal, urinary obstruction
Precautions: Pregnancy (C), lactation, impaired hepatic function, severe allergy, bronchial asthma, impaired renal function
Pharmacokinetics:
PO: Partially absorbed, peak 1½-6 hr, half-life 5-10 hr, excreted in urine as sulfasalazine (15%), sulfapyridine (60%), 5-aminosalicylic acid and metabolites (20%-33%), in breast milk; crosses placenta
Interactions:
• Decreased absorption of digoxin, folic acid
• Decreased effectiveness: oral contraceptives
• Increased hypoglycemic response: sulfonylurea agents
• Increased anticoagulant effects: oral anticoagulants
• Decreased renal excretion of methotrexate
• Decreased hepatic clearance of phenytoin
Lab test intereferences:
False positive: Urinary glucose test
NURSING CONSIDERATIONS
Assess:
• Kidney function studies: BUN, creatinine, urinalysis (long-term therapy)
• Blood dyscrasias: skin rash, fever, sore throat, bruising, bleeding, fatigue, joint pain
• Allergic reaction: rash, dermatitis, urticaria, pruritus, dyspnea, bronchospasm
Administer:
• With full glass of H_2O to maintain adequate hydration; increase fluids to 2 L/day to decrease crystallization in kidneys
• Medication after C&S; repeat C&S after full course of medication
• With resuscitative equipment available; severe allergic reaction may occur
• Total daily dose in evenly spaced doses and after meals to help minimize GI intolerance
Perform/provide:
• Storage in tight, light-resistant container at room temp
Evaluate:
• Therapeutic response: absence of fever, mucus in stools
Teach patient/family:
• To take each oral dose with full glass of H_2O to prevent crystalluria
• To complete full course of treatment to prevent superinfection
• To avoid sunlight or use sunscreen to prevent burns
• To avoid OTC medication (aspirin, vit C) unless directed by prescriber
• To use alternative contraceptive measures; decreased effectiveness of oral contraceptives may result

* Available in Canada only

• To notify prescriber of skin rash, sore throat, fever, mouth sores, unusual bruising, bleeding

sulfinpyrazone (℞)

(sul-fin peer′a-zone)

Antazone*, Antiple, Anturan*, Anturane, Apo-Sulfinpyrazone*, Novopyrazone

Func. class.: Uricosuric

Chem. class.: Pyrazolone

Action: Inhibits tubular reabsorption of urates, with increased excretion of uric acid; inhibits prostaglandin synthesis, which decreases platelet aggregation

Uses: Inhibition of platelet aggregation, gout

Dosage and routes:

Inhibition of platelet aggregation

• *Adult:* PO 200 mg qid

Gout/gouty arthritis

• *Adult:* PO 100-200 mg bid × 1 wk, then 200-400 mg bid, not to exceed 800 mg/day

Available forms: Tabs 100 mg; caps 200 mg

Side effects/adverse reactions:

CNS: Dizziness, ***convulsions, coma***

EENT: Tinnitus

GU: Renal calculi, hypoglycemia

GI: Gastric irritation, nausea, vomiting, anorexia, ***hepatic necrosis,*** GI bleeding

INTEG: Rash, dermatitis, pruritus, fever, photosensitivity

HEMA: ***Agranulocytosis*** (rare)

RESP: ***Apnea,*** irregular respirations

Contraindications: Hypersensitivity to pyrazolone derivatives, severe hepatic disease, blood dyscrasias, severe renal disease, CrCl <50 mg/min, active peptic ulcer, GI inflammation, renal calculi

Precautions: Pregnancy (C), lactation

Pharmacokinetics:

PO: Peak 1-2 hr, duration 4-6 hr, half-life 3 hr; metabolized by liver, excreted in urine

Interactions:

• Increased toxicity: sulfa drugs, dapsone, clofibrate, PAS, indomethacin, rifampin, naproxen, methotrexate, pantothenic acid, tolbutamide, warfarin

• Decreased effects of sulfinpyrazone: salicylates, xanthines

Lab test interferences:

Increase: PSP, aminohippuric acid

False positive: Clinitest

NURSING CONSIDERATIONS

Assess:

• Uric acid levels (3-7 mg/dl); joint mobility, pain, swelling

• Respiratory rate, rhythm, depth; notify prescriber of abnormalities

• Renal function

• Bleeding tendencies, RBC, Hct

• I&O

• Electrolytes, CO_2 before, during treatment

• Urine pH, output, glucose during beginning treatment

Administer:

• With glass of milk

• With food for GI symptoms

• Increased fluids to prevent calculi; alkalinization of urine may be required

Evaluate:

• Therapeutic response: absence of pain, stiffness in joints

Teach patient/family:

• To avoid aspirin, alcohol, high-purine diet

S

sulfisoxazole (℞)

(sul-fi-sox'a-zole)

Gantrisin, Novosoxazole*, sulfisoxazole

Func. class.: Antiinfective

Chem. class.: Sulfonamide, short acting

Combination products: Cantri, Vagilia: sulfisoxazole 10%, allantoin 2%, aminacrine 0.2%

Action: Interferes with bacterial biosynthesis of proteins by competitive antagonism of PABA

Uses: Urinary tract, systemic infections; chancroid; trachoma; toxoplasmosis; acute otitis media; lymphogranuloma venereum, eye infections

Dosage and routes:

- *Adult:* PO 2-4 g loading dose, then 1-2 g qid × 7-10 days
- *Child >2 mo:* PO 75 mg/kg or 2 g/m^2 loading dose, then 120-150 mg/kg/day or 4 g/m^2/day in divided doses q6h, not to exceed 6 g/day

Available forms: Tabs 500 mg; syr, pediatric susp 500 mg/5 ml

Side effects/adverse reactions:

SYST: ***Anaphylaxis***

GI: Nausea, vomiting, abdominal pain, stomatitis, ***hepatitis,*** glossitis, pancreatitis, diarrhea, ***enterocolitis,*** anorexia

CNS: Headache, insomnia, hallucinations, depression, vertigo, fatigue, anxiety, ***convulsions,*** drug fever, chills, drowsiness

HEMA: ***Leukopenia, thrombocytopenia, agranulocytosis, hemolytic anemia, aplastic anemia***

INTEG: Rash, dermatitis, urticaria, ***Stevens-Johnson syndrome,*** erythema, photosensitivity, alopecia

GU: ***Renal failure, toxic nephrosis,*** increased BUN, creatinine, crystalluria, hematuria, proteinuria

CV: ***Allergic myocarditis***

Contraindications: Hypersensitivity to sulfonamides and sulfonylureas, thiazide and loop diuretics, salicylates; pregnancy at term

Precautions: Pregnancy (C), lactation, impaired hepatic function, severe allergy, bronchial asthma

Pharmacokinetics:

PO: Rapidly absorbed, peak 2-4 hr, 85% protein bound; half-life 4-7 hr, excreted in urine, crosses placenta

Interactions:

- Decreased effectiveness of oral contraceptives
- Increased hypoglycemic response: sulfonylurea agents
- Increased anticoagulant effect: oral anticoagulants
- Decreased renal excretion of methotrexate
- Decreased hepatic clearance of phenytoin

Lab test interferences:

False positive: Urinary glucose test

NURSING CONSIDERATIONS

Assess:

- I&O ratio; note color, character, pH of urine if drug administered for UTIs; output should be 800 ml less than intake; if urine is highly acidic, alkalization may be needed
- Kidney function studies: BUN, creatinine, urinalysis (long-term therapy)
- Blood dyscrasias: skin rash, fever, sore throat, bruising, bleeding, fatigue, joint pain
- Allergic reaction: rash, dermatitis, urticaria, pruritus, dyspnea, bronchospasm

Administer:

- With full glass of H_2O to maintain adequate hydration; increase fluids to 2 L/day to decrease crystallization in kidneys

* Available in Canada only

• Medication after C&S; repeat C&S after full course of medication
• With resuscitative equipment available; severe allergic reaction may occur

Perform/provide:
• Storage in tight, light-resistant container at room temp

Evaluate:
• Therapeutic response: absence of pain, fever, C&S negative

Teach patient/family:
• Take each oral dose with full glass of H_2O to prevent crystalluria
• To complete full course of treatment to prevent superinfection
• To avoid sunlight or use sunscreen to prevent burns; avoid hazardous activities if dizziness occurs
• To avoid OTC medication (aspirin, vit C) unless directed by prescriber
• To use alternative contraceptive measures; decreased effectiveness of oral contraceptives may result
• To notify prescriber of skin rash, sore throat, fever, mouth sores, unusual bruising, bleeding

sulindac (℞)

(sul-in'dak)

Apo-Sulin*, Clinoril, NovoSundac*, sulindac

Func. class.: Nonsteroidal antiinflammatory

Chem. class.: Indeneacetic acid derivative

Action: Inhibits prostaglandin synthesis by decreasing an enzyme needed for biosynthesis; analgesic, antiinflammatory, antipyretic

Uses: Mild to moderate pain, osteoarthritis, rheumatoid, gouty arthritis, ankylosing spondylitis

Dosage and routes:

Arthritis
• *Adult:* PO 150 mg bid, may increase to 200 mg bid

Bursitis/acute arthritis
• *Adult:* PO 200 mg bid × 1-2 wk, then reduce dose

Available forms: Tabs 150, 200 mg

Side effects/adverse reactions:

GI: Nausea, anorexia, vomiting, diarrhea, jaundice, ***cholestatic hepatitis,*** constipation, flatulence, cramps, dry mouth, peptic ulcer, ***bleeding, ulceration, perforation***

CNS: Dizziness, drowsiness, fatigue, tremors, confusion, insomnia, anxiety, depression

CV: Tachycardia, peripheral edema, palpitations, dysrhythmias

INTEG: Purpura, rash, pruritus, sweating, photosensitivity

GU: ***Nephrotoxicity: dysuria, hematuria, oliguria, azotemia***

HEMA: ***Blood dyscrasias***

EENT: Tinnitus, hearing loss, blurred vision

Contraindications: Hypersensitivity, asthma, severe renal disease, severe hepatic disease, active ulcers

Precautions: Pregnancy (C), lactation, child, bleeding disorders, GI disorders, cardiac disorders, hypersensitivity to other antiinflammatory agents

Pharmacokinetics:

PO: Peak 2 hr, half-life 3-3½ hr; metabolized in liver; excreted in urine (metabolites), breast milk; 93% protein binding

Interactions:
• Increased action of coumarin, phenytoin, sulfonamides

NURSING CONSIDERATIONS

Assess:
• Renal, liver, blood studies: BUN, creatinine, AST, ALT, Hgb, before treatment, periodically thereafter
• Have BP checked qmo; drug causes Na retention

S

• Audiometric, ophthalmic exam before, during, after treatment
• For eye, ear problems: blurred vision, tinnitus may indicate toxicity

Administer:
• With food to decrease GI symptoms; best to take on empty stomach to facilitate absorption; tablet may be crushed

Perform/provide:
• Storage at room temp

Evaluate:
• Therapeutic response: decreased pain, stiffness, swelling in joints, ability to move more easily

Teach patient/family:
• To report blurred vision or ringing, roaring in ears (may indicate toxicity)
• To avoid driving, other hazardous activities if dizzy or drowsy
• To report change in urine pattern, weight increase, edema, pain increase in joints, fever, blood in urine (indicates nephrotoxicity)
• That therapeutic effects may take up to 1 mo
• To avoid alcohol and aspirin
• To take with full glass of water
• To use sunscreen

sumatriptan (℞)

(soo-ma-trip′tan)
Imitrex
Func. class.: Migraine agent
Chem. class.: 5HT-1-like receptor agonist

Action: Binds selectively to the vascular 5-HT-1 receptor subtype, exerts antimigraine effect; causes vasoconstriction in cranial arteries
Uses: Acute treatment of migraine with or without aura and cluster headache

Dosage and routes:
• *Adult:* SC 6 mg or less; may repeat in 1 hr; not to exceed 12 mg/24 hr

Available forms: Inj 6 mg (12 mg/ml); unit-of-use syringes (0.5 mg/ml); self-dosing system, 6-mg single-dose vial (0.5 ml in 2 ml)

Side effects/adverse reactions:
NEURO: Tingling, hot sensation, burning, feeling of pressure, tightness, numbness, dizziness, sedation, headache, anxiety, fatigue, cold sensation
CV: Flushing
RESP: Chest tightness, pressure
EENT: Throat, mouth, nasal discomfort, vision changes
GI: Abdominal discomfort
MS: Weakness, neck stiffness, myalgia
INTEG: Injection site reaction, sweating

Contraindications: Angina pectoris, history of MI, documented silent ischemia, Prinzmetal's angina, ischemic heart disease, IV use, concurrent ergotamine-containing preparations, uncontrolled hypertension, hypersensitivity, basilar or hemiplegic migraine

Precautions: Postmenopausal women, men >40 yr, risk factors for CAD, hypercholesterolemia, obesity, diabetes, impaired hepatic or renal function, pregnancy (C), lactation, children, elderly

Pharmacokinetics: Onset of pain relief 10 min-2 hr, peak 10-20 min, 10%-20% plasma protein binding, metabolized in the liver (metabolite), excreted in urine, feces

NURSING CONSIDERATIONS
Assess:
• Tingling, hot sensation, burning, feeling of pressure, numbness, flushing, infection site reaction
• For stress level, activity, recreation, coping mechanisms

* Available in Canada only

• Neurologic status: LOC, blurring vision, nausea, vomiting, tingling in extremities preceding headache
• Ingestion of tyramine foods (pickled products, beer, wine, aged cheese), food additives, preservatives, colorings, artificial sweeteners, chocolate, caffeine, which may precipitate these types of headaches

Administer:
• SC only; avoid IM or IV administration

Perform/provide:
• Quiet, calm environment with decreased stimulation for noise, bright light, excessive talking

Evaluate:
• Therapeutic response: decrease in frequency, severity of headache

Teach patient/family:
• Use of self-dosing system; not to exceed 12 mg/24 hr
• To report any side effects to prescriber
• To use contraception while taking drug

tacrine (tetrahydroaminoacridine, THA) (℞)

(tack'rin)
Cognex
Func. class.: Reversible cholinesterase

Action: Elevates acetylcholine concentrations (cerebral cortex) by slowing degradation of acetylcholine released in cholinergic neurons; does not alter underlying dementia

Uses: Treatment of mild to moderate dementia in Alzheimer's disease

Dosage and routes:
• *Adult:* PO 10 mg qid × 6 wk, then 20 mg qid × 6 wk, increase at 6-wk intervals if patient tolerating drug well and if transaminase is WNL
• ***Available forms:*** Caps 10, 20, 30, 40 mg

Side effects/adverse reactions:
CNS: ***Dizziness, confusion, insomnia,*** tremor, ***ataxia, somnolence, anxiety, agitation, depression, hallucinations, hostility, abnormal thinking,*** chills, fever
CV: Hypotension or hypertension
GI: ***Nausea, vomiting, anorexia, abdominal pain, constipation,*** dyspepsia, flatulence
GU: ***Frequency, UTI, incontinence***
INTEG: ***Rash,*** flushing
RESP: ***Rhinitis, URI, cough,*** pharyngitis

Contraindications: Hypersensitivity to this drug or acridine derivatives, patients treated with this drug who developed jaundice with a total bilirubin of >3 mg/dl

Precautions: Sick sinus syndrome, history of ulcers, GI bleeding, hepatic disease, bladder obstruction, asthma, pregnancy (C), lactation, children

Pharmacokinetics: Rapidly absorbed PO, 55% bound to plasma proteins, metabolized to metabolites, elimination half-life 2-4 hr

Interactions:
• Decreased activity of anticholinergics
• Increased elimination half-life of theophylline
• Synergistic effect: succinylcholine, cholinesterase inhibitors, cholinergic agonists

NURSING CONSIDERATIONS

Assess:
• B/P: hypotension, hypertension
• Mental status: affect, mood, behavioral changes, depression; complete suicide assessment; hallucinations, confusion
• GI status: nausea, vomiting, anorexia, constipation, abdominal pain; add bulk, increase fluids for constipation

T

• GU status: urinary frequency, incontinence

Administer:

• Between meals; may be given with meals for GI symptoms

• Dosage adjusted to response no more than q6wk

Perform/provide:

• Assistance with ambulation during beginning therapy; dizziness, ataxia may occur

Evaluate:

• Therapeutic response: decrease in confusion, improved mood

Teach patient/family:

• To report side effects: twitching, eye spasms; indicate overdose

• To use drug exactly as prescribed: at regular intervals, preferably between meals; may be taken with meals for GI upset

• To notify prescriber of nausea, vomiting, diarrhea (dose increase or beginning treatment) or rash, very dark or very light stools, jaundice (delayed onset)

• Not to increase or abruptly decrease dose; serious consequences may result

Treatment of overdose: Withdraw drug, administer tertiary anticholinergics, provide supportive care

tacrolimus (℞)

(tak-roe-li′mus)

Prograf

Func. class.: Immunosuppressant

Chem. class.: Macrolide

Action: Produces immunosuppression by inhibiting T-lymphocytes

Uses: Organ transplants to prevent rejection

Dosage and routes:

• *Adult, child:* IV 0.15 mg/kg/day × 3 days then PO 0.15 mg/kg bid

Available forms: Inj IV 5 mg/ml; caps 1, 5 mg

Side effects/adverse reactions:

HEMA: ***Anemia, leukocytosis, thrombocytopenia, purpura***

GI: Nausea, vomiting, diarrhea, constipation

CV: Hypertension

CNS: Tremors, headache, insomnia, paresthesia, chills, fever

GU: UTIs, ***albuminuria, hematuria, proteinuria, renal failure***

META: Hirsutism, hyperglycemia, hyperkalemia, hyperuricemia, hypokalemia, hypomagnesemia

RESP: ***Pleural effusion, atelectasis,*** dyspnea

INTEG: Rash, flushing, itching, alopecia

EENT: Blurred vision, photophobia

Contraindications: Hypersensitivity to this drug or to some kinds of castor oil

Precautions: Severe renal, hepatic disease, pregnancy (C), diabetes mellitus, hyperkalemia, hyperuricemia, lymphomas, lactation, children <12, hypertension

Pharmacokinetics: Extensively metabolized, half-life 10 hr, 75% protein binding

Interactions:

• Increased toxicity: aminoglycosides, cisplatin, cyclosporine

• Increased blood levels: antifungals, calcium channel blockers, cimetidine, danazol, erythromycin

• Decreased blood levels: carbamazepine, phenobarbitol, phenytoin, rifamycins

• Decreased effect of: vaccines

NURSING CONSIDERATIONS

Assess:

• Blood studies: Hgb, WBC, platelets during treatment qmo; if leukocytes <3000/mm^3 or platelets <100,000/mm^3, drug should be discontinued or reduced; decreased he-

* Available in Canada only

moglobulin level may indicate bone marrow suppression
• Liver function studies: alk phosphatase, AST (SGOT), ALT (SGPT), amylase, bilirubin, and for hepatotoxicity: dark urine, jaundice, itching, light-colored stools; drug should be discontinued
Administer:
• All medications PO if possible, avoiding IM injections; bleeding may occur
• With meals to reduce GI upset; nausea is common
• For several days before transplant surgery; patients should be placed in protective isolation
IV route: After diluting in 0.9% NaCl or D_5W to 0.004 to 0.02 mg/ml as a continuous infusion
Teach patient/family:
• To report fever, rash, severe diarrhea, chills, sore throat, fatigue; serious infections may occur; clay-colored stools, cramping (hepatotoxicity)
• To avoid crowds, persons with known infections to reduce risk of infection
Evaluate:
Therapeutic response: Absence of graft rejection; immunosuppression in autoimmune disorders

talbutal (℞)

(tal'byoo-tal)
Lotusate
Func. class.: Sedative/hypnotic barbiturate (intermediate acting)
Chem. class.: Barbitone

Controlled Substance Schedule II (USA), Schedule G (Canada)
Action: Depresses activity in brain cells, primarily in reticular activating system in brain stem; selectively depresses neurons in posterior hypothalamus, limbic structures
Uses: Insomnia, short-term only
Dosage and routes:
• *Adult:* PO 120 mg hs
Available forms: Tabs 120 mg
Side effects/adverse reactions:
CNS: Lethargy, drowsiness, hangover, dizziness, paradoxical stimulation in elderly and children, lightheadedness, dependency, CNS depression, mental depression, slurred speech
GI: Nausea, vomiting, diarrhea, constipation
INTEG: Rash, urticaria, pain, abscesses at injection site, angioedema, thrombophlebitis, ***Stevens-Johnson syndrome***
CV: Hypotension, bradycardia
RESP: Depression, apnea, ***laryngospasm, bronchospasm***
HEMA: ***Agranulocytosis, thrombocytopenia, megaloblastic anemia*** (long-term treatment)
Contraindications: Hypersensitivity to barbiturates, respiratory depression, addiction to barbiturates, severe liver impairment, porphyria, pregnancy (D), uncontrolled severe pain
Precautions: Anemia, lactation, hepatic disease, renal disease, hypertension, elderly, acute/chronic pain
Pharmacokinetics:
Onset 30-45 min, duration 4-6 hr; metabolized by liver, excreted by kidneys (metabolites)
Interactions:
• Increased CNS depression: alcohol, MAOIs, sedatives, narcotics
• Decreased effect of oral anticoagulants, corticosteroids, griseofulvin, quinidine
• Decreased half-life of doxycycline
Lab test interferences:
False increase: Sulfobromophthalein

T

NURSING CONSIDERATIONS

Assess:

• Blood studies: Hct, Hgb, RBCs, if blood dyscrasias are suspected

• Hepatic studies: AST, ALT, bilirubin, if hepatic damage has occurred

• Mental status: mood, sensorium, affect, memory (long, short)

• Physical dependency: frequent requests for medication, shakes, anxiety

• Barbiturate toxicity: hypotension; pupillary constriction; cold, clammy skin; cyanosis of lips; insomnia; nausea; vomiting; hallucinations; delirium; weakness; mild symptoms may occur in 8-12 hr without drug

• Respiratory dysfunction: respiratory depression, character, rate, rhythm; hold drug if respirations are <10/min or if pupils are dilated (rare)

• Blood dyscrasias: fever, sore throat, bruising, rash, jaundice, epistaxis (rare)

Administer:

• After removal of cigarettes to prevent fires

• After trying conservative measures for insomnia

• ½-1 hr before hs for sleeplessness

• On empty stomach for best absorption

• For <14 days; drug not effective after that; tolerance develops

• Crushed or whole

Perform/provide:

• Assistance with ambulation after receiving dose

• Safety measure: side rails, nightlight, call bell within easy reach

• Checking to see PO medication has been swallowed

• Storage in tight container in cool environment

Evaluate:

• Therapeutic response: ability to sleep at night, decreased amount of early morning awakening

Teach patient/family:

• That AM hangover is common

• That drug is indicated only for short-term treatment of insomnia, is probably ineffective after 2 wk

• That physical dependency may result when used for extended periods (45-90 days depending on dose)

• To avoid driving, other activities requiring alertness; sleep occurs within 45-60 min, lasts 6-8 hr

• To avoid alcohol ingestion, CNS depressants; serious CNS depression may result

• To tell all prescribers that barbiturate is being taken

• That withdrawal insomnia may occur after short-term use; not to start using drug again; insomnia will improve in 1-3 nights; may experience increased dreaming

• That effects may take 2 nights for benefits to be noticed

• Alternative measures to improve sleep (reading, exercise several hours before hs, warm bath, warm milk, TV, self-hypnosis, deep breathing)

Treatment of overdose: Lavage, activated charcoal, warming blanket, vital signs, hemodialysis, I&O ratio

tamoxifen (℞)

(ta-mox'i-fen)

Nolvadex Nolvadex-D*, Novo-Tamoxifen*, Tamofen*, Tamone*

Func. class.: Antineoplastic

Chem. class.: Antiestrogen hormone

Action: Inhibits cell division by binding to cytoplasmic estrogen receptors; resembles normal cell complex but inhibits DNA synthesis and estrogen response of target tissue

Uses: Advanced breast carcinoma not responsive to other therapy in

* Available in Canada only

estrogen-receptor-positive patients (usually postmenopausal)

Dosage and routes:

• *Adult:* PO 10-20 mg bid

Available forms: Tabs 10 mg

Side effects/adverse reactions:

HEMA: ***Thrombocytopenia, leukopenia***

GI: Nausea, vomiting, altered taste (anorexia)

GU: Vaginal bleeding, pruritus vulvae

INTEG: Rash, alopecia

CV: Chest pain

CNS: Hot flashes, headache, lightheadedness, depression

META: Hypercalcemia

EENT: Ocular lesions, retinopathy, corneal opacity, blurred vision (high doses)

Contraindications: Hypersensitivity, pregnancy (D)

Precautions: Leukopenia, thrombocytopenia, lactation, cataracts

Pharmacokinetics:

PO: Peak 4-7 hr, half-life 7 days (1 wk terminal), excreted primarily in feces

Lab test interferences:

Increase: Serum Ca

NURSING CONSIDERATIONS

Assess:

• CBC, differential, platelet count qwk; withhold drug if WBC is <3500 or platelet count is <100,000; notify prescriber

• Bleeding: hematuria, guaiac, bruising, petechiae, mucosa or orifices q8h

• Food preferences; list likes, dislikes

• Effects of alopecia on body image; discuss feelings about body changes

• Symptoms indicating severe allergic reactions: rash, pruritus, urticaria, purpuric skin lesions, itching, flushing

Administer:

• Antacid before oral agent; give drug after evening meal, before bedtime

• Antiemetic 30-60 min before giving drug to prevent vomiting

Perform/provide:

• Liquid diet, if needed including cola, Jell-O; dry toast or crackers may be added if patient is not nauseated or vomiting

• Increase fluid intake to 2-3 L/day to prevent dehydration

• Nutritious diet with iron, vitamin supplements as ordered

• Storage in light-resistant container at room temp

Evaluate:

• Therapeutic response: decreased tumor size, spread of malignancy

Teach patient/family:

• To report any complaints, side effects to prescriber

• That vaginal bleeding, pruritus, hot flashes are reversible after discontinuing treatment

• To report immediately decreased visual acuity, which may be irreversible; stress need for routine eye exams, who should be told about tamoxifen therapy

• To report vaginal bleeding immediately

• That tumor flare—increase in size of tumor, increased bone pain—may occur and will subside rapidly; may take analgesics for pain

• That premenopausal women must use mechanical birth control because ovulation may be induced

• That hair may be lost during treatment; a wig or hairpiece may make patient feel better; new hair may be different in color, texture

temazepam (℞)

(te-maz'e-pam)

Razepam, Restoril, temazepam

Func. class.: Sedative-hypnotic

Chem. class.: Benzodiazepine

Controlled Substance Schedule IV (USA), Schedule F (Canada)

Action: Produces CNS depression at limbic, thalamic, hypothalamic levels of the CNS; may be mediated by neurotransmitter γ-aminobutyric acid (GABA); results are sedation, hypnosis, skeletal muscle relaxation, anticonvulsant activity, anxiolytic action

Uses: Insomnia

Dosage and routes:

• *Adult:* PO 15-30 mg hs

Available forms: Caps 15, 30 mg

Side effects/adverse reactions:

HEMA: ***Leukopenia, granulocytopenia*** (rare)

CNS: Lethargy, drowsiness, daytime sedation, dizziness, confusion, lightheadedness, headache, anxiety, irritability

GI: Nausea, vomiting, diarrhea, heartburn, abdominal pain, constipation, anorexia

CV: Chest pain, pulse changes

Contraindications: Hypersensitivity to benzodiazepines, pregnancy (X), lactation, intermittent porphyria

Precautions: Anemia, hepatic disease, renal disease, suicidal individuals, drug abuse, elderly, psychosis, child <15 yr, acute narrow-angle glaucoma, seizure disorders

Pharmacokinetics:

PO: Onset 30-45 min, duration 6-8 hr, half-life 10-20 hr; metabolized by liver, excreted by kidneys, crosses placenta, excreted in breast milk

Interactions:

• Increased effects of cimetidine, disulfiram, oral contraceptives

• Increased action of both drugs: alcohol, CNS depressants

• Decreased effect of antacids, theophylline, smoking, rifampin

Lab test interferences:

Increase: ALT (SGPT), AST (SGOT), serum bilirubin

Decrease: RAI uptake

False increase: Urinary 17-OHCS

NURSING CONSIDERATIONS

Assess:

• Blood studies: Hct, Hgb, RBCs (long-term therapy)

• Hepatic studies: AST (SGPT), ALT (SGOT), bilirubin (long-term therapy)

• Mental status: mood, sensorium, affect, memory (long, short)

• Blood dyscrasias: fever, sore throat, bruising, rash, jaundice, epistaxis (rare)

• Type of sleep problem: falling asleep, staying asleep

Administer:

• After removal of cigarettes to prevent fires

• After trying conservative measures for insomnia

• ½-1 hr before hs for sleeplessness

• On empty stomach for fast onset, but may be taken with food if GI symptoms occur

Perform/provide:

• Assistance with ambulation after receiving dose

• Safety measures: side rails, nightlight, call bell within easy reach

• Checking to see PO medication has been swallowed

• Storage in tight container in cool environment

Evaluate:

• Therapeutic response: ability to sleep at night, decreased early morning awakening if taking drug for insomnia

* Available in Canada only

Teach patient/family:
- To avoid driving, other activities requiring alertness until stabilized
- To avoid alcohol ingestion, CNS depressants; serious CNS depression may result
- That effects may take 2 nights for benefits to be noticed
- Alternative measures to improve sleep: reading, exercise several hours before hs, warm bath, warm milk, TV, self-hypnosis, deep breathing
- That hangover, memory impairment are common in elderly but less common than with barbiturates

Treatment of overdose: Lavage, activated charcoal; monitor electrolytes, VS

teniposide (℞)

(ten-i-poe'side)

Vumon, VM 26

Func. class.: Antineoplastic

Chem. class.: Semisynthetic podophyllotoxin

Action: Inhibits mitotic activity through metaphase to mitosis; also inhibits cells from entering mitosis, depresses DNA, RNA synthesis; a vesicant

Uses: Childhood acute lymphoblastic leukemia (ALL)

Dosage and routes:
- *Child IV INF:* Combo teniposide 165 mg/m^2 and cytarabine 300 mg/m^2 2×/wk × 8-9 doses or combo teniposide 250 mg/m^2 and vincristine 1.5 mg/m^2 qwk × 4-8 wk and prednisone 40 mg/m^2 PO × 28 days

Available forms: Inj 10 mg/ml

Side effects/adverse reactions:

HEMA: ***Thrombocytopenia, leukopenia, neutropenia, myelosuppression, anemia***

GI: Nausea, vomiting, anorexia, ***hepatotoxicity,*** diarrhea, stomatitis

INTEG: Rash, alopecia, phlebitis

RESP: ***Bronchospasm***

CV: Hypotension

CNS: Headache, fever

GU: ***Nephrotoxicity***

SYST: ***Anaphylaxis***

Contraindications: Hypersensitivity, bone marrow depression, severe hepatic disease, severe renal disease, bacterial infection, pregnancy (D)

Precautions: Renal disease, hepatic disease, lactation, children, gout, depression

Pharmacokinetics:

Half-life terminal 1-5 hr, metabolized in liver, excreted in urine, crosses placenta

Interactions:
- Plasma clearance of methotrexate may be increased: methotrexate
- Increased toxicity: sodium salicylate, sulfamethizole, tolbutamide
- Avoid live virus vaccinations

NURSING CONSIDERATIONS

Assess:
- CBC, differential, platelet count qwk; withhold drug if WBC is <4000 or platelet count is <75,000; notify prescriber
- Renal function studies: BUN, serum uric acid, urine CrCl, electrolytes before, during therapy
- I&O ratio; report fall in urine output of 30 ml/hr
- Monitor temp q4h; may indicate beginning infection
- Liver function tests before, during therapy (bilirubin, AST [SGOT], ALT [SGPT], LDH) as needed or monthly
- RBC, Hct, Hgb since these may be decreased
- Bleeding: hematuria, guaiac stools, bruising or petechiae, mucosa or orifices q8h
- Food preferences; list likes, dislikes

T

• Effects of alopecia on body image; discuss feelings about body changes
• Yellow skin, sclera, dark urine, clay-colored stools, itchy skin, abdominal pain, fever, diarrhea
• Buccal cavity q8h for dryness, sores or ulceration, white patches, oral pain, bleeding, dysphagia
• Local irritation, pain, burning, discoloration at inj site
• Symptoms indicating severe allergic reaction: rash, pruritus, urticaria, purpuric skin lesions, itching, flushing
• Symptoms of anaphylaxis: flushing, restlessness, coughing, difficulty breathing
• Frequency of stools, characteristics: cramping, acidosis; signs of dehydration: rapid respirations, poor skin turgor, decreased urine output, dry skin, restlessness, weakness

Administer:
• Sol should be prepared by qualified personnel under controlled conditions; gloves, gown, mask should be worn
• Use Luer Loc tubing to prevent leakage, do not let sol come in contact with skin
• After diluting in D_5 or 0.9% NaCl to a concentration of 0.1, 0.2, 0.4, or 1 mg/ml; infuse over 30-60 min or longer; prepare and use glass or polyolefin plastic bags or containers
• Antiemetic 30-60 min before giving drug and prn to prevent vomiting
• Allopurinol or sodium bicarbonate to maintain uric acid levels, alkalinization of urine
• Hyaluronidase 150 U/ml to 1 ml NaCl to infiltration area, ice compress
• Transfusion for anemia
• Antispasmodic

Perform/provide:
• Storage in refrigerator of unopened amps; do not freeze
• Liquid diet: cola, Jell-O; dry toast or crackers may be added if patient is not nauseated or vomiting
• Increase fluid intake to 2-3 L/day to prevent urate deposits, calculi formation
• Diet low in purines: organ meats (kidney, liver), dried beans, peas, to maintain alkaline urine
• Nutritious diet with iron, vitamin supplements
• HOB raised to facilitate breathing

Evaluate:
• Therapeutic response: remission of ALL

Teach patient/family:
• To report any changes in breathing, coughing, fever, chills, rapid heartbeat
• That hair may be lost during treatment, a wig or hairpiece may make patient feel better; tell patient that new hair may be different in color, texture
• To make position changes slowly to prevent fainting
• To avoid vaccinations during treatment
• To avoid products containing aspirin or ibuprofen; to report signs of bleeding
• To report signs of anemia: fatigue, headache, irritability, faintness, shortness of breath

terazosin (℞)

(ter-ay′zoe-sin)
Hytrin
Func. class.: Antihypertensive
Chem. class.: Peripherally acting adrenergic blocker

Action: Decreases total vascular resistance, which is responsible for a

* Available in Canada only

decrease in B/P; this occurs by blockade of α_1-adrenoreceptors
Uses: Hypertension, as a single agent or in combination with diuretics or β-blockers, BPH
Dosage and routes:
• *Adult:* PO 1 mg hs, may increase dose slowly to desired response; not to exceed 20 mg/day
Available forms: Tabs 1, 2, 5 mg
Side effects/adverse reactions:
CV: Palpitations, orthostatic hypotension, tachycardia, edema, rebound hypertension
CNS: Dizziness, headache, drowsiness, anxiety, depression, vertigo, weakness, fatigue
GI: Nausea, vomiting, diarrhea, constipation, abdominal pain
GU: Urinary frequency, incontinence, impotence, priapism
EENT: Blurred vision, epistaxis, tinnitus, dry mouth, red sclera, nasal congestion, sinusitis
RESP: Dyspnea
Contraindications: Hypersensitivity
Precautions: Pregnancy (C), children, lactation
Pharmacokinetics:
Peak 1 hr, half-life 9-12 hr, highly bound to plasma proteins; metabolized in liver, excreted in urine, feces
Interactions:
• Increased hypotensive effects: β-blockers, nitroglycerin, verapamil, nifedipine
NURSING CONSIDERATIONS
Assess:
• B/P, pulse, jugular venous distention q4h
• BUN, uric acid if on long-term therapy
• Weight qd, I&O
• Skin turgor, dryness of mucous membranes for hydration status
• Rales, dyspnea, orthopnea q30 min
Perform/provide:
• Cool storage in tight container
Evaluate:
• Therapeutic response: decreased B/P, edema in feet, legs
Teach patient/family:
• That fainting occasionally occurs after first dose; not to drive or operate machinery for 4 hr after first dose or after an increase in dose; or take first dose hs
• To rise slowly from sitting/lying position

---

terbinafine (℞)

(ter-bin′a-feen)
Lamisil
Func. class.: Topical antifungal
Chem. class.: Synthetic allylamine derivative

Action: Interferes with cell membrane permeability in fungi such as *T. rubrum, T. mentagrophytes, T. tonsurans, E. floccosum, M. canis, M. audouinii, M. gypseum, Candida,* broad-spectrum antifungal
Uses: Tinea cruris, tinea corporis, tinea pedis
Dosage and routes: TOP/massage into affected area, surrounding area qd or bid, continue for 7-14 days, not to exceed 4 wk
Available forms: Cream 1%
Side effects/adverse reactions:
INTEG: Burning, stinging, dryness, itching, local irritation
Contraindications: Hypersensitivity
Precautions: Pregnancy (B), lactation, children
NURSING CONSIDERATIONS
Assess:
• For continuing infection: increased size, number of lesions
Administer:
• To affected area, surrounding area;

do not cover with occlusive dressings

Perform/provide:

• Storage below 30° C (86° F)

Evaluate:

• Therapeutic response: decrease in size, number of lesions

Teach patient/family:

• To wear cotton clothing

• To use clean towel, dry well

• To avoid contact with mucous membranes

• Not to cover areas unless directed by prescriber

• To report excessive itching, burning

• How to apply; massage cream into affected area and surrounding skin in AM, PM; effects observed within 1 wk, continue 1-2 wk after symptoms decrease

terbutaline (℞)

(ter-byoo'te-leen)

Brethaire, Brethine, Bricanyl

Func. class.: Selective β_2-agonist; bronchodilator

Chem. class.: Catecholamine

Action: Relaxes bronchial smooth muscle by direct action on β_2-adrenergic receptors through accumulation of cAMP at β-adrenergic receptor sites; bronchodilation, diuresis, CNS, cardiac stimulation occur

Uses: Bronchospasm, premature labor

Investigational uses: Premature labor

Dosage and routes:

Bronchospasm

• *Adult and child >12 yr:* INH 2 puffs q1min, then q4-6h; PO 2.5-5 mg q8h; SC 0.25 mg q8h

Premature labor

• *Adult:* IV INF: 10 µg/min, increased by 5 µg q10min, not to exceed 25 µg/min; SC 0.25 mg q1h; PO 5 mg q4h × 48 hr, then 5 mg q6h as maintenance

Available forms: Tabs 2.5, 5 mg; aerosol 0.2 mg/actuation; inj 1 mg/ml

Side effects/adverse reactions:

CNS: Tremors, anxiety, insomnia, headache, dizziness, stimulation

CV: Palpitations, tachycardia, hypertension, dysrhythmias, ***cardiac arrest***

GI: Nausea, vomiting

Contraindications: Hypersensitivity to sympathomimetics, narrow-angle glaucoma, tachydysrhythmias

Precautions: Pregnancy (B), cardiac disorders, hyperthyroidism, diabetes mellitus, prostatic hypertension, lactation, elderly, hypertension, glaucoma

Pharmacokinetics:

PO: Onset ½ hr, peak 1-2 hr, duration 4-8 hr

SC: Onset 6-15 min, peak ½-1 hr, duration 1½-4 hr

INH: Onset 5-30 min, peak 1-2 hr, duration 3-6 hr

Interactions:

• Increased effects of both drugs: other sympathomimetics

• Decreased action: β-blockers

• Hypertensive crisis: MAOIs

• Incompatible with bleomycin

Syringe compatibility: Doxapram

Y-site compatibility: Insulin

Additive compatibility: Aminophylline

NURSING CONSIDERATIONS

Assess:

• Respiratory function: vital capacity, forced expiratory volume, ABGs, B/P, pulse, respiratory pattern, lung sounds, sputum before and after treatment

• Tolerance over long-term therapy; dose may have to be changed; monitor for rebound bronchospasm

* Available in Canada only

Administer:
• With food; may be crushed
• IV after diluting each 5 mg/1 L D_5W for inf
• IV, run 5 μg/min; may increase 5 μg q10 min, titrate to response; after ½-1 hr taper dose by 5 μg; switch to PO as soon as possible
• 2 hr before hs to avoid sleeplessness

Perform/provide:
• Storage at room temp; do not use discolored sol

Evaluate:
• Therapeutic response: absence of dyspnea, wheezing

Teach patient/family:
• Not to use OTC medications; extra stimulation may occur
• Use of inhaler; review package insert with patient
• To avoid getting aerosol in eyes; burning, stinging, will occur
• To wash inhaler in warm water and dry qd, rinse mouth after use
• On all aspects of drug; avoid smoking, smoke-filled rooms, persons with respiratory infections
• To increase fluids >2 L/day; allow 15 min between inhalation of this drug and inhaler containing steroid
• Take on time; if missed, do not make up after 1 hr; wait till next dose

Treatment of overdose: Administer an α-blocker, then norepinephrine for severe hypotension

terconazole (℞)

(ter-kon′a-zole)
Terazol 3, Terazol 7
Func. class.: Local antiinfective
Chem. class.: Antifungal

Action: Interferes with fungal DNA replication; binds sterols in fungal cell membranes, which increases permeability, leaking of nutrients

Uses: Vaginal, vulval, vulvovaginal candidiasis (moniliasis)

Dosage and routes:
• *Adult:* Vag 5 g (1 applicator) hs × 7 days

Available forms: Vag cream 0.4%

Side effects/adverse reactions:
GU: Vulvovaginal burning, itching, pelvic cramps
INTEG: Rash, urticaria, stinging, burning
MISC: Headache, body pain

Contraindications: Hypersensitivity

Precautions: Children <2 yr, pregnancy, lactation

NURSING CONSIDERATIONS

Assess:
• Allergic reaction: burning, stinging, swelling, redness

Administer:
• Enough medication to cover lesions completely
• After cleansing with soap, water before each application; dry well

Perform/provide:
• Dry storage at room temp

Evaluate:
• Therapeutic response: decrease in size, number of lesions

Teach patient/family:
• To use medical asepsis (hand washing) before, after application
• To avoid use of OTC creams, ointments, lotions unless directed by prescriber
• To avoid contact with eyes
• To continue during menses even if symptoms subside; to refrain from sexual intercourse during treatment
• To complete full treatment regimen

T

terfenadine (℞)

(ter-fen′i-deen)

Seldane

Func. class.: Antihistamine

Chem. class.: Butyrophenone derivative

Action: Acts on blood vessels, GI, respiratory systems by competing with histamine for H_1-receptor site; decreases allergic response by blocking histamine

Uses: Rhinitis, allergy symptoms

Dosage and routes:

- *Adult, child >12 yr:* PO 60 mg bid
- *Child <12 yr:* PO 15-30 mg bid

Available forms: Tabs 60, 120* mg; oral susp 6 mg/ml*

Side effects/adverse reactions:

CV: Life-threatening dysrhythmias (rare)

CNS: Dizziness, poor coordination

RESP: Increased thick secretions

GI: Anorexia, increased liver function tests, dry mouth

GU: Retention

Contraindications: Hypersensitivity, severe hepatic disease

Precautions: Pregnancy (C)

Pharmacokinetics:

PO: Peak 1-2 hr, 97% bound to plasma proteins; half-life is biphasic 3½ hr, 16-23 hr

Interactions:

- Not to be taken with ketoconazole, erythromycin

Lab test interferences:

False negative: Skin allergy tests

NURSING CONSIDERATIONS

Assess:

- I&O ratio; be alert for urinary retention, frequency, dysuria; drug should be discontinued
- CBC during long-term therapy
- Respiratory status: rate, rhythm, increase in bronchial secretions, wheezing, chest tightness

Administer:

- With meals for GI symptoms; absorption may slightly decrease

Perform/provide:

- Hard candy, gum, frequent rinsing of mouth for dryness
- Storage in tight, light-resistant container

Evaluate:

- Therapeutic response: no running or congested nose, rash

Teach patient/family:

- To notify prescriber of confusion, sedation, hypotension
- Not to exceed recommended dose; dysrhythmias may occur

Treatment of overdose: Administer ipecac syrup or lavage, diazepam, vasopressors, barbiturates (short-acting)

terpin hydrate (OTC)

(ter′pin)

Func. class.: Expectorant

Combination products: Terpin Hydrate and Codeine: terpin hydrate 85 mg/5 ml with dextromethorphan hydrobromide 10 mg/5 ml (with alcohol 39%-44%); Prunicodeine: terpin hydrate 29 mg/5 ml, codeine sulfate 10 mg/5 ml

Action: Direct action on respiratory tract, which increases fluids, allows for expectoration

Uses: Bronchial secretions

Dosage and routes:

- *Adult:* ELIX 5-10 ml q4-6h

Available forms: Elix terpin hydrate codeine 10 mg codeine/85 mg terpin hydrate; elix, plain 85 mg/5 ml

Side effects/adverse reactions:

GI: Nausea, vomiting, anorexia

Contraindications: Hypersensitivity, child <12 yr

Precautions: Pregnancy (C)

* Available in Canada only

NURSING CONSIDERATIONS
Assess:
• Cough: type, frequency, character, including sputum
Administer:
• With glass of water or food to decrease GI irritation
Perform/provide:
• Storage at room temp
Evaluate:
• Therapeutic response: absence of thick secretions
Teach patient/family:
• To avoid driving, other hazardous activities until stabilized on this medication (if combined with codeine, drowsiness occurs)
• Not to exceed recommended dosage

testolactone (℞)
(tess-toe-lak'tone)
Teslac
Func. class.: Antineoplastic
Chem. class.: Androgen hormone

Action: Acts on adrenal cortex to suppress activity; reduces estrone synthesis
Uses: Advanced breast carcinoma in postmenopausal women; prostatic cancer
Dosage and routes:
• *Adult:* PO 250 mg qid
Available forms: Tabs 50 mg
Side effects/adverse reactions:
GI: Nausea, vomiting, anorexia, glossitis
GU: Urinary retention, ***renal failure***
INTEG: Rash, nail changes, facial hair growth
CV: Orthostatic hypertension, edema
CNS: Paresthesias, dizziness
EENT: Deepening voice
META: Hypercalcemia

Contraindications: Hypersensitivity, premenopausal women, carcinoma of male breast
Precautions: Renal disease, hypercalcemia, cardiac disease, pregnancy (C)
Pharmacokinetics: None known
Interactions:
• Enhanced effects of oral anticoagulants
Lab test interferences:
Increase: Urinary 17-OHCS
Decrease: Estradiol

NURSING CONSIDERATIONS
Assess:
• CA^+ levels
• B/P q4h; tell patient to rise slowly from sitting or lying down
• Food preferences; list likes, dislikes
• Edema in feet; joint, stomach pain; shaking
• Symptoms indicating severe allergic reaction: rash, pruritus, urticaria, purpuric skin lesions, itching, flushing
• Anorexia, nausea, vomiting, constipation, weakness, loss of muscle tone (indicating hypercalcemia)
Administer:
• For mo or longer for desired response
Evaluate:
• Therapeutic response: decreased tumor size, spread of malignancy
Teach patient/family:
• To recognize and report signs of hepatotoxicity, hypercalcemia, virilization (in females), bleeding if on anticoagulants

T

testosterone (℞)

Andro L.A. 200, Delatest, Delatestryl, Durathate-200, Everone 100, Everone 200, Testone LA 100, Testone LA 200, testosterone enanthate, Testrin PA, Andro-Cyp 100, Andro-Cyp 200, Andronate 100, Andronate 200, depAndro 100, depAndro 200, Depotest 100, Depotest 200, Depo-Testosterone, Duratest-100, Duratest-200, testosterone cypionate, Testred Cypionate, Testex, testosterone propionate

Func. class.: Androgenic anabolic steroid

Chem. class.: Halogenated testosterone derivative

Action: Increases weight by building body tissue, increases potassium, phosphorus, chloride, nitrogen levels, bone development

Uses: Female breast cancer, eunuchoidism, male climacteric, oligospermia, impotence, osteoporosis

Dosage and routes:

Oligospermia

• *Adult:* IM 100-200 mg q4-6wk (cypionate or enanthate)

Breast cancer

• *Adult:* IM 50-100 mg 3 ×/wk (propionate) or 200-400 mg q2-4wk (cypionate or enanthate)

Male climacteric/eunuchoidism/eunuchism

• *Adult:* IM 10-25 mg 2-4 × /wk (propionate)

Available forms: Propionate inj 25, 50, 100 mg/ml; enanthate inj 100, 200 mg/ml; cypionate inj 50, 100, 200 mg/ml

Side effects/adverse reactions:

INTEG: Rash, acneiform lesions, oily hair and skin, flushing, sweating, acne vulgaris, alopecia, hirsutism

CNS: Dizziness, headache, fatigue, tremors, paresthesias, flushing, sweating, anxiety, lability, insomnia, carpal tunnel syndrome

MS: Cramps, spasms

CV: Increased B/P

GU: Hematuria, amenorrhea, vaginitis, decreased libido, decreased breast size, clitoral hypertrophy, testicular atrophy

GI: Nausea, vomiting, constipation, weight gain, ***cholestatic jaundice***

EENT: Conjunctional edema, nasal congestion

ENDO: Abnormal GTT

Contraindications: Severe renal, severe cardiac, severe hepatic disease, hypersensitivity, pregnancy (X), lactation, genital bleeding (rare)

Precautions: Diabetes mellitus, CV disease, MI

Pharmacokinetics:

PO: Metabolized in liver, excreted in urine, breast milk; crosses placenta

Interactions:

• Increased effects of oral antidiabetics, oxyphenbutazone
• Increased PT: anticoagulants
• Edema: ACTH, adrenal steroids
• Decreased effects of insulin

Lab test interferences:

Increase: Serum cholesterol, blood glucose, urine glucose

Decrease: Serum Ca, serum K, T_4, T_3, thyroid ^{131}I uptake test, urine 17-OHCS, 17-KS, PBI

NURSING CONSIDERATIONS

Assess:

• Weight qd; notify prescriber if weekly weight gain is >5 lb
• B/P q4h
• I&O ratio; be alert for decreasing urinary output, increasing edema
• Growth rate in children; growth rate may be uneven (linear/bone growth) with extended use

* Available in Canada only

• Electrolytes: K, Na, Cl, Ca; cholesterol
• Liver function studies: ALT (SGPT), AST (SGOT), bilirubin
• Edema, hypertension, cardiac symptoms, jaundice
• Mental status: affect, mood, behavioral changes, aggression
• Signs of masculinization in female: increased libido, deepening of voice, decreased breast tissue, enlarged clitoris, menstrual irregularities; male: gynecomastia, impotence, testicular atrophy
• Hypercalcemia: lethargy, polyuria, polydipsia, nausea, vomiting, constipation; drug may have to be decreased
• Hypoglycemia in diabetics; oral antidiabetic action is increased

Administer:
• Titrated dose; use lowest effective dose
• IM deep into upper outer quadrant of gluteal muscle

Perform/provide:
• Diet with increased calories, protein; decrease Na if edema occurs

Evaluate:
• Therapeutic response: 4-6 wk in osteoporosis

Teach patient/family:
• That drug must be combined with complete health plan: diet, rest, exercise
• To notify prescriber if therapeutic response decreases
• Not to discontinue abruptly
• About changes in sex characteristics
• Women to report menstrual irregularities
• That 1-3-mo course is necessary for response in breast cancer
• Procedure for use of buccal tablets (requires 30-60 min to dissolve, change absorption site with each dose; not to eat, drink, chew, or smoke while tablet is in place)

tetanus toxoid, adsorbed; tetanus toxoid (℞)

Func. class.: Toxoid

Action: Produces specific antibodies to tetanus

Uses: Tetanus toxoid: used for prophylactic treatment of wounds

Dosage and routes:
• *Adult and child:* IM 0.5 ml q4-6 wk × 2 doses, then 0.5 ml 1 yr after dose 2 (adsorbed); SC/IM 0.5 ml q4-8wk × 3 doses, then 0.5 ml ½-1 yr after dose 3, booster dose 0.5 ml q10yr

Available forms: Inj adsorbed IM 5, 10 LfU/0.5 ml; inj IM, SC 4, 5 LfU/0.5 ml

Side effects/adverse reactions:
GI: Nausea, vomiting, anorexia
INTEG: Skin abscess, urticaria, itching, swelling, erythema, induration at injection site
CV: Tachycardia, hypotension
SYST: Lymphadenitis, ***anaphylaxis***
CNS: Crying, fretfulness, fever, drowsiness

Contraindications: Hypersensitivity, active infection, poliomyelitis outbreak, immunosuppression

Precautions: Pregnancy (C), elderly

NURSING CONSIDERATIONS

Assess:
• For skin reactions: swelling, rash, urticaria
• For history of allergies, skin conditions (eczema, psoriasis, dermatitis), reactions to vaccinations
• For anaphylaxis: inability to breathe, bronchospasm

Administer:
• At least 4 wk apart × 3 doses for children >6 wk old

T

• Only with epinephrine 1:1000 on unit to treat laryngospasm

Perform/provide:

• Written record of immunization

Teach patient/family:

• That doses are given at least 4 wk apart × 3 doses; booster needed at 10-yr intervals

---

tetracaine (℞)

(tet′ra-kane)

Pontocaine

Func. class.: Local anesthetic

Chem. class.: Ester

Action: Competes with calcium for sites in nerve membrane that control sodium transport across cell membrane; decreases rise of depolarization phase of action potential

Uses: Spinal anesthesia, epidural and peripheral nerve block, perineum, lower extremities

Dosage and routes:

Varies with route of anesthesia

Available forms: Inj 0.2%, 0.3%, 1%; powder

Side effects/adverse reactions:

CNS: Anxiety, restlessness, ***convulsions, LOC,*** drowsiness, disorientation, tremors, shivering

CV: ***Myocardial depression, cardiac arrest, dysrhythmias,*** bradycardia, hypotension, hypertension, fetal bradycardia

GI: Nausea, vomiting

EENT: Blurred vision, tinnitus, pupil constriction

INTEG: Rash, urticaria, allergic reactions, edema, burning, skin discoloration at injection site, tissue necrosis

RESP: ***Status asthmaticus, respiratory arrest, anaphylaxis***

Contraindications: Hypersensitivity, severe liver disease, heart block

Precautions: Elderly, severe drug allergies, pregnancy (C), lacation, children

Pharmacokinetics:

Onset 15 min, duration 3 hr; metabolized by liver, excreted in urine (metabolites)

Interactions:

• Dysrhythmias: epinephrine, halothane, enflurane

• Hypertension: MAOIs, tricyclic antidepressants, phenothiazines

• Decreased action of tetracaine: chloroprocaine

• Decreased action of sulfonamides

NURSING CONSIDERATIONS

Assess:

• B/P, pulse, respiration during treatment

• Fetal heart tones during labor

• Allergic reactions: rash, urticaria, itching

• Cardiac status: ECG for dysrhythmias, pulse, B/P, during anesthesia

Administer:

• Only if not cloudy, does not contain precipitate

• Only with crash cart, resuscitative equipment nearby

• Only without preservatives for epidural or caudal anesthesia

Perform/provide:

• Use of new sol, discard unused portions, store in refrigerator

Evaluate:

• Therapeutic response: anesthesia necessary for procedure

Treatment of overdose: Airway, O_2, vasopressor, IV fluids, anticonvulsants for seizures

---

tetracaine (ophthalmic) (℞)

(tet′ra-kane)

Pontocaine Eye, Pontocaine HCl, tetracaine, Supracaine*

Func. class.: Ophthalmic anesthetic

Chem. class.: Ester

Action: Decreases ion permeability by stabilizing neuronal membrane

Uses: Cataract extraction, tonometry, gonioscopy, removal of foreign objects, corneal suture removal, glaucoma surgery

Dosage and routes:

• *Adult and child:* INSTILL 1-2 gtt before procedure; oint ½-1 in to lower conjunctival fornix

Available forms: Sol, oint 0.5%

Side effects/adverse reactions:

EENT: Blurred vision, stinging, burning, lacrimation, photophobia, conjunctival redness

INTEG: Contact dermatitis

SYST: CNS stimulation, CNS and CV depression

Contraindications: Hypersensitivity to PABA

Precautions: Abnormal levels of plasma esterases, allergies, hyperthyroidism, hypertension, cardiac disease, pregnancy (C)

Pharmacokinetics:

Instill: Onset 13-30 sec, duration 15-20 min

Interactions:

• Decreases antibacterial action of sulfonamides

NURSING CONSIDERATIONS

Assess:

• Previous hypersensitivity to anesthetics

Perform/provide:

• Protective covering for eye

• Storage at room temp in tight, light-resistant container or refrigerate

Teach patient/family:

• To report change in vision, with blurring or loss of sight, trouble breathing, sweating, flushing

• Not to touch or rub eye, which may further damage eye

• That someone must drive the patient home after the appointment

tetracaine (topical) (OTC)

(tet′ra-cane)

Pontocaine

Func. class.: Topical anesthetic

Action: Inhibits nerve impulses from sensory nerves, which produces anesthesia

Uses: Pruritus, sunburn, toothache, sore throat, cold sores, oral pain, rectal pain and irritation, control of gagging

Dosage and routes:

• *Adult and child:* TOP apply to affected area 1 oz for adult, ¼ oz for child

Available forms: Sol 2%; aero spray, liq, 0.5%; oint, gel, cream 1%

Side effects/adverse reactions:

INTEG: Rash, irritation, sensitization, burning, stinging, tenderness

Contraindications: Hypersensitivity, infants <1 yr, application to large areas, PABA allergies

Precautions: Child <6 yr, sepsis, pregnancy (C), denuded skin

NURSING CONSIDERATIONS

Assess:

• Allergy: rash, irritation, reddening, swelling

• Infection: if affected area is infected, do not apply

Administer:

• After cleansing and drying of affected area

Evaluate:

• Therapeutic response: absence of pain, itching of affected area

T

Teach patient/family:
• To report rash, irritation, redness, swelling
• How to apply sol

tetracycline (℞)

(tet-ra-sye′kleen)

Achromycin, Achromycin V, Alatel, Apo-Tetra*, Nor-Tet, Novotetra*, Nu-Tetra*, Panmycin, Robitet, Sumycin 250, Sumycin 500, Sumycin Syrup, Teline, Teline 500, Tetracap, tetracycline HCl, tetracycline HCl Syrup, Tetracyn, Tetralan 250, Tetralan 500, Tetralan Syrup, Tetralean*, Tetram

Func. class.: Broad-spectrum antiinfective

Chem. class.: Tetracycline

Combination products: Mysteclin-F: tetracycline equivalent to 125 mg tetracycline HCl per 5 ml with amphotericin B 25 mg/5 ml; Mysteclin-F: tetracycline equivalent to 350 mg tetracycline HCl with amphotericin B 50 mg/5 ml; Mysteclin-F Syrup: tetracycline equivalent to 125 mg tetracycline HCl per 5 ml with amphotericin B 25 mg/5 ml

Action: Inhibits protein synthesis and phosphorylation in microorganisms; bacteriostatic

Uses: Syphilis, *Chlamydia trachomatis,* gonorrhea, lymphogranuloma venereum, uncommon gram-positive, gram-negative organisms, rickettsial infections

Dosage and routes:
• *Adult:* PO 250-500 mg q6h; IM 250 mg/day or 150 mg q12h; IV 250-500 mg q8-12h
• *Child >8 yr:* PO 25-50 mg/kg/day in divided doses q6h; IM 15-25 mg/kg/day in divided doses q8-12h; IV 10-20 mg/kg/day in divided doses q12h

Gonorrhea
• *Adult:* PO 1.5 g, then 500 mg qid for a total of 9 g × 7 days

Chlamydia trachomatis
• *Adult:* PO 500 mg qid × 7 days

Syphilis
• *Adult:* PO 2-3 g in divided doses × 10-15 days; if syphilis duration > 1 yr, must treat 30 days

Brucellosis
• *Adult:* PO 500 mg qid × 3 wk with 1 g streptomycin IM 2 × /day × 1 wk, and 1 × /day the second wk

Urethral syndrome in women
• *Adult:* PO 500 mg qid × 7 days

Acne
• *Adult:* 1 g/day in divided doses; maintenance 125-500 mg/day

Available forms: Oral susp 125 mg/5 ml; caps 100, 200, 500 mg; tabs 100, 250, 500 mg; powder for inj

Side effects/adverse reactions:

CNS: Fever, headache, paresthesia

HEMA: ***Eosinophilia, neutropenia, thrombocytopenia, leukocytosis, hemolytic anemia***

EENT: Dysphagia, glossitis, decreased calcification, discoloration of deciduous teeth, oral candidiasis, oral ulcers

GI: Nausea, abdominal pain, *vomiting, diarrhea,* anorexia, enterocolitis, ***hepatotoxicity,*** flatulence, abdominal cramps, epigastric burning, stomatitis

CV: Pericarditis

GU: Increased BUN

INTEG: Rash, urticaria, photosensitivity, increased pigmentation, ***exfoliative dermatitis,*** pruritus, ***angioedema***

Contraindications: Hypersensitivity to tetracyclines, children <8 yr, pregnancy (D), lactation

Precautions: Renal disease, hepatic disease

* Available in Canada only

Pharmacokinetics:
PO: Peak 2-3 hr, duration 6 hr, half-life 6-10 hr; excreted in urine, breast milk; crosses placenta; 20%-60% protein bound

Interactions:
• Decreased effect of tetracycline: antacids, $NaHCO_3$, dairy products, alkali products, iron, kaolin/pectin
• Increased effect: anticoagulants
• Decreased effect of penicillins, oral contraceptives
• Nephrotoxicity: methoxyflurane
• Incompatible in sol with amikacin, aminophylline, amobarbital, amphotericin B, Ca, carbenicillin, cefazolin, cephalothin, cephapirin, chloramphenicol, chlorothiazide, dimenhydrinate, erythromycin, heparin, hydrocortisone, methicillin, methohexital, methyldopate, methylprednisolone, metoclopramide, oxacillin, penicillins, pentobarbital, phenobarbital, phenytoin, polymyxin B, prochlorperazine, secobarbital, thiopental, warfarin, fat emulsion 10%

Lab test interferences:
False negative: Urine glucose with Clinistix or Tes-Tape
False increase: Urinary catecholamines

NURSING CONSIDERATIONS

Assess:
• Signs of anemia: Hct, Hgb, fatigue
• I&O ratio
• Blood studies: PT, CBC, AST (SGOT), ALT (SGPT), BUN, creatinine
• Allergic reactions: rash, itching, pruritus, angioedema
• Nausea, vomiting, diarrhea; administer antiemetic, antacids as ordered
• Overgrowth of infection: fever, malaise, redness, pain, swelling, drainage, perineal itching, diarrhea, changes in cough or sputum

Administer:
• IM: deep; no more than 2 ml/injection site
• IV after diluting 250 mg or less/5 ml of sterile H_2O; may be further diluted with 100 ml or more D_5W or NS; give 100 mg or less over 5 min or more; use sol within 12 hr
• After C&S obtained
• 2 hr before or after ferrous products; 3 hr after antacid or kaolin/pectin products

Perform/provide:
• Storage in tight, light-resistant container at room temp

Evaluate:
• Therapeutic response: decreased temp, absence of lesions, negative C&S

Teach patient/family:
• To avoid sun exposure; sunscreen does not seem to decrease photosensitivity
• Diabetic should avoid use of Clinistix, Diastix, or Tes-Tape for urine glucose testing
• That all prescribed medication must be taken to prevent superinfection
• To avoid milk products, antacids, or separate by 2 hr; take with a full glass of water

tetracycline (ophthalmic) (℞)

(tet-ra-sye'kleen)
Achromycin Ophthalmic
Func. class.: Antiinfective

Action: Inhibits bacterial protein synthesis

Uses: Infection of eye, ophthalmia neonatorum

Dosage and routes:
• *Adult and child:* INSTILL 1-2 gtt bid-qid as needed

Ophthalmia neonatorum
• *Neonate:* TOP 1-2 gtt each eye

immediately after delivery; SOL, 1 gtt q6-12h more frequently
Available forms: Oint, susp 1%
Side effects/adverse reactions:
EENT: Poor corneal wound healing, overgrowth of nonsusceptible organisms
Contraindications: Hypersensitivity, pregnancy (D), varicella, vaccinia, mycobacterial, fungal infections of the eye, epithelial herpes simplex keratitis
Precautions: Antibiotic hypersensitivity
NURSING CONSIDERATIONS
Assess:
- Allergy: itching, lacrimation, redness, swelling

Administer:
- After washing hands; cleanse crusts or discharge from eye before application

Perform/provide:
- Storage at room temp in light-resistant container

Evaluate:
- Therapeutic response: absence of redness, inflammation, tearing

Teach patient/family:
- To use drug exactly as prescribed, shake well before using
- Not to use eye make-up, towels, washcloths, or eye medication of others, or reinfection may occur
- That drug container tip should not be touched to eye
- To report itching, increased redness, burning, stinging, swelling; drug should be discontinued
- That drug may cause blurred vision when ointment is applied

tetracycline (topical) (℞)

(tet-ra-sye′kleen)
Achromycin, Topicycline
Func. class.: Local antiinfective
Chem. class.: Tetracycline

Action: Interferes with microorganism protein synthesis
Uses: Acne vulgaris, skin abrasions
Dosage and routes:
- *Adult and child >12 yr:* TOP apply to affected area bid

Available forms: Oint 3%; sol 0.22%
Side effects/adverse reactions:
INTEG: Rash, urticaria, stinging, burning, redness, swelling, photosensitivity
Contraindications: Hypersensitivity, pregnancy (D)
Precautions: Lactation, children, hepatic, renal disease
NURSING CONSIDERATIONS
Assess:
- Allergic reaction: burning, stinging, swelling, redness

Administer:
- Enough medication to cover lesions completely
- After cleansing with soap, water before each application; dry well

Perform/provide:
- Dry storage at room temp; use within 2 mo or discard

Evaluate:
- Therapeutic response: decrease in size, number of lesions

Teach patient/family:
- To apply with glove to prevent further infection
- To avoid use of OTC creams, ointments, lotions unless directed by prescriber
- To use medical asepsis (hand washing) before, after each application, avoid eyes, nose, mouth

• To notify prescriber if condition worsens
• That some stinging may occur
• To avoid sunlight, ultraviolet light, or burning may occur
• That clothing and skin may be stained

tetrahydrozoline (nasal) (OTC)

(tet-ra-hye-dro'zoe-leen)

Tyzine HCl, Tyzine Pediatric

Func. class.: Nasal decongestant

Chem. class.: Sympathomimetic amine

Action: Produces vasoconstriction (rapid, long-acting) of arterioles, decreasing fluid exudation, mucosal engorgement

Uses: Nasal congestion

Dosage and routes:

• *Adult and child >6 yr:* INSTILL 2-4 gtt or sprays q4-6h prn (0.1%)
• *Child 2-6 yr:* INSTILL 2-3 gtt q4-6h prn (0.05%)

Available forms: Sol 0.05%, 0.1%

Side effects/adverse reactions:

GI: Nausea, vomiting, anorexia

EENT: Irritation, burning, sneezing, stinging, dryness, rebound congestion

INTEG: Contact dermatitis

CNS: Anxiety, restlessness, tremors, weakness, insomnia, dizziness, fever, headache

Contraindications: Hypersensitivity to sympathomimetic amines

Precautions: Child <6 yr, elderly, diabetes, cardiovascular disease, hypertension, hyperthyroidism, increased ICP, prostatic hypertrophy, pregnancy (C), glaucoma

Interactions:

• Hypertension: MAOIs, β-adrenergic blockers
• Hypotension: methyldopa, mecamylamine, reserpine

NURSING CONSIDERATIONS

Assess:

• Redness, swelling, pain in nasal passages

Administer:

• No more than q4h
• For <4 consecutive days

Perform/provide:

• Environmental humidification to decrease nasal congestion, dryness
• Storage in light-resistant container; do not expose to heat

Evaluate:

• Therapeutic response: decreased nasal congestion

Teach patient/family:

• That stinging may occur for several applications; drying of mucosa may be decreased by environmental humidification
• To notify prescriber of irregular pulse, insomnia, dizziness, or tremors
• Proper administration to avoid systemic absorption

tetrahydrozoline (ophthalmic) (OTC)

(tet-ra-hye-dro'zoe-leen)

Collyrium Fresh Eye Drops, Eyesine, Murine Plus Eye Drops, Optigene 3 Eye Drops, Soothe Eye Drops, tetrahydrozoline HCl, Visine Eye Drops, Tyzine HCl, Tyzine Pediatric

Func. class.: Ophthalmic vasoconstrictor

Chem. class.: Direct sympathomimetic amine

Action: Vasoconstriction of eye arterioles; decreases eye engorgement by stimulation of α-adrenergic receptors

Uses: Ocular congestion, irritation,

itching, redness; adjunct in otitis media

Dosage and routes:

• *Adult, child >2 yr:* INSTILL 1-2 gtt bid or tid

Available forms: Sol 0.05%

Side effects/adverse reactions:

CNS: Headache, dizziness, weakness

CV: Reflex bradycardia, hypertension, dysrhythmias, tachycardia, ***CV collapse,*** palpitation

EENT: Stinging, lacrimation, blurred vision, conjunctival allergy

Contraindications: Hypersensitivity, narrow-angle glaucoma

Precautions: Severe hypertension, diabetes, hyperthyroidism, elderly, severe arteriosclerosis, cardiac disease, infants, pregnancy (C), lactation, diabetes, asthma, coronary artery disease

Pharmacokinetics:

Instill: Duration 2-3 hr

Interactions:

• Increased pressor effects: MAOIs, tricyclic antidepressants

• Increased side effects: β-blockers

• Sensitized myocardium: anesthetics

NURSING CONSIDERATIONS

Assess:

• B/P, pulse; systemic absorption does occur

Perform/provide:

• Storage in tight, light-resistant container; do not use discolored sol

Evaluate:

• Therapeutic response: decreased eye irritation, itching

Teach patient/family:

• To report change in vision, blurring, loss of sight; breathing trouble, sweating, flushing

• Method of instillation: tilt head backward, hold dropper over eye, drop medication inside lower lid, using pressure on inside corner of eye; hold 1 min; do not touch dropper to eye

• That blurred vision will decrease with repeated use of drug

• To notify prescriber of headache, spots, redness, pain; discontinue use

• To use sunglasses for photophobia

• To use exactly as prescribed

• Not to use for longer than 72 hr without prescriber's approval

---

theophylline (℞)

(thee-off'i-lin)

Accurbron, Aerolate III, Aerolate Jr., Aerolate Slo-Phyllin, Aerolate Sr., Aquaphyllin, Asmalix, Bronkodyl, Constant-T, Elixomin, Elixophyllin, Elixophyllin SR, Lanophyllin, Quibron-T Dividose, Quibron-T/SR Dividose, Respbid, Slo-Bid Gyrocaps, Slo-Phyllin Gyrocaps, Sustaire, Theolair-SR, Theo-24, Theobid Duracaps, Theobid Jr. Duracaps, Theochron, Theoclear-80, Theoclear L.A., Theo-Dur, Theo-Dur Sprinkle, Theolair, Theolair-SR, Theophylline, Theophylline and 5% Dextrose, Theophylline Extended Release, Theophylline Oral, Theophylline S.R., Theo-Sav, Theospan-SR, Theostat 80, Theovent, Theox, T-Phyl, Uniphyl

Func. class.: Spasmolytic

Chem. class.: Xanthine, ethylenediamide

Combination products: Theomax DF Syrup, Marax-DF Syrup: 97.5 mg theophylline, 18.75 mg ephedrine

---

Action: Relaxes smooth muscle of respiratory system by blocking

---

* Available in Canada only

phosphodiesterase, which increases cAMP
Uses: Bronchial asthma, bronchospasm of COPD, chronic bronchitis
Dosage and routes:
Bronchospasm, bronchial asthma
• *Adult:* PO 100-200 mg q6h; dosage must be individualized; REC 250-500 mg q8-12h
• *Child:* PO 50-100 mg q6h, not to exceed 12 mg/kg/24 hr
COPD, chronic bronchitis
• *Adult:* PO 330-660 mg q6-8h pc (sodium glycinate)
• *Child >12 yr:* PO 220-330 mg q6-8h pc (sodium glycinate)
• *Child 6-12 yr:* PO 330 mg q6-8h pc (sodium glycinate)
• *Child 3-6 yr:* PO 110-165 mg q6-8h pc (sodium glycinate)
• *Child 1-3 yr:* PO 55-110 mg q6-8h pc (sodium glycinate)
Available forms: Caps 50, 100, 200, 250 mg; tabs 100, 125, 200, 225, 250, 300 mg; tabs time-release 100, 200, 250, 300, 400, 500 mg; caps time-release 50, 65, 100, 125, 130, 200, 250, 260, 300, 400, 500 mg; elix 80, 11.25 mg/15 ml; sol 80 mg/15 ml; liq 80, 150, 160 mg/15 ml; susp 300 mg/15 ml
Side effects/adverse reactions:
CNS: Anxiety, restlessness, insomnia, dizziness, convulsions, headache, light-headedness, muscle twitching
CV: Palpitations, sinus tachycardia, hypotension, other dysrhythmias, fluid retention with tachycardia
GI: Nausea, vomiting, anorexia, diarrhea, bitter taste, dyspepsia, gastric distress
RESP: Increased rate
INTEG: Flushing, urticaria
Contraindications: Hypersensitivity to xanthines, tachydysrhythmias
Precautions: Elderly, CHF, cor pulmonale, hepatic disease, active peptic ulcer disease, diabetes mellitus, hyperthyroidism, hypertension, children, pregnancy (C)
Pharmacokinetics:
SOL: Peak 1 hr, metabolized in liver, excreted in urine and breast milk, crosses placenta
Interactions:
• Increased action of theophylline: cimetidine, propranolol, erythromycin, troleandomycin
• May increase effects of anticoagulants
• Cardiotoxicity: β-blockers
• Decreased effect of lithium

NURSING CONSIDERATIONS
Assess:
• Theophylline blood levels (therapeutic level is 10-20 μg/ml); toxicity may occur with small increase above 20 μg/ml
• Monitor I&O; diuresis occurs; elderly or child may be dehydrated
• Signs of toxicity: irritability, insomnia, restlessness, tremors, nausea, vomiting
• Respiratory rate, rhythm, depth; auscultate lung fields bilaterally; notify prescriber of abnormalities
• Allergic reactions: rash, urticaria; drug should be discontinued
Administer:
• PO after meals for GI symptoms; absorption may be affected
Evaluate:
• Therapeutic response: ability to breathe more easily
Teach patient/family:
• To check OTC medications, current prescription medications for ephedrine, which will increase stimulation; to avoid alcohol, caffeine
• To avoid hazardous activities; dizziness may occur
• That if GI upset occurs, to take drug with 8 oz H_2O; avoid food; absorption may be decreased

T

• Not to crush, dissolve, or chew slow-release products
• That contents of bead-filled capsule may be sprinkled over food for children's use
• To notify prescriber of toxicity: nausea, vomiting, anxiety, insomnia, convulsions
• To notify prescriber of change in smoking habit; dosage may have to be changed

thiabendazole (℞)

(thye-a-ben'da-zole)
Mintezol
Func. class.: Antihelminthic
Chem. class.: Benzimadazole derivative

Action: Inhibits anaerobic metabolism, disrupts microtubules
Uses: Pinworm, roundworm, threadworm, whipworm, trichinosis, hookworm, cutaneous larva migrans (creeping eruption)
Dosage and routes:
• *Adult and child:* PO 25 mg/kg in 2 doses qd × 2-5 days, not to exceed 3 g/day
Available forms: Tabs, chew 500 mg; oral susp 500 mg/5 ml
Side effects/adverse reactions:
SYST: ***Anaphylaxis***
GU: ***Hematuria, nephrotoxicity,*** enuresis, abnormal smell of urine
INTEG: Rash, pruritus, erythema, ***Stevens-Johnson syndrome***
CNS: Dizziness, headache, drowsiness, fever, flushing, ***convulsions,*** behavioral changes
EENT: Tinnitus, blurred vision, xanthopsia
GI: Nausea, vomiting, anorexia, diarrhea, jaundice, liver damage, epigastric distress
CV: Hypotension, bradycardia
Contraindications: Hypersensitivity
Precautions: Severe malnutrition, hepatic disease, renal disease, anemia, severe dehydration, child <14 kg, pregnancy (C)
Pharmacokinetics:
PO: Peak 1-2 hr, metabolized completely by liver, excreted in feces and urine
NURSING CONSIDERATIONS
Assess:
• Stools periodically during entire treatment
Administer:
• Susp after shaking
• PO after meals to avoid GI symptoms
Perform/provide:
• Storage in tight container
Evaluate:
• Therapeutic response: stools negative for helminths
Teach patient/family:
• Proper hygiene after BM, including hand-washing technique; tell patient not to put fingers in mouth
• That infected person should sleep alone; not to shake bed linen; to change bed linen qd
• To clean toilet qd with disinfectant (green soap solution)
• Need for compliance with dosage schedule, duration of treatment
• To drink fruit juice to remove mucus that intestinal tapeworms burrow in; aids in expulsion of worms
• To avoid hazardous activities if drowsiness occurs
Treatment of overdose: Induce emesis or gastric lavage

thiamine (vit B_1)

(PO-OTC, IM-℞)
Betaxin*, Betalin S, Biamine, Revitonus, Thiamilate, thiamine HCl
Func. class.: Vit B_1
Chem. class.: Water soluble

* Available in Canada only

Action: Needed for pyruvate metabolism, carbohydrate metabolism
Uses: Vit B_1 deficiency or polyneuritis, cheilosis adjunct with thiamine beriberi, Wernicke-Korsakoff syndrome, pellagra, metabolic disorders
Dosage and routes:
Beriberi
• *Adult:* IM 10-500 mg tid × 2 wk, then 5-10 mg qd × 1 mo
• *Child:* IM 10-50 mg qd × 4-6 wk
Anemia/alcoholism/pregnancy/pellagra
• *Adult:* PO 100 mg qd
• *Child:* PO 10-50 mg qd in divided doses
Beriberi with cardiac failure
• *Adult, child:* IV 100-500 mg
Wernicke's encephalopathy
• *Adult:* IV 500 mg or less, then 100 mg bid
Available forms: Tabs 50, 100, 250, 500 mg; inj 100 mg/ml; enteric coated tabs 20 mg
Side effects/adverse reactions:
CNS: Weakness, restlessness
GI: Hemorrhage, ***nausea, diarrhea***
CV: ***Collapse, pulmonary edema,*** hypotension
INTEG: ***Angioneurotic edema,*** cyanosis, sweating, warmth
SYST: ***Anaphylaxis***
EENT: Tightness of throat
Contraindications: Hypersensitivity
Precautions: Pregnancy (A)
Pharmacokinetics:
PO/INJ: Unused amounts excreted in urine (unchanged)
Y-site compatibility: Famotidine
NURSING CONSIDERATIONS
Assess:
• Thiamine levels throughout treatment
• Nutritional status: yeast, beef, liver, whole or enriched grains, legumes

Administer:
• IV undiluted over 5 min or diluted with IV sol and given as an inf at 100 mg or less/5 min or more
• By IM injection; rotate sites if pain and inflammation occur; do not mix with alkaline sols; Z-track to minimize pain
• Application of cold may decrease pain
Perform/provide:
• Storage in tight, light-resistant container
Evaluate:
• Therapeutic response: absence of nausea, vomiting, anorexia, insomnia, tachycardia, paresthesias, depression, muscle weakness
Teach patient/family:
• Necessary foods to be included in diet: yeast, beef, liver, legumes, whole grain

---

thiethylperazine (℞)

(thye-eth-il-per′a-zeen)
Norzine, Torecan
Func. class.: Antiemetic
Chem. class.: Phenothiazine, piperazine derivative

Action: Acts centrally by blocking chemoreceptor trigger zone, which in turn acts on vomiting center
Uses: Nausea, vomiting
Dosage and routes:
• *Adult:* PO/IM/REC 10 mg/qd-tid
Available forms: Tabs 10 mg; supp 10 mg; inj 5 mg/ml
Side effects/adverse reactions:
GU: Urinary retention, dark urine
CNS: Euphoria, depression, restlessness, tremor, EPS, ***convulsions,*** drowsiness
GI: Nausea, vomiting, anorexia, dry mouth, diarrhea, constipation, weight loss, metallic taste, cramps
CV: ***Circulatory failure, tachycar-***

dia, postural hypotension, ECG changes
RESP: ***Respiratory depression***
Contraindications: Hypersensitivity to phenothiazines, coma, seizure, encephalopathy, bone marrow depression
Precautions: Children <2 yr, pregnancy (C), elderly, lactation
Pharmacokinetics:
PO: Onset 45-60 min
REC: Onset 45-60 min, metabolized by liver, crosses placenta, excreted in urine, breast milk
Interactions:
• Decreased effect of thiethylperazine: barbiturates, antacids
• Increased anticholinergic action: anticholinergics, antiparkinson drugs, antidepressants
• Do not mix with other drug in syringe or sol
NURSING CONSIDERATIONS
Assess:
• VS, B/P; check patients with cardiac disease more often
• Respiratory status before, during, after administration of emetic; check rate, rhythm, character; respiratory depression can occur rapidly with elderly or debilitated patients
Administer:
• IM inj in large muscle mass; aspirate to avoid IV administration; patient should remain recumbent 1 hr after inj
Evaluate:
• Therapeutic response: absence of nausea, vomiting
Teach patient/family:
• To avoid hazardous activities, activities requiring alertness; dizziness may occur

thioguanine (6-TG) (℞)

(thye-oh-gwah'neen)
thioguanine, Lanvis*
Func. class.: Antineoplastic-antimetabolite
Chem. class.: Purine analog

Action: Interferes with synthesis, utilization of purine nucleotides; S phase of cell cycle specific
Uses: Acute leukemias, chronic granulocytic leukemia, lymphomas, multiple myeloma, solid tumors
Dosage and routes:
• *Adult, child:* PO 2 mg/kg/day, then increase slowly to 3 mg/kg/day after 4 wk
Available forms: Tabs 40 mg
Side effects/adverse reactions:
HEMA: ***Thrombocytopenia, leukopenia, myelosuppression, anemia***
GI: Nausea, vomiting, anorexia, diarrhea, stomatitis, ***hepatotoxicity,*** gastritis, jaundice
GU: ***Renal failure,*** hyperuricemia, oliguria
INTEG: Rash, dermatitis, dry skin
Contraindications: Prior drug resistance, leukopenia (<2500/mm^3), thrombocytopenia (<100,000/mm^3), anemia, pregnancy (D)
Precautions: Liver disease
Pharmacokinetics: Oral form absorbed only 30%, metabolized in liver, only small amounts excreted in urine (unchanged)
Interactions:
• Increased toxicity: radiation, other antineoplastics
Lab test interferences:
Increase: Uric acid (blood, urine)
NURSING CONSIDERATIONS
Assess:
• CBC, differential, platelet count qwk; withhold drug if WBC is <3500/mm^3 or platelet count is

* Available in Canada only

<100,000/mm^3; notify prescriber; drug should be discontinued
• Renal function studies: BUN, serum uric acid, urine CrCl, electrolytes before, during therapy
• I&O ratio; report fall in urine output to <30 ml/hr
• Monitor temp q4h; fever may indicate beginning infection
• Liver function tests before, during therapy: bilirubin, alk phosphatase, AST (SGOT), ALT (SGPT)
• Bleeding time, coagulation time during treatment
• Bleeding: hematuria, guaiac, bruising, petechiae, mucosa or orifices q8h
• Food preferences; list likes, dislikes
• Hepatotoxicity: yellow skin, sclera, dark urine, clay-colored stools, pruritus, abdominal pain, fever, diarrhea
• Buccal cavity q8h for dryness, sores, ulceration, white patches, oral pain, bleeding, dysphagia
• Symptoms indicating severe allergic reaction: rash, urticaria, itching, flushing

Administer:
• Antacid before oral agent; give drug after evening meal before bedtime
• Antiemetic 30-60 min before giving drug to prevent vomiting
• Allopurinol or sodium bicarbonate to maintain uric acid levels, alkalinization of urine
• Antibiotics for prophylaxis of infection
• Topical or systemic analgesics for pain
• Transfusion for anemia

Perform/provide:
• Strict medical asepsis, protective isolation if WBC levels are low
• Liquid diet: carbonated beverage, Jell-O; dry toast, crackers may be added when patient is not nauseated or vomiting
• Increase fluid intake to 2-3 L/day to prevent urate deposits, calculi formation, unless contraindicated
• Diet low in purines: no organ meats (kidney, liver), dried beans, peas to maintain alkaline urine
• Rinsing of mouth tid-qid with water, club soda, brushing of teeth bid-tid with soft brush or cotton-tipped applicators for stomatitis; use unwaxed dental floss
• Nutritious diet with iron, vitamin supplements as ordered
• Storage in tightly closed container in cool environment

Evaluate:
• Therapeutic response: decreased tumor size, spread of malignancy

Teach patient/family:
• Why protective isolation precautions are needed
• To report any complaints, side effects to prescriber: black tarry stools, chills, fever, sore throat, bleeding, bruising, cough, shortness of breath, dark, bloody urine
• To avoid foods with citric acid, hot or rough texture if stomatitis is present
• To report stomatitis: any bleeding, white spots, ulcerations in mouth; to examine mouth qd, report symptoms
• That contraceptive measures are recommended during therapy
• To drink 10-12 (8 oz) glasses of fluid/day

thiopental (℞)

(thye-oh-pen′tal)
Pentothal, thiopental sodium
Func. class.: General anesthetic
Chem. class.: Barbiturate

Controlled Substance Schedule III
Action: Acts in reticular-activating

system to produce anesthesia, raises seizure threshold

Uses: Short general anesthesia, narcoanalysis, induction anesthesia before other anesthetics

Investigational uses: Increased intracranial pressure

Dosage and routes:

Induction

• *Adult:* IV 210-280 mg or 3-5 ml/kg

General anesthetic

• *Adult:* IV 50-75 mg given at 20-40 sec intervals

Narcoanalysis

• *Adult:* IV 100 mg/min, not to exceed 50 ml/min

Sedation or narcosis

• *Adult:* REC 12-20 mg/lb

Available forms: Inj 250, 400, 500 mg, 1 g; rectal sus 400 mg/g

Side effects/adverse reactions:

RESP: ***Respiratory depression, bronchospasm***

CNS: Retrograde amnesia, prolonged somnolence

CV: Tachycardia, hypotension, ***myocardial depression, dysrhythmias***

EENT: Sneezing, coughing

INTEG: Chills, *shivering,* necrosis, pain at injection site

MS: Muscle irritability

Contraindications: Hypersensitivity, status asthmaticus, hepatic/intermittent porphyrias

Precautions: Severe cardiovascular disease, renal disease, hypotension, liver disease, myxedema, myasthenia gravis, asthma, increased intracranial pressure, pregnancy (C)

Pharmacokinetics:

IV: Onset 30-40 sec; half-life 11½ hr; crosses placenta

Interactions:

• Increased action: CNS depressants

Syringe compatibilities: Aminophylline, hydrocortisone sodium succinate, neostigmine, pentobarbital, scopolamine, tubocurarine

Additive compatibilities: Chloramphenicol, hydrocortisone sodium succinate, pentobarbital, potassium chloride

Solution compatibilities: D_5/0.45% NaCl, D_5W, multiple electrolyte sol, 0.45% NaCl, 0.9% NaCl, 1/6 M sodium lactate

NURSING CONSIDERATIONS

Assess:

• VS q3-5min during IV administration, after dose, q4h postoperatively

• Extravasation; if it occurs, use nitroprusside or chloroprocaine to decrease pain, increase circulation

• Dysrhythmias or myocardial depression

Administer:

• IV after diluting 500 mg/20 ml sterile H_2O for inj; give each 25 mg or less/min, titrate to response

• Only with crash cart, resuscitative equipment nearby

Evaluate:

• Therapeutic response: maintenance of anesthesia

thioridazine (℞)

(thye-or-rid'a-zeen)

Mellaril, Mellaril Concentrate, Mellaril-5, Novoridazine*, thioridazine HCl

Func. class.: Antipsychotic/neuroleptic

Chem. class.: Phenothiazine, piperidine

Action: Depresses cerebral cortex, hypothalamus, limbic system, which control activity, aggression; blocks neurotransmission produced by dopamine at synapse; exhibits strong α-adrenergic, anticholinergic blocking action; mechanism for antipsychotic effects is unclear

Uses: Psychotic disorders, schizophrenia, behavioral problems in chil-

* Available in Canada only

dren, alcohol withdrawal as adjunct, anxiety, major depressive disorders, organic brain syndrome

Dosage and routes:

Psychosis

• *Adult:* PO 25-100 mg tid, max dose 800 mg/day; dose is gradually increased to desired response, then reduced to minimum maintenance

Depression/behavioral problems/ organic brain syndrome

• *Adult:* PO 25 mg tid, range from 10 mg bid-qid to 50 mg tid-qid

• *Child 2-12 yr:* PO 0.5-3 mg/kg/ day in divided doses

Available forms: Tabs 10, 15, 25, 50, 100, 150, 200, 300 mg; conc 30, 100 mg/ml; susp 25, 100 mg/5 ml; syr 10 mg/15 ml

Side effects/adverse reactions:

RESP: ***Laryngospasm,*** dyspnea, ***respiratory depression***

CNS: EPS (rare): pseudoparkinsonism, akathisia, dystonia, tardive dyskinesia, ***seizures,*** *headache,* confusion

HEMA: Anemia, ***leukopenia, leukocytosis, agranulocytosis***

INTEG: Rash, photosensitivity, dermatitis

EENT: Blurred vision, glaucoma, dry eyes

GI: Dry mouth, nausea, vomiting, anorexia, constipation, diarrhea, jaundice, weight gain

GU: Urinary retention, urinary frequency, enuresis, impotence, amenorrhea, gynecomastia

CV: Orthostatic hypotension, ***cardiac arrest,*** ECG changes, ***tachycardia***

Contraindications: Hypersensitivity, blood dyscrasias, coma, child <2 yr, brain damage, bone marrow depression

Precautions: Pregnancy (C), lactation, seizure disorders, hypertension, hepatic disease, cardiac disease

Pharmacokinetics:

PO: Onset erratic, peak 2-4 hr; metabolized by liver, excreted in urine, breast milk; crosses placenta, half-life 26-36 hr

Interactions:

• Oversedation: other CNS depressants, alcohol, barbiturate anesthetics

• Toxicity: epinephrine

• Decreased absorption: aluminum hydroxide, magnesium hydroxide antacids

• Decreased effects of lithium, levodopa

• Increased effects of both drugs: β-adrenergic blockers, alcohol

• Increased anticholinergic effects: anticholinergics

Lab test interferences:

Increase: Liver function tests, cardiac enzymes, cholesterol, blood glucose, prolactin, bilirubin, PBI, cholinesterase, ^{131}I

Decrease: Hormones (blood, urine)

False positive: Pregnancy test, PKU

False negative: Urinary steroid, pregnancy test

NURSING CONSIDERATIONS

Assess:

• Mental status before first dose

• Swallowing of PO medication; check for hoarding or giving of medication to other patients

• I&O ratio; palpate bladder if low urinary output occurs

• Bilirubin, CBC, liver function studies qmo

• Urinalysis is recommended before and during prolonged therapy

• Affect, orientation, LOC, reflexes, gait, coordination, sleep pattern disturbances

• B/P standing and lying; also include pulse and respirations q4h during initial treatment; establish base-

T

line before starting treatment; report drops of 30 mm Hg
• Dizziness, faintness, palpitations, tachycardia on rising
• EPS including akathisia (inability to sit still, no pattern to movements), tardive dyskinesia (bizarre movements of jaw, mouth, tongue, extremities), pseudoparkinsonism (rigidity, tremors, pill rolling, shuffling gait)
• For neuroleptic malignant syndrome: altered mental status, muscle rigidity, increased CPK, hyperthermia
• Skin turgor qd
• Constipation, urinary retention qd; increase bulk, water in diet

Administer:
• Antiparkinsonian agent, on order from prescriber for EPS
• Concentrate mixed in citrus juices or distilled or acidified tap water

Perform/provide:
• Decreased sensory input by dimming lights, avoiding loud noises
• Supervised ambulation until stabilized on medication if needed; do not involve in strenuous exercise program because fainting is possible; patient should not stand still for long periods
• Increased fluids to prevent constipation
• Sips of water, candy, gum for dry mouth
• Storage in tight, light-resistant container; avoid contact with skin

Evaluate:
• Therapeutic response: decrease in emotional excitement, hallucinations, delusions, paranoia, reorganization of patterns of thought, speech

Teach patient/family:
• That orthostatic hypotension occurs frequently, to rise from sitting or lying position gradually; to avoid hazardous activities until stabilized on medication
• To remain lying down after IM injection for at least 30 min
• To avoid hot tubs, hot showers, tub baths; hypotension may occur
• To avoid abrupt withdrawal of thioridazine, or EPS may result; drug should be withdrawn slowly
• To avoid OTC preparations (cough, hay fever, cold) unless approved by prescriber; serious drug interactions may occur; avoid use with alcohol, CNS depressants; increased drowsiness may occur
• To use a sunscreen
• Regarding compliance with drug regimen
• About necessity for meticulous oral hygiene, since oral candidiasis may occur
• To report sore throat, malaise, fever, bleeding, mouth sores; if these occur, CBC should be drawn and drug discontinued
• In hot weather, heat stroke may occur; take extra precautions to stay cool

Treatment of overdose: Lavage if orally ingested, provide an airway; *do not induce vomiting*

thiotepa (℞)

(thye-oh-tep′a)
thiotepa
Func. class.: Antineoplastic
Chem. class.: Alkylating agent

Action: Responsible for cross-linking DNA strands leading to cell death; activity is not cell cycle specific

Uses: Hodgkin's disease, lymphomas; breast, ovarian, lung, bladder, cancer; neoplastic effusions

Dosage and routes:
• *Adult:* IV 50.2 mg/kg × 5 days, then 0.2 mg/kg q1-3 wk

Neoplastic effusions
• *Adult:* INTRACAVITY 10-15 mg
Bladder cancer
• *Adult:* INSTILL 60 mg/60 ml water for inj instilled in bladder for 2 hr once weekly × 4 wk
Available forms: Inj 15 mg, powder for inj
Side effects/adverse reactions:
CNS: Dizziness, headache
HEMA: ***Thrombocytopenia, leukopenia, pancytopenia***
GI: Nausea, vomiting, anorexia, stomatitis
GU: Hyperuricemia, ***hematuria, amenorrhea, azoospermia***
INTEG: Rash, pruritus
Contraindications: Hypersensitivity, pregnancy (D)
Precautions: Radiation therapy, bone marrow suppression, impaired renal or hepatic function
Pharmacokinetics:
Onset slow, metabolized in liver, excreted in urine
Interactions:
• Increased apnea: succinylcholine
Syringe compatibilities: Procaine HCl, (2%), epinephrine 1:1000

NURSING CONSIDERATIONS
Assess:
• CBC, differential, platelet count qwk; withhold drug if WBC is <4000 or platelet count is <75,000; notify prescriber
• Renal function studies: BUN, serum uric acid, urine CrCl before, during therapy
• I&O ratio, report fall in urine output of 30 ml/hr
• Monitor temp q4h (may indicate beginning infection)
• Liver function tests before, during therapy (bilirubin, AST [SGOT], ALT [SGPT], LDH) as needed or monthly
• Bleeding: hematuria, guaiac, bruising or petechiae, mucosa or orifices q8h
• Food preferences; list likes, dislikes
• Inflammation of mucosa, breaks in skin
• Yellow skin, sclera, dark urine, clay-colored stools, itchy skin, abdominal pain, fever, diarrhea
• Buccal cavity q8h for dryness, sores, ulceration, white patches, oral pain, bleeding, dysphagia
• Symptoms indicating severe allergic reaction: rash, pruritus, urticaria, itching, flushing
Administer:
• IV after diluting 15 mg/1.5 ml of sterile H_2O for inj; give over 1-3 min; may be further diluted in 50-100 ml compatible sol
• Antiemetic 30-60 min before giving drug to prevent vomiting
• Allopurinol or sodium bicarbonate to maintain uric acid levels, alkalinization of urine
• Antibiotics for prophylaxis of infection
• Local or systemic drugs for infection
Perform/provide:
• Storage in light-resistant container; refrigerate
• Strict medical asepsis, protective isolation if WBC levels are low
• Special skin care
• Increase fluid intake to 2-3 L/day to prevent urate deposits, calculi formation
• Diet low in purines: organ meats (kidney, liver), dried beans, peas, to maintain alkaline urine
• Rinsing of mouth tid-qid with water; brushing of teeth bid-tid with soft brush or cotton-tipped applicators for stomatitis; use unwaxed dental floss
• Warm compresses at injection site for inflammation
Evaluate:
• Therapeutic response: decreased tumor size, spread of malignancy

Teach patient/family:

- About protective isolation
- That azoospermia or amenorrhea can occur; reversible after discontinuing treatment
- To avoid foods with citric acid, hot or rough texture
- To report any bleeding, white spots or ulcerations in mouth to prescriber; to examine mouth qd
- To report signs of infection: fever, sore throat, flu symptoms
- To report signs of anemia: fatigue, headache, faintness, shortness of breath, irritability
- To avoid use of razors, commercial mouthwash
- To avoid use of aspirin products, ibuprofen

thiothixene (℞)

(thye-oh-thix'een)

Navane, thiothixene

Func. class.: Antipsychotic/neuroleptic

Chem. class.: Thioxanthene

Action: Depresses cerebral cortex, hypothalamus, limbic system, which control activity, aggression; blocks neurotransmission produced by dopamine at synapse; exhibits strong α-adrenergic blocking action; mechanism for antipsychotic effects is unclear

Uses: Psychotic disorders, schizophrenia, acute agitation

Dosage and routes:

- *Adult:* PO 2-5 mg bid-qid depending on severity of condition; dose gradually increased to 15-30 mg if needed; IM 4 mg bid-qid; max dose 30 mg qd; administer PO dose as soon as possible

Available forms: Caps 1, 2, 5, 10, 20 mg; conc 5 mg/ml; inj 2 mg/ml; powder for inj 5 mg/ml

Side effects/adverse reactions:

RESP: ***Laryngospasm,*** dyspnea, ***respiratory depression***

CNS: EPS: pseudoparkinsonism, akathisia, dystonia, tardive dyskinesia; seizures, *headache*

HEMA: Anemia, ***leukopenia, leukocytosis, agranulocytosis***

INTEG: Rash, photosensitivity, dermatitis

EENT: Blurred vision, glaucoma

GI: Dry mouth, nausea, vomiting, anorexia, constipation, diarrhea, jaundice, weight gain

GU: Urinary retention, urinary frequency, enuresis, impotence, amenorrhea, gynecomastia

CV: Orthostatic hypotension, hypertension, ***cardiac arrest,*** ECG changes, ***tachycardia***

Contraindications: Hypersensitivity, blood dyscrasias, child <12 yr, bone marrow depression, circulatory collapse, CNS depression, coma, alcoholism, CV disease, hepatic disease, Reye's syndrome, narrow-angle glaucoma

Precautions: Pregnancy (C), lactation, seizure disorders, hypertension, hepatic disease

Pharmacokinetics:

PO: Onset slow, peak 2-8 hr, duration up to 12 hr

IM: Onset 15-30 min, peak 1-6 hr, duration up to 12 hr; metabolized by liver, excreted in urine, breast milk; crosses placenta, half-life 34 hr

Interactions:

- Oversedation: other CNS depressants, alcohol, barbiturate anesthetics
- Toxicity: epinephrine
- Decreased absorption: aluminum hydroxide, magnesium hydroxide antacids
- Decreased effects of thiothixene: lithium, levodopa
- Increased effects of both drugs: β-adrenergic blockers, alcohol

* Available in Canada only

• Increased anticholinergic effects: anticholinergics

Lab test interferences:

Increase: Liver function tests, cardiac enzymes, cholesterol, blood glucose, prolactin, bilirubin, PBI, cholinesterase, ^{131}I

Decrease: Uric acid

NURSING CONSIDERATIONS

Assess:

• Mental status before initial administration
• Swallowing of PO medication; check for hoarding or giving of medication to other patients
• I&O ratio, palpate bladder if low urinary output occurs
• Bilirubin, CBC, liver function studies qmo
• Urinalysis is recommended before and during prolonged therapy
• Affect, orientation, LOC, reflexes, gait, coordination, sleep pattern disturbances
• B/P standing and lying; pulse and respirations q4h during initial treatment; establish baseline before starting treatment; report drops of 30 mm Hg
• Dizziness, faintness, palpitations, tachycardia on rising
• EPS including akathisia (inability to sit still, no pattern to movements), tardive dyskinesia (bizarre movements of jaw, mouth, tongue, extremities), pseudoparkinsonism (rigidity, tremors, pill rolling, shuffling gait)
• For neuroleptic malignant syndrome: muscle rigidity, altered mental status, increased CPK, hyperthermia
• Constipation, urinary retention daily; increase bulk, water in diet

Administer:

• Antiparkinsonian agent on order from prescriber for EPS
• Concentrate mixed in citrus juices or distilled or acidified tap water
• IM injection into large muscle mass

Perform/provide:

• Decreased sensory input by dimming lights, avoiding loud noises
• Supervised ambulation until stabilized on medication; do not involve in strenuous exercise program because fainting is possible; patient should not stand still for long periods
• Increased fluids to prevent constipation
• Sips of water, candy, gum for dry mouth
• Storage in tight, light-resistant container; keep reconstituted sol at room temp for up to 48 hr; avoid contact with skin

Evaluate:

• Therapeutic response: decrease in emotional excitement, hallucinations, delusions, paranoia, reorganization of patterns of thought, speech

Teach patient/family:

• That orthostatic hypotension occurs frequently, and to rise from sitting or lying position gradually; to avoid hazardous activities until stabilized on medication
• To remain lying down after IM inj for at least 30 min
• To avoid hot tubs, hot showers, tub baths; hypotension may occur
• To avoid abrupt withdrawal of this drug, or EPS may result; drug should be withdrawn slowly
• To avoid OTC preparations (cough, hay fever, cold) unless approved by prescriber; serious drug interactions may occur; avoid use with alcohol, CNS depressants; increased drowsiness may occur
• To use a sunscreen
• Regarding compliance with drug regimen
• About EPS
• Necessity for meticulous oral hy-

T

giene, since oral candidiasis may occur
• To report sore throat, malaise, fever, bleeding, mouth sores; if these occur, CBC should be drawn and drug discontinued
• In hot weather, heat stroke may occur; take extra precautions to stay cool
Treatment of overdose: Lavage if orally ingested; provide an airway; *do not induce vomiting*

thrombin (℞)

Thrombinar, Thrombogen, Thrombostat

Func. class.: Hemostatic
Chem. class.: Bovine thrombin

Action: Converts fibrinogen to fibrin, promotes clotting
Uses: GI hemorrhage, bleeding in dental, plastic, nasal, laryngeal surgery, skin grafting
Dosage and routes:
• *Adult:* TOP apply 100 U/1 ml sterile isotonic NaCl or distilled H_2O in light to moderate bleeding, or 1000-2000 U/ml sterile isotonic NaCl in severe bleeding; dry area before applying
Available forms: Powder 1000, 5000, 10,000, 20,000, 50,000 U
Side effects/adverse reactions:
INTEG: Rash, allergic reactions
HEMA: ***Intravascular clotting when entering large blood vessels***
Contraindications: Hypersensitivity to bovine products
Precautions: Pregnancy (C), children
NURSING CONSIDERATIONS
Assess:
• For allergic reactions: fever, rash, itching, changes in VS; thrombosis formation
Administer:
• Only to area sponged free of blood
• After preparing with NS, isotonic saline
• With blood available for transfusion
Perform/provide:
• Storage in refrigerator; use reconstituted sol within 3 hr; some can be administered up to 48 hr after reconstitution if refrigerated or preferably frozen shortly after reconstituted; discard unused portion
Evaluate:
• Therapeutic response: control of bleeding

thyroglobulin (℞)

(thye-roe-glob′yoo-lin)
Proloid

Func. class.: Thyroid hormone
Chem. class.: Combination of natural T_4/T_3; ratio 2.5 to 1

Action: Increases metabolic rates, cardiac output, O_2 consumption, body temp, blood volume, growth, development at cellular level
Uses: Hypothyroidism
Dosage and routes:
Adult: 32 mg/day increasing q2-3wk to desired response; maintenance 65-200 mg/day
Available forms: Tabs 32, 65, 100, 130, 200 mg
Side effects/adverse reactions:
INTEG: Sweating, alopecia
CNS: Anxiety, insomnia, tremors, headache, heat intolerance, fever, coma, thyroid storm
CV: Tachycardia, palpitations, angina, dysrhythmias, hypertension, ***CHF***
GI: Nausea, diarrhea, increased or decreased appetite, cramps
GU: Menstrual irregularities
Contraindications: Adrenal insufficiency, MI, thyrotoxicosis

* Available in Canada only

Precautions: Elderly, angina pectoris, hypertension, ischemia, cardiac disease, pregnancy (A), lactation

Pharmacokinetics:

PO: Peak 12-48 hr, half-life 6-7 days

Interactions:

• Decreased absorption of thyroglobulin: cholestyramine
• Increased effects of anticoagulants, sympathomimetics, tricyclic antidepressants, catecholamines
• Decreased effects of digitalis drugs, insulin, hypoglycemics
• Decreased effects of liothyronine: estrogens

Lab test interferences:

Increase: CPK, LDH, AST (SGOT), PBI, blood glucose

Decrease: TSH, ^{131}I uptake test, uric acid, triglycerides

NURSING CONSIDERATIONS

Assess:

• B/P, pulse before each dose
• I&O ratio
• Weight qd in same clothing, using same scale, at same time of day
• Height, growth rate of child
• T_3, T_4, which are decreased; radioimmunoassay of TSH, which is increased; radio uptake, which is decreased if dosage is too low
• Pro-time may require decreased anticoagulant; check for bleeding, bruising
• Increased nervousness, excitability, irritability, which may indicate too high dose of medication, usually after 1-3 wk of treatment
• Cardiac status: angina, palpitation, chest pain, change in VS

Administer:

• In AM if possible as a single dose to decrease sleeplessness
• At same time each day to maintain drug level
• Only for hormone imbalances; not to be used for obesity, male infertility, menstrual disorders, lethargy
• Lowest dose that relieves symptoms

Perform/provide:

• Removal of medication 4 wk before RAIU test

Evaluate:

• Therapeutic response: absence of depression; increased weight loss, diuresis, pulse, appetite; absence of constipation, peripheral edema, cold intolerance, pale, cool dry skin, brittle nails, alopecia, coarse hair, menorrhagia, night blindness, paresthesias, syncope, stupor, coma, rosy cheeks

Teach patient/family:

• To report excitability, irritability, anxiety, which indicate overdose
• Not to switch brands unless approved by prescriber
• That hypothyroid child will show almost immediate behavior/personality change
• That drug is not to be taken to reduce weight
• To avoid OTC preparations with iodine, to read labels
• To avoid iodine food, iodized salt, soybeans, tofu, turnips, some seafood, some bread

thyroid USP (desiccated) (℞)

(thye'roid)

Armour Thyroid, Cholaxin*, S-P-T, Thyrar, Thyroid Strong, Thyroid USP

Func. class.: Thyroid hormone

Chem. class.: Active thyroid hormone in natural state and ratio

Action: Increases metabolic rates, increases cardiac output, O_2 consumption, body temp, blood volume, growth, development at cellular level

T

Uses: Hypothyroidism, cretinism, myxedema

Dosage and routes:

Hypothyroidism

• *Adult:* PO 65 mg qd, increased by 65 mg q30d until desired response; maintenance dose 65-195 mg qd

• *Geriatric:* PO 7.5-15 mg qd, double dose q6-8wk until desired response

Cretinism/juvenile hypothyroidism

• *Child over 1 yr:* PO up to 180 mg qd titrated to response

• *Child 4-12 mo:* PO 30-60 mg qd

• *Child 1-4 mo:* PO 15-30 mg qd; may increase q2wk; titrated to response; maintenance dose 30-45 mg qd

Myxedema

• *Adult:* PO 16 mg qd, double dose q2wk, maintenance 65-195 mg/day

Available forms: Tabs 16, 32, 65, 98, 130, 195, 260, 325 mg; tabs enteric coated 32, 65, 130 mg; sugar-coated tabs 32, 65, 130, 195 mg; caps 65, 130, 195, 325 mg

Side effects/adverse reactions:

CNS: Insomnia, tremors, headache, thyroid storm

CV: Tachycardia, palpitations, angina, dysrhythmias, hypertension, ***cardiac arrest***

GI: Nausea, diarrhea, increased or decreased appetite, cramps

MISC: Menstrual irregularities, weight loss, sweating, heat intolerance, fever

Contraindications: Adrenal insufficiency, MI, thyrotoxicosis

Precautions: Elderly, angina pectoris, hypertension, ischemia, cardiac disease, pregnancy (A), lactation

Pharmacokinetics:

PO: Peak 12-48 hr, half-life 6-7 days

Interactions:

• Decreased absorption of thyroid: cholestyramine

• Increased effects of anticoagulants, sympathomimetics, tricyclic antidepressants, catecholamines

• Decreased effects of digitalis drugs, insulin, hypoglycemics

• Decreased effects of thyroid: estrogens

Lab test interferences:

Increase: CPK, LDH, AST (SGOT), PBI, blood glucose

Decrease: TSH, ^{131}I uptake test, uric acid, triglycerides

NURSING CONSIDERATIONS

Assess:

• B/P, pulse before each dose

• I&O ratio

• Weight qd in same clothing, using same scale, at same time of day

• Height, growth rate of child

• T_3, T_4, which are decreased; radioimmunoassay of TSH, which is increased; radio uptake, which is decreased if dosage is too low

• Pro-time may require decreased anticoagulant, check for bleeding, bruising

• Increased nervousness, excitability, irritability; may indicate too high dose of medication, usually after 1-3 wk of treatment

• Cardiac status: angina, palpitation, chest pain, change in VS

Administer:

• In AM if possible as a single dose to decrease sleeplessness

• At same time each day to maintain drug level

• Only for hormone imbalances; not to be used for obesity, male infertility, menstrual disorders, lethargy

• Lowest dose that relieves symptoms

Perform/provide:

• Removal of medication 4 wk before RAIU test

Evaluate:

• Therapeutic response: absence of depression; increased weight loss, diuresis, pulse, appetite; absence of

* Available in Canada only

constipation, peripheral edema, cold intolerance, pale, cool dry skin, brittle nails, alopecia, coarse hair, menorrhagia, night blindness, paresthesias, syncope, stupor, coma, rosy cheeks

Teach patient/family:

- That hair loss will occur in child, is temporary
- To report excitability, irritability, anxiety; indicates overdose
- Not to switch brands unless directed by prescriber
- That hypothyroid child will show almost immediate behavior/personality change
- That treatment drug is not to be taken to reduce weight
- To avoid OTC preparations with iodine; read labels
- To avoid iodine food, iodized salt, soybeans, tofu, turnips, some seafood, some bread

thyrotropin (thyroid-stimulating hormone, TSH) (℞)

(thye-roe-troe′pin)

Thytropar

Func. class.: Thyroid hormone

Chem. class.: TSH

Action: Increases uptake of iodine by thyroid gland, production and release of thyroid hormone

Uses: Diagnosis and treatment of thyroid cancer, diagnosis of primary/secondary hypothyroidism

Dosage and routes:

Diagnosis of hypothyroidism

- *Adult:* IM/SC 10 U qd × 1-3 days

Diagnosis of thyroid cancer

- *Adult:* IM/SC 10 IU qd × 3-7 days

Treatment of thyroid cancer

- *Adult:* IM/SC 10 U qd × 3-8 days

Available forms: Powder for inj 10 IU/vial

Side effects/adverse reactions:

INTEG: Urticaria

CNS: Headache, fever

CV: Tachycardia, angina, ***atrial fibrillation, CHF,*** hypotension

GI: Nausea, vomiting

SYST: ***Anaphylactic reactions***

Contraindications: Hypersensitivity, coronary thrombosis, untreated Addison's disease

Precautions: Angina pectoris, adrenal insufficiency, pregnancy (C), lactation, children

Pharmacokinetics:

IM/SC: Onset 8 hr, peak 24-48 hr

NURSING CONSIDERATIONS

Administer:

- After dilution with 2 ml sterile NS
- Three-day dose schedule for myxedema (pituitary)
- In combination with ^{131}I to treat thyroid cancer

Treatment of overdose: Discontinue drug, give supportive care

ticarcillin (℞)

(tye-kar-sill′in)

Ticar

Func. class.: Broad-spectrum antiinfective

Chem. class.: Extended-spectrum penicillin

Action: Interferes with cell wall replication of susceptible organisms; osmotically unstable cell wall swells, bursts from osmotic pressure.

Uses: Respiratory, soft tissue, urinary tract infections, bacterial septicemia; effective for gram-positive cocci *(S. aureus, S. faecalis, S. pneumoniae),* gram-negative cocci *(N. gonorrhoeae),* gram-positive bacilli *(C. perfringens, C. tetani),* gram-negative bacilli *(Bacteroides, F. nucleatum, E. coli, P. mirabilis, Salmonella, M. morganii, P. rettgeri, Enterobacter, P. aeruginosa, Serra-*

tia, Peptococcus, Peptostreptococcus, Eubacterium)

Dosage and routes:

• *Adult:* IV/IM 12-24 g/day in divided doses q3-6h; infuse over ½-2 hr

• *Child:* IV/IM 50-300 mg/kg/day in divided doses q4-8h

• *Neonates:* IV INF 75-100 mg/kg/8-12 hr

Available forms: Inj 1, 3, 6, 20, 30 g

Side effects/adverse reactions:

HEMA: Anemia, increased bleeding time, ***bone marrow depression, granulocytopenia***

GI: Nausea, vomiting, diarrhea, increased AST, ALT, abdominal pain, glossitis, colitis

GU: Oliguria, proteinuria, hematuria, *vaginitis, moniliasis,* ***glomerulonephritis***

CNS: Lethargy, hallucinations, anxiety, depression, twitching, ***coma, convulsions***

META: Hypokalemia

Contraindications: Hypersensitivity to penicillins

Precautions: Hypersensitivity to cephalosporins, pregnancy (B), lactation

Pharmacokinetics:

IM: Peak 1 hr, duration 4-6 hr

IV: Peak 30-45 min, duration 4 hr, half-life 70 min; small amount metabolized in liver; excreted in urine, breast milk

Interactions:

• Decreased antimicrobial effect of ticarcillin: tetracyclines, erythromycins, aminoglycosides IV

• Increased ticarcillin concentrations: aspirin, probenecid

• Incompatible in sol with aminoglycosides, tetracyclines, amphotericin B, gentamycin, amikacin, tobramycin

Lab test interferences:

False positive: Urine glucose, urine protein

NURSING CONSIDERATIONS

Assess:

• I&O ratio; report hematuria, oliguria, since penicillin in high doses is nephrotoxic

• Any patient with compromised renal system, since drug is excreted slowly in poor renal system function; toxicity may occur rapidly

• Liver studies: AST (SGOT), ALT (SGPT)

• Blood studies: WBC, RBC, Hgb, Hct, bleeding time

• Renal studies: urinalysis, protein, blood

• C&S before drug therapy; drug may be given as soon as culture is taken

• Bowel pattern before, during treatment

• Skin eruptions after administration of penicillin to 1 wk after discontinuing drug

• Respiratory status: rate, character, wheezing, tightness in chest

• Allergies before initiation of treatment, reaction of each medication; highlight allergies on chart

Administer:

• IV after diluting 1 g or less/4 ml sterile H_2O for inj; dilute further with 10-20 ml or more D_5W, NS, or sterile H_2O for inj sol; give 1 g or less/5 min or more or by intermittent inf over ½-2 hr or by continuous inf at prescribed rate

• Drug after C&S has been completed

Perform/provide:

• Adrenalin, suction, tracheostomy set, endotracheal intubation equipment

• Adequate fluid intake (2 L) during diarrhea episodes

• Scratch test to assess allergy on order from prescriber; usually done

* Available in Canada only

when penicillin is only drug of choice
• Storage at room temp, reconstituted sol 72 hr at room temp
Evaluate:
• Therapeutic response: absence of fever, purulent drainage, redness, inflammation
Teach patient/family:
• That culture may be taken after completed course of medication
• To report sore throat, fever, fatigue (may indicate superinfection)
• To wear or carry Medic Alert ID if allergic to penicillins
• To notify nurse of diarrhea
Treatment of overdose: Withdraw drug, maintain airway, administer epinephrine, aminophylline, O_2, IV corticosteroids for anaphylaxis

ticarcillin/ clavulanate (℞)

Timentin
Func. class.: Broad-spectrum antibiotic
Chem. class.: Extended-spectrum penicillin

Action: Interferes with cell wall replication of susceptible organisms; osmotically unstable cell wall swells, bursts from osmotic pressure
Uses: Respiratory, soft tissue, and urinary tract infections, bacterial septicemia; effective for gram-positive cocci *(S. aureus, S. faecalis, S. pneumoniae),* gram-negative cocci *(N. gonorrhoeae),* gram-positive bacilli *(C. perfringens, C. tetani),* gram-negative bacilli *(Bacteroides, F. nucleatum, E. coli, P. mirabilis, Salmonella, M. morganii, P. rettgeri, Enterobacter, P. aeruginosa, Serratia, Peptococcus, Peptostreptococcus, Eubacterium)*

Dosage and routes:
• *Adult:* IV INF 1 vial containing ticarcillin 3 g, clavulanate K 0.1 g q4-6h, infuse over 30 min
• *Child <60 kg:* IV INF 200-300 mg ticarcillin/kg/day in divided doses q4-6h
Available forms: Inj IM, IV 3 g ticarcillin, 0.1g clavulanate; IV INF 3 g ticarcillin, 0.1 g clavulanate
Side effects/adverse reactions:
HEMA: Anemia, increased bleeding time, ***bone marrow depression, granulocytopenia***
GI: Nausea, vomiting, diarrhea, increased AST, ALT, abdominal pain, glossitis, colitis
GU: Oliguria, proteinuria, hematuria, *vaginitis, moniliasis,* ***glomerulonephritis***
CNS: Lethargy, hallucinations, anxiety, depression, twitching, ***coma, convulsions***
META: Hyperkalemia, hypokalemia, alkalosis, hypernatremia
Contraindications: Hypersensitivity to penicillins; neonates
Precautions: Hypersensitivity to cephalosporins, pregnancy (B)
Pharmacokinetics:
IV: Peak 30-45 min, duration 4 hr, half-life 64-68 min; excreted in urine
Interactions:
• Decreased antimicrobial effect of ticarcillin: tetracyclines, erythromycins, aminoglycosides IV
• Increased ticarcillin concentrations: aspirin, probenecid
• Incompatible in sol with aminoglycosides, amikacin, $NaCO_3$
Lab test interferences:
False positive: Urine glucose, urine protein, Coombs' test
NURSING CONSIDERATIONS
Assess:
• I&O ratio; report hematuria, oliguria, since penicillin in high doses is nephrotoxic
• Any patient with compromised re-

T

nal system, since drug is excreted slowly in poor renal system function; toxicity may occur rapidly
• Liver studies: AST (SGOT), ALT (SGPT)
• Blood studies: WBC, RBC, Hct, Hgb, bleeding time
• Renal studies: urinalysis, protein, blood
• C&S before drug therapy; drug may be given as soon as culture is taken
• Bowel pattern before, during treatment
• Skin eruptions after administration of penicillin to 1 wk after discontinuing drug
• Respiratory status: rate, character, wheezing, and tightness in chest
• Allergies before initiation of treatment, reaction of each medication; highlight allergies on chart

Administer:
• IV after diluting 3.1 g or less/13 ml of sterile H_2O or NaCl (200 mg/ml), shake; may further dilute in 50-100 ml or more NS, D_5W, or LR sol and run over ½ hr
• Drug after C&S

Perform/provide:
• Adrenalin, suction, tracheostomy set, endotracheal intubation equipment
• Adequate fluid intake (2 L) during diarrhea episodes
• Scratch test to assess allergy on order from prescriber; usually done when penicillin is only drug of choice
• Storage at room temp, reconstituted sol 12-24 hr or 3-7 days refrigerated

Evaluate:
• Therapeutic response: absence of fever, purulent drainage, redness, inflammation

Teach patient/family:
• That culture may be taken after completed course of medication
• To report sore throat, fever, fatigue (may indicate superinfection)
• To wear or carry Medic Alert ID if allergic to penicillins

Treatment of overdose: Withdraw drug, maintain airway, administer epinephrine, aminophylline, O_2, IV corticosteroids for anaphylaxis

ticlopidine (℞)

(tye-cloe′pi-deen)
Ticlid
Func. class.: Platelet aggregation inhibitor

Action: Inhibits first and second phases of ADP-induced effects in platelet aggregation

Uses: Reducing the risk of stroke in high-risk patients

Dosage and routes:
• *Adult:* PO 250 mg bid with food

Available forms: Tabs 250 mg

Side effects/adverse reactions:
INTEG: Rash, pruritus
GI: Nausea, vomiting, diarrhea, GI discomfort, ***cholestatic jaundice, hepatitis,*** increased cholesterol, LDL, VLDL
HEMA: ***Bleeding (epistaxis, hematuria, conjunctival hemorrhage, GI bleeding), agranulocytosis, neutropenia, thrombocytopenia***

Contraindications: Hypersensitivity, active liver disease, blood dyscrasias

Precautions: Past liver disease, renal disease, elderly, pregnancy (B), lactation, children, increased bleeding risk

Pharmacokinetics: Peak 1-3 hr, metabolized by liver, excreted in urine, feces; half-life increases with repeated dosing

Interactions:
• Increased bleeding tendencies: anticoagulants, aspirin

* Available in Canada only

• Decreased plasma levels of ticlopidine: antacids
• Decreased plasma levels of digoxin
• Increased effects of ticlopidine: cimetidine
• Increased effects of theophylline

NURSING CONSIDERATIONS
Assess:
• Liver function studies: AST (SGOT), ALT (SGPT), bilirubin, creatinine (long-term therapy)
• Blood studies: CBC, Hct, Hgb, pro-time (long-term therapy)

Administer:
• With food to decrease gastric symptoms

Evaluate:
• Therapeutic response: absence of stroke

Teach patient/family:
• That blood work will be necessary during treatment
• To report any unusual bleeding to prescriber
• To take with food or just after eating to minimize GI discomfort
• To report side effects such as diarrhea, skin rashes, subcutaneous bleeding, signs of cholestasis (yellow skin and sclera, dark urine, light-colored stools)

timolol (℞)

(tye'moe-lole)
Blocadren, timolol maleate
Func. class.: Antihypertensive
Chem. class.: Nonselective β-blocker

Action: Competitively blocks stimulation of β-adrenergic receptor within vascular smooth muscle; produces chronotropic, inotropic activity (decreases rate of SA node discharge, increases recovery time), slows conduction of AV node, decreases heart rate, which decreases O_2 consumption in myocardium; also decreases renin-aldosterone-angiotensin system, at high doses inhibits β-2 receptors in bronchial system

Uses: Mild to moderate hypertension, sinus tachycardia, persistent atrial extrasystoles, tachydysrhythmias, prophylaxis of angina pectoris, reduction of mortality after MI

Investigational uses: Mitral valve prolapse, hypertrophic cardiomyopathy, thyrotoxicosis, tremors, anxiety, pheochromocytoma, tachyarrhythmias, angina pectoris

Dosage and routes:

Hypertension
• *Adult:* PO 10 mg bid, or 20 mg qd, may increase by 10 mg q2-3d, not to exceed 60 mg/day

Myocardial infarction
• *Adult:* 10 mg bid beginning 1-4 wks after MI

Migraine headache prevention
• *Adult:* PO 10 mg bid or 20 mg qd; may increase to 30 mg/day, 20 mg in AM, 10 mg in PM

Available forms: Tabs 5, 10, 20 mg

Side effects/adverse reactions:
CV: Hypotension, bradycardia, ***CHF,*** edema, chest pain, bradycardia, claudication
CNS: Insomnia, dizziness, hallucinations, anxiety
GI: Nausea, vomiting, ***ischemic colitis,*** diarrhea, *abdominal pain,* ***mesenteric arterial thrombosis***
INTEG: Rash, alopecia, pruritus, fever
HEMA: ***Agranulocytosis, thrombocytopenia, purpura***
EENT: Visual changes, sore throat, *double vision,* dry burning eyes
GU: Impotence, frequency
RESP: ***Bronchospasm,*** *dyspnea,* cough, rales
META: Hypoglycemia
MUSC: Joint pain, muscle pain

Contraindications: Hypersensitivity to β-blockers, cardiogenic shock, heart block (2nd, 3rd degree), sinus bradycardia, CHF, cardiac failure

Precautions: Major surgery, pregnancy (C), lactation, diabetes mellitus, renal disease, thyroid disease, COPD, well-compensated heart failure, CAD, nonallergic bronchospasm

Pharmacokinetics:

PO: Peak 2-4 hr; half-life 3-4 hr; excreted 30%-45% unchanged; 60%-65% metabolized by liver; excreted in urine, breast milk

Interactions:

- Increased hypotension, bradycardia: reserpine, hydralazine, methyldopa, prazosin, anticholinergics
- Decreased antihypertensive effects: idomethacin
- Increased hypoglycemic effects: insulin
- Decreased bronchodilation: theophyllines

Lab test interferences:

Increase: Liver function tests, renal function tests, K, uric acid

Decrease: Hct, Hgb, HDL

NURSING CONSIDERATIONS

Assess:

- I&O, weight qd
- B/P during initial treatment, periodically thereafter, pulse q4h; note rate, rhythm, quality
- Apical/radial pulse before administration; notify prescriber of any significant changes
- Baselines in renal, liver function tests before therapy begins
- Edema in feet, legs qd
- Skin turgor, dryness of mucous membranes for hydration status

Administer:

- PO ac, hs, tablet may be crushed or swallowed whole
- Reduced dosage in renal dysfunction

Perform/provide:

- Dry storage at room temp; do not freeze

Evaluate:

- Therapeutic response: decreased B/P after 1-2 wk

Teach patient/family:

- To take with or immediately after meals
- Not to discontinue drug abruptly; taper over 2 wk; may cause precipitate angina
- Not to use OTC products containing α-adrenergic stimulants (nasal decongestants, cold preparations) unless directed by prescriber
- To report bradycardia, dizziness, confusion, depression, fever, sore throat, shortness of breath to prescriber
- To take pulse at home; advise when to notify prescriber
- To avoid alcohol, smoking, sodium intake
- To comply with weight control, dietary adjustments, modified exercise program
- To carry Medic Alert ID to identify drug, allergies
- To avoid hazardous activities if dizziness is present
- To report symptoms of CHF: difficult breathing, especially on exertion or when lying down; night cough; swelling of extremities
- To take medication hs to minimize effect of orthostatic hypotension
- To wear support hose to minimize effects of orthostatic hypotension

Treatment of overdose: Lavage, IV atropine for bradycardia, IV theophylline for bronchospasm, digitalis, O_2, diuretic for cardiac failure, hemodialysis; administer vasopressor (norepinephrine)

* Available in Canada only

timolol (optic) (℞)

(tye'moe-lole)

Timoptic, Timoptic in Ocudose

Func. class.: β-Adrenergic blocker

Chem. class.: l-isomer

Action: Reduces production of aqueous humor by unknown mechanism

Uses: Ocular hypertension, chronic open-angle glaucoma, secondary glaucoma, aphakic glaucoma

Dosage and routes:

- *Adult:* INSTILL 1 gtt 0.25% sol in affected eye(s) bid, then 1 gtt for maintenance; may increase to 1 gtt 0.5% sol bid if needed

Available forms: Sol 0.25%, 0.5%

Side effects/adverse reactions:

CNS: Weakness, fatigue, depression, anxiety, headache, confusion

GI: Nausea, anorexia, dyspepsia

EENT: Eye irritation, conjunctivitis, keratitis

INTEG: Rash, urticaria

CV: Bradycardia, hyotension, dysrhythmias, syncope, heart block, ***CHF, CVA***

RESP: ***Bronchospasm,*** dyspnea

Contraindications: Hypersensitivity, asthma, 2nd or 3rd degree heart block, right ventricular failure, congenital glaucoma (infants), COPD

Precautions: Nonallergic bronchospasm, diabetes, pregnancy, children, lactation, myasthenia gravis

Pharmacokinetics:

INSTILL: Onset 15-30 min, peak 1-2 hr, duration 24 hr

Interactions:

- Toxicity: β-adrenergic blockers
- Increased effect: propranolol, metoprolol
- Bradycardia, asystole; verapamil

NURSING CONSIDERATIONS

Evaluate:

- Therapeutic response: decreased intraocular pressure

Teach patient/family:

- To report change in vision with blurring or loss of sight, trouble breathing, sweating, flushing; systemic absorption may occur
- Method of instillation, including pressure on lacrimal sac for 1 min, and not to touch dropper to eye
- That long-term therapy may be required
- That blurred vision will decrease with continued use of drug

tiopronin (℞)

(tye-o-pro'nen)

Thiola

Func. class.: Orphan drug

Chem. class.: Active reducing, complexing thiol compound

Action: Prevents cystine (kidney) stone formation by increasing amount of water-soluble cystine

Uses: Prevention of kidney stone formation in patients with severe homozygous cystinuria with urinary cystine greater than 500 mg/day, who are resistant to conservative treatment

Dosage and routes:

- *Adult:* PO 800-1000 mg/day, given in divided doses tid at least 1 hr before or 2 hr after meals
- *Child:* PO 15 mg/kg/day, given in divided doses tid at least 1 hr before or 2 hr after meals

Available forms: Tabs 100 mg

Side effects/adverse reactions:

MISC: Blunting of taste

INTEG: Erythema, maculopapular rash, wrinkling skin, lupuslike syndrome (fever, arthralgia, lymphadenopathy), pruritus

CNS: Drug fever

META: Vit B_6 deficiency
Contraindications: History of agranulocytosis, thrombocytopenia, aplastic anemia
Precautions: Pregnancy (C), lactation, myasthenia gravis, Goodpasture's syndrome, children <9 yr
Pharmacokinetics:
Reduction of urinary cystine of 250-500 mg on 1-2 g/day may be expected; excreted in urine 78% in 3 days
NURSING CONSIDERATIONS
Assess:
• I&O during treatment; check urine for stones; strain all urine, keep output at 2 L/day
• Diet for alkaline foods: dairy products; prevent overindulgence of Na, alkali foods, since hypercalciuria results
• Urine pH; notify prescriber of pH over 7
• Urinary cystine 1 mo after treatment, q3mo thereafter
Administer:
• After adequate hydration, conservative treatment: 3 L/day fluid, 16 oz fluid at meals and hs
Perform/provide:
• Storage at room temp
Evaluate:
• Therapeutic response: decrease in urinary cystine to <250 mg/L, absence of pain, hematuria
Teach patient/family:
• To watch for lupuslike syndrome: fever, joint pain, swollen lymph glands; drug may have to be discontinued

tobramycin (ophthalmic) (℞)

(toe-bra-mye'sin)
Tobrex
Func. class.: Antiinfective
Chem. class.: Aminoglycoside

Action: Inhibits bacterial protein synthesis
Uses: Infection of eye
Dosage and routes:
• *Adult, child:* INSTILL 1-2 gtt q1-4h depending on infection; OINT: 1 cm bid-tid
Available forms: Oint 0.3%; sol 0.3%
Side effects/adverse reactions:
EENT: Poor corneal wound healing, visual haze (temporary), overgrowth of nonsusceptible organisms
Contraindications: Hypersensitivity, varicella, vaccinia, mycobacterial/fungal infection, epithelial herpes, simplex keratitis
Precautions: Antibiotic hypersensitivity, pregnancy (D)
NURSING CONSIDERATIONS
Assess:
• Allergy: itching, lacrimation, redness, swelling
Administer:
• After washing hands; cleanse crusts or discharge from eye before application
• Apply pressure on lacrimal sac for 1 min
Perform/provide:
• Storage at room temp
Evaluate:
• Therapeutic response: absence of redness, inflammation, tearing
Teach patient/family:
• To use drug exactly as prescribed
• Not to use eye make-up, towels, washcloths, or eye medication of others, or reinfection may occur

• That drug container tip should not be touched to eye
• To report itching, increased redness, burning, stinging; drug should be discontinued
• That drug may cause blurred vision when ointment is applied

tobramycin (℞)

(toe-bra-mye'sin)

Nebcin, tobramycin sulfate, Tobrax

Func. class.: Antiinfective

Chem. class.: Aminoglycoside

Action: Interferes with protein synthesis in bacterial cell by binding to ribosomal subunit, causing inaccurate peptide sequence to form in protein chain, causing bacterial death

Uses: Severe systemic infections of CNS, respiratory, GI, urinary tract, bone, skin, soft tissues caused by *P. aeruginosa, E. coli, Enterobacter, Providencia, Citrobacter, Staphylococcus, Proteus, Klebsiella, Serratia*

Dosage and routes:

• *Adult:* IM/IV 3 mg/kg/day in divided doses q8h; may give up to 5 mg/kg/day in divided doses q6-8h
• *Child:* IM/IV 6-7.5 mg/kg/day in 3-4 equal divided doses
• *Neonates <1 wk:* IM up to 4 mg/kg/day in divided doses q12h; IV up to 4 mg/kg/day in divided doses q12h diluted in 50-100 mg NS or D_5W; give over 30-60 min

Available forms: Inj 10, 40 mg/ml; powder for inj 1.2 g; inj 20 mg/2 ml

Side effects/adverse reactions:

GU: ***Oliguria, hematuria, renal damage, azotemia, renal failure, nephrotoxicity***

CNS: Confusion, depression, numbness, tremors, ***convulsions,*** muscle twitching, ***neurotoxicity,*** dizziness, vertigo

EENT: ***Ototoxicity,*** deafness, visual disturbances, tinnitus

HEMA: ***Agranulocytosis, thrombocytopenia, leukopenia, eosinophilia,*** anemia

GI: Nausea, vomiting, anorexia, increased ALT (SGPT), AST (SGOT), bilirubin, hepatomegaly, ***hepatic necrosis,*** splenomegaly

CV: Hypotension, hypertension, palpitation

INTEG: Rash, burning, urticaria, dermatitis, alopecia

Contraindications: Severe renal disease, hypersensitivity to aminoglycosides

Precautions: Neonates, mild renal disease, pregnancy (D), myasthenia gravis, lactation, hearing deficits, Parkinson's disease

Pharmacokinetics:

IM: Onset rapid, peak 1 hr

IV: Onset immediate, peak 1 hr

Plasma half-life 2-3 hr; not metabolized, excreted unchanged in urine, crosses placental barrier

Interactions:

• Increased ototoxicity, neurotoxicity, nephrotoxicity: other aminoglycosides, amphotericin B, polymyxin, vancomycin, ethacrynic acid, furosemide, mannitol, methoxyflurane, cisplatin, cephalosporins, bacitracin, acyclovir

Y-site compatibilities: Acyclovir, amsacrine, amiodarone, ciprofloxacin, cyclophosphamide, enalaprilat, esmolol, fluconazole, fludarabine, foscarnet, furosemide, hydromorphone, insulin (regular), labetalol, magnesium sulfate, meperidine, morphine, perphenazine, tolazoline, zidovudine

Additive compatibilities: Aztreonam, bleomycin, calcium gluconate, cefoxitin, ciprofloxacin, clindamycin, furosemide, metronidazole, ranitidine, verapamil

T

NURSING CONSIDERATIONS

Assess:

- Weight before treatment; dosage is usually based on ideal body weight, but may be calculated on actual body weight
- I&O ratio, urinalysis qd for proteinuria, cells, casts; report sudden change in urine output
- VS during infusion; watch for hypotension, change in pulse
- IV site for thrombophlebitis, including pain, redness, swelling q30min; change site if needed; apply warm compresses to discontinued site
- Serum peak, drawn at 30-60 min after IV infusion or 60 min after IM injection, trough level <2 μg/ml; serum levels <12 mEq/ml
- Urine pH if drug is used for UTI; urine should be kept alkaline
- Renal impairment by securing urine for CrCl testing, BUN, serum creatinine; lower dosage should be given in renal impairment (CrCl <80 ml/min)
- Deafness by audiometric testing, ringing, roaring in ears, vertigo; assess hearing before, during, after treatment
- Dehydration: high specific gravity, decrease in skin turgor, dry mucous membranes, dark urine
- Overgrowth of infection: fever, malaise, redness, pain, swelling, perineal itching, diarrhea, stomatitis, change in cough, sputum
- C&S before starting treatment to identify infecting organism
- Vestibular dysfunction: nausea, vomiting, dizziness, headache; drug should be discontinued if severe
- Inj sites for redness, swelling, abscesses; use warm compresses at site

Administer:

- IV diluted in 50-100 ml NS or D_5W (adult), infuse over 20-60 min
- IM inj in large muscle mass; rotate inj sites
- Drug in evenly spaced doses to maintain blood level
- Bicarbonate to alkalinize urine if ordered in treating UTI, as drug is most active in an alkaline environment

Perform/provide:

- Adequate fluids of 2-3 L/day unless contraindicated to prevent irritation of tubules
- Flush of IV line with NS or D_5W after infusion
- Supervised ambulation, other safety measures with vestibular dysfunction

Evaluate:

- Therapeutic response: absence of fever, draining wounds, negative C&S after treatment

Teach patient/family:

- To report headache, dizziness, symptoms of overgrowth of infection, renal impairment
- To report loss of hearing, ringing, roaring in ears, feeling of fullness in head

Treatment of overdose: Hemodialysis; monitor serum levels of drug

tocainide (℞)

(toe-kay′nide)

Tonocard

Func. class.: Antidysrhythmic (Class IB)

Chem. class.: Lidocaine analog

Action: Decreases sodium and potassium, resulting in decreased excitability of myocardial cells

Uses: PVCs, ventricular tachycardia

Dosage and routes:

- *Adult:* PO 600 mg loading dose, then 400 mg q8h

Available forms: Tabs 400, 600 mg

Side effects/adverse reactions:
CNS: Headache, dizziness, involuntary movement, confusion, psychosis, restlessness, irritability, paresthesias, tremors, ***seizures***
EENT: Tinnitus, blurred vision, hearing loss
GI: Nausea, vomiting, anorexia, diarrhea, hepatitis
CV: Hypotension, bradycardia, angina, PVCs, ***heart block, cardiovascular collapse, arrest, CHF,*** chest pain, tachycardia
RESP: Dyspnea, ***respiratory depression, pulmonary fibrosis***
INTEG: Rash, urticaria, edema, swelling
HEMA: ***Blood dyscrasias: leukopenia, agranulocytosis, hypoplastic anemia, thrombocytopenia***
Contraindications: Hypersensitivity to amides, severe heart block
Precautions: Pregnancy (C), lactation, children, renal disease, liver disease, CHF, respiratory depression, myasthenia gravis, blood dyscrasias
Pharmacokinetics:
PO: Peak 0.5-3 hr; half-life 10-17 hr; metabolized by liver, excreted in urine
Interactions:
• Increased effects: propranolol, quinidine, all other antidysrhythmics
Lab test interferences:
Increase: CPK
Positive: ANA titer
NURSING CONSIDERATIONS
Assess:
• Chest x-ray film, pulmonary function tests, liver enzymes during treatment
• CBC during beginning treatment
• I&O ratio; check for decreasing output
• Blood levels (therapeutic level 4-10 µg/ml)
• B/P continuously for fluctuations
• Lung fields; bilateral rales may occur in CHF patient
• Increased respiration, increased pulse; drug should be discontinued
• Toxicity: fine tremors, dizziness
• Blood dyscrasias: fatigue, sore throat, fever, bruising
• Cardiac rate, respiration: rate, rhythm, character
Evaluate:
• Therapeutic response: decreased dysrhythmia
Treatment of overdose: O_2, artificial ventilation, ECG; administer dopamine for circulatory depression, diazepam or thiopental for convulsions

tolazamide (℞)

(tole-az'a-mide)
Tolamide, tolazimide, Tolinase
Func. class.: Antidiabetic
Chem. class.: Sulfonylurea (1st generation)

Action: Causes functioning β-cells in pancreas to release insulin, leading to drop in blood glucose levels; may improve binding to insulin receptors or increase the number of insulin receptors with prolonged administration; may also reduce basal hepatic glucose secretion; this drug not effective if patient lacks functioning β-cells
Uses: Type II (NIDDM) diabetes mellitus
Dosage and routes:
• *Adult:* PO 100 mg/day for FBS <200 mg/dl or 250 mg/day for FBS >200 mg/dl; dose should be titrated to response (1 g or less/day)
Available forms: Tabs 100, 250, 500 mg scored
Side effects/adverse reactions:
CNS: Headache, weakness, fatigue, lethargy, dizziness, vertigo, tinnitus

T

GI: Nausea, vomiting, diarrhea, constipation, gas, ***hepatotoxicity, jaundice,*** heartburn
HEMA: ***Leukopenia, thrombocytopenia, agranulocytosis, aplastic anemia, pancytopenia, hemolytic anemia***
INTEG: Rash, (rare) allergic reactions, pruritus, urticaria, eczema, photosensitivity, erythema
ENDO: ***Hypoglycemia***

Contraindications: Hypersensitivity to sulfonylureas, juvenile or brittle diabetes

Precautions: Pregnancy (C), elderly, cardiac disease, thyroid disease, severe hypoglycemic reactions, renal disease, hepatic disease, lactation

Pharmacokinetics:
PO: Completely absorbed by GI route; onset 4-6 hr, peak 4-8 hr, duration 12-24 hr; half-life 7 hr; metabolized in liver, excreted in urine (metabolites), breast milk, highly protein bound

Interactions:
- Increased hypoglycemic reaction: oral anticoagulants, chloramphenicol, cimetidine, MAOIs, insulin, guanethidine, methyldopa, nonsteroidal antiinflammatories, salicylates, probenecid, sulfonamides, ranitidine
- Mask symptoms of hypoglycemia: β-blockers
- Decreased effects of both drugs: diazoxide
- Decreased action of tolazamide: calcium channel blockers, corticosteroids, oral contraceptives, thiazide diuretics, thyroid preparations, estrogens, phenothiazines, phenytoin, rifampin, isoniazide, phenobarbital, sympathomimetics
- Disulfiram-like reaction: alcohol

NURSING CONSIDERATIONS
Assess:
- Hypoglycemic, hyperglycemic reaction; can occur soon after meals

Administer:
- Drug 30 min before meal

Perform/provide:
- Cool storage in tight container

Evaluate:
- Therapeutic response: decrease in polyuria, polydipsia, polyphagia, clear sensorium, absence of dizziness, stable gait

Teach patient/family:
- To check for symptoms of cholestatic jaundice (dark urine, pruritus, yellow sclera); notify prescriber
- To use a capillary blood glucose test while on this drug
- The symptoms of hypoglycemia, hyperglycemia, what to do about each; have glucagon emergency kit available
- That this drug must be taken daily; explain consequence of discontinuing drug abruptly
- To take drug in morning to prevent hypoglycemic reactions at night
- To avoid alcohol, OTC medications unless directed by prescriber; explain disulfiram reaction
- That diabetes is a lifelong illness; drug will not cure disease
- That all food in diet plan must be eaten to prevent hypoglycemia
- To carry a Medic Alert ID for emergency purposes

Treatment of overdose: Glucose 25g IV, via dextrose 50% sol, 50 ml or 1 mg glucagon

tolazoline (℞)

(toe-laz'a-leen)
Priscoline
Func. class.: Peripheral vasodilator
Chem. class.: Imidazoline derivative

Action: Peripheral vasodilation occurs by direct relaxation on vascular smooth muscle; also has weak α- and β-adrenergic properties

Uses: Persistent pulmonary hypertension of newborn

Dosage and routes:

• *Newborn:* IV 1-2 mg/kg via scalp vein; IV INF 1-2 mg/kg/hr

Available forms: Inj SC, IM, IV 25 mg/ml

Side effects/adverse reactions:

CV: Orthostatic hypotension, ***tachycardia,*** dysrhythmias, hypertension, ***cardiovascular collapse***

RESP: ***Pulmonary hemorrhage***

GU: Edema, oliguria, hematuria

GI: Nausea, vomiting, diarrhea, peptic ulcer, ***GI hemorrhage, hepatitis***

INTEG: Flushing, tingling, rash, chills, sweating, increased pilomotor activity

HEMA: ***Thrombocytopenia, leukopenia***

Contraindications: Hypersensitivity, CVA, CAD

Precautions: Pregnancy (C), active peptic ulcer, lactation, mitral stenosis

Pharmacokinetics:

IM/SC: Peak 30-60 min, duration 3-4 hr, excreted in urine, half-life 3-10 hr

Interactions:

• Increased effects with alcohol, β-blockers, antihypertensives

• Decreased B/P, rebound hypertension: epinephrine

• Incompatible with ethacrynic acid, hydrocortisone, methylprednisolone

NURSING CONSIDERATIONS

Assess:

• ABGs, electrolytes, VS in newborn

• B/P, pulse during treatment until stable; take B/P lying, standing; orthostatic hypotension is common

• Hepatic tests: AST, ALT, bilirubin; liver enzymes may increase

• Blood studies: CBC, platelets; watch for thrombocytopenia, agranulocytosis

• Hepatic involvement: nausea, vomiting, jaundice; drug should be discontinued

• For bleeding from GI tract: coffee grounds vomitus, increased pulse, pain in upper gastric area

• Affected areas for changes in temp, color

Administer:

• IV undiluted; give 10 mg or less over 1 min; in scalp vein may be diluted in D_5, D_5NS, LR, NS, ½NS, Ringer's sol; run over 1 hr

• Ordered analgesic for headache

• Intraarterially to patient in supine position

• To patient who is sitting or lying down during treatment

Perform/provide:

• Dark storage at room temp

Evaluate:

• Therapeutic response: decrease in pulmonary hypertension or pulse volume, increased temp in extremities, ability to walk without pain

Teach patient/family:

• To report jaundice, dark urine, joint pain, fatigue, malaise, bruising, easy bleeding; may indicate blood dyscrasias

• That it is necessary to quit smoking to prevent excessive vasoconstriction if prescribed for PVD

• To avoid hazardous activities until stabilized on medication; dizziness may occur

Treatment of overdose: Administer IV fluids, head-low position

T

tolbutamide (℞)

(tole-byoo'ta-mide)

Mobenol*, Novobutamide*, Orinase, tolbutamide, Tolbutone*

Func. class.: Antidiabetic

Chem. class.: Sulfonylurea (1st generation)

Action: Causes functioning β-cells in pancreas to release insulin, leading to drop in blood glucose levels; may improve binding to insulin receptors or increase the number of insulin receptors with prolonged administration; may also reduce basal hepatic secretion; not effective if patient lacks functioning β-cells

Uses: Type II (NIDDM) diabetes mellitus

Dosage and routes:

- *Adult:* PO 1-2 g/day in divided doses, titrated to patient response; IV 1 g (Fajans test)

Available forms: Tabs 250, 500 mg scored; inj IV

Side effects/adverse reactions:

CNS: Headache, weakness, paresthesia, tinnitus, dizziness, vertigo

GI: Nausea, fullness, heartburn, ***hepatotoxicity, cholestatic jaundice,*** taste alteration, diarrhea

HEMA: ***Leukopenia, thrombocytopenia, agranulocytosis, aplastic anemia,*** increased AST (SGOT), ALT (SGPT), alk phosphatase

INTEG: Rash, allergic reactions, pruritus, urticaria, eczema, photosensitivity, erythema

ENDO: ***Hypoglycemia***

MS: Joint pains

Contraindications: Hypersensitivity to sulfonylureas, juvenile or brittle diabetes

Precautions: Pregnancy (C), elderly, cardiac disease, thyroid disease, severe hypoglycemic reactions, renal disease, hepatic disease, lactation

Pharmacokinetics:

PO: Completely absorbed by GI route; onset 30-60 min, peak 3-5 hr, duration 6-12 hr; half-life 4-5 hr; metabolized in liver; excreted in urine (metabolites), breast milk; 90%-95% plasma protein bound

Interactions:

- Increased hypoglycemic reaction: oral anticoagulants, chloramphenicol, cimetidine, MAOIs, insulin, guanethidine, methyldopa, nonsteroidal antiinflammatories, salicylates, probenecid, sulfonamides, ranitidine
- Mask symptoms of hypoglycemia: β-blockers
- Decreased effects of both drugs: diazoxide
- Increased effects of tolbutamide: insulin, MAOIs
- Possible disulfiram (Antabuse) reaction
- Decreased action of tolbutamide: calcium channel blockers, corticosteroids, oral contraceptives, thiazide diuretics, thyroid preparations, estrogens, phenobarbital, phenytoin, rifampin, phenothiazines, sympathomimetics

Lab test interferences:

Decrease: RAIU test

Interfere: Urinary albumin

NURSING CONSIDERATIONS

Assess:

- Hypoglycemic, hyperglycemic reaction; can occur soon after meals

Administer:

- Drug 30 min before meals

Perform/provide:

- Storage in tight container in cool environment

Evaluate:

- Therapeutic response: decrease in polyuria, polydipsia, polyphagia, clear sensorium, absence of dizziness, stable gait

* Available in Canada only

Teach patient/family:
- To check for symptoms of cholestatic jaundice (dark urine, pruritus, yellow sclera); if these occur, a presciber should be notified
- To use a capillary blood glucose test while on this drug
- To test urine glucose levels with Chemstrip 3 × /day
- The symptoms of hypoglycemia, hyperglycemia, what to do about each; have glucagon emergency kit available
- That this drug must be taken daily; explain consequence of discontinuing drug abruptly
- To take drug in morning to prevent hypoglycemic reaction at night
- To avoid OTC medications and alcohol unless directed by prescriber; explain disulfiram reaction
- That diabetes is a lifelong illness; drug will not cure disease
- That all food in diet plan must be eaten to prevent hypoglycemia
- To carry a Medic Alert ID for emergency purposes

Treatment of overdose: 10%-50% glucose sol IV or 1 mg glucagon

---

tolmetin (℞)

(tole'met-in)

Tolectin DS, Tolectin 200, Tolectin 600, tolmetin sodium

Func. class.: Nonsteroidal antiinflammatory

Chem. class.: Pyrrole acetic acid derivative

Action: Inhibits prostaglandin synthesis by decreasing an enzyme needed for biosynthesis; analgesic, antiinflammatory, antipyretic

Uses: Mild to moderate pain, osteoarthritis, rheumatoid arthritis

Dosage and routes:
- *Adult:* PO 400 mg tid-qid, not to exceed 2 g/day
- *Child >2 yr:* PO 15-30 mg/kg/day in 3 or 4 divided doses

Available forms: Caps 400 mg; tabs 200, 600 mg

Side effects/adverse reactions:

GI: Nausea, anorexia, vomiting, diarrhea, jaundice, ***cholestatic hepatitis,*** constipation, flatulence, cramps, dry mouth, peptic ulcer, ulceration, bleeding, perforation

CNS: Dizziness, drowsiness, fatigue, tremors, confusion, insomnia, anxiety, depression

CV: Tachycardia, peripheral edema, palpitations, dysrhythmias, hypertension

INTEG: Purpura, rash, pruritus, sweating

GU: ***Nephrotoxicity: dysuria, hematuria, oliguria, azotemia, pseudoproteinuria***

HEMA: ***Blood dyscrasias***

EENT: Tinnitus, hearing loss, blurred vision

Contraindications: Hypersensitivity, asthma, severe renal disease, severe hepatic disease, ulcer disease

Precautions: Pregnancy (B), lactation, children, bleeding disorders, GI disorders, cardiac disorders, hypersensitivity to other antiinflammatory agents, peptic ulcer disease

Pharmacokinetics:

PO: Peak 2 hr, half-life 3-3½ hr; metabolized in liver, excreted in urine (metabolites), excreted in breast milk, 99% protein binding

Interactions:
- Increased action of coumarin, phenytoin, sulfonamides

NURSING CONSIDERATIONS

Assess:
- Renal, liver, blood studies: BUN, creatinine, AST (SGOT), ALT (SGPT), Hgb before treatment, periodically thereafter
- I&O ratio
- Audiometric, ophthalmic exam before, during, after treatment

T

• For eye, ear problems: blurred vision, tinnitus (may indicate toxicity)

Administer:

• With food to decrease GI symptoms; best to take on empty stomach to facilitate absorption; tab may be crushed

Perform/provide:

• Storage at room temp

Evaluate:

• Therapeutic response: decreased pain, stiffness, swelling in joints, ability to move more easily

Teach patient/family:

• To report blurred vision, ringing, roaring in ears (may indicate toxicity)
• To avoid driving, other hazardous activities if dizzy or drowsy
• To report change in urine pattern, weight increase, edema, pain increase in joints, fever, blood in urine (indicates nephrotoxicity)
• That therapeutic effects may take up to 1 mo
• To drink 8 glasses water daily

---

tolnaftate (topical) (OTC)

(tole-naf'tate)

Absorbine Antifungal, Absorbine Jock Itch, Absorbine Jr. Antifungal, Aftate For Athlete's Foot, Aftate For Jock Itch, Genaspor, NP-27, Quinsana Plus, Tinactin, Ting, Tolnaftate, Zeasorb-AF

Func. class.: Local antiinfective

Chem. class.: Antifungal

Action: Interferes with fungal cell membrane, which increases permeability, leaking of cell nutrients

Uses: Tinea pedis, tinea cruris, tinea corporis, tinea capitis, tinea unguium, tinea versicolor

Dosage and routes:

• *Adult and child:* TOP apply to affected area bid for 2-6 wk, rub in

Available forms: Cream, powder, aerosol powder, aerosol liq, gel, pump spray liq 1%

Side effects/adverse reactions:

INTEG: Rash, urticaria, stinging

Contraindications: Hypersensitivity, nail infections

Precautions: Pregnancy (C), lactation

NURSING CONSIDERATIONS

Assess:

• Allergic reaction: burning, stinging, swelling, redness

Administer:

• Aerosol powder after shaking
• Enough medication to cover lesions completely
• After cleansing with soap, water; dry well

Perform/provide:

• Dry storage at room temp; do not puncture or incinerate aerosol container

Evaluate:

• Therapeutic response: decrease in size, number of lesions

Teach patient/family:

• To use medical asepsis (hand washing) before, after application
• To apply with glove to prevent further infection
• To avoid use of OTC creams, ointments, lotions unless directed by prescriber
• To avoid contact with eyes
• To notify prescriber if condition worsens or does not improve in 10 days; continue even if symptoms improve
• To complete treatment regimen

torsemide (℞)

(tore-sa'mide)

Demadex

Func. class.: Loop diuretic

Chem. class.: Sulfonamide derivative

Action: Acts on loop of Henle by increasing excretion of chloride, sodium, water

Uses: Treatment of hypertension and edema in CHF, hepatic disease, renal disease

Dosage and routes:

• *Adult:* PO 2.5-5 mg qd; may gradually increase dose as needed

Available forms: Tabs 5, 10, 20, 100 mg; 10 mg/ml vials of 2, 5 ml

Side effects/adverse reactions:

CNS: Headache, fatigue, weakness, vertigo, paresthesias

CV: Orthostatic hypotension, chest pain, ECG changes, ***circulatory collapse***

EENT: ***Loss of hearing,*** ear pain, tinnitus, blurred vision

ENDO: Hyperglycemia

ELECT: Hypokalemia, hypochloremic alkalosis, hypomagnesemia, hyperuricemia, hypocalcemia, hyponatremia, metabolic alkalosis

GI: Nausea, diarrhea, dry mouth, vomiting, anorexia, cramps, oral and gastric irritations, pancreatitis

GU: Polyuria, ***renal failure,*** glycosuria

HEMA: ***Thrombocytopenia, agranulocytosis, leukopenia, neutropenia, anemia***

INTEG: Rash, pruritus, purpura, ***Stevens-Johnson syndrome,*** sweating, photosensitivity, urticaria

MS: Cramps, stiffness

Contraindications: Hypersensitivity to sulfonamides, anuria, hypovolemia, infants, lactation, electrolyte depletion

Precautions: Diabetes mellitus, dehydration, severe renal disease, pregnancy (C)

Pharmacokinetics:

PO: Rapidly absorbed; duration 6 hr; excreted in urine, feces, breast milk; crosses placenta; half-life 2-4 hr, plasma protein binding 97%-99%

Interactions:

• Increased toxicity: lithium, nondepolarizing skeletal muscle relaxants, digitalis

• Increased action of antihypertensives, oral anticoagulants, nitrates

• Increased ototoxicity: aminoglycosides, cisplatin, vancomycin

• Decreased antihypertensive effect of torsemide: indomethacin, metolazone

• Incompatible with acidic sol, Vit C, corticosteroids, diphenhydramine, dobutamine, esmolol, epinephrine, gentamicin, levarterenol, meperidine, milrione, netilmicin, reserpine, spironolactone, tetracyclines in sol

• Incompatible with any drug in syringe

Lab test interferences:

Interference: GTT

NURSING CONSIDERATIONS

Assess:

• Hearing when giving high doses

• Weight, I&O daily to determine fluid loss; effect of drug may be decreased if used qd

• Rate, depth, rhythm of respiration, effect of exertion

• B/P lying, standing; postural hypotension may occur

• Electrolytes: K, Na, Cl; include BUN, blood sugar, CBC, serum creatinine, blood pH, ABGs, uric acid, Ca, Mg

• Glucose in urine of diabetic

• Signs and symptoms of metabolic alkalosis: drowsiness, restlessness

• Signs and symptoms of hypokalemia: postural hypotension, malaise, fatigue, tachycardia, leg cramps, weakness
• Rashes, temp elevation qd
• Confusion, especially in elderly; take safety precautions if needed

Perform/provide:
• In AM to avoid interference with sleep if using drug as a diuretic
• K replacement if less than 3 mg/dl
• With food if nausea occurs; absorption may be decreased slightly

Evaluate:
• Therapeutic response: improvement in edema of feet, legs, sacral area qd if medication is being used in CHF

Teach patient/family:
• To rise slowly from lying, sitting position
• Adverse reactions: muscle cramps, weakness, nausea, dizziness
• To take food or milk for GI symptoms
• To take early in day to prevent nocturia

Treatment of overdose:
Lavage if taken orally; monitor electrolytes, administer dextrose in saline; monitor hydration, CV, renal status

trace elements (℞)

Concentrated Multiple Trace Elements, ConTE-PAK-4, M.T.E.-4, M.T.E.-4 Concentrated, M.T.E.-5, M.T.E.-5 Concentrated, M.T.E.-6, M.T.E.-6 Concentrated, M.T.E.-7, MulTE-PAK-4, MulTE-PAK-5, Multiple Trace Element, Multiple Trace Element Neonatal, Multiple Trace Element Pediatric, Neotrace 4, PedTE-PAK-4, Pedtrace-4, P.T.E.-4, P.T.E.5

Func. class.: Mineral supplements

Action: Needed for adequate absorption and synthesis of amino acids

Uses: Prevention of trace element deficiency

Dosage and routes:
Usual dosage may be given in TPN sol

Chromium
• *Adult:* IV 10-15 μg qd
• *Child:* IV 0.14-0.20 μg/kg/day

Copper
• *Adult:* IV 0.5-1.5 mg/day
• *Child:* IV .05-0.2 mg/kg/day

Iodine
• *Adult:* IV 1 μg/kg/day

Manganese
• *Adult:* IV 1-3 mg/day

Selenium
• *Adult:* 40-120 μg/day
• *Child:* 3 μg/kg/day

Zinc
• *Adult:* IV 2-4 mg/day
• *Child:* IV 0.05 mg/kg/day

Available forms: Many forms available—see particular elements

Side effects/adverse reactions: Depends on element

Precautions: Liver, biliary disease, pregnancy (C), lactation, vomiting, diarrhea

* Available in Canada only

NURSING CONSIDERATIONS
Assess:
• Trace element levels; notify prescriber if low; copper 0.07-0.15 mg/ml, zinc 0.05-0.15 mg/100 ml, manganese 4-20 μg/100 ml, selenium 0.1-0.19 μg/ml
• Trace element deficiency of patient receiving TPN for extended period
Administer:
• By IV infusion, often mixed with TPN solution
Evaluate:
• Therapeutic response: absence of element deficiency

tranylcypromine (℞)

(tran-ill-sip'roe-meen)
Parnate
Func. class.: Antidepressant-MAOI
Chem. class.: Nonhydrazine

Action: Increases concentrations of endogenous epinephrine, norepinephrine, serotonin, dopamine in storage sites in CNS by inhibition of MAO; increased concentration reduces depression
Uses: Depression, when uncontrolled by other means
Dosage and routes:
• *Adult:* PO 10 mg bid; may increase to 30 mg/day after 2 wk
Available forms: Tabs 10 mg
Side effects/adverse reactions:
HEMA: Anemia
CNS: Dizziness, drowsiness, confusion, headache, anxiety, tremors, stimulation, weakness, hyperreflexia, mania, insomnia, fatigue, weight gain
GI: Constipation, dry mouth, nausea, vomiting, *anorexia,* diarrhea, weight gain
GU: Change in libido, urinary frequency
INTEG: Rash, flushing, increased perspiration
CV: Orthostatic hypotension, hypertension, dysrhythmias, hypertensive crisis
EENT: Blurred vision
ENDO: ***SIADH-like syndrome***
Contraindications: Hypersensitivity to MAOIs, elderly, hypertension, CHF, severe hepatic disease, pheochromocytoma, severe renal disease, severe cardiac disease
Precautions: Suicidal patients, convulsive disorders, severe depression, schizophrenia, hyperactivity, diabetes mellitus, pregnancy (C), lactation
Pharmacokinetics:
Metabolized by liver, excreted by kidneys, crosses placenta, excreted in breast milk
Interactions:
• Increased pressor effects: guanethidine, clonidine, indirect acting sympathomimetics (ephedrine)
• Increased effects of direct-acting sympathomimetics (epinephrine), alcohol, barbiturates, benzodiazepines, CNS depressants, levodopa
• Hyperpyretic crisis, convulsions, hypertensive episode: tricyclic antidepressants, meperidine
• Hypoglycemic effect increased: insulin

NURSING CONSIDERATIONS
Assess:
• B/P (lying, standing), pulse; if systolic B/P drops 20 mm Hg, stop drug, notify prescriber
• Blood studies: CBC, leukocytes, cardiac enzymes (long-term therapy)
• Hepatic studies: ALT (SGPT), AST (SGOT), bilirubin; hepatotoxicity may occur
• Toxicity: increased headache, palpitation; discontinue drug immediately; prodromal signs of hypertensive crisis
• Mental status changes: mood, sen-

T

sorium, affect, memory (long, short), increase in psychiatric symptoms
• Urinary retention, constipation, edema: take weight weekly
• Withdrawal symptoms: headache, nausea, vomiting, muscle pain, weakness

Administer:
• Increased fluids, bulk in diet if constipation occurs
• With food or milk for GI symptoms
• Crushed if patient is unable to swallow medication whole
• Dosage hs if oversedation occurs during day
• Gum, hard candy, frequent sips of water for dry mouth
• Phentolamine for severe hypertension

Perform/provide:
• Cool storage in tight container
• Assistance with ambulation during beginning therapy for drowsiness/dizziness
• Safety measures including side rails
• Checking to see PO medication swallowed

Evaluate:
• Therapeutic response: decreased depression

Teach patient/family:
• That therapeutic effects may take 2-3 wk
• To avoid driving, other activities requiring alertness
• To avoid alcohol ingestion, CNS depressants, OTC medications: cold, weight loss, hay fever, cough syrup
• Not to discontinue medication quickly after long-term use
• To avoid high-tyramine foods: cheese (aged), sour cream, beer, wine, pickled products, liver, raisins, bananas, figs, avocados, meat tenderizers, chocolate, yogurt; increased caffeine
• To report headache, palpitation, neck stiffness

Treatment of overdose: Lavage, activated charcoal; monitor electrolytes, vital signs; diazepam IV, $NaHCO_3$

trazodone (℞)

(tray′zoe-done)
Desyrel, Desyrel Dividose, trazodone HCl
Func. class.: Antidepressant, miscellaneous
Chem. class.: Triazolopyridine

Action: Selectively inhibits serotonin uptake by brain, potentiates behavorial changes

Uses: Depression

Investigational uses: Chronic pain syndromes

Dosage and routes:
• *Adult:* PO 150 mg/day in divided doses; may increase by 50 mg/day q3-4d, not to exceed 600 mg/day

Available forms: Tabs 50, 100, 150, 300 mg

Side effects/adverse reactions:
HEMA: ***Agranulocytosis, thrombocytopenia, eosinophilia, leukopenia***
CNS: Dizziness, drowsiness, confusion, headache, anxiety, tremors, stimulation, weakness, insomnia, nightmares, EPS (elderly), increase in psychiatric symptoms
GI: Diarrhea, dry mouth, nausea, vomiting, ***paralytic ileus,*** increased appetite, cramps, epigastric distress, jaundice, ***hepatitis,*** stomatitis
GU: Retention, ***acute renal failure, priapism***
INTEG: Rash, urticaria, sweating, pruritus, photosensitivity
CV: Orthostatic hypotension, ECG changes, tachycardia, ***hypertension,*** palpitations

* Available in Canada only

EENT: Blurred vision, tinnitus, mydriasis

Contraindications: Hypersensitivity to tricyclic antidepressants, recovery phase of MI, convulsive disorders, prostatic hypertrophy

Precautions: Suicidal patients, severe depression, increased intraocular pressure, narrow-angle glaucoma, urinary retention, cardiac disease, hepatic disease, hyperthyroidism, electroshock therapy, elective surgery, pregnancy (C)

Pharmacokinetics:

Metabolized by liver, excreted by kidneys, feces; half-life 4.4-7.5 hr

Interactions:

- Decreased effects of guanethidine, clonidine, indirect-acting sympathomimetics (ephedrine)
- Increased effects of direct-acting sympathomimetics (epinephrine), alcohol, barbiturates, benzodiazepines, CNS depressants
- Hyperpyretic crisis, convulsions, hypertensive episode: MAOI (pargyline [Eutonyl])

Lab test interferences:

Increase: Serum bilirubin, blood glucose, alk phosphatase

False increase: Urinary catecholamines

Decrease: VMA, 5-HIAA

NURSING CONSIDERATIONS

Assess:

- B/P (lying, standing), pulse q4h; if systolic B/P drops 20 mm Hg, hold drug, notify prescriber; take vital signs q4h in patients with cardiovascular disease
- Blood studies: CBC, leukocytes, differential, cardiac enzymes if patient is receiving long-term therapy
- Hepatic studies: AST (SGOT), ALT (SGPT), bilirubin
- Weight qwk; appetite may increase with drug
- ECG for flattening of T wave, bundle branch block, AV block, dysrhythmias in cardiac patients
- EPS, primarily in elderly: rigidity, dystonia, akathisia
- Mental status changes: mood, sensorium, affect, suicidal tendencies, increase in psychiatric symptoms, depression, panic
- Urinary retention, constipation; constipation most likely in children
- Withdrawal symptoms: headache, nausea, vomiting, muscle pain, weakness; not usual unless drug discontinued abruptly
- Alcohol consumption; hold dose until morning

Administer:

- Increased fluids, bulk in diet if constipation occurs, especially in elderly
- With food, milk for GI symptoms
- Dosage hs for oversedation during day; may take entire dose hs; elderly may not tolerate qd dosing
- Gum, hard candy, frequent sips of water for dry mouth

Perform/provide:

- Storage in tight, light-resistant container at room temp
- Assistance with ambulation during beginning therapy for drowsiness/dizziness
- Safety measures, including side rails, primarily for elderly
- Checking to see PO medication swallowed

Evaluate:

- Therapeutic response: decreased depression

Teach patient/family:

- That therapeutic effects may take 2-3 wk
- To use caution in driving, other activities requiring alertness because of drowsiness, dizziness, blurred vision
- To avoid alcohol ingestion, other CNS depressants

T

• Not to discontinue medication quickly after long-term use; may cause nausea, headache, malaise
• To wear sunscreen or large hat, since photosensitivity occurs

Treatment of overdose: ECG monitoring; induce emesis; lavage, activated charcoal; administer anticonvulsant

---

tretinoin (vit A acid, retinoic acid) (℞)

(tret'i-noyn)

Retin-A, Stievaa*

Func. class.: Vit A acid/acne product

Chem. class.: Tretinoin derivative

Action: Decreases cohesiveness of follicular epithelium, decreases microcomedone formation

Uses: Acne vulgaris (grades 1-3)

Investigational uses: Skin cancer

Dosage and routes:

• *Adult and child:* TOP cleanse area, apply hs; cover lightly

Available forms: Cream 0.05%, 0.01%; gel 0.025%, 0.01%; liq 0.05%

Side effects/adverse reactions:

INTEG: Rash, stinging, warmth, redness, erythema, blistering, crusting, peeling, contact dermatitis, hypopigmentation, hyperpigmentation

Contraindications: Hypersensitivity

Precautions: Pregnancy (C), lactation, eczema, sunburn

Pharmacokinetics:

TOP: Poor systemic absorption

Interactions:

• Increase peeling: medication containing agents such as sulfur, benzoyl peroxide, resorcinol, salicylic acid
• Use with caution medicated, abrasive soaps, cleansers that have drying effect, products with high concentrations of alcohol astringents

NURSING CONSIDERATIONS

Assess:

• Area of body involved, including time, what helps or aggravates condition; cysts, dryness, itching; lesions may worsen at beginning of treatment

Administer:

• Once daily before hs; cover area lightly using gauze

Perform/provide:

• Storage at room temp
• Hand washing after application

Evaluate:

• Therapeutic response: decrease in size and number of lesions

Teach patient/family:

• To avoid application on normal skin, getting cream in eyes, nose, other mucous membranes
• To avoid sunlight, sunlamps or use protective clothing, sunscreen
• That treatment may cause warmth, stinging; dryness; peeling will occur
• That cosmetics may be used over drug; not to use shaving lotions
• That rash may occur during first 1-3 wk of therapy
• That drug does not cure condition; only relieves symptoms
• Therapeutic results may be seen in 2-3 wk but may not be optimal until after 6 wk

---

triamcinolone (℞)

(trye-am-sin'oh-lone)

Aristocort, Atolone, Kenacort, Azmacort, Cenocort A-40, Kenaject-40, Kenalog, Kenalog-10, Kenalog-40, Tac-3, Tac-40, Triam-A, triamcinolone acetonide, Triamonide 40, Amcort, Aristocort Forte, Aristocort Intralesional, Articulose L.A., Cenocort Forte, triamcinolone, Triam Forte, Triamolone 40, Trilone, Trisoject, Aristospan Intra-Articular, Aristospan Intralesional, Tri-Kort, Trilog

Func. class.: Corticosteroid

Chem. class.: Glucocorticoid, intermediate-acting

Action: Decreases inflammation by suppression of migration of polymorphonuclear leukocytes, fibroblasts, reversal to increase capillary permeability and lysosomal stabilization

Uses: Severe inflammation, immunosuppression, neoplasms, asthma (steroid dependent), collagen, respiratory, dermatologic disorders

Dosage and routes:

• *Adult:* PO 4-12 mg/day in divided doses qd-qid; IM 40 mg qwk (acetonide, or diacetate), 5-48 mg into neoplasms (diacetate, acetonide), 2-40 mg into joint or soft tissue (diacetate, acetonide), 0.5 mg/in^2 of affected intralesional skin (hexacetonide), 2-20 mg into joint or soft tissue (hexacetonide)

• *Child:* PO 117 μg/kg/day as a single or divided dose

Asthma

• *Adult:* INH 2 tid-qid, not to exceed 16 INH/day

• *Child 6-12 yr:* INH 1-2 tid-qid, not to exceed 12 INH/day

Available forms: Tabs 1, 2, 4, 8, 16 mg; syr 2 mg/5 ml, 4.85 mg/5 ml; inj 25, 40 mg/ml diacetate; inj 3, 10, 40 mg/ml acetonide; inj 20, 5 mg/ml hexacetonide

Side effects/adverse reactions:

INTEG: Acne, poor wound healing, ecchymosis, petechiae

CNS: Depression, flushing, sweating, headache, mood changes

CV: Hypertension, ***circulatory collapse, thrombophlebitis, embolism,*** tachycardia, edema

HEMA: ***Thrombocytopenia***

MS: Fractures, osteoporosis, weakness

GI: Diarrhea, nausea, abdominal distention, ***GI hemorrhage,*** *increased appetite,* ***pancreatitis***

EENT: Fungal infections, increased intraocular pressure, blurred vision

Contraindications: Psychosis, hypersensitivity, idiopathic thrombocytopenia, acute glomerulonephritis, amebiasis, fungal infections, nonasthmatic bronchial disease, child <2 yr, AIDS, TB

Precautions: Pregnancy (C), diabetes mellitus, glaucoma, osteoporosis, seizure disorders, ulcerative colitis, CHF, myasthenia gravis, renal disease, esophagitis, peptic ulcer

Pharmacokinetics:

PO/IM: Peak 1-2 hr, 2 days, 1-6 wk (IM), half-life 2-5 hr

Interactions:

• Decreased action of triamcinolone: cholestyramine, colestipol, barbiturates, rifampin, ephedrine, phenytoin, theophylline

• Decreased effects of anticoagulants, anticonvulsants, antidiabetics, ambenonium, neostigmine, isoniazid, toxoids, vaccines, anticholinesterases, salicylates, somatrem

• Increased side effects: alcohol, salicylates, indomethacin, amphotericin B, digitalis, cyclosporine, diuretics

T

• Increased action of triamcinolone: salicylates, estrogens, indomethacin, oral contraceptives, ketoconazole, macrolide antibiotics

Lab test interferences:

Increase: Cholesterol, Na, blood glucose, uric acid, Ca, urine glucose

Decrease: Ca, K, T_4, T_3, thyroid ^{131}I uptake test, urine 17-OHCS, 17-KS, PBI

False negative: Skin allergy tests

NURSING CONSIDERATIONS

Assess:

• K, blood sugar, urine glucose while on long-term therapy; hypokalemia and hyperglycemia

• Weight qd; notify prescriber if weekly gain >5 lb

• B/P q4h, pulse; notify prescriber if chest pain occurs

• I&O ratio; be alert for decreasing urinary output, increasing edema

• Plasma cortisol levels during long-term therapy (normal level: 138-635 nmol/L SI units when drawn at 8 AM)

• Infection: increased temp, WBC, even after withdrawal of medication; drug masks infection

• K depletion: paresthesias, fatigue, nausea, vomiting, depression, polyuria, dysrhythmias, weakness

• Edema, hypertension, cardiac symptoms

• Mental status: affect, mood, behavioral changes, aggression

Administer:

• After shaking suspension (parenteral)

• Titrated dose; use lowest effective dose

• IM injection deep in large muscle mass; rotate sites; avoid deltoid; use 21G needle

• In one dose in AM to prevent adrenal suppression; avoid SC administration; may damage tissue

• With food or milk to decrease GI symptoms

Perform/provide:

• Assistance with ambulation for patient with bone tissue disease to prevent fractures

Evaluate:

• Therapeutic response: ease of respirations, decreased inflammation

Teach patient/family:

• That ID as steroid user should be carried

• To notify prescriber if therapeutic response decreases; dosage adjustment may be needed

• Not to discontinue abruptly; adrenal crisis can result

• To avoid OTC products: salicylates, alcohol in cough products, cold preparations unless directed by prescriber

• About cushingoid symptoms

• Symptoms of adrenal insufficiency: nausea, anorexia, fatigue, dizziness, dyspnea, weakness, joint pain

triamcinolone (topical) (℞)

(trye-am-sin'oh-lone)

Aristocort, Aristocort A, Flutex, Kenalog, Kenalog-H, Triacet, Triamcinolone Acetonide, Triderm

Func. class.: Topical corticosteroid

Chem. class.: Synthetic fluorinated agent, group II potency (0.5%), group III potency (0.1%), group IV potency (0.025%)

Action: Antipruritic, antiinflammatory

Uses: Psoriasis, eczema, contact dermatitis, pruritus

Dosage and routes:

• *Adult and child:* TOP apply to affected area bid-qid

Available forms: Oint 0.025%, 0.1%, 0.5%; cream 0.025%, 0.1%, 0.5%; lotion 0.025%, 0.1%; aerosol 0.2 mg/2 sec; paste 0.1%
Side effects/adverse reactions:
INTEG: Burning, dryness, itching, irritation, acne, folliculitis, hypertrichosis, perioral dermatitis, hypopigmentation, atrophy, striae, miliaria, allergic contact dermatitis, secondary infection
Contraindications: Hypersensitivity to corticosteroids, fungal infections
Precautions: Pregnancy (C), lactation, viral infections, bacterial infections

NURSING CONSIDERATIONS
Assess:
- Temp; if fever develops, drug should be discontinued
- For systemic absorption: fever, inflammation, irritation

Administer:
- Only to affected areas; do not get in eyes
- Medication, then cover with occlusive dressing if prescribed, seal to normal skin, change q12h; use occlusive dressing with extreme caution (group II potency); systemic absorption may occur
- Only to dermatoses; do not use on weeping, denuded, or infected area

Perform/provide:
- Cleansing before application; apply to slightly moist skin; use gloves, a cotton-tipped applicator
- Treatment for a few days after area has cleared
- Storage at room temp

Evaluate:
- Therapeutic response: absence of severe itching, patches on skin, flaking

Teach patient/family:
- To avoid sunlight on affected area; burns may occur

triamcinolone (topical-oral) (OTC)
(trye-am-sin′oh-lone)
Kenalog in Orabase, Oralone Dental
Func. class.: Topical anesthetic
Chem. class.: Synthetic fluorinated adrenal corticosteroid

Action: Inhibits nerve impulses from sensory nerves
Uses: Oral pain
Dosage and routes:
- *Adult and child:* TOP press ¼ inch into affected area until film appears, repeat bid-tid

Available forms: Paste 0.1%
Side effects/adverse reactions:
INTEG: Rash, irritation, sensitization
Contraindications: Hypersensitivity, infants <1 yr, application to large areas, presence of fungal, viral, or bacterial infections of mouth or throat
Precautions: Child <6 yr, sepsis, pregnancy (C), denuded skin

NURSING CONSIDERATIONS
Assess:
- Allergy: rash, irritation, reddening, swelling
- Infection: if affected area is infected, do not apply

Administer:
- After cleansing oral cavity

Evaluate:
- Therapeutic response: absence of pain in affected area

Teach patient/family:
- To report rash, irritation, redness, swelling
- How to apply paste

triamterene (℞)

(trye-am′ter-een)

Dyrenium

Func. class.: Potassium-sparing diuretic

Chem. class.: Peridine derivative

Action: Acts on distal tubule to inhibit reabsorption of sodium, chloride; increase potassium retention

Uses: Edema; may be used with other diuretics, hypertension

Dosage and routes:

• *Adults:* PO 100 mg bid pc, not to exceed 300 mg/day

Available forms: Cap 50, 100 mg

Side effects/adverse reactions:

GI: Nausea, diarrhea, vomiting, dry mouth, jaundice, liver disease

ELECT: Hyperkalemia, hyponatremia, hypochloremia

CNS: Weakness, headache, dizziness

INTEG: Photosensitivity, rash

HEMA: ***Thrombocytopenia, megaloblastic anemia,*** low folic acid levels

GU: ***Azotemia, interstitial nephritis,*** increased BUN, creatinine, renal stones, bluish discoloration of urine

Contraindications: Hypersensitivity, anuria, severe renal disease, severe hepatic disease, hyperkalemia, pregnancy (D), lactation

Precautions: Dehydration, hepatic disease, CHF, renal disease, cirrhosis

Pharmacokinetics:

PO: Onset 2 hr, peak 6-8 hr, duration 12-16 hr; half-life 3 hr; metabolized in liver, excreted in bile and urine

Interactions:

• Nephrotoxicity: indomethacin

• Enhanced action of antihypertensives, lithium, amantadine

• Increased hyperkalemia: other K-sparing diuretics, K products, ACE inhibitors, salt substitutes

Lab test interferences:

Interference: Quinidine serum levels, LDH

NURSING CONSIDERATIONS

Assess:

• Weight, I&O qd to determine fluid loss; effect of drug may be decreased if used qd

• Electrolytes: K, Na, Cl; include BUN, blood sugar, CBC, serum creatinine, blood pH, ABGs, liver function tests

• Improvement in CVP q8h

• Signs of metabolic acidosis: drowsiness, restlessness

• Rashes, temp qd

• Confusion, especially in elderly; take safety precautions if needed

• Hydration: skin turgor, thirst, dry mucous membranes

Administer:

• In AM to avoid interference with sleep

• With food if nausea occurs; absorption may be decreased slightly

Evaluate:

• Therapeutic response: improvement in edema of feet, legs, sacral area qd if medication is being used in CHF

Teach patient/family:

• To take medication after meals for GI upset

• To avoid prolonged exposure to sunlight; photosensitivity may occur

• To avoid foods high in K: oranges, bananas, salt substitutes, dried apricots, dates

• To notify prescriber of weakness, headache, nausea, vomiting, dry mouth, fever, sore throat, mouth sores, unusual bleeding or bruising

Treatment of overdose: Lavage if taken orally; monitor electrolytes;

administer IV fluids, dialysis; monitor hydration, CV, renal status

---

triazolam (℞)
(trye-ay'zoe-lam)
Apo-Triazo*, Halcion, Novo-triolam*, Nu-Triazol*
Func. class.: Sedative-hypnotic
Chem. class.: Benzodiazepine

Controlled Substance Schedule IV (USA), Schedule F (Canada)
Action: Produces CNS depression at limbic, thalamic, hypothalamic levels of CNS; may be mediated by neurotransmitter γ-aminobutyric acid (GABA); results are sedation, hypnosis, skeletal muscle relaxation, anticonvulsant activity, anxiolytic action
Uses: Insomnia
Dosage and routes:
• *Adult:* PO 0.125-0.5 mg hs
• *Elderly:* PO 0.125-0.25 mg hs
Available forms: Tabs 0.125, 0.25, 0.5 mg
Side effects/adverse reactions:
HEMA: ***Leukopenia, granulocytopenia*** (rare)
CNS: Headache, lethargy, drowsiness, daytime sedation, dizziness, confusion, light-headedness, anxiety, irritability, amnesia, poor coordination
GI: Nausea, vomiting, diarrhea, heartburn, abdominal pain, constipation
CV: Chest pain, pulse changes
Contraindications: Hypersensitivity to benzodiazepines, pregnancy (X), lactation, intermittent porphyria
Precautions: Anemia, hepatic disease, renal disease, suicidal individuals, drug abuse, elderly, psychosis, child <15 yr, acute narrow-angle glaucoma, seizure disorders
Pharmacokinetics:
PO: Onset 30-45 min, duration 6-8 hr; metabolized by liver, excreted by kidneys (inactive metabolites), crosses placenta, excreted in breast milk; half-life 2-3 hr
Interactions:
• Increased effects of cimetidine, disulfiram, erythromycin, macrolides, probenecid, isoniazid, oral contraceptives
• Increased action of both drugs: alcohol, CNS depressants
• Decreased effect of antacids, theophylline, rifampin, smoking
Lab test interferences:
Increase: ALT (SGPT), AST (SGOT), serum bilirubin
Decrease: RAI uptake
False increase: Urinary 17-OHCS
NURSING CONSIDERATIONS
Assess:
• Blood studies: Hct, Hgb, RBC if blood dyscrasias suspected (rare)
• Hepatic studies: AST (SGOT), ALT (SGPT), bilirubin if liver damage has occurred
• Mental status: mood, sensorium, affect, memory (long, short)
• Blood dyscrasias: fever, sore throat, bruising, rash, jaundice, epistaxis (rare)
• Type of sleep problem: falling asleep, staying asleep
Administer:
• After removal of cigarettes to prevent fires
• After trying conservative measures for insomnia
• ½-1 hr before hs for sleeplessness
• On empty stomach for fast onset, but may be taken with food if GI symptoms occur
Perform/provide:
• Assistance with ambulation after receiving dose
• Safety measures: side rails, night-light, call bell within easy reach

T

- Checking to see PO medication has been swallowed
- Cool storage in tight container

Evaluate:
- Therapeutic response: ability to sleep at night, decreased amount of early morning awakening if taking drug for insomnia

Teach patient/family:
- That dependence is possible after long-term use
- To avoid driving, other activities requiring alertness until drug is stabilized
- To avoid alcohol ingestion, CNS depressants; serious CNS depression may result
- That effects may take 2 nights for benefits to be noticed
- Alternative measures to improve sleep: reading, exercise several hours before hs, warm bath, warm milk, TV, self-hypnosis, deep breathing
- That hangover is common in elderly but less common than with barbiturates; rebound insomnia may occur for 1-2 nights after discontinuing drug

Treatment of overdose: Lavage, activated charcoal; monitor electrolytes, VS

trientine (℞)

(trye-en'teen)

Syprine

Func. class.: Heavy-metal antagonist

Chem. class.: Chelating agent (thiol compound)

Action: Binds with ions of lead, mercury, copper, iron, zinc to form a water-soluble complex excreted by kidneys

Uses: Wilson's disease

Dosage and routes:
- *Adult:* PO 750-2000 mg in divided doses bid-qid
- *Child:* PO 500-1500 mg in divided doses bid-qid

Available forms: Caps 125, 250 mg; tabs 250 mg

Side effects/adverse reactions:

HEMA: Anemia, *iron deficiency*

INTEG: *Urticaria,* fever

SYST: Hypersensitivity

GI: Epigastric distress, anorexia, heartburn

Contraindications: Hypersensitivity, cystinuria, rheumatoid arthritis, biliary cirrhosis

Precautions: Pregnancy (C), lactation, children, iron deficiency anemia

Pharmacokinetics:

PO: Peak 1 hr, metabolized in liver, excreted in urine

Interactions:
- Decreased action of trientine: mineral supplements

NURSING CONSIDERATIONS

Assess:
- Monitor hepatic, renal studies: ALT (SGPT), AST (SGOT), alk phosphatase, BUN, creatinine, serum copper level
- Monitor I&O
- For anemia: fatigue, Hct, Hgb
- Allergic reactions (rash, urticaria); drug should be discontinued

Administer:
- On an empty stomach, ½-1 hr before meals or 2 hr after meals
- Vit B_6 daily; depleted by this drug

Evaluate:
- Therapeutic response: improvement in neurologic, psychiatric symptoms

Teach patient/family:
- That therapeutic effect may take 1-3 mo or longer
- To report urticaria, fever, fatigue

trifluoperazine (℞)

(trye-floo-oh-per'a-zeen)

Novoflurazine*, Solazine*, Stelazine, Suprazine, Terfluzine, trifluoperazine HCl, Triflurin

Func. class.: Antipsychotic/neuroleptic

Chem. class.: Phenothiazine, piperazine

Action: Depresses cerebral cortex, hypothalamus, limbic system, which control activity, aggression; blocks neurotransmission produced by dopamine at synapse; exhibits strong α-adrenergic, anticholinergic blocking action; mechanism for antipsychotic effects is unclear

Uses: Psychotic disorders, nonpsychotic anxiety, schizophrenia

Dosage and routes:

Psychotic disorders

• *Adult:* PO 2-5 mg bid, usual range 15-20 mg/day, may require 40 mg/day or more; IM 1-2 mg q4-6h

• *Child >6 yr:* PO 1 mg qd or bid; IM *not recommended for children,* but 1 mg may be given qd or bid

Nonpsychotic anxiety

• *Adult:* PO 1-2 mg bid, not to exceed 5 mg/day; do not give longer than 12 wk

Available forms: Tabs 1, 2, 5, 10, 20 mg; conc 10 mg/ml; inj 2 mg/ml

Side effects/adverse reactions:

RESP: ***Laryngospasm,*** dyspnea, ***respiratory depression***

CNS: EPS: pseudoparkinsonism, akathisia, dystonia, tardive dyskinesia, ***seizures,*** *headache*

HEMA: Anemia, ***leukopenia, leukocytosis, agranulocytosis***

INTEG: Rash, photosensitivity, dermatitis

EENT: Blurred vision, glaucoma, dry eyes

GI: Dry mouth, nausea, vomiting, anorexia, constipation, diarrhea, jaundice, weight gain

GU: Urinary retention, urinary frequency, enuresis, impotence, amenorrhea, gynecomastia

CV: Orthostatic hypotension, hypertension, ***cardiac arrest,*** ECG changes, ***tachycardia***

Contraindications: Hypersensitivity, cardiovascular disease, coma, blood dyscrasias, severe hepatic disease, child <6 yr, glaucoma

Precautions: Breast cancer, seizure disorders, pregnancy (C), lactation, diabetes mellitus, respiratory conditions, prostatic hypertrophy

Pharmacokinetics:

PO: Onset rapid, peak 2-3 hr, duration 12 hr

IM: Onset immediate, peak 1 hr, duration 12 hr

Metabolized by liver, excreted in urine, breast milk; crosses placenta

Interactions:

• Oversedation: other CNS depressants, alcohol, barbiturate anesthetics

• Toxicity: epinephrine

• Decreased absorption: aluminum hydroxide, magnesium hydroxide antacids

• Decreased effects of lithium, levodopa

• Increased effects of both drugs: β-adrenergic blockers, alcohol

• Increased anticholinergic effects: anticholinergics

Lab test interferences:

Increase: Liver function tests, cardiac enzymes, cholesterol, blood glucose, prolactin, bilirubin, PBI, cholinesterase, ^{131}I

Decrease: Hormones (blood, urine)

False positive: Pregnancy tests, PKU

False negative: Urinary steroids, 17-OHCS, pregnancy tests

T

NURSING CONSIDERATIONS

Assess:

- Mental status before initial administration
- Swallowing of PO medication; check for hoarding or giving of medication to other patients
- I&O ratio; palpate bladder if low urinary output occurs
- Bilirubin, CBC, liver function studies qmo
- Urinalysis is recommended before and during prolonged therapy
- Affect, orientation, LOC, reflexes, gait, coordination, sleep pattern disturbances
- B/P standing and lying; also include pulse, respirations q4h during initial treatment; establish baseline before starting treatment; report drops of 30 mm Hg
- Dizziness, faintness, palpitations, tachycardia on rising
- EPS including akathisia (inability to sit still, no pattern to movements), tardive dyskinesia (bizarre movements of jaw, mouth, tongue, extremities), pseudoparkinsonism (rigidity, tremors, pill rolling, shuffling gait)
- Skin turgor qd
- Constipation, urinary retention qd; if these occur increase bulk, water in diet

Administer:

- Antiparkinsonian agent on order from prescriber for EPS
- Conc in 120 ml of tomato or fruit juice, milk, orange, carbonated beverage, coffee, tea, water, or semisolid foods (soup, pudding)

Perform/provide:

- Decreased stimulus by dimming lights, avoiding loud noises
- Supervised ambulation until stabilized on medication if needed; do not involve in strenuous exercise program because fainting is possible; patient should not stand still for long periods
- Increased fluids to prevent constipation
- Sips of water, candy, gum for dry mouth
- Storage in tight, light-resistant container, oral sol in amber bottles; slight yellowing of inj or conc is common, does not affect potency

Evaluate:

- Therapeutic response: decrease in emotional excitement, hallucinations, delusions, paranoia, reorganization of patterns of thought, speech

Teach patient/family:

- That orthostatic hypotension occurs frequently, and to rise from sitting or lying position gradually; avoid hazardous activities until stabilized on medication
- To remain lying down after IM injection for at least 30 min
- To avoid hot tubs, hot showers, tub baths; hypotension may occur
- To avoid abrupt withdrawal of this drug, or EPS may result; drug should be withdrawn slowly
- To avoid OTC preparations (cough, hay fever, cold) unless approved by prescriber, since serious drug interactions may occur; avoid use with alcohol, CNS depressants; increased drowsiness may occur
- To use a sunscreen
- Regarding compliance with drug regimen
- About necessity for meticulous oral hygiene; oral candidiasis may occur
- To report sore throat, malaise, fever, bleeding, mouth sores; CBC should be drawn and drug discontinued
- In hot weather, that heat stroke may occur; take extra precautions to stay cool

---

Treatment of overdose: Lavage if orally ingested; provide an airway; *do not induce vomiting*

triflupromazine (℞)

(trye-floo-proe'ma-zeen)
Vesprin
Func. class.: Antipsychotic/neuroleptic
Chem. class.: Phenothiazine, aliphatic

Action: Depresses cerebral cortex, hypothalamus, limbic system, which control activity, aggression; blocks neurotransmission produced by dopamine at synapse; exhibits strong α-adrenergic, anticholinergic blocking action; mechanism for antipsychotic effects is unclear

Uses: Psychotic disorders, schizophrenia, acute agitation, nausea, vomiting

Dosage and routes:

Psychosis

- *Adult:* PO 10-50 mg bid-tid depending on severity of condition; dose is gradually increased to desired dose; IM 60 mg, not to exceed 150 mg/day
- *Child >2 yr:* PO 0.5-2 mg/kg/day in 3 divided doses; may increase to 10 mg if needed; IM 0.2 to 0.25 mg/kg to a maximum total dose of 10 mg/day

Nausea/vomiting

- *Adult:* PO 20-30 mg qd; IV 1-3 mg; IM 5-15 mg, q4h, max 60 mg qd
- *Child >2 yr:* PO/IM 0.2 mg/kg, max 10 mg qd

Acute agitation

- *Adult:* IM 60-150 mg/day in 3 divided doses
- *Child >2 yr:* IM 0.2-0.25 mg/kg/day in divided doses, max 10 mg/qd

Available forms: Tabs 10, 25, 50 mg*; inj IM, IV 10, 20 mg/ml

Side effects/adverse reactions:

RESP: ***Laryngospasm,*** dyspnea, ***respiratory depression***

CNS: EPS: pseudoparkinsonism, akathisia, dystonia, tardive dyskinesia; drowsiness, headache, ***seizures***

HEMA: Anemia, ***leukopenia, leukocytosis, agranulocytosis***

INTEG: Rash, photosensitivity, dermatitis

EENT: Blurred vision, glaucoma

GI: Dry mouth, nausea, vomiting, anorexia, constipation, diarrhea, jaundice, weight gain

GU: Urinary retention, urinary frequency, enuresis, impotence, amenorrhea, gynecomastia

CV: Orthostatic hypotension, hypertension, ***cardiac arrest,*** ECG changes, ***tachycardia***

Contraindications: Hypersensitivity, blood dyscrasias, coma, child <2½ yr, brain damage, bone marrow depression

Precautions: Pregnancy (C), lactation, seizure disorders, hepatic disease, cardiac disease

Pharmacokinetics:

PO: Onset erratic, peak 2-4 hr, duration 4-6 hr

IM: Onset 15-30 min, peak 1 hr, duration 4-6 hr

Metabolized by liver, excreted in urine, breast milk; feces, crosses placenta

Interactions:

- Oversedation: other CNS depressants, alcohol, barbiturate anesthetics
- Toxicity: epinephrine
- Decreased absorption: aluminum hydroxide, magnesium hydroxide antacids
- Decreased effects of lithium, levodopa
- Increased effects of both drugs: β-adrenergic blockers, alcohol

T

• Increased anticholinergic effects: anticholinergics

Lab test interferences:

Increase: Liver function tests, cardiac enzymes, cholesterol, blood glucose, prolactin, bilirubin, PBI, cholinesterase, ^{131}I

Decrease: Hormones (blood, urine)

False positive: Pregnancy tests, PKU

False negative: Urinary steroids, pregnancy tests

NURSING CONSIDERATIONS

Assess:

• Swallowing of PO medication; check for hoarding or giving of medication to other patients
• I&O ratio; palpate bladder if low urinary output occurs
• Bilirubin, CBC, liver function studies qmo
• Urinalysis is recommended before and during prolonged therapy
• Affect, orientation, LOC, reflexes, gait, coordination, sleep pattern disturbances
• B/P standing and lying; pulse, respirations q4h during initial treatment; establish baseline before starting treatment; report drops of 30 mm Hg
• For neuroleptic malignant syndrome: altered mental status, muscle rigidity, increased CPK, hyperthermia
• Dizziness, faintness, palpitations, tachycardia on rising
• EPS, including akathisia (inability to sit still, no pattern to movements), tardive dyskinesia (bizarre movements of jaw, mouth, tongue, extremities), pseudoparkinsonism (rigidity, tremors, pill rolling, shuffling gait)
• Constipation, urinary retention qd; if these occur, increase bulk, water in the diet

Administer:

• Reduced dose to elderly
• IV after diluting 10 mg/9 ml of NS; give 1 mg or less/2 min
• Antiparkinsonian agent on order from prescriber for EPS
• IM inj into large muscle mass; avoid contact with skin

Perform/provide:

• Decreased stimulus by dimming lights, avoiding loud noises
• Supervised ambulation until stabilized on medication; do not involve in strenuous exercise program because fainting is possible; patient should not stand still for long periods
• Increased fluids to prevent constipation
• Sips of water, candy, gum for dry mouth
• Storage in tight, light-resistant container

Evaluate:

• Therapeutic response: decrease in emotional excitement, hallucinations, delusions, paranoia, reorganization of patterns of thought, speech

Teach patient/family:

• That orthostatic hypotension occurs frequently, and to rise from sitting or lying position gradually; to avoid hazardous activities until stabilized on medication
• To remain lying down for at least 30 min after IM inj
• To avoid hot tubs, hot showers, tub baths; hypotension may occur
• To avoid abrupt withdrawal; or EPS may result; drug should be withdrawn slowly
• To avoid OTC preparations (cough, hay fever, cold) unless approved by prescriber; serious drug interactions may occur; avoid use with alcohol, CNS depressants; increased drowsiness may occur
• To use sunscreen
• Regarding compliance with drug regimen

• About necessity for meticulous oral hygiene, since oral candidiasis may occur
• To report sore throat, malaise, fever, bleeding, mouth sores; if these occur, CBC should be drawn and drug discontinued
• That in hot weather, heat stroke may occur; take extra precautions to stay cool

Treatment of overdose: Lavage if orally ingested; provide an airway; *do not induce vomiting*

trifluridine (ophthalmic) (℞)

(trye-floor'i-deen)
Viroptic
Func. class.: Antiviral
Chem. class.: Pyrimidine nucleoside

Action: Inhibits viral DNA synthesis and replication
Uses: Primary keratoconjunctivitis, recurring epithelial keratitis
Dosage and routes:
• *Adult and child:* INSTILL 1 gtt q2h, not to exceed 9 gtt/day, until corneal epithelium is regrown, then 1 gtt q4h × 1 wk

Available forms: Ophth sol 1%
Side effects/adverse reactions:
EENT: Burning, stinging, swelling, photophobia, irritation, pain
Contraindications: Hypersensitivity
Precautions: Antibiotic hypersensitivity, pregnancy (C), lactation

NURSING CONSIDERATIONS
Assess:
• Allergy: itching, lacrimation, redness, swelling

Administer:
• After washing hands; cleanse crusts or discharge from eye before application

Perform/provide:
• Storage in refrigerator

Evaluate:
• Therapeutic response: absence of redness, inflammation, tearing

Teach patient/family:
• To use drug exactly as prescribed
• Not to use eye make-up, towels, washcloths, or eye medication of others, or reinfection may occur
• That drug container tip should not be touched to eye
• To report itching, increased redness, burning, stinging; drug should be discontinued

trihexyphenidyl (℞)

(trye-hex-ee-fen'i-dill)
Artane, Artane Sequels, Novohexidyl*, Trihexy-2, Trihexy-5, trihexyphenidyl HCl, Trihexane
Func. class.: Cholinergic blocker
Chem. class.: Synthetic tertiary amine

Action: Blocks central muscarinic receptors, which decreases involuntary movements, sweating, salivation
Uses: Parkinson symptoms, drug-induced EPS
Dosage and routes:
Parkinson symptoms
• *Adult:* PO 1 mg, increased by 2 mg q3-5d to a total of 6-10 mg/day

Drug-induced EPS
• *Adult:* PO 1 mg/day; usual dose 5-15 mg/day

Available forms: Tabs 2, 5 mg; caps sus-rel 5 mg; elix 2 mg/5 ml
Side effects/adverse reactions:
CNS: Confusion, anxiety, restlessness, irritability, delusions, hallucinations, headache, sedation, depression, incoherence, dizziness, flushing, weakness

EENT: Blurred vision, photophobia, dilated pupils, difficulty swallowing, dry eyes, increased intraocular tension, angle-closure glaucoma
CV: Palpitations, tachycardia, postural hypotension
INTEG: Urticaria, rash
MISC: Suppression of lactation, nasal congestion, decreased sweating, increased temp, hyperthermia, heat stroke, numbness of fingers
MS: Weakness, cramping
GI: Dryness of mouth, constipation, nausea, vomiting, abdominal distress, ***paralytic ileus***
GU: Hesitancy, retention, dysuria

Contraindications: Hypersensitivity, narrow-angle glaucoma, myasthenia gravis, GI/GU obstruction, tachycardia, myocardial ischemia, unstable CV disease, prostatic hypertrophy

Precautions: Pregnancy (C), elderly, lactation, tachycardia, abdominal obstruction, infection, children, gastric ulcer

Pharmacokinetics:
PO: Onset 1 hr, peak 2-3 hr, duration 6-12 hr, excreted in urine

Interactions:
- Increased anticholinergic effects: antihistamines, phenothiazines, amantadine
- Decreased action of haloperidol

NURSING CONSIDERATIONS
Assess:
- I&O ratio; retention commonly causes decreased urinary output
- B/P, pulse frequently while dose is being determined
- Urinary hesitancy, retention; palpate bladder if retention occurs
- Constipation; increase fluids, bulk, exercise
- For tolerance over long-term therapy; dosage may have to be increased or medication changed
- Mental status: affect, mood, CNS depression, worsening of mental symptoms during early therapy

Administer:
- With or after meals for GI upset; may give with fluids other than water
- At hs to avoid daytime drowsiness in patient with parkinsonism

Perform/provide:
- Storage at room temp in light-resistant container
- Hard candy, frequent drinks, sugarless gum to relieve dry mouth

Evaluate:
- Therapeutic response: parkinsonism: shuffling gait, muscle rigidity, involuntary movements

Teach patient/family:
- Not to discontinue this drug abruptly; to taper off over 1 wk
- To avoid driving, other hazardous activities; drowsiness may occur
- To avoid OTC medications: cough, cold preparations with alcohol, antihistamines unless directed by prescriber
- To avoid sudden position changes
- To avoid hot climates; overheating may occur

trimeprazine (℞)

(trye-mep′ra-zeen)
Panectyl*, Temaril
Func. class.: Antihistamine
Chem. class.: Phenothiazine analog, H_1-receptor antagonist

Action: Acts on blood vessels, GI, respiratory system by competing with histamine for H_1-receptor site; decreases allergic response by blocking histamine

Uses: Pruritus

Dosage and routes:
- *Adult:* PO 2.5 mg qid; TIME-REL 5 mg bid

* Available in Canada only

• *Child 3-12 yr:* PO 2.5 mg tid or hs
• *Child 6 mo-1 yr:* PO 1.25 mg tid or hs
Available forms: Tabs 2.5 mg; spans 5 mg; syr 2.5 mg/5 ml
Side effects/adverse reactions:
CNS: Dizziness, drowsiness, fatigue, anxiety, euphoria, confusion, paresthesia, neuritis
CV: Hypotension, palpitations, tachycardia
RESP: Increased thick secretions, wheezing, chest tightness
HEMA: ***Thrombocytopenia, agranulocytosis, hemolytic anemia***
GI: Dry mouth, nausea, vomiting, anorexia, constipation, diarrhea
INTEG: Rash, urticaria, photosensitivity
GU: Retention, dysuria, frequency
EENT: Blurred vision, dilated pupils, tinnitus, nasal stuffiness, dry nose, throat, mouth
Contraindications: Hypersensitivity to H_1-receptor antagonist, acute asthma attack, lower respiratory tract disease
Precautions: Increased intraocular pressure, renal disease, cardiac disease, hypertension, bronchial asthma, seizure disorder, stenosed peptic ulcers, hyperthyroidism, prostatic hypertrophy, bladder neck obstruction, pregnancy (C)
Interactions:
• Increased CNS depression: barbiturates, narcotics, hypnotics, tricyclic antidepressants, alcohol
• Decreased effect of oral anticoagulants, heparin
• Increased effect of trimeprazine: MAOIs
Lab test interferences:
False negative: Skin allergy tests
NURSING CONSIDERATIONS
Assess:
• I&O ratio; be alert for urinary retention, frequency, dysuria; drug should be discontinued
• CBC during long-term therapy; blood dyscrasias
• Respiratory status: rate, rhythm, increase in bronchial secretions, wheezing, chest tightness
• Cardiac status: palpitations, increased pulse, hypotension
Administer:
• Coffee, tea, cola (caffeine) to decrease drowsiness
• With meals for GI symptoms; absorption may slightly decrease
• Sustained-release formulation only to adults
Perform/provide:
• Hard candy, gum, frequent rinsing of mouth for dryness
• Storage in tight container at room temp
Evaluate:
• Therapeutic response: decreased itching associated with pruritus
Teach patient/family:
• To notify prescriber of confusion, sedation, hypotension
• To avoid driving, other hazardous activity if drowsiness occurs
• To avoid concurrent use of alcohol, other CNS depressants
Treatment of overdose: Administer ipecac syrup or lavage, diazepam, vasopressors, barbiturates (short-acting)

trimethadione (℞)

(trye-meth-a-dye'one)
Tridione
Func. class.: Anticonvulsant
Chem. class.: Oxazolidinedione

Action: Decreases seizures in cortex, basal ganglia; decreases synaptic stimulation to low-frequency impulses
Uses: Refractory absence (petit mal) seizures

Dosage and routes:
• *Adult:* PO 300 mg tid, may increase by 300 mg/wk, not to exceed 600 mg qid
• *Child:* PO 20-50 mg/kg/day, may increase by 150-300 mg/wk
Available forms: Caps 300 mg; chew tabs 150 mg; sol 200 mg/5 ml; oral sol 40 mg/ml
Side effects/adverse reactions:
HEMA: ***Thrombocytopenia, agranulocytosis, leukopenia, neutropenia, hemolytic anemia,*** increased protime, ***eosinophilia, aplastic anemia***
CNS: Drowsiness, dizziness, fatigue, paresthesia, irritability, headache, insomnia
GU: Vaginal bleeding, albuminuria, nephrosis, abdominal pain, weight loss
GI: Nausea, vomiting, bleeding gums, abnormal liver function tests
INTEG: ***Exfoliative dermatitis,*** rash, alopecia, petechiae, erythema
EENT: Photophobia, diplopia, epistaxis, retinal hemorrhage
CV: Hypertension, hypotension
Contraindications: Hypersensitivity, blood dyscrasias, pregnancy (D)
Precautions: Hepatic disease, renal disease
Pharmacokinetics:
PO: Peak 30 min-2 hr, excreted by kidneys, half-life 6-13 days
NURSING CONSIDERATIONS
Assess:
• Blood studies: Hct, Hgb, RBC, serum folate, vit D; hepatic studies: AST (SGOT), ALT (SGPT), bilirubin, creatinine; drug should be stopped if neutrophil count falls below 2500/mm^3 on long-term therapy
• Mental status: mood, sensorium, affect, memory (long, short)
• Rash, alopecia, convulsions; discontinue drug if these occur
Administer:
• After diluting oral sol with H_2O, give slowly through lavage needle
• Oral with juice or milk to cover taste/smell; decreases GI symptoms
Perform/provide:
• Ventilation of room
Evaluate:
• Therapeutic response: decreased seizures
Teach patient/family:
• To notify prescriber of skin rash, alopecia, sore throat, fever, bruising, epistaxis or visual disturbances, particularly day blindness
• That physical dependency may result from extended use
• To avoid driving, other activities that require alertness
• Not to discontinue medication quickly after long-term use; convulsions may result
• Drug may take 1-4 wk to work; patient may still have seizures
• Report symptoms of renal damage: edema, urinary frequency, burning, cloudy urine

trimethobenzamide (℞)

(trye-meth-oh-ben'za-mide)
Arrestin, Benzacot, Brogan, Stemetic, T-Gen, Tebamide, Ticon, Tigan, Tiject-20, Triban, Trimazide, Trimethobenzamide, trimethobenzamide HCl
Func. class.: Antiemetic, anticholinergic
Chem. class.: Ethanolamine derivative

Action: Acts centrally by blocking chemoreceptor trigger zone, which in turn acts on vomiting center
Uses: Nausea, vomiting, prevention of postoperative vomiting
Dosage and routes:
Postoperative vomiting
• *Adult:* IM/REC 200 mg before

or during surgery; may repeat 3 hr after

Discontinuing anesthesia

• *Child 13-40 kg:* PO/REC 100-200 mg tid-qid

• *Child <13 kg:* PO/REC 100 mg tid-qid

Nausea/vomiting

• *Adult:* PO 250 mg tid-qid; IM/REC 200 mg tid-qid

Available forms: Caps 100, 250 mg; supp 100, 200 mg; inj 100 mg/ml

Side effects/adverse reactions:

CNS: Drowsiness, restlessness, headache, dizziness, insomnia, confusion, nervousness, tingling, *vertigo,* EPS

GI: Nausea, anorexia, diarrhea, vomiting, constipation

CV: Hypertension, hypotension, palpitation

INTEG: Rash, urticaria, fever, chills, flushing

EENT: Dry mouth, blurred vision, diplopia, nasal congestion, photosensitivity

Contraindications: Hypersensitivity to narcotics, shock, children (parenterally)

Precautions: Children, cardiac dysrhythmias, elderly, asthma, pregnancy (C), prostatic hypertrophy, bladder-neck obstruction, narrow-angle glaucoma, stenosing peptic ulcer, pyloroduodenal obstruction

Pharmacokinetics:

PO: Onset 20-40 min, duration 3-4 hr

IM: Onset 15 min, duration 2-3 hr

Metabolized by liver, excreted by kidneys

Interactions:

• Increased effect: CNS depressants

• May mask ototoxic symptoms associated with antibiotics

NURSING CONSIDERATIONS

Assess:

• For nausea, vomiting before, after treatment

• VS, B/P; check patients with cardiac disease more often

• Signs of toxicity of other drugs or masking of symptoms of disease: brain tumor, intestinal obstruction

• Observe for drowsiness, dizziness

Administer:

• IM inj in large muscle mass; aspirate to avoid IV administration

• Tablets may be swallowed whole, chewed, allowed to dissolve

Evaluate:

• Therapeutic response: decreased nausea, vomiting

Teach patient/family:

• To avoid hazardous activities, activities requiring alertness; dizziness may occur; to request assistance with ambulation

• To avoid alcohol, other depressants

• To keep out of children's reach

trimethoprim (℞)

(trye-meth′oh-prim)

Proloprim, Trimethoprim, Trimpex

Func. class.: Urinary antiinfective

Chem. class.: Folate antagonist

Action: Prevents bacterial synthesis by blocking enzyme reduction of dihydrofolic acid

Uses: *E.coli, P. mirabilis, Klebsiella, Enterobacter* UTIs

Dosage and routes:

• *Adult:* PO 100 mg q12h

Available forms: Tabs 100, 200 mg

Side effects/adverse reactions:

INTEG: ***Exfoliative dermatitis,*** pruritus, rash

HEMA: ***Thrombocytopenia, leukopenia, neutropenia, megaloblastic anemia*** (rare)

GI: Nausea, vomiting, abdominal pain, abnormal taste, increased AST

(SGOT), ALT (SGPT), bilirubin, creatinine
CNS: Fever
Contraindications: Hypersensitivity, CrCl <15 ml/min, renal disease, hepatic disease, megaloblastic anemia
Precautions: Folate deficiency, pregnancy (C), lactation, fragile X chromosome, child <12 yr old
Pharmacokinetics:
PO: Peak 1-4 hr, half-life 8-11 hr; metabolized in liver, excreted in urine (unchanged 60%), breast milk; crosses placenta
Interactions:
• Increased action of phenytoin
NURSING CONSIDERATIONS
Assess:
• Nocturia; may indicate drug resistance
• Signs of infection, anemia
• AST (SGOT), ALT (SGPT), BUN, bilirubin, creatinine, urine cultures
• C&S; drug may be given as soon as culture is obtained
• Skin eruptions
Administer:
• With full glass of water
Perform/provide:
• Storage in tight, light-resistant container
• Adequate intake of fluids (2 L) to decrease bacteria in bladder
Evaluate:
• Therapeutic response: absence of pain in bladder area, negative C&S
Teach patient/family:
• Aspects of drug therapy: need to complete entire course of medication to ensure organism death (10-14 days); culture may be taken after completed course of medication
• That drug must be taken in equal intervals around clock to maintain blood levels
• To notify nurse of nausea, vomiting

trimetrexate (℞)
(tri-me-trex′ate)
Neutrexin
Func. class.: Antineoplastic antimetabolite
Chem. class.: Nonclassical folic acid antagonist

Action: Inhibits an enzyme that reduces folic acid, which is needed for purine biosynthesis in all cells; result is disruption of RNA, DNA, cell death; leucovorin usually transported into cells by active, carrier-mediated process; however, *Pneumocystis carinii* organisms lack carrier system; trimetrexate must be given with leucovorin to protect normal cells
Uses: Moderate to severe *P. carinii* pneumonia as an alternative to TMP/SMZ; may be useful in treating non-small cell lung, prostate, colorectal cancer
Dosage and routes:
Leucovorin must be given concurrently and for 72 hr past last trimetrexate dose
• *Adult:* IV 45 mg/m^2 qd over 60-90 min; with leucovorin IV 20 mg/m^2 over 5-10 min q6h for a daily dose of 80 mg/m^2 or PO qid 20 mg/m^2 evenly spaced during the day; PO dose should be rounded to the next higher 25 mg; course is trimetrexate 21 days, leucovorin 24 days; modifications in dose must be based on hematologic toxicity
Available forms: Powder for inj lyophilized 25 mg
Side effects/adverse reactions:
CNS: Confusion, fatigue, fever
GI: Nausea, vomiting, ***hepatotoxicity,*** ulcer, stomatitis
GU: Increased serum creatinine
HEMA: ***Thrombocytopenia, anemia***
INTEG: Rash, pruritus

* Available in Canada only

META: Hyponatremia, hypocalcemia

Contraindications: Hypersensitivity to trimetrexate, leucovorin, methotrexate; thrombocytopenia (<25,000/mm^3), severe anemia, neutropenia (<500 mm^3) pregnancy (D)

Precautions: Renal disease, hepatic disease, lactation, children, seizures

Pharmacokinetics:
Terminal half-life 7-15 hr; may be 95%-98% protein bound

Interactions:
Specific interactions not known; these interactions may occur:

- Increased toxicity: aspirin, sulfa drugs, other antineoplastics, radiation
- Decreased effect of trimetrexate: erythromycin, ketoconazole, fluconazole, rifampin, rifabutin, cimetidine

NURSING CONSIDERATIONS

Assess:

- CBC, differential, platelet count qwk; withhold drug if neutrophils <500/mm^3 or platelet count <25,000/mm^3; notify prescriber; drug should be discontinued; hematologic toxicity should be graded 1-4, 4 most severe
- Renal function studies: BUN, serum uric acid, urine CrCl, electrolytes before, during therapy; treatment should be interrupted when creatinine >2.5 mg/dl
- I&O ratio; report urine output <30 ml/hr
- Monitor temp q4h; fever may indicate beginning infection; no rectal temps
- Liver function tests before, during therapy: bilirubin, alk phosphatase, AST (SGOT), ALT (SGPT); treatment should be interrupted when alk phosphatase or transaminase >5 × upper normal limit
- Bleeding time, coagulation time during treatment

Administer:

- Reconstitute with 2 ml D_5 or sterile H_2O (12.5 mg/ml) filter 0.22 micro prior to dilution; dilute reconstituted sol with D_5 for concentration of 0.25-2 mg/ml; give over 60 min; flush IV line thoroughly with 10 ml D_5 before, after dose
- Trimetrexate and leucovorin sol separately; leucovorin may be given before or after trimetrexate; IV line must be flushed between infusions
- If trimetrexate comes in contact with skin, wash with soap, water immediately
- Antiemetic 30-60 min before giving drug to prevent vomiting
- Topical or systemic analgesics for pain
- Transfusion for anemia

Perform/provide:

- Strict medical asepsis and protective isolation if WBC levels low
- Liquid diet: carbonated beverage, Jell-O; dry toast, crackers may be added when patient is not nauseated or vomiting
- Rinsing of mouth tid-qid with water, club soda; brushing of teeth bid-tid with soft brush or cotton-tipped applicators for stomatitis; use unwaxed dental floss
- Nutritious diet with iron, vitamin supplements
- Storage after reconstitution up to 24 hr refrigerated; do not freeze reconstituted sol; discard after 24 hr

Evaluate:

- Therapeutic response: decreased symptoms of pneumocystis
- Bleeding: hematuria, guaiac, bruising or petechiae, mucosa or orifices q8h
- Food preferences; list likes, dislikes

T

• Hepatotoxicity: yellow skin, sclera, dark urine, clay-colored stools, pruritus, abdominal pain, fever, diarrhea
• Buccal cavity q8h for dryness, sores, ulceration, white patches, oral pain, bleeding, dysphagia
• Symptoms of severe allergic reaction: rash, urticaria, itching, flushing

Teach patient/family:
• About protective isolation
• To report any complaints, side effects to nurse or prescriber: black tarry stools, chills, fever, sore throat, bleeding, bruising, cough, shortness of breath, dark or bloody urine
• To avoid foods with citric acid, hot or rough texture if stomatitis is present
• To report to prescriber stomatitis: any bleeding, white spots, ulcerations in mouth; to examine mouth qd, report symptoms to nurse
• To drink 10-12 glasses of fluid/day
• To avoid alcohol, salicylates
• To avoid use of razors, commercial mouthwash

trimipramine (℞)

(tri-mip′ra-meen)
Surmontil, Trimipramine Maleate, Trisoralen
Func. class.: Antidepressant—tricyclic
Chem. class.: Tertiary amine

Action: Selectively inhibits serotonin uptake by brain; potentiates behavioral changes
Uses: Depression, enuresis in children
Dosage and routes:
• *Adult:* PO 75 mg/day in divided doses, may be increased to 200 mg/day
• *Child >6 yr:* 25 mg hs, may increase to 50 mg in child <12 yr or 75 mg in child >12 yr
Available forms: Caps 25, 50, 100 mg
Side effects/adverse reactions:
HEMA: ***Agranulocytosis, thrombocytopenia, eosinophilia, leukopenia***
CNS: Dizziness, drowsiness, confusion, headache, anxiety, tremors, stimulation, weakness, insomnia, nightmares, EPS (elderly), increase in psychiatric symptoms
GI: Diarrhea, dry mouth, nausea, vomiting, ***paralytic ileus,*** increased appetite, cramps, epigastric distress, jaundice, ***hepatitis,*** stomatitis, constipation
GU: Retention, ***acute renal failure***
INTEG: Rash, urticaria, sweating, pruritus, photosensitivity
CV: Orthostatic hypotension, ECG changes, tachycardia, ***hypertension,*** palpitations
EENT: Blurred vision, tinnitus, mydriasis
Contraindications: Hypersensitivity to tricyclic antidepressants, recovery phase of MI, convulsive disorders, prostatic hypertrophy
Precautions: Suicidal patients, severe depression, increased intraocular pressure, narrow-angle glaucoma, urinary retention, cardiac disease, hepatic disease, hyperthyroidism, electroshock therapy, elective surgery, pregnancy (C)
Pharmacokinetics:
Metabolized by liver, excreted by kidneys, steady state 2-6 days; half-life 7-30 hr
Interactions:
• Decreased effects of: guanethidine, clonidine, indirect-acting sympathomimetics (ephedrine)
• Increased effects of direct-acting sympathomimetics (epinephrine), al-

cohol, barbiturates, benzodiazepines, CNS depressants
- Hyperpyretic crisis, convulsions, hypertensive episode: MAOI (pargyline [Eutonyl])

Lab test interferences:
Increase: Serum bilirubin, blood glucose, alk phosphatase
False increase: Urinary catecholamines
Decrease: VMA, 5-HIAA

NURSING CONSIDERATIONS

Assess:
- B/P (lying, standing), pulse q4h; if systolic B/P drops 20 mm Hg, hold drug, notify prescriber; take vital signs q4h in patients with cardiovascular disease
- Blood studies: CBC, leukocytes, differential, cardiac enzymes if patient is receiving long-term therapy
- Hepatic studies: AST (SGOT), ALT (SGPT), bilirubin, creatinine
- Weight qwk; appetite may increase with drug
- ECG for flattening of T wave, bundle branch block, AV block, dysrhythmias in cardiac patients
- EPS primarily in elderly: rigidity, dystonia, akathisia
- Mental status changes: mood, sensorium, affect, suicidal tendencies, increase in psychiatric symptoms, depression, panic
- Urinary retention, constipation; constipation is more likely to occur in children, elderly
- Withdrawal symptoms: headache, nausea, vomiting, muscle pain, weakness; not usual unless drug is discontinued abruptly
- Alcohol consumption; hold dose until morning

Administer:
- Increased fluids, bulk in diet for constipation, urinary retention
- With food, milk for GI symptoms
- Dosage hs for oversedation during day; may take entire dose hs; elderly may not tolerate once/day dosing
- Gum, hard candy, or frequent sips of water for dry mouth

Perform/provide:
- Storage in tight, light-resistant container at room temp
- Assistance with ambulation during beginning therapy for drowsiness/dizziness
- Safety measures, including side rails, primarily for elderly
- Checking to see PO medication swallowed

Evaluate:
- Therapeutic response: decreased depression or enuresis

Teach patient/family:
- That therapeutic effects may take 2-3 wk
- To use caution in driving, other activities requiring alertness because of drowsiness, dizziness, blurred vision
- To avoid alcohol ingestion, other CNS depressants
- Not to discontinue medication quickly after long-term use; may cause nausea, headache, malaise
- To wear sunscreen or large hat, since photosensitivity occurs

Treatment of overdose: ECG monitoring; induce emesis; lavage, activated charcoal; administer anticonvulsant

T

tripelennamine (℞)

(tri-pel-enn'a-meen)
PBZ, PBZ-SR, Pelamine, tripelennamine HCl
Func. class.: Antihistamine
Chem. class.: Ethylenediamine derivative

Action: Acts on blood vessels, GI, respiratory system by competing with histamine for H_1-receptor site;

decreases allergic response by blocking histamine

Uses: Rhinitis, allergy symptoms

Dosage and routes:

• *Adult:* PO 25-50 mg q4-6h, not to exceed 600 mg/day; TIME-REL 100 mg bid-tid, not to exceed 600 mg/day

• *Child >5 yr:* TIME-REL 50 mg q8-12hr, not to exceed 300 mg/day

• *Child <5 yr:* PO 5 mg/kg/day in 4-6 divided doses, not to exceed 300 mg/day

Available forms: Tabs 25, 50 mg; time-rel tabs 100 mg; elix 37.5 mg/5 ml

Side effects/adverse reactions:

CNS: Dizziness, drowsiness, poor coordination, fatigue, anxiety, euphoria, confusion, paresthesia, neuritis

CV: Hypotension, palpitations, tachycardia

RESP: Increased thick secretions, wheezing, chest tightness

HEMA: ***Thrombocytopenia, agranulocytosis, hemolytic anemia***

GI: Constipation, dry mouth, nausea, vomiting, anorexia, diarrhea

INTEG: Rash, urticaria, photosensitivity

GU: Retention, dysuria, frequency

EENT: Blurred vision, dilated pupils, tinnitus, nasal stuffiness, dry nose, throat, mouth

Contraindications: Hypersensitivity to H_1-receptor antagonist, acute asthma attack, lower respiratory tract disease

Precautions: Increased intraocular pressure, renal disease, cardiac disease, hypertension, bronchial asthma, seizure disorder, stenosed peptic ulcers, hyperthyroidism, prostatic hypertrophy, bladder neck obstruction, pregnancy (C)

Pharmacokinetics:

PO: Onset 15-30 min, duration 4-6 hr; detoxified in liver, excreted by kidneys

Interactions:

• Increased CNS depressants: barbiturates, narcotics, hypnotics, tricyclic antidepressants, alcohol

• Decreased effect of oral anticoagulants, heparin

• Increased effect of tripelennamine: MAOIs

Lab test interferences:

False negative: Skin allergy test

False positive: Urine pregnancy tests

NURSING CONSIDERATIONS

Assess:

• I&O ratio; be alert for urinary retention, frequency, dysuria; drug should be discontinued

• CBC during long-term therapy; blood dyscrasias

• Respiratory status: rate, rhythm, increase in bronchial secretions, wheezing, chest tightness

• Cardiac status: palpitations, increased pulse, hypotension

Administer:

• With meals for GI symptoms; absorption may slightly decrease

• Time-release tab to adults only

Perform/provide:

• Hard candy, gum, frequent rinsing of mouth for dryness

• Storage in tight container at room temp

Evaluate:

• Therapeutic response: decrease in itching associated with pruritus

Teach patient/family:

• All aspects of drug use; to notify prescriber of confusion, sedation, hypotension

• To avoid driving, other hazardous activity if drowsiness occurs

• To avoid concurrent use of alcohol, other CNS depressants

Treatment of overdose: Administer ipecac syrup or lavage, diazepam, vasopressors, barbiturates (short-acting)

* Available in Canada only

triprolidine (℞, OTC)

(trye-proe'li-deen)

Actidil, Alleract, Myidil, triprolidine HCl

Func. class.: Antihistamine

Chem. class.: Alkylamine, H_1-receptor antagonist

Action: Acts on blood vessels, GI, respiratory system by competing with histamine for H_1-receptor site; decreases allergic response by blocking histamine

Uses: Rhinitis, allergy symptoms

Dosage and routes:

- *Adult:* PO 2.5 mg tid-qid
- *Child >6 yr:* PO 1.25 mg tid-qid
- *Child 4-6 yr:* PO 0.9 mg tid-qid
- *Child 2-4 yr:* PO 0.6 mg tid-qid
- *Child 4 mo-2 yr:* 0.3 mg tid-qid

Available forms: Tab 2.5 mg; syr 1.25 mg/5 ml

Side effects/adverse reactions:

CNS: Dizziness, drowsiness, poor coordination, fatigue, anxiety, euphoria, confusion, paresthesia, neuritis

CV: Hypotension, palpitations, tachycardia

RESP: Increased thick secretions, wheezing, chest tightness

HEMA: ***Thrombocytopenia, agranulocytosis, hemolytic anemia***

GI: Constipation, dry mouth, nausea, vomiting, anorexia, diarrhea

INTEG: Rash, urticaria, photosensitivity

GU: Retention, dysuria, frequency

EENT: Blurred vision, dilated pupils, tinnitus, nasal stuffiness, dry nose, throat, mouth

Contraindications: Hypersensitivity to H_1-receptor antagonist, acute asthma attack, lower respiratory tract disease

Precautions: Increased intraocular pressure, renal disease, cardiac disease, hypertension, bronchial asthma, seizure disorder, stenosed peptic ulcers, hyperthyroidism, prostatic hypertrophy, bladder neck obstruction, pregnancy (C)

Pharmacokinetics:

PO: Onset 20-60 min, duration 8-12 hr; detoxified in liver, excreted by kidneys (metabolites/free drug), half-life 20-24 hr

Interactions:

- Increased CNS depressants: barbiturates, narcotics, hypnotics, tricyclic antidepressants, alcohol
- Decreased effect of oral anticoagulants, heparin
- Increased effect of triprolidine: MAOIs

Lab test interferences:

False negative: Skin allergy tests

NURSING CONSIDERATIONS

Assess:

- I&O ratio; be alert for urinary retention, frequency, dysuria; drug should be discontinued
- CBC during long-term therapy; blood dyscrasias
- Respiratory status: rate, rhythm, increase in bronchial secretions, wheezing, chest tightness
- Cardiac status: palpitations, increased pulse, hypotension

Administer:

- With meals for GI symptoms; absorption may slightly decrease

Perform/provide:

- Hard candy, gum, frequent rinsing of mouth for dryness
- Storage in tight container at room temp

Evaluate:

- Therapeutic response: decreased itching associated with pruritus

Teach patient/family:

- All aspects of drug use; to notify prescriber of confusion, sedation, hypotension

T

• To avoid driving, other hazardous activity if drowsiness occurs
• To avoid concurrent use of alcohol, other CNS depressants
Treatment of overdose: Administer ipecac syrup or lavage, diazepam, vasopressors, barbiturates (short-acting)

---

tromethamine (℞)
(troe-meth'a-meen)
Tham, Tham-E
Func. class.: Alkalinizer
Chem. class.: Amine

Action: Proton acceptor that corrects acidosis by combining with hydrogen ions to form bicarbonate and buffer; acts as diuretic (osmotic)
Uses: Acidosis (metabolic) associated with cardiac disease, COPD
Dosage and routes:
• *Adult:* IV 0.3 M required = kg of weight × HCO_3 deficit (mEq/L)
• *Child:* IV Same as above given over 3-6 hr, not to exceed 40 ml/kg
Available forms: Inj IV 36 mg/ml, powd for inj IV 36 g
Side effects/adverse reactions:
CV: Irregular pulse, ***cardiac arrest***
META: Alkalosis, hypoglycemia
RESP: Shallow, slow respirations, cyanosis, ***apnea***
GI: ***Hepatic necrosis***
INTEG: Infection at injection site, extravasation, phlebitis
Contraindications: Hypersensitivity, anuria, uremia
Precautions: Severe respiratory disease/respiratory depression, pregnancy (C), cardiac edema, renal disease, infants
Pharmacokinetics:
IV: Excreted in urine
NURSING CONSIDERATIONS
Assess:
• Respiratory rate, rhythm, depth; notify prescriber of abnormalities that may indicate acidosis
• Electrolytes, blood glucose, chloride; CO_2, before, during treatment
• Urine pH, urinary output, urine glucose during beginning treatment
• I&O ratio, report large increase or decrease
• IV site for extravasation, phlebitis, thrombosis
• For signs of K^+ depletion
Administer:
• IV slowly to avoid pain at infusion site and toxicity
• IV undiluted as inf or added to priming fluid or ACD blood; give 5 ml or less/min
Evaluate:
• Therapeutic response: decreased metabolic acidosis
Teach patient/family:
• To increase K^+ in diet: bananas, oranges, cantaloupe, honeydew, spinach, potatoes, dried fruit

---

tropicamide (optic) (℞)
(troe-pik'a-mide)
Mydriacyl Ophthalmic, Tropicacyl, tropicamide, I-Picamide
Func. class.: Mydriatic, cycloplegia, anticholingeric
Chem. class.: Belladonna alkaloid

Action: Blocks response of sphincter muscle of iris and ciliary body, producing dilation and paralysis of accommodation
Uses: Fundus exam, cycloplegic refraction, dilation of pupil in inflammatory conditions of the iris and uveal tract
Dosage and routes:
• *Adult, child:* INSTILL 1-2 gtt of 1% sol, repeat in 5 min (refraction)

---

* Available in Canada only

or 1-2 gtt of 0.5% sol 15-20 min before fundus examination
Available forms: Ophth sol 0.5%, 1%
Side effects/adverse reactions:
EENT: Blurred vision, photophobia, increased intraocular pressure, irritation, edema
SYST: Tachycardia, confusion, hallucinations, emotional changes in children, fever, flushing, dry skin, dry mouth, abdominal discomfort (infants: bladder distention, irregular pulse, drowsiness, blurred vision, ***respiratory depression***)
Contraindications: Hypersensitivity, infants <3 mo, glaucoma, conjunctivitis, elderly
Precautions: Pregnancy (C), lactation, children, Down syndrome
Pharmacokinetics:
Instill: Peak 20-40 min (mydriasis), 20-35 min (cycloplegia), duration 6 hr

NURSING CONSIDERATIONS
Evaluate:
• Eye pain; discontinue use
Teach patient/family:
• To report change in vision, with blurring or loss of sight, trouble breathing, flushing
• Method of instillation, including pressure on lacrimal sac for 1 min, and not to touch dropper to eye
• That blurred vision will decrease with repeated use of drug
• Not to engage in hazardous activities until able to see
• To wait 5 min to use other drops
• Not to blink more than usual
• That dark glasses may be worn if photophobia occurs

tubocurarine (℞)

(too-boe-kyoo-ar'een)
Tubarine*, Tubocuraine
Func. class.: Neuromuscular blocker
Chem. class.: Curare alkaloid

Action: Inhibits transmission of nerve impulses by binding with cholinergic receptor sites, antagonizing action of acetylcholine
Uses: Facilitation of endotracheal intubation, skeletal muscle relaxation during mechanical ventilation, surgery, or general anesthesia
Dosage and routes:
• *Adult:* IV BOL 0.4-0.5 mg/kg, then 0.08-0.10 mg/kg 20-45 min after 1st dose if needed for long procedures
Available forms: Inj 3 mg/ml, 20 U/ml
Side effects/adverse reactions:
CV: Bradycardia, tachycardia, increased, decreased B/P
RESP: ***Prolonged apnea, bronchospasm, cyanosis, respiratory depression***
EENT: Increased secretions
INTEG: Rash, flushing, pruritus, urticaria
Contraindications: Hypersensitivity
Precautions: Pregnancy (C), cardiac disease, lactation, children <2 yr, electrolyte imbalances, dehydration, neuromuscular disease, respiratory disease
Pharmacokinetics:
IV: Onset 15 sec, peak 2-3 min, duration ½-1½ hr; half-life 1-3 hr, degraded in liver, kidney (minimally), excreted in urine (unchanged) crosses placenta
Interactions:
• Increased neuromuscular blockade: aminoglycosides, clindamy-

T

cin, lincomycin, quinidine, local anesthetics, polymyxin antibiotics, lithium, narcotic analgesics, thiazides, enflurane, isoflurane, trimethophan, Mg salts
• Dysrhythmias: theophylline
Syringe compatibilities: Pentobarbital, thiopental
Solution compatibilities: D_5, $D_{10}W$, 0.9% NaCl, 0.45% NaCl , Ringer's, LR, dextrose/Ringer's or dextrose/LR combinations
NURSING CONSIDERATIONS
Assess:
• For electrolyte imbalances (K, Mg); may lead to increased action of this drug
• Vital signs (B/P, pulse, respirations, airway) q15min until fully recovered; rate, depth, pattern of respirations, strength of hand grip
• I&O ratio; check for urinary retention, frequency, hesitancy
• Recovery: decreased paralysis of face, diaphragm, leg, arm, rest of body; allow to recover fully before completing neurologic assessment
• Allergic reactions: rash, fever, respiratory distress, pruritus; drug should be discontinued
Administer:
• With diazepam or morphine when used for therapeutic paralysis; provides no sedation alone
• Using nerve stimulator by anesthesiologist to determine neuromuscular blockade
• Anticholinesterase to reverse neuromuscular blockade
• IV undiluted 3 mg/ml; give single dose over 1-1½ sec by qualified person; diluted to 4 ml in NS given 0.5 ml/2 min myasthenia testing
Perform/provide:
• Storage in light-resistant area; use only fresh sol
• Reassurance if communication is difficult during recovery from neuromuscular blockade
Evaluate:
• Therapeutic response: paralysis of jaw, eyelid, head, neck, rest of body
Treatment of overdose: Edrophonium or neostigmine, atropine, monitor VS; may require mechanical ventilation

undecylenic acid (topical) (OTC)

(un-de-sye'len-ik)
Caldesene, Cruex, Decylenes, Desenex, Desenex Maximum Strength, Protectol
Func. class.: Local antiinfective
Chem. class.: Antifungal, antibacterial

Action: Interferes with fungal cell membrane permeability
Uses: Tinea cruris, tinea pedis, diaper rash, minor skin irritations
Dosage and routes:
• *Adult and child:* TOP apply to affected areas bid
Available forms: Powder 10, 15, 19%; oint 22%; cream 8, 20%; foam 10%; soap 97.5 g/bar
Side effects/adverse reactions:
INTEG: Rash, urticaria, stinging, burning
Contraindications: Hypersensitivity
Precautions: Pregnancy (C), lactation; impaired circulation; diabetes mellitus; broken, pustular skin; puncture wounds
NURSING CONSIDERATIONS
Assess:
• Allergic reaction: burning, stinging, swelling, redness
Administer:
• Enough medication to cover lesions completely
• After cleansing with soap, water before each application; dry well

* Available in Canada only

Perform/provide:
• Dry storage at room temp
Evaluate:
• Therapeutic response: decrease in size, number of lesions
Teach patient/family:
• To use medical asepsis (hand washing) before, after each application
• To apply with glove to prevent further infection
• To avoid use of OTC creams, ointments, lotions unless directed by prescriber
• To avoid inhaling and contact with eyes or other mucous membranes; to seek medical attention if symptoms persist
• To complete treatment regimen

uracil mustard (℞)

(yoor'a-sill)

Func. class.: Antineoplastic alkylating agent
Chem. class.: Nitrogen mustard

Action: Responsible for cross-linking DNA strands leading to cell death; activity is not cell cycle specific

Uses: Hodgkin's disease, lymphomas; cervix, ovarian, lung cancer; chronic lymphocytic, myelocytic leukemia; reticulum cell sarcoma, mycosis fungoides; polycythemia vera

Dosage and routes:
• *Adult:* PO 1-2 mg/day × 3 mo or desired response, then 1 mg/day for 3 out of 4 wk until desired response or 3-5 mg × 7 days, not to exceed total dose of 0.5 mg/kg then 1 mg/day until desired response, then 1 mg/day 3 out of 4 wk

Available forms: Caps 1 mg

Side effects/adverse reactions:
HEMA: ***Thrombocytopenia, leukopenia,*** anemia
GI: Nausea, vomiting, diarrhea, ***hepatotoxicity***
GU: Amenorrhea, azoospermia
INTEG: Alopecia, dermatitis, pruritus, rash

Contraindications: Severe thrombocytopenia/leukopenia, hypersensitivity, pregnancy (X)

Precautions: Radiation therapy

Pharmacokinetics:
Excreted unchanged in urine

Interactions:
• Increased toxicity: antineoplastics, radiation

NURSING CONSIDERATIONS

Assess:
• CBC, differential, platelet count qwk; withhold drug if WBC is <4000 or platelet count is <75,000; notify prescriber
• Renal function studies: BUN, serum uric acid, urine CrCl before, during therapy
• I&O ratio; report fall in urine output of 30 ml/hr
• Monitor temp q4h (may indicate beginning infection)
• Liver function tests before, during therapy (bilirubin, AST [SGOT], ALT [SGPT], LDH) as needed or qmo
• Bleeding: hematuria, guaiac, bruising or petechiae, mucosa or orifices q8h
• Food preferences; list likes, dislikes
• Yellow skin, sclera, dark urine, clay-colored stools, itchy skin, abdominal pain, fever, diarrhea
• Effects of alopecia on body image; discuss feelings about body changes
• Inflammation of mucosa, breaks in skin
• Symptoms indicating severe allergic reaction: rash, pruritus, urticaria, itching
• Check for tartrazine dye allergy

Administer:
• Medications by oral route if possible; avoid IM, SC, IV routes to prevent infections
• Antacid before oral agent; give drug after evening meal, before bedtime
• Antiemetic 30-60 min before giving drug to prevent vomiting
• Antibiotics for prophylaxis of infection
• Topical or systemic analgesics for pain
• Local or systemic drugs for infection

Perform/provide:
• Storage in tight container at room temp
• Strict medical asepsis, protective isolation if WBC is low
• Special skin care
• Liquid diet, including cola, Jell-O; dry toast or crackers may be added if not nauseated or vomiting
• Increase fluid intake to 2-3 L/day to prevent urate deposits, calculi formation

Evaluate:
• Therapeutic response: decreased tumor size, spread of malignancy

Teach patient/family:
• About protective isolation
• That effect may take 3 mo
• To report signs of infection: fever, sore throat, flu symptoms
• To report signs of anemia: fatigue, headache, faintness, shortness of breath, irritability
• To avoid use of razors, commercial mouthwash
• To avoid use of aspirin products, ibuprofen
• That azoospermia, amenorrhea can occur, are reversible after discontinuing treatment
• That hair may be lost during treatment; a wig or hairpiece may make patient feel better; new hair may be different in color, texture
• To avoid foods with citric acid, hot or rough texture

urea (℞)

(yoor-ee'a)
Ureaphil, Carbamex*
Func. class.: Diuretic, osmotic
Chem. class.: Carbonic acid diamide salt

Action: Elevates plasma osmolality, increasing flow of water into the extracellular compartment
Uses: To decrease intracranial pressure, intraocular pressure
Dosage and routes:
• *Adult:* IV 1-1.5 g/kg of 30% sol over 1-3 hr; do not exceed 120 g/day
• *Child >2 yr:* IV 0.5-1.5 g/kg, not to exceed 4 ml/min
• *Child <2 yr:* IV 0.1 g/kg, not to exceed 4 ml/min
Available forms: Inj IV 40 g/150 ml
Side effects/adverse reactions:
CNS: Dizziness, disorientation, fever, syncope, *headache*
GI: Nausea, vomiting
INTEG: Venous thrombosis, phlebitis, extravasation
CV: Postural hypotension, tachycardia
Contraindications: Severe renal disease, active intracranial bleeding, marked dehydration, liver failure
Precautions: Hepatic disease, renal disease, pregnancy (C), electrolyte imbalances, lactation
Pharmacokinetics:
IV: Onset ½-1 hr, peak 1 hr, duration 3-10 hr (diuresis), 5-6 hr (intraocular pressure); half-life 1 hr; excreted in urine, breast milk; crosses placenta

* Available in Canada only

Interactions:
• Incompatible with whole blood, alkalies in sol or syringe
• Increased renal excretion of lithium

NURSING CONSIDERATIONS

Assess:
• Weight, I&O qd to determine fluid loss; effect of drug may be decreased if used qd; for hourly urinary output
• Rate, depth, rhythm of respiration, effect of exertion
• B/P lying, standing, postural hypotension may occur
• Electrolytes: K, Na, Cl; include BUN, blood sugar, CBC, serum creatinine, blood pH, ABGs, liver function tests
• Signs of metabolic acidosis: drowsiness, restlessness
• Signs of hypokalemia: postural hypotension, malaise, fatigue, tachycardia, leg cramps, weakness
• Fever, signs of extravasation
• Confusion, especially in elderly; take safety precautions if needed
• Hydration: skin turgor, thirst, dry mucous membranes

Administer:
• IV after diluting 30 g/100 ml diluent with D_5, D_{10}; run 30% sol over 1-2 hr; check for extravasation; do not exceed 4 ml/min; may cause bleeding; use IV filter
• Within minutes of reconstitution; sol becomes ammonia on standing

Evaluate:
• Therapeutic response: improvement in edema of feet, legs, sacral area daily in CHF

Teach patient/family:
• That drug will cause diuresis in ½ hr

Treatment of overdose: Lavage if taken orally; monitor electrolytes, administer IV fluids, monitor BUN, hydration, CV status

urofollitropin (℞)

(yoor-o-foll'i-tropin)
Metrodin
Func. class.: Ovulation stimulant
Chem. class.: Gonadotropin

Action: Stimulates ovarian follicular growth in primary ovarian failure

Uses: Induction of ovulation in polycystic ovarian disease in those who have elevated LH/FSH ratios and do not respond to other treatment, assisted reproductive technologies (in virto fertilization)

Dosage and routes:
• *Adult:* IM 75 IU/day × 7-12 days, then 5000-10,000 U HCG 1 day after last urofollitropin if pregnancy does not occur; may repeat for 2 courses before increasing dose to 150 IU/day 7-12 days then 5000-10,000 U HCG 1 day after last urofollitropin; may repeat for 2 more courses

Available forms: Powder for injection 0.83 mg (76 IU FSH)/amp, 1.66 mg (150 IU FSH)/amp

Side effects/adverse reactions:
CNS: Malaise
GI: Nausea, vomiting, constipation, increased appetite, abdominal pain
INTEG: Rash, dermatitis, urticaria, alopecia
GU: Polyuria, frequency, birth defects, spontaneous abortions, multiple ovulation, breast pain

Contraindications: Hypersensitivity, pregnancy (X), undiagnosed vaginal bleeding, intracranial lesion, ovarian cyst not caused by polycystic ovarian disease

Precautions: Lactation, arterial thromboembolism

U

Pharmacokinetics:
Detoxified in liver, excreted in feces, stored in fat

NURSING CONSIDERATIONS
Assess:
• At same time qd to maintain drug level

Administer:
• After dissolving contents of ampule in 1-2 ml of sterile saline, give immediately, discard unused portion

Evaluate:
• Therapeutic response: ovulation, pregnancy

Teach patient/family:
• That multiple births are common after taking this drug
• To notify prescriber of low abdominal pain; may indicate ovarian cyst, cyst rupture
• Method of taking, recording basal body temp to determine whether ovulation has occurred
• That if ovulation can be determined (there is a slight decrease, then a sharp increase for ovulation), to attempt coitus 3 days before and qod until after ovulation
• If pregnancy is suspected, notify prescriber immediately

urokinase (℞)
(yoor-oh-kin′ase)
Abbokinase, Abbokinase Open-Cath
Func. class.: Thrombolytic enzyme
Chem. class.: β-Hemolytic streptococcus filtrate (purified)

Action: Promotes thrombolysis by directly converting plasminogen to plasmin

Uses: Venous thrombosis, pulmonary embolism, arterial thrombosis, arterial embolism, arteriovenous cannula occlusion, lysis of coronary artery thrombi after MI

Dosage and routes:
Lysis of pulmonary emboli
• *Adult:* IV 4400 IU/kg/hr × 12-24 hr, not to exceed 200 ml; then IV heparin, then anticoagulants

Coronary artery thrombosis
• *Adult:* INSTILL 6000 IU/min into occluded artery for 1-2 hr after giving IV bol of heparin 2500-10,000 U
• May also give as IV inf 2 million-3 million U over 45-90 min

Venous catheter occlusion
• *Adult:* INSTILL 5000 IU into line, wait 5 min, then aspirate, repeat aspiration attempts q5min × ½ hr; if occlusion has not been removed, cap line and wait ½-1 hr, then aspirate; may need 2nd dose if still occluded

Available forms: Inj

Side effects/adverse reactions:
HEMA: Decreased Hct, ***bleeding***
INTEG: Rash, urticaria, phlebitis at IV infusion site, itching, flushing
CNS: Headache, fever
GI: Nausea
RESP: Altered respirations, SOB, ***bronchospasm***
MS: Low back pain
CV: Hypertension, dysrhythmias
EENT: Periorbital edema
SYST: ***GI, GU, intracranial, retroperitoneal bleeding,*** surface bleeding, ***anaphylaxis***

Contraindications: Hypersensitivity, active bleeding, intraspinal surgery, neoplasms of CNS, ulcerative colitis/enteritis, severe hypertension, renal disease, hepatic disease, hypocoagulation, COPD, subacute bacterial endocarditis, rheumatic valvular disease, cerebral embolism/thrombosis/hemorrhage, intraarterial diagnostic procedure or surgery (10 days), recent major surgery

Precautions: Arterial emboli from left side of heart, pregnancy (B)
Pharmacokinetics:
IV: Half-life 10-20 min; small amounts excreted in urine
Interactions:
• Bleeding potential: aspirin, indomethacin, phenylbutazone, anticoagulants
• Considered incompatible with any drug in sol or syringe
Lab test interferences:
Increase: PT, APTT, TT
NURSING CONSIDERATIONS
Assess:
• VS, B/P, pulse, resp, neurologic signs, temp at least q4h; temp >104° F (40° C) is an indicator of internal bleeding; cardiac rhythm following intracoronary administration
• For neurologic changes that may indicate intracranial bleeding
• Retroperitoneal bleeding: back pain, leg weakness, diminished pulses
• Peripheral pulses, lung sounds, respiratory function
• Allergy: fever, rash, itching, chills; mild reaction may be treated with antihistamines
• Bleeding during 1st hr of treatment (hematuria, hematemesis, bleeding from mucous membranes, epistaxis, ecchymosis)
• Blood studies (Hct, platelets, PTT, PT, TT, APTT) before starting therapy; PT or APTT must be less than 2 × control before starting therapy TT; or PT q3-4h during treatment
Administer:
• Using infusion pump, terminal filter (0.45 μm or smaller)
• IV; reconstitute only with 5.2 ml sterile water for inj (not bacteriostatic water), and roll (not shake) to enhance reconstitution; further dilute with 190 ml; give as intermittent inf or give to clear cannula by using 1 ml of diluted drug; inject into cannula slowly, clamp 5 min, aspirate clot
• As soon as thrombi identified; not useful for thrombi over 1 wk old
• Cryoprecipitate or fresh frozen plasma if bleeding occurs
• Loading dose at beginning of therapy; may require increased loading doses
• Heparin therapy after thrombolytic therapy is discontinued, TT or APTT less than 2 × control (about 3-4 hr)
Perform/provide:
• Storage in refrigerator; use immediately after reconstitution
• Bed rest during entire course of treatment; use caution in handling patients
• Avoidance of venous, arterial puncture procedures, inj, rectal temp
• Treatment of fever with acetaminophen or aspirin
• Placement of sign above patient's bed stating urokinase therapy
• Pressure for 30 sec to minor bleeding sites; 30 min to sites of arterial puncture followed by pressure dressing; inform prescriber if hemostasis not attained, apply pressure dressing
Evaluate:
• Therapeutic response: decreased clotting, thrombosis, embolism

ursodiol (℞)
(your-so'dee-ol)
Actigall
Func. class.: Gallstone solubilizing agent
Chem. class.: Ursodeoxycholic acid

Action: Suppresses hepatic synthesis, secretion of cholesterol; inhibits intestinal absorption of cholesterol

U

Uses: Dissolution of radiolucent, noncalcified gallbladder stones (less than 20 mm in diameter) in which surgery is not indicated

Dosage and routes:

• *Adult:* PO 8-10 mg/kg/day in 2-3 divided doses using gallbladder ultrasound q6mo; determine if stones have dissolved; if so, continue therapy, repeat ultrasound within 1-3 mo

Available forms: Caps 300 mg

Side effects/adverse reactions:

GI: Diarrhea, nausea, vomiting, abdominal pain, constipation, stomatitis, flatulence, dyspepsia, biliary pain

INTEG: Pruritus, rash, urticaria, dry skin, sweating, alopecia

CNS: Headache, anxiety, depression, insomnia, fatigue

MS: Arthralgia, myalgia, back pain

OTHER: Cough, rhinitis

Contraindications: Calcified cholesterol stones, radiopaque stones, radiolucent bile pigment stones, chronic liver disease, hypersensitivity

Precautions: Pregnancy (B), lactation, children

Pharmacokinetics: 80% excreted in feces, 20% metabolized, excreted into bile, lost in feces

Interactions:

• Reduced action of ursodiol: cholestyramine, colestipol, aluminum-based antacids

NURSING CONSIDERATIONS

Assess:

• GI status: diarrhea, abdominal pain, nausea, vomiting; drug may have to be discontinued if side effects are severe

• Skin for pruritus, rash, urticaria, dry skin; provide soothing lotion to lesions

• Musculoskeletal status: aches or stiffness in joints

Administer:

• For up to 9-12 mo; if no improvement is seen, discontinue drug

Evaluate:

• Therapeutic response: decreasing size of stones on ultrasound

Teach patient/family:

• That anxiety, depression, insomnia are side effects and are reversible after discontinuing drug

valproate/valproic acid, divalproex sodium (℞)

(val-proe'ate)

Depakene, Dalpro, Deproic, Epival*, Myproic acid/Depakote

Func. class.: Anticonvulsant

Chem. class.: Carboxylic acid derivative

Action: Increases levels of γ-aminobutyric acid (GABA) in brain, which decreases seizure activity

Uses: Simple, complex (petit mal) absence, mixed, tonic-clonic (grand mal) seizures, myoclonic seizures; mood stabilizer

Dosage and routes:

• *Adult and child:* PO 15 mg/kg/day divided in 2-3 doses, may increase by 5-10 mg/kg/day qwk, not to exceed 30 mg/kg/day in 2-3 divided doses

Available forms: Valproic acid caps 250 mg; divalproex tabs delayed rel 125, 250, 500 mg; valproate sodium syr 250 mg/5 ml

Side effects/adverse reactions:

HEMA: ***Thrombocytopenia, leukopenia, lymphocytosis,*** increased pro-time

CNS: Sedation, drowsiness, dizziness, headache, incoordination, paresthesia, depression, hallucinations,

* Available in Canada only

behavioral changes, tremors, aggression, weakness
GI: Nausea, vomiting, constipation, diarrhea, heartburn, anorexia, cramps, ***hepatic failure, pancreatitis, toxic hepatitis,*** stomatitis
INTEG: Rash, alopecia, bruising
GU: Enuresis, irregular menses
Contraindications: Hypersensitivity
Precautions: MI (recovery phase), hepatic disease, renal disease, Addison's disease, pregnancy (D), lactation
Pharmacokinetics:
PO: Onset 15-30 min, peak 1-4 hr, duration 4-6 hr
REC: Onset slow, duration 4-6 hr
Metabolized by liver, excreted by kidneys, in feces, breast milk; crosses placenta, half-life 6-16 hr
Interactions:
• Increased effects: CNS depressants
• Increased toxicity: salicylates, warfarin, sulfinpyrazone, carbamazepine, phenytoin
Lab test interferences:
False-positive: Ketones
NURSING CONSIDERATIONS
Assess:
• Blood studies: Hct, Hgb, RBC, serum folate, pro-time, Vit D if on long-term therapy
• Hepatic studies: AST (SGOT), ALT (SGPT), bilirubin, creatinine, failure
• Blood levels: therapeutic level 50-100 μg/ml
• Mental status: mood, sensorium, affect, memory (long, short)
• Respiratory dysfunction: respiratory depression, character, rate, rhythm; hold drug if respirations are <12/min or if pupils are dilated
Administer:
• Tablets or capsules whole
• Elixir alone; do not dilute with carbonated beverage; do not give syrup to patients on sodium restriction
• Give with food or milk to decrease GI symptoms
Evaluate:
• Therapeutic response: decreased seizures
Teach patient/family:
• That physical dependency may result from extended use
• To avoid driving, other activities that require alertness
• Not to discontinue medication quickly after long-term use; convulsions may result
• To report visual disturbances, rash, diarrhea, light-colored stools, jaundice, protracted vomiting to prescriber

vancomycin (℞)

(van-koe-mye'sin)
Lyphocin, Vancocin, Vancoled, vancomycin HCl
Func. class.: Antibacterial
Chem. class.: Tricyclic glycopeptide

Action: Inhibits bacterial cell wall synthesis
Uses: Resistant staphylococcal infections, pseudomembranous colitis, staphylococcal enterocolitis, endocarditis prophylaxis for dental procedures
Dosage and routes:
Serious staphylococcal infections
• *Adult:* IV 500 mg q6h or 1 g q12h
• *Child:* IV 40 mg/kg/day divided q6h
• *Neonates:* IV 15 mg/kg initially followed by 10 mg/kg q8-12h
Pseudomembranous/staphylococcal enterocolitis
• *Adult:* PO 500 mg -2 g/day in 3-4 divided doses for 7-10 days
• *Child:* PO 40 mg/kg/day divided q6h, not to exceed 2 g/day

V

Endocarditis prophylaxis
• *Adult:* IV 1 g over 1 hr, 1 hr before dental procedure
Available forms: Pulvules 125, 250 mg; powder for oral sol 1, 10 g; powder for inj IV 500 mg, 1 g
Side effects/adverse reactions:
CV: ***Cardiac arrest, vascular collapse***
EENT: ***Ototoxicity, permanent deafness,*** tinnitus
HEMA: ***Leukopenia, eosinophilia, neutropenia***
GI: ***Nausea***
RESP: Wheezing, dyspnea
SYST: ***Anaphylaxis***
GU: ***Nephrotoxicity,*** *increased BUN, creatinine, albumin,* ***fatal uremia***
INTEG: Chills, fever, rash, thrombophlebitis at injection site, urticaria, pruritus, necrosis (Redman's syndrome)
Contradindications: Hypersensitivity, decreased hearing
Precautions: Renal disease, pregnancy (C), lactation, elderly, neonates
Pharmacokinetics:
IV: Peak 5 min; half-life 4-8 hr; excreted in urine (active form); crosses placenta
Interactions:
• Ototoxicity or nephrotoxicity: aminoglycosides, cephalosporins, colistin, polymyxin, bacitracin, cisplatin, amphotericin B
• Incompatible with aminophylline, amobarbital, chloramphenicol, chlorothiazide, dexamethasone, heparin, hydrocortisone, methicillin, penicillins, pentobarbital, phenobarbital, phenytoin, prochlorperazine, secobarbital, warfarin

NURSING CONSIDERATIONS
Assess:
• I&O ratio; report hematuria, oliguria; nephrotoxicity may occur
• Any patient with compromised renal system; drug is excreted slowly in poor renal system function; toxicity may occur rapidly
• Blood studies: WBC
• C&S; drug may be given as soon as culture is taken
• Auditory function during, after treatment
• B/P during administration; sudden drop may indicate Redman's syndrome
• Signs of infection
• Hearing loss, ringing, roaring in ears; drug should be discontinued
• Skin eruptions
• Respiratory status: rate, character, wheezing, tightness in chest
• Allergies before treatment, reaction of each medication; place allergies on chart in bright red letters; notify all people giving drugs
Administer:
• After reconstitution with 10 ml sterile water for injection (500 mg/10 ml) further dilution is needed for IV, 500 mg/100 ml NS, D_5W given as int inf over 1 hr
• Antihistamine if Redman's syndrome occurs: decreased B/P, flushing of neck, face
• Dose based on serum concentration
Perform/provide:
• Storage at room temp for up to 2 wk after reconstitution
• Adrenalin, suction, tracheostomy set, endotracheal intubation equipment on unit; anaphylaxis may occur
• Adequate intake of fluids (2 L) to prevent nephrotoxicity
Evaluate:
• Therapeutic response: absence of fever, sore throat
Teach patient/family:
• Aspects of drug therapy: need to complete entire course of medication to ensure organism death (7-10

days); culture may be taken after completed course of medication
• To report sore throat, fever, fatigue; could indicate superinfection
• That drug must be taken in equal intervals around clock to maintain blood levels

vasopressin (℞)

(vay-soe-press'in)
Pitressin Synthetic
Func. class.: Pituitary hormone
Chem. class.: Lysine vasopressin

Action: Promotes reabsorption of water by action on renal tubular epithelium; causes vasoconstriction
Uses: Diabetes insipidus (nonnephrogenic/nonpsychogenic), abdominal distention postoperatively, bleeding esophageal varices
Dosage and routes:
Diabetes insipidus
• *Adult:* IM/SC 5-10 units bid-qid as needed; IM/SC 2.5-5 units q2-3 days (Pitressin Tannate) for chronic therapy
• *Child:* IM/SC 2.5-10 units bid-qid as needed; IM/SC 1.25-2.5 units q2 3 days (Pitressin Tannate) for chronic therapy
Abdominal distention
• *Adult:* IM 5 units, then q3-4h, increasing to 10 units if needed (aqueous)
Available forms: Inj 20, 5 U/ml (tannate), spray, cotton pledgets
Side effects/adverse reactions:
EENT: Nasal irritation, congestion, rhinitis
CNS: Drowsiness, headache, lethargy, flushing
GU: Vulval pain, uterine cramping
GI: Nausea, heartburn, cramps
CV: Increased B/P
MISC: Tremor, sweating, vertigo, urticaria, bronchial constriction
Contraindications: Hypersensitivity, chronic nephritis
Precautions: CAD, pregnancy (C)
Pharmacokinetics:
Nasal: Onset 1 hr, duration 3-8 hr, half-life 15 min; metabolized in liver, kidneys, excreted in urine

NURSING CONSIDERATIONS
Assess:
• Nasal mucosa if given by intranasal spray; for irritation
• Pulse, B/P, when giving drug IV or IM
• I&O ratio, weight daily; check for edema in extremities; if water retention is severe, diuretic may be prescribed
• H_2O intoxication: lethargy, behavioral changes, disorientation, neuromuscular excitability
Evaluate:
• Therapeutic response: absence of severe thirst, decreased urine output, osmolality

vecuronium (℞)

(vek-yoo-roe'nee-um)
Norcuron
Func. class.: Neuromuscular blocker
Chem. class.: Monoquaternary analog of pancuronium

Action: Inhibits transmission of nerve impulses by binding with cholinergic receptor sites, antagonizing action of acetylcholine
Uses: Facilitation of endotracheal intubation, skeletal muscle relaxation during mechanical ventilation, surgery, general anesthesia
Dosage and routes:
• *Adult and child >9 yr:* IV BOL 0.08-0.10 mg/kg, then 0.01-0.015 mg/kg for prolonged procedures
Available forms: 10 mg/5 ml vial

V

Side effects/adverse reactions:
CNS: Skeletal muscle weakness or paralysis (rare)
RESP: ***Prolonged apnea, possible respiratory paralysis***
Contraindications: Hypersensitivity
Precautions: Pregnancy (C), cardiac disease, lactation, children <2 yr, electrolyte imbalances, dehydration, neuromuscular disease, respiratory disease
Pharmacokinetics:
IV: Onset 15 min, peak 3-5 min, duration 45-60 min; half-life 65-75 min; not metabolized; excreted in feces; crosses placenta
Interactions:
- Increased neuromuscular blockade: aminoglycosides, clindamycin, lincomycin, quinidine, local anesthetics, polymyxin antibiotics, lithium, narcotic analgesics, thiazides, enflurane, isoflurane, succinylcholine
- Dysrhythmias: theophylline

Y-site compatibilities: Aminophylline, cefazolin, cefuroxime, cimetidine, cortimoxazole, dobutamine, dopamine, epinephrine, esmolol, fentanyl, gentamicin, heparin, hydrocortisone sodium succinate, isoproterenol, lorazepam, midazolam, morphine, nitroglycerin, ranitidine, sodium nitroprusside, vancomycin
NURSING CONSIDERATIONS
Assess:
- For electrolyte imbalances (K, Mg); may lead to increased action of this drug
- Vital signs (B/P, pulse, respirations, airway) q15min until fully recovered; rate, depth, pattern of respirations, strength of hand grip
- I&O ratio; check for urinary retention, frequency, hesitancy
- Recovery: decreased paralysis of face, diaphragm, leg, arm, rest of body; allow to recover fully before completing neurologic assessment
- Allergic reactions: rash, fever, respiratory distress, pruritus; drug should be discontinued

Administer:
- With diazepam or morphine when used for therapeutic paralysis; provides no sedation alone
- Using nerve stimulator by anesthesiologist to determine neuromuscular blockade
- Anticholinesterase to reverse neuromuscular blockade
- IV after diluting with diluent provided; give by direct IV over 1 min; may give as continuous inf 10-20 mg/100 ml; titrate to patient response (only by qualified person)

Perform/provide:
- Storage in refrigerator; discard in 24 hr
- Reassurance if communication is difficult during recovery from neuromuscular blockade

Evaluate:
- Therapeutic response: paralysis of jaw, eyelid, head, neck, rest of body

Treatment of overdose: Edrophonium or neostigmine, atropine, monitor VS; may require mechanical ventilation

---

venlafaxine (℞)
(ven-la-fax'een)
Effexor
Func. class.: Second-generation antidepressant

Action: Potent inhibitor of neuronal serotonin and norepinephrine uptake, weak inhibitor of dopamine; no muscarinic, histaminergic, or α-adrenergic receptors in vitro
Uses: Depression
Dosage and routes:
- *Adult:* PO 75 mg/day in 2 or 3 divided doses; taken with food, may

* Available in Canada only

be increased to 150 mg/day; if needed, may be further increased to 225 mg/day; increments of 75 mg/ day at intervals of no less than 4 days; some hospitalized patients may require up to 375 mg/day in 3 divided doses

Available forms: Tabs scored 25, 37.5, 50, 75, 100 mg

Side effects/adverse reactions:

CNS: Emotional lability, vertigo, apathy, ataxia, CNS stimulation, euphoria, hallucinations, hostility, increased libido, hypertonia, hypotonia, psychosis

CV: Migraine, angina pectoris, extrasystoles, hypotension, syncope, thrombophlebitis

EENT: Abnormal vision, ear pain, cataract, conjunctivitis, corneal lesions, dry eyes, otitis media, photophobia

GI: Dysphagia, eructation, colitis, gastritis, gingivitis, rectal hemorrhage, stomatitis, stomach and mouth ulceration

GU: Anorgasmia, dysuria, hematuria, metrorrhagia, vaginitis, impaired urination, albuminuria, amenorrhea, kidney calculus, cystitis, nocturia, breast and bladder pain, polyuria, uterine hemorrhage, vaginal hemorrhage, moniliasis

INTEG: Ecchymosis, acne, alopecia, brittle nails, dry skin, photosensitivity

META: Peripheral edema, weight gain, diabetes mellitus, edema, glycosuria, hyperlipemia, hypokalemia

MS: Arthritis, bone pain, bursitis, myasthenia tenosynovitis

RESP: Bronchitis, dyspnea, asthma, chest congestion, epistaxis, hyperventilation, laryngitis

SYST: Accidental injury, malaise, neck pain, enlarged abdomen, cyst, facial edema, hangover, hernia

Contraindications: Hypersensitivity

Precautions: Mania, pregnancy (C), lactation, children, elderly, hypertension, seizure disorder

Pharmacokinetics: Well absorbed, extensively metabolized in the liver to an active metabolite; 87% of drug recovered in urine; 27% protein binding; half-life 5-7, 11-13 hr respectively

Interactions:

Hyperthermia, rigidity, rapid fluctuations of vital signs, mental status changes: MAOIs

NURSING CONSIDERATIONS

Assess:

- B/P lying, standing; pulse q/4 h; if systolic B/P drops 20 mm Hg, hold drug, notify prescriber; take VS q4h in patients with cardiovascular disease
- Blood studies: CBC, leukocytes, differential cardiac enzymes if patient is receiving long-term therapy
- Hepatic studies: AST (SGOT), ALT (SGPT), bilirubin
- Weight qwk; appetite may increase with drug
- With food, milk for GI symptoms
- Gum, hard candy, frequent sips of water for dry mouth
- Mental status: mood, sensorium, affect, suicidal tendencies, increase in psychiatric symptoms; depression, panic
- Withdrawal symptoms: headache, nausea, vomiting, muscle pain, weakness; not usual unless drug is discontinued abruptly

Perform/provide:

- Storage in tight container at room temp; do not freeze
- Assistance with ambulation during beginning therapy, since drowsiness, dizziness occur
- Checking to see if PO medication swallowed

Evaluate:

- Therapeutic response; decreased depression

Teach patient/family:

- To dispense in small amounts because of suicide potential, especially in the beginning of therapy
- To use with caution when driving or other activities requiring alertness because of drowsiness, dizziness, blurred vision
- To avoid alcohol ingestion, other CNS depressants
- Not to discontinue medication quickly after long-term use; may cause nausea, headache, malaise
- To wear sunscreen or large hat, since photosensitivity occurs

Treatment of overdose: ECG monitoring; induce emesis; lavage, activated charcoal; administer anticonvulsant

verapamil (℞)

(ver-ap'a-mill)

Calan, Calan SR, Isoptin, Isoptin SR, verapamil HCl, verapamil HCl SR, Verelan

Func. class.: Calcium channel blocker; antihypertensive; antianginal

Chem. class.: Phenylalkylamine

Action: Inhibits calcium ion influx across cell membrane during cardiac depolarization; produces relaxation of coronary vascular smooth muscle; dilates coronary arteries; decreases SA/AV node conduction; dilates peripheral arteries

Uses: Chronic stable angina pectoris, vasospastic angina, dysrhythmias, hypertension

Investigational uses: Prevention of migraine headaches, ventricular outflow obstruction in hypertrophic cardiomyopathy

Dosage and routes:

- *Adult:* PO 80 mg tid or qid, increase qwk; IV BOL 5-10 mg >2 min, repeat if necessary in 30 min
- *Child 0-1 yr:* IV BOL 0.1-0.2 mg/kg >2 min with ECG monitoring, repeat if necessary in 30 min
- *Child 1-15 yr:* IV BOL 0.1-0.3 mg/kg over >2 min, repeat in 30 min, not to exceed 10 mg in a single dose

Available forms: Tabs 40, 80, 120 mg; sus rel tabs 120, 180, 240 mg; inj 2.5 mg/ml; sus rel caps 120, 180, 240 mg

Side effects/adverse reactions:

CV: Edema, ***CHF,*** bradycardia, hypotension, palpitations, AV block

GI: Nausea, diarrhea, gastric upset, constipation, increased liver function studies

GU: Nocturia, polyuria

CNS: Headache, drowsiness, dizziness, anxiety, depression, weakness, insomnia, confusion, light-headedness

Contraindications: Sick sinus syndrome, 2nd or 3rd degree heart block, hypotension less than 90 mm Hg systolic, cardiogenic shock, severe CHF

Precautions: CHF, hypotension, hepatic injury, pregnancy (C), lactation, children, renal disease, concomitant β-blocker therapy

Pharmacokinetics:

IV: Onset 3 min, peak 3-5 min, duration 10-20 min

PO: Onset variable, peak 3-4 hr, duration 17-24 hr, half-life (biphasic) 4 min, 3-7 hr (terminal)

Metabolized by liver, excreted in urine (96% as metabolites)

Interactions:

- Increased hypotension: prazosin, quinidine
- Increased effects: β-blockers, antihypertensives, cimetidine

Available in Canada only

• Decreased effects of lithium
• Increased levels of digoxin, theophylline, cyclosporine, carbamazepine, nondepolarizing muscle relaxants

Syringe compatibilities: Amrinone, heparin, milrinone

Y-site compatibilities: Amrinone, azlocillin, carbenicillin, dobutamine, dopamine, famotidine, hydralazine, meperidine, methicillin, milrinone, penicillin G potassium, piperacillin, ticarcillin

Lab test interferences:

Increase: Liver function tests

NURSING CONSIDERATIONS

Assess:

• Cardiac status: B/P, pulse, respiration, ECG intervals (PR, QRS, QT)

Administer:

• IV undiluted through Y-tube or 3-way stopcock of compatible sol; give over 2 min, or 3 min elderly
• Before meals, hs; sus rel give with food

Evaluate:

• Therapeutic response: decreased anginal pain, decreased B/P, dysrhythmias

Teach patient/family:

• How to take pulse before taking drug; to keep record or graph
• To avoid hazardous activities until stabilized on drug, dizziness no longer a problem
• To limit caffeine consumption; no alcohol products
• To avoid OTC drugs unless directed by prescriber
• To comply with all areas of medical regimen: diet, exercise, stress reduction, drug therapy
• To change positions slowly to prevent syncope

Treatment of overdose: Defibrillation, atropine for AV block, vasopressor for hypotension

vidarabine (ophthalmic) (℞)

(vye-dare'a-been)

Vira-A Ophthalmic

Func. class.: Antiviral

Chem. class.: Purine nucleoside

Action: Inhibits viral DNA synthesis by blocking DNA polymerase

Uses: Recurrent epithelial keratitis, superficial keratitis due to herpes simplex, cytomegalovirus, varicella zoster

Dosage and routes:

• *Adult, child:* TOP ½ inch oint into conjunctival sac q3h, 5 times daily

Available forms: Oint 3%

Side effects/adverse reactions:

EENT: Burning, stinging, photophobia, pain, temporary visual haze, edema

Contraindications: Hypersensitivity

Precautions: Antibiotic hypersensitivity, pregnancy (C)

NURSING CONSIDERATIONS

Assess:

• Allergy: itching, lacrimation, redness, swelling

Administer:

• After washing hands; cleanse crusts or discharge from eye before application

Perform/provide:

• Storage at room temp

Evaluate:

• Therapeutic response: absence of redness, inflammation, tearing

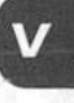

Teach patient/family:

• To use drug exactly as prescribed
• Not to use eye makeup, towels, washcloths, or eye medication of others, or reinfection may occur
• That drug container tip should not be touched to eye
• To report itching, increased red-

ness, burning, stinging, photophobia; drug should be discontinued
• That drug may cause blurred vision when ointment is applied
• To use sunglasses to prevent photophobia

vidarabine (℞)

(vye-dare'a-been)
Vira-A
Func. class.: Antibacterial, antiviral
Chem. class.: Purine nucleoside

Action: Inhibits bacterial/viral replication by preventing DNA synthesis
Uses: Herpes simplex virus encephalitis, varicella-zoster encephalomyelitis, herpes zoster in immunosuppressed
Dosage and routes:
Herpes simplex encephalitis
• *Adult, child:* IV INF 15 mg/kg/day × 10 days; infuse over 12-24 hr
Herpes zoster in immunocompromised patients
• *Adult, child:* IV 10 mg/kg/day × 5 day
Herpes simplex
• *Neonate:* IV 15 mg/kg/day × 10 days
Available forms: Susp for inj 200 mg/ml
Side effects/adverse reactions:
CNS: Psychosis, hallucinations, dizziness, weakness, tremors, ***fatal metabolic encephalopathy,*** confusion, malaise, headache
META: SIADH
HEMA: ***Anemia, thrombocytopenia, neutropenia***
GI: Nausea, vomiting, anorexia, diarrhea, weight loss
INTEG: Pain, thrombophlebitis at injection site
Contraindications: Hypersensitivity
Precautions: Renal disease, liver disease, lactation, pregnancy (C)
Pharmacokinetics: Crosses blood-brain barrier, excreted by kidneys (metabolites), crosses placenta, half-life 1½-3 hr
Interactions:
• Increased neurologic side effects: allopurinol
• Incompatible with blood, protein products
NURSING CONSIDERATIONS
Assess:
• Liver studies: AST (SGOT), ALT (SGPT)
• Blood studies: WBC, difficult differential, RBC, Hct, Hgb, platelets
• Renal studies: urinalysis, protein, blood
• C&S; drug may be given as soon as culture is taken; C&S may be taken after therapy
• Bowel pattern before, during treatment
• Fluid overload; drug requires large volume to stay in sol
• Weakness, tremors, confusion, dizziness, psychosis; drug may have to be decreased or discontinued
Administer:
• Shake sol; dilute to 450 mg/L IV; give fluid at constant rate over 12-24 hr, using in-line filter with mean pore diameter of 0.45 mm or less
Evaluate:
• Therapeutic response: decreased infection

vinblastine (VLB) (℞)

(vin-blast'een)
Velban, Velbe*, vinblastine sulfate
Func. class.: Antineoplastic
Chem. class.: Vinca rosea alkaloid

Action: Inhibits mitotic activity, arrests cell cycle at metaphase; inhib-

* Available in Canada only

its RNA synthesis, blocks cellular use of glutamic acid needed for purine synthesis; a vesicant

Uses: Breast, testicular cancer, lymphomas, neuroblastoma; Hodgkin's, non-Hodgkin's lymphomas; mycosis fungoides, histiocytosis, Kaposi's sarcoma

Dosage and routes:

• *Adult:* IV 0.1 mg/kg or 3.7 mg/m^2 qwk or q2wk, not to exceed 0.5 mg/kg or 18.5 mg/m^2 qwk

• *Child:* 2.5 mg/m^2 then 3.75, 5, 6.25, 7.5 at 7-day intervals

Available forms: Inj, powder 10 mg for 10 ml IV inj

Side effects/adverse reactions:

HEMA: ***Thrombocytopenia, leukopenia, myelosuppression***

GI: Nausea, vomiting, ileus, *anorexia, stomatitis,* constipation, abdominal pain, GI, rectal bleeding, ***hepatotoxicity,*** pharyngitis

GU: Urinary retention, ***renal failure***

INTEG: Rash, alopecia, photosensitivity

RESP: ***Fibrosis, pulmonary infiltrate***

CV: Tachycardia, orthostatic hypotension

CNS: Paresthesias, peripheral neuropathy, depression, headache, ***convulsions***

META: SIADH

Contraindications: Hypersensitivity, infants, pregnancy (D)

Precautions: Renal disease, hepatic disease

Pharmacokinetics: Half-life (triphasic) 35 min, 53 min, 19 hr, metabolized in liver, excreted in urine, feces, crosses blood-brain barrier

Interactions:

• Increased action of methotrexate
• Do not use with radiation
• Synergism: bleomycin
• Decreased phenytoin level: phenytoin
• Bronchospasm: mitomycin

Syringe compatibilities: Bleomycin, cisplatin, cyclophosphamide, droperidol, fluorouracil, leucovorin, methotrexate, metoclopramide, mitomycin, ondansetron, vincristine

Y-site compatibilities: Bleomycin, cisplatin, cyclophosphamide, doxorubicin, droperidol, fluorouracil, heparin, leucovorin, methotrexate, metoclopramide, mitomycin, ondansetron, sargramostim, vincristine

NURSING CONSIDERATIONS

Assess:

• CBC, differential, platelet count qwk; withhold drug if WBC is <4000 or platelet count is <75,000; notify prescriber
• Pulmonary function tests, chest x-ray studies before, during therapy; chest x-ray film should be obtained q2wk during treatment
• Neurologic status: sensory-vibratory evaluation if side effects occur
• Renal function studies: BUN, serum uric acid, urine CrCl, electrolytes before, during therapy
• I&O ratio; report fall in urine output of 30 ml/hr
• Monitor temp q4h; may indicate beginning infection
• Liver function tests before, during therapy (bilirubin, AST [SGOT], ALT [SGPT], LDH) as needed or qmo
• RBC, Hct, Hgb, since these may be decreased
• Bleeding: hematuria, guaiac, bruising or petechiae, mucosa of orifices q8h
• Dyspnea, rales, unproductive cough, chest pain, tachypnea, fatigue, increased pulse, pallor, lethargy
• Food preferences; list likes, dislikes

V

• Effects of alopecia on body image; discuss feelings about body changes
• Sensitivity of feet/hands, which precedes neuropathy
• Inflammation of mucosa, breaks in skin
• Yellow skin, sclera, dark urine, clay-colored stools, itchy skin, abdominal pain, fever, diarrhea
• Buccal cavity q8h for dryness, sores, or ulceration, white patches, oral pain, bleeding, dysphagia
• Local irritation, pain, burning, discoloration at injection site
• Symptoms indicating severe allergic reaction: rash, pruritus, urticaria, purpuric skin lesions, itching, flushing
• Frequency of stools and characteristics: cramping, acidosis; signs of dehydration: rapid respirations, poor skin turgor, decreased urine output, dry skin, restlessness, weakness

Administer:

• IV after diluting 10 mg/10 ml NaCl; give through Y-tube or 3-way stopcock or directly over 1 min
• Hyaluronidase 150 U/ml in 1 ml NaCl, warm compress for extravasation for vesicant activity treatment
• Antacid before oral agent; give drug after evening meal, before bedtime
• Antiemetic 30-60 min before giving drug and prn to prevent vomiting
• Local or systemic drugs for infection
• Transfusion for anemia
• Antispasmodic for GI symptoms

Perform/provide:

• Deep-breathing exercises with patient 3-4 × day; place in semi-Fowler's position
• Liquid diet: cola, Jell-O; dry toast or crackers may be added if patient is not nauseated or vomiting
• Increase fluid intake to 2-3 L/day to prevent urate deposits, calculi formation
• Rinsing of mouth tid-qid with water
• Brushing of teeth bid-tid with soft brush or cotton-tipped applicators for stomatitis; use unwaxed dental floss
• Nutritious diet with iron, vitamin supplements
• HOB raised to facilitate breathing

Evaluate:

• Therapeutic response: decreased tumor size, spread of malignancy

Teach patient/family:

• To report any complaints or side effects to nurse or prescriber
• To report any changes in breathing or coughing
• That hair may be lost during treatment, a wig or hairpiece may make patient feel better; tell patient that new hair may be different in color, texture
• To report change in gait or numbness in extremities; may indicate neuropathy
• To avoid foods with citric acid, hot or rough texture
• To report any bleeding, white spots or ulcerations in mouth to prescriber; to examine mouth qd

vincristine (VCR) (℞)

(vin-kris'teen)

Oncovin, Vincasar PFS, vincristine sulfate

Func. class.: Antineoplastic

Chem. class.: Vinca alkaloid

Action: Inhibits mitotic activity, arrests cell cycle at metaphase; inhibits RNA synthesis, blocks cellular

* Available in Canada only

use of glutamic acid needed for purine synthesis; a vesicant

Uses: Breast, lung cancer, lymphomas, neuroblastoma, Hodgkin's disease, acute lymphoblastic and other leukemias, rhabdomyosarcoma, Wilms' tumor, osteogenic and other sarcomas

Dosage and routes:

- *Adult:* IV 1-2 mg/m^2/wk, not to exceed 2 mg
- *Child:* IV 1.5-2 mg/m^2/wk, not to exceed 2 mg

Available forms: Inj 1 mg/ml

Side effects/adverse reactions:

INTEG: Alopecia

HEMA: ***Thrombocytopenia, leukopenia, myelosuppression, anemia***

GI: Nausea, vomiting, anorexia, stomatitis, constipation, ***paralytic ileus,*** *abdominal pain,* ***hepatotoxicity***

CV: Orthostatic hypotension

CNS: Decreased reflexes, numbness, weakness, motor difficulties, CNS depression, cranial nerve paralysis, ***seizures***

Contraindications: Hypersensitivity, infants, pregnancy (D)

Precautions: Renal disease, hepatic disease, hypertension, neuromuscular disease

Pharmacokinetics: Half-life (triphasic) 0.85 min, 7.4 min, 164 min; metabolized in liver; excreted in bile, feces; crosses placental barrier, blood-brain barrier

Interactions:

- Increased action of methotrexate, anticoagulants
- Do not use with radiation
- Neurotoxicity: peripheral nervous system drugs
- Decreased digoxin level: digoxin
- Decreased action of vincristine: L-asparaginase
- Acute pulmonary reactions: mitomycin-c

Syringe compatibilities: Bleomycin, cisplatin, cyclophosphamide, droperidol, fluorouracil, leucovorin, methotrexate, metoclopramide, mitomycin, ondansetron, vinblastine

Y-site compatibilities: Blemycin, cisplatin, cyclophosphamide, droperidol, fluorouracil, leucovorin, methotrexate, metoclopramide, mitomycin, ondansetron, sargramostim, vinblastine

NURSING CONSIDERATIONS

Assess:

- CBC, differential, platelet count qwk; withhold drug if WBC is <4000 or platelet count is <75,000; notify prescriber
- Renal function studies: BUN, serum uric acid, urine CrCl, electrolytes before, during therapy
- I&O ratio, report fall in urine output of 30 ml/hr
- Monitor temp q4h; may indicate beginning infection
- Liver function tests before, during therapy (bilirubin, AST [SGOT], ALT [SGPT], LDH) as needed or monthly
- RBC, Hct, Hgb; may be decreased
- Deep tendon reflexes; drug is neurotoxic
- Sensitivity of feet/hands, which precedes neuropathy
- Bleeding: hematuria, guaiac, bruising or petechiae, mucosa of orifices q8h
- Food preferences; list likes, dislikes
- Effects of alopecia on body image, discuss feelings about body changes
- Inflammation of mucosa, breaks in skin
- Yellow skin, sclera, dark urine, clay-colored stools, itchy skin, abdominal pain, fever, diarrhea
- Buccal cavity q8h for dryness, sores or ulceration, white patches, oral pain, bleeding, dysphagia

• Symptoms indicating severe allergic reaction: rash, pruritus, urticaria, purpuric skin lesions, itching, flushing
• Frequency of stools, characteristics: cramping, acidosis; signs of dehydration: rapid respirations, poor skin turgor, decreased urine output, dry skin, restlessness, weakness

Administer:
• Agents to prevent constipation
• Antiemetic 30-60 min before giving drug and prn
• IV after diluting with diluent provided or 1 mg/10 ml of sterile H_2O or NaCl; give through Y-tube or 3-way stopcock or directly over 1 min
• Hyaluronidase 150 U/ml in 1 ml NaCl; apply warm compress for extravasation
• Transfusion for anemia
• Antispasmodic for GI symptoms

Perform/provide:
• Liquid diet: cola, Jell-O; dry toast or crackers may be added if patient is not nauseated or vomiting
• Rinsing of mouth tid-qid with water
• Brushing of teeth bid-tid with soft brush or cotton-tipped applicators for stomatitis; use unwaxed dental floss
• Nutritious diet with iron, vitamin supplements

Evaluate:
• Therapeutic response: decreased tumor size, spread of malignancy

Teach patient/family:
• To report change in gait or numbness in extremities; may indicate neuropathy
• To report any complaints or side effects to nurse or prescriber
• To report any bleeding, white spots or ulcerations in mouth to prescriber; to examine mouth qd

vinorelbine (℞)
(vi-nor′el-bine)
Navelbine
Func. class.: Antineoplastic
Chem. class.: Semisynthetic vinca alkaloid

Action: Inhibits mitotic activity, arrests cell cycle at metaphase; inhibits RNA synthesis, blocks cellular use of glutamic acid needed for purine synthesis; a vesicant

Uses: Unresectable advanced non-small cell lung cancer (NSCLC) stage IV; may be used alone or in combination with cisplatin for stage III or IV NSCLC breast cancer

Dosage and routes:
• *Adult:* IV 30 mg/m^2 qwk

Breast cancer
• *Adult:* IV 30 mg/m^2 qwk

Available forms: Powder 10 mg for 10 ml IV inj

Side effects/adverse reactions:
CV: Chest pain
RESP: Shortness of breath
HEMA: ***Neutropenia, anemia, thrombocytopenia granulocytopenia***
GI: Nausea, vomiting, ileus, *anorexia, stomatitis,* constipation, abdominal pain, diarrhea, ***hepatotoxicity***
INTEG: Rash, alopecia, photosensitivity
CNS: Paresthesias, peripheral neuropathy, depression, headache, ***convulsions***, weakness, jaw pain
META: SIADH
MS: Myalgia

Contraindications: Hypersensitivity, infants, pregnancy (D), granulocyte count <1000 cells/mm^3 pretreatment

Precautions: Renal, hepatic disease, elderly, lactation, children

* Available in Canada only

Pharmacokinetics: Half-life 27-43 hr, peak 1-2 hr

Interactions:

- Possible increased toxicity: fluorouracil

NURSING CONSIDERATIONS

Assess:

- B/P, (baseline and q15min) during administration
- CBC, differential, platelet count weekly; withhold drug if WBC is <4000 or platelet count is <75,000; notify prescriber of results, recovery will take 3 wk
- For dyspnea, rales, unproductive cough, chest pain, tachypnea
- Renal function studies: BUN, serum uric acid, urine CrCl before, during therapy; I&O ratio; report fall in urine output of 30 ml/hr; for decreased hyperuricemia
- For cold, fever, sore throat (may indicate beginning infection); notify prescriber if these occur
- For bleeding: hematuria, guaiac, bruising or petechiae, mucosa or orifices q8h, no rectal temps; avoid IM injections; use pressure to venipuncture sites
- Nutritional status: an antiemetic may be needed
- For symptoms of severe allergic reactions: rash, pruritus, urticaria, itching, flushing, bronchospasm, hypotension, epinephrine and crash cart should be nearby

Administer:

- IV hyaluronidase 150 U/ml in 1 ml NaCl, warm compress for extravasation for vesicant activity treatment
- Antiemetic 30-60 min before giving drug and prn to prevent vomiting

By cont inf: 40 mg/m^2 q3wk after an IV bol of 8 mg/m^2; may be given in combination with doxorubicin, fluorouracil, cisplatin

Perform/provide:

- Liquid diet: cola, Jell-O; dry toast or crackers if patient not nauseated or vomiting
- Brushing of teeth bid-tid with soft brush or cotton-tipped applicators for stomatitis; unwaxed dental floss
- Nutritious diet with iron, vitamin supplements

Evaluate:

Therapeutic response: decreased tumor size, spread of malignancy

Teach patient/family:

- To report change in gait or numbness in extremities; may indicate neuropathy
- To report any complaints or side effects to nurse or prescriber
- To examine mouth qd for bleeding, white spots, ulcerations; notify prescriber

vitamin A (℞, OTC)

Aquasol A, Del-Vi-A, Vitamin A

Func. class.: Vitamin, fat soluble

Chem. class.: Retinol

Action: Needed for normal bone, tooth development, visual dark adaptation, skin disease, mucosa tissue repair, assists in production of adrenal steroids, cholesterol, RNA

Uses: Vit A deficiency

Dosage and routes:

- *Adult, child >8 yr:* PO 100,000-500,000 IU qd × 3 days, then 50,000 qd × 2 wk; dose based on severity of deficiency; maintenance 10,000-20,000 IU for 2 mo
- *Child 1-8 yr:* IM 5000-15,000 IU qd × 10 days
- *Infants <1 yr:* IM 5000-15,000 IU × 10 days

Maintenance

- *Child 4-8 yr:* IM 15,000 IU qd × 2 mo

V

• *Child <4 yr:* IM 10,000 IU qd × 2 mo

Available forms: Caps 10,000, 25,000, 50,000 IU; drops 5000 IU; inj 50,000 IU/ml; tabs 10,000, 25,000, 50,000 IU

Side effects/adverse reactions:

GI: Nausea, vomiting, anorexia, abdominal pain, ***jaundice***

CNS: Headache, ***increased intracranial pressure, intracranial hypertension,*** lethargy, malaise

EENT: Gingivitis, papilledema, exophthalmos, inflammation of tongue and lips

INTEG: Drying of skin, pruritus, increased pigmentation, night sweats, alopecia

MS: Arthralgia, retarded growth, hard areas on bone

META: Hypomenorrhea, hypercalcemia

Contraindications: Hypersensitivity to vit A, malabsorption syndrome (PO)

Precautions: Lactation, impaired renal function, pregnancy (A)

Pharmacokinetics:

PO/Inj: Stored in liver, kidneys, fat; excreted (metabolites) in urine, feces

Interactions:

• Decreased absorption of vit A: mineral oil, cholestyramine, colestipol

• Increased levels of vit A: corticosteroids, oral contraceptives

• Do not administer IV because of risk of anaphylactic shock

Lab test interferences:

False increase: Bilirubin, serum cholesterol

NURSING CONSIDERATIONS

Assess:

• Nutritional status: yellow and dark green vegetables, yellow/orange fruits, A-fortified foods, liver, egg yolks

• Vit A deficiency: decreased growth, night blindness, dry, brittle nails, hair loss, urinary stones, increased infection, hyperkeratosis of skin, drying of cornea

Administer:

• With food (PO) for better absorption

Perform/provide:

• Storage in tight, light-resistant container

Evaluate:

• Therapeutic response: increased growth rate, weight; absence of dry skin and mucous membranes, night blindness

Teach patient/family:

• Instruct patient that if dose is missed, it should be omitted

• Ophthalmic exams may be required periodically throughout therapy

• Not to use mineral oil while taking this drug

• To notify prescriber of nausea, vomiting, lip cracking, loss of hair, headache

• Not to take more than the prescribed amount

Treatment of overdose: Discontinue drug

vitamin D (cholecalciferol, vitamin D_3 or ergocalciferol, vitamin D_2) (℞, OTC)

Calciferol, Drisdol, Radiostol*, Radiostol Forte* Delta-D, Vitamin D, Vitamin D_3

Func. class.: Vit D

Chem. class.: Fat soluble

Action: Needed for regulation of calcium, phosphate levels, normal bone development, parathyroid activity, neuromuscular functioning

* Available in Canada only

Uses: Vit D deficiency, rickets, renal osteodystrophy, hypoparathyroidism, hypophosphatemia, psoriasis, rheumatoid arthritis

Dosage and routes:

Deficiency

- *Adult:* PO/IM 12,000 IU qd, then increased to 500,000 IU/day
- *Child:* PO/IM 1500/5000 IU qd × 2-4 wk, may repeat after 2 wk or 600,000 IU as single dose

Hypoparathyroidism

- *Adult and child:* PO/IM 200,000 IU given with 4 g Ca tab

Available forms: Tabs 400, 1000, 50,000 IU; caps 25,000, 50,000 IU; liq 8000 IU/ml; inj 500,000 IU/ml, 500,000 IU/5 ml

Side effects/adverse reactions:

GI: Nausea, vomiting, anorexia, cramps, diarrhea, constipation, metallic taste, dry mouth, decreased libido

CNS: Fatigue, weakness, drowsiness, ***convulsions,*** headache, psychosis

GU: Polyuria, nocturia, ***hematuria, albuminuria, renal failure***

CV: Hypertension, dysrhythmias

MS: Decreased bone growth, early joint pain, early muscle pain

INTEG: Pruritus, photophobia

Contraindications: Hypersensitivity, hypercalcemia, renal dysfunction, hyperphosphatemia

Precautions: Cardiovascular disease, renal calculi, pregnancy (A)

Pharmacokinetics:

PO/Inj: Half-life 7-12 hr; stored in liver, duration 2 mo; excreted in bile (metabolites) and urine

Interactions:

- Decreased effects of vit D: cholestyramine, colestipol, phenobarbital, phenytoin
- Increased toxicity: diuretics (thiazides), antacids, verapamil

NURSING CONSIDERATIONS

Assess:

- Vit D levels q2wk during treatment
- Ca, PO_4, Mg, BUN, alk phosphatase, urine Ca, creatinine
- In children, monitor height and weight
- Nutritional status: egg yolk, fortified dairy products, cod, halibut, salmon, sardines

Administer:

- IM inj deep in large muscle mass; administer slowly; aspirate carefully; rotate inj sites; avoid IV administration

Evaluate:

- Therapeutic response: absence of rickets/osteomalacia, adequate Ca/phosphate levels, decrease in bone pain

Teach patient/family:

- If dose is missed, omit
- Necessary foods in diet
- To avoid vitamin supplements unless directed by prescriber
- To keep doctor's appointments; line between therapeutic and toxic doses is narrow
- To report weakness, lethargy, headache, anorexia, loss of weight
- To report nausea, vomiting, abdominal cramps, diarrhea, constipation, excessive thirst, polyuria, muscle and bone pain
- To decrease intake of antacids and laxatives containing Mg

V

vitamin E (OTC)

Amino-Opti-E, Aquasol E, Daltose*, E-Complex-600, E-Ferol, E-Vitamin Succinate, E-200 I.U. Softgels, Gordo-Vite E, Tocopherol, Vitamin E, Vita-Plus E Softgells, Vitec

Func. class.: Vit E

Chem. class.: Fat soluble

Action: Needed for digestion and metabolism of polyunsaturated fats, decreases platelet aggregation, decreases blood clot formation, promotes normal growth and development of muscle tissue, prostaglandin synthesis

Uses: Vit E deficiency, impaired fat absorption, hemolytic anemia in premature neonates, prevention of retrolental fibroplasia, sickle cell anemia, supplement in malabsorption syndrome

Dosage and routes:

Deficiency

• *Adult:* PO 60-75 IU qd, not to exceed 300 IU/day

• *Child:* PO 1 mg/0.6 g of dietary fat

Prevention of deficiency

• *Adult:* PO 30 U/day; TOP apply to affected areas

Available forms: Caps 100, 200, 400, 500, 600, 1000 IU; tabs 100, 200, 400 IU; drops 50 mg/ml; chew tabs 400 U; ointment, cream, lotion, oil

Side effects/adverse reactions:

META: Altered metabolism of hormones, thyroid, pituitary, adrenal, altered immunity

MS: Weakness

CNS: Headache, fatigue

GI: Nausea, cramps, diarrhea

GU: Gonadal dysfunction

CV: Increased risk of thrombophlebitis

EENT: Blurred vision

INTEG: Sterile abscess, contact dermatitis

Contraindications: None significant

Precautions: Pregnancy (A)

Pharmacokinetics:

PO: Metabolized in liver, excreted in bile

Interactions:

• Increased action of oral anticoagulants

• Decreased absorption: cholestyramine, colestipol, mineral oil, sucralfate

NURSING CONSIDERATIONS

Assess:

• Vit E levels during treatment

• Nutritional status: wheat germ, dark green leafy vegetables, nuts, eggs, liver, vegetable oils, dairy products, cereals

Administer:

• *PO:* Administer with or after meals

• *Chewable tabs:* Chew well

• *Sol:* May be dropped in mouth or mixed with food

• Topically to moisturize dry skin

Perform/provide:

• Storage in tight, light-resistant container

Evaluate:

• Therapeutic response: absence of hemolytic anemia, adequate vit E levels, improvement in skin lesions, decreased edema

Teach patient/family:

• Necessary foods in diet

• To omit if dose missed

• To avoid vitamin supplements unless directed by prescriber

warfarin (℞)

(war'far-in)

Coumadin, Sofarin, warfarin sodium, Warfilone Sodium*

Func. class.: Anticoagulant

Action: Interferes with blood clot-

* Available in Canada only

ting by indirect means; depresses hepatic synthesis of vit K-dependent coagulation factors (II, VII, IX, X)

Uses: Pulmonary emboli, deep vein thrombosis, MI, atrial dysrhythmias, postcardiac valve replacement

Dosage and routes:

• *Adult:* PO/IV 10-15 mg/day × 3 days, then titrated to prothrombin time qd

Available forms: Tabs 1 mg, 2, 2.5, 5, 7.5, 10 mg; inj 50 mg/2 ml

Side effects/adverse reactions:

GI: Diarrhea, nausea, vomiting, anorexia, stomatitis, cramps, ***hepatitis***

GU: ***Hematuria***

INTEG: Rash, dermatitis, urticaria, alopecia, pruritus

CNS: Fever

HEMA: ***Hemorrhage, agranulocytosis, leukopenia, eosinophilia***

Contraindications: Hypersensitivity, hemophilia, leukemia with bleeding, peptic ulcer disease, thrombocytopenic purpura, hepatic disease (severe), severe hypertension, subacute bacterial endocarditis, acute nephritis, blood dyscrasias, pregnancy (D), eclampsia, preeclampsia, lactation

Precautions: Alcoholism, elderly

Pharmacokinetics:

PO: Onset 12-24 hr, peak 1½-3 days, duration 3-5 days, half-life 1½-2½ days; metabolized in liver, excreted in urine/feces (active/inactive metabolites), crosses placenta, 99% bound to plasma proteins

Interactions:

• Increased action of warfarin: allopurinol, chloramphenicol, amiodarone, diflunisal, heparin, steroids, cimetidine, disulfiram, thyroid, glucagon, metronidazole, quinidine, sulindac, sulfinpyrazone, sulfonamides, clofibrate, salicylates, ethacrynic acids, indomethacin, mefenamic acid, oxyphenbutazones, phenylbutazone, cefamondole, chloral hydrate, cotrimoxazole, erythromycin, quinolone antibiotics, isoniazid, thrombolytic agents, tricyclic antidepressants

• Decreased action of warfarin: barbiturates, griseofulvin, ethchlorvynol, carbamazepine, rifampin, oral contraceptives, phenytoin, estrogens, vit K, cholestyramine, corticosteroids, mercaptopurine, sucralfate, vit K foods, vit supplement

• Increased toxicity: oral sulfonylureas, phenytoin

• Incompatible with amikacin, dextrose, epinephrine, metaraminol, oxytocin, promazine, tetracycline, vancomycin

Lab test interferences:

Increase: T_3 uptake

Decrease: Uric acid

NURSING CONSIDERATIONS

Assess:

• Blood studies (Hct, platelets, occult blood in stools) q3mo

• Prothrombin time, which should be 1½-2 × control, PT; often done qd initially or INR (international normalized ratio)

• Bleeding gums, petecchiae, ecchymosis, black tarry stools, hematuria

• Fever, skin rash, urticaria

• Needed dosage change q1-2wk; when stable, PT q3wk

Administer:

• IV after diluting with diluent provided (50 mg/2 ml); rotate vial, give through Y-tube or 3-way stopcock at ≤25 mg/min

• At same time each day to maintain steady blood levels

• Tabs whole or crushed

• Avoiding all IM injections that may cause bleeding

Perform/provide:

• Storage in tight container

Evaluate:
• Therapeutic response: decrease of deep vein thrombosis

Teach patient/family:
• To avoid OTC preparations that may cause serious drug interactions unless directed by prescriber
• To use soft-bristle toothbrush to avoid bleeding gums, and to use electric razor
• To carry a Medic Alert ID identifying drug taken
• Importance of compliance
• To report any signs of bleeding: gums, under skin, urine, stools
• To avoid hazardous activities (football, hockey, skiing), dangerous work
• Importance of avoiding unusual changes in vitamin intake, diet or life-style
• To inform dentists and other physicians of anticoagulant intake
• That smoking increases dose requirements

Treatment of overdose: Administer vit K

xylometazoline (nasal) (OTC)

(xye-loe-met-az'oh-leen)
Otrivin, Otrivin Pediatric Nasal Drops, xylometazoline HCl

Func. class.: Nasal decongestant

Chem. class.: Sympathomimetic amine

Action: Dilates arterioles of nasal membrane, which decreases congestion

Uses: Nasal congestion

Dosage and routes:
• *Adult, child >12 yr:* INSTILL 2-3 gtt or 2 sprays q8-10h (0.1%)
• *Child <12 yr:* INSTILL 2-3 gtt or 1% spray q8-10h (0.05%)

Available forms: Sol 0.05%, 0.1%

Side effects/adverse reactions:
EENT: Irritation, burning, sneezing, stinging, dryness, rebound congestion
INTEG: Contact dermatitis

Contraindications: Hypersensitivity to sympathomimetic amines

Precautions: Pregnancy (C), glaucoma

Pharmacokinetics:
Instill: Onset 5-10 min, duration 5-6 hr

NURSING CONSIDERATIONS

Assess:
• Redness, swelling, pain in nasal passages

Administer:
• No more than q4h
• For <4 consecutive days

Perform/provide:
• Environmental humidification to decrease nasal congestion, dryness
• Storage in light-resistant containers; do not expose to heat

Evaluate:
• Therapeutic response: decreased nasal congestion

Teach patient/family:
• To avoid contamination of container
• That stinging may occur for a few applications; drying of mucosa may be decreased by environmental humidification
• To notify prescriber of irregular pulse, insomnia, dizziness, tremors
• Proper administration to avoid systemic absorption

* Available in Canada only

zalcitabine (℞)

(zal-sit'a-bin)

ddC, dideoxy-citidine, HIVID

Func. class.: Antiviral

Chem. class.: Synthetic pyrimidine nucleoside analog of 2'-deoxycytidine

Action: Inhibits HIV replication by the conversion of this drug by cellular enzymes to an active antiviral metabolite

Uses: Advanced HIV infections in adults, children >13 yr who cannot use zidovudine or who do not respond to treatment

Dosage and routes:

• *Adult:* PO combined with zidovudine in advanced HIV infection: 0.75 mg concomitantly with 200 mg zidovudine q8h; dosage reduction not necessary for patients weighing >30 kg; in presence of peripheral neuropathy initiate dose at 0.375 mg q8h of zalcitabine

Available forms: Tabs 0.375, 0.75 mg

Side effects/adverse reactions:

GI: Pancreatitis, diarrhea, nausea, vomiting, abdominal pain, constipation, stomatitis, dysplasia, liver abnormalities, oral ulcers, flatulence, taste perversion, dry mouth, oral thrush, melena, increased ALT (SGPT), AST (SGOT), alk phosphatase, amylase, increased bilirubin

GU: Uric acid, ***toxic nephropathy,*** polyuria

CNS: Headache, peripheral neuropathy, seizures, confusion, anxiety, hypertonia, abnormal thinking, asthenia, insomnia, CNS depression, pain, dizziness, chills, fever

RESP: Cough, pneumonia, dyspnea, asthma, hypoventilation

INTEG: Rash, pruritus, alopecia, sweating, acne

MS: Myalgia, arthritis, myopathy, muscular atrophy

CV: Hypertension, vasodilation, dysrhythmia, syncope, palpitation, tachycardia

EENT: Ear pain, otitis, photophobia, visual impairment

HEMA: ***Leukopenia, granulocytopenia, thrombocytopenia,*** anemia

Contraindications: Hypersensitivity

Precautions: Renal, hepatic disease, pregnancy (C), lactation, child <13 yr, peripheral neuropathy

Pharmacokinetics:

PO: Elimination half-life 1.62 hr; extensive metabolism is thought to occur; administration within 5 min of food will decrease absorption

Interactions:

• Increased risk of pancreatitis with agents that can cause pancreatitis

• Increased risk of peripheral neuropathy with other agents that can cause peripheral neuropathy: chloramphenicol, cisplatin, dapsone, disulfiram, ethionamide, glutethimide, gold, hydralazine, iodoquinol, isoniazid, metronidazole, nitrofurantoin, phenytoin, ribavirin, vincristine; use with didenosine is not recommended

• Decreased absorption: ketoconazole, dapsone, food

• Do not administer with tetacyclines

• Decreased concentrations of fluoroquinolone antibiotics

NURSING CONSIDERATIONS

Assess:

• Neuropathy: tingling or pain in hands and feet, distal numbness

• Pancreatitis: abdominal pain, nausea, vomiting, elevated liver enzymes; drug should be discontinued, since condition can be fatal

Z

• Children by dilated retinal examination q6mo to rule out retinal depigmentation
• CBC, differential, platelet count qwk; withhold drug if WBC is <4000 or platelet count is <75,000; notify prescriber
• Renal function studies: BUN, serum uric acid, urine CrCl before, during therapy
• Temp q4h; may indicate beginning infection
• Liver function tests before, during therapy (bilirubin, AST [SGOT], ALT [SGPT]) prn or qmo

Administer:
• Antibiotics: for prophylaxis of infection

Perform/provide:
• Strict medical asepsis, protective isolation if WBC levels are low
• Clean-up of powdered products; use wet mop or damp sponge

Evaluate:
• Therapeutic response: absence of infection; symptoms of HIV

Teach patient/family:
• To report signs of infection: fever, sore throat, flu symptoms
• To report signs of anemia: fatigue, headache, faintness, shortness of breath, irritability
• To report bleeding; avoid use of razors, commercial mouthwash
• That hair may be lost during therapy; a wig or hairpiece may make patient feel better

zidovudine (℞)

(zye-doe′-vue-deen)
Apo-Zidovudine*, Azidothymidine, AZT, Novo-AZT*, Retrovir
Func. class.: Antiviral
Chem. class.: Thymidine analog

Action: Inhibits replication of HIV virus by incorporating into cellular DNA by viral reverse transcriptase, thereby terminating the cellular DNA chain

Uses: Symptomatic HIV infections (AIDS, ARC), confirmed *P. carinii* pneumonia, or absolute CD4 lymphocytes of <200/mm^3

Dosage and routes:
• *Adult:* PO 200 mg q4h; may have to stop treatment if severe bone marrow depression occurs, and restart after bone marrow recovery; IV 1-2 mg/kg q4h, initiate PO as soon as possible

Available forms: Caps 100 mg; inj 200 mg/20 ml; oral syr 50 mg/5 ml

Side effects/adverse reactions:
HEMA: ***Granulocytopenia, anemia***
CNS: Fever, headache, malaise, diaphoresis, dizziness, *insomnia,* paresthesia, somnolence, chills, tremor, twitching, anxiety, confusion, depression, lability, vertigo, loss of mental acuity
GI: Nausea, vomiting, diarrhea, anorexia, cramps, *dyspepsia,* constipation, dysphagia, *flatulence,* rectal bleeding, mouth ulcer
RESP: Dyspnea
EENT: Taste change, hearing loss, photophobia
INTEG: Rash, acne, pruritus, urticaria
MS: Myalgia, arthralgia, muscle spasm
GU: Dysuria, polyuria, frequency, hesitancy

Contraindications: Hypersensitivity

Precautions: Granulocyte count <1000/mm^3 or Hgb <9.5 g/dl, pregnancy (C), lactation, child, severe renal disease, severe hepatic function

Pharmacokinetics:
PO: Rapidly absorbed from GI tract, peak ½-1½ hr, metabolized in liver (inactive metabolites), excreted by kidneys

* Available in Canada only

Interactions:

• Toxicity: amphotericin B, dapsone, flucytosine, adriamycin, interferon, vincristine, vinblastine, pentamidine, probenecid, experimental nucleoside analogs, benzodiazepines, cimetidine, morphine, sulfonamides

• Granulocytopenia: acetaminophen, aspirin, indomethacin

Y-site compatibilities: Acyclovir, amikacin, amphotericin B, aztreonam, ceftazidine, ceftriaxone, cimetidine, clindamycin, dexamethasone, dobutamine, dopamine, erythromycin lactobionate, fluconazole, fludarabine, gentamicin, heparin, imipenem/cilastatin, lorazepam, metoclopramide, morphine, nafcillin, ondansetron, oxacillin, pentamidine, phenylephrine, piperacillin, potassium chloride, ranitidine, sargramostim, tobramycin, trimethoprim-sulfamethoxazole, vancomycin

NURSING CONSIDERATIONS

Assess:

• Blood counts q2wk; watch for decreasing granulocytes, Hgb; if low, therapy may have to be discontinued and restarted after hematologic recovery; blood transfusions may be required

Administer:

• IV after diluting each 1 mg/0.25 ml or more D_5W to 4 mg/ml or less; give over 1 hr

• By mouth; capsules should be swallowed whole

• Trimethoprim-sulfamethoxazole, pyrimethamine, or acyclovir as ordered to prevent opportunistic infections; if these drugs are given, watch for neurotoxicity

Perform/provide:

• Storage in cool environment; protect from light

Evaluate:

• Blood dyscrasias (anemia, granulocytopenia): bruising, fatigue, bleeding, poor healing

Teach patient/family:

• That GI complaints and insomnia resolve after 3-4 wk of treatment

• That drug is not cure for AIDS but will control symptoms

• To notify prescriber of sore throat, swollen lymph nodes, malaise, fever; other infections may occur

• That patient is still infective, may pass AIDS virus on to others

• That follow-up visits must be continued since serious toxicity may occur; blood counts must be done q2wk

• That drug must be taken q4h around clock, even during night

• That serious drug interactions may occur if OTC products are ingested; check with prescriber before taking aspirin, acetaminophen, indomethacin

• That other drugs may be necessary to prevent other infections

• That drug may cause fainting or dizziness

zinc (ophthalmic) (OTC)

Eye-Sed Ophthalmic

Func. class.: Misc ophthalmic

Chem. class.: Zinc product

Action: Vasoconstriction occurs by action on conjunctiva

Uses: Ocular congestion, irritation, itching

Dosage and routes:

• *Adult, child >2 yr:* INSTILL 1-2 gtt bid or tid

Available forms: Sol 0.217%, 0.25%

Side effects/adverse reactions:

EENT: Eye irritation, burning

Contraindications: Hypersensitivity

Precautions: Narrow-angle glaucoma, pregnancy (C)

NURSING CONSIDERATIONS

Perform/provide:
- Storage in tight container

Evaluate:
- Therapeutic response: decreased ocular irritation, itching, congestion

Teach patient/family:
- To report change in vision, irritation
- Method of instillation; tilt head back, hold dropper over eye, drop medication inside lower lid, using pressure on inside corner of eye hold 1 min; not to touch dropper to eye
- If pain/irritation persists discontinue use, consult prescriber

---

zinc (℞, OTC)

Orazinc, PMS Egozine*, Verazinc, Zinca-Pak, Zincate, Zinc 15, Zinc-220, zinc sulfate

Func. class.: Trace element; nutritional supplement

Action: Needed for adequate healing, bone and joint development (23% zinc)

Uses: Prevention of zinc deficiency, adjunct to vit A therapy

Investigational uses: Wound healing

Dosage and routes:

Dietary supplement
- *Adult:* PO 25-50 mg/day

Nutritional supplement (IV)
- Adult IV 2.5-4 mg/day; may increase by 2 mg/day if needed
- *Child 1-5 yr:* IV 100 μg/kg/day
- *Infant <1.5-3 kg:* IV 300 μg/kg/day

Available forms: Tabs 66, 110 mg; caps 220 mg; inj 1 mg, 5 mg/ml

Side effects/adverse reactions:

GI: Nausea, vomiting, cramps, heartburn, ulcer formation

Overdose: Diarrhea, rash, dehydration, restlessness

Precautions: Pregnancy (A)

Interactions:
- Decreased absorption of other covalent cations

NURSING CONSIDERATIONS

Assess:
- Zinc levels during treatment

Administer:
- With meals to decrease gastric upset; to avoid dairy products

Evaluate:
- Therapeutic response: absence of zinc deficiency

Teach patient/family:
- That element must be taken for 2 mo to be effective
- To report immediately nausea, diarrhea, rash, severe vomiting, restlessness, abdominal pain, tarry stools

---

zolpidem (℞)

(zole-pi'dem)

Ambien

Func. class.: Sedative-hypnotic

Chem. class.: Nonbenzodiazepine of imidazopyridine class

Action: Produces CNS depression at limbic, thalamic, hypothalamic levels of CNS; may be mediated by neurotransmitter-aminobutyric acid (GABA); results are sedation, hypnosis, skeletal muscle relaxation, anticonvulsant activity, anxiolytic action

Uses: Insomnia, short-term treatment

Dosage and routes:
- *Adult:* PO 10 mg hs × 7-10 days only; total dose should not exceed 10 mg

Available forms: Tabs 5, 10 mg

Side effects/adverse reactions:

HEMA: ***Leukopenia, granulocytopenia*** (rare)

---

* Available in Canada only

CNS: Headache, lethargy, drowsiness, daytime sedation, dizziness, confusion, light-headedness, anxiety, irritability, amnesia, poor coordination
GI: Nausea, vomiting, diarrhea, heartburn, abdominal pain, constipation
CV: Chest pain, palpitation
Contraindications: Hypersensitivity to benzodiazepines
Precautions: Anemia, hepatic disease, renal disease, suicidal individuals, drug abuse, elderly, psychosis, child <18 yr, seizure disorders, pregnancy (B), lactation
Pharmacokinetics:
PO: Onset 1.5 hr, metabolized by liver, excreted by kidneys (inactive metabolites), crosses placenta, excreted in breast milk; half-life 2-3 hr
Interactions:
• Increased action of both drugs: alcohol, CNS depressants
Lab test interferences:
• *Increase:* ALT (SGPT), AST (SGOT), serum bilirubin
• *Decrease:* RAI uptake
• *False increase:* Urinary 17-OHCS

NURSING CONSIDERATIONS
Assess:
• Blood studies: Hct, Hgb, RBC, if blood dyscrasias are suspected (rare)
• Hepatic studies: AST (SGOT), ALT (SGPT), bilirubin if liver damage has occurred
• Mental status: mood, sensorium, affect, memory (long, short)
• Blood dyscrasias: fever, sore throat, bruising, rash, jaundice, epistaxis (rare)
• Type of sleep problem: falling asleep, staying asleep
Administer:
• After removal of cigarettes to prevent fires
• After trying conservative measures for insomnia
• ½-1 hr before hs for sleeplessness
• On empty stomach for fast onset but may be taken with food if GI symptoms occur
Perform/provide:
• Assistance with ambulation after receiving dose
• Safety measure: side rails, nightlight, call bell within easy reach
• Checking to see PO medication has been swallowed
• Storage in tight container in cool environment
Evaluate:
• Therapeutic response: ability to sleep at night, decreased amount of early morning awakening if taking drug for insomnia
Teach patient/family:
• That dependence is possible after long-term use
• To avoid driving or other activities requiring alertness until drug is stabilized
• To avoid alcohol ingestion, CNS depressants; serious CNS depression may result
• That effects may take 2 nights for benefits to be noticed
• Alternative measures to improve sleep: reading, exercise several hours before hs, warm bath, warm milk, TV, self-hypnosis, deep breathing
• That hangover is common in elderly but less common than with barbiturates; rebound insomnia may occur for 1-2 nights after discontinuing drug
Treatment of overdose: Lavage, activated charcoal; monitor electrolytes, vital signs

Appendix a

Selected new drugs

acarbose (℞)

(ay-car′bose)

Precose

Func. class.: Oral hypoglycemic

Chem. class.: α-Glucosidase inhibitor

Action: Delays digestion of ingested carbohydrates, results in smaller rise in blood glucose after meals; does not increase insulin production

Uses: Non-insulin-dependent diabetes mellitus (NIDDM) Type II

Dosage and routes:

- *Adult:* PO 25 mg tid initially, with first bite of meal; maintenance dose may be increased to 50 mg tid; may be increased to 100 mg tid if needed (only in patients >60 kg) with dosage adjustment at 4-9 wk intervals

Available forms: Tabs 50, 100 mg

Side effects/adverse reactions:

GI: Abdominal pain, diarrhea, flatulence

Contraindications: Hypersensitivity, diabetic ketoacidosis, cirrhosis, inflammatory bowel disease, colonic ulceration, partial intestinal obstruction, chronic intestinal disease

Precautions: Pregnancy (B), renal disease, lactation, children, hepatic disease

Pharmacokinetics:

Metabolized in GI tract, excreted as intact drug in urine, half-life 2 hr

Interactions:

- Effect of acarbose may be decreased: digestive enzymes, intestinal absorbents
- Increased hypoglycemia: sulfonylureas, insulin

Lab test interferences:

- *Decrease:* Hct
- *Increase:* AST

NURSING CONSIDERATIONS

Assess:

- Hypoglycemia, hyperglycemia; even though drug does not cause hypoglycemia, if patient is on sulfonylureas or insulin, hypoglycemia may be additive

Administer:

- Tid with first bite of each meal

Perform/provide:

- Storage in tight container in cool environment

Evaluate:

- Therapeutic response: decreased signs/symptoms of diabetes mellitus (polyuria, polydipsia, polyphagia, clear sensorium, absence of dizziness, stable gait)

Teach patient/family:

- Symptoms of hypo/hyperglycemia, what to do about each
- That medication must be taken as prescribed; explain consequences of discontinuing medication abruptly
- To avoid OTC medications unless approved by health-care provider
- That diabetes is life-long illness; that this drug is not a cure
- To carry a Medic Alert ID for emergency purposes

• That diet and exercise regimen must be followed

alendronate (℞)

(al-en-drone'ate)

Fosamax

Func. class.: Bone-resorption inhibitor

Chem. class.: Biphosphonate

Action: Absorbs calcium phosphate crystal in bone and may directly block dissolution of hydroxyapatite crystals of bone; inhibits bone resorption, apparently without inhibiting bone formation, mineralization

Uses: Osteoporosis in postmenopausal women, Paget's disease

Dosage and routes:

Osteoporosis in postmenopausal women

• *Adult and elderly:* PO 10 mg qd

Paget's disease

• *Adult and elderly:* PO 40 mg qd × 6 mo

Available forms: Tabs 10, 40 mg

Side effects/adverse reactions:

META: Anemia, hypokalemia, hypomagnesemia, hypophosphatemia

GI: Abdominal pain, anorexia, constipation, nausea, vomiting

MS: Bone pain

CV: Hypertension

GU: UTI, fluid overload

Contraindications: Hypersensitivity to biphosphonates

Precautions: Children, lactation, pregnancy (C), renal disease

Pharmacokinetics: Rapidly cleared from circulation, taken up mainly by bones, eliminated primarily through kidneys

NURSING CONSIDERATIONS

Assess:

• Electrolytes: renal function studies; Ca, P, Mg, K

• For hypercalcemia: paresthesia, twitching, laryngospasm, Chvostek's, Trousseau's signs

Administer:

• PO for 6 months to be effective in Paget's disease

Perform/provide:

• Storage in cool environment, out of direct sunlight

Evaluate:

• Therapeutic response: increased bone mass, absence of fractures

bicalutamide (℞)

(bye-kal-u'ta-mide)

Casodex

Func. class.: Antineoplastic

Chem. class.: Non-steroidal antiandrogen

Action: Binds to cytosol androgen in target tissue, which competitively inhibits the action to androgens

Uses: Prostate cancer in combination with luteinizing hormone-releasing hormone (LHRH) analog

Dosage and routes:

• *Adult:* PO 50 mg qd with LHRH

Available forms: Tabs 50 mg

Side effects/adverse reactions:

GI: Diarrhea, constipation, nausea, vomiting, increased liver enzyme test

CV: Hot flashes, hypertension

CNS: Dizziness, paresthesia, insomnia

INTEG: Rash, sweating

GU: Nocturia, hematuria, UTI, impotence, gynecomastia, urinary incontinence

MISC: Infection, anemia, dyspnea, bone pain, headache, asthenia, back pain, flu syndrome

Contraindications: Hypersensitivity, pregnancy (X)

Precautions: Renal, hepatic disease, elderly, lactation

Pharmacokinetics: Well absorbed, metabolized by liver, excreted in urine, feces

Interactions:

- May displace anticoagulants from their binding sites

Lab test interferences:

- *Increase:* AST, ALT, bilirubin, BUN, creatinine
- *Decrease:* Hgb, WBC

NURSING CONSIDERATIONS

Assess:

- For diarrhea, constipation, nausea, vomiting
- For hot flashes, gynecomastia (assure patient that these are common side effects)
- Prostate specific antigen (PSA), liver function studies

Administer:

- At same time each day, either AM or PM, with/without food
- With LHRH treatment

Evaluate:

- Therapeutic response: decreased tumor size, spread of malignancy

Teach patient/family:

- To recognize, report signs of anemia, hepatoxicity, renal toxicity

carvedilol (℞)

(kar-ved'i-lole)

Coreg

Func. class.: Alpha/beta-adrenergic blocker

Action: A mixture of nonselective α-and β-adrenergic blocking activity; decreases cardiac output, exercise-induced tachycardia, reflex orthostatic tachycardia; causes vasodilation, reduction in peripheral vascular resistance

Uses: Essential hypertension alone or in combination with other antihypertensives

Investigational uses: CHF, angina pectoris, idiopathic cardiomyopathy

Dosage and routes:

Essential hypertension

- *Adult:* PO 6.25 mg bid × 7-14 days; if tolerated well, then increase to 12.5 mg bid × 7-14 days; if tolerated well, may be increased (if needed) to 25 mg bid; not to exceed 50 mg qd

Congestive heart failure

- *Adult:* PO 12.5-50 mg bid

Angina pectoris

- *Adult:* PO 25-50 mg bid

Idiopathic cardiomyopathy

- *Adult:* PO 6.25-25 mg bid

Available forms: Tabs 6.25, 12.5, 25 mg

Side effects/adverse reactions:

CNS: Dizziness, somnolence, insomnia, ataxia, hyperesthesia, paresthesia, vertigo, depression

GI: Diarrhea, abdominal pain

CV: Bradycardia, postural hypotension, dependent edema, peripheral edema, ***AV block,*** extrasystoles, hypertension, hypotension, palpitations, peripheral ischemia

RESP: Rhinitis, pharyngitis, dyspnea

MISC: Fatigue, injury, back pain, UTI, viral infection, hypertriglyceridemia, ***thrombocytopenia***

Contraindications: Hypersensitivity, bronchial asthma, class IV decompensated cardiac failure, 2nd- or 3rd-degree heart block, cardiogenic shock, severe bradycardia

Precautions: Cardiac failure, hepatic injury, peripheral vascular disease, anesthesia, major surgery, diabetes mellitus, thyrotoxicosis, elderly, pregnancy (C), lactation, children, emphysema, chronic bronchitis

Pharmacokinetics: Readily and extensively absorbed PO, >98% bound to plasma proteins, extensively metabolized by liver, excreted through bile into feces, terminal half-life 5-9 hr with increases in elderly, hepatic disease

Interactions:

• Increased hypoglycemia: antidiabetic agents
• Decreased heart rate, b/p: clonidine
• Increased concentrations of digoxin
• Increased levels of carvedilol: cimetidine
• Decreased levels of carvedilol: rifampin

NURSING CONSIDERATIONS

Assess:

• Renal studies, including protein, BUN, creatinine; watch for increased levels that may indicate nephrotic syndrome; obtain baselines in renal, liver function studies before beginning treatment
• I&O, weight daily
• B/P during beginning treatment, periodically thereafter; pulse q4h, note rate, rhythm, quality
• Apical/radial pulse before administration; notify prescriber of significant changes
• Edema in feet, legs daily

Administer:

• PO ac, hs; tablets may be crushed or swallowed whole
• Reduced dosage in renal dysfunction

Evaluate:

• Therapeutic response: decreased B/P in hypertension

Teach patient/family:

• To comply with dosage schedule, even if feeling better
• To rise slowly to sitting or standing position to minimize orthostatic hypotension
• To report bradycardia, dizziness, confusion, depression, fever
• To take pulse at home; advise when to notify prescriber
• Not to discontinue drug abruptly

dirithromycin (℞)

(dye-rith-roe-mye'sin)
Dynabac
Func. class.: Antiinfective
Chem. class.: Macrolide

Action: Binds to 50S ribosomal subunits of susceptible bacteria, suppresses protein synthesis

Uses: Infections of the respiratory tract caused by *Moraxella catarrhalis, Streptococcus* sp., *(S. pneumoniae, S. agalactiae, S. viridans), Legionella pneumophilia, Mycoplasma pneumoniae, S. pyogenes, Staphylococcus aureus, Bordetella pertussis, Propionibacterium acnes*

Dosage and routes:

• *Adult:* PO 500 mg qd, given for 7-14 days depending on infections

Available forms: Tabs, enteric coated 250 mg

Side effects/adverse reactions:

GI: Abdominal pain, nausea, diarrhea, vomiting, dyspepsia, GI disorders, flatulence, abnormal stools, anorexia, constipation, ***pseudomembranous colitis***

CNS: Headache, dizziness, insomnia

HEMA: Increased platelet count, increased eosinophils

RESP: Cough, dyspnea

INTEG: Pruritus, urticaria

Contraindications: Hypersensitivity to this drug or any other macrolide, or erythromycin, bacteremias

Precautions: Elderly, pregnancy (C), lactation, children, hepatic, renal disease

Pharmacokinetics: Rapidly absorbed, widely distributed, no hepatic metabolism, excreted in bile, feces (up to 97%), plasma half-life 8 hr, terminal 44 hr

Interactions:

• Absorption of dirithromycin slightly enhanced: antacids, H_2 antagonists

NURSING CONSIDERATIONS

Assess:

• I&O ratio; report hematuria, oliguria in renal disease

• Liver studies: AST, ALT

• Renal studies: Urinalysis, protein, blood

• C&S before drug therapy; drug may be given as soon as culture is taken; C&S may be repeated after treatment

• Bowel pattern before, during treatment; pseudomembranous colitis may occur

• Skin eruptions, itching

• Respiratory status: rate, character, wheezing, tightness in chest; discontinue drug

• Allergies before treatment, reaction of each medication; place allergies on chart, notify all people giving drugs

Administer:

• Adequate intake of fluids (2 L) during diarrhea episodes

• Whole; do not cut, crush, chew tablets

• With food or within 1 hr of food

Perform/provide:

• Storage at room temp, in tight container

Evaluate:

• Therapeutic response: C&S negative for infection

Teach patient/family:

• To take with full glass of water; to give with food

• To report sore throat, fever, fatigue; may indicate superinfection

• To notify nurse of diarrhea stools, dark urine, pale stools, yellow discoloration of eyes or skin, severe abdominal pain

• To take at evenly-spaced intervals; complete dosage regimen

Treatment of hypersensitivity: Withdraw drug, maintain airway, administer epinephrine, aminophylline, O_2, IV corticosteroids

lamivudine (3TC) (℞)

(lam-i-voo'deen)

Epivir

Func. class.: Antiviral

Action: Inhibits replication of HIV virus by incorporating into cellular DNA by viral reverse transcriptase, thereby terminating cellular DNA chain

Uses: HIV infection in combination with zidovudine

Dosage and routes:

• *Adult and adolescents:* (12-16 yr): PO 150 mg bid with zidovudine; <50 kg (110 lbs): PO 2 mg/kg bid with zidovudine

• *Child:* 3 months-12 yr: PO 4 mg/kg bid, may be given 150 mg bid with zidovudine

Dosage adjustment is required in renal function impairment

Available forms: Tabs 150 mg; oral sol 10 mg/ml

Side effects/adverse reactions:

HEMA: ***Neutropenia, anemia, thrombocytopenia***

CNS: Fever, headache, malaise, dizziness, insomnia, depression

GI: Nausea, vomiting, diarrhea, anorexia, cramps, dyspepsia

RESP: Cough

EENT: Taste change, hearing loss, photophobia

INTEG: Rash

MS: Myalgia, arthralgia, pain

Contraindications: Hypersensitivity

Precautions: Granulocyte count $<1000/mm^3$ or Hgb <9.5 g/dl, pregnancy (C), lactation, child, severe renal disease, severe hepatic function, pancreatitis

Pharmacokinetics: Rapidly absorbed, distributed to extravascular space, excreted unchanged in urine

Interactions:

• Increased level of zidovudine when given with lamivudine

• Increased level of lamivudine: trimethoprim-sulfamethoxazole

NURSING CONSIDERATIONS

Assess:

• Blood counts q2wk; watch for neutropenia, thrombocytopenia, Hgb; if low, therapy may have to be discontinued and restarted after hematologic recovery; blood transfusions may be required

Administer:

• PO bid

• With zidovudine only

Perform/provide:

• Storage in cool environment; protect from light

Evaluate:

• Blood dyscrasias: bruising, fatigue, bleeding, poor healing

Teach patient/family:

• That GI complaints, insomnia resolve after 3-4 wk of treatment

• That drug is not a cure for AIDS, but will control symptoms

• To notify prescriber of sore throat, swollen lymph nodes, malaise, fever; other infections may occur

• That patient is still infective, may pass HIV virus on to others

• That follow-up visits must be continued since serious toxicity may occur; blood counts must be done q2wk

• That drug must be taken twice a day, even if patient feels better

• That other drugs may be necessary to prevent other infections

• That drug may cause fainting or dizziness

lansoprazole (℞)

(lan-so-prey'zole)

Prevacid

Func. class.: Antisecretory compound-proton pump inhibitor

Chem. class.: Benzimidazole

Action: Suppresses gastric secretion by inhibiting hydrogen/potassium ATPase enzyme system in gastric parietal cell; characterized as gastric acid pump inhibitor, since it blocks final step of acid production

Uses: Gastroesophageal reflux disease (GERD), severe erosive esophagitis, poorly-responsive systemic GERD, pathologic hypersecretory conditions (Zollinger-Ellison syndrome, systemic mastocytosis, multiple endocrine adenomas); possibly effective for treatment of duodenal ulcers

Dosage and routes:

Duodenal ulcer

• *Adult:* PO 15 mg qd before eating for 4 wk

Erosive esophagitis

• *Adult:* PO 30 mg qd before eating for up to 8 wks, may use another 8 wk course if needed

Pathological hypersecretory conditions

• *Adult:* PO 60 mg qd, may give up to 90 mg bid

Available forms: Caps, delayed rel 15, 30 mg

Side effects/adverse reactions:

CNS: Headache, dizziness, confusion, agitation, amnesia, depression

GI: Diarrhea, abdominal pain, vomiting, nausea, constipation, flatulence, acid regurgitation, anorexia, irritable colon

RESP: Upper respiratory infections, cough, epistaxis, asthma, bronchitis, dyspnea

INTEG: Rash, urticaria, pruritus, alopecia
META: Weight gain/loss, gout
EENT: Tinnitus, taste perversion, deafness, eye pain, otitis media
CV: Chest pain, angina, tachycardia, bradycardia, palpitations, ***CVA,*** hypertension/hypotension, ***MI, shock,*** vasodilation
GU: ***Hematuria,*** glycosuria, impotence, kidney calculus, breast enlargement
HEMA: ***Hemolysis,*** anemia
Contraindications: Hypersensitivity
Precautions: Pregnancy (B), lactation, children
Pharmacokinetics: Absorption after granules leave stomach, rapid, plasma half-life 1.5 hr, protein binding 97%, extensively metabolized in liver, excreted in urine, feces; clearance decreased in the elderly, renal and hepatic impairment
Interactions:
• Decreased clearance of theophylline when given with lansoprazole
• Delayed absorption of lansoprazole: sucralfate
• May be decreased absorption of: ketoconazole, ampicillin iron, digoxin
NURSING CONSIDERATIONS
Assess:
• GI system: bowel sounds q8h, abdomen for pain, swelling, anorexia
• Hepatic enzymes: AST (SGOT), ALT (SGPT), alk phosphatase during treatment
Administer:
• Before eating; swallow capsule whole; do not open, chew, or crush caps
Evaluate:
Therapeutic response: absence of epigastric pain, swelling, fullness
Teach patient/family:
• To report severe diarrhea; drug may have to be discontinued
• That diabetic patient should know that hypoglycemia may occur
• To avoid hazardous activities; dizziness may occur
• To avoid alcohol, salicylates, ibuprofen; may cause GI irritation

moexipril (℞)

(moe-ox'a-prile)
Univasc
Func. class.: Antihypertensive
Chem. class.: Angiotensin-converting enzyme inhibitor

Action: Selectively suppresses renin-angiotensin-aldosterone system; inhibits ACE; prevents conversion of angiotensin I to angiotensin II; results in dilation of arterial, venous vessels
Uses: Hypertension, alone or in combination with thiazide diuretics
Dosage and routes:
• *Adult:* PO 7.5 mg 1 hr ac initially, may be increased or divided depending on B/P response; maintenance dosage; 7.5-30 mg qd in 1-2 divided doses 1 hr ac
Available forms: Tabs 7.5, 15 mg
Side effects/adverse reactions:
CV: Hypotension, postural hypotension
GU: Impotence, dysuria, nocturia, proteinuria, nephrotic syndrome, acute reversible renal failure, polyuria, oliguria, frequency
HEMA: ***Neutropenia***
INTEG: Rash
RESP: ***Bronchospasm,*** dyspnea, cough
META: Hypokalemia
GI: Loss of taste
CNS: Fever, chills
SYST: ***Angioedema***
Contraindications: Hypersensitivity, children, lactation, heart block, bilateral renal stenosis, K-sparing diuretics

Precautions: Dialysis patients, hypovolemia, leukemia, scleroderma, lupus erythematosus, blood dyscrasias, CHF, diabetes mellitus, renal disease, thyroid disease, COPD, asthma, pregnancy (C)
Pharmacokinetics: Metabolized by liver (metabolites), excreted in urine; crosses placenta; excreted in breast milk
Interactions:
• Increased hypotension: diuretics, other antihypertensives, ganglionic blockers, adrenergic blockers
• Do not use with potassium-sparing diuretics, sympathomimetics, potassium supplements
Lab test interferences:
• *False positive:* Urine acetone
NURSING CONSIDERATIONS
Assess:
• Blood studies: neutrophils, decreased platelets
• B/P
• Renal studies: protein, BUN, creatinine; watch for increased levels that may indicate nephrotic syndrome
• Baselines in renal, liver function test before therapy begins
• K levels, although hyperkalemia rarely occurs
• Edema in feet, legs daily
• Allergic reaction: rash, fever, pruritus, urticaria; drug should be discontinued if antihistamines fail to help
• Symptoms of CHF; edema, dyspnea, wet rales, B/P
• Renal symptoms: polyuria, oliguria, frequency
Administer:
• PO 1 hr before meals
Perform/provide:
• Storage in tight container at 86° F or less
Evaluate:
• Therapeutic response: decrease in B/P in hypertension
Teach patient/family:
• To take 1 hr ac
• Not to discontinue drug abruptly
• Not to use OTC (cough, cold, or allergy) products unless directed by prescriber
• To comply with dosage schedule, even if feeling better
• To rise slowly to sitting or standing position to minimize orthostatic hypotension
• To notify prescriber of mouth sores, sore throat, fever, swelling of hands or feet, irregular heartbeat, chest pain, signs of angioedema
• That excessive perspiration, dehydration, vomiting, diarrhea may lead to fall in blood pressure; consult prescriber if these occur
• That dizziness, fainting, lightheadedness may occur during first few days of therapy
• That skin rash or impaired perspiration may occur
• How to take B/P
Treatment of overdose: 0.9% NaCl IV inf, hemodialysis

mycophenolate mofetil (℞)

(mye-koe-phen′oh-late)
CellCept
Func. class.: Immunosuppressive

Action: Inhibits inflammatory responses that are mediated by the immune system; prolongs the survival of allogenic transplants
Uses: Organ transplants (to prevent rejection)
Dosage and routes:
• *Adult:* PO give initial dose 72 hr prior to transplantation; 1 g bid given to renal transplant patients in combination with corticosteroids, cyclosporine

Available forms: Caps 250 mg
Side effects/adverse reactions:
GI: Nausea, vomiting, stomatitis
HEMA: ***Leukopenia, thrombocytopenia, anemia, pancytopenia***
INTEG: Rash
MS: Arthralgia, muscle wasting
RESP: Dyspnea, respiratory infection, increased cough, pharyngitis, bronchitis, pneumonia
CNS: Tremor, dizziness, insomnia, headache, fever
META: Peripheral edema, hypercholesteremia, hypophosphatemia, edema, hyperkalemia, hypokalemia, hyperglycemia
GU: UTI, hematuria, ***renal tubular necrosis***
Contraindications: Hypersensitivity to this drug or mycophenolic acid
Precautions: Lymphomas, malignancies, neutropenia, renal disease, pregnancy (C), lactation
Interactions:
- Increased concentration of both drugs: acyclovir, ganciclovir
- Increased levels of mycophenolate: probenecid, salicylate
- Decreased levels of mycophenolate: antacids, cholestyramine
- Decreased binding of phenytoin, theophylline

Pharmacokinetics: Rapidly, completely absorbed, metabolized to active metabolite (MPA), excreted in urine, feces

NURSING CONSIDERATIONS
Assess:
- Blood studies: CBC during treatment monthly
- Liver function studies: alk phosphatase, AST (SGOT), ALT (SGPT), bilirubin

Administer:
- 72 hr prior to transplantation; may be given in combination with corticosteroids, cyclosporine
- Give alone for better absorption

Evaluate:
- Therapeutic response: absence of graft rejection

Teach patient/family:
- To report fever, rash, severe diarrhea, chills, sore throat, fatigue, since serious infections may occur
- To reduce risk of infection by avoiding crowds

nalmefene
(nal'mah-feen)
Revex
Func. class.: Opioid antagonist
Chem. class.: Analog of naltrexone

Action: Competes with opioids at opioid receptor sites; prevents or reverses the effects of opioids
Uses: Reversal of opioid effects, management of known or suspected opioid overdose
Dosage and routes:
Opioid overdose
- *Adult (green label):* Titrate to reverse effects of opioids; 0.5 mg/70 kg, may give 1 mg/70 kg at 2-5 min intervals; since this drug is longer acting, use incremental dosing to avoid over-reversal

Postoperative opioid depression
- *Adult (blue label):* 0.25 µ/kg, then 0.25 µg/kg at 2-5 min ntervals

Available forms: Inj 1 mg/ml
Side effects/adverse reactions:
CNS: Drowsiness, nervousness, dizziness, headache, chills, fever
CV: Tachycardia, hypertension, hypotension, vasodilation, bradycardia
GI: Nausea, vomiting, diarrhea
Contraindications: Hypersensitivity
Precautions: Pregnancy (B), children, opioid dependency, lactation, respiratory depression, renal or hepatic disease, elderly

Pharmacokinetics: Complete bioavailability, rapidly distributed, metabolized by liver, excreted in urine, terminal half-life approx 40 min, 10-15 hr

Interactions:

- Seizures: flumazenil

NURSING CONSIDERATIONS

Assess:

- Withdrawal: cramping, hypertension, anxiety, vomiting
- VS q3-5min
- ABGs, including Po_2, Pco_2
- Cardiac status: tachycardia, hypertension; monitor ECG
- Respiratory dysfunction: respiratory depression, character, rate, rhythm; if respirations are <10/min, administer this drug; probably due to opioid overdose; monitor LOC

Administer:

- Only with resuscitative equipment, O_2 nearby

Perform/provide:

- Storage at room temperature

Evaluate:

- Therapeutic response: reversal of respiratory depression; LOC-alert

tramadol (℞)

(tram'a-dole)

Ultram

Func. class.: Central analgesic

Action: Not completely understood, binds to opioid receptors, inhibits reuptake of norepinehprine, serotonin; does not cause histamine release or affect heart rate

Uses: Management of moderate to severe pain

Dosage and routes:

- *Adult:* PO 50-100 mg prn q4-6 h; not to exceed 400 mg/day
- *Elderly (>75 years):* PO <300 mg/day in divided dose

Hepatic impairment: PO 50 mg q12h

Available forms: Tabs 50 mg

Side effects/adverse reactions:

CNS: Dizziness, CNS stimulation, somnolence, headache, anxiety, confusion, euphoria, ***seizure,*** hallucinations

GI: Nausea, constipation, vomiting, dry mouth, diarrhea, abdominal pain, anorexia, flatulence, ***GI bleeding***

CV: Vasodilation, orthostatic hypotension, tachycardia, hypertension, abnormal ECG

INTEG: Pruritus, rash, urticaria, vesicles

GU: Urinary retention/frequency, menopausal symptoms, dysuria, menstrual disorder

Interactions:

- Decreased levels of tramadol: carbamazepine
- Inhibition of norepinephrine and serotonin reuptake: MAO inhibitors, use together with caution

Lab test interferences:

- *Increase:* Creatinine, liver enzymes
- *Decrease:* Hgb

Contraindications: Hypersensitivity, acute intoxication with any CNS depressant

Precautions: Seizure disorder, pregnancy (C), lactation, children, elderly, renal or hepatic disease, respiratory depression, head trauma, increased intracranial pressure, acute abdominal condition, drug abuse

Pharmacokinetics: Rapidly and almost completely absorbed, steady state 2 days, may cross blood-brain barrier, extensively metabolized, 30% excreted in the urine as unchanged drug

NURSING CONSIDERATIONS

Assess:

- Pain: location, type, character; give before pain becomes extreme
- I&O ratio: check for decreasing output; may indicate urinary retention
- Need for drug

- For constipation: increase fluids, bulk in diet
- CNS changes: dizziness, drowsiness, hallucinations, euphoria, LOC, pupil reaction
- Allergic reactions: rash urticaria

Administer:

- With antiemetic for nausea, vomiting
- When pain is beginning to return; determine dosage interval by patient response

Perform/provide:

- Storage in cool environment, protected from sunlight
- Assistance with ambulation
- Safety measures: side rails, night light, call bell within easy reach

Evaluate:

- Therapeutic response: decrease in pain

Teach patient/family:

- To report any symptoms of CNS changes, allergic reactions
- That drowsiness, dizziness, and confusion may occur, to call for assistance
- To make position changes slowly, orthostatic hypotension may occur
- To avoid OTC medications and alcohol unless approved by prescriber

Appendix b

Controlled substance chart

Drugs	United States	Canada
Heroin, LSD, peyote, marijuana, mescaline	Schedule I	Schedule H
Opium (morphine), meperidine, amphetamines, cocaine, short-acting barbiturates (secobarbital)	Schedule II	Schedule G
Glutethimide, paregoric, phen-dimetrazine	Schedule III	Schedule F
Chloral hydrate, chlordiazepox-ide, diazepam, mazindol, mep-robamate, phenobarbital (Canada-G)	Schedule IV	Schedule F
Antidiarrheals with opium (Canada-G), antitussives	Schedule V	Schedule F

Appendix c

FDA pregnancy categories

A No risk demonstrated to the fetus in any trimester

B No adverse effects in animals, no human studies available

C Only given after risks to the fetus are considered; animal studies have shown adverse reactions, no human studies available

D Definite fetal risks, may be given in spite of risks if needed in life-threatening conditions

X Absolute fetal abnormalities; not to be used anytime during pregnancy

Appendix d

Commonly used antibiotics in adults and children

amoxicillin

Adult: PO 750 mg-1.5 g qd in divided doses q8h
Child: PO 20-40 mg/kg/day in divided doses q8h

ampicillin

Adult: PO 1-2 g qd in divided doses q6h
IM/IV 2-8 g qd in divided doses q4-6h
Child: PO 50-100 mg/kg/day in divided doses q6h
IM/IV 100-200 mg/kg/day in divided doses q6h

cefaclor

Adult: PO 250-500 mg q8h
Child: PO 24-40 mg/kg/day in divided doses q8h

cephalexin

Adult: PO 250-500 mg q6h
Child: PO 25-50 mg/kg/day in 4 equal doses

chloramphenicol

Adult and child >3 mo: 50-100 mg/kg/day in divided doses q6h

clindamycin

Adult: PO 150-450 mg q6h
IM/IV 300 mg q6-12h
Child >1 mo: PO 8-25 mg/kg/day in divided doses q6-8h
IM/IV 15-40 mg/kg/day in divided doses q6-8h

erythromycin

Adult: 250-500 mg q6h
Child: 30-50 mg/kg/day in divided doses q6h

gentamicin

Adult: IV INF 3-5 mg/kg/day in divided doses q8h
Child: IV/IM 2-2.5 mg/kg q8h
Neonates and infants: IV/IM 2.5 mg/kg q8h

kanamycin

Adult and child: IV INF/IM 15 mg/kg/day in divided doses q8-12h

methicillin

Adult: IM/IV 4-12 g/day in divided doses q4-6h
Child: IM/IV 50-300 mg/kg/day in divided doses q4-12h
PO 25-50 mg/kg/day in divided doses q6h
Neonates: IM 10 mg/kg q12h

nafcillin

Adult: PO/IM/IV 2-6 g/day in divided doses q4-6h
Child: IM 25 mg/kg q12h

oxacillin

Adult: PO 2-6 g/day in divided doses q4-6h
IM/IV 2-12 g/day in divided doses q4-6h
Child: PO/IM/IV 50-100 mg/kg/day in divided doses q6h

penicillin G benzathine

Adult: IM 1.2 million U

penicillin G potassium

Adult: PO 400,000-500,000 U q6-8h
Child <12 yr: PO 25,000-90,000 U/kg/day in 3-6 divided doses

penicillin G procaine

Adult and child: IM 600,000-1.2 million U in 1-2 doses/day
Newborn: IM 50,000 U/kg qd

nitrofurantoin

Adult and child >12 yr: PO 50-100 mg qid pc

sulfisoxazole

Adult: PO 2-4 g loading dose, then 1-2 g qid
Child >2 mo: PO 75 mg/kg or 2 g/m^2 loading dose, then 150 mg/kg/day or 4 g/m^2/day in divided doses q6h

ticarcillin

Adult: IV/IM 12-24 g/day in divided doses q3-6h
Child: IV/IM 50-300 mg/kg/day in divided doses q4-8h
Neonates: IV INF 75-100 mg/kg q8-12h

APPENDIX

Appendix e

Formulas for drug calculations

Surface area rule:

$$\text{Child dose} = \frac{\text{Surface area (m}^2\text{)}}{1.73\text{m}^2} \times \text{Adult dose}$$

Calculating strength of a solution:

Solution Strength: *Desired Solution:*

$$\frac{x}{100} = \frac{\text{Amount of drug desired}}{\text{Amount of finished solution}}$$

Calculating flow rate for IV:

$$\text{Rate of flow} = \frac{\text{Amount of fluid} \times \text{Administration set calibration}}{\text{Running time}}$$

$$\frac{x}{1} = \frac{\text{(ml) (gtt/min)}}{\text{min}}$$

Calculation of medication dosages:

Formula method:

$$\frac{\text{Amount ordered}}{\text{Amount on hand}} \times \text{Vehicle} = \text{Number of tablets, capsules, or amount of liquid}$$

Vehicle is the drug form or amount of liquid containing the dosage. Amounts used in calculation by formula must be in same system.

Ratio—proportion method:

1 tablet:tablet in mg on hand: :x tablet order in mg

Know or have: :Want to know or order

Multiply means and extremes, divide both sides by known amount to get X. Amounts used in equation must be in same system.

Dimensional analysis method:

$$\text{Order in mg} \times \frac{\text{1 tablet or capsule}}{\text{What 1 tablet or capsule is in mg}} = \text{Tablets or capsules to be given}$$

If amounts are in different systems:

$$\text{Order in mg} \times \frac{\text{1 tablet or capsule}}{\text{What 1 tablet or capsule is in g}} \times \frac{1}{\text{1000 mg}} = \text{Tablets or capsules to be given}$$

Appendix f

Nomogram for calculation of body surface area

Place a straight edge from the patient's height in the left column to the patient's weight in the right column. The point of intersection on the body surface area column indicates the body surface area (BSA). (Reproduced from Behrman RE, and Vaughn VC (editors): *Nelson's textbook of pediatrics,* ed 12, Philadelphia, 1983, WB Saunders.)

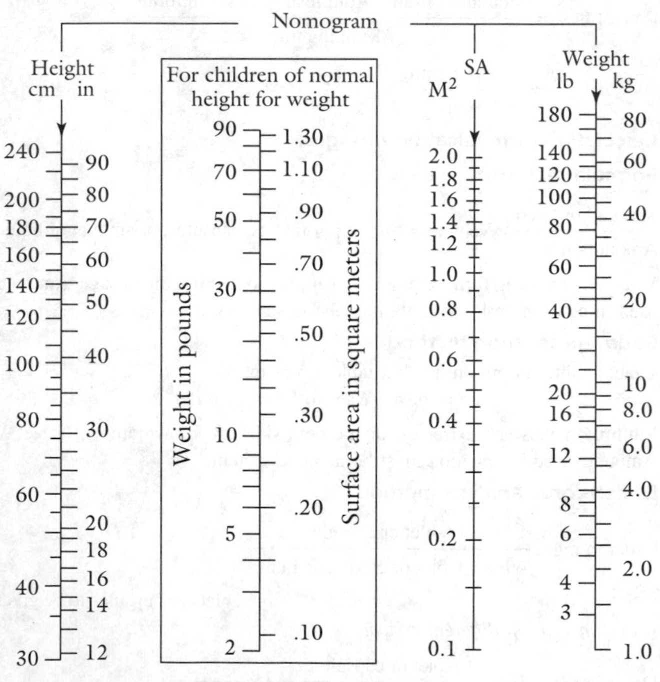

Appendix g

Weights and equivalents

METRIC SYSTEM

Weight

kilogram	= kg	=	1000 grams
gram	= g	=	1 gram
milligram	= mg	=	0.001 gram
microgram	= µg	=	0.001 milligram

Volume

liter	= L	=	1 L
milliliter	= ml	=	0.001 L

AVOIRDUPOIS WEIGHT

1 ounce (oz)= 437.5 grains
1 pound (lb)= 16 ounces = 7000 grains

METRIC AND APOTHECARY EQUIVALENTS

Exact weight equivalents

Metric	*Apothecary*
1 mg	1/64.8 grain
64.8 mg	1 grain
324 mg	5 grains
1 g	15.432 grains
31.103 g	1 ounce = 480 grains

Exact volume equivalents

Metric	*Apothecary*		
1.00 ml	16.23 minims		
3.69 ml	1 fluidram	=	60 minims
29.57 ml	1 fluidounce	=	480 minims
473.16 ml	1 pint	=	7680 minims
946.33 ml	1 quart	=	15,360 minims

Appendix h

Home care medication record

Home care medication record

Patient's Name Age	Sex Allergies	
Pharmacy	Caffeine	Smoking
Physician	Alcohol	Herb tea/home rem.
OTC medications: Name, dose, route, regiment	Tube feeding: Ostomy?	Difficulty swallowing?
Antacids, antidiarrheals/laxatives, hemorrhoidal, emetic/antemetic, cough/cold, analgesics, vitamins/minerals/iron, sleep aids, ophthalmic/otic, topical/lotion/ointments, other	COMMENTS:	

PRESCRIPTION MEDICATIONS MT = Medication teaching sheet requested? Yes (Y) or No (N)

Date ordered	Medication—strength, route, frequency of administration	N/C	MT	Indication	Side effects discussed with patient	Date given	Date return

COMMENTS TO PHARMACIST		
White—chart Yellow—pharmacist Pink—nurse	NURSE	DATE

Appendix i

Bibliography

Clark JB, Queener SF, Karb VB: *Pharmacological basis of nursing practice,* ed 4, St Louis, 1994, Mosby–Year Book.

Drug Information 94: Bethesda, 1994, American Hospital Formulary Service.

Facts and Comparisons: Philadelphia, updated monthly, JB Lippincott.

Gahart BL: *Intravenous medications,* ed 11, St Louis, 1995, Mosby-Year Book.

Goodman A and others: *Goodman and Gilman's The pharmacological basis of therapeutics,* ed 9, New York, 1994, Pergamon Press.

McKenry LM, Salerno E: *Mosby's pharmacology in nursing,* ed 18, St Louis, 1992, Mosby–Year Book.

Mediphor Editorial Group: *Drug interaction facts,* Philadelphia, updated quarterly, JB Lippincott.

Appendix j

Abbreviations

abd abdomen
ABG arterial blood gas
ac before meals
ACE angiotensin-converting enzyme
ADA American Diabetes Association
ADH antidiuretic hormone
ALT alanine aminotransferase
ANA antinuclear antibody
AP anteroposterior
APTT activated partial thromboplastin time
ASA acetylsalicylic acid, aspirin
ASHD arteriosclerotic heart disease
AST aspartate aminotransferase (SGOT)
AV atrioventricular
bid twice a day
BM bowel movement
BMR basal metabolic rate
B/P blood pressure
BPH benign prostatic hypertrophy
BPM beats per minute
BS blood sugar
BUN blood urea nitrogen
C Celsius (centigrade)
Ca cancer
CAD coronary artery disease
cap capsule
Cath catheterization or catheterize
CBC complete blood cell count
CC chief complaint
cc cubic centimeter
CHF congestive heart failure
cm centimeter
CNS central nervous system
CO_2 carbon dioxide
CONT continuous
COPD chronic obstructive pulmonary disease
CPAP continuous positive airway pressure
CPK creatinine phosphokinase
CPR cardiopulmonary resuscitation
CrCl creatinine clearance
C&S culture and sensitivity
C sect cesarean section
CSF cerebrospinal fluid
CV cardiovascular
CVA cerebrovascular accident
CVP central venous pressure
D&C dilatation and curettage
DIR INF direct infusion
dr dram
D_5W 5% glucose in distilled water
ECG electrocardiogram (EKG)
EDTA ethylenediamine tetraacetic acid
EEG electroencephalogram
EENT ear, eye, nose, and throat
EPS extrapyramidal symptom
ESR erythrocyte sedimentation rate
EXT
REL extended release
EXTRA
STREN
SUSP extra strength suspension
FBS fasting blood sugar
FHT fetal heart tones
FSH follicle-stimulating hormone
g gram
GABA γ-aminobutyric acid
GI gastrointestinal
gr grain
GTT glucose tolerance test
gtt drops
GU genitourinary
H_2 histamine$_2$

HCG human chorionic gonadotropin
Hct hematocrit
HDCV human diploid cell rabies vaccine
Hgb hemoglobin
H & H hematocrit and hemoglobin
5-HIAA 5-hydroxyindoleacetic acid
HIV human immunodeficiency virus (AIDS)
H_2O water
HOB head of bed
HR heart rate
hr hour
hs at bedtime
IgG immunolobulin G
IM intramuscular
INF infusion
INH inhalation
inj injection
I&O intake and output
IPPB intermittent positive-pressure breathing
ITP idiopathic thrombocytopenic purpura
IUD intrauterine device
IV intravenous
IVP intravenous pyelogram
K potassium
kg kilogram
L liter
lb pound
LDH lactic dehydrogenase
LE lupus erythematosus
LH luteinizing hormone
LLQ left lower quadrant
LMP last menstrual period
LOC level of consciousness
LR lactated Ringer's solution
LUQ left upper quadrant
M meter
m minim
m^2 square meter
MAOI monoamine oxidase inhibitor
mEq milliequivalent
mg milligram
μg microgram
MI myocardial infarction
min minute
ml milliliter
mm millimeter
mo month
Na sodium
neg negative
NPO nothing by mouth (Lat. *nulla per os*)
NS normal saline
O_2 oxygen
OBS organic brain syndrome
OD right eye
OR operating room
os left eye
OTC over-the-counter
OU each eye
oz ounce
p̄ after
P56 plasma-lyte 56
$PaCO_2$ arterial carbon dioxide tension (pressure)
PaO_2 arterial oxygen tension (pressure)
PAT paroxysmal atrial tachycardia
PBI protein-bound iodine
PCWP pulmonary capillary wedge pressure
PEEP positive end-expiratory pressure
PERRLA pupils equal, round, react to light and accommodation
pH hydrogen ion concentration
PO by mouth
postop postoperative
PP postprandial
preop preoperative
prn as required
PT prothrombin time
PTT partial thromboplastin time
PVC premature ventricular contraction
q every
qAM every morning
qd every day
qh every hour
q2h every 2 hours
q3h every 3 hours
q4h every 4 hours
q6h every 6 hours
q12h every 12 hours
qid four times daily
qod every other day
qPM every night

qs sufficient quantity
qt quart
R right
RAIU radioactive iodine uptake
RBC red blood count or cell
RLQ right lower quadrant
ROM range of motion
RUQ right upper quadrant
SC subcutaneous
SIMV synchronous intermittent mandatory ventilation
SL sublingual
SLE systemic lupus erythematosus
SOB shortness of breath
sol solution
ss one half
suppos suppository
sus rel sustained release
Syr syrup
T&A tonsillectomy and adenoidectomy
tab tablet
tbsp tablespoon
temp temperature
tid three times daily
tinc tincture
TPN total parenteral nutrition
top topical
TRANS transdermal
TSH thyroid-stimulating hormone
tsp teaspoon
TT thrombin time
U unit
UA urinalysis
UTI urinary tract infection
UV ultraviolet
vag vaginal
VMA vanillylmandelic acid
vol volume
VS vital sign
WBC white blood cell count
wk week
wt weight
yr year
> greater than
< less than
= equal
° degree
% percent
γ gamma
β beta

Index

A
Abbokinase, 1074-1075
Abenol, 69-72
Absorbine, 1040
acarbose, 1101-1102
Accupril, 920-922
Accurbron, 1010-1012
Accutane, 587-588
acebutolol, 67-68
Aceon, 829-830
Aceta, 69-72
acetaminophen, 69-72
Acetaminophen Uniserts, 69-72
Acetazolam, 72-73
acetazolamide, 72-73
acetohexamide, 74-75
Acetonide, 1048-1049
acetylcysteine, 75-76
acetylsalicylic acid, 136-138
Aches-N-Pain, 549-550
Achromycin, 1006-1007
Achromycin Ophthalmic, 1007-1008
Achromycin (topical), 1008
Acne-10, 166-167
Acne-Aid, 166-167
acrivastine/pseudoephedrine, 76-77
Acrocillin, 815-816
ACT, 474-475
Acta-Char, 77-78
Acta-Char Liquid-A, 77-78
Actamin, 69-72
ACTH, 304-306
Acthar, 304-306
Acti-B_{12}, 541-542
Acticort 100, 535-536
Actidil, 1067-1068
Actidose-Aqua, 77-78
Actigall, 1075-1076
Actimmune, 574-575
Actinex, 642
Actiprofen, 549-550
Activase, 92-93
Activase rt-PA, 92-93
activated charcoal, 77-78
Actrapid, 565-566
Acu-Dyne, 874
Acular, 596-597
acyclovir, 79-81
acyclovir (topical), 78
Adalat, 760-761
Adavite, 731-732
Adenocard, 81
adenosine, 81
Adipex-P, 843-844
Adipost, 835-836
A-D Kaopectate II Caplets, 625-626
Adrenalin Chloride, 412-415
Adriamycin, 395-397
Adrucil, 476-478
Adsorbocarpine, 854-855
Adsorbonac Ophthalmic Solution, 959
Advil, 549-550
Advil Cold and Sinus, 910
AeroBid, 473-474
Aerolate, 1010-1012
Aerolone, 583-584
Aeroseb-Dex, 339-341
Aeroseb-HC, 535-536
Aerosporin, 868-869
Afrin, 791
Afrin Children's Nose Drops, 791
Aftate, 1040
Agoral Plain, 716-717

Entries can be identified as follows: generic name, Trade Name, DRUG CATEGORY, *Combination Product.*

A-Hydrocort, 536-538
a-2-interferon, 571-572
Airbron, 75-76
Akarpine, 854-855
AK-Chlor, 253-254
AK-Con Ophthalmic, 745
AK-Dex, 342
AK-Dilate Ophthalmic, 848-849
Akineton, 176-177
AK-Mycin, 420-421
AK-NaCl, 959
AK-Nefrin Ophthalmic, 848-849
Akne-Mycin, 421
AK-Pentolate, 314-315
AK-Pred, 882-883
AK-Sulf, 977-978
AK-Tracin, 157
AK-Zol, 72-73
Ala-Cort, 535-536
Ala-Scalp, 535-536
Alatel, 1006-1007
Alazine, 530-532
Albalon Liquifilm Ophthalmic, 745
albumin, normal serum, 82-83
Albuminar, 82-83
Albutein, 82-83
albuterol, 83-84
Alcomicin, 499-500
Alconefrin, 847-848
Aldactone, 966-967
aldesleukin, 84-86
Aldomet, 690-691
alendronate, 1102
Aleve, 745-746
Alfenta, 86-87
alfentanil, 86-87
Alferon N, 572-573
alglucerase, 87-88
Alka-Mints, 200-201
Alkeran, 654-656
Alleract, 1067-1068
Aller-Chlor, 261-262
Allerdryl, 378-380
Allerest Eye Drops, 745
Allerest 12-Hour Nasal, 791
Allerid, 910-911
AllerMax, 378-380
allopurinol, 88-89
Aloe Extra, 611
Alophen, 840
ALPHA-ADRENERGIC BLOCKERS, 1
Alpha-Baclofen, 158-159
Alphaderm, 535-536
Alphamin, 541-542
Alpha-Nine SD, 448-449
Alphatrex, 171-173
alprazolam, 89-90
alprostadil, 91-92
Altace, 927-928
alteplase, 92-93
AlternaGEL, 95-96
altretamine, 93-94
Alu-Cap, 95-96
Alugel, 95-96
aluminum acetate, 94-95
aluminum hydroxide, 95-96
Alupent, 670-671
Alu-Tab, 95-96
Alzapam, 627-629
amantadine, 96-97
amantadine HCl, 96-97
Ambien, 1098-1099
Amcill, 124-125
amcinonide, 97
Amcort, 1047-1048
Amen, 650-651
Amersol, 549-550
amethopterin, 683-685
Amicar, 103-104
Amidate, 445
Amigesic, 942-943
amikacine, 98-99
amikacin sulfate, 98-99
Amikin, 98-99
amiloride, 99-101
amiloride HCl, 99-101
amino acid injection, 101-102

Entries can be identified as follows: generic name, Trade Name, DRUG CATEGORY, *Combination Product.*

amino acid solution, 102-103
aminocaproic acid, 103-104
Aminofen, 69-72
aminoglutethimide, 104-105
Amino-Opti-E, 1092
aminophylline, 105-107
Aminosyn, 102-103
amiodarone, 107-109
amiodipine, 110-111
Amitone, 200-201
Amitril, 109-110
amitriptyline, 109-110
amitriptyline HCl, 109-110
ammonium chloride, 111-112
amobarbital, 113-115
amobarbital sodium, 113-115
Amodopal, 690-691
Amoline, 105-107
Amonidrin, 512-513
amoxapine, 115-116
amoxicillin, 118-119
amoxicillin/clavulanate potassium, 117-118
Amoxil, 118-119
amphetamine, 120-121
amphetamine sulfate, 120-121
Amphojel, 95-96
amphotericin B, 121-123
amphotericin B (topical), 123
ampicillin, 124-125
ampicillin, sulbactam, 125-127
Ampicin, 124-125
amrinone, 127-128
amyl nitrite, 128-129
Amyl Nitrite Aspirols, 128-129
Amyl Nitrite Vaporole, 128-129
Amytal, 113-115
Anacin-3 Infant's Drops, 69-72
Anacin-3 Maximum Strength, 69-72
Anadrol-50, 792-793
Anafranil, 290-291
Anapolon 50, 792-793
Anaprox DS, 745-746
Anaspaz, 548-549
Anbesol Maximum Strength, 164
Ancasal, 136-138
Ancef, 221-222
Ancobon, 468-469
Ancotil, 468-469
Andro-Cyp, 1002-1003
Andro L.A. 200, 1002-1003
Androlone-D 200, 742-744
Andronate, 1002-1003
Anectine, 974-976
Anergan, 898-899
Anestacon, 611-613
ANESTHETICS-GENERAL/LOCAL, 2-3
aniosoylated plasminogen, 129-130
anistreplase (APSAC), 129-130
Anorex, 835-836
Ansaid, 485-486
Antabuse, 384-385
ANTACIDS, 3-4
Antazone, 985
ANTIANGINALS, 5-6
ANTICHOLINERGICS, 6-8
ANTICOAGULANTS, 8-9
ANTICONVULSANTS, 10-11
ANTIDEPRESSANTS, 11-13
ANTIDIABETICS, 13-15
ANTIDIARRHEALS, 15-16
ANTIDYSRHYTHMICS, 16-18
Antiflux, 634-635
ANTIFUNGALS (SYSTEMIC), 18-20
antihemophilic factor (AHF), 130-132
ANTIHISTAMINES, 20-21
ANTIHYPERTENSIVES, 21-23
ANTIINFECTIVES, 23-25
Antilirium, 852
Antiminth, 912-913
ANTINEOPLASTICS, 25-27
ANTIPARKINSON AGENTS, 28-29
Antiple, 985

Entries can be identified as follows: generic name, Trade Name, DRUG CATEGORY, *Combination Product.*

ANTIPSYCHOTICS, 29-31
Antispas, 359-360
antithrombin III, human, 132
ANTITUBERCULARS, 31-32
Anti-tuss, 512-513
ANTITUSSIVES/
EXPECTORANTS, 32-34
Antivert, 648-649
ANTIVIRALS, 34-35
Antrizine, 648-649
Anturan, 985
Anturane, 985
Anxanil, 546-547
Apacet, 69-72
APL, 271-272
Apo-Acetaminophen, 69-72
Apo Allopurinol, 88-89
Apo-Alpraz, 89-90
Apo-Amitriptylin, 109-110
Apo-Amoxi, 118-119
Apo-Ampi, 124-125
Apo-ASA, 136-138
Apo-Asen, 136-138
Apo-Atenol, 139-141
Apo-Benztropin, 167-169
Apo-Bisacodyl, 177-178
Apo-C, 133-134
Apo-Carbamazepine, 207-208
Apo-Chlordiazepoxide, 255-257
Apo-Chlorthalidone, 266-267
Apo-Cimetidine, 273-275
Apo Cloxi, 297-298
Apo-Diltiaz, 373-374
Apo-Dipyridamole, 382-383
Apo-Doxy, 397-398
Apo-Erythro-EC, 422-424
Apo-Folic, 487-488
Apogen, 499-500
Apo-Guanethidine, 515-516
Apo-Haloperidol, 521-523
Apo-Hydroxyzine, 546-547
Apo-Ibuprofen, 549-550
Apo-Imipramine, 555-557
Apo-Indomethacin, 560-561
Apo-ISDN, 585-586
Apo-Lorazepam, 627-629
Apo-Methyldopa, 690-691
Apo-Metoprolol, 704-706
Apo-Metronidazole, 706-707
Apo-Napro-Na, 745-746
Apo-Naproxen, 745-746
Apo-Nifed, 760-761
Apo-Nitrofurantoin, 761-762
Apo-Oxazepam, 786-787
Apo-Oxtriphylline, 788-789
Apo-Pen-VK, 820-821
Apo-Perphenazine, 831-834
Apo-Piroxicam, 863-864
Apo-Prednisone, 883-884
Apo-Primidone, 885-886
Apo-Propanolol, 904-906
Apo-Quinidine, 923-924
Apo-Ranitidine, 929-930
Apo-Sulfamethoxazole, 980-982
Apo-Sulfatrim, 982-983
Apo-Sulfinpyrazone, 985
Apo-Sulin, 987-988
Apo-Tetra, 1006-1007
Apo-Triazo, 1051-1052
Apo-Zidovudine, 1096-1097
Apresoline, 530-532
APSAC, 129-130
A-200 Pyrinate, 913-914
Aquachloral Supprettes, 249-250
AquaMEPHYTON, 853-854
Aquaphyllin, 1010-1012
Aquasol A, 1089-1090
Aquasol E, 1092
Aqueous-Charcodote, 77-78
Aquest, 432-433
Aralen HCl, 258-259
Aralen Phosphate, 258-259
Arduran, 857-858
Aredia, 800
Argesic-SA, 942-943
Argyrol, 954
Aristocort, 1047-1048
Aristocort A, 1048-1049

Entries can be identified as follows: generic name, Trade Name, DRUG CATEGORY, *Combination Product.*

Aristocort (topical), 1048-1049
Aristospan, 1047-1048
Arm & Hammer Pure Baking Soda, 957-958
Arm-a-Med, 580-581
Arm-A-Med Metaproterenol Sulfate, 670-671
Armour Thyroid, 1023-1024
Arrestin, 1060-1061
Artane, 1057-1058
Arthra-G, 942-943
Arthrinol, 136-138
Arthrisin, 136-138
Arthropan, 270-271
Articulose-50, 880-882
Articulose L.A., 1047-1048
A.S.A., 136-138
A.S.A. and Codeine Compound No. 3 Pulvules, 136
Asacol, 667-668
Ascorbic Acid Caplets, 133-134
ascorbic acid (vitamin C), 133-134
Ascorbicap, 133-134
Ascriptin with Codeine, 136
Asendin, 115-116
Asmalix, 1010-1012
asparaginase, 134-136
Aspergum, 136-138
aspirin, 136-138
Aspirin-Free Pain Relief, 69-72
astemizole, 138-139
AsthmaHaler, 412-414
Asthma Nefrin, 412-414
Astramorph PF, 728-729
Atabrine HCl, 919-920
Atarax, 546-547
Atasol, 69-72
atenolol, 139-141
Ativan, 627-629
ATnativ, 132
Atolone, 1047-1048
atovaquone, 141-142
Atozine, 546-547
atracurium, 142-143
Atria S.R., 136-138
Atrohist Pediaetric, 910
Atromid-S, 288-289
Atropair, 143-145
Atro-Pen, 143-145
atropine, 143-145, 364-365
Atropine, 145-146
Atropine, Demerol Injection, 143
atropine (optic), 145-146
Atropine Sulfate, 145-146
atropine sulfate diphenoxylate, 364-365
Atropine Sulfate Injection, 728
Atropisol, 143-145
Atropisol (optic), 145-146
Atrovent, 577
A/T/S, 421
Augmentin, 117-118
auranofin, 146-147
aurothioglucose, 147-148
Aventyl, 770-772
Avitene, 713-714
Avlosulfon, 330-331
Axid, 765-766
Axotal, 136
Azactam, 153-154
azatadine, 148-149
azathioprine, 149-150
Azidothymidine, 1096-1097
azithromycin, 150-151
Azlin, 152-153
azlocillin, 152-153
Azmacort, 1047-1048
Azo Gantanol, 980
Azo-Standard, 834-835
Azo Sulfamethoxazole, 980
AZT, 1096-1097
aztreonam, 153-154
Azulfidine, 983-985

B

Baby Anbesol, 164
B-A-C, 136
bacampicillin, 154-156

Entries can be identified as follows: generic name, Trade Name, DRUG CATEGORY, *Combination Product.*

Bacarate, 835-836
Baciguent, 157-158
Baci-IM, 156
Bacitin, 157-158
bacitracin, 156
bacitracin (ophthalmic), 157
bacitracin (topical), 157-158
Bacitracin U.S.P., 156
baclofen, 158-159
B-A-C No. 3, 136
Bactine Hydrocortisone, 535-536
Bactocill, 781-783
Bactrim, 982-983
Bactroban, 732
BAL in Oil, 376-377
Balminil, 512-513
Balminil DM, 348-350
Bancap, 69-72
Bancap HC, 533
Banesin, 69-72
Banflex, 780-781
Banophen, 378-380
Banthine, 674-675
Barbidonna, 161
Barbita, 838-840
BARBITURATES, 35-36
Barc, 913-914
Baridium, 834-835
Basaljel, 95-96
Bayer, 136-138
Bayer Children's Aspirin, 136-138
Bayer Select Head Cold Caplets, 910
Bayer Select Maximum Strength Sinus Pain Relief Caplets, 910
Baylocaine, 611-613
b-Capsa 1, 517-518
BCNU, 213-214
BC Powder, 136
Beclo disk, 159-160
Becloforte Inhaler, 159-160
beclomethasone, 159-160
beclomethasone (nasal), 160-161
Beclovent Rotocaps, 159-160
Beconase, 160-161
Bedoz, 310-311
Beesix, 916
Belap, 161
Belix, 378-380
Belladenal-S, 161
belladonna alkaloids, 161-162
Bellafoline, 161-162
Bellalphen, 161
Bellans, 957-958
Bellergal-S, 418
Bena-D, 378-380
Benadryl, 378-380
Benahist, 378-380
Ben-Allergin-50, 378-380
Ben-Aqua, 166-167
benazepril, 162-164
Benemid, 886-887
Benisone, 173-174
Benoject, 378-380
Benophene, 903-904
Benoxyl, 166-167
Bensylate, 167-169
Bentyl, 359-360
Bentylol, 359-360
Benuryl, 886-887
Benylin, 378
Benylin Cough, 378-380
Benylin DM, 348-350
Benzac, 166-167
Benzacot, 1060-1061
Benzagel, 166-167
benzocaine (oral), 164
BENZODIAZEPINES, 37-38
benzonatate, 165
benzoyl peroxide, 166
benzquinamide, 167
benztropine, 167-169
benztropine mesylate, 167-169
bepridil, 169
beractant, 170-171
BETA-ADRENERGIC BLOCKERS, 38-40
Betacort, 171-173

Entries can be identified as follows: generic name, Trade Name, DRUG CATEGORY, *Combination Product.*

Beta Cort, 174
Betaderm, 171-173, 174
Betadine, 874
Betalin S, 1012-1013
Betaloc, 704-706
betamethasone, 173-174
betamethasone acetate, 171-173
Betamethasone Dipropionate, 171-173
betamethasone disodium phosphate, 171-173
betamethasone sodium phosphate, 171-173
betamethasone valerate, 174
Betapace, 962-964
Betapen-VK, 820-821
Betaseron, 573-574
Betatrex, 171-173, 174
Beta-2, 580-581
Beta-Val, 174
Beta-Val Betnelan, 171-173
Betaxin, 1012-1013
bethanechol, 174-175
bethanechol chloride, 174-175
Bethaprim, 982-983
Biamine, 1012-1013
Biaxin, 281-282
bicalutamide, 1102-1103
Bicillin, 813-815
Bicillin C-R, 813-815
BiCNU, 213-214
Biltricide, 878
Biocef, 242-243
Biodine Topical 1%, 874
biperiden, 176-177
Biphetamine, 347
bisacodyl, 177-178
Bisacodyl Uniserts, 177-178
Bisacolax, 177-178
Bisco-Lax, 177-178
Bismtral Pepto-Bismol, 178
bismuth subsalicylate, 178
bisoprolol, 179-180
bitolterol, 180-181
Bitrate, 821
Black Draught, 951-952
Blanex, 267
Blenoxane, 181-183
bleomycin, 181-183
Bleph-10, 977-978
BLM, 181-183
Blocadren, 1029-1030
Bluboro Powder, 94-95
Bonamine, 648-649
Bonine, 648-649
Bontril, 835-836
Boropak Powder, 94-95
Breonesin, 512-513
B_{12} Resin, 310-311
Brethaire, 998-999
Brethine, 998-999
Bretylate, 183-184
bretylium, 183-184
bretylium tosylate, 183-184
Bretylol, 183-184
Brevibloc, 424-425
Brevital Sodium, 682-683
Brevoxyl, 166-167
Bricanyl, 998-999
Brietal Sodium, 682-683
British Anti-Lewisite, 376-377
Brogan, 1060-1061
Bromfed PD, 910
bromocriptine, 184-185
bromopheniramine, 185-186
Bromo-seltzer, 69
Bromphen, 185-186
BRONCHODILATORS, 40-41
Broncho-Grippol-DM, 348-350
Bronitin Mist, 412-414
Bronkaid Mist, 412-414
Bronkephrine, 441-442
Bronkodyl, 1010-1012
Bronkometer, 580-581
Bronkosol, 580-581
Bucladin-S, 187
buclizine, 187
budesonide, 187-188

Entries can be identified as follows: generic name, Trade Name, DRUG CATEGORY, *Combination Product.*

bumetanide, 188-189
Bumex, 188-189
Buminate, 82-83
Buprenex, 189-190
buprenorphine, 189-190
bupropion, 191-192
Burcillin-G, 815-816
Burn Relief, 611
Burow's Solution, 94-95
BuSpar, 192-193
buspirone, 192-193
busulfan, 193-194
Butazolidin, 845-846
Butibel, 161
Butibel Elixir, 161
butoconazole, 194-195
butorphanol, 195-196
Byclomine, 359-360
Bydramine, 378-380

C
Cafergot, 418
Cafergot suppositories, 418
Caladryl, 300
Calan, 1082-1083
Cal Carb-HD, 200-201
Calci-Chew, 200-201
Calciday 667, 200-201
Calcidrine, 300
calcifediol, 196-197
Calciferol, 1090-1091
Calcijex, 199-200
Calcilean, 524-526
Calcimar, 198-199
Calci-Mix, 200-201
Calciparine, 524-526
calcitonin (human), 197-198
calcitonin (salmon), 198-199
calcitriol, 199-200
Calcium 600, 200-201
calcium carbonate, 200-201
CALCIUM CHANNEL BLOCKERS, 41-43
calcium chloride, 201-202
calcium disodium versenate, 403-404
calcium EDTA, 403-404
calcium gluceptate, 201-202
calcium gluconate, 201-202
calcium lactate, 201-202
calcium polycarbophil, 203
Caldecort Anti-Itch, 535-536
Calderol, 196-197
Caldesene, 1070-1071
Cal-Guard, 200-201
Calicylic Creme, 940-941
Calm-X, 375-376
Cal-Plus, 200-201
Caltrate, 200-201
CAM-AP-ES, 532
Campain, 69-72
camphorated opium tincture, 778-779
Canesten, 296-297
Cantil, 657-658
Cantri, 986
Capastat Sulfate, 203-204
Capital and Codeine, 300
Capital with Codeine, 69
Caposide, 204
Capoten, 204-206
capreomycin, 203-204
captopril, 204-206
Carafate, 976
carbachol, 206-207
carbamazepine, 207-208
Carbamex, 1072-1073
carbidopa-levodopa, 208-209
Carbocaine, 663-664
Carbocaine with Neo-Cobefrin, 663-664
Carbolith, 621-622
carboplatin, 209-211
carboprost, 211-212
Carboptic, 206-207
Cardene, 756-757
CARDIAC GLYCOSIDES, 43-44
Cardilate, 419-420

Entries can be identified as follows: generic name, Trade Name, DRUG CATEGORY, *Combination Product.*

Cardioquin, 923-924
Cardizem, 373-374
Cardura, 392-393
carisoprodol, 212-213
carmustine, 213-214
carteolol, 214-216
Cartrol, 214-216
carvedilol, 1103-1104
cascara sagrada, 216
Casodex, 1102-1103
Cataflam, 357-358
Catapres, 293-295
Catozym, 801-802
Caverject, 91-92
CCNU, 623-625
C-Crystals, 133-134
CdA, 279-280
CDDP Platinol, 277-279
Cebid Timecelles, 133-134
Ceclor, 217-218
Cecon, 133-134
Cedocard-SR, 585-586
CeeNU, 623-625
cefactor, 217-218
cefadroxil, 218-219
Cefadyl, 245-246
cefamandole, 219-221
cefazolin, 221-222
cefazolin sodium, 221-222
cefixime, 222-223
Cefizox, 237-239
cefmetazole, 223-225
Cefobid, 226-227
cefonicid, 225-226
cefoperazone, 226-227
ceforanide, 227-229
Cefotan, 230-231
cefotaxime, 229-230
cefotetan, 230-231
cefoxitin, 232-233
cefpodoxime, 233-234
cefprozil, 235-236
ceftazidime, 236-237
Ceftin, 240-242
ceftizoxime, 237-239
ceftriaxone, 239-240
cefuroxime, 240-242
Cefzil, 235-236
Celestone/Alphatrex, 171-173
Celestone Phosphate, 171-173
CellCept, 1108-1109
Celontin, 688-689
Cel-U-Jec, 171-173
Cena-K, 870-872
Cenocort, 1047-1048
Cenolate, 133-134
Centrax, 877-878
cephalexin, 242-243
cephalothin, 243-245
cephalothin sodium, 243-245
cephaprin, 245-246
cephaprin sodium, 245-246
cephradine, 247-248
Cephulac, 600
Ceporacin, 243-245
Ceporex, 242-243
Ceptaz, 236-237
Ceredase, 87-88
Cerespan, 803-804
Cermill, 133-134
Cerubidine, 331-333
Cervidil, 377-378
C.E.S., 430-432
Cetacort, 535-536
Cetane, 133-134
Cevalin, 133-134
Cevi-Bid, 133-134
Ce-Vi-Sol, 133-134
Charac-50, 77-78
Charcoaide, 77-78
Charcocaps, 77-78
Charcodote, 77-78
Charcotabs, 77-78
Chardonna-2, 161
Chealamide, 404-405
Checkmate, 474-475
Chemet, 974
Chenix, 248-249

Entries can be identified as follows: generic name, Trade Name, DRUG CATEGORY, *Combination Product.*

chenodiol, 248-249
Cherapas, 530
Chibroxin, 768-769
Children's Advil, 549-550
Children's Chloraseptic, 164
Children's Feverall, 69-72
Children's Hold, 348-350
Children's Hold 4 Hour, 348
Children's Sudafed, 910-911
Chlo-Amine, 261-262
chloral hydrate, 249-250
chlorambucil, 250-252
chloramphenicol, 252-253
chloramphenicol (ophthalmic), 253-254
chloramphenicol (otic), 254
chloramphenicol palmitate, 252-253
chloramphenicol sodium succinate, 252-253
chloramphenicol (topical), 254-255
Chlorate, 261-262
chlordiazepoxide, 255-257
chlordiazepoxide HCl, 255-257
Chlorofon-F, 267
Chloromycetin, 252-253, 254-255
Chloromycetin Ophthalmic, 253-254
Chloromycetin Otic, 254
Chloronase, 265-266
chloroprocaine, 257-258
Chloroptic, 253-254
chloroquine, 258-259
chloroquine phosphate, 258-259
Chloroserp, 930
Chloroserpine-250, 930
chlorothiazide, 259-261
Chlorpazine, 892-893
Chlorphed-LA, 791
chlorpheniramine, 261-262
chlorpheniramine maleate, 261-262
Chlor-Pro, 261-262
Chlorpromanyl, 262-265
chlorpromazine, 262-265
chlorpromazine HCl, 262-265
chlorpropamide, 265-266
Chlorspan-12, 261-262
Chlortab-4, 261-262
Chlortab-B, 261-262
chlorthalidone, 266-267
ChlorTrimeton, 261-262
Chlor-Trimeton Repetabs, 261-262
Chlorzone Forte, 267
chlorzoxazone, 267-268
Cholac, 600
Cholaxin, 1023-1024
cholecalciferol, 1090-1091
Choledyl, 788-789
cholestyramine, 269
CHOLINERGICS, 44-45
CHOLINERGIC BLOCKERS, 46-47
choline salicylate, 270-271
Cholybar, 269
Chooz, 200-201
Chorex, 271-272
chorionic gonadotropin, human, 271-272
Choron 10, 271-272
Chronulac, 600
Chymodiactin, 272-273
chymopapain, 272-273
Cibacalcin, 197-198
Cibalith-S, 621-622
ciclopirox, 273
Ciclosporine, 318-319
Cidomycin, 499-500
cilastatin/imipenem, 554-555
Cillium, 911-912
Ciloxan, 275-276
cimetidine, 273-275
Cin-Quin, 923-924
Cipro, 275-276
ciprofloxacin, 275-276
cisapride, 276-277
cisplatin, 277-279
Citrocarbonate, 957-958
Citrucel, 689-690
cladribine (CdA), 279-280
Claforan, 229-230

Entries can be identified as follows: generic name, Trade Name, DRUG CATEGORY, *Combination Product.*

Claripen, 288-289
Claripex, 288-289
clarithromycin, 281-282
Claritin, 627
clavulanate/amoxicillin, 117-118
clavulanate/ticarcillin, 1027-1028
Clavulin, 117-118
Clearasil, 166-167
Clear Away, 940-941
Clear Away Plantar, 940-941
Clear By Design, 166-167
Clear Eyes, 745
clemastine, 282-283
Cleocin, 284-285
clidinium, 283-284
Climestrone, 426-428
clindamycin, 284-285
Clindamycin HCl, 284-285
Clindamycin Phosphate, 284-285
Clindex, 255, 283
Clinoril, 987-988
Clinoxide, 255, 283
clioquinol, 285-286
Clipoxide, 255, 283
clobetasol, 286-287
clocortolone, 287
Cloderm, 287
clofazimine, 287-288
clofibrate, 288-289
Clomid, 289-290
clomiphene, 289-290
clomiphene citrate, 289-290
clomipramine, 290-291
clonazepam, 291-293
clonidine, 293-295
clonidine HCl, 293-295
Clopra, 700-701
clorazepate, 295-296
clorazepate dipotassium, 295-296
clotrimazole, 296-297
cloxacillin, 297-298
cloxacillin sodium, 297-298
Cloxapen, 297-298
clozapine, 298-300
Clozaril, 298-300
Cobex, 310-311
Cocrema Mercolized, 541
Codalan, 69
codeine, 300-301
Codimal-A, 185-186
Codoxy, 790
Cogentin, 167-169
Co-Gesic, 533
Cognex, 989-990
colchicine, 301-302
Colestid, 302-303
colestipol, 302-303
colfosceril, 303-304
Collyrium Fresh Eye Drops, 1009-1010
Combantrin, 912-913
Combipres, 293
Comfort Eye Drops, 745
Comoxol, 982-983
Compa-Z, 892-893
Compazine, 892-893
Compound W, 940-941
Compoz, 378-380
Comtrex, 348
Conar, 348-349
Concentraid, 337-338
Concentrated Aluminum Hydroxide, 95-96
Concentrated Multiple Trace Elements, 1042-1043
Concentrated Phillip's Milk of Magnesia, 638-639
Congespirin, Aspirin-Free, 69
conjugated estrogens, 430-432
Constant-T, 1010-1012
Constilac, 600
Constulose, 600
Contac Jr., 349
Contac Severe Cold Formula, 349
ConTE-PAK-4, 1042-1043
Contranzine, 892-893
Copavin Pulvules, 300
Cophene-B, 185-186

Entries can be identified as follows: generic name, Trade Name, DRUG CATEGORY, *Combination Product.*

Cordarone, 107-109
Cordran, 483-484
Coreg, 1103-1104
Corgard, 734-735
Coricidin Nasal Mist, 791
Coronex, 585-586
Corophyllin, 105-107
Correctol, 840
Correctol Extra Gentle, 387-388
Cortaid, 535-536
Cortamed, 535
Cort-Dome, 535-536
Cortef, 536-538
Cortef Feminine Itch, 535-536
Cortenema, 536-538
CORTICOSTEROIDS, 47-49
corticotropin, 304-306
cortisone, 306-307
Cortizone, 535-536
Cortone, 306-307
Cortril, 535-536
Cortrosyn, 307-308
Cosmegen, 324-325
cosyntropin, 307-308
Cotanal, 903-904
Cotane, 133-134
Cotazym, 801-802
Cotrim, 982-983
CoTylenol, 349
CoTylenol Cold Medication Tablets, 349
Coumadin, 1092-1094
Cozaar, 629
Cremacoat, 349
Creon Capsules, 801-802
cromolyn, 308-309
crotamiton, 309-310
Cruex, 1070-1071
Crystamine, 310-311
Crystapen, 818-820
Crysti-12, 310-311
Crysticillin A.S., 817-818
Crystodign, 367-368
C-Solve 2, 421
Cuprimine, 398-399
Curretab, 650-651
Cuticura Acne, 166-167
Cyanabin, 310-311
cyanocobalamin (vitamin B_{12}), 310-311
Cyanoject, 310-311
Cyclan, 311-312
cyclandelate, 311-312
cyclizine, 312-313
cyclobenzaprine, 313-314
cyclobenzaprine HCl, 313-314
Cyclocort, 97
Cycloflex, 313-314
Cyclogyl, 314-315
Cyclomen, 327-328
Cyclomydril Ophthalmic, 314
cyclopentolate, 314-315
cyclophosphamide, 315-317
cycloserine, 317-318
Cyclospasmol, 311-312
Cyclosporin A, 318-319
cyclosporine, 318-319
Cycrin, 650-651
Cylert, 812-813
Cyomin, 310-311
Cypionate, 428-429
cyproheptadine, 319-320
cyproheptadine HCl, 319-320
Cystex, 674
Cystospaz, 548-549
Cytadren, 104-105
cytarabine, 320-322
Cytomel, 617-618
Cytosar, 320-322
Cytotec, 719-720
Cytovene, 496-498
Cytoxan, 315-317

D

dacarbazine, 322-324
dactinomycin, 324-325
Dalacin C, 284-285
Dalalone, 340-341

Entries can be identified as follows: generic name, Trade Name, DRUG CATEGORY, *Combination Product.*

Dalcaine, 613-614
Dalgan, 351-352
Dallergy-JR, 910
Dalmane, 484-485
Dalpro, 1076-1077
dalteparin, 325-326
Daltose, 1092
Damacet-P, 533
Damason-P, 533-534
D-Amp, 124-125
danazol, 327-328
Danocrine, 327-328
Dantrium, 328-329
dantrolene, 328-329
Dapa Extra Strength, 69-72
dapiprazole, 329-330
dapsone, 330-331
Daraprim, 917-918
Darvocet-N, 903-904
Darvon, 903-904
Darvon Compound-65, 903-904
Darvon Compound Pulvules, 136
Darvon-N and A.S.A., 136
Darvon-N Compound, 903-904
Darvon with A.S.A. Pulvules, 136
Datril Extra Strength, 69-72
daunorubicin, 331-333
Dayalets, 731-732
Daypro, 785-786
Dazamide, 72-73
DC Softgels, 387-388
DDAVP, 337-338
ddC, 1095-1096
ddI, 360-362
DDS, 330-331
Decabid, 559-560
Decaderm, 339-341
Decadron-LA, 340-341
Decadron Phosphate, 340-341, 342-343
Decadron Phosphate Respihaler, 340-341
Decadron Phosphate Turbinaire, 343-344
Decadron with Xylocaine, 340
Deca-Durabolin, 742-744
Decaject, 340-341
Decaspray, 339-341
Declomycin, 334-335
Decofed Syrup, 910-911
Decylenes, 1070-1071
DeFed-60, 910-911
deferoxamine, 333-334
Degest 2, 745
Dehist, 185-186
Delacort, 535-536
Delalutin, 544-545
Del Aqua, 166-167
Delatest, 1002-1003
Delatestryl, 1002-1003
Delaxin, 681-682
Delcort, 535-536
Delestrogen, 428-429
Delsym, 348-350
Delta-Cortef, 880-882
Delta-D, 1090-1091
Deltapen, 815-816
Deltapen-VK, 820-821
Deltasone, 883-884
Del-Vi-A, 1089-1090
Demadex, 1041-1042
demeclocycline, 334-335
Demerol, 658-660
Demser, 708
Depakene, 1076-1077
Depen, 398-399
depGynogen, 428-429
Depo Estadiol, 428-429
Depogen, 428-429
Depo-Medrol, 697
Deponit, 762-764
Depo-Provera, 650-651
Depotest, 1002-1003
Depo-Testosterone, 1002-1003
Deproic, 1076-1077
Deprol, 664
Dermacort, 535-536
Derma Flex, 611

Entries can be identified as follows: generic name, Trade Name, DRUG CATEGORY, *Combination Product.*

Dermamycin, 378-380
Dermatop, 880
Dermicort, 535-536
Dermolate Anti-Itch, 535-536
Dermtex HC, 535-536
DES, 363-364
Desenex, 1070-1071
Desferal, 333-334
desipramine, 335-337
desipramine HCl, 335-337
desmopressin, 337-338
desonide, 338
DesOwen, 338
desoximetasone, 338-339
Desoxyn, 673-674
desoxyribonuclease/fibrinolysin, 462
Desquam, 166-167
Desyrel, 1044-1046
Detensol, 904-906
Dexacen, 340-341
dexamethasone, 339-340, 340-344
dexamethasone acetate, 340-341
Dexamethasone Ophthalmic Suspension, 342
dexamethasone sodium phosphate, 340-341, 342-343
dexamethasone sodium phosphate (nasal), 343-344
Dexasone, 340-341
Dexchlor, 344-345
dexchlorpheniramine, 344-345
Dexchlorpheniramine Maleate, 344-345
Dexedrine, 347-348
Dexone, 340-341
dextran 40, 345-346
dextran 70/75, 346-347
dextroamphetamine, 347-348
dextroamphetamine sulfate, 347-348
dextromethorphan, 348-350
dextrose, 350-351
Dey-Pak Sodium Chloride, 959
dezocine, 351-352
D-glucose, 350-351
D.H.E. 45, 371-372
DHPG, 496-498
DHT, 372-373
DiaBeta, 504-506
Diabinese, 265-266
Diachlor, 259-261
Diahist, 378-380
Diamine T.D., 185-186
Diamox, 72-73
Diapid, 633
Diaqua, 532-533
diazepam, 352-354
Diazepam Intensol, 352-354
diazoxide, 354-355
diazoxide (oral), 355-356
diazoxide parenteral, 354-355
Dibent, 359-360
Dibenzyline, 841
dibucaine HCl (topical), 356
Dicarbosil, 200-201
diclofenac, 357-358
dicloxacillin, 358-359
dicloxacillin sodium, 358-359
dicyclomine, 359-360
dicyclomine HCl, 359-360
didanosine, 360-362
dideoxy-citidine, 1095-1096
dideoxyinosine, 360-362
Didronel, 443-444
dienestrol, 362-363
diethylstilbestrol, 363-364
diethylstilbestrol diphosphate, 363-364
difenoxin HCl, 364-365
diflorasone, 365-366
Diflucan, 467-468
diflunisal, 366-367
Digestalin, 77-78
Digibind, 370-371
digitoxin, 367-368
digoxin, 368-370
digoxin immune FAB (ovine), 370-371
dihydroergotamine, 371-372

Entries can be identified as follows: generic name, Trade Name, DRUG CATEGORY, *Combination Product.*

dihydrotachysterol, 372-373
dihydroxyaluminum sodium carbonate, 373
1,25-dihydroxycholecalciferol, 199-200
Dilacor-XR, 373-374
Dilantin, 849-850
Dilantin with Phenobarbital, 849
Dilatrate-SR, 585-586
Dilaudid, 538-540
Dilaudid Cough Syrup, 540
Dilocaine, 613-614
Dilor, 401-402
diltiazem, 373-374
Dimelor, 74-75
dimenhydrinate, 375-376
dimercaprol, 376-377
dimercaptopropanol, 376-377
Dimetabs, 375-376
Dimetane, 185-186
Dimetane-DX Cough Syrup, 349
Dimetapp Sinus, 910
Dimycor, 821
Dinate, 375-376
dinoprostone, 377-378
Diocto, 387-388
Diodoquin, 575-576
Dioeze, 387-388
Dioval, 428-429
Dipentum, 775
Di Phen, 849-850
Diphenacen-50, 378-380
Diphenatol, 364-365
Diphen Cough, 378-380
Diphenhist, 378-380
diphenhydramine, 378-380
diphenhydramine HCl, 378-380
diphenidol, 380
Diphenylan, 849-850
diphenylhydantoin, 849-850
diphtheria and tetanus toxoids and pertussis vaccine (DTP), 380-381
dipivefrin, 381
Diprivan, 901-902
Diprolene AF/Betamethasone Sodium Phosphate, 171-173
Diprosone, 171-173
dipyridamole, 382-383
dirithromycin, 1104-1105
Disalcid, 942-943
Disodium EDTA, 404-405
Disonate, 387-388
Disoprofol, 901-902
disopyramide, 383-384
Disotate, 404-405
Di-Spaz, 359-360
Dispos-a-Med Isoproterenol HCl, 583-584
disulfiram, 384-385
Ditall, 835-836
Ditropan, 789
Diuchlor H, 532-533
Diulo, 703-704
Diupres, 259, 930
DIURETICS, 49-51
Diuril, 259-261
divalproex sodium, 1076-1077
Dividose, 1010-1012
Dixarit, 293-295
Dizmiss, 648-649
DNase, 385-386
Doan's pills, 637-638
dobutamine, 386-387
Dobutrex, 386-387
docusate calcium, 387-388
docusate potassium, 387-388
docusate sodium, 387-388
DOK, 387-388
Dolacet, 533
Dolane, 69-72
Dolane AP, 903-904
Dolene, 903-904
Dolene Compound-65, 136, 903
Dolobid, 366-367
Dolophine HCl, 672-673
Domeboro, 94-95
Dommanate, 375-376

Entries can be identified as follows: generic name, Trade Name, DRUG CATEGORY, *Combination Product.*

Donnagel-PG, 778
Donnagel Suspension, 593
Donnatal, 161
Donnatal Elixir, 161
Donnatal Extentabs, 161
Dopamet, 690-691
dopamine, 388-389
dopamine HCl, 388-389
Dopar, 605-606
Dopastat, 388-389
Dopram, 391-392
Doral, 918-919
Doraphen, 903-904
Doraphen Compound, 903-904
Dorcol Children's Cough Syrup, 349
Dorcol Children's Decongestant, 910-911
Dorcol Children's Fever and Pain Reducer, 69-72
Doriden, 503-504
Dormarex 2, 378-380
Dormin, 378-380
Doryx, 397-398
dorzolamide, 389-390
DOS Softgel, 387-388
doxacurium, 390-391
Doxapap-N, 903-904
Doxaphene, 903-904
Doxaphene Compound, 903
doxapram, 391-392
doxazosin, 392-393
doxepin, 393-395
doxepin HCL, 393-395
Doxinate, 387-388
doxorubicin, 395-397
doxorubicin HCl, 395-397
Doxy, 397-398
Doxy-Caps, 397-398
Doxychel Hyclate, 397-398
Doxycin, 397-398
doxycycline, 397-398
D-penicillamine, 398-399
Dramamine, 375-376
Dramanate, 375-376
Dramocen, 375-376
Dramoject, 375-376
Dr. Caldwell Senna Laxative, 951-952
Drenison, 483-484
D-Rex, 903-904
Drisdol, 1090-1091
Dristan Cold Caplets, 910
Dristan Long Lasting, 791
Dristan Sinus, 910
Drixoral Non-Drowsy Formula, 910-911
droperidol, 399-400
droperidol/fentanyl combination, 458-459
Drotic, 751
Dry and Clear, 166-167
D-S-S, 387-388
DTIC, 322-324
DTIC-Dome, 322-324
DTP, 380-381
D-Tran, 352-354
Dulcagen, 177-178
Dulcolax, 177-178
Dull-C, 133-134
Duofilm, 940-941
DUO-Medihaler, 583
Duo-Trach Kit, 613-614
Duotrate, 821-822
Duphalac, 600
Durabolin, 742-744
Duracillin A.S., 817-818
Duradyne, 533
Dura-Estrin, 428-429
Duragen, 428-429
Duragesic, 459-460
Duralith, 621-622
Duralone, 695-696
Duralutin, 544-545
Duramist Plus, 791
Duramorph, 728-729
Duranest HCl, 442-443
Duratest, 1002-1003

Entries can be identified as follows: generic name, Trade Name, DRUG CATEGORY, *Combination Product.*

Durathate-200, 1002-1003
Duration, 791, 847-848
Durel, 546-547
Duricef, 218-219
Duri-Tap/PD, 910
Durrex, 546-547
Duvoid, 174-175
DV, 362-363
Dyazide, 532
Dycill, 358-359
Dyflex, 401-402
Dylline, 401-402
Dymelor, 74-75
Dymenate, 375-376
Dynabac, 1104-1105
DynaCirc, 589
Dynafed Tablets, Maximum Strength, 910
Dynapen, 358-359
dyphylline, 401-402
Dyrenium, 1050-1051
Dyrexan-OD, 835-836
Dyrexin, 378-380

E

E-200 I.U. Softgels, 1092
EACA, 103-104
Easprin, 136-138
E-Base, 422-424
echothiophate, 402-403
E-Complex-600, 1092
econazole, 403
Econopred, 882-883
Ecostigmine Iodide, 402-403
Ecotrin, 136-138
edathamil calcium disodium, 403-404
Edecrin, 433-434
edetate calcium disodium, 403-404
edetate disodium, 404-405
edrophonium, 405-407
E.E.S. 400, 422-424
E-Ferol, 1092
Effer-K, 870-872
Effer-Syllium, 911-912
Effexor, 1080-1082
Efidac/24, 910-911
Efo-Dine, 874
Efudex, 476
8-Hour Bayer Timed Release, 136-138
Elavil, 109-110
Eldepryl, 950-951
Eldopaque, 541
Eldoquin, 541
Elimite, 830-831
Elixomin, 1010-1012
Elixophyllin, 1010-1012
E-Lor, 903-904
Elspar, 134-136, 810-812
Eltor, 910-911
Elzyme 303 Enseals, 800-801
Emcyt, 429-430
Emete-Con, 167
Emex, 700-701
Eminase, 129-130
Emitrip, 109-110
Empirin, 136-138
Empirin with Codeine, 136
Empracet with Codeine Phosphate, 69
Emulose, 600
E-Mycin, 422-424
enalapril, 407-408
enalaprilat, 407-408
Endecon, 69
Endep, 109-110
Endrate, 404-405
Ener-B, 310-311
Enlon, 405-407
Enovil, 109-110
enoxacin, 408-409
enoxaparin, 409-410
Entex, 512-513
Entex LA, 513
Entrophen, 136-138
Enulose Lactulax, 600
E-Pam, 352-354

Entries can be identified as follows: generic name, Trade Name, DRUG CATEGORY, *Combination Product.*

ephedrine, 411-412
ephedrine sulfate, 411-412
ephedrine (nasal), 410-411
E-Pilo, 412
Epimorph, 728-729
Epinal, 412-414
epinephrine, 412-414
epinephrine bitartrate, 412-414
epinephrine bitartrate (optic), 414-415
epinephrine HCl, 412-414
epinephrine (nasal), 415
epinephrine HCl (optic), 414-415
Epinephrine Pediatric, 412-414
epinephryl borate (optic), 414-415
Epipen Jr., 412-414
Epitol, 207-208
Epitrate, 412-415
Epival, 1076-1077
Epivir, 1105-1106
EPO, 415-416
epoetin alpha, 415-416
Epogen, 415-416
Eppy, 414-415
Eppy/N, 412-414
Epromate, 664
Equagesic, 136, 664
Equanil, 664-665
Equazine-M, 136, 664
Equilet, 200-201
Ergamisol, 603-605
Ergocaff, 418
ergocalciferol, 1090-1091
ergoloid, 416-417
ergonovine, 417-418
ergonovine maleate, 417-418
Ergostat Ergomar, 418-419
ergotamine, 418-419
Ergotrate Maleate, 417-418
Eridium, 834-835
Erybid, 422-424
Eryc, 422-424
Erycette, 421
Eryderm, 421
Erygel, 421
Erymax, 421
Eryped, 422-424
Ery Ped Drops, 422-424
Ery-Tab, 422-424
erythrityl, 419-420
erythromycin base, 422-424
erythromycin estolate, 422-424
erythromycin ethylsuccinate, 422-424
Erythromycin Filmtabs, 422-424
erythromycin gluceptate, 422-424
erythromycin lactobionate, 422-424
erythromycin (ophthalmic), 420-421
erythromycin stearate, 422-424
erythromycin (topical), 421
Esgic, 69
Esidrix, 532-533
Esimil, 515
Eskalith, 621-622
esmolol, 424-425
E-Solve 2, 421
Esoterica, 541
Espotabs, 840
estazolam, 425
esterified estrogens, 426-428
Estinyl, 437-438
Estivin II, 745
Estra-D, 428-429
Estraderm/Deladiol-40, 428-429
Estraderm TTS, 428-429
estradiol, 428-429
estradiol cypionate, 428-429
estradiol transdermal system, 428-429
estradiol valerate, 428-429
Estra-L, 428-429
estramustine, 429-430
Estratab, 426-428
Estratest, 426
Estro-Cyp, 428-429
estrogenic substances, conjugated, 430-432
estrogens, esterified, 426-428

Entries can be identified as follows: generic name, Trade Name, DRUG CATEGORY, *Combination Product.*

Estroject-LA, 428-429
estrone, 432-433
Estrone-5, 432-433
Estrone Aqueous, 432-433
Estronol, 432-433
Estronol-LA/Estrace, 428-429
Estrovis, 922-923
ethacrynate, 433-434
ethacrynic, 433-434
ethambutol, 435
ethchlorvynol, 435-437
ethinyl estradiol, 437-438
ethionamide, 438-439
Ethmozine, 727-728
ethosuximide, 439-440
ethotoin, 440-441
ethylnorepinephrine, 441-442
Etibi, 435
etidocaine, 442-443
etidronate, 443-444
etodolac, 444-445
etomidate, 445
etoposide, 446-447
Etrafon, 831
Etrafon-Forte, 831
etretinate, 447-448
ETS-2%, 421
Eulexin, 486
Eurax, 309-310
Euthroid, 609, 618-620
Evac-U-Gen, 840
Evac-U-Lax, 840
Everone, 1002-1003
E-Vista, 546-547
E-Vitamin Succinate, 1092
Excedrin, 69
Excedrin Extra Strength, 69
Excedrin IS, 549-550
Excedrin P.M., 69
Exdol, 69-72
Ex-Lax, 840
Exosurf Neonatal, 303-304
Exsel, 951
Extra Strength Gas-X, 955
Eye-Sed Ophthalmic, 1097-1098
Eyesine, 1009-1010
Ezide, 532-533

F

factor IV (human), 448-449
factor IX complex (human), 448-449
Factrel, 509-510
famciclovir, 450
famotodine, 450-452
Famvir, 450
Fansidar with sulfadoxine, 917-918
Fastin, 843-844
fat emulsions, 452-453
Feen-A-Mint, 840
felbamate, 453-454
Felbatol, 453-454
Feldene, 863-864
felodipine, 454-455
Femazole, 706-707
FemCare, 296-297
Feminone, 437-438
Femiron, 460-462
Femogen Forte, 432-433
Femotrone, 894-895
Femstat, 194-195
Fenesin, 512-513
Fenicol, 253-254
fenofibrate, 455-456
fenoprofen, 456-457
fentanyl, 457-458
fentanyl/droperidol combination, 458-459
fentanyl transdermal, 459-460
Feosol, 460-462
Feostat, 460-462
Feratab, 460-462
Fergon, 460-462
Fer-In-Sol, 460-462
Fer-Iron, 460-462
Fermalox, 460
Ferndex, 347-348
Ferocyl, 460

Entries can be identified as follows: generic name, Trade Name, DRUG CATEGORY, *Combination Product.*

Fero-Gradumet, 460-462
Ferospace, 460-462
Ferralet, 460-462
Ferralyn, 460-462
Ferra-TD, 460-462
Ferrets, 460-462
Ferro-Sequels, 460
ferrous fumarate, 460-462
ferrous gluconate, 460-462
ferrous sulfate, 460-462
Festal II Tablets, 801-802
Fiberall, 911-912
Fiber Norm, 203
fibrinolysin/desoxyribonuclease, 462
filgrastin, 463
finasteride, 463-464
Fioricet, 69
Fiorinal, 136
Fiorinal with Codeine, 136
Fisostin, 851
Flagyl, 706-707
Flamazine, 954-955
Flarex, 475-476
Flatulex Gas Relief, 955
Flavorcee, 133-134
flavoxate, 464-465
Flaxedil, 495-496
flecainide, 465-466
Fleet Babylax, 506
Fleet Bisacodyl Laxit, 177-178
Fleet Enema, 958-959
Fleet Mineral Oil Enema, 716-717
Fletcher's Castoria, 951-952
Flexeril, 313-314
Flexoject, 780-781
Flexon, 780-781
Florinef Acetate, 471-472
Florone, 365-366
Floropryl, 581-582
Floxin, 774-775
floxuridine, 466-467
Flucinolone, 474
fluconazole, 467-468
flucytosine, 468-469
Fludara, 469-471
fludarabine, 469-471
fludrocortisone, 471-472
Flumadine, 935-936
flumazenil, 472-473
flunisolide, 473-474
Fluocinolone Acetonide, 474
fluocinonide, 474
Fluogen, 561-562
Fluonid, 474
Fluor-A-Day, 474-475
fluoride, 474-475
Fluorigard, 474-475
Fluorinse, 474-475
Fluoritab, 474-475
fluorometholone, 475-476
Fluor-Op, 475-476
Fluoroplex, 476
fluorouracil, 476
5-fluorouracil, 476-478
Fluotic, 474-475
fluoxetine, 478-480
fluoxymesterone, 480-481
fluphenazine, 481-483
fluphenazine decanoate, 481-483
fluphenazine HCl, 481-483
Flura, 474-475
Flura-Drops, 474-475
Flura-Loz, 474-475
flurandrenolide, 483-484
flurazepam, 484-485
flurbiprofen, 485-486
Flurosyn, 474
FluShield, 561-562
flutamide, 486
Flutex, 1048-1049
Fluviral, 561-562
Fluvirin, 561-562
fluvoxamine, 486-487
Fluzone, 561-562
FML, 475-476
Folate, 487-488
Folex PFS, 683-685
folic acid, 487-488

Entries can be identified as follows: generic name, Trade Name, DRUG CATEGORY, *Combination Product.*

Folvite, 487-488
Formula Q, 924-925
Formulex, 359-360
Fortaz, 236-237
Fosamax, 1102
foscarnet, 488-490
Foscavir, 488-490
fosinopril, 490-491
Fostex, 166-167
4-Way Long Acting Nasal, 791
Fragmin, 325-326
FreAmine HBC, 101-102
FreAmine III, 102-103
Freezone, 940-941
Froben, 485-486
5-FU, 476-478
FUDR, 466-467
Fulvicin, 511-512
Fumasorb, 460-462
Fumerin, 460-462
Fumide, 492-493
Fungizone, 123
Fungizone IV, 121-123
Furacin, 762
Furadantin, 761-762
Furalan, 761-762
Furomide M.D., 492-493
furosemide, 492-493

G
gabapentin, 494-495
gallamine, 495-496
gallium, 496
Gamastan, 557-558
Gamimune N, 557-558
Gammagard, 557-558
Gammagee, 526-527
gamma globulin IG, 557-558
Gammar, 557-558
Gamulin Rh, 931-932
ganciclovir, 496-498
Ganite, 496
Gantanol, 980-982
Gantrisin, 986-987
Garamycin, 499-500, 501-502
Garamycin Ophthalmic, 501
Gastrocrom, 308-309
Gastrosed, 548-549
Gas-X, 955
GBH, 616-617
G-CSF, 463
Gee-Gee, 512-513
Gelcalc 600, 200-201
Gel II, 474-475
Gel-Kam, 474-475
Gel-Tin, 474-475
gemfibrozil, 498
Gemnisyn, 69
Genabid, 803-804
Genagesic, 903-904
Genahist, 378-380
Genapap Extra Strength, 69-72
Genapap Infant's Drops, 69-72
Genaphed, 910-911
Genasal, 791
Genaspor, 1040
Genatuss, 512-513
Geners Extra Strength, 69-72
Gen-K, 870-872
Genoptic, 501
Genpril, 549-550
Genprin, 136-138
Gen-Salbutamol, 83-84
Gentacidin, 501
Gentak, 501
Gent-AK, 501
Gentamicin Ophthalmic Liquifilm, 501
gentamicin, 499-500
gentamicin sulfate, 499-500
gentamicin (ophthalmic), 501
gentamicin (topical), 501-502
Gentlax, 951-952
Gentran 40, 345-346
Gentran 75, 346-347
Gen-Xene, 295-296
Geridium, 834-835
Gerimal, 416-417

Entries can be identified as follows: generic name, Trade Name, DRUG CATEGORY, *Combination Product.*

Gesterol 50, 894-895
Gesterol L.A. 250, 544-545
GG-Cen, 512-513
Glaucon, 412-414
Glaucon/Epinal, 414-415
glipizide, 502-503
Glucophage, 671-672
Glucose, 350-351
Glucotrol, 502-503
glutethimide, 503-504
Glutose, 350-351
Glyate, 512-513
glyburide, 504-506
glycerin, 506
glycerin, anhydrous, 506-507
Glycerin USP, 506
Glycerol, 506
glycopyrrolate, 507-508
Glycotuss, 512-513
Glynase Prestab, 504-506
Glytuss, 512-513
G-Myticin, 501-502
gold sodium thiomalate, 147-148
gonadorelin acetate, 508-509
gonadorelin HCl, 509-510
Gonic, 271-272
Gordofilm, 940-941
Gordo-Vite E, 1092
goserelin, 510
granisetron, 511
granulocyte colony stimulator, 463
Gravol, 375-376
Grifulvin V, 511-512
Grisactin, 511-512
griseofulvin microsize, 511-512
griseofulvin ultramicrosize, 511-512
Gris-PEG, 511-512
guaifenesin, 512-513
guanabenz, 513-514
guanadrel, 514-515
guanethidine, 515-516
guanethidine sulfate, 515-516
guanfacine, 516-517
Guiatuss, 512-513
G-Well, 616-617
Gyne-Lotrimin, 296-297
Gynergen, 418-419
Gynogen L.A., 428-429

H

Habitrol, 759-760
haemophilus b vaccines, 517-518
halazepam, 518-519
halcinonide, 519-520
Halcion, 1051-1052
Haldol, 521-523
Haldrone, 807-808
Halenol Children's, 69-72
Halfan, 520-521
halofantrene, 520-521
Halofed, 910-911
Halog, 519-520
haloperidol, 521-523
Haloperidol 100, 521-523
Haloperidol Decanoate 50, 521-523
haloprogin, 523-524
Halotestin, 480-481
Halotex, 523-524
Halotussin, 512-513
Haltran, 549-550
H-BIG, 526-527
1% HC, 535-536
Head and Shoulders Intensive Treatment, 951
Heet Relief, 875-876
Hemabate, 211-212
Hemocyte, 460-462
Hemofil M, 130-132
Hepalean, 524-526
heparin, 524-526
Heparin Leo, 524-526
Heparin Lock Flush, 524-526
Heparin Sodium and Sodium Chloride, 524-526
HepatAmine, 101-102
hepatitis B vaccine, 526-527
Hep-B, 526-527
Hep-Lock, 524-526

Entries can be identified as follows: generic name, Trade Name, DRUG CATEGORY, *Combination Product.*

Hepto-M, 664
Herplex, 552-553
Hespan, 527-528
hetastarch, 527-528
Hexa-Betalin, 916
Hexadrol Phosphate, 340-341
Hexalen, 528-529, 93-94
Hexalol, 674
hexamethylmelamine, 528-529, 93-94
Hib-Imune, 517-518
HibVAX (polysaccharide), 517-518
Hi-Cor, 535-536
Hiprex, 677-678
Hip-Rex, 677-678
Histaject, 185-186
HISTAMINE H_2 ANTAGONISTS, 51-52
Histanil, 898-899
HIVID, 1095-1096
Hold DM, 348-350
homatropine, 529-530
Homatropine HBr Ophthalmic, 529-530
Honvol, 363-364
H.P. Acthar Gel, 304-306
Humate-P, 130-132
Humatin, 808-809
Humatrope, 961-962
Humegon, 657
Humibid, 512-513
Humulin 70/30, 563-564
Humulin L, 568-569
Humulin N, 562-563
Humulin R, 565-566
hyaluronidase, 530
Hybephen, 161
Hybolin Decanoate, 742-744
Hybolin Improved, 742-744
Hycodan, 533-535
Hycort, 535-536
Hydeltrasol, 880-882
Hydeltra-T.B.A., 880-882
Hydergine, 416-417
hydralazine, 530-532
hydralazine HCl, 530-532
Hydramine, 378-380
Hydramyn, 378-380
Hydrate, 375-376
Hydrazol/Diamox Parenteral, 72-73
Hydrea, 545-546
Hydrisalic, 940-941
Hydrobexan, 541-542
Hydrocet, 533
Hydro-Chlor, 532-533
hydrochlorothiazide, 532-533
Hydrochlorothiazide Tablets, 904
Hydrocil Instant Powder, 911-912
hydrocodone, 533-535
hydrocortisone, 535, 536-538
hydrocortisone acetate, 535, 536-538
hydrocortisone acetate (topical), 535-536
hydrocortisone sodium phosphate, 536-538
hydrocortisone sodium succinate, 536-538
hydrocortisone (topical), 535-536
hydrocortisone valerate (topical), 535-536
Hydrocortone/Cortef Acetate, 536-538
Hydrocortone Phosphate, 536-538
Hydro-Crysti 12, 541-542
HydroDiuril, 532-533
Hydrogesic, 534
Hydromal, 532-533
hydromorphone, 538-540
hydromorphone/guaifenesin/alcohol, 540
hydromorphone HCl, 538-540
Hydromox R, 930
Hydro-Par, 532-533
Hydropres, 930
hydroquinone, 541
Hydro-Reserpine, 930
Hydro Rho-D Mini-Dose, 931-932

Entries can be identified as follows: generic name, Trade Name, DRUG CATEGORY, *Combination Product.*

Hydroserp, 930
Hydroserpalan, 930
Hydroserpine, 930
Hydrosine, 930
Hydro-T, 532-533
Hydrotensin, 930
HydroTex, 535-536
Hydroxo-12, 541-542
hydroxocobalamin (vitamin B_{12}), 310-311, 541-542
Hydroxyacen, 546-547
hydroxychloroquine, 542-543
hydroxymagnesium aluminate, 634-635
hydroxyprogesterone, 544-545
hydroxyurea, 545-546
hydroxyzine, 546-547
hydroxyzine HCl, 546-547
hydroxyzine pamoate, 546-547
Hydrozide, 532-533
Hygroton, 266-267
Hylidone, 266-267
Hylorel, 514-515
Hylutin, 544-545
hyoscyamine, 548-549
Hyosophen, 161
Hyosophen Elixir, 161
Hyperab, 925-926
HyperHep, 526-527
Hyperstat IV, 354-355
Hy-Phen, 533
Hypo-Rho-D, 931-932
Hyprogest 250, 544-545
Hyproval PA, 544-545
Hyrexin-50, 378-380
Hytakerol, 372-373
Hytone, 535-536
Hytrin, 996-997
Hytuss, 512-513
Hyzine-50, 546-547

I

^{131}I, 926-927
Ibuprin, 549-550
ibuprofen, 549-550
Ibuprohm, 549-550
IBU-Tab, 549-550
Idamycin, 550-552
idarubicin, 550-552
idoxuridine-IDU, 552-553
Ifex, 553-554
ifosfamide, 553-554
IGIV, 557-558
IL-2, 84-86
Iletin I, 565-566
Iletin II, 565-566
Iletin NPH, 562-563
Ilosone, 422-424
Ilotycin, 420-421
Ilotycin Gluceptate, 422-424
Ilozyme, 801-802
Imferon, 577-579
imipenem/cilastatin, 554-555
imipramine, 555-557
imipramine HCl, 555-557
Imitrex, 988-989
immune globulin, 557-558
immune serum globulin, 557-558
IMMUNOSUPPRESSANTS, 52-53
Imodium, 625-626
Imogam, 925-926
Impril, 555-557
Imuran, 149-150
Inapsine, 399-400
Indameth, 560-561
indapamide, 558-559
indecainide, 559-560
Inderal, 904-906
Inderide, 904
Indocid, 560-561
Indocin, 560-561
indomethacin, 560-561
In Fed, 577-579
Inflamase, 882-883
influenza virus vaccine, trivalent A & B (whole virus/split virus), 561-562
Infumorph, 728-729

Entries can be identified as follows: generic name, Trade Name, DRUG CATEGORY, *Combination Product.*

INH, 582-583
Innovar, 458-459
Inocor, 127-128
Insomnal, 378-380
Insta-Char, 77-78
Insta-Glucose, 350-351
Insulatard NPH, 562-563
insulin, isophane suspension and regular insulin, 563-564
insulin, isophane suspension (NPH), 562-563
insulin, regular, 565-566
insulin, regular concentrated, 566-567
insulin, zinc suspension, prompt (Semilente), 570-571
insulin, zinc suspension extended (Ultralente), 569-570
insulin, zinc suspension (Lente), 568-569
Insulin Reaction, 350-351
Intal, 308-309
interferon alfa-2a, 571-572
interferon alfa-2b, 571-572
interferon alfa-n 3, 572-573
interferon β-1b, 573-574
interferon gamma-1b, 574-575
interleukin-2, 84-86
Intralipid, 452-453
Intropin, 388-389
Inversine, 645-646
Iodex Regular, 874
iodoquinol, 575-576
Ionamin, 843-844
Iophen DM, 349
Iosat, 873-874
ipecac, 576-577
I-Picamide, 1068-1069
ipratropium, 577
Ircon, 460-462
iron dextran, 577-579
ISDN, 585-586
ISG, 557-558
Ismelin, 515-516
ISMO, 586-587
Ismotic, 584-585
Iso-Bid, 585-586
Isocaine HCl, 663-664
isocarboxazid, 579-580
isoetharine, 580-581
isoetharine HCl, 580-581
isoflurophate, 581-582
Isonate, 585-586
isoniazid, 582-583
isoproterenol, 583-584
isoproterenol HCl, 583-584
Isoptin, 1082-1083
Isopto, 529-530
Isopto-Atropine, 143-145
Isopto Atropine, 145-146
Isopto Carbachol, 206-207
Isopto Carpine, 854-855
Isopto Cetamide, 977-978
Isopto Eserine Solution/Eserine Sulfate Ointment, 851
Isopto Fenical, 253-254
Isopto Frin, 848-849
Isopto-Hyoscine, 946
Isorbid, 585-586
Isordil, 585-586
isosorbide, 584-585
isosorbide dinitrate, 585-586
isosorbide mononitrate, 586-587
Isotamine, 582-583
Isotrate Timecelles, 585-586
isotretinoin, 587-588
isoxsuprine HCl, 588-589
isradipine, 589
Isuprel, 583-584
itraconazole, 590-591
I-Tropina, 143-145
Iveegam, 557-558

J

Janimine, 555-557
Jenamicin, 499-500
Junior Strength Feverall, 69-72

Entries can be identified as follows: generic name, Trade Name, DRUG CATEGORY, *Combination Product.*

K

K^+10, 870-872
Kabikinase, 969-971
kanamycin, 591-593
kanamycin sulfate, 591-593
Kantrex, 591-593
Kaochlor, 870-872
kaolin, pectin, 593
Kaon-Cl, 870-872
Kao-Nor, 870-872
Kaopectate II Caplets, 625-626
Kapseals, 688-689, 841-842
Karacil, 911-912
Karidium, 474-475
Karigel, 474-475
Kasof/Colace, 387-388
Kato, 870-872
Kay Ciel, 870-872
Kayexalate, 959-960
Kaylixir, 870-872
K^+ Care, 870-872
K-Dur, 870-872
Keflex, 242-243
Keflin, 243-245
Keftab, 242-243
Kefurox, 240-242
Kefzol, 221-222
Kemadrin, 893-894
Kenacort, 1047-1048
Kenaject-40, 1047-1048
Kenalog, 1047-1048
Kenalog-H, 1048-1049
Kenalog in Orabase, 1049
Kenalog (topical), 1048-1049
Keralyt, 940-941
Kestrone-5, 432-433
Ketalar, 593-594
ketamine, 593-594
ketoconazole, 594-595
ketoprofen, 595-596
ketorolac, 596-597
Key-Pred, 880-882
K-G Elixir, 870-872
Kidrolase, 134-136
Kinesed, 161
K-Lease, 870-872
Klonopin, 291-293
Klor, 870-872
Klor-Con, 870-872
Klortrix, 870-872
Klorvess, 870-872
K-Lyte, 870-872
K-Lyte/Cl, 870-872
K-Norm, 870-872
Koate, 130-132
Koffex, 348-350
Kogenate, 130-132
Konakion, 853-854
Kondremul, 716-717
Konsyl-D, 911-912
Konyne 80, 448-449
Kronofed-A Jr., 910
Kryobulin VH, 130-132
K-Tab, 870-872
Ku-Zyme HP Capsules, 801-802
Kwell, 616-617
Kwellada, 616-617
Kwildane, 616-617
Kybernin, 132
Kytril, 511

L

LA-12, 541-542
labetalol, 598-599
Lacticare-HC, 535-536
Lactisol, 940-941
lactulose, 600
L.A.E. 20, 428-429
Lamictal, 600-601
Lamisil, 997-998
lamivudine, 1105-1106
lamotrigine, 600-601
Lamprene, 287-288
Laniazid, 582-583
Lanophyllin, 1010-1012
Lanoxicaps, 368-370
Lanoxin, 368-370
lansoprazole, 1106-1107

Entries can be identified as follows: generic name, Trade Name, DRUG CATEGORY, *Combination Product.*

Lansoyl, 716-717
Lanvis, 1014-1015
Largactil, 262-265
Lariam, 653
Larodopa, 605-606
Lasix, 492-493
LAXATIVES, 53-55
Lax-Pills, 840
L-Caine, 611-614
L-Dopa, 605-606
Ledercillin-VK, 820-821
Legatrin, 924-925
Lentard, 562-563
Lentard Monotard, 568-569
Lente Iletin I, 568-569
Lente Iltein II, 568-569
Lente Insulin, 568-569
Lente Purified Pork Insulin, 568-569
leucovorin, 601-602
leucovorin calcium, 601-602
Leukeran, 250-252
Leukine, 943-944
leuprolide, 602-603
Leupron Depo Ped, 602-603
Leustatin, 279-280
levamisole, 603-605
Levarterenol, 766-767
Levate, 109-110
levodopa, 605-606
Levo-Dromoran, 608-609
levomethydyle, 606-607
levonorgestrel implant, 607-608
Levophed, 766-767
Levoprome, 685-686
levorphanol, 608-609
Levothroid, 609-611
levothyroxine, 609-611
levothyroxine sodium, 609-611
Levoxine, 609-611
Levsin, 548-549
Levsinex Timecaps, 548-549
Levsinex with Phenobarbital Elixir, 548
Levsinex with Phenobarbital Time-caps, 548
Levsin-PB, 548
Levsin with Phenobarbital Tablets, 548
Librax, 255, 283
Libritabs, 255-257
Librium, 255-257
Lidemol, 474
Lidex, 474
lidocaine, 611-613
lidocaine (local), 613-614
lidocaine HCl (local), 613-614
lidocaine (topical), 611
lidocaine HCl (topical), 611
lidocaine viscous, 611
Lidoject, 613-614
Lidopen Auto-Injector, 611-613
Lidox, 255, 283
Lidoxide, 283
Limbitrol, 255
Lincocin, 614-615
lincomycin, 614-615
Lincorex, 614-615
lindane, 616-617
Lioresal, 158-159
liothyronine sodium, 617-618
liothyronine (T_3), 617-618
liotrix, 618-620
Lipidil, 455-456
Liposyn, 452-453
Liquaemin Sodium, 524-526
Liqu-Char, 77-78
Liqui-Char, 77-78
Liqui-doss, 716-717
Liquid Pred, 883-884
Liquiprin Elixir, 69-72
Liquiprin Infant Drops, 69-72
lisinopril, 620-621
Listermint with Fluoride, 474-475
Lithane, 621-622
lithium, 621-622
lithium carbonate, 621-622
Lithizine, 621-622

Entries can be identified as follows: generic name, Trade Name, DRUG CATEGORY, *Combination Product.*

Lithonate, 621-622
Lithotabs, 621-622
LKV Drops, 731-732
LMD 10%, 345-346
Lobac, 268
Lodine, 444-445
Lofene, 364-365
Logene, 364-365
Lomanate, 364-365
lomefloxacin, 622-623
Lomotil, 364-365
lomustine, 623-625
Loniten, 718-719
loperamide, 625-626
Lopid, 498
Lopresor, 704-706
Lopressor, 704-706
Lopressor HCT, 704
Loprox, 273
Lopurin, 88-89
Lorabid, 626-627
loracarbef, 626-627
loratadine, 627
Loraz, 627-629
lorazepam, 627-629
Lorelco, 887-888
losartan, 629-630
Losec, 776-777
Lotensin, 162-164
Lotrimin, 296-297
Lo-Trol, 364-365
Lotusate, 991-992
lovastatin, 630-631
Lovenox, 409-410
Lowsium, 634-635
Loxapac, 631-633
loxapine, 631-633
loxapine succinate, 631-633
Loxitane, 631-633
Lozide, 558-559
Lozol, 558-559
Loz-Tabs, 474-475
L-PAM, 654-656
L-Sarcolysin, 654-656
Ludiomil, 640-642
Lufyllin, 401-402
Lufyllin-EPG, 401
Lupron, 602-603
Luramide, 492-493
Luride, 474-475
Luroxide Oxy 5, 166-167
Lutrepulse, 508-509
Luvox, 486-487
Lyphocin, 1077-1079
lypressin, 633
Lysodren, 722-723

M

Maalox Antidiarrheal Caplets, 625-626
Macpac, 761-762
Macrobid, 761-762
Macrodantin, 761-762
Macrodex, 346-347
mafenide (topical), 633-634
magaldrate (hydromagnesium aluminate), 634-635
Magan, 637-638
Magnacef, 236-237
magnesium, 635-636
magnesium oxide, 636-637
magnesium salicylate, 637-638
magnesium salts, 638-639
Mag-Ox, 636-637
Major Con, 955
Mallamint, 200-201
Mallergan Pentazine, 898-899
Mallisol, 874
Mallopress, 930
Malotuss, 512-513
Mandameth, 677-678
Mandelamine, 677-678
Mandol, 219-221
mannitol, 639-640
Maox, 636-637
maprotiline, 640-642
Marax-DF Syrup, 1010
Marbaxin 750, 681-682

Entries can be identified as follows: generic name, Trade Name, DRUG CATEGORY, *Combination Product.*

Marezine, 312-313
Marflex, 780-781
Margesic A-C, 903-904
Marmine, 375-376
Marplan, 579-580
masoprocol, 642
Matulane, 890-892
Maxair, 862-863
Maxaquin, 622-623
Maxeran, 700-701
Maxidex, 342
Maxiflor, 365-366
Maximum Bayer, 136-138
Maximum Strength Dynafed Tablets, 910
Maximum Strength Ornex Caplets, 910
Maximum Strength Sine-Aid Tablets, Gelcaps, Caplets, 910
Maxivate, 171-173
Maxolon, 700-701
Maxzide, 532
Mazanor, 643-644
Mazepine, 207-208
Mazicon, 472-473
mazindol, 643-644
MCT Oil, 650
measles, mumps, and rubella vaccine, 644
Mebaral, 662-663
mebendazole, 645
mecamylamine, 645-646
mechlorethamine, 646-648
meclizine, 648-649
meclizine HCl, 648-649
meclofen, 649-650
meclofenamate, 649-650
Meclomen, 649-650
Meda Cap, 69-72
Medamint, 164
Medihaler-Epi, 412-414
Medihaler Ergotamine, 418-419
Medihaler-Iso, 583-584
Medilax, 840
Medilium, 255-257
Mediplast, 940-941
Medipren, 549-550
Mediqueall, 349
Meditran, 664-665
medium-chain triglycerides, 650
Medralone, 695-696
Medrol/Depo-Medrol, 695-696
medroxyprogesterone, 650-651
medroxyprogesterone acetate, 650-651
mefenamic acid, 652
mefloquine, 653
Mefoxin, 232-233
Megacc, 653-654
Megacillin, 813-815, 815-816
megestrol, 653-654
megestrol acetate, 653-654
Melanex, 541
Melfiat-105 Unicelles, 835-836
Mellaril, 1016-1018
melphalan, 654-656
menadiol sodium diphosphate, 656
menadione, 656
Menadol, 549-550
Menest, 426-428
Meni-D, 648-649
menotropins, 657
Menrium, 255
mepenzolate, 657-658
Mepergan, 658
Mepergan Fortis, 658-659
meperidine, 658-660
mephentermine, 660-661
mephenytoin, 661-662
mephobarbital, 662-663
Mephyton, 853-854
mepivacaine, 663-664
mepivacaine HCl, 663-664
Mepor Compound, 136
Mepro-Analgesic, 136
meprobamate, 664-665
Mepro Compound, 664
Meprogesic, 664

Entries can be identified as follows: generic name, Trade Name, DRUG CATEGORY, *Combination Product.*

Mepron, 141-142
Meprospan, 664-665
Meravil, 109-110
mercaptopurine, 665-667
mesalamine, 667-668
Mesantoin, 661-662
mesoridazine, 668-670
Mestinon, 914-915
Mesylates, 416-417
Metamucil, 911-912
Metaprel, 670-671
metaproterenol, 670-671
metformin, 671-672
methadone, 672-673
methadone HCl Intensol, 672-673
methamphetamine, 673-674
methantheline, 674-675
methazolamide, 675-677
methenamine, 677-678
methenamine mandelate, 677-678
Methergine, 692-693
methicillin, 678-679
Methidate, 693-694
methimazole, 679-680
methocarbamol, 681-682
methohexital, 682-683
methotrexate, 683-685
Methotrexate LPF, 683-685
methotrimeprazine, 685-686
methoxsalen, 686-687
methscopolamine, 687-688
methsuximide, 688-689
methylcellulose, 689-690
methyldopa, 690-691
methyldopate, 690-691
methyldopate HCl, 690-691
methylene blue, 692
Methylergobasine, 692-693
methylergonovine, 692-693
methylphenidate, 693-694
methylprednisolone, 695-696, 697
methylprednisolone acetate, 695-696
methylprednisolone sodium succinate, 695-696
methyprylon, 697-698
methysergide, 699-700
Meticorten, 883-884
metipranolol, 700
metoclopramide, 700-701
metoclopramide HCl, 700-701
metocurine, 702-703
metolazone, 703-704
metoprolol, 704-706
Metra, 835-836
Metreton Ophthalmic, 882-883
Metrodin, 1073-1074
Metro IV, 706-707
metronidazole, 706-707
Metronidazole Redi-Infusion, 706-707
Metryl, 706-707
Metubine, 702-703
metyrosine, 708
Mevacor, 630-631
Meval, 352-354
mexiletine, 709-710
Mexitil, 709-710
Mezlin, 710-711
mezlocillin, 710-711
Miacalcin, 198-199
Micatin, 713
miconazole, 711-712
miconazole nitrate (topical), 713
Micrainin, 136, 664
MICRhoGAM, 931-932
microfibrillar collagen hemostat, 713-714
Micro-K, 870-872
Micro KLS, 870-872
Micronase, 504-506
Micro-Nefrin, 412-414
Micronor, 767-768
Midamor, 99-101
midazolam, 714-715
Midol-200, 549-550
Midol Caplets, 136

Entries can be identified as follows: generic name, Trade Name, DRUG CATEGORY, *Combination Product.*

Midol PMS Caplets, 69
Migral, 418
Milkinol, 716-717
Milk of Magnesia, 638-639
Milontin, 841-842
Milophene, 289-290
Milprem, 664
milrinone, 715-716
Miltown, 664-665
mineral oil, 716-717
Mini-Gamulin RH, 931-932
Minims Atropine, 143-145
Minipress, 879
Minitran, 762-764
Minizide, 879
Minocin, 717-718
minocycline, 717-718
Minodyl, 718-719
minoxidil, 718-719
Mintezol, 1012
Minute-Gel, 474-475
Miostat, 206-207
misoprostol, 719-720
Mithracin, 865-867
mithramycin, 865-867
mitomycin, 720-722
mitotane, 722-723
mitoxantrone, 723-724
Mitran, 255-257
Mitrolan, 203
Mivacron, 724-725
mivacurium, 724-725
Mixtard, 563-564
M-Kya, 924-925
M-M-R-II, 644
Moban, 725-727
Mobenol, 1038-1039
Mobidin, 637-638
Modane, 840
Modane Bulk, 911-912
Modane Soft, 387-388
Modified Burow's Solution, 94-95
moexipril, 1107-1108
molindone, 725-727
Mol-Iron, 460-462
Monistat, 711-712, 713
Monistat-Derm, 713
Monistat Dual-Pak, 713
Monitan, 67-68
Monocid, 225-226
Monoclate, 130-132
Monodox, 397-398
Mono-Gesic, 942-943
Mononine, 448-449
Monopril, 490-491
8-MOP, 686-687
moricizine, 727-728
morphine, 728-729
Morphine, Atropine Sulfate Injection, 728
morphine sulfate, 728-729
Morphitec, 728-729
M.O.S., 728-729
Mosco, 940-941
M.O.S.-S.R., 728-729
Motofen, 364-365
Motrin, 549-550
Motrin IB Sinus, 910
moxalactam, 729-731
Moxam, 729-731
6-MP, 665-667
MS Contin, 728-729
M.T.E., 1042-1043
MTX, 683-685
Mucomyst, 75-76
Mucosal, 75-76
MulTE-PAK, 1042-1043
Multi-75, 731-732
Multiday, 731-732
Multipax, 546-547
Multiple Trace Element, 1042-1043
Multiple Trace Element Neonatal, 1042-1043
Multiple Trace Element Pediatric, 1042-1043
multivitamins, 731-732
mupirocin, 732

Entries can be identified as follows: generic name, Trade Name, DRUG CATEGORY, *Combination Product.*

Murine Plus Eye Drops, 1009-1010
Murocoll-2, 945
muromonab-CD3, 732-733
Muro-128 Ophthalmic, 959
Muroptic-S, 959
Mus-Lax, 268
Mustargen, 646-648
Mutamycin, 720-722
Myambutol, 435
Myapap Drops, 69-72
Mycelex, 296-297
Mycifradin Sulfate, 749-750
Myciguent, 751-752
Mycobutin, 933-934
mycophenolate mofetil, 1108-1109
Mycostatin, 772-773
Mycostatin (topical), 773
Mydfrin Ophthalmic, 848-849
Mydriacyl Ophthalmic, 1068-1069
Myfedrine, 910-911
Myidil, 1067-1068
myidone, 885-886
My-K Elixir, 870-872
Mykrox, 703-704
Mylanta Gas, 955
Myleran, 193-194
Mylicon, 955
Myochrysine, 147-148
Myolin, 780-781
Myotonachol, 174-175
Myproic acid/Depakote, 1076-1077
Mysoline, 885-886
Mysteclin-F, 121, 1006
Mytrate/Epifrin, 414-415
Mytussin, 512-513

N
nabumetone, 733-734
Nadastine, 773
nadolol, 734-735
Nadostine, 772-773
nafarelin, 735-736
Nafazair, 745
Nafcil, 736-738
nafcillin, 736-738
nafcillin sodium, 736-738
Nafrine, 791
naftifine, 738
Naftin, 738
nalbuphine, 738-739
nalbuphine HCl, 738-739
Naldecon-DX Adult, 349
Naldecon-DX Children's Syrup, 349
Naldecon Senior EX, 512-513
Naldegisic, 69
Nalfon, 456-457
nalidixic acid, 740
Nallpen, 736-738
nalmefene, 1109-1110
naloxone, 741
naloxone HCl, 741
naltrexone, 741-742
Nandrobolic, 742-744
nandrolone decanoate, 742-744
nandrolone phenpropionate, 742-744
Napamide, 383-384
naphazoline, 744, 745
naphazoline HCl, 745
Naphcon, 745
Naprosyn Anaprox, 745-746
naproxen, 745-746
Narcan, 741
NARCOTICS, 55-56
Nardil, 837-838
Nasahist-B, 185-186
Nasalcrom, 308-309
Nasalide, 473-474
Natacyn, 746-747
natamycin (ophthalmic), 746-747
Natulan, 890-892
Natural Vegetable Reguloid, 911-912
Nauseal, 375-376
Nauseatol, 375-376
Navane, 1020-1022
Navelbine, 1088-1089

Naxen, 745-746
ND Stat, 185-186
Nebcin, 1033-1034
Nebupent, 822-823
nedocromil inhaler, 747-748
nefazodone, 748-749
NegGram, 740
Nemasole, 645
Nembutal, 825-827
Neo-Codema, 532-533
Neo-Cultol, 716-717
Neocyten, 780-781
Neo-DM, 348-350
Neo-Durabolic, 742-744
Neo-Estrone, 426-428
Neo-Metric, 706-707
neomycin, 749-750
neomycin (otic), 751
Neomycin Sulfate, 751-752
neomycin (topical), 751-752
Neoquess, 359-360, 548-549
Neorespin, 411-412
Neosar, 315-317
Neosporin G.U. Irrigant, 868
neostigmine, 752-753
neostigmine bromide, 752-753
neostigmine methylsulfate, 752-753
Neo-Synephrine, 846-847
Neo-Synephrine (nasal), 847-848
Neo-Synephrine (optic), 848-849
Neo-Synephrine 12 Hour, 791
Neothylline, 401-402
Neotrace 4, 1042-1043
Neo-Tran, 664-665
Nephro-Calci, 200-201
Nephro-Fer, 460-462
Nephronex, 761-762
Nephron Inhalant, 412-414
Neptazane, 675-677
Nervocaine, 613-614
Nesacaine, 257-258
Nestrex, 916
netilmicin, 753-755
Netromycin, 753-755
Neupogen, 463
NEUROMUSCULAR BLOCKING AGENTS, 57-58
Neurontin, 494-495
Neutrexin, 1062-1064
Nia-Bid, 755-756
Niac, 755-756
Niacels, 755-756
niacin, 755-756
niacinamide, 755-756
nicardipine, 756-757
N'ice Vitamin C Drops, 133-134
Niclocide, 757-758
niclosamide, 757-758
Nico-400, 755-756
Nicobid, 755-756
Nicoderm, 759-760
Nicolar, 755-756
Nicorette, 758-759
nicotinamide, 755-756
nicotine resin complex, 758-759
nicotine transdermal system, 759-760
Nicotinex, 755-756
nicotinic acid, 755-756
Nicotrol, 759 760
NicoVert, 375-376
Nidryl, 378-380
nifedipine, 760-761
Nilstat, 773
Nipent, 827-828
Nitro-Bid, 762-764
Nitro-Bid Plateau Caps, 762-764
Nitrocine, 762-764
Nitrodisc, 762-764
Nitro-Dur, 762-764
Nitrofuracot, 761-762
nitrofurantion, 761-762
nitrofurazone (topical), 762
Nitrogard, 762-764
nitrogen mustard, 646-648
nitroglycerin, 762-764
nitroglycerin transdermal, 762-764

Entries can be identified as follows: generic name, Trade Name, DRUG CATEGORY, *Combination Product.*

Nitroglyn, 762-764
Nitrol, 762-764
Nitrolingual, 762-764
Nitrong, 762-764
Nitropress, 764-765
nitroprusside, 764-765
Nitrostat, 762-764
Nitrotym Plus, 762-763
Nix, 830-831
nizatidine, 765-766
Nizoral, 594-595
Noctec, 249-250
No Drowsiness Sinarest Tablets and Caplets, 910
Noludar, 697-698
Nolvadex, 992-993
NONSTEROIDAL ANTIINFLAMMATORIES, 58-59
Norcet, 533
Norcuron, 1079-1080
Nordryl, 378-380
norepinephrine, 766-767
norethindrone, 767-768
Norflex, 780-781
norfloxacin, 768-769
Norgesic, 780
norgestrel, 769-770
Norlutin, 767-768
Nor-Mil, 364-365
Normodyne, 598-599
Normozide, 598
Noroxin, 768-769
Norpace, 383-384
Norpanth, 900-901
Norplant System, 607-608
Norpramin, 335-337
Nor-QD, 767-768
Nor-Tet, 1006-1007
nortriptyline, 770-772
Norvasc, 110-111
Norwich Extra-Strength, 136-138
Norzine, 1013-1014
Nostril, 847-848
Nostrilla, 791
Novafed, 910-911
Novahistine Cough and Cold Formula, 349
Novamedopa, 690-691
Novamine, 102-103
Novamobarb, 113-115
Novamoxin, 118-119
Novaniacin, 755-756
Novantrone, 723-724
Novapropoxyn, 903-904
Nova-Rectal, 825-827
Novasen, 136-138
Novasorbide, 585-586
Novo-Alprazol, 89-90
Novo Ampicillin, 124-125
Novo-Atenol, 139-141
Novo-AZT, 1096-1097
Novobutamide, 1038-1039
Novocain, 889-890
Novo Carbamaz, 207-208
Novochlorhydrate, 249-250
Novochlorocap, 252-253
Novochloroquine, 258-259
Novo-Chlorpromazine, 262-265
Novocimetine, 273-275
Novoclopate, 295-296
Novocloxin, 297-298
Novodimenate, 375-376
Novodipam, 352-354
Novodoxyclin, 397-398
Novoflurazine, 1053-1055
Novofolacid, 487-488
Novofuran, 761-762
Novohexidyl, 1057-1058
Novohydrazide, 532-533
Novohydroxyzine, 546-547
novo-Hylazin, 530-532
Novolexin, 242-243
Novolin 70/30, 563-564
Novolin L, 568-569
Novolin N, 562-563
Novolin R, 565-566
Novolorazem, 627-629
Novomepro, 664-665

Entries can be identified as follows: generic name, Trade Name, DRUG CATEGORY, *Combination Product.*

Novomethacin, 560-561
Novometoprol, 704-706
Novonaprox sodium, 745-746
Novonidazole, 706-707
Novo-Nifedin, 760-761
Novopen G, 815-816
Novopen-VK, 820-821
Novoperidol, 521-523
novopirocam, 863-864
Novopoxide, 255-257
Novo-Pramine, 555-557
Novo-Pranol, 904-906
Novoprofen, 549-550
Novopropamide, 265-266
Novopropoxy Compound, 903-904
Novopyrazone, 985
Novoquine, 924-925
Novoquinidin, 923-924
Novoreserpine, 930-931
Novoridazine, 1016-1018
Novorythro, 422-424
Novosalmol, 83-84
Novosemide, 492-493
Novosoxazole, 986-987
Novospiroton, 966-967
NovoSundac, 987-988
Novo-Tamoxifen, 992-993
Novotetra, 1006-1007
Novothalidone, 266-267
Novotriolam, 1051-1052
Novotriphyl, 788-789
Novotriptyn, 109-110
Novoxapam, 786-787
Nozinan, 685-686
NP-27, 1040
NPH Iletin II, 562-563
NPH Insulin, 562-563
NPH Purified, 562-563
NTZ Long-Acting Nasal, 791
Nu-Alpraz, 89-90
Nu-Amoxi, 118-119
Nu-Ampi, 124-125
Nubain, 738-739
Nu-Cephalex, 242-243
Nu-Clox, 297-298
Nujol, 716-717
Numorphan, 793-794
Nu N. Sed, 760-761
Nupercainal, 356
Nuprin, 549-550
Nuromax, 390-391
Nu-Tetra, 1006-1007
Nutracort, 535-536
Nu-Triazol, 1051-1052
Nutropin, 961-962
Nydrazid, 582-583
Nyoderm, 773
Nyquil Nighttime Cold Medicine, 349
nystatin, 772-773
nystatin (topical), 773
Nystex, 773
Nytime Cold Medicine, 349
Nytol, 378-380

O

Obalan, 835-836
Obe-Nix, 843-844
Obephen, 843-844
Obeval, 835-836
Occlusal, 940-941
Occuflox, 774-775
Octamide PFS, 700-701
Octocaine HCl, 613-614
Ocu-Carpine, 854-855
Ocufen, 485-486
Ocupress, 214-216
Ocusert Pilo, 854-855
Ocu-Tropine, 143-145
Off-Ezy Wart Remover, 940-941
O-Flex, 780-781
ofloxacin, 774-775
olsalazine, 775
omeprazole, 776-777
Omnipen, 124-125
OMS Concentrate, 728-729
Oncaspar, 810-812
Oncovin, 1086-1088

ondansetron, 777-778
One-A-Day, 731-732
Opcon, 745
Operand Povidone-Iodine, 874
Ophthacet, 977-978
Ophthalgan Ophthalmic, 506-507
Opium and Belladonna, 778
opium tincture, 778-779
Opium Tincture Deodorized, 778-779
Optigene 3 Eye Drops, 1009-1010
Optilets, 731-732
Optimine, 148-149
Optipranolol, 700
Orabase Baby, 164
Oracin, 164
Ora-Jel, 164
oral contraceptives, 779-780
Oralone Dental, 1049
Oramorph SR, 728-729
Oraphen-PD, 69-72
Orasone, 883-884
Oratect, 164
Orazinc, 1098
Orbenin, 297-298
Oretic, 532-533
Oreticyl, 532
Orex DM, 348-350
Orimune, 868
Orinase, 1038-1039
ORLAMM, 606-607
Ormazine, 262-265
Ornex Caplets, Maximum Strength, 910
orphenadrine, 780-781
Orphenadrine Citrate, 780-781
Orphenate, 780-781
Orthoclone OKT3, 732-733
Ortho Dienestrol, 362-363
Orthoxicol Cough Syrup, 349
OR-Tyl, 359-360
Orudis, 595-596
Oruvail, 595-596
Os-Cal, 200-201
Osmitrol, 639-640
Osmoglyn, 506
Ostercal, 200-201
Otall, 535
Otocort, 751
Otrivin, 1094
Ovol, 955
Ovral, 769-770
Ovrette, 769-770
O-V Statin, 773
oxacillin, 781-783
oxacillin sodium, 781-783
oxamniquine, 783-784
Oxandrin, 784-785
oxandrolone, 784-785
oxaprozin, 785-786
oxazepam, 786-787
oxidized cellulose, 787-788
Ox-Pam, 786-787
Oxsoralen, 686-687
oxtriphylline, 788-789
Oxy 5, 166-167
Oxy 10, 166-167
Oxybutazone, 794-795
oxybutynin, 789
oxybutynin chloride, 789
Oxycel, 787-788
Oxycocet, 790-791
Oxycodan, 790-791
oxycodone, 790-791
Oxycodone/Acetaminophen Endocet, 790-791
Oxycodone/Aspirin Endodan, 790-791
Oxydess II, 347-348
oxymetazoline HCl, 791
oxymetazoline (nasal), 791
oxymetholone, 792-793
oxymorphone, 793-794
oxyphenbutazone, 794-795
oxytetracycline, 795-796
Oxytetracycline HCl, 795-796
oxytocin, synthetic injection, 797-798

Entries can be identified as follows: generic name, Trade Name, DRUG CATEGORY, *Combination Product.*

oxytocin, synthetic nasal, 798
Oysco 500, 200-201
Oyst-Cal 500, 200-201
Oyster Shell Calcium 500, 200-201

P

paclitaxel, 798-800
Palaron, 105-107
Pamelor, 770-772
pamidronate, 800
Pamine, 687-688
Pamprin, 69
Pamprin-IB, 549-550
Pamprin Maximum Cramp Relief, 69
Panadol, 69-72
Panadol Infant's Drops, 69-72
Panasol-S, 883-884
Pancet Propacet, 903-904
Pancrease, 801-802
pancreatin, 800-801
pancrelipase, 801-802
pancuronium, 802-803
pancuronium bromide, 802-803
Panectyl, 1058-1059
Panex 500, 69-72
Panmycin, 1006-1007
Pan Oxyl, 166-167
Panscol, 940-941
Pantopan, 778-779
papaverine, 803-804
papaverine HCl, 803-804
Paplex Ultra, 940-941
Paracet Forte, 69, 267
Paradione, 806-807
Paraflex, 267-268
Parafon Forte, 267
Parafon Forte DSC, 267-268
Paral, 804-806
paraldehyde, 804-806
paramethadione, 806-807
paramethasone, 807-808
Paraplatin, 209-211
Paregoric, 778-779
Paregorique, 778-779
Parepectolin, 778
Parlodel, 184-185
Parnate, 1043-1044
paromomycin, 808-809
paroxetine, 809-810
Parten, 69-72
Pathibamate-200, 778
Pathocil, 358-359
Pavabid, 803-804
Pavarine Spancaps, 803-804
Pavased, 803-804
Pavatine, 803-804
Pavatym, 803-804
Paveral, 300-301
Paverolan Lanacaps, 803-804
Pavulon, 802-803
Paxil, 809-810
Paxipam, 518-519
PBZ, 1065-1066
PCE Dispertab, 422-424
p′-DDD, 722-723
Pedia Care Allergy Formula, 261-262
Pedia Care Infant's Decongestant, 910-911
Pediaflor, 474-475
Pediapatch, 940-941
Pediapred, 880-882
Pediatric Gentamicin Sulfate, 499-500
Pediazole, 422
Pedi-boro Soak Paks, 94-95
Pedric, 69-72
PedTE-PAK-4, 1042-1043
Pedtrace-4, 1042-1043
Peganone, 440-441
pegaspargase, 810-812
Pelamine, 1065-1066
pemoline, 812-813
Penapar-VK, 820-821
Penecort, 535-536
Penetrex, 408-409
Penglobe, 154-156

Entries can be identified as follows: generic name, Trade Name, DRUG CATEGORY, *Combination Product.*

D-penicillamine, 398-399
penicillin G benzathine, 813-815
penicillin G potassium, 815-816
penicillin G procaine, 817-818
penicillin G sodium, 818-820
penicillin V potassium, 820-821
Penntuss, 300
Pentacarinat, 822-823
Pentacef, 236-237
pentaerythritol, 821-822
Pentam 300, 822-823
pentamidine, 822-823
Pentamycin, 253-254
pentazocine, 823-825
Pentids, 815-816
pentobarbital, 825-827
pentobarbital sodium, 825-827
Pentogen, 825-827
Pentolair, 314-315
pentostatin, 827-828
Pentothal, 1015-1016
pentoxifylline, 828-829
Pentusa, 667-668
Pentylan, 821-822
Pen-Vee K, 820-821
Pepcid, 450-452
Pepto-Bismol Maximum Strength, 178
Pepto Diarrhea Control, 625-626
Peptol, 273-275
Perbuzem, 821
Percocet, 790-791
Percodan, 790-791
Percodan-Demi, 136, 790-701
Percogesic, 69
Perdiem, 911-912
Pergonal, 657
Peri-Colace, 387
Peridol, 521-523
perindopril, 829-830
Peritrate, 821-822
Perlactin, 319-320
Permapen, 813-815
permethrin, 830-831
Permitil, 481-483
Pernavite, 310-311
perphenazine, 831-834
Persa-Gel, 166-167
Persantine, 382-383
Persistin, 387
Pertofrane, 335-337
Pertussin, 348-350
Pethadol, 658-660
Pethidine, 658-660
P.E.T.N., 821-822
Petrogalar Plain, 716-717
Pfeiffer's Allergy, 261-262
Pfizerpen, 815-816, 818-820
Pfizerpen-AS, 817-818
PGEI, 91-92
Pharmadine, 874
Pharmaflur, 474-475
Phazyme, 955
Phena-Bella, 161
phenacemide, 834
Phenameth, 898-899
Phenapap No. 2, 69
Phenaphen Caplets, 69-72
Phenaphen with Codeine, 69-70
Phenaphen-650 with Codeine, 70
Phenazine, 831-834, 898-899
Phenazine-35, 835-836
Phenazo, 834-835
Phenazodine, 834-835
phenazopyridine, 834-835
phenazopyridine HCl, 834-835
phendimetrazine, 835-836
phendimetrazine tartrate, 835-836
Phendry, 378-380
phenelzine, 837-838
Phenergan, 898-899
Phenergan VC Syrup, 898
Phenergan with Dextromethorphan, 349
Phenetron, 261-262
phenobarbital, 838-840
Phenobarbital Sodium, 838-840
Phenoject-50, 898-899

Entries can be identified as follows: generic name, Trade Name, DRUG CATEGORY, *Combination Product.*

Phenolax, 840
phenolphthalein, 840
Phenoptic, 848-849
phenoxybenzamine, 841
phensuximide, 841-842
phentermine, 843-844
phentermine HCl, 843-844
Phentermine Resin, 843-844
phentolamine, 844-845
Phentrol, 843-844
Phenurone, 834
phenylbutazone, 845-846
phenylephrine, 846-847
Phenylephrine HCl, 848-849
phenylephrine (nasal), 847-848
phenylephrine (optic), 848-849
phenytoin, 849-850
phenytoin oral suspension, 849-850
Phenzine, 835-836
Phillip's Milk of Magnesia, 638-639
pHisoAc BP, 166-167
Phos-Flur, 474-475
Phospholine Iodide, 402-403
Phospho-Soda, 958-959
Phrenilin, 70
Phrenilin Forte, 70
Phrenilin with Codeine, 70
Phyllocontin, 105-107
physostigmine, 852
physostigmine (ophthalmic), 851
phytonadione, 853-854
Pilagan, 854-855
Pilocar, 854-855
pilocarpine, 854-855
pilocarpine HCl, 854-855
Pilopine HS, 854-855
Piloptic, 854-855
Pilopto-Carpine, 854-855
Pilostat, 854-855
Pima, 872-873
pinacidil, 855-856
Pindac, 855-856
pindolol, 856-857
Pin-X, 912-913
pipecuronium, 857-858
piperacillin, 858-860
piperacillin and tazobactam, 860-861
piperazine, 861-862
Pipracil, 858-860
pirbuterol, 862-863
piroxicam, 863-864
Pitocin, 797-798
Pitressin Synthetic, 1079
Placidyl, 435-437
Plaquenil Sulfate, 542-543
Plasbumin, 82-83
Plasmanate, 864-865
Plasma Plex, 864-865
plasma protein fraction, 864-865
Plasmatein, 864-865
Platinol-AQ, 277-279
Plegine, 835-836
Plendil, 454-455
plicamycin, 865-867
PMB, 664
PMS Egozine, 1098
PMS-Isoniazid, 582-583
PMS-Metronidazole, 706-707
PMS Perphenazine, 831-834
PMS Promethazine, 898-899
PMS Pyrazinamide, 913
Pneumopent, 822-823
Pod-Ben-25, 867-868
Podocon-25, 867-868
Podofilm, 867-868
Podofin, 867-868
podophyllum resin, 867-868
Point-Two, 474-475
Poladex, 344-345
Polaramine, 344-345
poliovirus vaccine, live, oral, trivalent, 868
Polocaine, 663-664
Polycillin, 124-125
Polydine, 874
Polyflex, 268

Entries can be identified as follows: generic name, Trade Name, DRUG CATEGORY, *Combination Product.*

Polymox, 118-119
polymyxin B, 868-869
polymyxin B (ophthalmic), 869-870
polymyxin B sulfate, 868-869
Poly-Vi-Sol, 731-732
Ponstel, 652
Pontocaine, 1004
Pontocaine Eye, 1004-1005
Pontocaine HCl, 1004-1005
Pontocaine (topical), 1005
Porcelana, 541
Potachlor, 870-872
Potage, 870-872
Potasalan, 870-872
potassium acetate, 870-872
potassium bicarbonate, 870-872
potassium chloride, 870-872
potassium gluconate, 870-872
potassium iodide, 872-873
potassium iodide (SSKI), 873-874
potassium phosphate, 870-872
povidone iodine, 874
PPF Protenate, 864-865
pralidoxime, 874-875
Pralzine, 530-532
pramoxine (topical), 875-876
Pravachol, 876
pravastatin, 876
Prax, 875-876
prazepam, 877-878
praziquantel, 878
prazosin, 879
Precef, 227-229
Precose, 1101-1102
Predalone-T.B.A., 880-882
Predcor, 880-882
Pred-Forte, 882-883
Pred-Mild, 882-883
prednicarbate, 880
Prednicen-M, 883-884
prednisolone, 880-882
prednisolone acetate, 880-882
prednisolone acetate (suspension), 882-883
prednisolone phosphate, 880-882
prednisolone sodium phosphate (solution), 882-883
prednisolone tebutate, 880-882
Prednisol TBA, 880-882
prednisone, 883-884
Prefrin, 848-849
Pregnyl, 271-272
Prelone, 880-882
Prelu-2, 835-836
Premarin, 430-432
Prepidil, 377-378
Prevacid, 1106-1107
Prevident, 474-475
Prilosec, 776-777
Primacor, 715-716
primaquine, 884-885
Primatene Mist, 412-414
Primaxin, 554-555
primidone, 885-886
Prinivil, 620-621
Priscoline, 1036-1037
Privine, 744
Pro 50, 898-899
Probalan, 886-887
Pro-Banthine, 900-901
probenecid, 886-887
probucol, 887-888
procainamide, 888-889
procaine, 889-890
Pro-Cal-Sof, 387-388
Procan SR, 888-889
procarbazine, 890-892
Procardia, 760-761
prochlorperazine, 892-893
Procrit, 415-416
ProctoFoam, 875-876
Procyclid, 893-894
procyclidine, 893-894
Procytox, 315-317
Pro-Depo, 544-545
Prodiem Plain, 911-912
Prodrox, 544-545
Profasi, 271-272

Entries can be identified as follows: generic name, Trade Name, DRUG CATEGORY, *Combination Product.*

Profene, 903-904
Profilate HP, 130-132
profilate OSD, 130-132
Profilnine Heat-Treated/Alpha Nine, 448-449
Progestasert, 894-895
progesterone, 894-895
Progesterone in Oil, 894-895
Progestillin, 894-895
Proglycem, 355-356
Prograf, 990-991
ProHIBIT (conjugate), 517-518
Prokine, 943-944
Pro-Lax, 911-912
Prolixin, 481-483
Prolixin Decanoate, 481-483
Prolixin Enanthate, 481-483
Proloid, 1022-1023
Proloprim, 1061-1062
Promanyl, 895-897
promazine, 895-897
Prometh-50, 898-899
promethazine, 898-899
promethazine HCl, 898-899
Promethazine HCl VC, 898
Promine, 888-889
Pronestyl, 888-889
Propacet 100, 903
propafenone, 899-900
Propanthel, 900-901
propantheline, 900-901
propantheline bromide, 900-901
Propa P.H. Liquid Acne Soap, 166-167
Propine, 381
Proplex SX-T, 448-449
Proplex T, 448-449
propofol, 901-902
Pro-Pox, 903-904
Pro-Pox Plus, 903-904
Pro-Pox with APAP, 903-904
Propoxycon, 903-904
Propoxyphene-AC, 903
propoxyphene, 903-904
propoxyphene/acetaminophen, 903-904
propoxyphene/aspirin/caffeine, 903-904
Propoxyphene Compound-65, 903
propoxyphene HCl, 903-904
Propoxyphene Napyslate with Acetaminophen Tablets, 903
Propoxyphene with APAP, 903-904
propranolol, 904-906
Propranolol HCl, 904
Propranolol Intensol, 904-906
Propulsid, 276-277
propylthiouracil, 906-908
Propyl-Thyracil, 906-908
Prorex, 898-899
Proscar, 463-464
ProSom, 425
prostaglandin E_1, 91-92
Prostaphilin, 781-783
Prostep, 759-760
Prostigmin, 752-753
Prostin E_2, 377-378
Prostin/15M, 211-212
Prostin VR, 91-92
protamine, 908
Protectol, 1070-1071
Prothazine Plain, 898-899
Protopam Chloride, 874-875
Protophylline, 401-402
Protostat, 706-707
protriptyline, 908-910
Provacin, 892-893
Proval, 69
Proventil, 83-84
Provera, 650-651
Proviodine, 874
Prozac, 478-480
Prozine, 895-897
Prulet, 840
Prunicodeine, 1000
pseudoephidrine, 910-911
pseudoephedrine/acrivastine, 76-77
pseudoephedrine HCl, 910-911

Entries can be identified as follows: generic name, Trade Name, DRUG CATEGORY, *Combination Product.*

Pseudogest Decongestant, 910-911
Pseudomonic Acid A, 732
Pseudo Syrup, 910-911
Psorcon, 365-366
psyllium, 911-912
P.T.E., 1042-1043
PTU, 906-908
Pulmozyme, 385-386
Purimol, 88-89
Purinethol, 665-667
PVFK, 820-821
pyrantel, 912-913
pyrazinamide, 913
pyrethrins, 913-914
Pyridiate, 834-835
Pyridium, 834-835
pyridostigmine, 914-915
pyridoxine, 916
pyridoxine HCl, 916
pyrimethamine, 917-918
Pyrinyl, 913-914

Q

Quarzan, 283-284
quazepam, 918-919
Quelicin, 974-976
Questran, 269
Quibron-T, 1010-1012
Quiess, 546-547
Quiet Nite, 349
quinacrine, 919-920
Quinaglute, 923-924
Quinalan, 923-924
Quinamm, 924-925
quinapril, 920-922
quinestrol, 922-923
Quinidex Extentabs, 923-924
quinidine, 923-924
quinidine gluconate, 923-924
quinidine sulfate, 923-924
quinine, 924-925
Quinine Sulfate, 924-925
Quinora, 923-924
Quinsana Plus, 1040
Quin tabs, 731-732
Quiphile, 924-925
Q-Vel, 924-925

R

rabies immune globulin, human, 925-926
radioactive iodine, 926-927
Radiostol, 1090-1091
ramipril, 927-928
ranitidine, 929-930
Rapifen, 86-87
Razepam, 994-995
Reclomide, 700-701
recombinant human deoxyribonuclease I, 385-386
recombinant human GM-CSF, 943-944
Recombinate, 130-132
Redisol, 310-311
Redoxon, 133-134
Redutemp, 69-72
Reese's Pinworm, 912-913
Regitine, 844-845
Reglan, 700-701
Regonol, 914-915
Regroton, 930
Regular (concentrated) Iltein II U-500, 566-567
Regulex SS, 387-388
Reguloid, 911-912
Regutol, 387-388
Rela, 212-213
Relafen, 733-734
Relief, 848-849
Remsed, 898-899
Remular-S, 267-268
Renese-R, 930
Renormax, 964-966
Rep-Pred/A-Methapred, 695-696
Rescon Jr., 910
Resectial, 639-640
Reserfia, 930-931
reserpine, 930-931

Entries can be identified as follows: generic name, Trade Name, DRUG CATEGORY, *Combination Product.*

Respbid, 1010-1012
Resposans-10, 255-257
Restoril, 994-995
Resyl, 512-513
Retin-A, 1046
retinoic acid, 1046
Retrovir, 1096-1097
Reversol, 405-407
Revex, 1109-1110
Rev-Eyes, 329-330
Revimine, 388-389
Revitonus, 1012-1013
Rexolate, 960-961
Rheomacrodex, 345-346
Rhesonatre Rho-Gam, 931-932
Rheumatrex Dose Pack, 683-685
Rhinall-10, 847-848
Rhinocort, 187-188
RH_o (D) immune globulin, human, 931-932
Rhotral, 67-68
rhu GM-CSF, 943-944
Rhythmin, 888-889
Rhythmodan, 383-384
riboflavin, 932-933
RID, 913-914
Ridaura, 146-147
rifabutin, 933-934
Rifadin, 934-935
Rifamate, 582
Rifampicin, 934-935
rifampin, 934-935
Rimactane, 582, 934-935
rimantadine, 935-936
rimexolone, 936
Riopan, 634-635
Risperdal, 937-938
risperidone, 937-938
Ritalin, 693-694
ritodrine, 938-939
Rivoiril, 291-293
RMS, 728-729
Robaxin, 681-682
Robaxisal, 664
Robicillin-VK, 820-821
Robidex, 348-350
Robidone, 533-535
Robigesic, 69-72
Robimycin Robitabs/Erythromid, 422-424
Robinul, 507-508
Robitet, 1006-1007
Robitussin, 512-513
Robitussin Cough Calmers, 348-350
Robitussin-DM, 349
Robitussin Pediatric Sedatuss, 348-350
Robomol, 681-682
Robomol/ASA, 664
Rocaltrol Vitamin D_3, 199-200
Rocephin, 239-240
rocuronium, 939-940
Rodex TD, 916
Rofact, 934-935
Roferon-a/Intron-a, 571-572
Rogaine, 718-719
Rogitine, 844-845
Rolaids Antacid, 373
Rolaids Calcium Rich, 200-201
Rolavil, 109-110
Rolzine, 530-532
Ronazicon, 472-473
Rounax, 69-72
Rowasa Salofalk, 667-668
Roxanol, 728-729
Roxicet, 790-791
Roxicodone, 790-791
Roxilox, 790-791
Roxiprin, 790-791
Rubesol-1000, 310-311
Rubex, 395-397
Rubion, 310-311
Rubramin PC, 310-311
Rufen, 549-550
Ru-Lets, 731-732
Rum-K, 870-872
Ru-Vert-M, 648-649

Entries can be identified as follows: generic name, Trade Name, DRUG CATEGORY, *Combination Product.*

Rynacrom, 308-309
Rythmol, 899-900

S

St. Joseph Aspirin-free Infant Drops, 69-72
St. Joseph Children's, 136-138
St. Joseph Cough Suppressant, 348-350
St. Joseph Measured Dose, 847-848
Salacid, 940-941
Sal-Acid, 940-941
Salactic Film, 940-941
Sal-Adult, 136-138
Salazopyrin, 983-985
Salbutamol, 83-84
Saleto, 549-550
Salflex, 942-943
SALICYLATES, 59-61
salicylic acid, 940-941
Salicylic Acid Creme 60%, 940-941
Sal-Infant, 136-138
salmeterol, 941-942
Sal Plant, 940-941
salsalate, 942-943
Salsitab, 942-943
Sandimmune, 318-319
Sandoglobulin, 557-558
Sani-Supp, 506
Sanorex, 643-644
Sansert, 699-700
sargramostim, 943-944
Saronil, 664-665
Satric, 706-707
Scabene, 616-617
scopolamine, 945-946
scopolamine (optic), 946
scopolamine (transdermal), 947
Scot-Tussin Allergy, 378-380
Scot-Tussin Expectorant, 512-513
SD-Deprenyl, 950-951
secobarbital, 947-949
Secobarbital Sodium, 947-949
Secogen Sodium, 947-949
Seconal Sodium, 947-949
Secretin-Ferring, 947-949
Sectral, 67-68
Sedabamate, 664-665
Seffin Neutral, 243-245
Seldane, 1000
selegiline, 950-951
selenium, 951
Selenium Sulfide, 951
Selestoject, 171-173
Selsun, 951
Selsun Blue, 951
Semilente Iletin I, 570-571
Semilente Insulin, 570-571
Senexon, 951-952
senna, 951-952
Senna-Gen, 951-952
Senokot, 951-952
Senokotxtra, 951-952
Senolax, 951-952
Septra, 982-983
Ser-a-Gen, 530
Seral, 947-949
Ser-Ap-Es, 530
Serathide, 530
Serax, 786-787
Sereen, 255-257
Serentil, 668-670
Serevent, 941-942
Seromycin Pulvules, 317-318
Serophene, 289-290
Serpasil, 930-931
Serpasil-Apresoline HCl, 530
Serpasil-Esidrix, 930
Serpazide, 530
Sertan, 885-886
sertraline, 952-953
Serutan, 911-912
Sesame Street Vitamins, 731-732
Siblin, 911-912
Silphen Cough, 378-380
Silvadene, 954-955
silver nitrate, 953-954
silver nitrate 1% (ophthalmic), 954

silver protein, mild, 954
silver sulfadiazine (topical), 954-955
simethicone, 955
Simron, 460-462
simvastatin, 956
Sinarest 12-Hour, 791
Sincomen, 966-967
Sine-Aid, 70
Sine-Aid Extra Strength Caplets, 70
Sine-Aid IB, 910
Sine-Aid, Maximum Strength, 910
Sinemet, 208-209
Sine-Off Extra Strength, 70
Sinequan, 393-395
Sinex, 847-848
Sinex Long-Acting, 791
S-2 Inhalant, 412-414
Sinubid, 70
Sinumist-SR, 512-513
Sinustat, 910-911
Sinutab, 70
Sinutab II Maximum, 70
Sinutab Maximum Nighttime, 70
SK-APAP with Codeine, 70
SK-65-Compound, 136
Skelez, 268
SK-Pramine, 555-557
Sleep-Eze 3, 378-380
Sleepinal, 378-380
Slo-Bid Gyrocaps, 1010-1012
Slo-Niacin, 755-756
Slo-Phyllin Gyrocaps, 1010-1012
Slow-Fe, 460-462
Slow-K, 870-872
Slyn-LL, 835-836
Soda Mint, 957-958
sodium bicarbonate, 957-958
sodium biphosphate, 958-959
sodium calcium edetate, 403-404
sodium chloride, hypertonic, 959
Sodium Fluoride, 474-475
sodium iodide, 926-927
sodium nitroprusside, 764-765
sodium phosphate, 958-959
sodium polystyrene sulfonate, 959-960
Sodium Sulamyd, 977-978
sodium sulfacetamide, 977-978
sodium thiosalicylate, 960-961
Sofarin, 1092-1094
Softabs, 187
Solaquin, 541
Solarcaine, 611
Solazine, 1053-1055
Solfoton, 838-840
Solganal, 147-148
Solium, 255-257
Solu-Cortef, 536-538
Solu-Medrol, 695-696
Solurex, 340-341
Soma, 212-213
Soma Compound, 212
Soma Compound with Codeine, 300
somatotropin, 961-962
Sominex, 378-380
Somnol, 484-485
Soothe Eye Drops, 1009-1010
Sopamycetin, 254
Soprodol, 212-213
Sorbitrate, 585-586
Soridol, 212-213
SOSS-10, 977-978
Sotacar, 962-964
sotalol, 962-964
Soyacal 20%, 452-453
Spancap 1, 347-348
Span-FF, 460-462
SpaN Niacin, 755-756
Sparine, 895-897
Spasmoject, 359-360
Spec-T Anesthetic, 164
Spectazole, 403
spectinomycin, 964
Spectrobid, 154-156
Spec-T Sore Throat Cough Suppressant, 349
spirapril, 964-966
Spironazide, 532

Entries can be identified as follows: generic name, Trade Name, DRUG CATEGORY, *Combination Product.*

spironolactone, 966-967
Spirozide, 532
Sporanox, 590-591
Sprx-105, 835-836
SPS Suspension, 959-960
S-P-T, 1023-1024
SSD, 954-955
SSKI, 872-874
Stadol, 195-196
stanozolol, 967-968
Staphcillin, 678-679
Staticin, 421
stavudine, 968-969
S-T Cort, 535-536
Stelazine, 1053-1055
Stemetic, 1060-1061
Stemetil, 892-893
Sterapred, 883-884
Stievaa, 1046
Stilphostrol, 363-364
Stop, 474-475
Stoxil, 552-553
Streptase, 969-971
streptokinase, 969-971
streptomycin, 971-972
streptozocin, 972-973
Stress-Pam, 352-354
Sublimaze, 457-458
succimer, 974
succinylcholine, 974-976
succinylcholine chloride, 974-976
Sucostrin, 974-976
sucralfate, 976
Sucrets Cough Control, 348-350
Sudafed, 910-911
Sudafed Cough Syrup, 349
Sudrin, 910-911
Sufenta, 967-977
sufentanil, 967-977
Sulcrate, 976
sulfacetamide (ophthalmic), 977-978
sulfadiazine, 978-979
Sulfair 15, 977-978
Sulfalax Calcium, 387-388
sulfamethizole, 979-980
sulfamethoxazole, 980-982
sulfamethoxazole and trimethoprim, 982-983
Sulfamylon, 633-634
sulfasalazine, 983-985
Sulfasol, 979-980
Sulfatrim, 982-983
sulfinpyrazone, 985
sulfisoxazole, 986-987
sulindac, 987-988
sumatriptan, 988-989
Sumycin, 1006-1007
Sunkist Vitamin C, 133-134
Supasa, 136-138
Supen, 124-125
Superchar, 77-78
Supeudol, 790-791
Suppress, 348-350
Supracaine, 1004-1005
Suprax, 222-223
Suprazine, 1053-1055
Surfak/Dialose, 387-388
Surgicel, 787-788
Surmontil, 1064-1065
Survanta, 170-171
Sus-Phrine, 412-414
Sustaire, 1010-1012
Suxamethonium, 974-976
Syllact, 911-912
Symadine, 96-97
Symmetrel, 96-97
Synacort, 535-536
Synacthen, 307-308
Synalar, 474
Synarel, 735-736
Synemol, 474
Synflex, 745-746
Synkavite, 656
Synkayvite, 656
Synthroid, 609-611
Syntocinon, 797-798

Syprine, 1052
Sytobex, 310-311

T

T_3, 617-618
T_4, 609-611
Tab-A-Vite, 731-732
Tac-3, 1047-1048
Tac-40, 1047-1048
tacrine, 989-990
tacrolimus, 990-991
Tagamet, 273-275
Talacen, 823
talbutal, 991-992
Talwin, 823-825
Tambocor, 465-466
Tamofen, 992-993
Tamone, 992-993
tamoxifen, 992-993
Tapanol Extra Strength, 69-72
Tapazole, 679-680
Tarabine PFS, 320-322
Tavist, 282-283
Taxol, 798-800
Tazicef, 236-237
Tazidime, 236-237
tazobactam and piperacillin, 860-861
T-Caine, 164
Tebumide, 1060 1061
Tebrazid, 913
Tega-Cort, 535-536
Tegison, 447-448
Tegopen, 297-298
Tegretol, 207-208
Telachlor, 261-262
Teladar/Diprolene, 171-173
Teldrin, 261-262
Teline, 1006-1007
Temaril, 1058-1059
temazepam, 994-995
Temovate, 286-287
Tempra, 69-72
Tenex, 516-517
teniposide, 995-996
Ten-K, 870-872
Tenoretic, 139
Tenormin, 139-141
Tensilon, 405-407
Terazol, 999
terazosin, 996-997
terbinafine, 997-998
terbutaline, 998-999
terconazole, 999
terfenadine, 1000
Terfluzine, 1053-1055
terpin hydrate, 1000-1001
Terpin Hydrate and Codeine, 1000
Terramycin, 795-796
Terramycin Intramuscular Solution, 795
Teslac, 1001
Tessalon Perles, 165
Testex, 1002-1003
testolactone, 1001
Testone LA, 1002-1003
testosterone, 1002-1003
testosterone cypionate, 1002-1003
testosterone enanthate, 1002-1003
testosterone propionate, 1002-1003
Testred Cypionate, 1002-1003
Testrin PA, 1002-1003
tetanus toxoid, 1003-1004
tetanus toxoid, adsorbed, 1003-1004
tetracaine, 1004
tetracaine (ophthalmic), 1004-1005
tetracaine (topical), 1005
Tetracap, 1006-1007
Tetracosactrin, 307-308
tetracycline, 1006-1007
tetracycline HCl, 1006-1007
tetracycline (ophthalmic), 1007-1008
tetracycline (topical), 1008
Tetracyn, 1006-1007
tetrahydroaminoacridine, 989-990
tetrahydrozoline (nasal), 1009

Entries can be identified as follows: generic name, Trade Name, DRUG CATEGORY, *Combination Product.*

tetrahydrozoline (ophthalmic), 1009-1010
Tetralan, 1006-1007
Tetralean, 1006-1007
Tetram, 1006-1007
Texacort, 535-536
6-TG, 1014-1015
T-Gen, 1060-1061
T-Gesic, 534
THA, 989-990
Thalitone, 266-267
Tham, 1068
Tham-E, 1068
Theelin Aqueous, 432-433
Theo-24, 1010-1012
Theobid Duracaps, 1010-1012
Theochron, 1010-1012
Theoclear, 1010-1012
Theo-Dur, 1010-1012
Theolair, 1010-1012
Theomax DF Syrup, 1010
theophylline, 1010-1012
Theophylline and Dextrose, 1010-1012
Theophylline Extended Release, 1010-1012
Theophylline Oral, 1010-1012
Theophylline S.R., 1010-1012
Theo-Sav, 1010-1012
Theospan-SR, 1010-1012
Theostat 80, 1010-1012
Theovent, 1010-1012
Theox, 1010-1012
Therabid, 731-732
Thera-Flur, 474-475
Theragram, 731-732
Theramycin Z, 421
Therapy Bayer, 136-138
Thermazene, 954-955
Theroxide, 166-167
thiabendazole, 1012
Thiacide, 674
Thiamilate, 1012-1013
thiamine, 1012-1013
thiamine HCl, 1012-1013
thiethylperazine, 1013-1014
thioguanine (6-TG), 1014-1015
Thiola, 1031-1032
Thionex, 616-617
thiopental, 1015-1016
thiopental sodium, 1015-1016
thioridazine, 1016-1018
thioridazine HCl, 1016-1018
Thiosulfil, 979-980
thiotepa, 1018-1020
thiothixene, 1020-1022
Thiuretic, 532-533
Thorazine, 262-265
Thor-prom, 262-265
3TC, 1105-1106
Thrombate III, 132
thrombin, 1022
Thrombinar, 1022
Thrombogen, 1022
THROMBOLYTICS, 61-62
Thrombostat, 1022
Thyrar, 1023-1024
Thyro-Block, 872-874
thyroglobulin, 1022-1023
THYROID HORMONES, 63-64
thyroid-stimulating hormone, 1025
Thyroid Strong, 1023-1024
thyroid USP (desiccated), 1023-1024
Thyrolar, 609, 619-620
thyrotropin, 1025
Thytropar, 1025
Ticar, 1025-1027
ticarcillin, 1025-1027
ticarcillin/clavulanate, 1027-1028
Ticlid, 1028-1029
ticlopidine, 1028-1029
Ticon, 1060-1061
Tigan, 1060-1061
Tiject-20, 1060-1061
Tilade, 747-748
Timentin, 1027-1028
Timolide 10/25, 532

Entries can be identified as follows: generic name, Trade Name, DRUG CATEGORY, *Combination Product.*

timolol, 1029-1030
timolol maleate, 1029-1030
timolol (optic), 1031
Timoptic, 1031
Tinactin, 1040
Ting, 1040
tiopronin, 1031-1032
TISIT, 913-914
tissue plasminogen activator, 92-93
tobramycin (ophthalmic), 1032-1033
tobramycin, 1033-1034
tobramycin sulfate, 1033-1034
Tobrax, 1033-1034
Tobrex, 1032-1033
tocainide, 1034-1035
Tocopherol, 1092
Tofranil, 555-557
Tolamide, 1035-1036
tolazamide, 1035-1036
tolazoline, 1036-1037
tolbutamide, 1038-1039
Tolbutone, 1038-1039
Tolectin, 1039-1040
Tolinase, 1035-1036
tolmetin, 1039-1040
tolmetin sodium, 1039-1040
tolnaftate (topical), 1040
Tonocard, 1034-1035
Topicort, 338-339
Topicycline, 1008
Toprol XL, 704-706
Toradol, 596-597
Torecan, 1013-1014
Tornalate, 180-181
torsemide, 1041-1042
Totacillin, 124-125
t-Pa, 92-93
T-Phyl, 1010-1012
trace elements, 1042-1043
Tracrium, 142-143
Trac Tabs 2X, 674
tramadol, 1110-1111
Trandate, 598-599
Tranhep, 664-665
Transderm-Nitro, 762-764
Transderm-Scop, 947
Trans-Plantar, 940-941
Trans-Ver-Sal, 940-941
Tranxene, 295-296
tranylcypromine, 1043-1044
Travamine, 375-376
Travasol, 102-103
trazodone, 1044-1046
trazodone HCl, 1044-1046
Trecator-SC, 438-439
Trendar, 70, 549-550
Trental, 828-829
Tresortil, 681-682
tretinoin, 1046
Trexan, 741-742
Triacet, 1048-1049
Triadapin, 393-395
Triam-A, 1047-1048
triamcinolone, 1047-1048
triamcinolone acetonide, 1047-1048
triamcinolone (topical), 1048-1049
triamcinolone (topical-oral), 1049
Triam Forte, 1047-1048
Triaminic-DM Cough Formula, 349
Triaminicol, 349
Triamolone 40, 1047-1048
Triamonide-40, 1047-1048
triamterene, 1050-1051
Triavil, 831
triazolam, 1051-1052
Tri-B, 755-756
Triban, 1060-1061
Tri-Barb Capsules, 838
Triderm, 1048-1049
Tridesilon, 338
Tridil, 762-764
Tridione, 1059-1060
trientine, 1052
trifluoperazine, 1053-1055
trifluoperazine HCl, 1053-1055
triflupromazine, 1055-1057
trifluridine (ophthalmic), 1057

Entries can be identified as follows: generic name, Trade Name, DRUG CATEGORY, *Combination Product.*

Triflurin, 1053-1055
Trigesic, 136
triglycerides, medium-chain, 650
Trihexane, 1057-1058
Trihexy, 1057-1058
trihexyphenidyl, 1057-1058
trihexyphenidyl HCl, 1057-1058
Tri-Hydroserpine, 530
Tri-Immunol, 380-381
Tri-K, 870-872
Trikacide, 706-707
Tri-Kort, 1047-1048
Trilafon, 831-834
Trilog, 1047-1048
Trilone, 1047-1048
Trimax, 118-119
Trimazide, 1060-1061
Trimegen, 261-262
trimeprazine, 1058-1059
trimethadione, 1059-1060
trimethobenzamide, 1060-1061
trimethobenzamide HCl, 1060-1061
trimethoprim, 1061-1062
trimethoprim and sulfamethoxazole, 982-983
trimetrexate, 1062-1064
trimipramine, 1064-1065
Trimipramine Maleate, 1064-1065
Trimpex, 1061-1062
Trimstat, 835-836
TrimTabs, 835-836
Triostat, 617-618
tripelennamine, 1065-1066
tripelennamine HCl, 1065-1066
Triple X, 913-914
Tripramine, 555-557
triprolidine, 1067-1068
triprolidine HCl, 1067-1068
Triptil, 908-910
Triptone Caplets, 375-376
Trisoject, 1047-1048
Trisoralen, 1064-1065
Trivalent, 561-562
Trobicin, 964
Trocal, 348-350
tromethamine, 1068
Tronolane, 875-876
Tronothane, 875-876
Trophmine, 102-103
Tropicacyl, 1068-1069
tropicamide (optic), 1068-1069
Truphylline, 105-107
Truscopt, 389-390
TSH, 1025
T-Stat, 421
T_3/T_4, 618-620
Tubarine, 1069-1070
Tubizid, 582-583
Tubocuraine, 1069-1070
tubocurarine, 1069-1070
Tums, 200-201
Tusal, 960-961
Tussi-Organidin DM, 349
Tusstat, 378-380
Twice-A-Day Nasal, 791
Twilite, 378-380
Twin-K, 870-872
Tylenol, 69-72
Tylenol Infant's Drops, 69-72
Tylenol Maximum Strength Sinus, 70
Tylenol Sinus Maximum Strength Caplets, 70
Tylenol with Codeine, 70
Tylox, 70, 790-791
Ty-Pap, 69-72
Tyrobenz, 164
Ty-Tab, 69-72
Tyzine (nasal), 1009
Tyzine (ophthalmic), 1009-1010

U

ULTRAbrom PD, 910
Ultralente, 569-570
Ultralente Iletin I, 569-570
Ultralente Insulin, 569-570
Ultram, 1110-1111
Ultrase, 801-802
Ultrazine, 892-893

Entries can be identified as follows: generic name, Trade Name, DRUG CATEGORY, *Combination Product.*

undecylenic acid (topical), 1070-1071
Uni-Bent Cough, 378-380
Unicaine, 889-890
Unicaps, 731-732
Unipen, 736-738
Uniphyl, 1010-1012
Unipres, 530, 532
UniTussin, 512-513
Univasc, 1107-1108
uracil mustard, 1071-1072
urea, 1072-1073
Ureaphil, 1072-1073
Urebeth, 174-175
Urecholine, 174-175
Urex, 677-678
Uridon, 266-267
Urisedamine, 532
Urispas, 464-465
Uri-Tet, 795-796
Uritol, 492-493
Urobiotic-250, 795
Urocit-K, 870-872
Urodine, 834-835
urofollitropin, 1073-1074
Uro Gantanol, 980
Urogesic, 834-835
urokinase, 1074-1075
Urolene Blue, 692
Uro-Mag, 636-637
Uroquid-Acid No. 2, 674
Urozide, 532-533
ursodiol, 1075-1076
Uticillin-VK, 820-821
Uticort, 173-174

V

Vagilia, 986
Valadol, 69-72
Valergen, 428-429
Valergen 40/Estace, 428-429
Valisone, 174
Valium, 352-354
Valorin, 69-72
valproate, 1076-1077
valproic acid, 1076-1077
Valrelease, 352-354
Vamate, 546-547
Vancenase Nasal, 160-161
Vancenase Nasal Inhaler, 159-160
Vanceril, 159-160
Vancocin, 1077-1079
Vancoled, 1077-1079
vancomycin, 1077-1079
vancomycin HCl, 1077-1079
Vanoxide, 166-167
Vanquish Caplets, 136
Vansil, 783-784
Vantin, 233-234
Vapo-Iso, 583-584
Vaponefrin, 412-414
Vascor, 169
Vaseretic, 407
Vasoclear, 745
Vasocon Regular, 745
Vasoderm, 474
Vasodilan, 588-589
VASODILATORS, 64-65
vasopressin, 1079
Vasotec, 407-408
Vatronol Nose Drops, 410-411
Vazepam, 352-354
V-Cillin K, 820-821
VCR, 1086-1088
vecuronium, 1079-1080
Veetids, 820-821
Velban, 1084-1086
Velbe, 1084-1086
Velosef, 247-248
Velosulin, 565-566
venlafaxine, 1080-1082
Venoglobulin-S, 557-558
Ventodisk, 83-84
Ventolin, 83-84
VePesid, 446-447
verapamil, 1082-1083
verapamil HCl, 1082-1083
Verazinc, 1098

Entries can be identified as follows: generic name, Trade Name, DRUG CATEGORY, *Combination Product.*

Verelan, 1082-1083
Vergogel Duoplant for Feet, 940-941
Vermox, 645
Versed, 714-715
Verukan HP Paplex, 940-941
Vesprin, 1055-1057
Vexol, 936
V-Gan, 898-899
Vibramycin, 397-398
Vibra-Tabs, 397-398
Vicks Childrens Cough Syrup, 349
Vicks Cough Silencers, 349-350
Vicks Daycare, 350
Vicks Formula 44, 348-350
Vicks Formula 44 Cough Control Discs, 350
Vicks Formula 44 Cough Mixture, 350
Vicks Formula 44D, 350
Vicks Formula 44M, 350
Vicodin, 533
vidarabine, 1084
vidarabine (ophthalmic), 1083-1084
Videx, 360-362
vinblastine, 1084-1086
vinblastine sulfate, 1084-1086
Vincasar PFS, 1086-1088
vincristine, 1086-1088
vincristine sulfate, 1086-1088
vinorelbine, 1088-1089
Vioform, 285-286
Viokase, 801-802
Vira-A, 1084
Vira-A Ophthalmic, 1083-1084
Viranol, 940-941
Viranol Gel Ultra, 940-941
Viridium, 834-835
Viroptic, 1057
Viserol, 359-360
Visine Eye Drops, 1009-1010
Visken, 856-857
Vistacon, 546-547
Vistaject, 546-547
Vistaquel 50, 546-547
Vistaril, 546-547
Vistazine 50, 546-547
Vita-Bob, 731-732
Vita-C, 133-134
Vita-Kid, 731-732
vitamin A, 1089-1090
vitamin A acid, 1046
vitamin B_1, 1012-1013
vitamin B_2, 932-933
vitamin B_3, 755-756
vitamin B_6, 916
vitamin B_9, 487-488
vitamin B_{12}, 310-311, 541-542
vitamin C, 133-134
vitamin D, 1090-1091
vitamin D_2, 1090-1091
vitamin D_3, 199-200
vitamin D_3, 1090-1091
vitamin E, 1092
vitamin K_1, 853-854
vitamin K_3, 656
VITAMINS, 66
Vita-Plus E Softgells, 1092
Vitec, 1092
Vivactil, 908-910
Vivol, 352-354
V-Lax, 911-912
VLB, 1084-1086
VM 26, 995-996
Volmax, 83-84
Voltaren, 357-358
Vontrol, 380
Vovox, 397-398
Voxsuprine, 588-589
Vumon, 995-996

W

warfarin, 1092-1094
warfarin sodium, 1092-1094
Warfilone Sodium, 1092-1094
Wart-Off, 940-941
Wart Remover, 940-941
Wehamine, 375-376
Wehdryl, 378-380

Entries can be identified as follows: generic name, Trade Name, DRUG CATEGORY, *Combination Product.*

Weh-Less, 835-836
Wehless Timecelles, 835-836
Weightrol, 835-836
Wellbutrin, 191-192
Wellcovorin, 601-602
Westcort, 535-536
Wigraine, 418
Wigraine Suppositories, 418
Winpred, 883-884
Winstrol, 967-968
Wyamine, 660-661
Wyanoids, 161
Wycillin, 817-818
Wydase, 530
Wygesic, 903-904
Wytensin, 513-514

X
Xanax, 89-90
Xerac BP, 166-167
X-Trozine, 835-836
Xylocaine, 611
Xylocaine HCl, 613-614
Xylocaine HCl for Cardiac Arrhythmias, 611-613
xylometazoline, 1094
xylometazoline HCl, 1094
xylometazoline (nasal), 1094

Y
Yodoxin, 575-576
Yutopar, 938-939

Z
zalcitabine, 1095-1096
Zanosar, 972-973
Zantac, 929-930
Zapex, 786-787
Zarontin, 439-440
Zaroxolyn, 703-704
Zeasorb-AF, 1040
Zebeta, 179-180
Zefazone, 223-225
Zemuron, 939-940
Zerit, 968-969
Zeroxin, 166-167
Zestril, 620-621
Zetran, 352-354
zidovudine, 1096-1097
Zilactin-L, 611
Zinacef, 240-242
Zinc 15, 1098
Zinc-220, 1098
Zinca-Pak, 1098
Zincate, 1098
zinc, 1098
zinc (ophthalmic), 1097-1098
zinc sulfate, 1098
Ziradyl, 378
Zithromax, 150-151
Zocor, 956
Zofran, 777-778
Zoladex, 510
Zolicef, 221-222
Zoloft, 952-953
zolpidem, 1098-1099
ZORprin, 136-138
Zosyn, 860-861
Zovirax, 78, 79-81
Zoxaphen, 267, 268
Zydone, 533
Zyloprim, 88-89
Zymase, 801-802
Zymenol, 716-717

Entries can be identified as follows: generic name, Trade Name, DRUG CATEGORY, *Combination Product.*

IV Drug/Solution Compatibility Chart

			D_5					
	D_5	D_{10}	½S	S	NS	R	LR	OTHER
Acetazolamide	C	C	C	C	C	C	C	
Acyclovir	C							
Alpha$_1$-proteinase inhibitor								Sterile water for inj
Alprostadil	C	C			C			
Alteplase								Sterile water for inj
Amdinocillin	C	C	C	C	C	C	C	D_5 in R
Amikacin	C				C			
Aminocaproic acid			C	C	C	C		D in distilled water
Ammonium Cl					C			May add KCl to solution
Amphotericin B	C							
Ampicillin	C				C			
Amrinone lactate					C			0.45% saline
Antithrombin III	C				C			Sterile water for inj
Ascorbic acid	C				C	C	C	Sodium lactate
Atenolol	C				C			0.45% saline
Azlocillin	C		C		C			
Aztreonam	C	C			C	C	C	Normosol-R
Bretylium tosylate	C				C			
Cefamandole	C				C			
Cefazolin	C				C			
Cefotetan	C				C			
Cefoxitin	C	C			C	C	C	Aminosol
Ceftazidime	C		C	C	C	C	C	M/G Sodium lactate

This chart is not inclusive and is based on manufacturers' recommendations.

Key

C = Compatible
C_5 = Dextrose 5%
D_{10} = Dextrose 10%
D_5½S = Dextrose 5% in saline 0.45%
D_5S = Dextrose 5% in saline 0.9%
NS = Sodium chloride 0.9% (normal saline)
R = Ringer's solution
LR = Lactated Ringer's solution